Psychoneuroimmunology

THIRD EDITION

Volume 1

Psychoneuroimmunology

THIRD EDITION

Volume 1

Edited by

Robert Ader

Department of Psychiatry
Center for Psychoneuroimmunology Research
University of Rochester Medical Center
Rochester, New York

David L. Felten

Center for Neuroimmunology
Loma Linda University School of Medicine
Loma Linda, California

Nicholas Cohen

Department of Microbiology and Immunology
Center for Psychoneuroimmunology Research
University of Rochester Medical Center
Rochester, New York

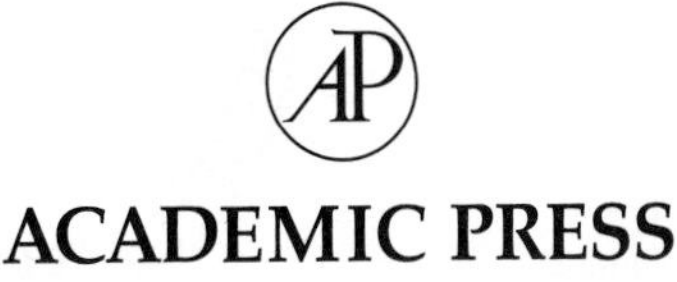

ACADEMIC PRESS

A Harcourt Science and Technology Company

San Diego San Francisco New York Boston London Sydney Tokyo

This book is printed on acid-free paper. 

Academic Press
A Harcourt Science and Technology Company
525 B Street, Suite 1900, San Diego, California 92101-4495, USA
http://www.academicpress.com

Academic Press
Harcourt Place, 32 Jamestown Road, London NW1 7BY, UK
http://www.academicpress.com

Library of Congress Catalog Card Number: 00-102888

International Standard Book Number: 0-12-044314-7 (Set)
International Standard Book Number: 0-12-044315-5 Volume 1
International Standard Book Number: 0-12-044316-3 Volume 2

PRINTED IN THE UNITED STATES OF AMERICA
00 01 02 03 04 05 WP 9 8 7 6 5 4 3 2 1

For Gayle,
Deb,
Janet,
Rini, and
Leslie;
Mary,
Mike,
Matt, and
Brannon;
Inike,
Jamie,
Jessica,
Mischa, and
Mark

Contents

PART
III
IMMUNE SYSTEM EFFECTS ON THE NERVOUS SYSTEM

VOLUME 2

PART IV

BEHAVIORAL EFFECTS ON IMMUNITY

PART V

STRESS AND IMMUNITY

Contributors

Numbers in parentheses indicate the volume number and pages on which the authors' contributions begin.

Abdul Abanomy (2:645) Department of Oral Rehabilitation, King Abdulaziz University Hospital, Jeddah 21452, Saudi Arabia

Robert Ader (2:3) Department of Psychiatry, Center for Psychoneuroimmunology Research, University of Rochester Medical Center, Rochester, New York 14642

Jack P. Antel (2:433) Department of Neurology and Neurosurgery, and Neuroimmunology Unit, Montreal Neurological Institute, McGill University, Montreal, Quebec, Canada H3A 2B4

William A. Banks (1:483) GRECC, Veteran Affairs Medical Center, St. Louis, and Department of Internal Medicine, Division of Geriatrics, Saint Louis University School of Medicine, St. Louis, Missouri 63104

C. J. Barnard (2:35) School of Life and Environmental Sciences, University of Nottingham, Nottingham NG7 2RD, United Kingdom

Andrew Baum (2:335) University of Pittsburgh Cancer Institute, University of Pittsburgh, Pittsburgh, Pennsylvania 15213

J. M. Behnke (2:35) School of Life and Environmental Sciences, University of Nottingham, Nottingham NG7 2RD, United Kingdom

Denise L. Bellinger (1:55; 1:113; 1:241) Center for Neuroimmunology, Loma Linda University School of Medicine, Loma Linda, California 92352

Shamgar Ben-Eliyahu (2:545) Department of Psychology, Tel Aviv University, Tel Aviv 69978, Israel

Gary G. Berntson (2:317) Department of Psychology and Institute of Behavioral Medicine Research, The Ohio State University, Columbus, Ohio 43210

Hugo O. Besedovsky (1:1) Division of Immunophysiology, Institute of Physiology, Phillips-Universitat Marburg, Marburg D-35032, Germany

Massimo Biondi (2:189) 3rd Psychiatric Clinic, University of Rome "La Sapienza," 00185 Rome, Italy

Rose-Marie Bluthé (1:703) Neurobiologie Intégrative, INRA-INSERM U394, 33077 Bordeaux Cedex, France

Robert H. Bonneau (2:483) Department of Microbiology and Immunology, The Pennsylvania State University College of Medicine, Milton S. Hershey Medical Center, Hershey, Pennsylvania 17033

Chad S. Boomershine (1:289) Department of Molecular Virology, Immunology, and Medical Genetics, The Ohio State University, Columbus, Ohio 43210

Torbjørn Breivik (2:627) Department of Periodontology, Faculty of Dentristry, University of Oslo, 0216 Oslo, Norway

Elizabeth B. Brooks (2:399) University of Pittsburgh School of Medicine, Pittsburgh, Pennsylvania15213

Suzanne R. Broussard (1:339) Laboratory of Immunophysiology, Department of Animal Sciences, University of Illinois at Urbana-Champaign, Urbana, Illinois 61801

John T. Cacioppo (2:317) Department of Psychology and Institute of Behavioral Medicine Research, The Ohio State University, Columbus, Ohio 43210

Salvatore Caniglia (1:363) Department of Neuropharmacology, OASI Institute for Research and Care on Mental Retardation and Brain Aging, Troina, Italy

Sonia L. Carlson (1:231) Department of Anatomy and Neurobiology, University of Kentucky Medical Center, Lexington, Kentucky 40536

Daniel J. J. Carr (1:405) Department of Ophthalmology, Dean McGee Eye Institute, The University of Oklahoma Health Sciences Center, Oklahoma City, Oklahoma 73104

Nathalie Castanon (1:703) Neurobiologie Intégrative, INRA-INSERM U394, 33077 Bordeaux Cedex, France

Lucile Chapuron (1:703) Neurobiologie Intégrative, INRA-INSERM U394, 33077 Bordeaux Cedex, France

Irshad H. Chaundry (2:291) Department of Surgery, University of Alabama at Birmingham, Birmingham, Alabama 35294

Nathalie Chauvet (1:703) Neurobiologie Intégrative, INRA-INSERM U394, 33077 Bordeaux Cedex, France

Francesco Chiappelli (2:49) Department of Neurobiology, University of California, Los Angeles, School of Medicine, and Division of Oral Biology and Medicine and Dental Research Institute, University of California, Los Angeles, School of Dentistry, Los Angeles, California 90095

Francesco Chiappelli (2:645) University of California, Los Angeles, School of Dentistry, Los Angeles, California 90095

Nicholas Cohen (1:21; 2:3; 2:525) Department of Microbiology and Immunology, Center for Psychoneuroimmunology Research, University of Rochester Medical Center, Rochester, New York 14642

Sheldon Cohen (2:499) Department of Psychology, Carnegie Mellon University, Pittsburgh, Pennsylvania 15213

Steve W. Cole (2:583) Department of Medicine, University of California, Los Angeles, School of Medicine, Los Angeles, California 90095

Robert Dantzer (1:339; 1:703) Department of Integrative Neurobiology, INRA-INSERM U394, 33077 Bordeaux Cedex, France

Adriana del Rey (1:1) Division of Immunophysiology, Institute of Physiology, Phillips-Universitat Marburg, Marburg D-35032, Germany

Douglas L. Delahanty (2:335) Department of Psychology, Kent State University, Kent, Ohio 44242

Firdaus S. Dhabhar (1:301) College of Dentristry, The Ohio State University, Columbus, Ohio 43210

Angela Liegey Dougall (2:335) University of Pittsburgh Cancer Institute, University of Pittsburgh, Pittsburgh, Pennsylvania 15213

Adrian J. Dunn (1:649) Department of Pharmacology and Therapeutics, Louisiana State University Health Sciences Center, Shreveport, Louisiana 71130

Ilia J. Elenkov (2:421) Inflammatory Joint Diseases Section, National Institute of Arthritis and Musculoskeletal and Skin Diseases, National Institutes of Health, Bethesda, Maryland 20892

Fredrik Eriksson (1:391) Department of Immunology, Wilhelmina Children's Hospital, The University Medical Center of Utrecht, 3584 EA Utrecht, The Netherlands

Jidong Fang (1:667) Department of Veterinary and Comparative Anatomy, Pharmacology, and Physiology, Washington State University, Pullman, Washington 99164

Eugene M. Farber (2:471) Psoriasis Research Institute, Palo Alto, California 94301

David L. Felten (1:55; 1:241) Center for Neuroimmunology, Loma Linda University School of Medicine, Loma Linda, California 92352

Stefan Fernandez (1:217) Department of Microbiology and Immunology, University of Kentucky College of Medicine, Lexington, Kentucky 40536

Gregory G. Freund (1:339) Laboratory of Immunophysiology, Department of Animal Sciences, University of Illinois at Urbana-Champaign, Urbana, Illinois 61801

Herman Friedman (1:415) Department of Medical Microbiology and Immunology, University of South Florida, College of Medicine, Tampa, Florida 33612

Francesco Gallo (1:363) Institute of Pharmacology, University of Catania Medical School, Catania, Italy

Gaetano Garozzo (1:363) Institute of Gynecology, University of Catania Medical School, Catania, Italy

Glyn Goodall (1:703) Neurobiologie Intégrative, INRA-INSERM U394, 33077 Bordeaux Cedex, France

Nicholas R. S. Hall (2:161) Saddlebrook Resort Wellness Center and Institute for Health and Human Performance, Wesley Chapel, Florida 33543

Uwe-Karsten Hanisch (1:585) Department of Cellular Neurosciences, Max Delbrück Center for Molecular Medicine, D-13092 Berlin-Buch, Germany

Cobi J. Heijnen (1:391) Wilhelmina Children's Hospital, The University Medical Center of Utrecht, 3584 EA Utrecht, The Netherlands

Deborah Hodgson (2:645) School of Behavioral Sciences, Laboratory of Neuroimmunology, University of Newcastle, Callaghan, New South Wales 2308, Australia

Laurie Hoffman-Goetz (2:123) Department of Health Studies and Gerontology, Faculty of Applied Health Sciences, University of Waterloo, Waterloo, Ontario, Canada N2L 3G1

Julianne Holt-Lunstad (2:317) Department of Psychology and Health Psychology Program, The University of Utah, Salt Lake City, Utah 84112

Tetsuro Hori (1:517) Department of Integrative Physiology, Kyushu University, Graduate School of Medical Sciences, Fukuoka 812-8582, Japan

Michael Irwin (2:383) Department of Psychiatry, San Diego VA Medical Center and University of California, San Diego, La Jolla, California 92093

Deborah J. Kasprowicz (1:161) Department of Microbiology and Immunology, Loyola University Medical Center, Maywood, Illinois 60153

Toshihiko Katafuchi (1:517) Department of Integrative Physiology, Kyushu University, Graduate School of Medical Sciences, Fukuoka 812-8582, Japan

Annemieke Kavelaars (1:391) Department of Immunology, Wilhelmina Children's Hospital, The University Medical Center of Utrecht, 3584 EA Utrecht, The Netherlands

Keith W. Kelley (1:339; 1:703) Laboratory of Immunophysiology, Department of Animal Sciences, University of Illinois at Urbana-Champaign, Urbana, Illinois 61801

Margaret E. Kemeny (2:87; 2:583) Departments of Psychology and Psychiatry and Biobehavioral Sciences, University of California, Los Angeles, California 90095

Kevin S. Kinney (1:21; 2:279) Department of Biological Sciences, DePauw University, Greencastle, Indiana 46135

Thomas W. Klein (1:415) Department of Medical Microbiology and Immunology, University of South Florida, College of Medicine, Tampa, Florida 33612

Matthew J. Kluger (1:687) Medical College of Georgia, Augusta, Georgia 30912

Melissa A. Knopf (1:217) Department of Microbiology and Immunology, University of Kentucky College of Medicine, Lexington, Kentucky 40536

Adam P. Kohm (1:161) Department of Cell Biology, Neurobiology, and Anatomy, Loyola University Medical Center, Maywood, Illinois 60153

Jan-Peter Konsman (1:703) Neurobiologie Intégrative, INRA-INSERM U394, 33077 Bordeaux Cedex, France

Willem J. Kop (2:525) Department of Medical and Clinical Psychology, Uniformed Services University of the Health Sciences, Bethesda Maryland 20814

Wieslaw Kozak (1:687) Medical College of Georgia, Augusta, Georgia 30912

James M. Krueger (1:667) Department of Veterinary and Comparative Anatomy, Pharmacology, and Physiology, Washington State University, Pullman, Washington 99164

Alexander W. Kusnecov (2:265) Department of Psychology, Rutgers University, Piscataway, New Jersey, 08855

Mark L. Laudenslager (2:73; 2:87) Department of Psychiatry, University of Colorado Health Sciences Center, Denver, Colorado 80220

Sophie Layé (1:703) Neurobiologie Intégrative, INRA-INSERM U394, 33077 Bordeaux Cedex, France

Jeongmin Lee (2:687) University of Arizona, College of Public Health, Tucson, Arizona 85724

Sophie Ligier (2:449) Section on Neuroendocrine Immunology and Behavior, Clinical Neuroendocrinology Branch, National Institute of Mental Health, National Institutes of Health, Bethesda, Maryland 20892

Emilio Lomeo (1:363) Institute of Gynecology, University of Catania Medical School, Catania, Italy

Dianne Lorton (1:55; 1:113; 1:241) Hoover Arthritis Research Center, Sun Health Research Institute, Sun City, Arizona 85372

Cheri Lubahn (1:55; 1:113) Hoover Arthritis Research Center, Sun Health Research Institute, Sun City, Arizona 85372

Donald T. Lysle (2:251) Department of Psychology, University of North Carolina at Chapel Hill, Chapel Hill, North Carolina 27599

Halina Machelska (2:111) Klinik für Anaesthesiologie und Operative Intensivmedizin, Klinikum Benjamin Franklin, Freie Universität Berlin, D-12200 Berlin, Germany

Kelley S. Madden (1:197; 1:241) Department of Psychiatry, Center for Psychoneuroimmunology Research, University of Rochester Medical Center, Rochester, New York 14642

Georges J. M. Maestroni (1:433) Center for Experimental Pathology, Instituto Cantonale de Patologia, 6601 Locarno, Switzerland

Steven F. Maier (1:563) Department of Psychology, University of Colorado, Boulder, Colorado 80309

Jeannine A. Majde (1:667) Office of Naval Research, Arlington, Virginia 22217

Bianca Marchetti (1:363) Department of Pharmacology and Gynecology, University of Sassary Medical School, Sassari, Italy; and Department of Neuropharmacology, OASI Institute for Research and Care on Mental Retardation and Brain Aging, Troina, Italy

Phillip T. Marucha (2:613) Institute for Behavioral Medicine Research, College of Medicine and Public Health, The Ohio State University, Columbus, Ohio 43210

Kimberly P. Mayfield (1:687) Medical College of Georgia, Augusta, Georgia 30912

Kenneth A. Mazey (2:645) University of California, Los Angeles, School of Dentistry, Los Angeles, California 90095

Bruce S. McEwen (1:301) Laboratory of Neuroendocrinology, The Rockefeller University, New York, New York 10021

Joseph P. McGillis (1:217) Department of Microbiology and Immunology, University of Kentucky College of Medicine, Lexington, Kentucky 40536

Jean E. Merrill (1:547) CNS Division, Aventis Pharmaceutical, Inc., Bridgewater, New Jersey 08807

Diana V. Messadi (2:645) University of California, Los Angeles, School of Dentistry, Los Angeles, California 90095

George E. Miller (2:499) Department of Psychology, Carnegie Mellon University, and Department of Psychiatry, University of Pittsburgh, Pittsburgh, Pennsylvania 15213

Ronald S. Mito (2:645) University of California, Los Angeles, School of Dentistry, Los Angeles, California 90095

Maria C. Morale (1:363) Department of Neuropharmacology, OASI Institute for Research and Care on Mental Retardation and Brain Aging, Troina, Italy

John E. Morley (2:701) Division of Geriatric Medicine, Department of Medicine, St. Louis University, and Geriatric Research, Education, and Clinical Center, St. Louis VA Medical Center, St. Louis, Missouri 63104

Shaaban A. Mousa (2:111) Klinik für Anaesthesiologie und Operative Intensivmedizin, Klinikum Benjamin Franklin, Freie Universität Berlin, D-12200 Berlin, Germany

Jan A. Moynihan (2:227) Department of Psychiatry, University of Rochester Medical Center, Rochester, New York 14642

Norbert Müller (2:373) Department of Psychiatry, Ludwig-Maximilian University, Munich, Germany

Dwight M. Nance (1:563) Department of Pathology, University of Manitoba, Manitoba, Canada

Cathy Newton (1:415) Department of Medical Microbiology and Immunology, University of South Florida, College of Medicine, Tampa, Florida 33612

Ichiro Nishimura (2:645) The Jane and Jerry Weintraub Center for Reconstructive Biotechnology, University of California, Los Angeles, School of Dentistry, Los Angeles, California 90095

Takakazu Oka (1:517) Department of Integrative Physiology, Kyushu University, Graduate School of Medical Sciences, Fukuoka 812-8582, Japan

David A. Padgett (2:483; 2:613) Neuroendocrine Immunology Program, Section of Oral Biology, College of Dentristry and the Institute for Behavioral Medicine Research, College of Medicine and Public Health, The Ohio State University, Columbus, Ohio 43210

Patricia Parnet (1:703) Neurobiologie Intégrative, INRA-INSERM U394, 33077 Bordeaux Cedex, France

Bente K. Pedersen (2:123) Department of Infectious Diseases, Copenhagen Muscle Research Centre, University of Copenhagen, DK-2200 Copenhagen, Denmark

John M. Petitto (2:173) Departments of Psychiatry, Neuroscience, Pharmacology, and the Brain Institute, University of Florida College of Medicine, Gainesville, Florida 32610

Florence Pousset (1:703) Neurobiologie Intégrative, INRA-INSERM U394, 33077 Bordeaux Cedex, France

Alexandre Prat (2:433) Neuroimmunology Unit, Montreal Neurological Institute, McGill University, Montreal, Quebec, Canada H3A 2B4

Bruce S. Rabin (2:265) Department of Pathology, University of Pittsburgh, Pittsburgh, Pennsylvania 15213

Mark Hyman Rapaport (2:373) Department of Psychiatry, University of California, San Diego, School of Medicine and Department of Psychiatric Service, San Diego Veteran's Affairs Health System, La Jolla, California 92037

Siba Prasad Raychaudhuri (2:471) Psoriasis Research Institute, Palo Alto, California 94301

Seymour Reichlin (1:499) Department of Medicine, University of Arizona College of Medicine, Tucson, Arizona 85724

Catherine Rivier (1:633) The Clayton Foundation Laboratories for Peptide Biology, The Salk Institute, La Jolla, California 92037

Malcolm P. Rogers (2:399) Department of Psychiatry, Brigham and Women's Hospital, Boston, Massachusetts 02115

Beatrice Roitman-Johnson (1:445) R & D Systems, Inc., Minneapolis, Minnesota 55418

Virginia M. Sanders (1:161) Department of Cell Biology, Neurobiology, and Anatomy, Loyola University Medical Center, Maywood, Illinois 60153

Martin G. Schwacha (2:291) Department of Surgery, University of Alabama at Birmingham, Birmingham, Alabama 35294

Suzanne C. Segerstrom (2:87) Department of Psychology, University of Kentucky, Lexington, Kentucky 40506

Sandra E. Sephton (2:565) Department of Psychiatry and Behavioral Science, University of Louisville School of Medicine, Louisville, Kentucky 40202

Tomas Sepulveda (2:687) University of Arizona, College of Public Health, Tucson, Arizona 85724

Guy Shakhar (2:545) Department of Psychology, Tel Aviv University, Tel Aviv 69978, Israel

Alvin P. Shapiro[†] (2:671) University of Pittsburgh, School of Medicine, Pittsburgh, Pennsylvania 15232

Pang N. Shek (2:511) Defense and Civil Institute of Environmental Medicine, Toronto, Ontario, Canada M3M 3MB9

Roy J. Shephard (2:511) Faculty of Physical Education and Health, University of Toronto, Toronto, Ontario, Canada M5S 2W6

John F. Sheridan (2:483; 2:613) Neuroendocrine Immunology Program, Section of Oral Biology, College of Dentistry and the Institute for Behavioral Medicine Research, College of Medicine and Public Health, The Ohio State University, Columbus, Ohio 43210

Elizabeth Snella (1:415) Department of Medical Microbiology and Immunology, University of South Florida, College of Medicine, Tampa, Florida 33612

George Freeman Solomon (2:701) Department of Psychiatry and Biobehavioral Sciences, University of California, Los Angeles, Los Angeles, California 90024

Gerald Sonnenfeld (2:279) Department of Microbiology and Immunology, Morehouse School of Medicine, Atlanta, Georgia 30310

Robert B. Sothern (1:445) Department of Biorhythmometry, College of Biological Sciences, University of Minnesota, St. Paul, Minnesota 55455

David Spiegel (2:565) Department of Psychiatry and Behavioral Sciences, Stanford University School of Medicine, Stanford, California 94305

Igor Spigelman (2:645) University of California, Los Angeles, School of Dentistry, Los Angeles, California 90095

Christoph Stein (2:111) Klinik für Anaesthesiologie und Operative Intensivmedizin, Klinikum Benjamin Franklin, Freie Universität Berlin, D-12200 Berlin, Germany

Esther M. Sternberg (2:449) Section on Neuroendocrine Immunology and Behavior, Clinical Neuroendocrinology Branch, National Institute of Mental Health, National Institutes of Health, Bethesda, Maryland 20892

Suzanne Y. Stevens (2:227) Department of Psychiatry, University of Rochester Medical Center, Rochester, New York 14642

Alan Sved (2:265) Department of Neuroscience, University of Pittsburgh, Pittsburgh, Pennsylvania 15213

Michelle A. Swanson (1:161) Department of Microbiology and Immunology, Loyola University Medical Center, Maywood, Illinois 60153

Elisabeth Tarkowski (2:349) Departments of Neurology, Clinical Immunology, and Rheumatology, University of Göteborg, Sahlgrenska University Hospital, S-413 46 Göteborg, Sweden

Anna N. Taylor (2:49) Department of Neurobiology, University of California, Los Angeles, School of Medicine, Los Angeles, California 90095

Gerald R. Taylor (2:279) NASA Johnson Space Center, Houston, Texas 77058

Nuccio Testa (1:363) Department of Neuropharmacology, OASI Institute for Research and Care on Mental Retardation and Brain Aging, Troina, Italy

Per Stanley Thrane (2:627) Department of Pathology and Forensic Odontology, Faculty of Dentristry, University of Oslo, 0216 Oslo, Norway

Srinivasan ThyagaRajan (1:241) Center for Neuroimmunology, Loma Linda University School of Medicine, Loma Linda, California 92352

Cataldo Tirolo (1:363) Department of Neuropharmacology, OASI Institute for Research and Care on Mental Retardation and Brain Aging, Troina, Italy

[†]Deceased.

Julie M. Turner-Cobb (2:565) Department of Psychology, University of Kent at Canterbury, Canterbury, Kent CT2 7LZ, United Kingdom

Bert N. Uchino (2:317) Department of Psychology and Health Psychology Program, The University of Utah, Salt Lake City, Utah 84112

Homer D. Venters (1:339) Laboratory of Immunophysiology, Department of Animal Sciences, University of Illinois at Urbana-Champaign, Urbana, Illinois 61801

Tianyi Wang (1:289) Department of Microbiology, The Ohio State University, Columbus, Ohio 43210

Linda R. Watkins (1:563) Department of Psychology, University of Colorado, Boulder, Colorado 80309

Ronald R. Watson (2:687) University of Arizona, College of Public Health, Tucson, Arizona 85724

Richard J. Weber (1:405) Department of Biomedical and Therapeutic Sciences, University of Illinois, College of Medicine at Peoria, Peoria, IL 61656

Herbert Weiner (2:671) Neuropsychiatric Institute and Brain Research Institute, University of California, Los Angeles, Los Angeles, California 90024

Ronald L. Wilder (2:421) Inflammatory Joint Diseases Section, National Institute of Arthritis and Muscoloskeletal and Skin Diseases, National Institutes of Health, Bethesda, Maryland 20892

Julie M. Worlein (2:73) Washington Regional Primate Research Center, University of Washington, Seattle, Washington 98195

Raz Yirmiya (2:49) Department of Psychology, The Hebrew University of Jerusalem, Mount Scopus, Jerusalem 91905, Israel

Robert Zachariae (2:133) Psychooncology Research Unit, Aarhus University Hospital, DK8000 Aarhus C, Denmark

René Zellweger (2:291) Department of Trauma Surgery, University of Zurich, 8091 Zurich, Switzerland

Bruce S. Zwilling (1:289) Department of Microbiology, The Ohio State University, Columbus, Ohio 43210

Preface

The first edition of *Psychoneuroimmunology* was published in 1981. It was a collection of only 17 chapters describing the relatively meager amount of ongoing research that bore directly or indirectly on the relationship between the brain and the immune system. It was also, as one reviewer prophesied, the signature volume of a new field of research. *Psychoneuroimmunology* gave a name to the temporally and conceptually unrelated research efforts that, for brief times in the past, had occupied the attention of a few researchers but, at that time, was becoming the focus of attention for several investigators from different disciplines.

The first sustained program of research on brain–immune system interactions began in the 1920s and concerned the Pavlovian conditioning of "immune" reactions. In the 1950s, there was a short-lived, but later revived, interest in the immunologic effects of lesioning and electrical stimulation of the hypothalamus. At the same time, Fred Rasmussen, Jr., a virologist, and Norma Brill, a psychiatrist (the first such interdisciplinary collaboration), initiated studies on the effects of stressful life experiences on susceptibility to experimentally induced infectious diseases.

Interest in this interdisciplinary research was rejuvenated when, in the 1970s, several independent lines of research converged to provide verifiable evidence of interactions between the brain and the immune system. John Hadden linked the immune system to the sympathetic nervous system by documenting the existence of β-adrenergic receptors on lymphocytes; Robert Ader and Nicholas Cohen demonstrated behaviorally conditioned suppression of the immune system, providing a functional link between the brain and the immune system; Roger Bartrop and his associates described immunologic changes associated with the bereavement that followed the death of a spouse; Hugo Besedovsky began to piece together a neuroendocrine–immune system network with his studies of the effects of immune responses on neural and endocrine function; the sympathetic innervation of lymphoid tissues was documented by David and Suzanne Felten and connections to the thymus were documented by Karen Bulloch; and Edwin Blalock and Eric Smith showed that lymphocytes, themselves, were capable of producing neuropeptides. These seminal studies precipitated new research on the receptors for hormones and neurotransmitters that existed on lymphocytes, the effects of sympathetic nervous system activity on immunity, conditioned immune responses, depression and immunity, the influence of stressful life experiences on immune function and resistance to disease, psychosocial factors in the progression of AIDS, and immunologic effects on behavior. Thus, the very meaning of "neuroimmunology" was changing and, most conspicuously, a behavioral component was becoming a prominent feature in the study of brain–immune system interactions.

Psychoneuroimmunology is, then, the study of the interactions among behavior, neural, and endocrine function and immune system processes. The basic premise underlying this interdisciplinary field is that adaptation is the product of a single, integrated network of defenses. Each component of this defensive network serves specialized functions and, at the same time, monitors and responds to information derived from the others. Thus, in contrast to disciplinary analyses of the mechanisms governing the functions of a singe system, psychoneuroimmunology studies the relationship among these systems. This integrative strategy, intended as a supplement to rather than as a substitute for traditional approaches, is necessary because, as this volume demonstrates, it is not possible to obtain a full understanding of immunoregulatory processes without considering the organism and the internal and external environment in which immune responses take place.

Two pathways bridge the brain and the immune system: autonomic nervous system activity and neuroendocrine outflow from the pituitary. Primary and secondary lymphoid organs are sympathetically innervated, and these nerve fibers form neuroeffector junctions with lymphocytes, monocytes/macrophages, and granulocytes that possess receptors for these neurotransmitters. Neural and neuroendocrine effects on immune processes are the subjects of the opening sections of this volume. Several of these chapters are substantive updates or more detailed additions to material presented in the second edition of *Psychoneuroimmunology* necessitated by the progress that has been made in elaborating the nature of neural–immune interactions. Other chapters, such as those describing the phylogenetic history of neural–immune interactions, biological rhythms in immune function, or the role of sleep or fever in immunity and health, have not been covered in previous editions. Immune system effects on the nervous system—the central and peripheral action of cytokines on neural, neuroendocrine, and immunologic processes and on behavior—are described in the entirely new third section of the book.

The following two sections document the effects of behaviors and stressful life experiences on immune function. A few of the chapters dealing with behavioral influences update earlier reviews. The chapter on conditioning, for example, is an "update" but, in this instance, the focus is on the conditioned enhancement rather than on the suppression of immunity. The majority of the contributions cover new material of conceptual, methodological, or practical significance. The same is true for the section on stress. Following up-to-date overviews, contributors consider the immunologic effects of acute and chronic physical or psychosocial stressors introduced under laboratory conditions or as the result of naturally occurring circumstances.

The behavioral and emotional states that accompany the appraisal and attempt to adapt to potentially stressful circumstances are associated with complex patterns of neuroendocrine changes capable of modulating immune functions. Thus, changes in immune function would constitute a critical link between psychosocial factors and an altered susceptibility to or progression of disease. This chain of psychophysiological events, however, has not yet been firmly established. That is, it remains to be conclusively demonstrated in different model systems that an altered resistance to disease is a direct result of biologically relevant changes in immune function induced by psychosocial or stressful life experiences. Such data are being collected and are described in the final section of the book. This series of chapters deals with the biologic impact of behaviorally induced alteration in immune function. Animal and human studies of immune changes associated with certain normal (e.g., aging) and pathophysiological (e.g., depression) conditions are described. Several other chapters deal with psychosocial and/or neuroendocrine influences on disease processes that are thought to involve immunologic mechanisms (e.g., autoimmune and infectious disease) or those in which data now suggest the immune system might be involved (e.g., schizophrenia, cardiovascular disease). These chapters confront some of the issues that need to be addressed to document the clinical import of psychoneuroimmunologic research.

The first edition of *Psychoneuroimmunology* attempted to collate what little information was available implicating neural and endocrine processes in the modulation of immunity. *Psychoneuroimmunology II* reflected an adolescence characterized by rapid growth along several dimensions that, taken together, provided unequivocal evidence of behavior–neural–endocrine–immune system interactions. Judging by this third edition, the previous volume attained its goal of stimulating interdisciplinary research by behavioral and neuroscientists, immunologists, and others who, as anticipated, have learned to communicate with each other and found such communication to be mutually rewarding. If not yet fully mature, this current edition of *Psychoneuroimmunology* reflects an increasing sophistication and a very considerable expansion of the research and the researchers who are now devoting attention to what has become a fully accepted interdisciplinary field of research. A paradigm shift (not our words) is occurring; immunoregulatory processes can no longer be studied as the independent activity of an autonomous immune system. That realization, the essential message of *Psychoneuroimmunology*, Third Edition, is the reader's invitation to contribute to a new understanding of the relationships between the brain and the immune system and their implications for health and disease.

Putting such a series of books together, especially an edition as large and with as many contributors as this one, has not been a labor of love. It's been more like sticking to an exercise regime that you don't really enjoy, but know that it needs to be done—and you do feel better when you stick to it. Besides, the aches and the pain go away while the good feeling stays with you. Having acknowledged the pain, our first thanks must go to the several contributors, many of whom, in the face of repeated badgering and requests for revisions, maintained their composure, their good humor—and our friendship. You should never even consider an undertaking of this magnitude unless you have the interpersonal skills, the organizational talents, and the good natured assistance of a Patricia Farrell. Pat's equivalent in California was Jo Verhelle. They were our primary accomplices and we cannot thank either of them enough for their efforts on our behalf. We are also grateful to Lee Grota, Gary Boehm, Sandra Lee, and Mark Larson, who did such an excellent job of preparing the subject index. Nikki Levy at Academic Press, who instigated this third edition, was supportive, helpful, and, most of all, patient in the face of repeated delays and missed deadlines. We appreciate all her efforts in furthering this field, as well as in the production of this book.

R.A.
D.L.F.
N.C.

About the Editors

ROBERT ADER, Ph.D., M.D. (HC)

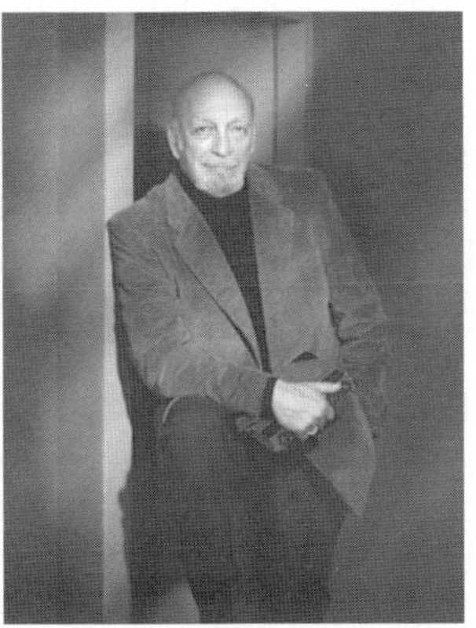

Dr. Ader received his B.S. from Tulane University in 1953 and his Ph.D. in experimental psychology from Cornell University in 1957. He joined the University of Rochester faculty in 1957 as an instructor in psychiatry and psychology. He became a professor of psychiatry and psychology in 1968 and also holds a secondary appointment as a professor of medicine. In 1983, Dr. Ader became the George L. Engel Professor of Psychosocial Medicine and is currently Director of the Division of Behavioral and Psychosocial Medicine and Director of the Center for Psychoneuroimmunology Research. From 1969 until 1999, Dr. Ader held a continuing Research Scientist Award from the National Institute of Mental Health. In 1992, he was awarded an honorary M.D. from the University of Trondheim in Norway. During the 1992–1993 academic year, Dr. Ader was a fellow at the Center for Advanced Study in the Behavioral Sciences at Stanford.

Dr. Ader edited *Psychoneuroimmunology* (1981), referred to as "the signature volume of a new field of research," and coedited the second edition in 1991. He serves on the editorial boards of several journals, was an associate editor of *Psychosomatic Medicine*, and is the Editor-in-Chief of *Brain, Behavior, and Immunity*. Dr. Ader is a past president of the American Psychosomatic Society, the International Society for Developmental Psychobiology, and the Academy of Behavioral Medicine Research and the founding president of the Psychoneuroimmunology Research Society.

DAVID L. FELTEN, M.D., Ph.D.

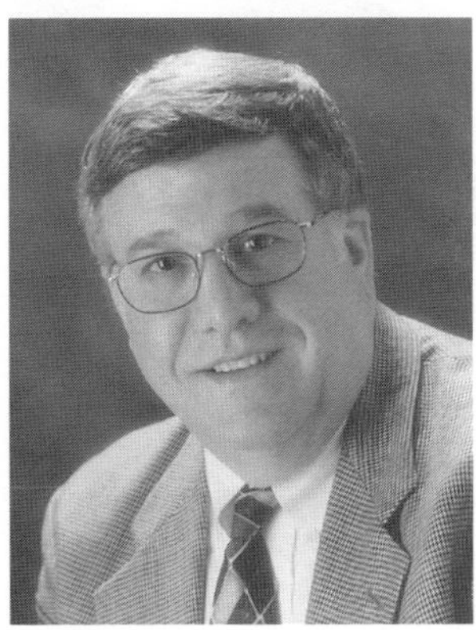

Dr. David Felten received a B.S. from the Massachusetts Institute of Technology in 1969, an M.D. from the University of Pennsylvania in 1973, and a Ph.D. in anatomy through the Institute of Neurological Sciences at the University of Pennsylvania in 1974. He joined the University of Rochester in 1983 as professor of neurobiology and anatomy with a secondary appointment as professor of psychiatry. He became Kilian J. and Caroline F. Schmitt Professor and Chair of the Department of Neurobiology and Anatomy in 1995. He was also Director of the Neurosciences Graduate Program and an associate director of the Center for Psychoneuroimmunology Research.

Dr. Felten has received an Alfred P. Sloan Foundation Fellowship, a John D. and Catherine T. MacArthur Foundation Prize Fellowship, an Andrew W. Mellon Foundation Fellowship, and the Norman Cousins Award in Mind–Body Health from The Fetzer Institute. Dr. Felten has held 10-year MERIT Awards from the National Institute on Aging and the National Institute of Mental Health. Dr. Felten was a coeditor of *Psychoneuroimmunology* (second edition) and associate editor of *Brain, Behavior, and Immunity*. Dr. Felten is currently a professor in the Department of Anatomy and Pathology and Director of the Center for Neuroimmunology at the Loma Linda University School of Medicine.

NICHOLAS COHEN, Ph.D.

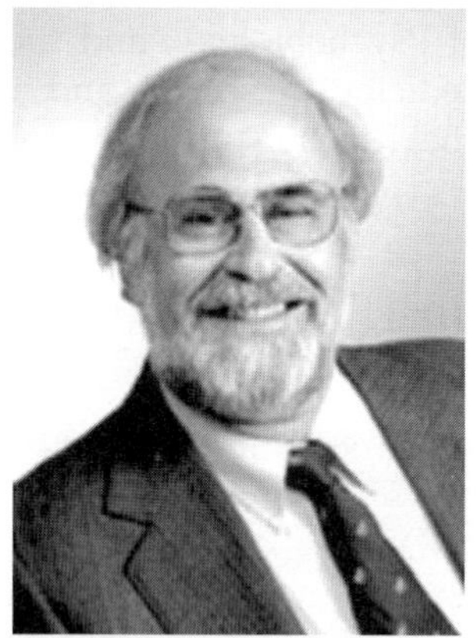

Nicholas Cohen received an A.B. (*cum laude*) from Princeton University in 1959 and his Ph.D. in biology from the University of Rochester in 1965. In 1967, he joined the University of Rochester faculty, where he is currently professor of microbiology and immunology and Director of the Immunology, Microbiology, and Vaccine Biology Graduate Program. He holds secondary appointments as professor of psychiatry and oncology and is an associate director of the Center for Psychoneuroimmunology Research. Dr. Cohen is a former member of the Basel Institute of Immunology in Switzerland and a Fulbright scholar and visiting professor at the Agricultural University in The Netherlands.

Dr. Cohen has served on the editorial board of *Immunogenetics* and is currently an associate editor of *Developmental and Comparative Immunology* and *Brain, Behavior, and Immunity*. He has coedited four books in immunology and coauthored a monograph on graduate education in the sciences. He was a member of the Immunobiology Study Section of the National Institutes of Health (NIH) and the recipient of an NIH Research Career Development Award. Currently, he is Principal Investigator of two NIH research grants and is Program Director of an NIH Pre- and Postdoctoral Training grant in immunology.

Dr. Cohen was Vice President of the International Society for Developmental and Comparative Immunology (Western Hemisphere) and a past president of the Division of Comparative Immunology of the American Society of Zoologists and was a councilor of the PsychoNeuroImmunology Research Society.

Cytokines as Mediators of Central and Peripheral Immune–Neuroendocrine Interactions

HUGO O. BESEDOVSKY, ADRIANA DEL REY

I. INTRODUCTION

For many years, the first two editions of *Psychoneuroimmunology* have been reference books in the field of interactions among the nervous, endocrine, and immune systems. This field has expanded enormously in a relatively short time. This is probably due not only to the need to understand how immune mechanisms are controlled by the brain, but also to the need to integrate, within a conceptual biological framework, knowledge that is the product of analytical, sometimes reductionist, approaches. In our opinion, the study of interactions among the immune, nervous, and endocrine systems constitutes one of the most rigorous attempts being made at present to face the problem of complexity in biological systems by reestablishing the balance between synthesis and analysis, the classical methodological approaches in natural sciences. The adequate combination of these approaches is providing clear information about how interactions between the immune and neuroendocrine systems are mediated, and about the relevance of such interactions for the operation of the immune system during health and disease.

We have chosen to emphasize in this Foreword the role of cytokines on immune–neuroendocrine interactions. Interactions imply reciprocity. On one hand, the mediators of the nervous and endocrine systems—hormones, neurotransmitters, and neuropeptides—are well-defined, and their effects on the immune system are discussed in several chapters of this book. On the other hand (and without dismissing that other immune-derived products also may play a similar role!), increasing evidence indicates that cytokines are the main messengers from the immune system to the brain. The use of the term "cytokine" has been extended during the last years practically to any protein released by a cell that can, in turn, affect itself or other cells. This denomination, however, is restricted here to those products originally described as being produced by immune cells and that can affect immune mechanisms in an autocrine or paracrine fashion. Because it has been shown that many of these cytokines can also elicit immunoregulatory neuroendocrine responses, and may even play a role in brain physiology, they appear as relevant protagonists in almost all chapters of this book. This is the main reason to concentrate this Foreword on cytokines. However, the amount of work published on this subject during the last years makes it impossible to include here a complete review of this literature. We shall concentrate instead on certain aspects, using examples derived mainly from our own work. More detailed discussions and references can be found in other chapters of this book.

II. THE IMMUNE SYSTEM AND THE BRAIN TALK TO EACH OTHER

The understanding of intrinsic mechanisms that underlie the immune response constitutes one of the most remarkable advances in biological sciences of the second half of this century. The structure of the main molecules (e.g., antibodies, T-cell receptor) that recognize the huge universe of antigens from inside and outside the organism is known. The molecular and genetic bases of the differentiation and diversification of immune cells, as well as the types and subtypes of cells that participate in an immune response, are largely understood. The biochemical pathways of immune cell activation and how these cells interact and receive information from antigen-presenting cells have also been clarified to a great extent. This knowledge showed that immune cells are extremely complex, and that refined interactions between them constitute the basis of different types of immune responses.

Under appropriate conditions, immune responses remarkably similar to those elicited in vivo can be triggered in culture. This evidence, together with the identification of efficient autoregulatory mechanisms, may suggest that, compared with other physiologic systems, the immune system displays a privileged autonomy. However, a "real" immune response in an integral organism depends on mechanisms that are under neuroendocrine control. The most obvious level of such dependence (and probably because of its obviousness generally neglected) is the need to control the highly demanding metabolic processes that underlie immune cell functions. Another example of dependence that cannot be mimicked in vitro is related to the circulatory systems. Indeed, no effective immune response would be possible if immune cells could not circulate and reach the places where antigens are presented. It could still be argued that these levels of dependence, although necessary for an efficient immune response, are too "elemental." However, hormones, neurotransmitters, and neuropeptides, the messengers that affect these "elemental" processes, can also influence more subtle mechanisms underlying immune cell activity (for review see Homo-Delarche & Durant, 1994). For example, neuroendocrine agents can affect processes that range from the expression of MHC molecules (necessary for antigen presentation), and the production of cytokines (e.g., Th1/Th2 cytokines, whose balance is decisive in developing a predominantly cellular or humoral immune response), to the generation and action of effector cells. Although most of these effects have been detected in vitro, there is much evidence that the in vivo manipulation of neuroendocrine mechanisms can also profoundly affect immune functions. Altogether, the information available shows that immune processes need the support of neuro-endocrine mechanisms, and indicate that these mechanisms can control essential steps of the immune response. However, a level of neuroendocrine control operating unidirectionally would not be efficient enough for a system that is permanently being challenged and responding to antigens from inside and outside the organism. The question is how the brain and neuroendocrine structures are informed about dynamic changes in the functioning of the immune system. The neuroendocrine regulation of different steps of inflammatory and immune responses would require an active exchange of signals between immune cells and mechanisms directly under brain control. This exchange of information is specially relevant in pathological conditions during which several body functions are altered, and, despite that, the immune system is expected to operate efficiently. We and others have proposed and provided experimental evidence that neuroendocrine responses mediated by immune-derived products are elicited following activation of the immune system (Besedovsky, del Rey, & Sorkin, 1981; Besedovsky, del Rey, Sorkin, Da Prada, Burri, & Honegger, 1983; Besedovsky, del Rey, Sorkin, Lotz, & Schwulera, 1985; Besedovsky & Sorkin, 1977; Besedovsky, Sorkin, Felix, & Haas, 1977; Besedovsky, Sorkin, Keller, & Mueller, 1975; for review see Besedovsky & del Rey, 1996). Such responses imply that the brain receives information from the immune system and responds to immune-derived signals. Studies showing that the immune process can be behaviorally conditioned also indicate that the brain is informed about the effects of the unconditioned stimulus on the immune system (Ader & Cohen, 1991).

In the following sections, we shall discuss briefly the responses of the brain and of systems under brain control to immune-derived cytokines that convey afferent signals from the immune system. We shall also refer to the influence of these mediators on the activity of peripheral nerves. Finally, the possibility that local actions of cytokines produced by neural cells play a role in brain physiology and in the coordination of neuroendocrine responses will be analyzed.

III. THE NERVOUS AND ENDOCRINE SYSTEMS RECEIVE AND RESPOND TO PERIPHERAL IMMUNE SIGNALS: LONG-LOOP INTERACTIONS

There is abundant evidence that neuroendocrine and metabolic alterations parallel infectious, inflammatory, autoimmune, and neoplastic diseases. These alterations could be directly caused by the infectious agent or neoplastic cells and/or their products, or by the tissue injury that they induce, and be, therefore, the consequence of the disease. Alternatively, the changes in neuroendocrine functions and intermediate metabolism observed during certain pathologies may be caused by mediators released when the immune system is activated. In support of this is the evidence obtained in our and other laboratories that, when the immune response to innocuous antigens is strong enough, several neuro and endocrine parameters are affected (for review see Besedovsky & del Rey, 1996) . This evidence indicates that mediators released during the immune response can trigger the activation of mechanisms integrated at brain level. Thus, at least some of the neuroendocrine responses observed during certain pathological conditions may be caused by immune-derived products rather than being the consequence of the disease itself.

An example of the operation of a regulatory immune-neuroendocrine circuit is seen in our recent study showing that the protective stimulation of the hypothalamus-pituitary-adrenal (HPA) axis during experimental autoimmune encephalomyelitis (EAE) is mainly immune mediated (del Rey, Klusman, & Besedovsky, 1998). It is well established that the increase in corticosterone output observed during EAE, an animal model of multiple sclerosis, is essential for the survival of animals affected with this disease (Levine, Sowinski, & Steinetz, 1980; MacPhee, Antoni, & Mason, 1989). Indeed, injection of myelin basic protein (MBP) in complete Freund's adjuvant into Lewis rats induces an autoimmune encephalomyelitis that is characterized by a paralytic attack from which all rats finally recover. However, the disease is lethal when the increase in the levels of corticosterone that parallels EAE is impeded (Levine et al., 1980; MacPhee et al., 1989). It is reasonable to assume that the HPA axis is stimulated by the stress caused by the paralytic attack. Alternatively, an increase in corticosterone blood levels during EAE could, at least in part, be immune mediated if the immune response to MBP, as to other antigens (for review see Besedovsky & del Rey, 1996), would trigger the stimulation of the HPA. We have shown that inoculation of MBP to PVG rats, which recognize and respond immunologically to MBP but do not develop the disease, also leads to an increase in corticosterone blood level (Figure 1). This endocrine response contributes to the resistance of PVG rats to develop EAE, since the disease is manifested in these animals when they are adrenalectomized. These results allow us to conclude that, following MBP immunization, the stimulation of the HPA axis is dissociable from the stress of a paralytic attack, and largely triggered by the immune response to this antigen.

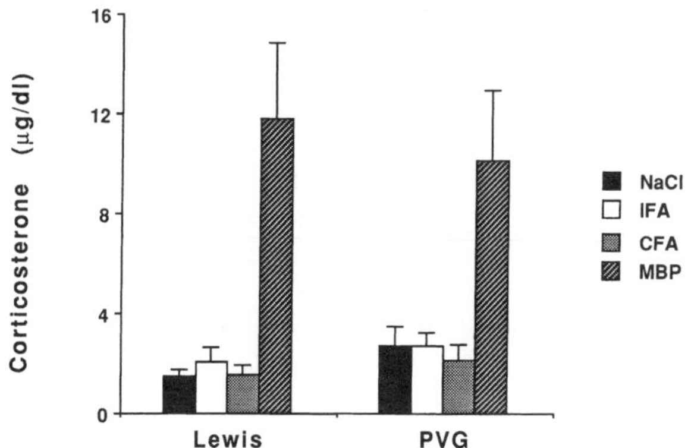

FIGURE 1 Blood corticosterone levels following MBP-administration to Lewis and PVG rats. Chronically cannulated rats received either MBP in Complete Freund's adjuvant (MBP, Lewis n = 14, PVG n = 10), Complete Freund's adjuvant (CFA, Lewis n = 13; PVG n = 8), Incomplete Freund's adjuvant (IFA, Lewis n = 6, PVG n = 7) or saline (NaCl, Lewis n = 9; PVG n = 6) injected subcutaneously. Blood samples were obtained daily via the implanted cannula. The results shown in the figure represent the mean ± SE of peak corticosterone levels in blood detected on day 13 in Lewis rats and on day 14 in PVG rats after injection. Adapted with permission from del Rey, Klusman, et al., 1998.

A. Effects of Cytokines on Neuroendocrine Mechanisms

More than 20 years ago, when the first neuroendocrine changes that parallel a specific immune response were detected, we reasoned that these changes should be mediated by immune cell products because the antigens used do not themselves cause any pathology. The first approach to search for these factors was to study whether stimulation of immune cells in vitro results in the production of mediators capable of stimulating the HPA axis. The conditioned medium from cultures of allogeneic and/or mitogenic stimulated human or murine lymphocytes evoked an increase in ACTH and corticosterone output when administered to normal rats and mice (Besedovsky et al., 1981; Besedovsky et al., 1985). The products that mediate these effects were generically termed glucocorticoid-increasing factors (GIF). The fact that one million lymphocytes stimulated in culture produce enough GIF to induce a several-fold increase in blood ACTH and corticosterone levels in adult animals illustrated the potency of these factors. This in vitro–in vivo approach, which was necessary at that time because few purified and no recombinant cytokines were available, is still useful in studying whether, and if so which, cytokines mediate a neuroendocrine change during a given immune response, as well as possible synergism between these mediators. We have recently used this approach to show that splenic cells obtained from Lewis rats undergoing EAE and further stimulated in vitro with MBP, produce factors that increase blood corticosterone levels when injected into normal rats (del Rey, Klusman, et al., 1998). This strongly suggests that in Lewis rats, as in PVG rats, the stimulation of the HPA axis is, at least in part, mediated by cytokines released during the immune response to MBP. This view is reinforced by studies showing that endogenous IL-1 is involved in the mediation of the corticosterone response in these animals (see following paragraph).

The availability of pure or recombinant immune cytokines allowed a more direct exploration of their capacity to influence endocrine and neural functions. The capacity of IL-1 to stimulate the HPA axis is the most extensively studied example of the influence of cytokines on endocrine functions. Both natural and recombinant forms of IL-1 can stimulate ACTH and corticosterone output in mice and rats, and IL-1 appears as the most likely mediator of the glucocorticoid changes induced by certain viruses (Besedovsky, del Rey, Sorkin, & Dinarello, 1986) and endotoxin (Rivier, Chizzonite, & Vale, 1989). Using the natural IL-1 receptor antagonist (IL-1ra), we have recently shown that endogenous IL-1 also is involved in the mediation of the stimulation of the HPA axis during EAE (del Rey, Klusman, et al., 1998) (Figure 2). Considered with the studies mentioned above, these results show for first time that cytokines released during the immune response to an antigen that induces an autoimmune disease mediate the activation of the HPA axis, an endocrine response that is essential for recovery from the disease. This example illustrates the relevance of a feedback circuit integrated by immune cytokines and the HPA axis for the control of mechanisms that lead to autoimmunity.

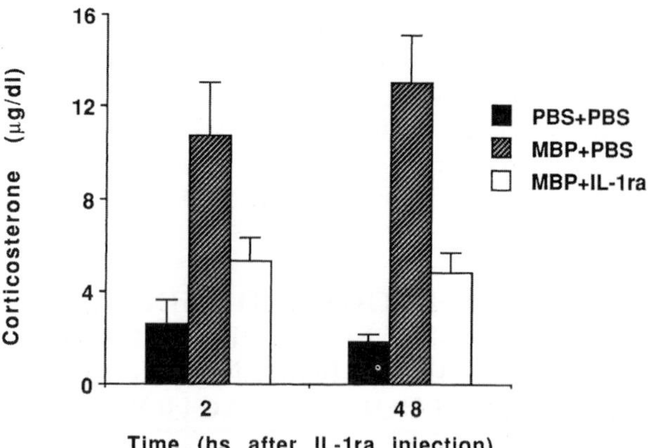

FIGURE 2 Blockade of IL-1 receptors interferes with the increase in corticosterone levels during EAE. Chronically cannulated Lewis rats received MBP or PBS. Blood samples were obtained 1 day before inoculation and once daily from day 5 after injection until day 20. Immediately after obtaining the blood sample corresponding to day 13, when all MBP-injected rats already showed clinical signs of EAE, IL-1ra was administered to a group of these animals (MBP + IL-1ra, n = 8). The other group of MBP-injected rats (n = 12) and the PBS-injected animals (n = 8) received the vehicle alone (MBP + PBS and PBS + PBS, resp.). The figure shows the levels of corticosterone (mean ± SE) determined on blood samples collected 2 and 48 hours later. Adapted with permission from del Rey, Klusman, et al., 1998.

Other authors have reached a similar conclusion by showing that the response of the HPA following antigen or cytokine challenge is defective in animals prone to autoimmune diseases (Schauenstein, Faessler, Dietrich, Schwarz, Kroemer, & Wick, 1987; Sternberg et al., 1989).

The stimulatory effect of IL-1 on the HPA axis seems to be rather specific since it is not paralleled by changes in other "stress hormones," such as somatotrophin, prolactin, and α-melanocyte-stimulating hormone (α-MSH), and the levels of catecholamines in blood are only modestly increased following IL-1 injection (Berkenbosch, de Goeij, del Rey & Besedovsky, 1989). Although IL-1β can affect ACTH release during long-term cultures of normal pituitary cells, the main site of action of IL-1 in vivo seems to be the hypothalamus. Other cytokines such as IL-6, TNFα, IFNγ and IL-12, and thymosin fraction 5 also stimulate the HPA axis (Holsboer, Stalla, von Bardeleben, Hammann, Muller, & Muller, 1988; Naitoh et al., 1988; Sacco et al., 1997; Sharp, Matta, Peterson, Newton, Chao, & Mcallen, 1989). However, comparative studies showed that IL-1 is more potent than TNFα and IL-6 (Besedovsky et al., 1991) in its capacity to increase blood corticosterone levels.

Following this initial evidence that lymphokines and monokines can affect the pituitary-adrenal axis, further studies on this and other neuroendocrine mechanisms have been reported. Generally, IL-1, TNF, and IL-6 exert an inhibitory action on the hypothalamus-pituitary-thyroid axis (Hermus et al., 1992; Rettori, Jurcovicova, & McCann, 1987). Regarding the hypothalamus-pituitary-gonadal axis, it is worth mentioning that IL-1 induces a decrease in LHRH and LH concentrations only when the cytokine is administered centrally (Rivest, Lee, Attardi, & Rivier, 1993). This indicates that the actions of IL-1 on plasma LH levels are most likely mediated within the brain (Rivier & Vale, 1989). However, IL-1 may also affect sexual steroid production by acting directly on the gonads. Another effect of IL-1 and IL-6 that is observed only when the cytokines are injected intracerebroventricularly is an increase in prolactin and growth hormone plasma levels (Lyson & McCann, 1991; Rettori et al., 1987; Rotiroti et al., 1993).

Although these in vivo experiments are pharmacological, they are valuable for assessing the potentially physiological neuroendocrine effects of cytokines. Many studies also have been performed in vitro (Nash, Brandon, & Bello, 1992; Smith, Brown, & Blalock, 1989; Yamaguchi et al., 1991; for review see Besedovsky & del Rey, 1996). The evidence reported is sometimes contradictory, for example with respect to the effects of IL-1 on ACTH and prolactin release, and of TNF on growth hormone and prolactin release. This is probably mainly due to the different in vitro systems used and to different culture conditions. However, as a whole, the evidence indicates that IL-1, IL-2, IL-6, TNFα, and IFNγ can also directly affect the pituitary gland. Pituitary-like peptides can also be produced by lymphoid cells following cytokine stimulation (Carr & Blalock, 1991; Heijnen, Kavelaars, & Ballieux, 1991). Since hypophysectomy profoundly affects immune functions (Berczi & Nagy, 1991; Kelley, 1991), it seems that these peptides cannot replace pituitary hormones. However, pituitary-like peptides produced by lymphoid cells are expected to act in a paracrine/autocrine fashion, and may therefore contribute to fine tuning the effects of hormones produced by the hypophysis.

B. Effect of Cytokines on Brain Neurotransmitters and Neuronal Activity

Administration of conditioned media from stimulated immune cells results in decreased noradrenaline (NA) content in the brain (Besedovsky, del Rey, Sorkin, Da Prada et al., 1983). Also, natural purified or recombinant cytokines affect brain neurotransmitters and central neuronal activity (Araujo, Lapchak, Collier, & Quirion, 1989; De Sarro, Ascioti, Audino, Rispoli, & Nistico, 1989; Dunn, 1988; Ericsson, Kovacs, & Sawchenko, 1994; Gemma, Ghezzi, & De Simoni, 1991; Kabiersch, del Rey, Honegger, & Besedovsky, 1988; Linthorst, Flachskamm, Holsboer, & Reul, 1994; Muller, Fontana, Zbinden, & Gahwiler, 1993; Reyes Vazquez, Prieto Gomez, Georgiades, & Dafny, 1984). IL-1 reduces NA content and increases the ratio 3-methoxy-4-hydroxyphenylethylene glycol (MHPG)/NA, which reflects an increased NA metabolism. This effect is observed in the hypothalamus, hippocampus, brain stem, and spinal cord. The fact that catecholaminergic fibers in the spinal cord are stimulated by IL-1 may indicate one possible neural pathway for the effect of this cytokine in the central nervous system (CNS). The stimulation of noradrenergic neurons in the CNS by IL-1 is consistent with evidence indicating that catecholaminergic neurons are involved in the response of the HPA axis to this cytokine (Chuluyan, Saphier, Rohn, & Dunn, 1992; Matta, Singh, Newton, & Sharp, 1990; Weidenfeld, Abramsky, & Ovadia, 1989). IL-1 and IL-6 stimulate dopamine metabolism in the striatum, hippocampus and prefrontal cortex. These cytokines also stimulate serotonin metabolism and release, but the effect is observed predominantly in the hippocampus. IL-1, however, induces an increase in the content of tryptophan, the amino acid precursor of serotonin, in most brain regions (Dunn, 1988; Kabiersch et al., 1988). IL-2 inhibits potassium-induced release of acetylcholine from hippocampal slices (Araujo et al., 1989), and IL-3, IFNγ, G-CSF, and GM-CSF augment choline-acetylcholine transferase (CHAT) activity in septal neurons in vitro (Konishi, Chui, Hirose, Kunishita, & Tabira, 1993).

Studies performed in vivo show that IL-1 administration stimulates neurons of the paraventricular and supraoptic nucleus of the hypothalamus and of the stria terminalis (Chang, Ren, & Zadina, 1993; Ericsson et al., 1994; Saphier & Ovadia, 1990). IL-2 and IFNγ stimulate neuronal activity in the cortex and hippocampus (De Sarro et al., 1989; Reyes Vazquez et al., 1984). In brain slices, IL-1 stimulates neurons of the supraoptic nucleus of the hypothalamus, an effect that is modulated by GABAergic inputs (Miller, Galpern, Dunlap, Dinarello, & Turner, 1991). IFNγ exerts an excitatory effect in CA3 pyramidal cells and decreases evoked inhibitory potential amplitude (Muller et al., 1993). TNF stimulates neurons of the organum vasculosum of the lamina terminalis (OVLT) (Shibata & Blatteis, 1991). In vitro, IL-1 inhibits long-term potentiation (LTP) in the hippocampus, and decreases voltage-gated calcium currents in dissociated CA1 neurons (Bellinger, Madamba, & Siggins, 1993). TNF (Tancredi et al., 1992) and IFNγ (Muller et al., 1993) also inhibit LTP. However, as we shall discuss later, LTP itself induces cytokine production. Therefore, the in vitro experiments mentioned above may not be comparable to what occurs spontaneously during this process.

C. Effects of Cytokines on Thermoregulation, Sleep, Food Intake, and Behavior

Immune cytokines influence complex mechanisms that involve a variety of neuronal circuits, such as thermoregulation, food intake, sleeping patterns, and behavior. These effects will not be discussed in detail since they have been previously reviewed (Rothwell & Hopkins, 1995) and several chapters of this book address this issue. We shall only mention a few examples here.

The existence of an endogenous pyrogen, as proposed 50 years ago, is now fully established, with the exception that not one but several endogenous substances, such as IL-1, IL-6, IL-8, IFNγ, IFNβ, and GM-CSF, possess the capacity of inducing fever (Blatteis, 1992; Kluger, 1991). Also, several cytokines, among which are IL-1, IL-6, IL-8, and TNFα inhibit food intake (Plata-Salaman, 1989; Rothwell, 1991). The capacity of increasing slow wave sleep is also shared by IL-1, IL-2, IFNγ, and TNFα (Nistico & De Sarro, 1991; Opp, Postlethwaite, Seyer, & Krueger, 1992). A dual role of cytokines in the sensitivity to pain has been described. IL-1 and IL-6, acting at sites of inflammation, sensitize afferent fibers through stimulating the release of prostaglandins (Dray & Bevan, 1993). However, when IL-1 is given systemically, it mediates an antinociceptive response (Kita, Imano, & Nakamura, 1993). Several cytokines are known to exert profound effects on behavior, e.g., learning and explorative and avoidance behavior (Dyck & Greenberg, 1991; Kent, Bluthé, Kelley, & Dantzer, 1992). Some effects of IL-1 on behavior are likely to occur at CNS levels, since i.c.v. administration of IL-1ra blocks such effects (Kent et al., 1992). There is also some evidence that cytokines may be involved in central mechanisms of learning and memory (Patterson & Nawa, 1993).

D. Pathways Followed by Cytokines to Affect Brain Functions

As discussed above, cytokines released during the immune response are the main messengers of afferent signals to the brain. Cytokines could follow humoral or neural routes to affect brain functions. Which of these routes predominate under different conditions is at present subject to intense investigation. It will only be mentioned here that there is evidence that both of these routes can be used to convey information to the brain. Circulating cytokines could enter the brain through areas with a poorly developed blood–brain barrier (BBB), such as the circumventricular organs, or can be actively transported (Gutierrez, Banks, & Kastin, 1993, 1994). Other possibilities are that cytokines induce the production of mediators that can cross the BBB, or that they induce their own production or other factors at the endothelial interface between the brain and the blood.

The evidence that neural pathways may mediate effects of cytokines on the brain derives from studies in animals in which subdiaphragmatic vagotomy abrogates behavioral changes, fever, and some of the neuroendocrine responses induced by lipopolysaccharid (LPS) (Bret-Dibat, Bluthe, Kent, Kelley, & Dantzer, 1995; Maier, Goehler, Fleshnwe, & Watkins, 1998; Sehic & Blatteis, 1996; Watkins et al., 1995). However, some of the effects of the endotoxin are not affected when only the afferent vagal fibers are cut (Schwartz, Plata-Salaman, & Langhans, 1997). Furthermore, in many cases, vagotomy significantly blocks LPS effects on the brain only if the endotoxin is administered intraperitoneally (Ericsson, Arias, & Sawchenko, 1997; Goldbach, Roth, & Zeisberger, 1997).

In general, the data available at present suggest that the humoral route to the CNS may be followed by circulating cytokines, while the neural route seems to predominate when these mediators are released locally in tissues with vagal innervation.

IV. SHORT-LOOP INTERACTIONS BETWEEN CYTOKINES AND PERIPHERAL NERVE FIBERS

Immune-neural interactions may also occur at local levels in the periphery, since neurotransmitters released by autonomic nerves can affect the immune process (for review see Besedovsky & del Rey, 1996, and Homo-Delarche & Durant, 1994). However, effects of cytokines on peripheral nerves have not been explored so broadly as those on the central nervous system. In vivo evidence showing effects of cytokines on peripheral nerve activity indicate that such effects are primarily exerted at central level. For example, systemic administration of IL-1 increases the rate of firing of splenic nerve fibers and stimulates peripheral NA release by acting on CRH-producing neurons in the brain (Niijima, Hori, Aou, & Oomura, 1991; Shimizu, Hori, & Nakane, 1994). However, peripheral nerve terminals may be affected by cytokines endogenously produced in their vicinity.

Data from in vitro experiments suggest this possibility (Bognar, Albrecht, Farasaty, & Fuder, 1995; Hart, Shadiack, & Jonakait, 1991; Hurst & Collins, 1993; Shadiack, Hart, Carlson, & Jonakait, 1993; Soliven & Wang, 1995).

An in vivo evidence for local effects of IL-1β on sympathetic nerve fibers is provided by our studies showing that the increase in splenic blood flow induced by this cytokine is exerted at a postganglionic level. We have previously shown that exogenously administered IL-1 causes a marked increase in splenic blood flow, and that this effect depends on an intact splenic innervation (Rogausch, del Rey, Kabiersch, & Besedovsky, 1995). More recently, we also found that increased endogenous IL-1 production induced by a low dose of LPS causes a similar effect (Rogausch, del Rey, Kabiersch, Reschke, Örtel, & Besedovsky, 1997). Surgical denervation or NA depletion by reserpine abrogates the IL-1 induced increase in splenic blood flow, indicating that the cytokine acts on sympathetic nerve fibers (Figure 3). Furthermore, using two approaches, we have shown that this effect of IL-1 is exerted at a postganglionic level. First, ganglionic blockade with hexamethonium does not interfere with the increase in splenic blood flow induced by LPS. Second, LPS administration completely antagonizes the decrease in blood flow induced by electrical stimulation of the splenic nerve, but does not interfere with the vasoconstrictor effects of NA. The most likely interpretation of these results is that, in vivo, endogenous IL-1 inhibits NA release by sympathetic nerve fibers rather than exerting an effect at postjunctional level (Figure 4). This conclusion is further supported by studies performed in vitro (Hurst & Collins, 1993).

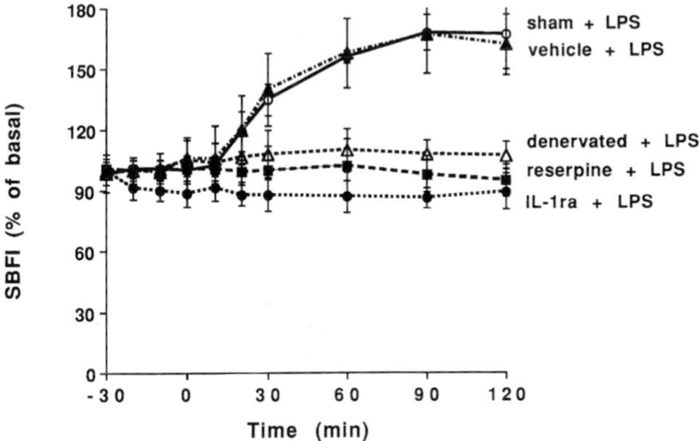

FIGURE 3 Effect of denervation, noradrenaline depletion and blockade of IL-1 receptors on LPS-induced increase in splenic blood flow. Rats were prepared for recording of splenic blood flow, heart rate and arterial blood pressure. When these parameters were stable for 1 hour, LPS (10 g/kg b.w.) was injected i.v. (time 0), and the recordings were continued for a further 2 hours. Groups of animals received the following treatments: 1) IL-1ra (1 mg/kg b.w.) or isotonic saline (vehicle) injected i.p. 30 min before LPS; 2) the splenic nerve was surgically interrupted (denervated) or a sham-operation was performed (sham) five days before LPS; 3) reserpine (10 mg/kg) injected i.p. 24 hours before LPS. The splenic blood flow index (SBFI) is expressed as % of the basal SBFI of each individual animal for each treatment. Values represent the mean ± SE of 4-8 animals per group. Adapted with permission from Rogausch, del Rey, Kabiersch, Reschke, et al., 1997.

Since blood vessels are the only circulatory system in the spleen, the increase in splenic blood flow caused by local interactions between IL-1 and sympathetic nerve fibers is expected to have immunoregulatory implications. Antigens are trapped in the spleen, and immune cells that reside in this organ are derived from the circulation and recirculate via the blood. Therefore, the control of splenic blood flow is relevant for these essential steps of the immune responses to circulating antigens. Collectively, the evidence discussed constitutes a clear example of short-loop immunoregulatory interactions between a product released by activated immune cells and peripheral nerve fibers.

V. DUAL IMMUNE AND NEURAL CONTROL OF CYTOKINE PRODUCTION IN THE BRAIN: THE "RELAY SYSTEM" HYPOTHESIS

In this section, evidence showing that receptors for some cytokines are expressed in the CNS, and also that certain brain cells can produce these cytokines will be discussed. We shall also refer to studies showing that peripheral immune signals and signals derived from brain neurons can both induce cytokine production in the CNS, indicating a dual control of this process. The hypothesis that cytokine-producing cells in the brain form part of a "relay system" that integrates neural and immune signals acting in the brain will be advanced.

A. Receptors for Immune Cytokines in the Nervous System

Following the finding that administration of certain cytokines can induce pronounced changes in endocrine parameters that are under neural control, a large number of reports became available showing that receptors for some of these cytokines are present in the central nervous system. Different techniques such as autoradiography, immunoautoradiography, in situ histochemistry, and in situ hybridization histochemistry, sometimes also combined with reverse transcriptase-polymerase chain reaction, have been used. As a whole, the evidence indicates the presence in the brain of receptors (or of the corresponding mRNAs) for IL-1 α and β (Ban, Milon, Prudhomme, Fillion, & Haour, 1991; Cunningham, Wada, Carter, Tracey,

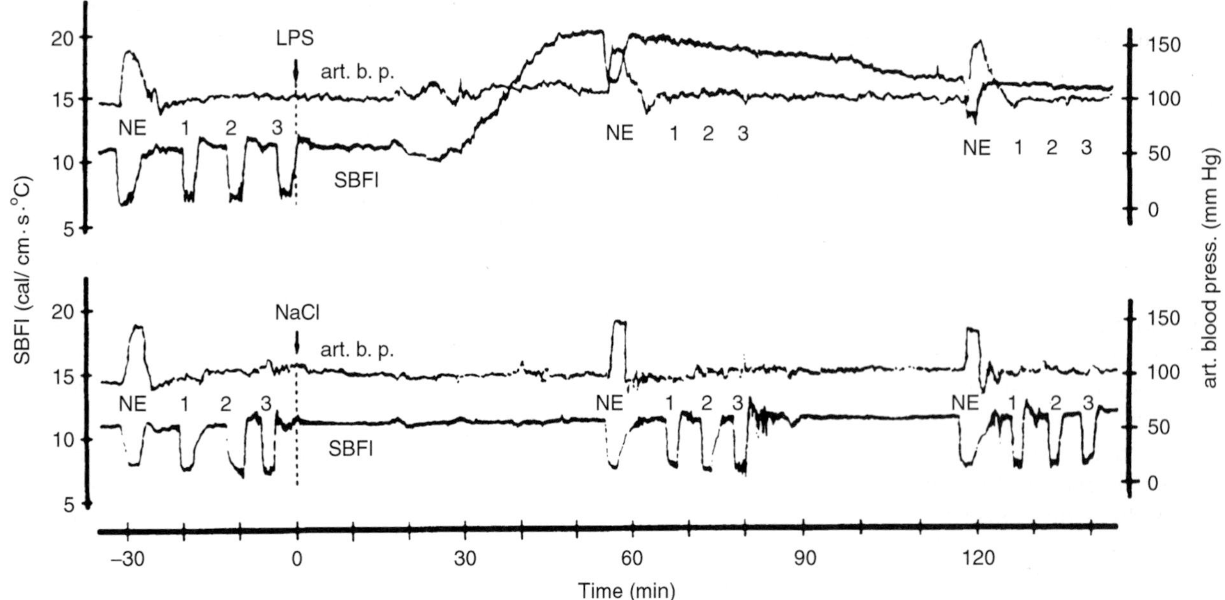

FIGURE 4 LPS interferes with the decrease in splenic blood flow induced by electrical stimulation of the splenic nerve. Rats were prepared for recording of splenic blood flow, heart rate and arterial blood pressure. Thirty minutes after all recorded parameters were stable, noradrenaline (NE, 0.5 μg/kg.) was injected i.v. When splenic blood flow index (SBFI) and arterial blood pressure (art. b. p.) returned to the basal values, the splenic nerve was electrically stimulated for three consecutive times (indicated by numbers in the figure). When the measured parameters returned again to the basal values, LPS (10 μg/kg) or isotonic saline (NaCl) was injected i.v. One and two hours later, the same procedures of NE administration and nerve stimulation were performed. The figure illustrates the results of a representative experiment. Reprinted with permission from Rogausch, del Rey, Kabiersch, Reschke, et al., 1997.

Battey, & De Souza, 1992; Deyerle, Sims, Dower, & Bothwell, 1992), IL-2 (Araujo et al., 1989), IL-4 (Lowenthal, Castle, Christiansen, Schreurs, Rennick, Arai, Hoy, Takebe, & Howard, 1988), IL-6 (Schöbitz, de Kloet, Sutanto, & Holsboer, 1993), TNFα (Kinouchi, Brown, Pasternak, & Donner, 1991), IFNγ (Tada, Diserens, Desbaillets, & de Tribolet, 1994), M-CSF, and SCF (Chang, Albright, & Lee, 1994). Probably the most studied receptors are those for IL-1. Although not all studies completely agree on the localization of specific binding sites for cytokines in the brain, there seems to be a general consensus that, in adult mice and rats, IL-1 receptors are mainly located or more concentrated in the hippocampus. Most authors have found that these receptors are present constitutively (for review see Besedovsky & del Rey, 1996), while others have detected them following endotoxin administration (Takao, Culp, & De Souza, 1993). The possibility that glucocorticoids or adrenalectomy modulate IL-1 receptors in the brain has also been addressed (Ban et al., 1993). This issue will not be discussed further here. More detailed information can be obtained in a relatively recent review (Besedovsky & del Rey, 1996) and in other chapters of this book.

B. Stimulation of Peripheral Immune Cells Induces Cytokine Expression in the Brain

Astrocytes and microglial cells were the brain cells first shown to produce several cytokines (Fontana, Kristensen, Dubs, Gemsa, & Weber, 1982; for review see Fabry, Raine, & Hart, 1994). Later, it was reported that certain neurons can also produce cytokines such as IL-1 (Breder, Dinarello, & Saper, 1988). The abundant evidence about cytokine induction during encephalopathies, such as those caused by brain infections, is not discussed here. Although these studies are, of course, vital for understanding the importance of cytokines for brain pathophysiology, it is usually difficult to determine whether under these circumstances, cytokines in the brain are produced by resident cells or are derived from invading peripheral immunocompetent cells. Furthermore, in most cases, it is not clear whether locally induced immune cytokines contribute to the regulation of the immune response in the CNS by affecting neural mechanisms.

Several cytokines, such as IL-1, its natural receptor antagonist (IL-1ra), IL-2, IL-3, IL-6, IL-8, IL-12, and IFNγ have been found in the brain (for review see

Besedovsky & del Rey, 1996), and most reports agree that peripheral administration of LPS results in further expression of cytokines in the brain (Buttini & Boddeke, 1995; Gabellec, Griffais, Fillion, & Haour, 1995; Gatti & Bartfai, 1993; Layé, Parnet, Goujon, & Dantzer, 1994; Quan, Sundar, & Weiss, 1994; van Dam, Bauer, Tilders, & Berkenbosch, 1995). However, the doses of LPS administered were rather high. Because this endotoxin can disturb the BBB in mice (Lustig, Danenberg, Kafri, Kobiler, & Ben-Nathan, 1992), these studies did not exclude the possibility that the increased expression of cytokines in the brain resulted from a direct action of LPS in the CNS. In addition, the possible contribution of endothelial cells or of the blood as a source of cytokines in the brain has in general not been excluded. Thus, we have studied the possibility that stimulation of peripheral immune cells triggers cytokine induction in the brain using a low dose of LPS known not to disrupt the BBB, and well below those that can induce septic shock. This is also a relevant issue, since cardiovascular and respiratory derangements could induce cytokine expression in the CNS nonspecifically. Since we expected that low amounts of cytokines would be produced in a "healthy" brain, a sensitive semiquantitative RT-PCR technique was used to study IL-1β, IL-6, TNFα, and IFNγ mRNA expression in defined brain areas. An eventual contribution of the blood to the cytokine signals detected was experimentally ruled out (Pitossi, del Rey, Kabiersch, & Besedovsky, 1997). Some of the results obtained are shown in Figure 5.

Constitutive expression of IL-1β, IL-6, and TNFα but not of IFNγ, was detected in the brain. However, cytokine mRNA transcripts were not evenly distributed since a three- to fourfold variation between the regions studied was noticed. The gene expression of the four cytokines studied was increased following peripheral administration of LPS. The onset of

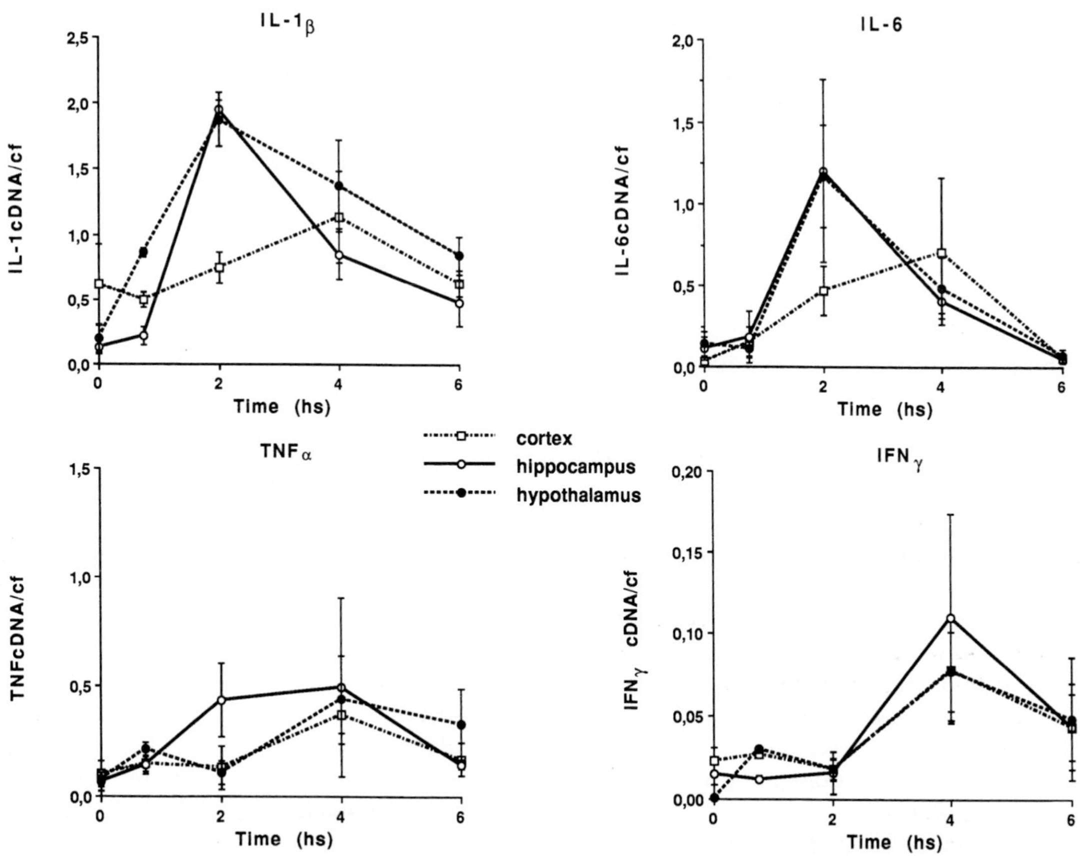

FIGURE 5 LPS induces cytokine expression in the brain Male C57Bl/6J mice received saline (indicated in the figure as time 0) or LPS (20 μg/kg) injected i.p., and groups of animals were killed by cervical dislocation after 45 minutes, and 2, 4, and 6 hours. The brain was dissected into six different regions and immediately frozen. The figure shows the results of semiquantitative RT-PCR determinations of IL-1β, IL-6, TNFα and IFNγ mRNAs in the cortex, hippocampus and hypothalamus expressed as the mean cDNA/competitive fragment (cf) ratio for each cytokine ± SEM. Adapted from with permission Pitossi et al., 1997. Copyright © 1997 Wiley-Liss, Inc., a subsidiary of John Wiley & Sons, Inc.

transcription varied from 45 minutes (IL-1β and TNFα) to 2 hours (IFNγ), and the peak of mRNA accumulation was observed at different times depending on the cytokine and the brain region studied. IL-1β and IL-6 were preferentially expressed in the hypothalamus and hippocampus, while TNFα expression was more marked in the thalamus-striatum. The brain cortex was the region in which cytokines were less inducible. No correlation between cytokine expression and the density of vascular structures in a given brain area was detected, indicating a low contribution of endothelial cell-derived mRNA transcripts to the levels of cytokine expression detected. Furthermore, no preferential or earlier cytokine expression was detected in brain areas that include circumventricular organs. This suggests that even if some LPS would have crossed the BBB at these sites, it did not significantly contribute to the induction of cytokines in regions near to the circumventricular organs. Taken together, the results show that stimulation of peripheral immune cells induces cytokine expression in the brain. The particular pattern of regional expression of cytokines in the hypothalamus and hippocampus suggests that, during activation of the immune system, brain-born cytokines may affect neuroendocrine mechanisms controlled in these areas.

C. Neuronal Stimuli Increase Cytokine Expression in the CNS

As discussed above, cytokines can be produced by glial cells and certain neurons, and can affect the activity of these cells by acting on specific receptors. The question that arises is whether effects of cytokines produced in the brain on brain functions are exerted only under pathological conditions when massive amounts are produced by resident or invading cells. Is it possible that cytokines produced by neurons or glial cells also play a physiologic, neuromodulatory role in the "healthy brain"? Apart from acting as growing factors during neuronal development, differentiation and repair, brain-born cytokines could also play an active role in supporting neuronal activity during different physiologic processes. For this to be possible, it must be demonstrated that (1) changes in the activity of neurons during a given physiological process result in the production of particular cytokines; and (2) such an increased cytokine production should in turn affect the activity of these and/or other interconnected neurons, and in this way, contribute to control the physiological process in which they are involved. We have recently approached this issue using as a model the LTP of synaptic activity in the hippocampus, a process that underlies certain forms of learning and memory. The hallmark of LTP is a sustained enhancement in synaptic transmission and postsynaptic neuronal activity following a high frequency stimulation of afferent fibers. Due to these characteristics, LTP makes it possible to explore whether a long-lasting increase in the activity of a defined population of neurons results in an increased production of a given cytokine, and whether, in turn, this cytokine can affect these neurons. We have found a clear accumulation of IL-1β transcripts during the course of LTP in hippocampal slices, the highest level of expression being detected 3 hours after induction of this process. A several-fold increase in IL-1β transcripts was also observed in freely moving rats undergoing LTP (Figure 6) (Schneider et al., 1998). This increased expression of IL-1β gene is triggered by glutaminergic neurons through NMDA receptors. These data constitute the first evidence that IL-1β gene expression in the brain can be triggered by a discrete population of neurons. Furthermore, the induction of this gene occurs, as expected during physiologic conditions, following stimulation of these neurons at a presynaptic level.

In the experimental model chosen, the second requirement mentioned above implies the demonstration that the IL-1β produced during LTP can affect the activity of the potentiated neurons. For this purpose, the specific IL-1 receptor antagonist IL-1ra was used to block the effects of endogenous IL-1β. The results obtained, both in vivo and in hippocampal slices, showed that blockade of IL-1 receptors resulted in the inhibition of LTP maintenance. This effect was reversible and occurred only when the antagonist was given 90 minutes after LTP was triggered, that is, at a time when, according to the previous studies, it was expected that the gene is translated and resulted in the production of biologically significant amounts of the cytokine (Figure 7). Thus, LTP was affected by the increased production of IL-1β triggered by potentiated neurons, rather than by basal levels of the cytokine. Collectively, these results strongly suggest that IL-1β is a key mediator for the maintenance of LTP, a process that is assigned a role in memory formation and in certain types of learning. Furthermore, these studies provide evidence for a physiologic, neuromodulatory role in the brain for a cytokine originally described as an immune mediator.

D. Cytokine-Producing Cells in the Brain Form Part of a "Relay System" in the Immune-CNS Circuitry

In previous sections, evidence showing that cytokines can convey signals from the immune system to

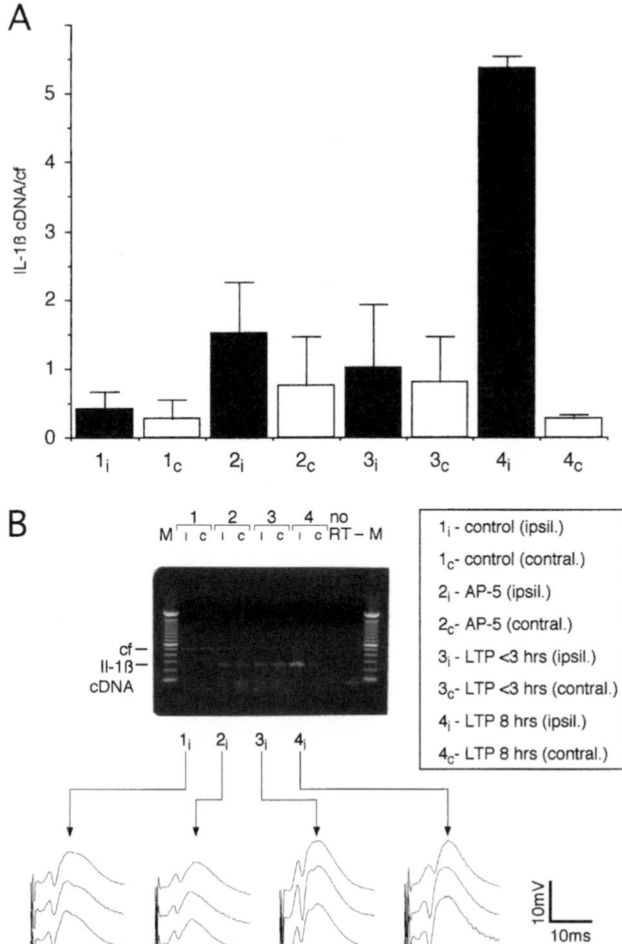

FIGURE 6 IL-1β gene expression during LTP in vivo. (A) IL-1β mRNA expression 8 hours after tetanization. Thirty minutes prior to tetanization, animals received either physiological saline (groups 1, 3 and 4) or AP-5 (group 2) administered i.c.v. Black bars indicate measurements performed in ipsilateral (i) and white bars in contralateral (c) hippocampi. Group 1: hippocampi of animals recorded under baseline conditions without tetanic stimulation. Group 2: hippocampi of animals in which the expression of LTP after tetanization was blocked by AP-5. Group 3: hippocampi of animals showing a potentiation that returned to baseline within 3 hours. Group 4: hippocampi of animals with a robust LTP lasting for 8 hours. Results of RT-PCR are expressed as mean $\pm$ SEM of the ratio IL-1β cDNA and the competitive fragment (cf). $n=4$ per group. Group 4i differs significantly from all other groups (ANOVA followed by Fisher's test for multiple comparisons). (B) Representative ethidium bromide-stained agarose gel showing the amplified transcripts of a RT-PCR obtained from ipsi- and contralateral hippocampi which were subjected to different experimental conditions (lane numbers correspond to the groups shown in A). The line graphs display representative analogue traces recorded during baseline (top), immediately after tetanization (middle) and 8 hours after tetanus (bottom). M: 100 bp ladder molecular weight marker, no RT: RT-PCR without addition of reverse transcriptase, - : RT-PCR without addition of cDNA. Reprinted from Schneider et al., 1998.

the CNS, and the neuroendocrine responses to these signals, were discussed. We have also referred to the fact that some of the same cytokines that mediate peripheral immune signals can be produced in the CNS. Furthermore, examples were provided showing that both peripheral immune and central neuronal signals can induce the production of certain cytokines in the brain. We have also mentioned that during pathological conditions, neuroendocrine, metabolic, and behavioral alterations occur, and that at least some of these alterations are triggered by immune cytokines rather than by the agent that causes the disease or by the disease itself. Thus, it appears that the immune system can affect, and, in advanced stages of different diseases, even control crucial homeostatic mechanisms integrated at brain levels. Because cytokines injected directly into the brain can induce neuroendocrine changes, it is reasonable to postulate that brain-born cytokines could also be involved in the mediation of neuroendocrine adjustments during processes in which the immune system is stimulated. An example is that the stimulation of the HPA axis that occurs during peripheral inflammation induced by turpentine can be blocked by interfering with TNFα produced in the brain (Turnbull et al., 1997). There is also evidence that brain-born cytokines influence behavioral effects of peripheral cytokines (Kent, Bluthe, Dantzer, et al., 1992; Linthorst, Flachskamm, Muller-Preuss, Holsboer, & Reul, 1995). On the other hand, it has been shown that cytokines such as IL-1 acting locally in the brain influence peripheral immune functions by affecting neuroendocrine mechanisms (Brown et al., 1991; Sundar, Cierpial, Kilts, Ritchie, & Weiss, 1990). Thus, an increased cytokine production in the brain triggered by peripheral stimulation of the immune system may contribute to mediation of the neuroendocrine alterations that accompany certain pathologies and also affect the activity of the immune system.

It is worth noting that effects of cytokines, when injected or induced either peripherally or centrally, are, in many cases, remarkably similar. Are these similarities just an expression of "redundancy" in cytokine actions? In our opinion, a valid alternative is that the production of both peripheral and central cytokines underlie well-programmed steps of responses integrated at brain levels. Under basal conditions, the release of low amounts of cytokines by brain cells could be one of the various inputs that control the activity of neurons involved in the regulation of adaptive functions integrated at hypothalamic and limbic system levels. In conditions during which changes in the activity of the immune system occur, peripheral cytokines and other mediators would

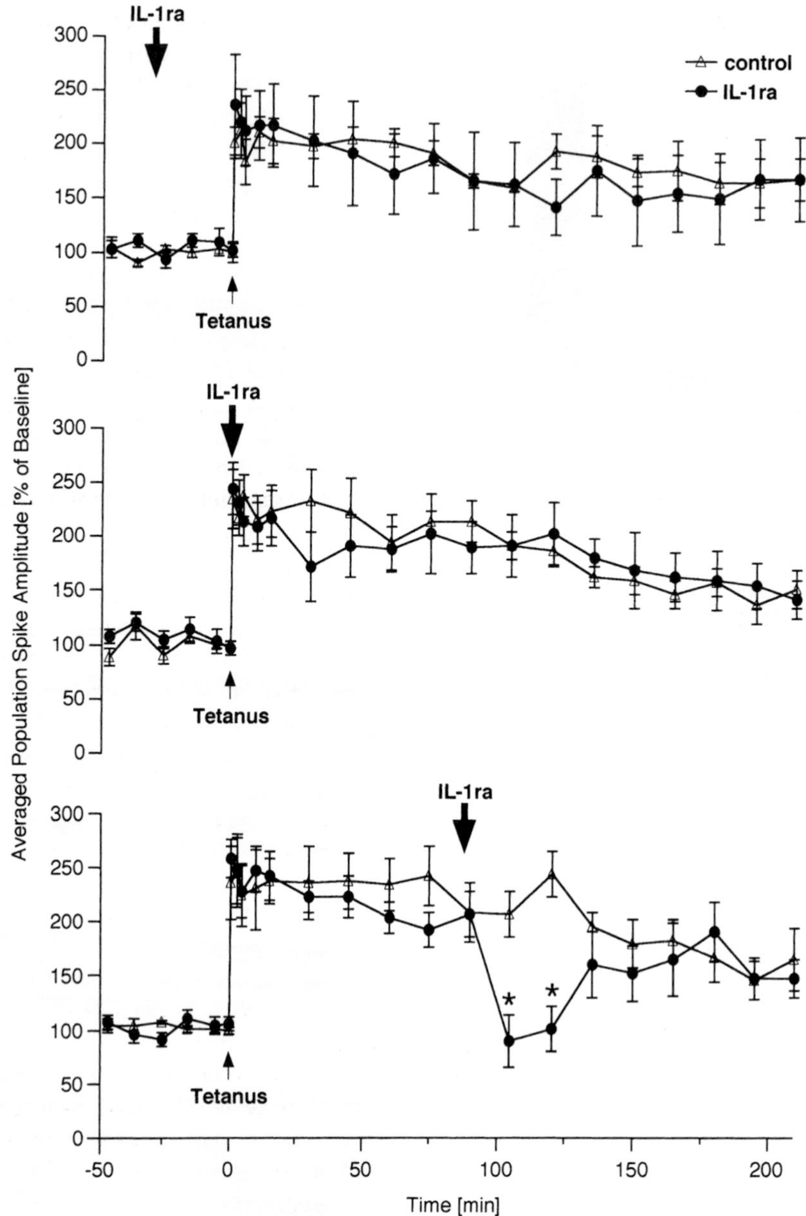

FIGURE 7 Blockade of IL-1 receptors causes a reversible inhibition of LTP maintenance in vivo. Either physiological saline (control) or IL-1ra was administered i.c.v. Data are plotted as average change from baseline response (mean±SEM). The times of tetanization and of drug application are indicated by an arrow. (Top). Application of IL-1ra 30 min prior to tetanization did not affect subsequent LTP (n = 6). (Middle) When IL-ra was applied immediately after tetanus no statistically significant effects could be observed (n = 7). (Bottom) IL-ra infused 90 min post-tetanus caused a marked decrease of potentiation (n = 8, *p < 0.05, ANOVA, followed by the Fisher's test for multiple comparisons) which lasted for about 40 min. Reprinted from Schneider et al., 1998.

trigger the initial step of neuroendocrine responses to immune cell stimulation. The quick neuroendocrine response observed when certain cytokines are administered peripherally may indicate that this initial step does not involve the de novo synthesis of cytokines in the brain. However, peripheral immune mediators and neurons activated during this initial step would trigger an increased expression of cytokines in the brain. This confluence of signals may contribute to determine a defined pattern of central cytokine expression during an immune response. As we have shown, during LTP these cytokines are expected to feed back on the neurons originally affected. Cytokine-producing cells (glial cells, neurons) located in brain regions where neuroendocrine mechanisms capable of affecting immune functions are controlled, may also be influenced by neurons stimulated by other sensorial inputs, e.g., during stress conditions. We therefore postulate a "relay system" based on interactions between neurons and cytokine-producing brain cells that would integrate peripheral immune and central neural signals and modulate neuroendocrine responses to these stimuli (Figure 8).

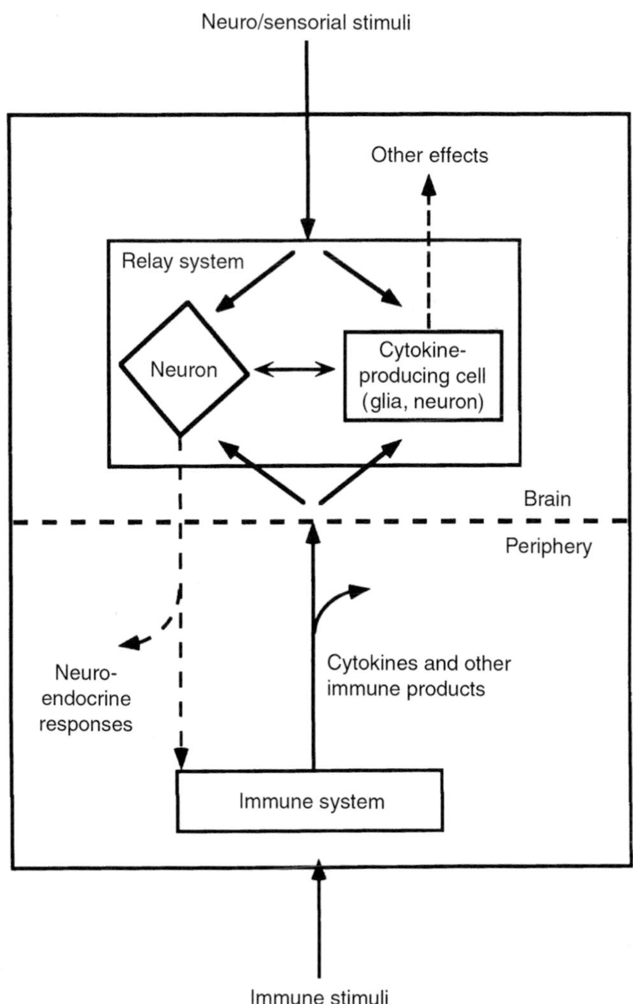

FIGURE 8 A relay system that integrates peripheral immune and neural/sensorial signals, and induces a re-setting of neuroendocrine functions is postulated. This relay system is based on interactions between cytokine-producing brain cells and neurons located in their close vicinity. When increased cytokine production is induced in areas such as the hypothalamus and the hippocampus as consequence of immune and/or neuronal signals, a re-setting of homeostatic functions would occur (themoregulation, glucose homeostasis, neuroendocrine feed-back, etc). This re-setting of homeostasis is expected to be specially relevant for neuro-endocrine adjustments needed during conditions in which primarily the immune system (e.g. infections) or the CNS (e.g. stress) is affected.

Cytokines produced in the brain under the control of such a relay system and acting in an autocrine/paracrine fashion, may change the "set point" for the control of those neuroendocrine variables that need to be adjusted. This would explain why neuroendocrine and metabolic effects of cytokines administered systemically are more prolonged than expected from the half-life of cytokines in the circulation. For example, a single injection of a low dose of IL-1β induces a long-lasting hypoglycemia and changes the set point for glucoregulation during several hours (del Rey & Besedovsky, 1987, 1989). Since peripheral IL-1 administration results in IL-1 gene expression in the CNS, and IL-1-induced hypoglycemia can be abrogated to large extent by i.c.v. administration of IL-1ra (del Rey, Monge-Arditi, & Besedovsky, 1998), these results suggest that the de novo produced cytokine in the brain contributes to hypoglycemia. Thus, not only thermoregulatory mechanisms but also glucose homeostasis can be centrally reset by cytokines. The existence of a relay system that integrates immune and neuronal signals and that, by controlling cytokine production in the brain, mediates a resetting of essential physiological variables, would provide an answer to critical questions such as (1) how the immune system can mediate long-lasting neuroendocrine adjustments of mechanisms controlled in many different brain regions; and (2) how these adjustments are coordinated with other needs of the organism and with the response to other sensorial signals.

Based on evidence that neuroendocrine changes occur during the immune response and that cytokines can mediate such changes, it was proposed that the immune system behaves as a sensorial receptor organ that conveys information to the brain about the type of immune response in operation (Besedovsky, del Rey, & Sorkin, 1983; Besedovsky, del Rey, Sorkin, Da Prada et al., 1983; Blalock, 1984). The relay system proposed above is intimately linked to this concept. The knowledge that cytokine-producing cells in the brain can be stimulated by peripheral immune signals suggests that these cells represent the immune system in the CNS. The preferential expression of cytokines and/or their receptors in the hypothalamus and hippocampus indicate these areas as main sites of immune representation in the CNS. However, because immune cells are sources of noncognitive signals to these primitive brain regions and these cells are mobile and spread out in the body, a somatotopic homunculus-like representation of the immune system in the brain is unlikely. If different types of peripheral immune responses would induce distinct patterns of cytokine expression in defined brain regions, this would instead suggest that a sort of functional immune homunculus is represented at central level.

VI. OVERVIEW

Some data and views on immune–neuroendocrine interactions were discussed in this chapter, and examples mainly derived from our work were included to illustrate the relevance of these interactions. However, psychoneuroimmunology is much more than what could be discussed in the Foreword of a book because this new discipline has "invaded" many fields in medical and biological sciences. The variety of aspects opened for investigation by the simultaneous analysis of parameters that were the exclusive domain of either neuroscience or immunology embraces almost all types of tissues, organs, and pathologies. The identification of a neuroendocrine level of immunoregulation implies the need to search for interplays between almost every immune cell product and hormone, neurotransmitter and neuropeptide. This field has broken the boundaries between different body systems by showing, for example, that a cytokine can behave as a neurotransmitter and a hormone as a cytokine. This explains the tremendous (we are tempted to write, with all respect, "biblical"!) amount of information that is provided in this third edition of *Psychoneuroimmunology*, which, as reflection of the glamorous expansion of the field, is at least three times bigger than the first one.

Acknowledgments

The authors wish to acknowledge the support of the Volkswagen Stiftung and the Deutsche Forschungsgemeinschaft (SFB 297).

References

Ader, R., & Cohen, N. (1991). The influence of conditioning on immune responses. In R. Ader, D. L. Felten, and N. Cohen (eds.), *Psychoneuroimmunology* (pp. 609–646). New York: Academic Press.

Araujo, D. M., Lapchak, P. A., Collier, B., & Quirion, R. (1989). Localization of interleukin-2 immunoreactivity and interleukin-2 receptors in the rat brain: Interaction with the cholinergic system. *Brain Research, 498*, 257–266.

Ban, E., Marquette, C., Sarrieau, A., Fitzpatrick, F., Fillion, G., Milon, G., Rostene, W., & Haour, F. (1993). Regulation of interleukin-1 receptor expression in mouse brain and pituitary by lipopolysaccharide and glucocorticoids. *Neuroendocrinology, 58*, 581–587.

Ban, E., Milon, G., Prudhomme, N., Fillion, G., & Haour, F. (1991). Receptors for interleukin-1 (alpha and beta) in mouse brain: Mapping and neuronal localization in hippocampus. *Neuroscience, 43*, 21–30.

Bellinger, F. P., Madamba, S., & Siggins, G. R. (1993). Interleukin 1 beta inhibits synaptic strength and long-term potentiation in the rat CA1 hippocampus. *Brain Research, 628*, 227–234.

Berczi, I., & Nagy, E. (1991). Effect of hypophysectomy on immune function. In R. Ader, D. L. Felten, and N. Cohen (Eds.), *Psychoneuroimmunology* (pp. 337–375). New York: Academic Press.

Berkenbosch, F., de Goeij, D. E. C., del Rey, A., & Besedovsky, H. O. (1989). Neuroendocrine, sympathetic, and metabolic responses induced by Interleukin-1. *Neuroendocrinology, 50*, 570–576.

Besedovsky, H. O. & del Rey, A. (1996). Immune-Neuro-Endocrine Interactions: Facts and Hypotheses. *Endocrine Reviews, 17*, 64–102.

Besedovsky, H. O., del Rey, A., Klusman, I., Furukawa, H., Monge Arditi, G., & Kabiersch, A. (1991). Cytokines as modulators of the hypothalamus-pituitary-adrenal axis. *Journal of Steroid Biochemistry and Molecular Biology, 40*, 613–618.

Besedovsky, H. O., del Rey, A., & Sorkin, E. (1981). Lymphokine containing supernatants from Con A-stimulated cells increase corticosterone blood levels. *Journal of Immunology, 126*, 385–387.

Besedovsky, H. O., del Rey, A., & Sorkin, E. (1983). What do the immune system and the brain know about each other? *Immunology Today, 4*, 342–346.

Besedovsky, H. O., del Rey, A., Sorkin, E., Da Prada, M., Burri, R., & Honegger, C. G. (1983). The immune response evokes changes in brain noradrenergic neurons. *Science, 221*, 564–566.

Besedovsky, H. O., del Rey, A., Sorkin, E., Lotz, W., & Schwulera, U. (1985). Lymphoid cells produce an immunoregulatory glucocorticoid increasing factor (GIF) acting through the pituitary gland. *Clinical and Experimental Immunology, 59*, 622–628.

Besedovsky, H., del Rey, A., Sorkin, E., & Dinarello, C. A. (1986). Immunoregulatory feedback between interleukin-1 and glucocorticoid hormones. *Science, 233*, 652–654.

Besedovsky, H. O., & Sorkin, E. (1977). Network of immune-neuroendocrine interactions. *Clinical and Experimental Immunology, 27*, 1–12.

Besedovsky, H. O., Sorkin, E., Felix, D., & Haas, H. (1977). Hypothalamic changes during the immune response. *European Journal of Immunology, 7*, 323–325.

Besedovsky, H. O., Sorkin, E., Keller, M., & Mueller, J. (1975). Hormonal changes during the immune response. *Proceedings of the Society for Experimental Biology and Medicine, 150*, 466–479.

Blalock, J. E. (1984). The immune system as a sensory organ. *Journal of Immunology, 132*, 1067–1070.

Blatteis, C. M. (1992). The OVLT: The interphase between the brain and circulating pyrogens? In O. D. Bartfai T (eds.), *Neuroimmunology of Fever* (pp. 167–176). New York: Pergamon Press.

Bognar, I. T., Albrecht, S. A., Farasaty, M., & Fuder, H. (1995). Inhibition by interleukin-1 beta of noradrenaline release in the rat spleen: Involvement of lymphocytes, NO and opioid receptors. *Naunyn-Schmiederbergs Archives of Pharmacology, 351*, 433–438.

Breder, C. D., Dinarello, C. A., & Saper, C. B. (1988). Interleukin-1 immunoreactive innervation of the human hypothalamus. *Science, 240*, 321–324.

Bret-Dibat, J. L., Bluthe, R. M., Kent, S., Kelley, K. W., & Dantzer, R. (1995). Lipopolysaccharide and interleukin-1 depress food-motivated behavior in mice by a vagal-mediated mechanism. *Brain, Behavior, and Immunity, 9*, 242–246.

Brown, R., Li, Z., Vriend, C. Y., Nirula, R., Janz, L., Falk, J., Nance, D. M., Dyck, D. G., & Greenberg, A. H. (1991). Suppression of splenic macrophage interleukin-1 secretion following intracerebroventricular injection of interleukin-1 beta: Evidence for pituitary-adrenal and sympathetic control. *Cellular Immunology, 132*, 84–93.

Buttini, M., & Boddeke, H. (1995). Peripheral lypopolysaccharide stimulation induces interleukin-1β messenger RNA in rat microglial cells. *Neuroscience, 65*, 523–530.

Carr, D. J., & Blalock, J. E. (1991). Neuropetide hormones and receptors common to the immune and neuroendocrine systems:

Bidirectional pathway of intersystem communication. In R. Ader, D. L. Felten, and N. Cohen (Eds.), *Psychoneuroimmunology* (pp. 573–588). New York: Academic Press.

Chang, S. L., Ren, T., & Zadina, J. E. (1993). Interleukin-1 activation of FOS proto-oncogene protein in the rat hypothalamus. *Brain Research, 617*, 123–130.

Chang, Y., Albright, S., & Lee, F. (1994). Cytokines in the central nervous system: Expression of macrophage colony stimulating factor and its receptor during development. *Journal of Neuroimmunology, 52*, 9–17.

Chuluyan, H. E., Saphier, D., Rohn, W. M., & Dunn, A. J. (1992). Noradrenergic innervation of the hypothalamus participates in adrenocortical responses to interleukin-1. *Neuroendocrinology, 56*, 106–111.

Cunningham, E. T. J., Wada, E., Carter, D. B., Tracey, D. E., Battey, J. F., & De Souza, E. B. (1992). In situ histochemical localization of type I interleukin-1 receptor messenger RNA in the central nervous system, pituitary, and adrenal gland of the mouse. *Journal of Neuroscience* 12, 1101–1114.

De Sarro, G. B., Ascioti, C., Audino, M. G., Rispoli, V., & Nistico, G. (1989). Behavioural and ECoG spectrum changes induced by intracerebral microinfusion of interferons and interleukin-2 in rats are antagonnized by naloxone. In J. W. Hadden, K. Masek and G. Nistico (Eds.), *Interactions among CNS, Neuroendocrine and Immune Systems* (pp. 351–364). Rome: Pythagora Press.

del Rey, A., & Besedovsky, H. (1987). Interleukin-1 affects glucose homeostasis. *American Journal of Physiology, 253*, R794–R798.

del Rey, A., & Besedovsky, H. O. (1989). Antidiabetic effects of Interleukin-1. *Proceedings of the National Academy of Sciences of the United States of America, 86*, 5943–5947.

del Rey, A., Klusman, I., & Besedovsky, H. (1998). Cytokines mediate the protective stimulation of glucocorticoids output during autoimmunity: Involvement of IL-1. *American Journal of Physiology, 275*, R1146–R1151.

del Rey, A., Monge-Arditi, G., & Besedovsky, H. O. (1998). Central and peripheral mechanisms contribute to the hypoglycemia induced by Interleukin-1. *Annals of the New York Academy of Sciences, 840*, 153–161.

Deyerle, K. L., Sims, J. E., Dower, S. K., & Bothwell, M. A. (1992). Pattern of IL-1 receptor gene expression suggests role in noninflammatory processes. *Journal of Immunology, 149*, 1657–1665.

Dray, A., & Bevan, S. (1993). Inflammation and hyperalgesia: Highlighting the team effort. *Trends in Pharmacological Sciences, 14*, 287–290.

Dunn, A. J. (1988). Systemic interleukin-1 administration stimulates hypothalamic norepinephrine metabolism parallelling the increased plasma corticosterone. *Life Sciences, 43*, 429–435.

Dyck, D. G., & Greenberg, A. H. (1991). Immunological tolerance as conditioned response: Dissecting the brain-immune pathways. In R. Ader, D. Felten, and N. Cohen (Eds.), *Psychoneuroimmunology* (pp. 663–684). New York: Academic Press.

Ericsson, A., Arias, C., & Sawchenko, P. E. (1997). Evidence for an intramedullary prostaglandin-dependent mechanism in the activation of stress-related neuroendocrine circuitry by intravenous interleukin-1. *Journal of Neuroscience, 17*, 7166–7179.

Ericsson, A., Kovacs, K. J., & Sawchenko, P. E. (1994). A functional anatomical analysis of central pathways subserving the effects of interleukin-1 on stress-related neuroendocrine neurons. *Journal of Neuroscience, 14*, 897–913.

Fabry, Z., Raine, C. S., & Hart, M. N. (1994). Nervous tissue as an immune compartment: The dialect of the immune response in the CNS. *Immunology Today, 15*, 218–224.

Fontana, A., Kristensen, F., Dubs, R., Gemsa, D., & Weber, E. (1982). Production of prostaglandin E and interleukin 1-like factors by cultured astrocytes and C-6 glioma cells. *Journal of Immunology, 129*, 2413–2419.

Gabellec, M., Griffais, R., Fillion, G., & Haour, F. (1995). Expression of interleukin-1α and interleukin-1β, and interleukin-1 receptor antagonist mRNA in mouse brain: Regulation by bacterial lipipolysaccharide (LPS) treatment. *Molecular Brain Research, 31*, 122–130.

Gatti, S., & Bartfai, T. (1993). Induction of tumor necrosis factor-alpha mRNA in the brain after peripheral endotoxin treatment: Comparison with interleukin-1 family and interleukin-6. *Brain Research, 624*, 291–294.

Gemma, C., Ghezzi, P., & De Simoni, M. G. (1991). Activation of the hypothalamic serotoninergic system by central interleukin-1. *European Journal of Pharmacology, 209*, 139–140.

Goldbach, J. M., Roth, J., & Zeisberger, E. (1997). Fever suppression by subdiaphragmatic vagotomy in guinea pigs depends on the route of pyrogen administration. *American Journal of Physiology, 272*, R675–R681.

Gutierrez, E. G., Banks, W. A., & Kastin, A. J. (1993). Murine tumor necrosis factor alpha is transported from blood to brain in the mouse. *Journal of Neuroimmunology, 47*, 169–176.

Gutierrez, E. G., Banks, W. A., & Kastin, A. J. (1994). Blood-borne interleukin-1 receptor antagonist crosses the blood brain barrier. *Journal of Neuroimmunology, 55*, 153–160.

Hart, R. P., Shadiack, A., & Jonakait, G. M. (1991). Substance P gene expression is regulated by interleukin 1 in cultured sympathetic ganglia. *Journal of Neuroscience Research, 29*, 282–291.

Heijnen, C. J., Kavelaars, A., & Ballieux, R. (1991). Corticotropin-releasing hormone and proopiomelanocortin-derieved peptides in the modulation of immune functions. In R. Ader, D. L. Felten, and N. Cohen (Eds.), *Psychoneuroimmunology* (pp. 429–446). New York: Academic Press.

Hermus, R. M., Sweep, C. G., van der Meer, M. J., Ross, H. A., Smals, A. G., Benraad, T. J., & Kloppenborg, P. W. (1992). Continuous infusion of interleukin-1 beta induces a nonthyroidal illness syndrome in the rat. *Endocrinology, 131*, 2139–2146.

Holsboer, F., Stalla, G. K., von Bardeleben, U., Hammann, K., Muller, H., & Muller, O. A. (1988). Acute adrenocortical stimulation by recombinant gamma interferon in human controls. *Life Sciences, 42*, 1–5.

Homo-Delarche, F., & Durant, S. (1994). Hormones, neurotransmitters and neuropeptides as modulators of lymphocyte functions. In M. Rola-Pleszczynski (Ed.), *Immunopharmacology of lymphocytes* (pp. 169–240). London: Academic Press.

Hurst, S., & Collins, S. M. (1993). Interleukin-1β modulation of norepinephrine release from rat myenteric nerves. *American Journal of Physiology, 264*, G30–G35.

Kabiersch, A., del Rey, A., Honegger, C. G., & Besedovsky, H. O. (1988). Interleukin-1 induces changes in norepinephrine metabolism in the rat brain. *Brain, Behavior, and Immunity, 2*, 267–274.

Kelley, K. W. (1991). Growth hormone in immunobiology. In R. Ader, D. L. Felten, & N. Cohen (Eds.), *Psychoneuroimmunology* (pp. 377–402). New York: Academic Press.

Kent, R. M., Bluthé, R. M., Dantzer, R., Hardwick, A. J., Kelley, K. W., Rothwell, N. J., & Vannice, J. L. (1992). Different receptor mechanisms mediate the pyrogenic and behavioral effects of interleukin 1. *Proceedings of the National Academy of Sciences of the United States of America, 89*, 9117–9120.

Kent, S., Bluthé, R. M., Kelley, K. W., & Dantzer, R. (1992). Sickness behavior as a new target for drug development. *Trends in Pharmacological Sciences, 13*, 24–28.

Kinouchi, K., Brown, G., Pasternak, G., & Donner, D. B. (1991). Identification and characterization of receptors for tumor necrosis factor-alpha in the brain. *Biochemical and Biophysical Research Communications, 18*, 1532–1538.

Kita, A., Imano, K., & Nakamura, H. (1993). Involvement of corticotropin-releasing factor in the antinociception produced by interleukin-1 in mice. *European Journal of Pharmacology, 237*, 317–322.

Kluger, M. J. (1991). Fever: Role of pyrogens and cryogens. *Physiological Reviews, 71*, 93–127.

Konishi, Y., Chui, D. H., Hirose, H., Kunishita, T., & Tabira, T. (1993). Trophic effect of erythropoietin and other hematopoietic factors on central cholinergic neurons in vitro and in vivo. *Brain Research, 609*, 29–35.

Layé, S., Parnet, P., Goujon, E., & Dantzer, R. (1994). Peripheral administration of lipopolysaccharide induces the expression of cytokine transcripts in the brain and pituitary of mice. *Molecular Brain Research, 27*, 157–162.

Levine, S., Sowinski, R., & Steinetz, B. (1980). Effects of experimental allergic encephalomyelitis on thymus and adrenal: Relation to remission and relapse. *Proceedings of the Society for Experimental Biology and Medicine, 165*, 218–224.

Linthorst, A. C., Flachskamm, C., Holsboer, F., & Reul, J. M. (1994). Local administration of recombinant human interleukin-1 beta in the rat hippocampus increases serotonergic neurotransmission, hypothalamic-pituitary-adrenocortical axis activity, and body temperature. *Endocrinology, 135*, 520–532.

Linthorst, A. C., Flachskamm, C., Muller-Preuss, P., Holsboer, F., & Reul, J. M. (1995). Effect of bacterial endotoxin and interleukin-1 beta on hippocampal serotonergic neurotransmission, behavioral activity, and free corticosterone levels: An in vivo microdialysis study. *Journal of Neuroscience, 15*, 2920–2934.

Lowenthal, J. W., Castle, B. E., Christiansen, J., Schreurs, J., Rennick, D., Arai, N., Hoy, P., Takebe, Y., & Howard, M. (1988). Expression of high affinity receptors for murine interleukin 4 (BSF-1) on hemopoietic and nonhemopoietic cells. *Journal of Immunology, 140*, 456–464.

Lustig, S., Danenberg, H. D., Kafri, Y., Kobiler, D., & Ben-Nathan, D. (1992). Viral neuroinvasion and encephalitis induced by lipopolysaccharide and its mediators. *Journal of Experimental Medicine, 176*, 707–712.

Lyson, K., & McCann, S. M. (1991). The effect of interleukin-6 on pituitary hormone release in vivo and in vitro. *Neuroendocrinology, 54*, 262–266.

MacPhee, I. A. M., Antoni, F. A., & Mason, W. D. (1989). Spontaneous recovery of rats from experimental allergic encephalomyelitis is dependent on regulation of the immune system by endogenous adrenal corticosteroids. *Journal of Experimental Medicine, 169*, 431–445.

Maier, S. F., Goehler, L. E., Fleshnwe, M., & Watkins, L. R. (1998). The role of the vagus nerve in cytokine-to-brain communication. *Annals of the New York Academy of Sciences, 840*, 289–300.

Matta, S., Singh, J., Newton, R., & Sharp, B. M. (1990). The adrenocorticotropin response to interleukin-1 beta instilled into the rat median eminence depends on the local release of catecholamines. *Endocrinology,* 127, 2175–2182.

Miller, L. G., Galpern, W. R., Dunlap, K., Dinarello, C. A., & Turner, T. J. (1991). Interleukin-1 augments gamma-aminobutyric acid A receptor function in brain. *Molecular Pharmacology, 39*, 105–108.

Muller, M., Fontana, A., Zbinden, G., & Gahwiler, B. H. (1993). Effects of interferons and hydrogen peroxide on CA3 pyramidal cells in rat hippocampal slice cultures. *Brain Research, 619*, 157–162.

Naitoh, Y., Fukata, J., Tominaga, T., Nakai, Y., Tamai, S., Mori, K., & Imura, H. (1988). Interleukin-6 stimulates the secretion of adrenocorticotropic hormone in conscious, freely-moving rats. *Biochemical and Biophysical Research Communications, 155*, 1459–1463.

Nash, A. D., Brandon, M. R., & Bello, P. A. (1992). Effects of tumour necrosis factor-alpha on growth hormone and interleukin 6 mRNA in ovine pituitary cells. *Molecular and Cellular Endocrinology, 84*, R31–R37.

Niijima, A., Hori, T., Aou, S., & Oomura, Y. (1991). The effects of interleukin-1 beta on the activity of adrenal, splenic and renal sympathetic nerves in the rat. *Journal of the Autonomic Nervous System, 36*, 183–192.

Nistico, G., & De Sarro, G. (1991). Behavioral and electrocortical spectrum power effects after microinfusion of lymphokines in several areas of the rat brain. *Annals of the New York Academy of Sciences, 621*, 119–134.

Opp, M. R., Postlethwaite, A. E., Seyer, J. M., & Krueger, J. M. (1992). Interleukin 1 receptor antagonist blocks somnogenic and pyrogenic responses to an interleukin 1 fragment. *Proceedings of the National Academy of Sciences of the United States of America, 89*, 3726–3730.

Patterson, P. H., & Nawa, H. (1993). Neuronal differentiation factors/cytokines and synaptic plasticity. *Cell, 72*, 123–137.

Pitossi, F., del Rey, A., Kabiersch, A., & Besedovsky, H. O. (1997). Induction of cytokine transcripts in the CNS and pituitary following peripheral administration of endotoxin to mice. *Journal of Neuroscience Research, 46*, 287–298.

Plata-Salaman, C. R. (1989). Immunomodulators and feeding regulation: A humoral link between the immune and nervous system. *Brain, Behavior, and Immunity, 3*, 193–213.

Quan, N., Sundar, S. K., & Weiss, J. M. (1994). Induction of interleukin-1 in various brain regions after peripheral and central injections of lipopolysaccharide. *Journal of Neuroimmunology, 49*, 125–134.

Rettori, V., Jurcovicova, J., & McCann, S. M. (1987). Central action of interleukin-1 in altering the release of TSH, growth hormone, and prolactin in the male rat. *Journal of Neuroscience Research, 18*, 179–183.

Reyes Vazquez, C., Prieto Gomez, B., Georgiades, J. A., & Dafny, N. (1984). Alpha and gamma interferons effects on cortical and hippocampal neurons. Microiontophoretic application and single cell recording. *International Journal of Neuroscience, 25*, 113–121.

Rivest, S., Lee, S., Attardi, B., & Rivier, C. (1993). The chronic intracerebroventricular infusion of interleukin-1 beta alters the activity of the hypothalamic-pituitary-gonadal axis of cycling rats. I. Effect on LHRH and gonadotropin biosynthesis and secretion. *Endocrinology, 133*, 2424–2430.

Rivier, C., Chizzonite, R., & Vale, W. (1989). In the mouse, the activation of the hypothalamic-pituitary-adrenal axis by a lipopolysaccharide (endotoxin) is mediated through interleukin-1. *Endocrinology, 125*, 2800–2805.

Rivier, C., & Vale, W. (1989). In the rat, interleukin-1 alpha acts at the level of the brain and the gonads to interfere with gonadotropin and sex steroid secretion. *Endocrinology, 124*, 2105–2109.

Rogausch, H., del Rey, A., Kabiersch, A., & Besedovsky, H. O. (1995). Interleukin-1 increases splenic blood flow by affecting the sympathetic vasoconstrictor tonus. *American Journal of Physiology, 268*, R902–R908.

Rogausch, H., del Rey, A., Kabiersch, A., Reschke, W., Örtel, J., Besedovsky, H. O. (1997). Endotoxin impedes vasoconstriction in the spleen: Role of endogenous interleukin-1 and sympathetic innervation. *American Journal of Physiology, 272*, R2048–R2054.

Rothwell, N. J. (1991). Functions and mechanisms of interleukin 1 in the brain. *Trends in Pharmacological Sciences, 12*, 430–436.

Rothwell, N. J., & Hopkins, S. J. (1995). Cytokines and Nervous Sytem: II. Actions and Mechanisms of action. *Trends in Neuroscience, 18*, 130–136.

Rotiroti, D., Ciriaco, E., Germana, G. P., Naccari, F., Gratteri, S., Laura, R., Abbate, F., & Germana, G. (1993). Stimulatory effects on lactotrophs and crop-sac of interleukin-1 and interleukin-2 in pigeons (*Columba livia*). *Functional Neurology, 8*, 205–210.

Sacco, S., Heremans, H., Echtenacher, B., Buurman, W. A., Amraoui, Z., Goldman, M., & Ghezzi, P. (1997). Protective effect of a single interleukin-12 (IL-12) predose against the toxicity of subsequent chronic IL-12 in mice: Role of cytokines and glucocorticoids. *Blood, 90*, 4473–4479.

Saphier, D., & Ovadia, H. (1990). Selective facilitation of putative corticotropin-releasing factor-secreting neurons by interleukin-1. *Neuroscience Letters, 114*, 283–288.

Schauenstein, K., Faessler, R., Dietrich, H., Schwarz, S., Kroemer, G., & Wick, G. (1987). Disturbed immune-endocrine communication in autoimmune disease. Lack of corticosterone response to immune signals in Obese Strain chickens with spontaneous autoimmune thyroiditis. *Journal of Immunology, 139*, 1830–1833.

Schneider, H., Pitossi, F., Balschun, D., Wagner, A., del Rey, A., Besedovsky, H. O. (1998). A neuromodulatory role of interleukin-1β in the hippocampus. *Proceedings of the National Academy of Sciences of the United States of America, 95*, 7778–7783.

Schöbitz, B., de Kloet, E. R., Sutanto, W., & Holsboer, F. (1993). Cellular localization of interleukin 6 mRNA and interleukin 6 receptor mRNA in rat brain. *European Journal of Neuroscience, 5*, 1426–1435.

Schwartz, G. J., Plata-Salaman, C. R., & Langhans, W. (1997). Subdiaphragmatic vagal deafferentation fails to block feeding-suppressive effects of LPS and IL-1 beta in rats. *American Journal of Physiology, 273*, R1193–R1198.

Sehic, E., & Blatteis, C. M. (1996). Blockade of lipopolysaccharide-induced fever by subdiaphragmatic vagotomy in guinea pigs *Brain Research, 726*, 160–166.

Shadiack, A. M., Hart, R. P., Carlson, C. D., & Jonakait, G. M. (1993). Interleukin-1 induces substance P in sympathetic ganglia through the induction of leukemia inhibitory factor (LIF). *Journal of Neuroscience, 13*, 2601–2609.

Sharp, B. M., Matta, S. G., Peterson, P. K., Newton, R., Chao, C., & Mcallen, K. (1989). Tumor necrosis factor-alpha is a potent ACTH secretagogue: comparison to interleukin-1 beta. *Endocrinology, 124*, 3131–3133.

Shibata, M., & Blatteis, C. M. (1991). Human recombinant tumor necrosis factor and interferon affect the activity of neurons in the organum vasculosum laminae terminalis. *Brain Research, 562*, 323–326.

Shimizu, N., Hori, T., & Nakane, H. (1994). An interleukin-1 beta-induced noradrenaline release in the spleen is mediated by brain corticotropin-releasing factor: An in vivo microdialysis study in conscious rats. *Brain, Behavior, and Immunity, 8*, 14–23.

Smith, L. R., Brown, S. L., & Blalock, J. E. (1989). Interleukin-2 induction of ACTH secretion: Presence of an interleukin-2 receptor alpha-chain-like molecule on pituitary cells. *Journal of Neuroimmunology, 21*, 249–254.

Soliven, B., & Wang, N. (1995). Tumor necrosis factor-alpha regulates nicotinic responses in mixed cultures of sympathetic neurons and nonneuronal cells. *Journal of Neurochemistry, 64*, 883–894.

Sternberg, E. M., Hill, J. M., Chrousos, G. P., Kamilaris, T., Listwak, S. J., Gold, P. W., & Wilder, R. L. (1989). Inflammatory mediator-induced hypothalamic-pituitary-adrenal axis activation is defective in streptococcal cell wall arthritis-susceptible Lewis rats. *Proceedings of the National Academy of Sciences of the United States of America, 86*, 2374–2378.

Sundar, S. K., Cierpial, M. A., Kilts, C., Ritchie, J. C., & Weiss, J. M. (1990). Brain IL-1-induced immunosuppression occurs through activation of both pituitary-adrenal axis and sympathetic nervous system by corticotropin-releasing factor. *Journal of Neuroscience, 10*, 3701–3706.

Tada, M., Diserens, A. C., Desbaillets, I., & de Tribolet, N. (1994). Analysis of cytokine receptor messenger RNA expression in human glioblastoma cells and normal astrocytes by reverse-transcription polymerase chain reaction. *Journal of Neurosurgery, 80*, 1063–1073.

Takao, T., Culp, S. G., & De Souza, E. B. (1993). Reciprocal modulation of interleukin-1 beta (IL-1 beta) and IL-1 receptors by lipopolysaccharide (endotoxin) treatment in the mouse brain-endocrine-immune axis. *Endocrinology, 132*, 1497–1504.

Tancredi, V., D'Arcangelo, G., Grassi, F., Tarroni, P., Palmieri, G., Santoni, A., & Eusebi, F. (1992). Tumor necrosis factor alters synaptic transmission in rat hippocampal slices. *Neuroscience Letters, 146*, 176–178.

Turnbull, A. V., Pitossi, F. J., Lebrun, J., Lee, S., Meltzer, J., Nance, D., del Rey, A., Besedovsky, H. O., & Rivier, C. (1997). Inhibition of tumor necrosis factor-α (TNFα) action within the central nervous system markedly reduces the ACTH response to peripheral local inflammation in rats. *Journal of Neuroscience, 17*, 3262–3273.

Vahouny, G. V., Kyeyune-Nyombi, E., McGillis, J. P., Tare, N. S., Huang, K. Y., Tomes, R., Goldstein, A. L., & Hall, N. R. (1983). Thymosin peptides and lymphomonokines do not directly stimulate adrenal corticosteroid production in vitro. *Journal of Immunology, 130*, 791–794.

van Dam, A. M., Bauer, J., Tilders, F. J. H., & Berkenbosch, F. (1995). Endotoxin-induced appearance of immunoreactive interleukin-1β in ramified microglia in rat brain: A light and electron microscopic study. *Neuroscience, 65*, 815–826.

Watkins, L. R., Goehler, L. E., Relton, J. K., Tartaglia, N., Silbert, L., Martin, D., & Maier, S. F. (1995). Blockade of interleukin-1 induced hyperthermia by subdiaphragmatic vagotomy: Evidence for vagal mediation of immune-brain communication. *Neuroscience Letters, 183*, 27–31.

Weidenfeld, J., Abramsky, O., & Ovadia, H. (1989). Evidence for the involvement of the central adrenergic system in interleukin 1-induced adrenocortical response. *Neuropharmacology, 28*, 1411–1414.

Yamaguchi, M., Koike, K., Matsuzaki, N., Yoshimoto, Y., Taniguchi, T., Miyake, A., & Tanizawa, O. (1991). The interferon family stimulates the secretion of prolactin and interleukin-6 by the pituitary gland in vitro. *Journal of Endocrinological Investigation, 14*, 457–461.

PART

I

NERVOUS SYSTEM EFFECTS ON IMMUNITY

CHAPTER

1

Exploring the Phylogenetic History of Neural–Immune System Interactions

NICHOLAS COHEN, KEVIN S. KINNEY

I. INTRODUCTION

Psychoneuroimmunology, the study of behaviorally associated immunological changes, and immunologically associated behavioral changes, that result from reciprocal interactions among the neural, endocrine, and immune systems has emerged as a new field of scientific inquiry within the past two decades (Ader, 1981, 1995). It is a field that has been defined phenomenologically, and is currently being explored mechanistically, by studying rodents and primates. Although hundreds of investigators are using mammals to address basic and clinical facets of psychoneuroimmunology, we are aware of only a handful of laboratories worldwide in which ectothermic (cold-blooded) vertebrate and invertebrate species are serving, or have served, as living tools to probe the evolutionary origins of neural–immune system interactions.

In this review we will first briefly summarize some of the relevant knowledge base of psychoneuroimmunology to provide the mammalian "gold standard." We will then comprehensively review what is known about neural–immune system interactions in avian, reptilian, amphibian, teleostean, and finally, invertebrate species. We are aware that at best, this descriptive comparative approach can allow us to make only educated guesses about the true evolutionary history of the integration of two complex physiological systems. We also recognize that our discussion of neural–immune system interactions in mammals is redundant with what appears elsewhere in this latest edition of *Psychoneuroimmunology*. We have included it because some comparative immunologists and physiologists who read our chapter may have only a minimal background in the research discipline of psychoneuroimmunology.

II. NEURAL–IMMUNE SYSTEM INTERACTIONS IN MAMMALS

Evidence revealing bidirectional communication between the neuroendocrine and immune systems has been derived from interdisciplinary studies in mammals (Ader, Cohen, & Felten, 1994; Ader, Felten, & Cohen, 1990, 1991; Madden & Felten, 1995; Maier, Watkins, & Fleshner, 1994). For example, behavioral and immunological studies using human and animal subjects have demonstrated that a variety of physical and psychosocial stressors can alter immune responsiveness (Ader et al., 1990, 1991, 1994; Glaser & Kiecolt-Glaser, 1994; Keller, Schleifer, & Demetrikopoulos, 1991; Kiecolt-Glaser & Glaser, 1991). Further, as reviewed in this book (Ader & Cohen, 2000), several laboratories have shown that clinically relevant immunopharmacologic effects (Ader et al., 1994), and even immune responses themselves, can be conditioned classically (Ader, Kelly, Moynihan, Grota, & Cohen, 1993; Gorczynski, Macrae, & Kennedy, 1984; Ramirez-Amaya & Bermudez-Rattoni, 1999). Additional evidence for the bidirectionality of this communication is exemplified by observations that central nervous system (CNS) nuclei exhibit altered activity and metabolism during an immune response (Felten et al., 1991), and that cells of the immune system can synthesize and secrete several immunomodulatory hormones (e.g., lutenizing hormone, prolactin (PRL), growth hormone (GH), corticotropin releasing hormone (CRH), adrenocorticotropin hormone (ACTH)) and neuropeptides (e.g., enkephalins [enk], endorphins [END]; Blalock, 1994; Carr and Blalock, 1991).

A. Avenues of Interaction between the Neuroendocrine and Immune Systems

One pathway by which psychosocial or physical stressors perceived by the CNS may be communicated to the cells of the immune system involves endocrine outflow from the CNS (i.e., hormones under control of the hypothalamus and pituitary) to the periphery. Probably the best known example of a behaviorally initiated endocrine influence on immunity involves hormones of the hypothalamo-pituitary-adrenal (HPA) axis and the resulting immunomodulatory effects of elevated levels of glucocorticoids (Munck & Guyre, 1991). In addition to hormones of the HPA axis (e.g., CRH, ACTH, glucocorticoids), many other hormones also may act directly on cells of the immune system; indeed, lymphocytes and macrophages express receptors for such hormones (Carr & Blalock, 1991). Additionally, as just mentioned, lymphocytes can produce some neuroendocrine hormones, and may regulate the production of hormones in an autocrine or paracrine fashion. A detailed description of this avenue of neural–immune system communication (see reviews by Ader et al., 1994; Madden & Felten, 1995) is beyond the scope of this paper.

A second pathway by which the central nervous system communicates with cells of the immune system is via the more "hard-wired" circuitry of the autonomic nervous system. Indeed, norepinephrine (NE), found in sympathetic nerve terminals, meets the following four critical criteria for neurotransmission with cells of the immune system serving as targets (Felten, Olschowka, Ackerman, & Felten, 1988): (1) Noradrenergic nerve fibers are found in specific compartments of both primary and secondary lymphoid organs, including the parenchyma; (2) NE is released from sympathetic nerve fibers of the spleen in response to sympathetic stimulation (Shimizu, Hori, & Nakane, 1994), allowing for paracrine effects; (3) a variety of cells of the mammalian immune system (e.g., T- and B-lymphocytes, monocytes/macrophages, natural killer cells) possess adrenoreceptors (Fuchs, Albright, & Albright, 1986; Felten et al., 1991; Madden, Sanders, & Felten, 1995; Roszman & Carlson, 1991); and (4) altering catecholamine levels, either by stimulation with NE or other catecholamines, or by denervation (see below), may result in altered immune function (Ackerman, Bellinger, Felten, & Felten, 1991; Madden & Livnat, 1991). With respect to criterion 2, it is worth noting that Th1, but not Th2, clones of resting murine $CD4^+$ T-cells express β-adrenergic receptors (Sanders et al., 1997).

CNS–immune system communication is bidirectional. One fundamental pathway by which the activated immune system communicates with the CNS involves cytokines that include interleukin (IL)-1, IL-6, and tumor necrosis factor alpha (TNF-α). Indeed, some of the earliest evidence for reciprocal interactions between the immune and nervous systems stemmed from the finding that "soluble factors" (i.e., cytokines) released into the circulation during the in vivo immune response to antigen stimulated neuronal activity such as an increase in electrical activity in the ventromedial hypothalamus (Besedovsky & Sorkin, 1977). Subsequent studies by many investigators revealed that IL-1 can activate the HPA axis, thereby stimulating production of immunomodulatory glucocorticoids, ACTH, and END (Berkenbosch, Oers, del Rey, Tilders, & Besedovsky, 1987; Besedovsky & del Rey, 1996; Besedovsky, Sorkin, & Mueller, 1975; Sapolsky, Rivier, Yamamoto, Plotsky, & Vale, 1987). We also know that the intraperitoneal (i.p.) injection of either IL-1β or an inducer of IL-1 (lipopolysaccharide [LPS]) can cause central effects such as fever, loss of appetite, and changes in slow wave sleep. Obviously, before such cytokine-triggered events can occur, the cytokines must first be able to reach neuronal cells in the brain. In this regard, mechanisms exist that allow cytokines produced in the periphery to cross the blood-brain barrier into the CNS (Banks & Kastin, 1985). Also, immune cells that produce cytokines can themselves cross the blood-brain barrier to release their mediators centrally (Weller, Engelhardt, & Phillips, 1996). Finally the vagus nerve provides another very important pathway by which peripherally generated cytokines (or cytokine-activated signals) reach the brain (Fleshner et al., 1995; Gaykema, Dijkstra, & Tilders, 1995; Goehler et al., 1997). Production of proinflammatory cytokines is not restricted to cells of the immune system. Microglia residing in the CNS produce several proinflammatory cytokines (Hopkins & Rothwell, 1995; Trunbull & Rivier, 1995). Furthermore, mRNA for IL-1β and TNF-α has been demonstrated in anterior pituitary cells (Abraham & Minton, 1997; Gatti & Bartfai, 1993; Koenig et al., 1990), and anterior pituitary cells from several mammalian species secrete IL-6 (Spangelo, MacLeod, & Isakson 1991; Vankelecom et al., 1993). The fact that, in mammals, the CNS and immune system communicate with each other by using a common language of cytokines and their receptors as well as neuroendocrine signal molecules and their receptors is a phylogenetically critical theme in this review.

B. Innervation of Lymphoid Organs

Noradrenergic sympathetic nerve fibers have been identified in both primary and secondary lymphoid organs of rodents by using sucrose-potassium phosphate-glyoxylic acid-induced (SPG) histofluorescence (de la Torre, 1980) for catecholamines (NE and dopamine) and immunocytochemical detection of tyrosine hydroxylase (TH), the rate limiting enzyme in the synthesis of catecholamines (Felten & Olschowka, 1987). In such preparations, fluorescence microscopy reveals fibers around the central artery that extend beyond the smooth muscle of the vasculature into the white pulp, the focus of lymphocyte accumulation in the mammalian spleen (Felten, Ackerman, Wiegand, & Felten, 1987; Felten, Felten, Carlson, Olschowka, & Livnat, 1985). Felten & Olschowka (1987) have provided electron microscopic evidence of nerve terminals in direct synaptic-like contact with lymphocytes. Such noradrenergic innervation is regionally specific, associating with lymphocytes and macrophages in specific compartments of the lymphoid organs (Felten et al., 1985; Felten et al., 1987; Felten & Olschowka, 1987).

In addition to the substantial body of evidence for noradrenergic neurotransmission with cells of the immune system, there is also more circumstantial (i.e., not all of the criteria for neurotransmission have been satisfied) evidence for a neuropeptidergic link with cells of the immune system. As shown immunocytochemically (Felten et al., 1985; Bellinger et al., 1990; Romano, Felten, Felten, & Olschowka, 1991; Fried et al., 1986), several neuropeptides are also located in nerve terminals innervating primary and secondary lymphoid organs (e.g., vasoactive intestinal peptide (VIP), cholecystokinin (CCK), substance P (SP), and neuropeptide Y (NPY). Many of these neuropeptides are co-localized with NE (e.g. NPY, enk), other monoamines (SP, enk, CCK), or other neuropeptides (enk, VIP, SP).

C. Effects of Sympathectomy on Immune Function[1]

Early studies by Besedovsky, del Rey, Sorkin, Da Prada, and Keller (1979) demonstrated that local surgical denervation of the spleen of 2–3-month-old rats, or chemical sympathectomy (SyX) of perinatal rats with 6-hydroxydopamine (6-OHDA), a neurotoxin that destroys adrenergic nerve terminals, resulted in enhanced numbers of antisheep red blood cell (SRBC) antibody producing plaque forming cells (PFCs). In the surgical denervation experiments, adult animals were immunized 5 days after SyX with an i.p. injection of SRBC, and PFCs were enumerated after an additional 5 days. The chemical SyX experiments were performed by injecting neonatal mice with 6-OHDA daily for their first 5 days of life, a protocol that results in a profound, long-lasting central and peripheral denervation (Ackerman, Madden, Livnat, Felten, & Felten, 1991). They were then immunized at 2 months of age and PFCs were counted 5 days later. The increase in PFCs was more marked when SyX was accompanied by adrenalectomy to eliminate adrenal compensation

Livnat, Felten, Carlson, Bellinger, and Felten (1985) reviewed additional studies involving 6-OHDA SyX and immune function. Their studies confirmed the earlier observation that local surgical denervation or neonatal chemical SyX results in enhanced anti-SRBC PFC responses, but additional studies involving immunization of *adult* mice shortly after 6-OHDA treatment resulted in unaltered (Miles, Quintans, Chelmicka-Schorr, & Arnason, 1981) or reduced (Livnat et al., 1985) responses to thymus-dependent (T-dependent) antigens. Further studies revealed considerable interstrain variability of the effects of chemical SyX on immune function (Livnat et al., 1985) that correlated with different susceptibilities of the strains to the neurotoxic effects of 6-OHDA. Subsequent investigations on the effects of 6-OHDA

[1]Interpretation of the effects of SyX on immune function in adult rodents must consider regeneration of peripheral sympathetic nerve fibers following treatment with 6-OHDA (Lorton, Hewitt, Bellinger, Felten, & Felten, 1990).

denervation on delayed-type hypersensitivity (DTH) responses (Madden, Felten, Felten, Sundaresan, & Livnat, 1989) revealed that SyX of C3H/HeJ and BALB/c mice was associated with reduced ear swelling induced by antigen challenge of sensitized animals. This effect was seen regardless of whether SyX occurred before or after sensitization. Based on these DTH studies, the investigators concluded that SyX alters at least the efferent phase of the cell-mediated immune response. The reduction in DTH was, in part, a result of reduced antigen-specific T-cell response, since lymphocytes harvested from draining lymph nodes (LN) of sympathectomized animals 5 days after contact sensitization exhibited reduced antigen-specific IL-2 production and cytotoxic T-lymphocyte activity. Since these effects of SyX were prevented by pretreatment of the animals with desmethylimipramine (DMI), which blocks uptakes of 6-OHDA into noradrenergic nerve terminals, the possibility that 6-OHDA may be acting directly on the lymphocytes was ruled out.

Madden, Felten, Felten, Hardy, and Livnat (1994a) reported that chemical SyX of nonimmune adult BALB/cByJ mice resulted in an increased weight and cellularity of inguinal and axillary LN; increased cellular proliferation in vivo in these organs; transient increases in cellular proliferation in spleen and bone marrow; enhanced migration of normal lymphocytes into LN of SyX animals; and decreased migration of lymphocytes from SyX animals into LN of normal animals. In a companion paper, Madden, Moynihan, and colleagues (1994) pointed out that SyX resulted in other changes in the LN including reduced concanavalin A (Con A)-induced proliferation in vitro; enhanced Con A-induced interferon (IFN)-γ production (but unaltered IL-2 production); enhanced mitogenic response to LPS; decreased LPS-induced IgM secretion; and dramatically enhanced IgG secretion. In the spleen, both LPS- and Con A-induced lymphoproliferation were decreased after SyX, as was production of IL-2 and IFN-γ. In all instances, the effects of 6-OHDA could be blocked with DMI. More recently, Kruszewska, Felten, and Moynihan (1995) reported that 6-OHDA treatment of adult mice (BALB/cJ and C57Bl/6J), followed 2 days later by immunization with KLH, resulted in elevated in vitro production of both IL-2 and IL-4, augmented KLH-induced cellular proliferation in vitro, and increased anti-KLH antibody production in vivo. SyX, which effects central activation (Callahan, Moynihan, & Piekut, 1998), is also associated with a transitory increase in plasma glucocorticoids systems (Kruszewska, Felten, and Moynihan, 1998). However, blocking glucocorticoid receptor binding in vivo with RU486 slow-release pellets did not abrogate the sympathectomy-associated enhancement of immune reactivity seen in antigen-driven systems (Kruszewska et al., 1998). In summary, it seems clear that SyX alters immune responses. Whether these changes are increases or decreases in the particular immune parameter being measured appears to depend on the species and strain being studied; the timing of SyX relative to immunization; the immune parameter being examined; and whether one is examining mitogen or antigen-specific stimulation.

III. NEURAL–IMMUNE SYSTEM INTERACTIONS IN BIRDS

The study of neural–immune system interactions in birds, like the study of avian immunity itself (Sharma, 1991), has lagged behind comparable studies in mammals. Nevertheless, several lines of evidence (Marsh & Scanes, 1994) are totally consistent with neuroendocrine regulation of immune processes in the few commercially important avian species that have been studied.

A. Innervation of Lymphoid Organs and Immunomodulation by Neuropeptides

The earliest indication that the bursa of Fabricius, the primary lymphoid organ involved in B-lymphocyte ontogeny in birds, is innervated was provided by observations of Pintea, Constantinescu, and Radu (1967), Cordier (1969), and Inue (1971). More recently, Zentel and colleagues (1991) have described peptidergic innervation of the chicken bursa. Specifically, immunoreactivity for tachykinins, VIP, calcitonin gene-related peptide (CGRP), and NPY was described in proximity to bursal vasculature and specific cell populations, primarily B-cells. Although some T-lymphocytes are found in the bursa, these investigators did not find peptidergic fibers near labeled T-cells. Although Zentel and Weihe (1991) were unable to directly demonstrate sympathetic innervation of the bursa, they associated the NPY staining with sympathetic innervation, since at least in mammals NPY and NE are colocalized in sympathetic fibers (Bellinger et al., 1990).

More recently, Ciriaco, Ricci, Bronzetti, Mammola, Germanà, and Vega (1995) investigated innervation of the pigeon bursa of Fabricius from hatching to 4 months of age by histochemically staining for noradrenergic (NA) and acetylcholinesterase (AChE)-reactive nerve fibers. NA nerve fibers were largely perivascular, but a small number were also seen in interfollicular connective tissue. In bursas from 30–75 day-old animals, fibers were occasionally observed beneath the bursal epithelium, in the cortex, and at the corticomedullary border, but not the medullary portion, of the lymphoid follicles. Although no age-associated changes in the density of NA innervation were observed in the vascular areas, there was a progressive increase in the density of nonvascular NA nerve fibers for the first 30 days of life, no variation from 30–75 days, and an apparent regional increase during bursal involution. The distribution and density of perivascular ACh-E-positive nerve fibers was similar to that for NA fibers. AChE-reactive fibers were also observed in the capsule of the bursa and in the interfollicular septa, and ACh-E-reactive dendritic-like cells and cell processes were seen subepithelially, in the cortex and at the corticomedullary border of the lymphoid follicles. No age-dependent changes in AChE-staining were noted.

Other suggestive evidence for sympathetic modulation of immunity in chickens has been provided by Brown-Borg and Edens (1992). These investigators administered 6-OHDA to chicks in ovo on day 18 postfertilization, immunized the birds with SRBC 25 days posthatching, and observed a small but statistically significant increase in hemagglutinating antibody titers (relative to vehicle-injected controls) at 6, 8, and 10 days postimmunization. No change, however, was observed in a cutaneous cell-mediated response to PHA measured at the same times as anti-SRBC antibody responses. This suggests that their manipulation of the sympathetic nervous system may differentially affect different arms of the immune system. SyX of adult mice causes an increase in glucocorticoids (Callahan et al., 1998). Although this does not appear to be responsible for the SyX-associated immune changes seen in such mice (Kruszewska et al., 1998), this may not be the case in birds. That young chickens exhibit a corticosterone-unresponsive phase during the first 2–3 weeks posthatching (Guellati, Ramade, Le Nguyen, Ibos, & Bayle, 1991) also needs to be considered in the context of differential effects of SyX on cellular and humoral immunity described by Brown-Borg and Edens (1992).

As mentioned earlier, neonatal SyX of rodents results in a profound and long-lasting drop in splenic NE (Ackerman, Bellinger et al., 1991) that is accompanied by increased antibody response to T-dependent antigens (Ackerman, Bellinger et al., 1991; Besedovsky et al., 1979) and changes in a variety of other in vivo and in vitro immune system parameters (Ackerman, Madden et al., 1991; Chelmicka-Schorr, Kwasniewski, & Wollmann, 1992; Madden, Ackerman, Livnat, Felten, & Felten, 1993). Although in chickens, the injection of 6-OHDA in ovo causes central as well as peripheral denervation (Spooner & Winters, 1966), Brown-Borg and Edens (1992) did not directly demonstrate denervation in their 6-OHDA study. Indeed, they could not detect NE (the principal sympathetic neurotransmitter in the chick [Rome & Bell, 1983]), in the thymus or bursa at the time of hatching, and NE was detected in the brainstem and spleens of fewer than 30% of the control and experimental chicks examined. Moreover, similar levels of epinephrine and serotonin (5HT) were found in the brainstem, thymus, bursa, and spleen of both control and 6-OHDA-treated animals. Although the levels of splenic NE increased during the course of the antibody response, at the time of each antibody titration, no differences among levels of splenic NE, DA, and 5HT in controls and experimental birds were seen. The significance of their observation that the peak splenic NE and DA response in 6-OHDA-treated chicks lagged a few days behind that of vehicle-injected controls is unclear. Further studies are needed to clarify the developmental time course of innervation of lymphoid tissues in chicks as well as to provide definitive HPLC, immunohistochemical, and immunocytochemical evidence of peripheral denervation by 6-OHDA treatment in ovo.

In chickens, suppression of a PHA-induced cell-mediated immune reaction in the wattle (Kelsius, Johnson, & Kramer, 1977) was depressed following a single injection of NE, 5HT, and DA (Lukas, McCorkle, & Taylor, 1987). In vivo DA and 5HT administration also suppressed PFC responses (McCorkle, Lukas, & Taylor, 1986) and enhanced migration of peripheral blood lymphocytes (PBLs) following in vitro exposure of chicken leukocytes to each of these monoamines (McCorkle, Taylor, Denno, & Jabe, 1990).

B. Endocrine Regulation of Immunity[2]

In addition to modulation of immunity by peripheral nerves and neurotransmitters, hormones (e.g., corticosterone, thyroid hormone, growth hormone, PRL, and gonadal steroids) all affect in vivo and in vitro immune function in fowl (Bachman & Mashaly, 1996, 1997; Glick, 1984; Haddad & Mashaly, 1990, 1991; Marsh & Scanes, 1994; Mashaly, Trout, al-Dokhi, & Gehad, 1998; Skwarlo-Sonta, 1992; Trout & Mashaly, 1995). A few examples should suffice:

(1) CRF stimulates chicken macrophages, and to a lesser extent, lymphocytes, to secrete ACTH, and

[2]Given their economic importance, it is somewhat surprising that there is so little published on the effects of stressors on immunity in domestic fowl. What little there is, however, appears to hold no surprises (Cunnick, Kojic, & Hughes, 1994; Gross & Siegel, 1983).

concentrations of circulating corticosterone increase following antigen challenge (Hendricks & Mashaly, 1998; Hendricks, Siegel, & Mashaly, 1991; Mashaly, Trout, & Hendricks, 1993). The increased corticosterone causes a redistribution of different lymphocyte subpopulations from the blood to spleen (Mashaly et al., 1993, 1998). (2) In mallards the size of the thymus and bursa are reduced following corticosteroid treatment or blockade of thyroid hormone production (Glick, 1984). In vivo treatment of mallards with dexamethasone (DEX) suppresses primary antibody responses to SRBC. At the same concentration of DEX, NK cell activity is increased, apparently resulting from the decreased production of PGE-2 by macrophages included in the cultures (Fowles, Fairbrother, Fix, Schiller, & Kerkvliet (1993). (3) Castrated chickens, or chickens with early lesions of the anterior pituitary, display decreased T-cell-mediated immunity such as GVH in vivo and PHA-induced lymphoproliferation in vitro (Mashaly, 1984; Glick, 1984). (4) Chickens with either a genetic thyroid hormone deficiency (SLD dwarf chickens) or a thyroid hormone deficiency induced by synthesis blockade, exhibit depressed anti-SRBC antibody responses (Glick, 1984). The genetic deficiency and its associated immune dysfunction can be reversed by administration of thyroxine and growth hormone (Marsh, Gause, Sandhu, & Scanes, 1984). (5) PRL has a stimulatory effect on avian immunity in that it is associated with increased bursal mitotic activity in leghorns (Glick, 1984); increased bursa weight in hypophysectomized pigeons; enhanced chicken anti-SRBC responses; and enhanced mitogenic activity of chicken thymocytes and splenocytes (Skwarlo-Sonta, 1992). (6) Feeding thyrotropin releasing hormone (TRH) or triiodothyronine (T3) to 1-day-old chicks for 8 weeks is associated with an increase in bursal weight; T3 but not TRH also increases splenic weight and numbers of white blood cells (Haddad & Mashaly, 1990). (7) The bursa of Fabricius, like the thymus, has an endocrine as well as a critical immunological function. Surgical bursectomy (BsX) of 1-day-old chickens reduces the subsequent in vitro corticosterone response of adrenal glands exposed to ACTH (el Far, Mashaly, & Kamar, 1994). BsX is also associated with a reduction in testosterone production by Leydig cells (el Far et al., 1994).

One of the most thoroughly examined roles of neuroendocrine regulation of immunity in birds comes from investigations by a group of Austrian workers (Hu, Dietrich, Herold, Heinrich, & Wick, 1993) who studied the Obese Strain (OS) of chicken. This strain is characterized by the spontaneous onset of an autoimmune thyroiditis and hypothyroidism (Wick et al., 1990). OS birds exhibit increased corticosteroid binding globulin, decreased free corticosteroid, and an impaired or even absent increase in plasma glucocorticoids in response to either the intravenous (i.v.) administration of antigen, IL-1, or a conditioned medium from Con-A-stimulated splenocytes that is known to contain factors that increase glucocorticoid levels (GIFs) in birds (i.e., IL-1 but not IL-6 or TNF). This impaired glucocorticoid response is not seen in either normal birds or in the UCD 200 strain of chickens that spontaneously develops a different autoimmune pathology from OS chickens. Given that there is no strain-associated difference in the ability of mitogen-stimulated splenocytes from the OS and UCD 200 strain to produce conditioned medium with GIF activity (Schauenstein et al., 1987), the reduced glucocorticoid synthesis in OS chickens may well be referable to a neuroendocrine immunoregulatory defect in the HPA axis (Brezinschek et al., 1990; Wick, Hu, Schwarz, & Kroemer, 1993) such as that associated with induced or spontaneous autoimmune diseases in certain strains of rats and mice (Wick et al., 1993; Wilder, 1995). The situation for OS birds, however, is not as clear-cut as it might seem since hypothyroidism itself causes blunted HPA axis responses (Kamilaris et al., 1991).

IV. NEURAL–IMMUNE INTERACTIONS IN REPTILES

Our very limited knowledge of the interactions of the neuroendocrine and immune systems in reptiles is derived primarily from the following three lines of research by an Egyptian and a Spanish group of investigators: (1) lymphoid tissue innervation; (2) seasonal influences on several immunological parameters; and (3) effects of steroids on immunity. Much of what has been accomplished following the last 2 approaches is the focus of reviews by Zapata, Varras, and Torroba (1992), and Saad and Plytycz (1994).

A. Innervation of Lymphoid Organs

Saad (1993) described, in turtles, the presence of nerve endings in close proximity to lymphocytes in the spleen, as well as changes in brain catecholamine levels during the course of an immune response. Brain epinephrine levels were increased 10 hours after immunization with SRBC; they then decreased to below control levels at 48 hours, after which time they returned to baseline. DA was elevated at 4 hours, decreased at 2 to 4 days, then returned to normal values by day 10 (Saad, 1993). Clearly more details are needed about innervation of lymphoid organs in representatives of various reptilian orders. It is also unknown whether the seasonal waxing and waning of immune reactivity in reptiles described below is associated with seasonal changes in the pattern of innervation of lymphoid tissues.

B. Seasonal influences on Immunity

In the snake (*Natrix natrix*), a seasonal cyclicity in circulating leukocytes has been reported, with females showing lymphocytopenia and neutrophilic granulocytosis during the time of egg-laying, and males also showing similar, but less marked, white cell count cycling (Wojtaszek, 1992). Thymic involution in the turtle, *Mauremys caspica*, occurs in April-May as do diminished antibody responses and delayed graft rejection (Zapata et al., 1992; Zapata & Leceta, 1986). In the lizards *Eumeces schneideri* and *Chalcides ocellatus* (Saad, Nabil, & Raheem, 1993), numbers of lymphocytes in the peripheral blood, bone marrow, thymus, and spleen are lower during the fall and winter than in spring and summer. There also appears to be a trend toward increased humoral immunity (both in vivo and in vitro) in the summer relative to winter (Zapata et al., 1992; Saad et al., 1993). Lizards also have been reported to show seasonal variability in their ability to reject skin allografts in that animals grafted in winter months did not reject until the warmer spring months (Afifi, Mohamed, & el Ridi, 1993). These winter-spring responses, however, were still slower than those seen in warmer summer months.

Reptiles are ectotherms and high and low environmental temperatures are immunomodulatory in such species (Clem, Faulmann, Miller & Ellsaesser, 1984; Clem, Miller & Bly, 1991). Therefore, interpretation of data describing seasonal effects on the immune system is confounded by the possibility that variation in ambient temperature, rather than (or in addition to) neuroendocrine changes associated with seasonality and altered photoperiod, is the important variable. The fact that antibody titers in the turtle (*Mauremys capsica*) are higher in autumn than summer in turtles kept at the 27 °C and at a constant photoperiod (Zapata et al., 1983) argues against this interpretation. Comparable data presented below for a ranid frog (Bigaj & Plytycz, 1984), and for fish (Nakanishi, 1986; Yamaguchi, Teshima, Kurashige, Saito, & Mitsuhasi, 1981), also support some sort of seasonal cue (e.g., photoperiod?) other than temperature as an important component of this cyclicity of immune responses and lymphoid system changes. The impact of different photoperiods at a constant temperature on immune system parameters still needs to be determined at all seasons.

C. Effects of Steroids on Immunity

Correlational data on seasonal levels of testosterone, glucocorticoids, and changes in the reptilian immune system are worth highlighting (Zapata, Garrido, Leceta, & Gomariz, 1983; Zapata et al., 1992). Based on observations of a sexual dimorphism in immunity in a snake (Saad & Shoukrey, 1988), and of an increase in testosterone levels in the blood of *Chalcides ocellatus* during the spring, Saad, Abdel-Khalek, and el Ridi (1990) and Saad, Mansour, el Yazji, and Badir (1992) investigated the impact of adult orchiectomy and testosterone treatment on antibody production in *Chalcides*. Five injections of testosterone propionate (each separated by 5 days) during the summer (animals maintained at ambient, and therefore, fluctuating, temperatures), followed by immunization with SRBC, did not affect in vitro PFC responses but was associated with a significantly diminished serum antibody at some, but not all times, postimmunization. Orchiectomy during the spring effected a marked and long-lived reduction in serum levels of testosterone and was associated with an increased primary PFC and serum antibody response to SRBC. Although antibody responses in orchiectomized lizards that received a course of testosterone did not differ from responses of orchiectomized animals, this reconstitution experiment would have been strengthened had the investigators confirmed the efficacy of the orchiectomy itself by including a group of unmanipulated animals in their protocol.

A single injection of testosterone priopricnate also results in thymic involution and depletion of splenic and PBLs in the turtle *Mauremys caspica* (Saad, Torroba, Varas, & Zapata, 1991a, 1991b; Varas, Torroba , & Zapata, 1992).

In an earlier series of studies, the Egyptian group studied the histological, cytological, and immunological consequences of exogenously administered pharmacological concentrations of hydrocortisone acetate in *Chalcides* during the summer. As would be predicted from studies with mammals, exogenous hydrocortisone acetate caused profound, but seemingly nonselective, loss of both T- and B-lymphocytes in the thymus, peripheral blood, and spleen. Physiological concentrations of 10^{-3} M hydrocortisone also led to in vitro destruction of thymocytes, PBLs, and to a lesser extent, splenic lymphocytes (Saad, & Bassiouni, 1991; Saad, El Ridi, Zada, & Badir, 1984a, 1984b). Also in *Chalcides*, a single injection of 1.0 mg/g body weight of hydrocortisone acetate "caused" a 3-week-long physiological increase in serum corticosterone (peak 2×10^{-7}M) and cortisol (peak 1×10^{-6}M). This was associated with a suppression of the primary antibody response to rat RBC in vivo and in vitro, a delay in allograft rejection, and a reduction in proliferation in mixed leukocyte culture (Saad, El Ridi, El Deeb, & Soliman, 1986). An obvious confounding factor in this study is the extent to which the impaired immune response reflects the exogenously administered steroid rather than, or in addition to, endogenously synthesized glucocorticoid. Also, an increase in endogenous steroids in response to exogenous steroids is puzzling if the HPA axis of turtles, like that of mammals, has a characteristic feedback loop.

An important caveat in interpreting studies in which a correlation is being made between seasonally, associated alterations in immune function and putative seasonally associated alterations in levels of endogenous hormones is whether levels of given hormone have been determined sequentially during a 24-hour period in each season. In instances of the single time-of-day measurements that appear typical of the immunological studies in reptiles, amphibians, and teleosts reviewed in this chapter, a possible seasonal phase shift in the diurnal rhythm associated with a given hormones (Spieler, 1979) could significantly alter interpretation of the published data regarding mechanisms responsible for seasonal changes in immune function. Regardless of the underlying mechanisms, however, seasonal changes in lymphoid tissue architecture and cellularity remain real events.

V. NEURAL–IMMUNE INTERACTIONS IN AMPHIBIANS

Based on a variety of morphological and physiological characteristics that distinguish amphibia from fish and reptiles, this class of vertebrates is generally thought of as a phylogenetically pivotal group. As such, the immune systems of a few (hopefully representative) amphibian species have been exhaustively studied. Recently, a few "amphibian immunologists" have broadened their research focus to include neural–immune interactions in both frogs and salamanders. Areas being investigated include innervation of lymphoid tissues; neuropeptide/neurotransmitter regulation of immunity; seasonal/neuroendocrine effects on immunity in adults, and neuroendocrine regulation of immunity during metamorphosis.

A. Innervation of Lymphoid Organs

Several lines of evidence point to catecholamines as "neuroimmune transmitters" in amphibians. Prior to the published observations in mammals by the Feltens in the 1980s, Nilsson (1978) had used fluorescence histochemistry to reveal sympathetic innervation of the spleen of the cane toad, *Bufo marinus*, and Zapata, Villena, and Cooper (1982) published electron microscopic evidence of direct contacts between nerve endings and lymphoid cells in the jugular body of the leopard frog, *Rana pipiens* (Manning & Horton, 1982). More recently, Kinney, Cohen, and Felten, (1994a) described noradrenergic and peptidergic innervation of the spleen of the adult South African clawed frog, *Xenopus laevis*, using SPG histofluorescence and immunocytochemistry for TH, PGP 9.5 (a general neuronal antigen), and NPY. Spleens of this species, like those of other anurans, have a clearly defined red and white pulp (Manning, 1991; Manning & Horton, 1982). Noradrenergic fibers are almost exclusively restricted to the white pulp in association with the central artery. These fibers have occasional varicosities in the parenchyma, and additional fibers are present in the boundary cell/perifollicular areas where they may come into contact with B-cells and macrophages of the white pulp; nonlymphoid dendritic cells involved in trapping and retention of soluble antigen (Manning, 1991); and possibly the T-cells at the extreme boundary of the white pulp. In some instances, fibers also were noted in the splenic capsule. In short, this innervation pattern in *Xenopus* is similar to that described for the murine spleen (Felten et al., 1987).

The profile of fine varicose nerve fibers staining for NPY in the white pulp of the *Xenopus* spleen was similar to, but less abundant than, TH^+ fibers, an observation that may reflect a difference in sensitivity of the antibody used rather than an actual difference in amount of neurotransmitter present. SP-staining fibers also were found around vessels in the splenic white pulp (Kinney et al., 1994a).

Although frogs (Anura) and salamanders (Urodela) are all amphibians, the 2 orders differ immunologically in several interesting ways such as the delayed kinetics of antibody production and allograft rejection characteristic of salamanders (Cohen & Koniski, 1994). In addition, and in sharp contrast to the mammalian-type pattern of innervation that characterizes the compartmentalized *Xenopus* spleen, SPG histofluorescence analysis of the noncompartmentalized spleens of the salamanders *Taricha torosa, Notophthalmus viridescens*, and *Ambystoma mexicanum* revealed a diffuse pattern of innervation associated with the reticular network (Kinney et al., 1994a).

The third order of amphibians, the Gymniophiona (Apoda or caecelian) has received only limited attention from immunologists, perhaps because they are relatively difficult to obtain for laboratory research. The spleen of one such apodan, *Typhlonectes* sp., is elongate like that of salamanders. Unlike salamander spleens, however, the *Typhlonectes* spleen exhibits some aggregation of lymphocytes into white pulp-like regions that are less organized than the white pulps of the anuran or mammalian spleen (Manning, 1991). The spleen of this species is also characterized by less abundant innervation than the urodele spleen, both in immediate proximity to blood vessels and also in areas removed from blood vessels, as shown by SPG histofluorescence. PGP 9.5 staining of the *Typhlonectes* spleen revealed occasional individual fibers and fiber bundles in a pattern similar to that seen with histofluorescence (Kinney et al., 1994a).

The ontogeny of splenic innervation during the larval life of *Xenopus* has also received some attention. Clothier, Ruben, Balls, and Greenhalgh (1991) reported changes in splenic innervation during the period shortly before metamorphic climax. Specifically, they described a drop in the levels of splenic NE, as assessed by HPLC and SPG histofluorescence, at Nieuwkoop and Faber (1967) larval stage 58, a time when lymphocyte mitogen responsiveness is also significantly decreased (Rollins-Smith, Parsons, & Cohen, 1984). Unfortunately, this reported developmental loss of splenic NE was not accompanied by micrographic documentation of a loss of sympathetic nerve fibers in the spleen. The lack of such documentation becomes important in view of our observations (Kinney, Felten, & Cohen, 1996) that the larval *Xenopus* spleen is innervated earlier than stage 58 (i.e., from stage 54 onward), and that the appearance of innervation is very sensitive to the environmental conditions (e.g., temperature, animal density) under which the larvae are reared. We have also reported that SyX during larval life prior to the appearance of splenic compartmentation does not affect the subsequent development of the demarcation into a red and white pulp (Kinney et al., 1996), and that early larval thymectomy that renders animals T-cell deficient does not influence the normal development of innervation (Kinney, Felten, Horton, & Cohen, 1993; Rollins-Smith & Cohen, 1995).

B. Sympathetic and Neuroendocrine Regulation of Immunity

Chemical SyX of adult *Xenopus* is associated with a significant increase in the in vitro proliferative response by splenocytes cultured with the mitogens, LPS, Con A, and phorbol myristate acetate (Kinney, 1995). A similar increased proliferation was noted when splenocytes from frogs that had been immunized with KLH 2 days after chemical SyX were cultured with KLH (Kinney, 1995). This SyX-associated enhancement of polyclonal- and antigen-driven proliferation of *Xenopus* splenocytes is similar to observations in mice discussed previously (Kruszewska et al., 1995, 1998). Unlike these murine studies, however, our (Kinney, 1995) preliminary SyX experiments did not reveal an alteration in serum anti-KLH IgM antibody (assayed 1-55 days postimmunization) in frogs immunized 2 days after 6-OHDA treatment). Although we did not determine IgY antibody levels to KLH, we do know that SyX does not affect the time course of skin allograft rejection (Kinney, Cohen, & Felten, 1994b; Kinney, 1995), a T-dependent immune process in *Xenopus* (Manning, Donnelly, & Cohen, 1976). Specifically, injection of 6-OHDA 2 days before transplantation (and repeated weekly during the course of the experiment) did not affect skin graft survival, regardless of whether donor and hosts differed by major histocompatibility complex (MHC) plus minor histocompatibility (H) locus antigens or by minor H antigens only. There was also no effect of SyX on the accelerated second-set rejection of minor H locus disparate grafts. In confirmation of these data, Jozefowski, Jozefowski, Antkiewicz-Michaluk, Plytycz, and Seljelid (1996) reported that chronic in vivo administration of β-adrenergic (propranolol) or muscarinic (atropine) antagonists had no effect on skin allograft survival in *R. esculenta* and *R. temporaria*. Morphine too, was without effect. The picture was slightly different, however, when the fate of xenografts rather than allografts was investigated using *R. esculenta* as hosts. Specifically, repeated injections of propranolol increased the survival time of xenogeneic skin grafts from *R. temporaria* and *B. bomina*; injections of atropine significantly accelerated rejection of skin from *B. bomina* but not *R. temporaria*; and injections of morphine had no effects regardless of the donor species used. Interestingly, binding of radiolabeled ligands to muscarinic and adrenergic receptors on PBLs was increased significantly in xenografted animals but not on cells from recipients of allografts. It is also noteworthy that unlike classic T-cell mediated rejection of allografts, xenograft rejection in anurans is thought to involve primarily innate and antibody-mediated immunity (Horton, Horton, Ritchie, & Varley, 1992; Józkowicz, 1995).

In *Xenopus*, immunological tolerance characterizes the alloimmune response of perimetamorphic animals to skin grafts from adult donors that differ from the hosts only by minor H-antigens (DiMarzo & Cohen, 1982). SyX of newly metamorphosed recipients of such grafts had no effect on either the induction or maintenance of this tolerance (Kinney, 1995).

As in so-called higher vertebrates, immunological effects of sympathectomy suggest that cells involved in amphibian immunity express receptors for noradrenergic ligands. Indeed, in the late 1970s an English group (Hodgson, Clothier, & Balls, 1979; Hodgson, Clothier, Ruben, & Balls, 1978) reported that antigen-binding splenocytes from several species of SRBC-immunized salamanders (*T. cristatus, T. alpestris, Cynops hongkongensis, C. pyrrhogaster, N. viridescens*) were decreased following their in vitro exposure to both α- and β-adrenergic receptor (AR) stimulation.[3] In immunized frogs (*R. temporaria, X. laevis, R. esculenta, Bufo bufo*), α-AR stimulation decreased, whereas β-AR stimulation increased the number of antigen-binding splenocytes. In these early studies it was assumed, perhaps erroneously, that all antigen-binding cells were antibody-producing cells. Subsequently, this group (Clothier, Ruben, Tran, & Balls, 1989; Clothier et al., 1992) used an enzyme-linked immunosorbent assay to examine the effects of in vivo NE administration on in vitro antibody responses to T-dependent and T-independent antigens. They reported differential effects based on the thymus dependency of the antigen and the timing of immunization relative to NE administration. Implantation of an NE-containing pellet prior to priming with a T-dependent antigen resulted in increased antibody production, whereas pellet implantation at some (unstated) time after priming was without effect. The influence of NE on antibody responses to T-independent antigens was studied by injecting NE rather than implanting an NE-containing pellet. A single injection of an (unspecified) amount of NE at the time of immunization with TNP-LPS effected a reduction of the splenic anti-TNP antibody response. Unfortunately, the difference in routes of administration of the NE between the two experiments makes a general conclusion difficult. Addition of NE (10^{-6}–10^{-8} M) to cultures of splenocytes from animals primed in vivo with TNP-LPS also reduced the in vitro anti-TNP antibody response. Interestingly, an increase was seen if the cells were exposed to 10^{-12} M NE, a finding apparent from the data but not pointed out in the text. A low concentration (10^{-12}–10^{-15} M) of the β-AR agonist, isoproterenol, also enhanced in vitro antibody production when it was added on day 7 in culture. In contrast, the α2-agonist, clonidine (10^{-9}–10^{-15} M) resulted in a reduced response, an effect that was blocked by the α-antagonist, yohimbine. β-AR stimulation with 10^{-10}–10^{-12} M isoproterenol was also reported to reduce Phytohemagglutinin-stimulated T-cell mitogenesis, a finding we have been unable to replicate using physiological or even subpharmacological (i.e., less than 10^{-4} M) concentrations of isoproterenol (Cohen & Kinney, unpublished). Although Clothier and colleagues (1992) also claimed that immunization resulted in a depletion of NE in the spleen, an unexplained decrease in splenic NE was also seen in animals injected only with PBS.

In these same studies, Clothier et al. (1989, 1992) suggested reciprocal interactions between splenic NE content and processes involved in antibody production. Treatment with 6-OHDA reduced primary antihapten antibody responses to TNP-SRBC. When TNP was coupled to a T-independent carrier (LPS or Ficoll), the primary antihapten response was increased.

Most recently, Haberfeld, Johnson, Ruben, Clothier, and Shiigi (1999) reported that adrenoceptor agonists modulate in vitro apoptosis of lymphocytes. Although α-2 and β-2 receptor agonists themselves could not induce apoptosis of *Xenopus* splenocytes cultured for 4 or 20 hours, they did modulate apoptosis of *Xenopus* splenocytes that were cultured with a calcium ionophore. More specifically, clonidine (α-2 agonist) enhanced ionophore-induced apoptosis of lymphocytes cultured for 4 but not for 20 hours, whereas isoproterenol (β-2 agonist) decreased apoptosis in 4-hour cultures but enhanced this programmed cell death when lymphocytes were cultured for the longer period. By itself, the synthetic glucocorticoid, DEX (10^{-4}–10^{-6} M) also induced apoptosis of frog lymphocytes cultured for 4 or 20 hours. Whereas clonidine did not affect cell death caused by this synthetic steroid at either time point, isoproterenol enhanced apoptosis after 4, but not after 20, hours of coculture. Haberfeld et al. (1999) suggested that their data could reflect a different apoptotic pathway induced by the ionophore and the synthetic steroid.

All the aforementioned experiments dealing with noradrenergic modulation of immunity in amphibians were based on the assumption that the agonists and antagonists used were actually binding to bona fide β-AR receptors. Jozefowski and Plytycz (1998) used radiolabeled ligand binding to actually characterize β-AR receptors on splenocytes and activated peritoneal leukocytes from frogs (*R. temporaria* and *B. bufo*) and splenocytes from the salamander (*Salamandra salamandra*). Saturation, competition, and kinetic studies revealed a single site with a similar binding capacity. These investigators also estimated that there were about 4,000 and 14,000 receptors per frog splenocyte and peritoneal cell, respectively (the difference prob-

[3]To stimulate α receptors, either the specific α-agonist, phenylephrine, or a combination of epinephrine plus the β receptor antagonist, timolol were used; to stimulate β receptors, either the specific β-agonist isoproterenol, or a combination of epinephrine plus the α receptor antgonist thymoxamine, was used.

ably reflects the larger number of phagocytic adherent cells in the peritoneal exudate), and as many as of 183,000 on salamander splenocytes (consistent with their greater cell size). Although leukocytes from amphibians and goldfish (discussed later) all have β-AR receptors with similar affinities for the ligands [^{3}H]CGP-12177 and [^{3}H]DHA, competition experiments (Jozefowski & Plytycz, 1998) suggest that there may be taxa (class)-specific differences, not only for cells of the amphibians and teleosts studied, but also relative to birds and mammals. Radiolabeled ligand binding studies have also revealed cholingeric muscarinic receptors on elicited peritoneal leukocytes from 2 species of anurans (Jozefowski et al., 1996).

In a series of studies published throughout the 1990s, Ottaviani and co-workers used immunocytochemical procedures to investigate whether neuropeptides, neurohormones, and cytokines are produced by vertebrate and invertebrate cells and tissues involved in adaptive and innate immunity, respectively; these reports are considered in their phylogenetic context in this and subsequent sections of our review. With respect to the amphibia, pro-opiomelanocortin (POMC)-derived ACTH, β-endorphin, and α-melanocyte-stimulating hormone (α-MSH), as well as molecules that show antigenic cross-reactivity with antibodies directed against mammalian IL-1α, IL-1β, IL-2, IL-6, and TNF-α were revealed in PAS-positive epithelial cells of the thymus of the anuran amphibian *R. esculenta*. Three groups of PAS-positive epithelial cells were identified in subcapsular cortex, inner cortex, and medulla. The cells containing ACTH-, α-MSH- and cytokine-like molecules were distributed in the cortex, whereas those containing β-endorphin-like molecules were found in the medulla and inner cortex. Thymic lymphocytes were always negative for POMC-derived peptides and "cytokines." This does not appear to be the case for peripheral lymphocytes, however, since immunocytochemistry, cytofluometry (Ottaviani, Franchini, Cossarizza, & Frenceschi, 1992), and more recently, in situ hybridization with a digoxigenin-labeled human DNA probe (Ottaviani, Capriglione, & Franceschi, 1995), detected POMC (or POMC mRNA) in peripheral blood lymphocytes as well as in phagocytic leukocytes from this same species. Recently, Ottaviani, Franchini, and Franceschi (1998) also detected CRH and cortisol-like molecules immunocytochemically in the epithelial cells, interdigitating cells, and macrophages, but not lymphocytes, in thymuses from the fish, frog, chicken, and rat. These data suggest that throughout vertebrate evolution, the thymus can function as a neuroendocrine organ that is fully capable of displaying characteristics of a "stress response." In a 1992 study, the presence of immunoreactive ACTH and beta-endorphin molecules in phagocytic basophils and neutrophils of salamanders (*Salamandra salamandra, Triturus carnifex, Speleomantes imperialis*) was established (Ottaviani, Trevisan, & Pederzoli, 1992); ACTH increased phagocytic activity of these cells.

C. Seasonal Influences on Immunity

The amphibian immune system, like that of reptiles, is influenced by seasonal variations (Plytycz & Seljelid, 1996, 1997). Several examples are worth noting: (1) The inguinal lymphoid bodies of toads undergo seasonal cyclic changes in morphology (Plytycz & Szarski, 1987). (2) Gut-associated lymphoid tissues of some anuran species also undergo seasonal changes (Saad & Plytycz, 1994). In a recent study, for example, Wojtowicz and Plytycz (1997) found that the number of lymphoid nodules in the gut was negligible in field-collected *B. bufo* that were emerging from hibernation. This number increased in spring, reached its highest level in the summer, and declined in autumn. (3) The magnitude of the anti-SRBC response and the number of splenic lymphocytes in the toad, *B. regularis*, are high in spring, low in summer, high in autumn, and low again in winter (Hussein, Badir, Zada, el Ridi, & Zahran, 1984; Saad & Ali, 1992). (4) The percentage of lymphocytes in peripheral blood and hematopoiesis in the perihepatic subcapsular tissue is strikingly reduced in winter relative to summer in two species of newts (*T. carnifex, T. alpestris*; Barni, Nano, & Vignola, 1993). (5) The thymus of the frog, *R. temporaria*, undergoes cyclical changes with maximal development occurring during the summer and involution in the winter (Bigaj & Plytycz, 1984; Plytycz, Dulak, Bigaj, & Janeczko, 1991; Miodonski, Bigai, Mika, & Plytycz, 1996).

Surprisingly, only a few investigators have examined seasonal effects on amphibian immunity by modeling the normal winter hibernation of amphibians in the laboratory. In an early study of this kind, Green (Donnelly) and Cohen (1977) found that complement CH50 titers of *Rana pipiens* kept at 4 °C for several months in a hibernaculum decreased to undetectable levels. This finding was recently confirmed and extended to other components of the immune system by Maniero and Carey (1997). Cooper, Wright, Klempau, and Smith (1992) performed a more comprehensive study of hibernation-associated changes in the anuran immune system. Leopard frogs (acclimated to 22 °C) were placed in a hibernaculum (in the dark) in late autumn. Animals, sampled at days 45 and 90 after initiation of hibernation, underwent a progressive 9- to 10-fold loss of leukocytes in the blood, thymus, spleen, jugular bodies, and to a much lesser extent (1- to 2-fold), in the hematopoietic bone marrow. These changes were reflected by marked aplastic changes in these organs. By the end of the experimental hibernation period (day 135), however, numbers of leukocytes in these organs had begun to increase, even though the photoperiod was unchanged and the temperature remained at 4 °C. At day 30 after the frogs had been returned to room temperature, cell numbers had returned to, or were greater than, prehibernation values, and the architecture of the organs again appeared normal.

Although skin graft rejection by anurans grafted during different seasons appears reflective of temperature rather than neuroendocrine changes (Saad & Plytycz, 1994; Plytycz, personal communication), at least in the case of the *R. temporaria* thymus, manipulation of the environmental temperature during the period of winter involution and summer growth did not override the endogenous seasonal rhythms (Bigaj & Plytycz, 1984; Zapata et al., 1992). These morphological and functional changes may result from seasonal changes in levels of circulating hormones such as corticosteroids, sex steroids, GH, PRL, and/or thyroxine (Mosconi et al., 1994; Plytycz, Kusina, & Józkowicz, 1993; Saad & Ali, 1992; Zapata et al., 1992). Indeed, Holzapfel (1937) reported changes in the gross and histological changes in the adrenals, pituitary, gonads, pancreas, and thyroid during winter hibernation.

This yearly pattern of thymic involution and loss of lymphocytes followed by expansion of thymocytes and peripheral lymphocytes in the spring may offer a unique model for studying repertoire development and self-tolerance in the context of neuroendocrine regulation. Regardless of whether cold and/or neuroendocrine changes are responsible for the striking winter-associated depression of lymphoid tissues and specific immune responses (Plytycz & Seljelid, 1997), immunologists still have to contend with the issue of how such immunosuppressed amphibians survive during such periods. Several possibilities come to mind. First, at least some animals might not survive. Second, at least for amphibians living in temperate climates, low temperature may also suppress the growth of potential pathogens. Third, immunological memory (i.e., memory cells) to pathogens to which amphibians were exposed during the spring, summer, and fall may persist during the winter (Cooper et al., 1992). Finally, components of the nonspecific innate immune system may not be depressed during the winter, or may recover more rapidly after hibernation than specific adaptive immune responses. With respect to this last possibility, Maniero and Carey (1997) noted that complement activity increased within 2 days after *R. pipiens* were brought from artificial hibernation to room temperature. Moreover, complement levels continued to increase until, in some instances, they were significantly greater than those of controls held at room temperature. Similarly, Plytycz and Józkowicz (1994) reported that endocytosis of peritoneal macrophages from fish as well as anuran and urodele amphibians was effective in vitro over a wide temperature range and was actually enhanced in cells obtained from cold-acclimated animals.

D. Glucorticoid Effects on Amphibian Immunity

Exogenous administration of a single injection of DEX in *Rana perezi* effected thymic involution with massive destruction of cortical lymphocytes, diminution in white pulp, and lymphocyte redistribution to the bone marrow from blood and spleen (Garrido, Gomariz, Leceta, & Zapata, 1987). The nature and extent of these changes depended on whether DEX was administered in autumn or winter (Garrido, Gomariz, Leceta, & Zapata, 1989). Pharmacologic concentrations of hydrocortisone suppress antibody responses in *Xenopus* and cause massive cell death in vivo and in vitro in the thymuses and jugular bodies, but not the spleen, of *Rana temporaria* (Plytycz et al., 1993). Haberfield et al. (1999) have reported that 10^{-4}–10^{-6} M DEX induces in vitro apoptosis of splenocytes from *Xenopus*. In the Plytycz et al. (1993) study, the number of viable cells in the thymus and jugular body returned to normal within 1 week after a single injection of hydrocortisone.[4] Rollins-Smith and Blair (1993) also reported that physiological (10^{-5} M–10^{-9} M) rather than pharmacological concentrations of corticosterone inhibited PHA-induced proliferation of adult *Xenopus* splenocytes.

E. Neuroendocrine–Immune System Interactions during Metamorphosis

Thyroxine (T_4) and triiodothyronine (T_3) play major roles in driving amphibian metamorphosis (Kikuyama, Kawamura, Tanaka, & Yamamoto, 1993; Leloup & Buscaglia, 1977; White & Nicoll, 1981). Circulating levels of these hormones are low at premetamorphic stages, increase during prometamorphosis, peak during climax, and decline at the end of metamorphosis. Metamorphosis is also accompanied by increases in circulating levels of corticosteroids

[4]It should also be noted that thymic and splenic morphology may be affected by laboratory and/or husbandry conditions regardless of season (Dulak & Plytycz, 1989).

(Jaudet & Hatey, 1984; Kikuyama, Suzuki, & Iwamuro, 1986), PRL, and GH (Buckbinder & Brown, 1993; Clemons & Nicoll, 1977; White & Nicoll, 1981). Each of these hormones has immunomodulatory effects in mammalian species (Felten et al., 1991; Madden, & Felten, 1995); manipulation of at least some of these hormones also influences immune function in amphibians (Rollins-Smith & Cohen, 1995; Rollins-Smith, 1998).

1. *Thyroid Hormones*

Since metamorphosis is strictly regulated by the availability of thyroid hormones, manipulating their levels makes it possible to inhibit or accelerate metamorphosis and thereby determine the extent to which development of an adult parameter of immunity in frogs requires a normal metamorphic transition. *Xenopus* larvae reared in the water containing the goitrogen, sodium perchlorate, to inhibit iodine uptake by thyroid follicle cells (Capen, 1994), undergo arrested development and do not metamorphose. Such blocked animals reveal that development of some structural and functional components of the adult *Xenopus* immune system are dependent on thyroid hormones and a normal metamorphic transition, whereas others are metamorphosis-independent. Specifically, perchlorate-blocked larvae lack the adult pattern of antibody responses to a specific hapten (Hsu & Du Pasquier, 1984), and adult-type MHC class II^+ T-lymphocytes do not appear in the periphery (Rollins-Smith & Blair, 1990a). Moreover, the thymus does not assume an adult-type morphology (Clothier & Balls, 1985); lymphocytes in the thymus and spleen do not achieve the expanded cell numbers characteristic of postmetamorphic adults (Rollins-Smith & Blair, 1990a, 1990b); adult-type skin allograft rejection does not replace the typical tolerogenic responses of larvae (Cohen & Crosby, unpublished); and, as pointed out previously, splenic innervation and compartmentation of the spleen into a clearly defined red and white pulp is dramatically delayed (Kinney et al., 1996).

Immune system changes that occur in perchlorate-blocked tadpoles (i.e., are independent of thyroxine levels) include the expression of MHC class I antigens (Rollins-Smith, Flajnik, Blair, Davis, & Green, 1994; Rollins-Smith, 1998); the immigration and expansion of T-cell precursors in the thymus (Rollins-Smith, Blair, & Davis, 1992); and the development of high titer IgY antibody production (Hsu & Du Pasquier, 1984).

Just how thyroid hormones are related to the maturation of some facets of the *Xenopus* immune system is unknown. Thyroxine appears to drive the terminal maturation of larval erythrocytes (Galton & St. Germain, 1985) and the expansion of a separate adult erythrocyte population (Flajnik & Du Pasquier, 1988). However, since thyroid hormones have no deleterious effects on lymphocyte viability and inconsistent effects on proliferation (Rollins-Smith & Blair, 1993), the direct action of thyroid hormones does not appear to be responsible for the dramatic loss of larval lymphocytes at metamorphosis. In this regard, it is noteworthy that thyroid hormone deprivation initiated after metamorphosis does not appear to affect lymphocyte populations of postmetamorphic animals or the ability of T-cells from such animals to respond to mitogens (Rollins-Smith, Davis, & Blair, 1993).

2. *Corticosteroid Hormones*

In short-term in vitro studies, both adult and larval lymphocytes are killed by concentrations of corticosterone that are comparable to those occurring at metamorphosis (Rollins-Smith, 1998; Rollins-Smith, Barker, & Davis, 1997; Rollins-Smith & Blair, 1993). Corticosterone and aldosterone significantly inhibit PHA-induced proliferation of larval and adult spleen cells (Marx, Ruben, Nobis & Duffy, 1987; Rollins-Smith & Blair, 1993; Rollins-Smith & Cohen, 1995), and corticosterone induces apoptotic death of larval splenocytes at concentrations as low as 1–10 nM (Rollins-Smith et al., 1997; Rollins-Smith, 1998). Adult lymphocytes may be protected in vivo from the destructive effects of corticosterone since there is less total corticosterone in the circulation after metamorphosis, and most is in a bound state (Jolivet-Jaudet & Leloup-Hatey, 1986).

Since aldosterone levels do not appear to be affected by specific serum binding factors, the observed elevated levels of aldosterone in plasma of metamorphosing and adult frogs reflect the level of freely available aldosterone. Because larval lymphocyte function is affected by aldosterone at these physiologically relevant concentrations (Rollins-Smith & Cohen, 1995), aldosterone could play a role in the loss of larval lymphocytes.

Based on in vitro sensitivities of *Xenopus* lymphocytes to corticosterone and aldosterone, it is reasonable to propose that the naturally increasing concentrations of these hormones during metamorphosis are causally related to the death of significant numbers of larval splenic lymphocytes (Rollins-Smith & Cohen, 1995). This hypothesis is supported by evidence that the in vitro inhibition of PHA-stimulated splenocyte proliferation by corticosteroid hormones (CH) can be blocked by the CH-receptor antagonist, RU486 (Rollins-Smith, 1998; Rollins-Smith, & Cohen, 1995;

Rollins-Smith et al., 1997), and that in vivo treatment of stage 57–58 larvae with RU486 reveals a dose-dependent inhibition of the loss of splenocytes that normally occurs during metamorphosis (Rollins-Smith, 1998). Thus, corticosterone and/or aldosterone appear to be important regulators of peripheral splenocyte populations at metamorphosis in *Xenopus*. The putative hormonally induced loss of splenic lymphocytes during metamorphosis is quite important, for if these immunocompetent larval cells were not eliminated, they could be activated by newly emerging adult-specific self-molecules.

The role of increasing levels of CH on the viability and development of thymocytes is more difficult to evaluate. Viability of larval thymocytes cultured in 1–10 μg/mL corticosterone is significantly reduced (Rollins-Smith & Blair, 1993); this reduction can be inhibited by RU486 in vitro (Rollins-Smith et al., 1997; Rollins-Smith, 1998). However, other recent studies have reported significant apoptosis of *Xenopus* cultured thymocytes from all larval and metamorphic that does not appear to be increased by culture with DEX (Haberfeld et al., 1999; Ruben et al., 1994). Regardless of their outcome, these in vitro studies are difficult to interpret because thymocyte development is critically dependent on stromal/epithelial microenvironmental influences. For example, in mammalian systems thymic epithelial components can synthesize corticosteroids (Vacchio, Papadopoulos, & Ashwell, 1994). Thus, thymocytes may constantly receive local corticosteroid signals that influence their viability.

3. *Growth Hormone and Prolactin*

Although a role for growth hormone (GH) and Prolactin (PRL) in mammalian immunity is now well-established (Kelly, Arkins, & Li, 1992), very little is known about the involvement of these hormones in the development and function of cells of the amphibian immune system. Hypophysectomized tadpoles continue to grow, can usually reject skin or organ allografts differing by presumed or defined MHC antigens (Maéno & Katagiri, 1984; Rollins & Cohen, 1980, 1982), and as with control tadpoles, do not reject minor H-locus disparate grafts or grafts expressing organ-specific antigens (Maéno & Katagiri, 1984; Rollins-Smith & Cohen, 1982).

In preliminary studies, we (Cohen, unpublished) and Rollins-Smith (personal communication) have independently observed that anti-PRL antibodies suppress proliferation of mitogen-stimulated (LPS, PHA, Con A) larval and adult splenic lymphocytes. Thus, PRL may be an essential lymphocyte growth factor that developed early in vertebrate evolution (see discussion in Kelly et al., 1992). Although PRL can be provided by serum sources, lymphocytes cultured in serum-free conditions, or with a serum supplement that lacks PRL, demonstrate significant proliferation that can be inhibited with anti-PRL antibodies (Rollins-Smith, personal communication). This suggests that *Xenopus* leukocytes, like mammalian leukocytes (Pellegrini, Lebrun, Ali, & Kelly, 1992), may produce PRL.

VI. NEURAL–IMMUNE INTERACTIONS IN TELEOST FISH

Given the phylogenetic success of the teleosts (Hickman, Roberts & Larson, 1993), it would not be unreasonable to propose that fish, like all other ectotherms discussed thus far, display coordinated and integrated immune and neuroendocrine responses to environmental challenges. The information reviewed in this section and elsewhere (Weyts, Flik, Cohen, & Verburg-van Kemenade, 1999) clearly support this hypothesis.

A. Innervation of Lymphoid Organs

The spleens of cod (Nilsson, & Grove, 1974), coho salmon (Flory, 1989), and rainbow trout (Flory, 1990) have autonomic innervation. At least in the case of coho salmon, however, splenic innervation appears to be largely associated with the vasculature, with some branching out into the parenchyma (Flory, 1989). Chemical SyX of salmon with 6-OHDA depletes NA innervation as measured either by HPLC for NE, or by the absence of fluorescent NA nerve fibers using the SPG histofluorescence (Flory, 1989). Chemical SyX also has been reported to increase the number and percentage of splenic anti-SRBC PFCs in fish denervated prior to immunization; no effect was seen if immunization preceded SyX. These data are consistent with the augmented antibody response seen following SyX of neonatal rats (Besedovsky et al., 1979) and adult mice (Kruszewska et. al., 1995; 1998), but contrast with the decreased antibody and cell-mediated responses seen after SyX in adult mice (Livnat et al., 1985; Madden, Ackerman, Livnat, Felten, & Felten, 1989; Madden, Felten et al., 1989).

Flory (1990) also has demonstrated for rainbow trout that adrenergic and cholinergic agents can alter in vitro antibody response to TNP-LPS. Specifically, the in vitro induction of a primary anti-TNP-LPS PFC response was suppressed by the β-adrenergic agonist, isoproterenol (10^{-4}–10^{-7} M), whereas it was enhanced by the α-adrenergic agonist, phenylephrine. The β-

agonist effect was blockable by propranolol, consistent with receptor mediation, and the α effect was blocked by yohimbine, but not phentolamine. This suggestion of an α-2 adrenoreceptor was confirmed by the demonstration that clonidine (10^{-7}–10^{-11} M), an α-2 specific agonist, enhanced antibody responses. A cholinergic agonist also enhanced PFC responses over a dose range of 10^{-5}–10^{-11} M; this was blockable by the muscarinic antagonist, atropine. Subsequent studies have revealed an influence of adrenergic and cholinergic agents on the chemiluminescent and mitogenic responses of trout leukocytes (Bayne & Levy, 1991; Flory, & Bayne, 1991). Recently, Plytycz and co-workers (Jozefowski, Gruca., Józkowicz, & Plytycz, 1995; Jozefowski & Plytycz, 1998) extended Flory's studies by demonstrating first, that there are adrenergic and cholinergic receptors on head kidney leukocytes of the goldfish, *Carassius auratus*, and second, that high concentrations of the β-adrenergic agonist, isoproteronol (10^{-4} M) and the cholinergic agonist, carbachol (10^{-5} M), enhanced PMA-induced oxidative burst of goldfish macrophages, effects that could be blocked by equimolar concentrations of propranolol and atropine, respectively. Both epinephrine and norepinephrine enhance the respiratory burst activity of carp anterior kidney macrophages and neutrophils (Verburg van Kemenade, personal communication). Finally, Narnaware and colleagues (Narnaware & Baker, 1996; Narnaware, Baker, & Tomlinson, 1994) observed that both α- and β-adrenergic agonists depress in vitro phagocytosis of yeast by rainbow trout macrophages, and that injection of the adrenergic blocker phentolamine can prevent the depressive effects of "stress" on the phagocytic index of cells from the same species.

Serotonin (5-HT) is also immunomodulatory in fish. According to a set of detailed experiments (Ferriere, Khan, Troutaud, & Deschaux, 1996), 5-HT suppressed LPS- and PHA-induced proliferation of trout PBLs. This inhibitory effect could be mimicked by an agonist of 5-HT1A receptors (8-OH-DPAT) and was reversed by an antagonist of 5-HT1A and 5-HT1B receptors (spiperone). Scatchard plot analyses confirmed the existence of specific serotonin receptors on lymphocytes. In a competition study, serotonin inhibited the binding of ^{3}H-5HT to receptors in both resting and mitogen-stimulated lymphocytes. However, the agonists (8-OH-DPAT and buspirone) and antagonist (NAN-190) of the 5-HT1A receptor subtype failed to displace ^{3}H-5HT binding to receptor sites in resting cells, but they did inhibit ^{3}H-5HT binding in LPS- and PHA-stimulated lymphocytes. Based on these observations, the authors propose that 5-HT1A receptors are only expressed on activated lymphocytes after mitogenic stimulation. An agonist of 5-HT1B receptors (CGS-12066B) failed to affect ^{3}H-5HT binding on either resting or mitogen-stimulated lymphocytes, suggesting that this 5-HT receptor subtype is absent on lymphocytes. A subsequent pharmacological study from the same group (Meyniel, Khan, Ferriere, & Deschaux, 1997), using additional antagonists of mammalian 5-HT receptors (ICS-205-930 and metoclopramide), suggested that fish 5-HT3 lymphocyte receptors may differ pharmacologically from mammalian receptors.

B. Neuropeptide Production by Cells of the Teleost Immune System

Recently, investigators have begun to explore whether fish leukocytes synthesize hormones typically associated the hypothalamo-pituitary-interrenal gland (HPI) axis.[5] POMC-derived peptides (ACTH, α-MSH, and β-endorphin) have been detected immunocytochemically in goldfish thymic epithelial cells (Ottaviani, Franchini, & Franceschi, 1995), and constitutive and mitogen-stimulated production of immunoreactive POMC products by catfish lymphocytes also has been reported (Arnold & Rice, 1997). Since both studies were based on antibody detection of antigenic cross-reactivities, their interpretation may be questioned. However, Ottaviani, Capriglione, et al. (1995) have also reported that goldfish (*C. auratus*) phagocytic leukocytes express POMC mRNA as determined by in situ hybridization with a digoxigenin-labeled human DNA probe. The same probe also detected POMC mRNA in phagocytic leukocytes and peripheral blood lymphocytes from the frog, *R. esculenta*; but lymphocytes from goldfish did not express this gene. A study of different teleost and amphibian species, however, seems necessary before endorsing these authors' suggestion that expression of this gene in vertebrate lymphocytes first occurred in the amphibia.

Information regarding the impact of cytokines on the neuroendocrine system of fish is limited owing to the absence of purified or recombinant cytokines of the species in question. There are some hints, however, that such cytokine-mediated communication may exist at the teleost level of phylogeny. For example, injection of LPS into fish appears to stimulate the HPI axis (Balm, 1997). Further, direct exposure of pituitary tissue to LPS in vitro blunted ACTH and α-MSH release (Balm, van Lieshout, Lokate, & Wendelaar Bonga, 1995). Although it is reasonable to assume

[5]In fish the interrenal glands serve the function provided by the adrenal cortex in mammals (Chester Jones, Mosley, Henderson, & Garland, 1980).

that these changes resulted from an increase in cytokine secretion following LPS treatment, LPS can also affect endocrine tissues directly (Milton, Self, & Hillhouse, 1993; Brunetti, Preziosi, Ragazzon, & Vacca, 1994).

A study in tilapia showed that murine IL-1α inhibited α-MSH release by the HPI axis (Balm, Pepels, van Lieshout, & Wendelaar Bonga, 1993). This contrasts with reports that in mammals IL-1 activates the HPA axis. It is, of course, premature to conclude from these results that the fish HPI axis does, in fact, respond to mammalian IL-1. In functional studies, mammalian IL-1 is without apparent effect on teleost lymphocytes (see review by Haynes & Cohen 1991; Ellsaesser & Clem, 1994; Verburg-van Kemenade, Weyts, Begets, & Flik, (1995) and has minimal sequence identity with fish IL-1 at the DNA and amino acid sequence levels (Secombes, Zou, Daniels, Cunningham, Koussounadis, & Kemp, 1998). Clearly, availability of recombinant fish cytokines (Secombes et al., 1998) will greatly facilitate studying both comparative immunology and neural–immune system interactions.

C. Glucocorticoids, Neuropeptides, and Stressor Effects on Immunity

The neuroendocrine stress response of fish (Wendelaar Bonga, 1997) is quite similar to that of mammals (Chrousos & Gold, 1992) in that it consists, in part, of a stressor-sensitive HPI axis. Cortisol, the major glucocorticoid in fish, is produced by the interrenal gland. Primary mediators of cortisol in teleosts are ACTH (apparently for acute stress situations) and α-MSH (in more chronic situations [Donaldson, 1981; Lamers, Flik, & Wendelaar Bonga, 1994; Sumpter, Pottinger, Rand-Weaver, & Campbell, 1994]. These, hormones, in turn, are under hypothalamic control, via CRF for ACTH (Olivereau & Olivereau, 1991) or via both CRF and TRH α-MSH (Lamers et al., 1994). It is noteworthy that in a recent in vitro study, Harris and Bird (1998) demonstrated that a 1-hour exposure to α-MSH increases the phagocytic ability of head kidney macrophages and neutrophils from rainbow trout.

Perhaps owing to intense economic interests in fish aquaculture, there have been several studies exploring the effects of stressors on mortality and, to a lesser extent, on immune function in various teleost species (Barton & Iwama, 1991; Ellis, 1981; Ndoye, Troutaud, Rougier, & Dechaux, 1991; Pickering, 1981; Wendelaar Bonga, 1997). For example, a 30-second dip net removal of chinook salmon from the water temporarily elevated plasma cortisol, increased leukocyte numbers in the thymus and anterior kidney, decreased blood and spleen leukocytes, and altered resistance to the fish pathogen, *Vibrio anguillarum* (Maule, Tripp, Kaattari, & Schreck, 1989). Altered resistance was manifested by an increased mortality and decreased time-to-death in salmon exposed to *Vibrio* 4 hours after stressor exposure, and by a decreased mortality (relative to controls) and longer survival times in fish exposed 1 day after this acute stressor (Maule & Schreck, 1990a; Maule et al., 1989). Altered immune function also was reflected by a decreased in vitro anti-TNP antibody production (relative to unstressed fish) by anterior kidney leukocytes 4 hours and 7 days after stressor exposure. At this later time point, plasma cortisol levels had returned to normal (Maule et al., 1989) indicating that the effects of the stressor persist beyond the time of cortisol elevation. A similar observation was made by Betoulle, Troutaud, Khan, & Deschaux (1995) who subjected trout to hyperosmotic shock for 7 days or 30 days and measured cortisol, PRL, and anti-*Yersinia ruckeri* antibodies in the serum. Relatively short-term "stress" was associated with a correlation between high levels of both stress hormones and a delayed production and lower titers of antibody. More chronically exposed animals had no increase in stress hormones but still had low antibody titers. These two reports, then, are consistent with the idea that the putative immunomodulatory effects of stress hormones impact the earlier phases of antibody production.

Stressors also can modify various aspects of the nonspecific or innate immune system of teleosts. For example, in vitro respiratory burst activity of fish anterior kidney phagocytes was diminished following handling and exposure to anoxic shock, as well as by crowding (Angelidis, Baudin-Laurencin, & Youinou, 1987; Pulsford, Lemaire-Gony, Tomlinson, Collingwood, & Glynn, 1994; Yin, Lam, & Sin, 1995), but it was increased in trout following transfer from fresh to sea water (Marc, Quentel, Severe, Le Baile, & Boeuf (1995), indicating a variance across species and/or stress modalities. A social stress paradigm in rainbow trout led to increased in vivo phagocytosis of bacteria by peripheral blood phagocytes (Peters, Nüßgen, Raabe, & Möck, 1991). Transition from fresh to seawater, however, had no effect on natural cytotoxicity cell (NCC) activity of cells isolated from brown trout (Marc et al., 1995). Although decreasing the water temperature in which carp were held enhanced their NCC activity (Le Morvan-Rocher, Troutead, & Deschaux, 1995), the in vitro assay were all performed at 28 °C, which could have different consequences for cells isolated from fish adapted to different temperatures (Clem et al., 1984, 1991). A social stress paradigm in aggressive fish (*Tilapia*) resulted in depressed NCC and mitogenic responses in the subordinate fish (Ghoneum, Faisal, Peters, Ahmed, & Cooper, 1988); this effect seems to be mediated, at least in part, by endogenous opioids, as determined by blocking studies with naltrexone (Faisal, Chiappelli, Ahmed, Cooper, & Weiner, 1989). A group of Polish investigators demonstrated that endogenous opioids (i. e, morphine) also appear to be involved in reducing numbers, but increasing respiratory burst activity, of thioglycollate-elicited inflammatory cells in peritoneal exudates from goldfish (Gruca, Chadzinska, Lackowska, & Plytycz, 1996; Chadzinska, Jozefowski, Bigaj, & Plytycz, 1997) and salmon (Chadzinska, Kolaczkowska, Seljelid & Plytycz, 1999). This morphine-induced increase in respiratory burst activity did not occur if the exudate cells were harvested from stressed salmon (Plytycz, Chadzinska, Józkowicz, Gruca, & Seljelid, 1996). As would be predicted by the results from these studies involving the parenteral administration of morphine and naltrexone, opioid receptors have been identified on teleost head kidney leukocytes and characterized by radiolabeled ligand binding (Jozefowski & Plytycz, 1997).

As in mammals, lysozyme plays a nonspecific antibacterial defense role in fish. Plasma lysozyme levels (as well as plasma cortisol and epinephrine) in rainbow trout increased following 30 seconds of handling (Demers & Bayne, 1997). Lysozyme levels also were increased in brown trout following their transition from fresh to sea water (Marc et al., 1995) but were unaffected by parr-smolt transformation (see later discussion) in Atlantic salmon (Olsen, Reitan, & Roed, 1993), and were actually decreased in carp following 30 days of crowding (Yin et al., 1995). These differences may well relate to the duration and severity of the stressor, as was shown by Möck and Peters (1990) who observed that 30 minutes of handling increased lysozyme levels in rainbow trout, whereas a 2-hour transport stressor decreased their levels.

It seems clear that many of the effects of stressors on nonspecific and specific defense modalities in fish involve the HPI axis and glucocorticoids. Fish leukocytes possess receptors for corticosteroids (Maule & Schreck, 1990a, 1990b; Weyts, Verburg-van Kemenade, & Flik, 1998a; Weyts, Flik, Rombout, & Verburg-van Kemenade, 1998b). In coho salmon, receptor-like binding of a synthetic corticosteroid analogue (triamcinolone acetonide) to cells isolated from spleen and head kidney was reported (Maule & Schreck, 1990b). Carp peripheral blood cells also express cortisol receptors with a high binding affinity (Kd 3.8 nM). Neutrophilic granulocytes isolated from the carp head kidney contain cortisol-binding sites with the same characteristics (Weyts, Flik, et al., 1998b; Weyts et al., 1988a), suggesting that both PBL and head kidney neutrophils express the same glucocorticoid receptor. Basal receptor densities in both cell types are approximately 500 per cell. Following cortisol treatment in vivo, receptor numbers in carp PBL decrease (Weyts, Verburg-van Kemenade, Flik, Lambert, & Wendelaar Bonga, 1997), whereas numbers of corticosteroid receptors in coho salmon spleen and head kidney leukocytes increase following exposure to an acute or chronic stressor or by cortisol treatment in vivo (Maule & Schreck, 1991). These changes in receptor densities have been explained by a stress- or cortisol-induced trafficking of receptor-rich leukocyte subtypes from the circulation into lymphoid organs. However, since corticosteroid receptors in coho salmon head kidney leukocytes are also increased following an in vitro exposure to cortisol (Maule & Schreck, 1991), an actual upregulation of receptor numbers resulting from the cortisol treatment also seems reasonable.

The immunosuppressive effects of glucocorticoids have been demonstrated in several studies with teleosts. Anderson, Roberson, and Dixon (1982) injected rainbow trout with a synthetic glucocorticoid 24 hours after immunizing them with the O-antigen of *Yersinia ruckeri* and observed depressed in vitro and in vivo antibody production and a reduced number of splenic lymphocytes. A similar reduction in numbers of antibody-producing cells has been described in flounder (Carlson, Anderson, & Bodammer, 1993). Ellsaesser and Clem (1987) injected channel catfish i.v. with cortisol (6.7 μg/kg body weight), which resulted in a plasma level of cortisol 30 minutes following injection equivalent to that seen 30 minutes following "transport stress" in this species. This increase correlated with decreased numbers of circulating leukocytes, increased neutrophils, and decreased LPS- and Con A-induced lymphoproliferation. This last observation also has been made for salmon by Espelid, Lokken, Steiro, and Bogwald (1996). Since these Norwegian investigators noted that the addition of physiologic levels of cortisol to normal fish leukocytes in vitro did not alter mitogen responses, they suggested that an indirect mechanism was involved in the observed effects. However, Tripp, Maule, Schreck, and Kaattari (1987) found that physiological concentrations of cortisol in vitro did, in fact, depress both LPS-induced mitogenesis and the primary anti-TNP-LPS antibody responses of splenic and head kidney lymphocytes from coho salmon. In this paradigm, pronephric lymphocytes were sensitive early in the antibody response, whereas splenic lymphocytes were sensitive throughout the culture period. Although it is unknown whether the aforementioned differences in the in vitro effects of cortisol on salmon and catfish lymphocyte mitogenesis are related to the species used or to methodological considerations, others also have shown that in vitro cortisol inhibits teleost lymphocyte proliferation (Grimm, 1985; Pulsford, Crampe, Langston, & Glynn, 1995; Tripp et al., 1987), and reduces antibody production (Tripp et al., 1987; Wechsler, McAllister Hetrick, & Anderson, 1986).

It has been suggested that cortisol may act on fish lymphocytes through inhibition of cytokine production as it does in mammalian cells (Kaattari & Tripp, 1987; Tripp et al., 1987). On the other hand, the observation that in vivo cortisol treatment resulting in plasma concentrations of 400 ng/mL, enhances the numbers of apoptotic lymphocytes in the skin of rainbow trout (Iger, Balm, Jenner, & Wendelaar Bonga, 1995) suggests that apoptosis may be regulated by cortisol. Indeed, apoptosis appears to have been conserved as an immune regulatory mechanism in fish as well as other ectothermic vertebrates including frogs (Haberfeld, et al., 1999; Rollins-Smith, 1998; Rollins-Smith & Blair, 1993; Rollins-Smith et al., 1997; Ruben, et al., 1994), and salamanders (Ducoroy, Lesourd, Padros, & Tournefier, 1999). Cortisol-induced apoptosis of fish leukocytes is mediated by a glucocorticosteroid receptor since the glucocorticoid receptor antagonist RU486 (Weyts, Verburg-van Kemenade, et al., 1998; Weyts, Flik et al., 1998; Weyts, Flik, & Verburg-van Kemenade, 1998), could block apoptosis. The low concentration of cortisol (0.1 μM) that was effective in inducing B-cell apoptosis contrasts with the lack of effects of cortisol's natural conversion product, cortisone. Since the conversion of cortisol to cortisone in fish is highly preferred over the reverse reaction (Donaldson & Fagerlund, 1972), this conversion may provide the fish with a mechanism to regulate the effects of corticosteroids on cells of the immune system. The lack of apoptosis induction by cortisone correlates with the low affinity of the glucocorticosteroid receptor in carp PBL for cortisone (250 times lower than that for cortisol; Weyts, Verburg-van Kemenade, et al., 1998).

Effects of cortisol on leukocyte viability are cell-type-specific. For example, B-cells from carp are especially sensitive to cortisol, whereas thrombocytes and T-cells are insensitive. Induction of apoptosis depends on the developmental state and/or activation state of the lymphocyte. In the periphery, only activated B-cells appear sensitive, whereas in head kidney and spleen apoptosis induction in B-cells is independent of the activation state (Verburg-van Kemenade, Nowak, Engelsma, & Weyts, 1999).

Interestingly, in vitro apoptosis of carp head kidney neutrophils was reduced when cells were cultured with cortisol, and this effect of cortisol was also mediated by a glucocorticoid receptor (Weyts, Flik, & Verburg-van Kemenade, 1998). Analysis of the glucocorticoid receptors in these cells revealed that they may be the same as those detected in PBLs since both have the same affinity and specificity (Weyts, Verburg-van Kemenade, et al., 1998a). The inhibition of neutrophil apoptosis by cortisol, combined with the observation that neutrophil respiratory burst activity was not affected by cortisol, would augment the supply of functional neutrophils in stressful conditions. Taking into account that neutrophils, together with macrophages, form the first line of defense against invading microorganisms (Dalmo, Ingebrigtsen, & Bfgwald, 1997), mobilization of these cells under stressful conditions may be important for survival.

Although cortisol can trigger apoptosis of leukocytes, and stressors elevate this steroid in fish, Alford, Tomasso, Bodine, and Kendall (1994) observed that confinement stress of channel catfish was associated with a decrease in apoptotic PBLs, and in vitro culture of lymphoid cells with cortisol failed to induce apoptosis. This apparent discrepancy with some of the previously cited literature may relate to the fact these investigators used unstimulated cells in their experiments, and, at least in carp, only mitogen-stimulated PBLs are sensitive to cortisol-induced apoptosis (Weyts, Flik, & Verburg-van Kemenade, 1998).

Plasma cortisol concentrations in stressed salmonids and cyprinids range between 100–500 ng/mL (Barton & Iwama, 1991), of which approximately 25–125 ng/mL is present in an unbound configuration (Flik & Perry, 1988; Caldwell, Kattesh, & Strange, 1991). Therefore, concentrations in the micromolar range or higher may not be physiological. It appears that, in vitro, cortisol does not affect phagocytosis or respiratory burst activity (Narnaware et al., 1994; Weyts, Flik, & Verburg-van Kemenade, 1998) unless unphysiological concentrations in the micromolar range (or higher) are used (Stave & Roberson, 1985; Ainsworth, Dexiang, & Waterstat, 1991; Pulsford et al., 1995). Accordingly, respiratory burst activity of a goldfish macrophage cell line was unaffected by up to 10 μM cortisol (Wang & Belosevic, 1995). The inhibition of phagocytosis of SRBC that was described in the same study again was detected only at relatively high (1 μM) cortisol concentrations.

Studies of cellular immune functions associated with either stressor administration or in vivo cortisol treatment often fail to consider leukocyte trafficking and redistribution as an explanation of the apparent immunosuppression observed in vitro. A wealth of information reveals that many stressors (e.g., transport, anoxia, social conflict, handling, injection) cause decreased numbers of circulating B-lymphocytes and increased numbers of circulating neutrophils in several fish species (Ainsworth et al., 1991; Angelidis et al., 1987; Bly, Miller, & Clem, 1990; Ellsaesser & Clem, 1987; Espelid et al., 1996; Faisal et al., 1989; Pulsford et al., 1994; Salonius & Iwama, 1993). These effects are mimicked by in vivo corticosteroid treatment (Ellsaesser & Clem, 1987; Ainsworth et al., 1991; Espelid et al., 1996; Weyts et al., 1997). Increased infiltration of leukocytes into the thymus, head kidney, skin, and gill (Maule & Schreck, 1990a; Peters et al., 1991; Balm, & Pottinger, 1993; Iger et al., 1995) also has been observed following either stress or in vivo cortisol administration. Thus, interpretation of data obtained from in vitro functional analysis of leukocytes from stressed fish or from fish injected with cortisol needs to take into consideration the possible dis(appearance) of cell populations rather than simply changes in cell activity.

Although there are more data supporting a neuroendocrine–immune link in fish than there are for in any other nonmammalian vertebrate, studies to date have used many different species and many different types of stressor. Thus, no "best use" model has emerged to allow an in-depth study of the effects of various sorts of stressor on several immune parameters of a single species. Effects are leukocyte type-dependent, and the final outcome may depend on the severity and duration of the stressor, as it does in mammals (Moynihan, Ader, & Cohen, 1994). The cortisol-mediated rescue of neutrophils from apoptosis shows that cortisol does not suppress all aspects of the fish defense system. Rather, cortisol acts as a regulator, inhibiting some parts of the (specific) immune response and enhancing other (nonspecific) components that may be functional in stressful situations. Stimulation of an innate immune response may be part of an adaptive response necessary to combat potential pathogens under stressful condition (Weyts et al., 1999).

D. Seasonal Influences on Immunity

Smolting, a series of profound physiological changes that prepare juvenile freshwater salmon for entry into salt water, is characterized by increases in plasma thyroxine and cortisol levels (Maule, Schreck, & Kaattari, 1987). These hormonal changes correlate with decreased numbers of splenic PFCs in salmon immunized with the O-antigen from *V. anguillarum*, and also with decreased numbers of PBL (although there was an increase in the proportion of small lymphocytes) relative to either erythrocytes or fish body weight. Such changes, together with increased mortality to *Vibrio* infection, have also been seen following implantation of cortisol-containing pellets (Maule et al., 1987).

Like reptiles and amphibians, immune reactivities and lymphoid tissues of teleosts undergo seasonal changes in fish that are unrelated to smolting. For example, Yamaguchi and Colleagues (1981) found that the agglutinating and cytotoxic antibody responses of trout immunized in the spring with the pathogen *Aeromonas salmonicida* were higher and increased more rapidly than those of fish immunized in the winter, even though animals were held at a constant temperature of 18 °C. Seasonal modulation in antibody production in relation to the state of lymphoid tissue development also has been studied in the ovoviviparous marine fish, *Sebastiscus marmoratus* (Nakanishi, 1986). Fish immunized in summer with SRBC after having been acclimated for at least 2 weeks to 23 °C had higher antibody titers than fish immunized in winter, even when the environmental temperature of acclimation and immunization was constant. A sexual dimorphism was noted in that anti-SRBC antibody titers of mature females were lower than that of either males or immature females in the winter spawning season. In addition, the thymus of pregnant, and especially postspawning females, was entirely involuted, showing a marked decrease in the number of lymphocytes in both the cortex and medulla. The neuroendocrine regulation of such dramatic changes seems well worth further study.

Circadian rhythms have been shown to influence immune responses in fish. The gulf killifish, *Fundulus grandis*, exhibits a circadian variation in immune reactivity during scale allograft rejection. Specifically, a two- to threefold higher level of immune activity and cellular destruction occurs during the dark period, resulting in a longer survival time for grafts transplanted at light onset than for those grafted at lights off (Nevid & Meier, 1993, 1994). Phase relationships between two circadian neuroendocrine oscillations (daily photoperiod and nonphotic daily stimuli) appear to be involved (Nevid & Meier 1995a), as do levels of hormones and neuropeptides/neurotransmitters (Nevid & Meier, 1995b). For example, daily rhythms of alloimmune reactivity could be abrogated by treating fish with naloxone or propranolol at light offset only, GH or atropine at light onset only, or PRL at either light onset or light offset. Timed treatments with PRL or GH reduced the length of time needed to completely destroy scale grafts, whereas timed treatments with propranolol or naloxone prolonged graft survival (Nevid & Meier, 1995b).

VII. NEURAL–DEFENSE SYSTEM INTERACTIONS IN INVERTEBRATES

By all current definitions, invertebrates display features of innate immunity in the complete absence of adaptive immunity (e.g., MHC, immunoglobulin genes, rearranging T-cell receptor genes, immunological specificity, and memory). In recent years, two major research groups, one in Italy, the other in New York, have become interested in the possibility that communication between the neuroendocrine and innate defense systems exists in invertebrates as well as vertebrates. These investigators have used four basic interrelated approaches to address this phylogenetically critical issue. In the following review of their work, the generic term *hemocyte* refers to the invertebrate equivalent of vertebrate blood leukocyte.

A. Synthesis of Neuroendocrine and Neurotransmitter Molecules by Invertebrate Hemocytes

The first approach focused on whether endogenous neuroendocrine and/or neurotransmitter substances are synthesized by, and can affect the behavior of, invertebrate blood cells. Hemocytes from several molluscan species (*Planorbarius corneus*, *Lymnaea stagnalis*, *Mytilus edulis*) exhibit immunoreactivity for several vertebrate neuropeptides including met-enkephalin, oxytocin, somatostatin, SP, VIP (Ottaviani, & Cossarizza, 1990), ACTH (Ottaviani, Caselgrandi, Fontanili, & Franceschi, 1992; Ottaviani, Cossarizza, Ortolani, Monti, & Franceschi, 1991; Smith, Hughes, Leung, & Stefano, 1991), and β-endorphin (Ottaviani, Petraglia, et al., 1993b). ACTH- and TNF-α-like molecules are also found in some types of leukocytes residing in the hemolymph of the dipteran *Calliphora vomitoria*; staining for both ACTH and TNF-α of the mitotically active plasmacytes was related to their activated state during the formation of capsules to wall-off foreign substances (Franchini, Miyan, & Ottaviani, 1996). Immunoreactive met-enkephalin also has been detected in the coelomic fluid of earthworms, and treatment of earthworm coelomocytes with the synthetic enkephalin analogue, DAMA (D-Ala^2, met^5-enkephalinamide), stimulates coelomocyte migration, much as is seen in human granulocytes and molluscan hemocytes (Cooper et al., 1993). Recently, Ottaviani, Capriglione, et al. (1995) reported that hemocytes from freshwater snails, *Planorbarius corneus* and *Viviparus ater*, express POMC mRNA as assessed by in situ hybridization with a digoxigenin-labeled human DNA probe. Interestingly, this probe did not detect POMC mRNA in another morphologically distinct hemocyte from these species, a hemocyte that Ottaviani (1992) believes has features of the vertebrate T-cell. This is the same probe mentioned previously in connection with detection of POMC mRNA in phagocytic leukocytes from both the edible frog and goldfish, and in lymphocytes from frogs but not fish (Ottaviani, Capriglione, et al., 1995).

It also appears that stress stimulates invertebrate hemocytes to produce endogenous neural–immune mediators. For example, Stefano, Leung, Zhao, and Scharrer (1989) found elevated levels of endogenous morphine-like material in the hemolymph of *Mytilus* that had been subjected to electrical shock combined with mechanically preventing closure of their shells. Concurrent with this rise was a substantial increase in the proportion of activated (ameboid, as opposed to rounded or resting) hemocytes (Stefano et al., 1993).

B. Effects of Mammalian Neuroendocrine and Neurotransmitter Molecules on Invertebrate Hemocytes

A second group of studies has examined possible influence of exogenous neuroendocrine, neuropeptide, and/or neurotransmitter messenger molecules on the behavior of invertebrate hemocytes. Franchini and Ottaviani (1994) and Ottaviani, Caselgrandi, Petraglia, and Franceschi (1992) found that ACTH induces cytoskeletal and motility changes of phagocytic hemocytes from snails. Genedani, Bernardi, Ottaviani, Franceschi, Leung, and Stefano (1994) basically confirmed these studies for CRF. They also reported that ACTH fragments (1-24), (1-4), (4-9), (1-13), (1-17), and (11-24) stimulate molluscan hemocytemigration, whereas the entire sequence (1-39) and the fragment (4-11) have an inhibitory effect. Differences between species were noted with respect to the response to individual fragments. Additionally, the (4-11) fragment could antagonize some of the stimulatory fragments (4-9) as well as TNF-α-induced chemotaxis.

ACTH also causes molluscan hemocytes to release biogenic amines (NE, epinephrine, and dopamine) that influence chemotactic and phagocytic activities of hemocytes (Franchini & Ottaviani, 1994; Ottaviani, Caselgrandi, Petraglia, & Franceschi, 1992). The greatest release occurred after 15 minutes, whereas after 45 minutes the values were similar to those of the controls. Culturing hemocytes with CRF also provoked release of biogenic amines, suggesting that this release was mediated by their releasing endogenous

ACTH. These experiments also suggest that molluscan hemocytes have the capacity to bind and respond to CRH in a manner reminiscent of the way mammalian leukocytes respond to this releasing factor (Ottaviani, Caselgrandi, Franchini, & Franceschi, 1993). These authors further demonstrated immunoreactive tyrosine hydroxylase and dopamine beta-hydroxylase (enzymes involved in biogenic amine biosynthesis) in these hemocytes. Ottaviani, Franchini, Caselgrandi, Cossarizza, and Franceschi (1994) found a similar but less significant catecholamine response when IL-2 rather than ACTH was added to cultures of hemocytes. Interestingly, preincubation of hemocytes with IL-2 or with anti-IL-2 monoclonal antibody significantly reduced or completely eliminated the CRF-induced release of biogenic amines. Further direct evidence of competition between CRF and IL-2 was revealed by immunocytochemical and cytofluorimetric analysis. One explanation favored by these investigators (at least at that time) was the presence of a unique (ancestral?) receptor on molluscan hemocytes that was capable of binding both CRF and IL-2. If this is indeed the case, it would have significant implications for understanding the evolution of neural–immune system interactions. At the very least, these and other observations suggest that, in terms of catechol biosynthesis, the invertebrate hemocyte may be a major player in an ancestral stress response that is associated with the HPA axis in mammals.

Stefano and colleagues (Dureus, Louis, Grant, Bilfinger, & Stefano, 1993) also found that administration of mammalian NPY to either molluscan hemocytes or to human granulocytes inhibited both spontaneous activation and chemotaxis in response to the chemoattractant synthetic peptide, N-formyl-methionyl-leucyl-phenylalanine.

In a more recent investigation, Sassi, Kletsas, & Ottaviani (1998) confirmed that ACTH (1-24) induces cell shape changes in the immunocytes of the mollusk *Mytilus galloprovincialis*. Using computer-assisted microscopic image analysis, they reported that the G protein antagonist suramin sodium, the adenylate cyclase inhibitor 2′,5′-dideoxyadenosine, and the protein kinase inhibitor staurosporine inhibited this effect. The highly specific inhibitors H-89 (for protein kinase A) and calphostin C (for protein kinase C) only partially inhibited the morphological alterations, whereas the simultaneous action of H-89 and calphostin C completely blocked them. Thus, mammalian ACTH-induced cell shape changes appears to involve adenylate cyclase/cAMP/protein kinase A pathway, as well as the activation of protein kinase C. In a related paper (Ottaviani, Franchinim, & Hanukoglu, 1998), ACTH receptor-like messenger RNA was localized in molluscan hemocytes (and, as a control, in human lood mononuclear cells) using a digoxigenin-labeled bovine cDNA probe. These findings imply that the ACTH receptor gene has been highly conserved during evolution, and according to these investigators, support their hypothesis that there is a phylogenetic relationship between the immune and neuroendocrine systems in invertebrates.

Stefano et al. (1989) reported that opioids can also affect the behavior of hemocytes of the mussel *Mytilus edulis*. Specifically, they found that the synthetic enkephalin analogue DAMA modulated locomotion, adherence, and conformation of a subset of hemocytes, which resulted in their assuming a flattened and elongated conformation with extended pseudopodia. These morphological characteristics of hemocyte activation are similar to those seen following similar treatment of human granulocytes (Hughes, Smith, Barnett, Charles, & Stefano, 1991; Stefano, Cadet, & Scharrer, 1989; Stefano, Leung, Zhao, & Scharrer, 1989; Stefano, Shipp, & Scharrer, 1991).

C. Effects of Mammalian Cytokines on Invertebrate Hemocytes

The third approach to studying invertebrate neural–innate immune system interactions has involved exploring the impact of molecules purported to be homologues of mammalian proinflammatory cytokines on hemocyte locomotion and phagocytosis, and on the production of nitric oxide synthase (NOS) and biogenic amines (Ottaviani, Franchini, Cassenelli, & Genedani, 1995; Ottaviani, Caselgrandi, & Kletsas, 1997). Some of these studies provide suggestive evidence that the cytokines tested can bind to, and compete with, CRF for the same membrane receptor (Ottaviani & Franchini, 1995). However, given the known lack of cross-reactivity of most mammalian cytokines with cells from different mammalian species (Haynes & Cohen, 1991), these results with mammalian cytokines and invertebrate blood cells are more provocative than definitive.

D. Production of Cytokine-Like Molecules by Invertebrate Hemocytes

The final approach taken by these investigators addresses the production of cytokine-like molecules by invertebrate hemocytes in response to signals that clearly elicit cytokine production by mammalian leukocytes. Like human granulocytes, molluscan hemocytes respond to LPS stimulation by assuming the active conformation changes described above (Hughes et al.,

1990; Hughes, Chin, Smith, Leung, & Stefano, 1991; Hughes, Smith, Barnett, Charles, & Stefano, 1991b). Similar LPS-induced changes of hemocytes from the insect *Leucophaea maderae* also have been published (Ottaviani, Franchini, Sonetti, & Stefano, 1995). At least in molluscks, this effect could be blocked by anti-mammalian TNF-α and/or anti-IL-1 antibodies. DAMA also is able to induce molluscan hemocytes to produce immunoreactive (ir)IL-1 (Stefano, Smith, & Hughes, 1991). Administration of naloxone blocked the DAMA-induced conformational change by hemocytes, but these cells could still be activated by administration of recombinant human (rh) IL-1-α, suggesting that opioid activation may act through an IL-1-like molecule (Stefano, Smith, et al., 1991).

As mentioned earlier, molluscan hemocytes release biogenic amines when they are cultured with CRF, a phenomenon that Ottaviani and co-workers (1991) have described as a prototypic stress response. This response is significantly reduced when hemocytes are preincubated with IL-1α, IL-1β, TNF-α or TNF-β prior to adding CRF to the incubation mixture (Ottaviani, Caselgrandi, & Franceschi, 1995).

Ottaviani and Franchini (1995) and Franchini, Kletsas, and Ottaviani (1996) used immunocytochemistry to detect immunoreactive platelet-derived growth factor α and β (PDGFα/β) and transforming growth factor (TGF)-β in phagocytic invertebrate leukocytes. The presence of PDGF-α/β–like receptors and TGF-β receptor (type II)-like molecules on the plasma membranes of the immunocytes of the mollusk *Mytilus galloprovincialis* was also suggested by immunocytochemistry (Kletsas, Sassi, Franchini, & Ottaviani, 1998). This latter study also revealed that PDGF-α/β and TGF-β1 provoke changes in the shape of the molluscan hemocytes following interactions of these mammalian ligands with their putative receptors, and that these extracellular signals are transduced along the phosphoinositide-signaling pathway. Ottaviani, Caselgrandi, and Kletsas (1998) suggest that in the mussel the major pathway followed by PDGFα/β and TGFβ in provoking the release of norepinephrine, epinephrine, and dopamine into cell-free hemolymph is mediated by a (CRH-ACTH) biogenic amine axis.

In mammals microglial cells, like macrophages, are phagocytic and synthesize proinflammatory cytokines. Sonetti, Ottaviani, and Stefano (1997) argue that the snail *Planorbius corneus* also has a class of glial cells that resemble vertebrate microglia. Interestingly, these cells can be identified by their immunopositivity to anti-POMC-derived peptide antibodies. As in vertebrates, snail microglia exhibit macrophage-like mobility, and when they are exposed in vitro to LPS or bacteria, they undergo conformational and mobility changes and also become phagocytic. Moreover, when activated, they also express TNF-α-like molecules and increase production of NOS as shown immunocytochemically. Morphine (which appears to bind these cells via a μ3 receptor) inhibits this mobility and phagocytic activity of invertebrate microglia, suggesting to these investigators that opiate-like compounds may influence invertebrate microglia as well as hemocytes. Similar microglial-like cells also have been described in the mussel and in the insect *Leucophaea maderae* (Sonetti et al., 1994). Excitability of a population of nociceptive sensory neurons in aplysia can be influenced by neighboring hemocytes (Clatworthy, 1998), and Clatworthy and Grose (1999) suggest that in vitro activation of these hemocytes by LPS causes them to produce cytokine-like factors that modulate expression of injury-induced sensory nerve hyperexcitability.

These aforementioned studies with invertebrates are clearly provocative in that they suggest a common evolutionary origin of the immune and neuroendocrine systems with their attendant inflammatory and stress responses (Ottaviani & Franchini, 1995; Ottaviani & Franceschi, 1996, 1997, 1998). However, before accepting the validity of this hypothesis, or even some of the data that led to its formulation, we must emphasize the importance of characterizing all the immunoreactive molecules and their receptors described in the previous paragraphs at the structural and genomic levels to determine if they are true homologues of their mammalian counterparts rather than, for example, an artifact of the detection methods used to identify them (Hahn, Fryer, & Bayne, 1996).

VIII. CONCLUDING REMARKS AND FUTURE RESEARCH DIRECTIONS

Although there have been only limited analyses of components of the neural–immune system communication network in a few favorite nonmammalian species, enough data exist to support the proposition that the phylogenetic emergence of a link between these two systems was not a recent event. To find the earliest origins of the integration of these systems, and to determine whether the neuroendocrine and immune systems evolved from a "common ancestor" (Ottaviani & Franceschi, 1997) prior to the appearance of a blood-brain barrier (Cserr & Bundgaard, 1984), studies are needed that exploit the most primitive extant vertebrates, the agnatha (hagfish and lampreys) that lack MHC, Ig, and TCR genes, the elasmobranchs (sharks and rays) where these critical hallmarks of adaptive immunity emerge for the first time (Du

Pasquier & Flajnik, 1999), and the invertebrates. In this regard, recent studies of innate immunity have revealed several noncytokine molecules that are common to the innate defense systems of both invertebrates and vertebrates. Indeed, these data (see reviews by Hoffman, Kafatos, Janeway, & Ezekowitz, 1999; Medzhitov & Janeway, 1998) provide strong evidence of evolutionary parallels and conservation of ancient host defense pathways involving Toll receptors and NF-κB signaling in organisms (e.g., drosophilia) that have been separated from mammals by more than a billion years. Given the availability of the molecular tools that allowed this new information to be generated, it would seem worthwhile to determine whether such receptors and signaling pathways might be subject to regulation by those mammalian-like neuroendocrine mediators that also appear to have been phylogenetically conserved in invertebrates.

Although it is clear that the basic pathways by which the nervous system can regulate the immune system in mammals are operative in teleosts, amphibians, reptiles, and birds, the extent to which products of the immune system can affect the brain and behavior of ectothermic vertebrates is virtually unexplored. Clearly, one of the more exciting developments in our understanding of neural–immune networks in mammals has been the reproducible demonstration that proinflammatory cytokines (e.g., IL-1) induced, for example, by microbial products, act as bidirectional communication signal molecules between the immune system and the CNS (Felten et al., 1991; Fleshner et al., 1995; Krueger & Majde, 1994). There are reports that deliberate infection of lizards (Kluger, Ringler, & Anver, 1975) or amphibians (Lefcort & Eiger, 1993) with pathogens can evoke behavioral responses consistent with IL-1 mediation (e.g., thermoregulatory behavior resulting in the selection of a higher temperature in the classic study of Kluger and colleagues [Kluger et al., 1975]). Although the direct involvement of cytokines in such CNS responses has yet to be determined, such studies are now in the foreseeable future. A few years ago, Verburg-van Kemenade et al., (1995) demonstrated an IL-1-like factor in carp, one of the prime candidates for this function. Recent cloning of carp and trout IL-1 (Secombes, et al., 1998) suggests that recombinant cytokine molecules and anticytokine antibodies will be available to explore the possible bidirectionality of the immune–endocrine interactions not only in fish but also in other ectothermic vertebrates. That such reagents are invaluable for addressing fundamental questions about the phylogeny of neural immune system interactions is sharply revealed by a report that in the frog *Xenopus* IL-β and its type 1 receptor, as detected by immunohistochemistry using polyclonal antihuman antibodies, are expressed in neural tissue prior to the development of cells of the immune system (Jelaso, Acevedo, Dang, Lepere, & Ide, 1998). Although these investigators performed Western blotting to confirm the IL-1 and IL-1 receptor specificity of the antihuman polyclonal antibodies they used in their *Xenopus* system, the availability of monoclonal antibodies directed against recombinant *Xenopus* IL-1 would have eliminated "putative" as a decriptor of the frog "IL-1" they were examining. Until such reagents are available, the issue of whether IL-1 and other proinflammatory cytokines were first used (phylogenetically speaking) as regulatory molecules by the nervous system and were subsequently coopted by the adaptive immune system, or vice versa, remains purely speculative. This issue might best be addressed in invertebrates and agnathans where no adaptive immune system exists. As previously pointed out, some authors have written extensively about hemocyte-derived homologues of IL-1α and IL-1β, IL-2, IL-6, and TNF-α and β (Ottaviani & Franchini, 1995. Their reports are primarily, if not exclusively, based on cross-reactions with anti-mammalian cytokine antibodies. Although these mediators do appear to affect cell migration, phagocytosis, and the induction of biogenic amines and nitric oxide synthase in the species of origin (e.g., freshwater snails), we must reiterate that the appropriate molecular studies confirming that these invertebrate mediators are really cytokine homologues are lacking. Similarly, we are unaware of substantive reports that these hemocyte-derived mediators, whatever they are, can affect the nervous system and behavior in the homologous (or even heterologous) invertebrate species. Clearly, appropriate studies in invertebrates and ectothermic vertebrates could prove extremely interesting with respect to the evolution of these mediators themselves as well as to the phylogeny of neural–immune interactions. Information in this area may come from unexpected areas of research. For example, axons of the central nervous system in adult mammals do not regenerate spontaneously after injury, partly because of the presence of oligodendrocytes that inhibit axonal growth (Eitan, Zisling, Cohen, Belkin & Hirschberg, 1992). This is not the case in fish, where spontaneous regeneration of the optic nerve has been correlated with the presence of factors cytotoxic to oligodendrocytes. This cytotoxic factor from the fish optic nerve has been described by Eitan et al. as an IL-2-like cytokine.

One important outcome of fully understanding neural–immune interactions is the development of behavioral and/or psychopharmacological strategies to maintain optimal health status in humans. There is, however, another related but largely overlooked application of understanding the impact of psychosocial and physical stressors on immune function, namely that eliminating, or "controlling," or simply understanding stressors that may be encountered by feral animals may prove important for the health of both captive and wild populations. The following few examples should bring this point home.

- Briggs, Yoshida, and Gershwin. (1996) reviewed the impact of potential immunomodulatory effects of handling stress on the morbidity and mortality of seabirds that were cleaned after having suffered the misfortune of being contaminated by an oil spill.
- An important method for tracking avian species during their migrations involves capturing the birds (e.g., with mist nets) and then banding them before release. Trapping and handling wild birds clearly influences glucocorticoid levels (Romero & Wingfield, 1999; Romero, Ramenofsky, & Wingfield, 1997); the short- and long-term consequences of these well-intentioned manipulations on immune functions of these birds (many of whom are weakened by the flight and lack of feeding) certainly needs to be considered by those directing this information-gathering conservation effort.
- In their article describing the innervation of the spleen of the beluga whale, Romano, Felten, Olschowka, & Felten (1994) point out that in general the incidence of cetacean strandings, on the rise in recent years, is thought to be associated with an intense but as yet unidentified stressor. As such, the capacity of the immune system to respond to cues from the CNS may prove critical not only for understanding the reasons for such strandings, but also in the rehabilitation of stranded animals.
- Consequent to certain behavioral circumstances, individual subdominant male wolves may be ostracized from the pack to spend the rest of their lives as solitary animals. Whether this naturally occurring, but forced, isolation of a social animal is accompanied by immunomodulation, and whether the resulting solitary life is then shortened by opportunistic pathogens, is an intriguing scenario that begs to be written.
- Amphibians are exhibiting a worldwide decline that has been attributed to viral and fungal pathogens (reviewed in Carey, Cohen, & Rollins-Smith, 1999). Carey (1993) and colleagues (Carey et al., 1999) have proposed that environmental "stressors" (e.g., ultraviolet radiation, water pH) may modulate the immune response capacity of amphibians to render them more susceptible to opportunistic pathogens. In a related vein, Herbst and Klein (1995) have speculated that the relationship between environmental contaminants and the increasing prevalence of green turtle fibropapillomatosis (an epizootic, apparently virally induced, disease) may involve immunosuppression associated with environmental contaminants (e.g., endocrine disruptors) or "stressors" such as altered temperature or salinity. These speculations certainly provide an ecologically valid rationale for better understanding the mechanisms underlying neural–immune system cross talk in the amphibia and reptilia.

As a final note, captivity can impose potentially stressful environmental conditions (e.g., crowding, isolation, handling, and possible disturbances in circadian activity [Dulak & Plytycz, 1989; Worley & Jurd, 1979]) that are immunomodulatory in laboratory animals (Moynihan et al., 1994). Given that zoological specimens are similarly affected by these and other stressors, an understanding of the physiological impact of these conditions would be of benefit to both the animals bred and/or maintained in captivity and to the institutions involved in maintaining them. Min-imizing events detrimental to the animals' self-maintenance of health status also would minimize the necessity for intervention by animal handlers. As more species from more taxa are being represented by captive specimens, ensuring the individuals' continued health becomes more critical; one way to ensure this may be to understand better how to enable the organism to maintain its own defense against pathogens.

Acknowledgments

Research cited from the authors' laboratory was supported by grants R37 HD-07901 from the National Institutes of Health (NC) and by a National Science Foundation predoctoral fellowship #GER-9253919 (KSK). Preparation of this review was supported, in part, by grant RO1 AI-44022 from the NIH (NC).

References

Abraham, E. J. & Minton, J. E. (1997). Cytokines in the hypophysis: A comparative look at interleukin-6 in the porcine anterior pituitary gland. *Comparative Biochemistry and Physiology A. Physiology, 116*, 203–207.

Ackerman, K. D., Bellinger, D. L., Felten, S. Y., & Felten, D. L. (1991). Ontogeny and senescence of noradrenergic innervation of the rodent thymus and spleen. In R. Ader, D. L. Felten, D. L., & Cohen, N. (Eds.), *Psychoneuroimmunology* (2nd ed.), (pp. 72–125). San Diego: Academic Press.

Ackerman, K. D., Madden, K. S., Livnat, S., Felten, S. Y., & Felten, D. L. (1991). Neonatal sympathetic denervation alters the development of in vitro spleen cell proliferation and differentiation. *Brain, Behavior, and Immunity, 5*, 235–261.

Ader, R. (1995). Historical perspectives on psychoneuroimmunology. In H. Friedman, T. W. Klein, & A. L. Friedman (Eds.), *Stress, the immune system and infection*. Boca Raton, Fl: CRC Press.

Ader, R. (Ed.). (1981). *Psychoneuroimmunology.* San Diego: Academic Press.

Ader, R., & Cohen, N. (2000). Conditioning and immunity. In R. Ader, D. L. Felten, D. L., & Cohen, N. (Eds.), *Psychoneuroimmunology*, (3rd ed.), San Diego: Academic Press.

Ader, R., Cohen, N., & Felten, D. L (1994). Psychoneuroimmunology: Interactions between the nervous system and the immune system. *Lancet, 345*, 99–103.

Ader, R., Felten, D. L., & Cohen, N. (1990). Interactions between the brain and the immune system. *Annual Reviews of Pharmacology and Toxicology, 30*, 561–602.

Ader, R., Felten, D. L., & Cohen, N. (Eds.). (1991). *Psychoneuroimmunology*, (2nd ed.) San Diego: Academic Press.

Ader, R., Kelly, K., Moynihan, J. A., Grota, L., & Cohen, N. (1993). Conditioned enhancement of antibody production using antigen as the unconditioned stimulus. *Brain, Behavior, and Immunity, 7*, 334–343.

Afifi, A., Mohamed, E. R., & el Ridi, R. (1993). Seasonal conditions determine the manner of skin rejection in reptiles. *Journal of Experimental Zoology, 265*, 459–468.

Ainsworth, A. J., Dexiang, C., & Waterstat, P. R. (1991). Changes in peripheral blood leukocyte percentages and function of neutrophils in stressed channel catfish. *Journal of Aquatic Animal Health, 3*, 41–41.

Alford III, P. B., Tomasso J. R., Bodine, A. B., & Kendall, C. (1994). Apoptotic death of peripheral leukocytes in channel catfish: Effect of confinement-induced stress. *Journal of Aquatic Animal Health, 5*, 64–69.

Altmann, D. (1986) Soziale Funktionen im Wolfsrudel, *Canis lupus lupus. Linnaeus Wissenschaftliche Zeitschrift der Humbol, 35*, 292–295

Anderson, D. P., Roberson, B. S., & Dixon, O. W. (1982). Immunosuppression induced by a corticosteroid or an alkylating agent in rainbow trout (*Salmo gairdneri*) administered a *Yersinia ruckeri* bacteria. *Developmental and Comparative Immunology, 2*, 197–204.

Angelidis, P., Baudin-Laurencin, F., & Youinou, P. (1987). Stress in rainbow trout, *Salmo gairdneri*: Effect upon phagocyte chemiluminescence, circulating leukocytes and susceptibility to *Aeromonas salmonicida. Journal of Fish Biology, 31*(suppl. A), 113–122.

Arnold, R. E., & Rice, C.D. (1997). Channel catfish lymphocytes secrete ACTH in response to corticotropic releasing factor. *Developmental and Comparative Immunology, 21*, 152.

Bachman, S. E. & Mashaly, M. M. (1987). Relationship between circulating thyroid hormones and cell-mediated immunity in immature male chickens. *Developmental and Comparative Immunology, 11*, 203–213.

Bachman, S. E. & Mashaly, M. M. (1986). Relationship between circulating thyroid hormones and humoral immunity in immature male chickens. *Developmental and Comparative Immunology, 10*, 395–403.

Balm, P. H. M. (1997). Immuno-endocrine interactions. In G. K. Iwama, A. D. Pickering, J. P. Sumpter, & C. B. Schreck, (Eds.), *Fish stress and health in aquaculture* Cambridge, UK; Cambridge University Press.

Balm, P. H. M., Pepels, P., Lieshout, E. van, & Wendelaar Bonga, S.E. (1993). Neuroimmunological regulation of α-MSH release in tilapia (*Oreochromis mossambicus*). *Fish Physiology and Biochemistry, 11*, 125–130.

Balm, P. H. M., & Pottinger, T. G. (1993). Acclimation of rainbow trout (*Onchorhynchus mykiss*) to low environmental pH does not involve an activation of the pituitary-interrenal axis, but evokes adjustments in branchial ultrastructure. *Canadian Journal of Fish and Aquatic Science, 50*, 2532–2541.

Balm, P. H. M, van Lieshout, M. E., Lokate, J., & Wendelaar Bonga, S. E. W. (1995), Bacterial lipopolysaccharide (LPS) and interleukin-1 (IL-1) exert multiple physiological effects in the tilapia *Oreochromis mossambicus* (Teleostei). *Journal of Comparative Physiology B, 165*, 85–92.

Banks, W. A. & Kastin, A. J. (1985). Permeability of the blood-brain barrier to neuropeptides: The case for penetration. *Psychoneuroendocrinology, 10*, 385–399.

Barni, S., Nano, R., & Vignola, C. (1993). Changes in the hemopoietic activity and characteristics of circulating blood cells in *Triturus carnifex* and *Triturus alpestris* during the winter period. *Comparative Haematology International, 3*, 159–163.

Barton, B. A., & Iwama, G.K. (1991). Physiological changes in fish from stress in aquaculture with emphasis on the response and effects of corticosteroids. *Annual Review of Fish Diseases, 1*, 3–26.

Bayne, D. J., & Levy, S. (1991). Modulation of the oxidative burst in trout myeloid cells by adrenocorticotropic hormone and catecholamines: Mechanisms of action. *Journal of Leukocyte Biology, 50*, 554–560.

Berkenbosch, F., Oers, J. van, Del Rey, A., Tilders, F., & Besedovsky, H. (1987). Corticotropin-releasing factor-producing neurons in the rat activated by interleukin-1. *Science, 238*, 524–526.

Bellinger, D. L., Lorton, D., Romano, T. A., Olschowka, J. A., Felten, S. Y., & Felten, D. L. (1990). Neuropeptide innervation of lymphoid organs. *Annals of the New York Academy of Sciences, 594*, 17–33.

Besedovsky, H. G., & del Rey, A. (1996). Immune-neuro-endocrine interactions: Facts and hypothesis. *Endocrine Reviews, 17*, 64–102.

Besedovsky, H. G., & Sorkin, E. (1977). Network of immune-neuroendocrine interactions. *Clinical and Experimental Immunology, 27*, 1–12.

Besedovsky, H. O., del Rey, A., Sorkin, E., Da Prada, M., & Keller, H. H. (1979). Immunoregulation mediated by the sympathetic nervous system. *Cellular Immunology, 48*, 346–355.

Besedovsky, H. G. Sorkin, E., & Mueller, J. (1975). Hormonal changes during the immune response. *Proceedings of the Society for Experimental Biology and Medicine, 150*, 466–470.

Betoulle, S., Troutaud, D., Khan, N. & Deschaux, P. (1995). Antibody response, cortisolemia and prolactinemia in rainbow trouts. *Comptes Rendus de L'Academie des Sciences — Serie Iii, Sciences de la Vie. 318*, 677–681.

Bigaj, J., & Plytycz, B. (1984). Endogenous rhythm in the thymus gland of *Rana temporaria* (morphological study). *Thymus, 6*, 369–373.

Bly, J. E., Miller, N. W., & Clem, L. W. (1990). A monoclonal antibody specific for neutrophilic granulocytes in normal and stressed channel catfish. *Developmental and Comparative Immunology, 14*, 211–221.

Brezinschek, H. P., Fässler, R., Klocker, H., Krömer, G., Sgonc, R., Dietrich, H., Jakober, R., & Wick, G. (1990). Analysis of the immune-endocrine feedback loop in the avian system and its alteration in chickens with spontaneous autoimmune thyroiditis. *European Journal of Immunology, 20*, 2155–2159.

Briggs, K.T., Yoshida, S. H., & Gershwin M. E. (1996). The influence of petrochemicals and stress on the immune system of seabirds. *Regulatory Toxicology, and Pharmacology, 23*, 145–155,

Brown-Borg, H. M., & Edens, F. W. (1992). In vivo neurotoxin administration alters immune response in chickens (*Gallus domesticus*). *Comparative Biochemistry and Physiology, 102C*, 177–183.

Brunetti, L., Preziosi, P., Ragazzon, E., & Vacca, M. (1994). Effects of lipopolysaccharide on hypothalamic-pituitary-adrenal axis in vitro. *Life Sciences, 54*, 165–171.

Buckbinder, L., & Brown, D. D. (1993). Expression of *Xenopus laevis* prolactin and thyrotropin genes during metamorphosis. *Proceed-*

ings of the National Academy of Sciences of the United States of America, 90, 3820–3824.

Caldwell, C. A., Kattesh, H. G., & Strange, R. J. (1991). Distribution of cortisol among its free and protein-bound fractions in rainbow trout (*Oncorhynchus mykiss*): Evidence of control by sexual maturation. *Comparative Biochemistry and Physiology, 99A*, 593–595.

Callahan, T. A., Moynihan, J. A., & Piekut, D. T. 1998. Consequences of peripheral sympathetic denervation following injection of 6-hydroxydopamine: Activation of the central nervous system. *Brain, Behavior, and Immunity, 12*, 230–241.

Capen, C. C. (1994). Mechanisms of chemical injury of thyroid gland. *Progress in Clinical and Biological Research, 387*, 173–191.

Carey, C. (1993). Hypothesis concerning the causes of the disappearance of boreal toads from the mountains of Colorado. *Conservation Biology, 7*, 355–362.

Carey, C., Cohen, N. & Rollins-Smith, L. A. (1999). Amphibian declines: An immunological perspective. *Developmental and Comparative Immunology, 23*, 459–472.

Carlson, R. E., Anderson, D. P., & Bodammer, J. E. (1993). In vivo cortisol administration suppresses the in vitro primary immune response of winter flounder lymphocytes. *Fish and Shellfish Immunology, 3*, 299–312.

Carr, D., & Blalock, J. E. (1991). Neuropeptide hormones and receptors common to both the immune and neuroendocrine systems: A bidirectional pathway of intersystem communication. In R. Ader, D. L. Felten, D. L., & Cohen, N. (Eds.), *Psychoneuroimmunology* (2nd ed.). (pp. 573–588). San Diego: Academic Press.

Chadzinska, M., Jozefowski, S., Bigaj, J., & Plytycz, B. (1997). Morphine modulation of thioglycollate-elicited peritoneal inflammation in the goldfish, *Carassius auratus. Archivum Immunologiae et Therapiae Experimentalis, 45*, 321–327.

Chadzinska, M., Kolaczkowska, Seljelid, R., & Plytycz, B. (1999). Morphine modulation of peritoneal inflammation in Atlantic salmon and CB6 mice. *Journal of Leukocyte Biology, 65*, 590–596.

Chelmicka-Schorr, E., Kwasniewski, M. N., & Czlonkowska, A. (1992). Sympathetic nervous system modulates macrophage function. *International Journal of Immunopharmacology, 14*, 841–846.

Chelmicka-Schorr, E., Kwasniewski, M. N., & Wollmann, R. L. (1992). Sympathectomy augments adoptively transferred experimental allergic encephalomyelitis. *Journal of Neuroimmunology, 37*, 99–103.

Chester Jones, I., Mosley, W., Henderson, I. W., & Garland, H. O. (1980). The interrenal gland in pisces. In I. Chester Jones & I. W. Henderson (eds.), *General, comparative and clinical endocrinology of the adrenal cortex*, vol. III, (pp. 396–523). London: Academic Press.

Chrousos, G. P., & Gold, P. W. (1992). The concepts of stress and stress disorders. Overview of physical and behavioral homeostasis. *Journal of the American Medical Association, 267*, 1244–1252.

Ciriaco, E., Ricci, A., Bronzetti, E., Mammola, C. L., Germanà, G, & Vega, J.A. (1995). Age-related changes of the noradrenergic and acetylcholinesterase reactive nerve fibres innervating the pigeon bursa of Fabricius. *Annals of Anatomy, 177*, 237–242.

Clatworthy, A. L. (1998), Neural-immune interactions—an evolutionary perspective. *Neuroimmunomodulation, 5*, 136–142.

Clatworthy, A. L., & Grose, E. (1999). Immune-mediated alterations in nociceptive sensory function in *Alyssa. Journal of Experimental Biology, 202*, 623–630.

Clem, L., Faulmann, E., Miller, N., & Ellsaesser, E. (1984). Temperature-mediated processes in teleost immunity: Differential effects of and in vitro and in vivo temperatures on mitogenic responses of channel catfish lymphocytes. *Developmental and Comparative Immunology, 8*, 313–322.

Clem, L. W., Miller, N. W., & Bly, J. E. (1991). Evolution of lymphocyte subpopulations, their interactions and temperature sensitivities. In: G. W. Warr & N. Cohen (Eds.), *Phylogenesis of immune functions* (pp. 191–213). Boca Raton, FL: CRC Press.

Clemons, G., & Nicoll, C. S. (1977). Development and preliminary application of a homologous radioimmunoassay for bullfrog prolactin. *General and Comparative Endocrinology, 32*, 531–535.

Clothier, R. H., & Balls, M. (1985). Structural changes in the thymus glands of *Xenopus laevis* during development. In M. Balls, & M. Bownes (Eds.), *Metamorphosis*, (pp. 332–359). Oxford: Clarendon Press.

Clothier, R. H., Ruben, L. N., Balls, M., & Greenhalgh, L. (1991). Morphological and immunological changes in the spleen of *Xenopus laevis* during metamorphosis. *Research in Immunology, 142*, 360–362.

Clothier, R. H., Ruben, L. N., Johnson, R. O., Parker, K., Sovak, M., Greenhalgh, L., Ooi, E., & Balls, M. (1992). Neuroendocrine regulation of immunity: The effects of noradrenaline in *Xenopus laevis*, the South African clawed toad. *International Journal of Neuroscience, 62*, 123–140.

Clothier, R. H., Ruben, L. N., Tran, K., & Balls, M. (1989). Catecholamine regulation of and by immunity in *Xenopus laevis. Developmental and Comparative Immunology, 13*, 441–442.

Cohen, N., & Koniski, A. (1994). Axolotl immunology: Lymphocytes, cytokines, and alloincompatibility reactions. *Axolotl Newsletter 23*, 24–33.

Cooper, E. L., Leung, M. K., Suzuki, M. M., Vicki, K., Cadet, P., & Stefano, G. B. (1993). An enkephalin-like molecule in earthworm coelomic fluid modifies leukocyte behavior. *Developmental and Comparative Immunology, 17*, 201–209.

Cooper, E. L., Wright, R. K., Klempau, A. E., & Smith, C. T. (1992). Hibernation alters the frog's immune system. *Cryobiology, 29*, 616–631.

Cordier, A. (1969). L'innervation de la bourse de Fabricius durant l'embryogenèse et de la vie adulte. *Acta Anatomica, 73*, 38–47.

Cserr, H. F., & Bundgaard, M. (1984). Blood-brain interfaces in vertebrates: A comparative approach. *American Journal of Physiology, 146*, 277–288.

Cunnick, J. E., Kojic, L. D., & Hughes, R. A. (1994). Stress-induced changes in immune function are associated with increased production of an interleukin-1-like factor in young domestic fowl. *Brain, Behavior, and Immunity, 8*, 123–136.

de la Torre, J. C. (1980). Standardization of the sucrose-potassium phosphate-glyoxylic acid histofluorescence method for tissue monoamines. *Neuroscience Letters, 17*: 339–340.

Dalmo, R. A., Ingebrigtsen, K., & Bfgwald, J. (1997). Non-specific defence mechanisms in fish, with particular reference to the reticuloendothelial system (RES). *Journal of Fish Diseases, 20*, 241–273.

Demers, N. E., & Bayne, C. J. (1997). The immediate effects of stress on hormones and plasma lysozyme in rainbow trout. *Developmental and Comparative Immunology, 21*, 363–373.

DiMarzo, S. J., & Cohen, N. (1982). Immunogenetic aspects of in vitro tolerance induction during the ontogeny of *Xenopus laevis. Immunogenetics, 16*, 103–116.

Donaldson, E. M., (1981). The pituitary-interrenal axis as an indicator of stress in fish. In A. D. Pickering (Ed.), *Stress in fish*. (pp. 11–47). London: Academic Press.

Donaldson, E. M., & Fagerlund, U. H. M. (1972). Corticosteroid dynamics in Pacific salmon. *General and Comparative Endocrinology*, (Suppl. 3), 254–265.

Ducoroy, P., Lesourd, M., Padros, M. R., & Tournefier, A. (1999). Natural and induced apoptosis during lymphocyte development in the axolotl. *Developmental and Comparative Immunology, 23*, 241–252.

Dulak, J., & Plytycz, B. (1989). The effect of laboratory environment on the morphology of the spleen and the thymus in the yellow-bellied toad, *Bombina variegata* (L.). *Developmental and Comparative Immunology, 13*, 49–55.

Du Pasquier, L., & Flajnik, M. (1999). Origin and evolution of the vertebrate immune system. In: W. E. Paul (Ed.), *Fundamental immunology*, (4th ed., pp. 605–649). New York: Raven Press.

Dureus, P., Louis, D., Grant, A. V., Bilfinger, T. V., & Stefano, G. B. (1993). Neuropeptide Y inhibits human and invertebrate immunocyte chemotaxis, chemokinesis, and spontaneous activation. *Cellular and Molecular Neurobiology, 13*, 541–546.

Eitan, S., Zisling, R., Cohen, A., Belkin, M., & Hirschberg, D. L. (1992). Identification of an interleukin 2-like substance as a factor cytotoxic to oligodendrocytes and associated with central nervous system. *Proceedings of the National Academy of Sciences of the United States of America, 89*, 5424–5428.

el-Far A. A., Mashaly, M. M., & Kamar, G. A. (1994). Bursectomy and in vitro response of adrenal gland to adrenocorticotropic hormone and testis to human chorionic gonadotropin in immature male chickens. *Poultry Science, 73*, 113–117.

Ellsaesser, C. F., & Clem, L. W. (1994). Functionally distinct high and low molecular weight species of channel catfish and mouse IL-1. *Cytokine, 5*, 10–20.

Ellis, A. E. (1981). Stress and the modulation of defence mechanisms in fish. In A. D. Pickering (Ed.), *Stress in fish*, (pp. 147–169). London: Academic Press.

Ellsaesser, C. F., & Clem, L. W. (1987). Cortisol-induced hematologic and immunologic changes in channel catfish (*Ictalurus punctatus*). *Comparative and Biochemical Physiology, 87A*, 405–408.

Espelid, S., Lokken, G. B., Steiro, K., & Bogwald, J. (1996). Effects of cortisol and stress on the immune system in Atlantic salmon (*Salmo salar* L.). *Fish and Shellfish Immunology, 6*, 95–110.

Faisal, M., Chiappelli, F., Ahmed, I., Cooper, E. L., & Weiner, H. (1989). Social confrontation "stress" in aggressive fish is associated with an endogenous opioid-mediated suppression of proliferative response to mitogens and nonspecific cytotoxicity. *Brain, Behavior, and Immunity, 3*, 223–233.

Felten, S. Y., & Olschowka, J. A. (1987). Noradrenergic sympathetic innervation of the spleen: II. Tyrosine hydroxylase (TH)-positive nerve terminals form synaptic-like contacts on lymphocytes in the splenic white pulp. *Journal of Neuroscience Research, 18*, 37–48.

Felten, D. L., Ackerman, K. D., Wiegand, S. J., & Felten, S. Y. (1987). Noradrenergic sympathetic innervation of the spleen: I. Nerve fibers associate with lymphocytes and macrophages in specific compartments of the splenic white pulp. *Journal of Neuroscience Research, 18*, 28–36.

Felten, D. L., Cohen, N. Ader, R., Felten, S. Y., Carlson, S. L, & Roszman. T. L. (1991). Central neural circuits involved in neural-immune interactions. In R. Ader, D. L. Felten, & N. Cohen, (Eds.), *Psychoneuroimmunology* (2nd ed., pp. 3–25). San Diego: Academic Press.

Felten, S. Y., Felten, D. L., Bellinger, D. L., & Olschowka, J. A. (1992). Noradrenergic and peptidergic innervation of lymphoid organs. *Cellular Immunology, 52*, 25–48.

Felten, D. L., Felten, S. Y., Carlson, S. L., Olschowka, J. A., & Livnat, S. (1985). Noradrenergic and peptidergic innervation of lymphoid tissue. *Journal of Immunology, 135*, 755s–765s.

Felten, S. Y., Olschowka, J. A., Ackerman, K. D., & Felten, D. L. (1988). Catecholaminergic innervation of the spleen: Are lymphocytes targets of noradrenergic nerves? In *Progress in catecholamine research, part A: Basic aspects and peripheral mechanisms* (pp. 525–531). New York: Alan R. Liss.

Ferriere, F., Khan, N. A., Troutaud, D., & Deschaux, P. (1996) Serotonin modulation of lymphocyte proliferation via 5-HT1A receptors in rainbow trout (*Oncorhynchus mykiss*). *Developmental and Comparative Immunology, 20*, 273–283.

Flajnik, M. F., & Du Pasquier, L. (1988). MHC class I antigens as surface markers of adult erythrocytes during the metamorphosis of *Xenopus*. *Developmental Biology, 128*, 198–206.

Fleshner, M., Goehler, L. E., Hermann, J., Relton, J. K., Maier, S. F., & Watkins, L. R. (1995). Interleukin-1β induced corticosterone elevation and hypothalamic NE depletion is vagally mediated. *Brain Research Bulletin, 37*, 605–610.

Flik, G., & Perry, S. F. (1989). Cortisol stimulates whole body calcium uptake and the branchial calcium pump in fresh water rainbow trout. *Journal of Endocrinology, 120*, 75–82.

Flory, C. M. (1989). Autonomic innervation of the spleen of the coho salmon, *Oncorhynchus kisutch*: A histochemical demonstration and preliminary assessment of its immunoregulatory role. *Brain, Behavior, and Immunity, 3*, 331–334.

Flory, C. M. (1990). Phylogeny of neuroimmunoregulation: Effects of adrenergic and cholinergic agents on the in vitro antibody response of the rainbow trout, *Onchorynchus mykiss*. *Developmental and Comparative Immunology, 14*, 283–294.

Flory, C. M., & Bayne C. J. (1991). The influence of adrenergic and cholinergic agents on the chemiluminescent and mitogenic responses of leukocytes from the rainbow trout, *Oncorhynchus mykiss*. *Developmental and Comparative Immunology, 15*, 135–142.

Fowles, J. R., Fairbrother, A., Fix, M., Schiller, S., & Kerkvliet, N. I. (1993). Glucocorticoid effects on natural and humoral immunity in mallards. *Developmental and Comparative Immunology, 17*, 165–177.

Franchini, A., Ottaviani, E. (1994) Modification induced by ACTH in hemocyte cytoskeleton of the freshwater snail *Viviparus ater* (Gastropoda, Prosobranchia). *European Journal of Histochemistry, 38*, 145–150.

Franchini, A., Kletsas, D., & Ottaviani, E. (1996). Immunocytochemical evidence of PDGF- and TGF-beta-like molecules in invertebrate and vertebrate immunocytes: An evolutionary approach. *Histochemical Journal, 28*, 599–605.

Franchini, A., Miyan, J. A., & Ottaviani, E. (1996). Induction of ACTH- and TNF-alpha-like molecules in the hemocytes of *Calliphora vomitoria* (Insecta, Diptera). *Tissue and Cell, 28*, 587–592.

Franchini, A., Ottaviani, E., & Franceschi, C. (1995). Presence of immunoreactive pro-opiomelanocortin-derived peptides and cytokines in the thymus of an anuran amphibian (*Rana esculenta*). *Tissue and Cell, 27*, 263–267.

Fried, G., Terenius, L., Brodin, E., Efendic, S., Dockray, G., Fahrenkrug, J., Goldstein, M., & Hokfelt, T. (1986). Neuropeptide Y, enkephalin and noradrenaline coexist in sympathetic neurons innervating the bovine spleen: Biochemical and immunohistochemical evidence. *Cell and Tissue Research, 243*, 495–508.

Fuchs, B. A., Albright, J. W., & Albright, J. F. (1986). β-adrenergic receptors on murine lymphocytes: Density varies with cell maturity and lymphocyte subtype and is decreased after antigen administration. *Cellular Immunology, 243*, 495–508.

Galton, V. A., & St. Germain, D. (1985). Putative nuclear triiodothyronine receptors in tadpole erythrocytes during metamorphic climax. *Endocrinology, 116*, 99–104.

Garrido, E., Gomariz, R. P., Leceta, J., & Zapata, A. (1987). Effects of dexamethasone on the lymphoid organs of *Rana perezi*. *Developmental and Comparative Immunology, 11*, 375–384.

Garrido, E., Gomariz, R. P., Leceta, J., & Zapata, A. (1989). Differential sensitivity to the dexamethasone treatment of the lymphoid organs of *Rana perezi* in two different seasons. *Developmental and Comparative Immunology, 13*, 57–64.

Gatti, S., & Bartfai, T. (1993). Induction of tumor necrosis factor-alpha mRNA in the brain after peripheral endotoxin treatment: comparison with interleukin-1 family and interleukin-6. *Brain Research, 624*, 291–294.

Gaykema, R. P., Dijkstra, P. I, & Tilders, R. J. (1995). Subdiaphragmatic vagotomy suppresses endotoxin-induced activation of hypothalamic corticotropin-releasing hormone neurons and ACTH secretion. *Endocrinology, 136*, 4717–4720.

Genedani, S., Bernardi M., Ottaviani, E., Franceschi, C., Leung, M. K., & Stefano, G. B. (1994). Differential modulation of invertebrate hemocyte motility by CRF, ACTH, and its fragments. *Peptides 15*, 203–206.

Ghoneum, M., Faisal, M., Peters, G., Ahmed, I., & Cooper, E. L. (1988). Suppressionofnaturalcytotoxiccellactivitybysocialaggressiveness in tilapia. *Developmental and Comparative Immunology, 12*, 595–602.

Glaser, R., & Kiecolt-Glaser, J. (Eds.). (1994). *Handbook of human stress and immunity*. New York: Academic Press.

Glick, B. (1984). Interrelation of the avian immune and neuroendocrine systems. *Journal of Experimental Zoology, 232*, 671–682.

Goehler, L. E., Relton, J. K., Dripss, D., Kiechle, R., Tartaglia, N., Maier, S. F., & Watkins, L. R. (1997). Vagal paraganglia bind biotinylated interleukin-1 receptor antagonist: A possible mechanism for immune-to-brain communication. *Brain Research Bulletin, 43*, 357–364.

Gorczynski, R. M., Macrae, S., & Kennedy, M. (1984). Factors involved in classical conditioning of antibody response in mice. In: R. Ballieux, R. Fielding, & A. L'Abbate (Eds.). *Breakdown in human adaptation to stress: Toward a multidisciplinary approach* (pp. 704–712). Boston: Martinus Nijhof.

Green (Donnelly), N., & Cohen, N. (1977). The effect of temperature on serum complement levels in the leopard frog, *Rana pipiens*. *Developmental and Comparative Immunology, 1*, 59–64.

Grimm, A. S. (1985). Suppression by cortisol of the mitogen-induced proliferation of peripheral blood leucocytes from plaice, *Pleuronectes platessa* L. In M. J. Manning & M. F. Tatner (Eds.), *Fish Immunology.*, (pp. 263–271). London: Academic Press.

Gross, W. B., & Siegel, H. S. (1983) Evaluation of heterophil:lymphocyte ratio as a measure of stress in chickens. *Avian Diseases, 27*, 972–979.

Gruca, P., Chadzinska, M., Lackowska, B., Plytycz, B (1996). Analysis of peritoneal and head kidney phagocytes during thioglycollate-elicited peritoneal inflammation in the goldfish, *Carassius auratus*. *Folia Biologica (Krakow) 44*, 137–142.

Guellati, M., Ramade, F., Le Nguyen, D., Ibos, F., & Bayle, J. D. (1991). Effects of early embryonic bursectomy and opotherapic substitution on the functional development of the adrenocorticotropic axis. *Journal of Developmental Physiology, 15*, 357–363.

Haberfeld, M., Johnson, R. O., Ruben, L. N., Clothier, R. H., & Shiigi, S. (1999). Adrenergic modulation of apoptosis in splenocytes of *Xenopus laevis* in vitro. *Neuroimmunomodulation, 6*, 175–181.

Haddad, E. E., & Mashaly, M. M. (1990). Effect of thyrotropin-releasing hormone, triiodothyronine, and chicken growth hormone on plasma concentrations of thyroxine, triiodothyronine, growth hormone, and growth of lymphoid organs and leukocyte populations in immature male chickens. *Poultry Science, 69*, 1094–1102.

Haddad, E. E., & Mashaly, M. M. (1991). Chicken growth hormone, triiodothyronine and thyrotropin releasing hormone modulation of the levels of chicken natural cell-mediated cytotoxicity. *Developmental and Comparative Immunology, 15*, 65–71.

Hahn, U. K., Fryer, S. E., & Bayne, C. J. (1996). An invertebrate (molluscan) plasma protein that binds to vertebrate immunoglobulins and its potential for yielding false-positives in antibody-based detection systems. *Developmental and Comparative Immunology, 20*, 39–50.

Harris, J., & Bird, D. J. (1998). Alpha-melaocyte stimulating hormone (α-MSH) and melanin-concentrating hormone (MCH) stimulate phagocytosis by head kidney leucocytes of rainbow trout (*Oncorhynchus mykiss*) in vitro. *Fish and Shellfish Immunology, 8*, 631–638.

Haynes, L., & Cohen, N. (1991) Phylogenetic conservation of cytokines. In G. W. Warr, & N. Cohen, (Eds.), *Phylogenesis of immune functions* (pp. 241–268). Boca Raton, Fl: CRC Press.

Hendricks, G. L., & Mashaly, M. M. (1998). Effects of corticotropin releasing factor on the production of adrenocorticotropic hormone by leukocyte populations. *British Poultry Science, 39*, 123–127.

Hendricks, G. L., Siegel, H. S., & Mashaly, M. M. (1991). Ovine corticotropin-releasing factor increases endocrine and immunologic activity of avian leukocytes in vitro. *Proceedings of the Society for Experimental Biology and Medicine, 196*, 390–395.

Herbst, L. H., & Klein, P. A. (1995). Green turtle fibropapillomatosis: Challenges to assessing the role of environmental cofactors. *Environmental Health Perspectives, 103*, 27–30.

Hickman, C. P., Roberts, L. S., & Larson, A. (1993). *Integrated principles of zoology* (9th ed, pp. 603–657). St. Louis; Mosby-Year Book.

Hodgson, R., Clothier, R. H., & Balls, M. (1979). Adrenoreceptors, cyclic nucleotides, and the regulation of spleen cell antigen binding in urodele and anuran amphibians. *European Journal of Immunology, 9*, 289–293.

Hodgson, R., Clothier, R. H., Ruben, L. N., & Balls, M. (1978). The effects of α and β adrenergic agents on spleen cell antigen binding in four amphibian species. *European Journal of Immunology, 8*, 348–351.

Hoffmann, J. A., Kafatos, F. C., Janeway, C. A., & . Ezekowitz, R. A. (1999). Phylogenetic perspectives in innate immunity, *Science. 284*, 1313–1318,

Holzapfel, R. A. (1937). The cyclic character of hibernation in frogs. *Quarterly Review of Biology, 12*, 64–83.

Hopkins, S. J., & Rothwell, N. J. (1995). Cytokines and the nervous system. I.: Expression and recognition. *Trends in Neurosciences, 18*, 83–88.

Horton, J. D., Horton, T. L., Ritchie, P., & Varley, C.A. (1992) Skin xenograft rejection in *Xenopus*: Immunohistology and effect of thymectomy. *Transplantation, 53*, 473–476.

Hu, Y., Dietrich, H., Herold, M., Heinrich, P. C., & Wick, G. (1993). Disturbed immuno-endocrine communication via the hypothalamo-pituitary-adrenal axis in autoimmune disease. *International Archives of Allergy, 102*, 232–241.

Hughes, T., Smith, E., Barnett, J., Charles, R., & Stefano, G. B. (1991a). Lipopolysaccharide and opioids activate distinct populations of *Mytilus edulis* immunocytes. *Cell and Tissue Research, 264*, 317–320.

Hughes, T., Smith, E., Barnett, J., Charles, R., & Stefano, G. B. (1991b). LPS stimulated invertebrate hemocytes: A role for immunoreactive TNF and IL-1. *Developmental and Comparative Immunology, 15*, 117–122.

Hughes, T., Chin, R., Smith, E., Leung, M., & Stefano, G. B. (1991). Similarities of signal systems in vertebrates and invertebrates: Detection, action, and interactions of immunoreactive monokines in the mussel, *Mytilus edulis*. *Advances in Neuroimmunology, 6*, 59–69.

Hughes, T., Smith, E., Chin, R., Cadet, P., Sinisterra, J., Leung, M., Shipp, M., Scharrer, B., & Stefano, G. B. (1990). Interaction of immunoactive monokines (interleukin 1 and tumor necrosis factor) in the bivalve mollusc *Mytilus edulis*. *Proceedings of the National Academy of Science of the United States of America, 87*, 4426–4429.

Hussein, M., Badir, N., Zada, S., el Ridi, R., & Zahran, W. (1984). Effect of seasonal changes on immune system of the toad, *Bufo regularis*. *Bulletin of the Faculty of Sciences of Cairo University, 52*, 181–192.

Hsu, E., & Du Pasquier, L. (1984). Ontogeny of the immune system in *Xenopus*: II. Antibody repertoire differences between larvae and adults. *Differentiation, 28*, 116–122.

Iger, Y., Balm, P. H. M., Jenner, H. A., & Wendelaar Bonga, S. E. (1995). Cortisol induces stress-related changes in the skin of rainbow trout (*Oncorhynchus mykiss*). *General and Comparative Endocrinology, 97*, 188–189.

Inue, K. (1971). Innervation of the bursa of Fabricius in the domestic fowl. *Acta Anatomica, Nippon, 46*, 403–415.

Jaudet, G., & Hatey, J. (1984). Variations in aldosterone and corticosterone plasma levels during metamorphosis in *Xenopus laevis* tadpoles. *General and Comparative Endocrinology, 56*, 59–65.

Jelaso, A. M., Acevedo, S., Dang, T., Lepere, A., & Ide, C. F. (1998). Interleukin-1β and its type 1 receptor are expressed in developing neural circuits in the frog, *Xenopus laevis*. *Journal of Comparative Neurology, 394*, 242–251.

Jolivet-Jaudet, G., & Leloup-Hatey, J. (1986). Corticosteroid binding in plasma of *Xenopus laevis*: Modifications during metamorphosis and growth. *Journal of Steroid Biochemistry, 25*, 343–350.

Jozefowski, S. J., & Plytycz, B. (1997). Characterization of opiate binding sites on the goldfish (*Carassius auratus L.*) pronephric leukocytes. *Polish Journal of Pharmacology, 49*, 229–237.

Jozefowski, S. J., & Plytycz, B. (1998). Characterization of β-adrenergic receptors in fish and amphibian lymphoid organs. *Developmental and Comparative Immunology, 22*, 587–604.

Jozefowski, S., Gruca, P., Józkowicz, A., & Plytycz, B. (1995). Direct detection and modulatory effects of adrenergic and cholinergic receptors on goldfish leukocytes. *Journal of Marine Biotechnology, 3*, 171–173.

Jozefowski, S., Jozefowski, A., Antkiewicz-Michaluk, L., Plytycz, B., & Seljelid, R. (1996). Neurotransmitter and opioid modulation of the amphibian transplantation immunity. In J.S. Stolen, T. C. Fletcher, C. J. Bayne, C. J. Secombes, Zelikoff, J. T., Twerdok, & D. P. Anderson (Eds.), *Modulators of immune responses: The evolutionary trail.* (pp. 281–290). Fair Haven, N.J: SOS Publications.

Józkowicz, A. (1995). Mechanisms involved in allograft and xenograft rejection in anuran amphibians. Herpetopathologia. In P. Zwart & G. Matz (Eds.), *Proceedings of the Fifth International Colloquium on Pathology of Reptiles and Amphibians*, 31.03-01.04 (pp. 155–160). The Netherlands: NRG Repro Facility BV's-Hertogenbosch.

Kaattari, S. L., & Tripp, R. A. (1987). Cellular mechanism of glucocorticoid suppression in salmon. *Journal of Fisheries Biology, 31*(suppl. A), 129–132.

Kamilaris, T. C., Debold, C. R., Johnson, E. Q., Mamalaki, E., Listwak, S. J., Calogero, A. E., Kalogeras, K. T., Gold, P. W., & Orth, D. N. (1991). Effects of short and long duration hypothyroidism and hyperthyroidism on the plasma adrenocorticotropin and corticosterone responses to ovine corticotropin-releasing hormone in rats. *Endocrinology, 128*, 2567–2576.

Keller, S. E., Schleifer, S. J., & Demetrikopoulos, M. K. (1991). Stress-induced changes in immune function in animals: Hypothalamo-pituitary-adrenal influences. In R. Ader, D. L., Felten, & N. Cohen (Eds.), *Psychoneuroimmunology, Second Edition*, 771–787. Academic Press: San Diego.

Kelly, K. W., Arkins, S., & Li, Y. M. (1992). Growth hormone, prolactin and insulin-like growth factor; new jobs for old players. *Brain, Behavior, and Immunity, 6*, 317–326.

Kiecolt-Glaser, J., & Glaser, R. (1991). Stress and immune function in humans. In R. Ader, D. L Felten, & N. Cohen (Eds.), *Psychoneuroimmunology* (2nd ed., pp. 849–867). San Diego: Academic Press.

Kikuyama, S., Kawamura, K., Tanaka, S., & Yamamoto, (1993). Aspects of amphibian metamorphosis: hormonal control. *International Review of Cytology, 145*, 105–148.

Kikuyama, S., Suzuki, M. R., & Iwamuro, S. (1986). Elevation of plasma aldosterone levels in tadpoles at metamorphic climax. *General and Comparative Endocrinology, 63*, 186–190.

Kinney, K. S., Felten, S. Y., & Cohen, N. (1996). Sympathetic innervationof *the amphibian spleen: Developmental studies in Xenopus laevis.Developmental and Comparative Immunology, 20*, 51–59.

Kinney, K. S. (1995). Sympathetic innervation of the amphibian spleen: *Structural and functional studies*, Doctoral dissertation, University of Rochester, Rochester, NY.

Kinney, K. S., Cohen, N., & Felten, S. Y. (1994a). Noradrenergic and peptidergic innervation of the amphibian spleen: Comparative studies. *Developmental and Comparative Immunology, 18*, 511–521.

Kinney, K. S., Cohen, N., and Felten, S. Y. (1994b). Chemical sympathectomy with 6-OHDA does not alter skin graft rejection in the frog, *Xenopus laevis*. *Abstract of the Society for Neuroscience, 20*, 105.

Kinney, K. S., Felten, S. Y., Horton, J. D., & Cohen, N. (1993). Chemical sympathectomy and thymectomy effects on splenic anatomy in the frog *Xenopus laevis*. *Abstract of the Society for Neuroscience*, Part 2, 945.

Klesius, P., Johnson, W., & Kramer, T. (1977). Delayed wattle reaction as a measure of cell-mediated immunity in the chicken. *Poultry Science, 56*, 249–256.

Kletsas, D., Sassi, D., Franchini, A., & Ottaviani, E. (1998). PDGF and TGF-beta induce cell shape changes in invertebrate immunocytes via specific cell surface receptors. *European Journal of Cell Biology, 75*, 362–366.

Kluger, M. J., Ringler, D. H., & Anver, M. R. (1975). Fever and survival. *Science, 188*, 166–168.

Koenig, J. I., Snow, K., Clark, B. D., Toni, R., Cannon, J. G., Shaw, A. R., Dinarello, C. A., Reichlin, S., Lee, S. L., & Lechan, R. M. (1990). Intrinsic pituitary interleukin-1 beta is induced by bacteria. *Endocrinology, 126*, 3053–3058.

Krueger, J. M., & Majde, J. A (1994). Microbial products and cytokines in sleep and fever regulation. *Critical Reviews in Immunology, 14*, 355–379.

Kruszewska, B., Felten, S. Y., & Moynihan, J. A. (1995). Alterations in cytokine and antibody production following chemical sympathectomy in two strains of mice. *Journal of Immunology, 155*, 4613–4620.

Kruszewska, B., Felten, D.L., & Moynihan, J. A. (1998). Changes in cytokine production and proliferation following chemical sympathectomy: Interactions with glucocorticoids. *Brain, Behavior, and Immunity, 12*, 181–200.

Lamers, A. E., Flik, G., & Wendelaar Bonga, S.E. (1994). A specific role for TRH in release of diacetyl α-MSH in tilapia stressed by acid water. *American Journal of Physiology, 267* (*Regulatory, Integrative, and Comparative Physiology*, 36), R1302–R1308.

Lefcort, H., & Eiger, S. M. (1993). Antipredatory behaviour of feverish tadpoles: Implications for pathogen transmission. *Behaviour, 126*, 13–27.

Leloup, J., & Buscaglia, M. (1977). La triiodothyronine, hormone de la métamorphose des Amphibiens. *Compte Rendu de L'Academie des Sciences, Paris, 84D*, 2261–2263.

Le Morvan-Rocher, C., Troutead, D., & Deschaux, P. (1995). Effects of temperature on carp leukocyte mitogen-induced proliferation and nonspecific cytotoxic activity. *Developmental and Comparative Immunology, 19*, 87–95.

Livnat, S., Felten, S. Y., Carlson, S. L., Bellinger, D. L., & Felten, D. L. (1985). Involvement of peripheral and central catecholamine systems in neural-immune interactions. *Journal of Neuroimmunology, 10*, 5–30.

Lorton, D., Hewitt, D., Bellinger, D. L., Felten, S. Y., & Felten, D. L. (1990). Noradrenergic reinnervation of the rat spleen following chemical sympathectomy with 6-hydroxydopamine: Pattern and time course of reinnervation. *Brain, Behavior, and Immunity, 4*, 198–222.

Lukas, N. W., McCorkle, F. M., & Taylor, R. L. Jr. (1987). Monoamines suppress the phytohemagglutinin wattle response in chickens. *Developmental and Comparative Immunology, 11*, 759–768.

Madden, K. S., & Felten, D. L. (1995). Experimental basis for neural-immune interactions. *Physiological Reviews, 75*, 77–105.

Madden, K. S., & Livnat, S. (1991). Catecholaminergic influences on immune reactivity. In R. Ader, D. L. Felten, & N. Cohen (Eds.), *Psychoneuroimmunology*, (2nd ed., 283–310). San Diego: Academic Press.

Madden, K. S., Ackerman, K. D., Livnat, S., Felten, S. Y., & Felten, D. L. (1993). Neonatal sympathetic denervation alters developments of natural killer (NK) cell activity in F344 rats. *Brain, Behavior, and Immunity, 7*, 344–351.

Madden, K. S., Ackerman, K. D., Livnat, S., Felten, S. Y., & Felten, D. L. (1989). Patterns of noradrenergic innervation of lymphoid organs and immunological consequences of denervation. In *Neuroimmune networks: Physiology and diseases* (pp. 1–8). New York: Alan R. Liss.

Madden, K. S., Felten, S. Y., Felten, D. L., Hardy, C. A., & Livnat, S. (1994). Sympathetic nervous system modulation of the immune system II: Induction of lymphocyte proliferation and migration in vivo by chemical sympathectomy. *Journal of Neuroimmunology, 49*, 67–75.

Madden, K. S., Felten, S. Y., Felten, D. L., Sundaresan, P. R., & Livnat, S. (1989). Sympathetic neural modulation of the immune system: I. Depression of T-cell immunity in vivo and in vitro following chemical sympathectomy. *Brain, Behavior, and Immunity, 3*, 72–89.

Madden, K. S., Moynihan, J. A., Brenner, G. J., Felten, S. Y., Felten, D. L., & Livnat, S. (1994). Sympathetic nervous system modulation of the immune system III: Alterations in T and B cell proliferation and differentiation in vitro following chemical sympathectomy. *Journal of Neuroimmunology, 49*, 77–87.

Madden, K. S., Sanders, V. M., & Felten, D. L. (1995). Catecholamine influences and sympathetic neural modulation of immune responsiveness. *Annual Review of Pharmacology and Toxicology, 35*, 417–448.

Maéno, M. & Katagiri, C. (1984). Elicitation of weak immune response in larval and adult *Xenopus laevis* by allografted pituitary. *Transplantation, 38*, 251–255.

Maier, S. F., Watkins, L. R., & Fleshner, M. (1994). Psychoneuroimmunology: the interface between brain, behavior, and immunity, *American Psychologist, 49*, 1004–1017.

Maniero, G. D., & Carey, C. (1997). Changes in selected aspects of immune function in the leopard frog, *Rana pipiens*, associated with exposure to cold. *Journal of Comparative Physiology, Biochemical, Systemic, and Environmental Physiology, 167*, 256–263.

Manning, M. J. (1991). Histological organization of the spleen: Implications for immune functions in amphibians. *Research in Immunology, 142*, 355–359.

Manning, M. J., & Horton, J. D. (1982). RES structure and function of the amphibia. In N. Cohen & M. M. Sigel (Eds.), *The reticuloendothelial system: Phylogeny and ontogeny* (pp. 423–459). New York: Plenum Press.

Manning, M. J., Donnelly, N., & Cohen, N. (1976). Thymus dependent and thymus independent components of the amphibian immune system. In R. K. Wright, & E. L. Cooper (Eds.), *Phylogeny of thymus and bone marrow-bursa cells* (pp. 123–132). Amsterdam: North Holland Publishing Co.

Marc, A. M., Quentel, C., Severe, A., Le Bail, P. Y., & Boeuf, G. (1995). Changes in some endocrinological and non-specific immunological parameters during seawater exposure in the brown trout. *Journal of Fish Biology, 46*, 1065–1081.

Marsh, J. A., & Scanes, C. G. (1994). Neuroendocrine-immune interactions. *Poultry Science, 73*, 1049–1061.

Marsh, J. A., Gause, W. C., Sandhu, S., & Scanes, C. G. (1984). Enhanced growth and immune development in dwarf chickens treated with mammalian growth hormone and thyroxine. *Proceedings of the Society for Experimental Biology and Medicine, 175*, 351–360.

Marx, M., Ruben, L. N., Nobis, C., & Duffy, D. (1987). Compromised T-cell regulatory functions during anuran metamorphosis: The role of corticosteroids. *Developmental and Comparative Immunology*, 129–140.

Mashaly, M. M. (1984). Effect of caponization on cell-mediated immunity of immature cockerels. *Poultry Science, 63*, 369–372.

Mashaly, M. M., Trout, J. M., & Hendricks, G. L., 3d (1993). The endocrine function of the immune cells in the initiation of humoral immunity. *Poultry Science, 72*, 1289–1293.

Mashaly, M. M., Trout, J. M., Hendricks, G., 3rd, al-Dokhi, L. M., & Gehad, A. (1998). The role of neuroendocrine immune interactions in the initiation of humoral immunity in chickens. *Domestic Animal Endocrinology, 15*, 409–422.

Maule, A. G., & Schreck, C. B. (1990a). Changes in the numbers of leukocytes in immune organs of juvenile coho salmon after acute stress or cortisol treatment. *Journal of Aquatic Animal Health, 2*, 298–304.

Maule, A. G., & Schreck, C. B. (1990b). Glucocorticoid receptors in leukocytes and gill of juvenile coho salmon (*Oncorhynchus kisutch*). *General and Comparative Endocrinology, 77*, 448–455.

Maule, A. G., & Schreck, C. B. (1991). Stress and cortisol treatment changes affinity and number of glucocorticoid receptors in leukocytes and gill of coho salmon. *General and Comparative Endocrinology, 84*, 83–93.

Maule, A. G., Schreck, C., & Kaattari, S. (1987). Changes in the immune system of coho salmon (*Oncorhynchus kisutch*) during the parr-to-smolt transformation and after implantation of cortisol. *Canadian Journal of Fish and Aquatic Science, 44*, 161–166.

Maule, A. G., Tripp, R., Kaattari, S., & Schreck, C. (1989). Stress alters immune function and disease resistance in Chinook salmon (*Oncorhynchus tshawytscha*). *Journal of Endocrinology, 120*, 135–142.

McCorkle, R. M. Lukas, N., & Taylor, R. L., Jr. (1986). Effect of serotonin on plaque-forming cells in chickens. *Poultry Science, 65*, 90.

McCorkle, R. M., Taylor, R. L., Denno, K. M., & Jabe, H. M. (1990). Monoamines alter in vitro migration of chicken leukocytes. *Developmental and Comparative Immunology, 14*, 85–93.

Medzhitov, R., & Janeway, C. A., Jr. (1998). An ancient system of host defense. *Current Opinion in Immunology, 10*, 12–15.

Meyniel, J. P., Khan, N.A., Ferriere, F., & Deschaux, P. (1997). Identification of lymphocyte 5-HT3 receptor subtype and its implication in fish T-cell proliferation. *Immunology Letters, 55*, 151–160.

Miles, K., Quintans, J., Chelmicka-Schorr, E., & Arnason, B. G. W. (1981). The sympathetic nervous system modulates antibody response to thymus-independent antigens. *Journal of Neuroimmunology, 1*, 101–105.

Milton, N.G., Self, S.H., & Hillhouse, E.W. (1993). Effects of pyrogenic immunomodulators on the release of corticotropic-factor 41 and prostaglandin E2 from the intact rat hypothalamus in vitro. *British Journal of Pharmacology, 109*, 88–93.

Miodonski, A. J., Bigai, J., Mika, J., & Plytycz, B. (1996). Season-specific thymic architecture in the frog *Rana temporaria*: SEM studies. *Developmental and Comparative Immunology, 20*, 129–137.

Möck, A., & Peters, G. (1990). Lysozyme activity in rainbow trout, *Oncorhynchus mykiss* (Waldbaum), stressed by handling, transport and water pollution. *Journal of Fisheries Biology, 37*, 873–885.

Mosconi, G., Yamamoto, K., Carnevali, O., Nabissi, M., Polzonetti-Magni, A., & Kikuyama, S. (1994). Seasonal changes in plasma growth hormone and prolactin concentrations of the frog *Rana esculenta. General and Comparative Endocrinology, 93*, 380–387.

Moynihan, J. A., Ader, R., & Cohen, N (1994). Stress and immunity: Animal studies. In B. Scharrer, E. M. Smith, & G. B. Stefano (Eds), *Neuropeptides and immunoregulation* (pp. 120–138). Berlin: Springer-Verlag.

Munck, A., & Guyre, P. M. (1991). Glucocorticoids and immune function. In R. Ader, N. Cohen, & D. L. Felten. (Eds.), *Psychoneuroimmunology*, (2nd ed., pp. 447–493). San Diego: Academic Press.

Nakanishi, T. 1986. Seasonal changes in the humoral immune response and the lymphoid tissues of the marine teleost, *Sebastiscus marmoratus. Veterinary Immunology and Immunopathology, 12*, 336–342.

Narnaware, Y. K., & Baker, B. I. (1996). Evidence that cortisol may protect against the immediate effects of stress on circulating leukocytes in the trout. *General and Comparative Endocrinology, 103*, 359–366.

Narnaware, Y. K., Baker, B. I., & Tomlinson, M .G. (1994). The effect of various stresses, corticosteroids and adrenergic agents on phagocytosis in the rainbow trout *Oncorhynchus mykiss. Fish Physiology and Biochemistry, 13*, 31–40.

Ndoye, A., Troutaud, D., Rougier, F., & Dechaux, P. (1991). Neuroimmunology in fish. *Advances in Neuroimmunology, 1*, 242–251.

Nevid, N. J., & Meier, A. H. (1993). A day-night rhythm of immune activity during scale allograft rejection in the gulf killifish, *Fundulus grandis. Developmental and Comparative Immunology, 17*, 221–228.

Nevid, N. J., & Meier, A. H. (1994). Nonphotic stimuli alter a day-night rhythm of allograft rejection in gulf killifish. *Developmental and Comparative Immunology, 18*, 495–509.

Nevid, N. J., & Meier, A. H. (1995a). Time-dependent effects of daily thermoperiods, feeding, and disturbances on scale allograft survival in the gulf killifish, *Fundulus grandis. Journal of Experimental Zoology, 272*, 46–53.

Nevid, N. J., & Meier, A. H. (1995b). Timed daily administration of hormones and antagonists of neuroendocrine receptors alter day-night rhythms of allograft rejection in the gulf killifish, *Fundulus grandis. General and Comparative Endocrinology, 97*, 327–339.

Nieuwkoop, P. D., & Faber, J. (1967). *Normal table of Xenopus laevis* (Daudin). Amsterdam: North-Holland Publishing.

Nilsson, S. (1978). Sympathetic innervation of the spleen of the cane toad, *Bufo marinus. Comparative Biochemistry and Physiology, 61C*, 133–139.

Nilsson, S., & Grove, D. J. (1974). Adrenergic and cholinergic innervation of the cod *Gadus morhua. European Journal of Pharmacology, 28*, 135–143.

Olivereau, M., & Olivereau, J. M. (1991). Responses of brain and pituitary immunoreactive cortisotropin-releasing factor in surgically interrenalectomised eels: Immunocytochemical study. *General and Comparative Endocrinology, 81*, 295–303.

Olsen, Y. A., Reitan, L. J., & Roed, K. H. (1993). Gill Na+, K+-ATPase activity, plasma cortisol level, and non-specific immune response in Atlantic salmon (*Salmo salar*) during parr-smolt transformation. *Journal of Fisheries Biology, 43*, 559–573.

Ottaviani, E. (1992). Immunorecognition in the gastropod molluscs with particular reference to the freshwater snail *Planorbarius corneus* (*L.*) (Gastropoda, Pulmonata). *Boll. Zoologica, 59*, 129–139.

Ottaviani, E., & Cossarizza, A. (1990). Immunocytochemical evidence of vertebrate bioactive peptide-like molecules in the immuno cell types of the freshwater snail *Planorbarius corneus* (L.) (Gastropoda, Pulmonata). *FEBS Letters, 267*, 250–252.

Ottaviani, E., & Franceschi, C. (1998). A new theory on the common evolutionary origin of natural immunity, inflammation and stress response: The invertebrate phagocytic immunocyte as an eyewitness. *Domestic Animal Endocrinology, 15*, 291–296.

Ottaviani E., & Franceschi, C. (1997). The invertebrate phagocytic immunocyte: Clues to a common evolution of immune and neuroendocrine systems. *Immunology Today, 18*, 169–174.

Ottaviani E., & Franceschi C. (1996). The neuroimmunology of stress from invertebrates to man. *Progress in Neurobiology*, 421–440. [Published erratum appears *in Progress in Neurobiology, 49*, 285.]

Ottaviani, E., & Franchini A. (1995), Immune and neuroendocrine responses in molluscs: the role of cytokines. *Acta Biologica Hungarica, 46*, 341–349.

Ottaviani, E., Capriglione, & Francheschi, D. (1995). Invertebrate and vertebrate immune cells express pro-opiomelanocortin (POMC) mRNA. *Brain, Behavior, and Immunity, 9*, 1–8.

Ottaviani, E., Caselgrandi E., Fontanili, P., & Franceschi, C. (1992). Evolution, immune responses and stress: Studies on molluscan cells. *Acta Biologica Hungarica, 43*, 293–298.

Ottaviani, E., Caselgrandi, E., & Franceschi C. (1995). Cytokines and evolution: In vitro effects of IL-1 alpha, IL-1 beta, TNF-alpha and TNF-beta on an ancestral type of stress response. *Biochemical & Biophysical Research Communications, 207*, 288–292.

Ottaviani, E., Caselgrandi, E., Franchini, A., & Franceschi, C. (1993). CRF provokes the release of norepinephrine by hemocytes of *Viviparus ater* (*Gastropoda, prosobranchia*): Further evidence in favour of the evolutionary hypothesis of the "mobile immune-brain." *Biochemical and Biophysical Research Communication, 193*, 446–452.

Ottaviani, E., Caselgrandi, E., & Kletsas, D. (1997). Effect of PDGF and TGF-beta on the release of biogenic amines from invertebrate immunocytes and their possible role in the stress response. *FEBS Letters, 403*, 236–238.

Ottaviani, E., Caselgrandi, E., & Kletsas D. (1998). The CRH-ACTH-biogenic amine axis in invertebrate immunocytes activated by PDGF and TGF-beta. *FEBS Letters, 427*, 255–258.

Ottaviani, E., Caselgrandi, E., Petraglia, F., & Franceschi, C. (1992). Stress response in the freshwater snail Planorbarius corneus (L.) (Gastropoda, Pulmonata): Interaction between CRF, ACTH, and biogenic amines. *General and Comparative Endocrinology, 87*, 354–360.

Ottaviani, E., Cossarizza, A., Ortolani, C., Monti, D., & Franceschi, C. (1991). ACTH-like molecules in gastropod molluscs: A possible role in ancestral immune response and stress. *Proceedings of the Royal Society of London, 245*, 215–218.

Ottaviani, E., Franchini, A., Caselgrandi, E., Cossarizza, A., & Franceschi, C. (1994). Relationship between corticotropin-releasing factor and interleukin-2: Evolutionary evidence. *FEBS Letters, 351*, 19–21.

Ottaviani, E., Franchini, A., Cassenelli, S., & Genedani, S. (1995). Cytokines and invertebrate immune responses. *Biology of the Cell, 85*, 87–91.

Ottaviani, E., Franchini, A., Cossarizza, A., & Frenceschi, C. (1992). ACTH-like molecules in lymphocytes. A study in different vertebrate classes. *Neuropeptides, 23*, 215–219.

Ottaviani, E., Franchini, A., & Franceschi, C. (1995). Evidence for the presence of immunoreactive POMC-derived peptides and cytokines in the thymus of the goldfish (*Carassius c. auratus*). *Histochemical Journal, 27*, 597–601.

Ottaviani E., Franchini, A., & Franceschi, C. (1998). Presence of immunoreactive corticotropin-releasing hormone and cortisol molecules in invertebrate haemocytes and lower and higher vertebrate thymus. *Histochemical Journal, 30,* 61–67.

Ottaviani, E., Franchini, A., & Hanukoglu, I. (1998). In situ localization of ACTH receptor-like mRNA in molluscan and human immunocytes. *Cellular and Molecular Life Sciences, 54,* 139–142.

Ottaviani, E., Franchini, A., Sonetti, D. & Stefano, G. B. (1995). Antagonizing effect of morphine on the mobility and phagocytic activity of invertebrate immunocytes. *European Journal of Pharmacology, 276,* 35–39.

Ottaviani, E., Petraglia, F., Genedani, S., Bernardi, M., Bertolini, A., Cossarizza, A., Monti, D., & Franceschi, C. (1993b). Phagocytosis and ACTH-like and β-endorphin-like molecules in invertebrate (molluscan) and in vertebrate (human) cells. *Annals of the New York Academy of Science,* 454–457.

Ottaviani, E., Trevisan, P., & Pederzoli, A. (1992). Immunocytochemical evidence for ACTH- and beta-endorphin-like molecules in phagocytic blood cells of urodelean amphibians. *Peptides, 13,* 227–231.

Pickering, A. D. (Ed.). (1981). *Stress and fish.* New York: Academic Press.

Pintea V., Constantinescu, B. M., & Radu, C. (1967). Vascular and nerve supply of bursa of Fabricius in hen. *Acta Veterinaria Academiae Scientiarum Hungaricae, 17,* 263–268.

Pellegrini, I., Lebrun, J. J., Ali, S., & Kelly, P. A. (1992). Expression of prolactin and its receptor in human lymphoid cells. *Molecular Endocrinology, 6,* 1023–1031.

Peters, G., Nüβgen, A., Raabe, A., & Möck, A. (1991). Social stress induces structural and functional alterations of phagocytes in rainbow trout (*Oncorhynchus mykiss*). *Fish and Shellfish Immunology, 1,* 17–31.

Plytycz, B., & Józkowicz, A. (1994). Differential effects of temperature on macrophages of ectothermic vertebrates. *Journal of Leukocyte Biology, 56,* 729–731.

Plytycz, B., & Seljelid, R. (1996). Nervous-endocrine-immune interactions in vertebrates. In J.S. Stolen, T. C. Fletcher, C. J. Bayne, C. J. Secombes, J. T. Zelikoff, Twerdok, L. E., & D. P. Anderson (Eds.), *Modulators of immune responses: The evolutionary trail.* (pp. 119–130) . Fair Haven, NJ: SOS Publications.

Plytycz, B., & Seljelid, R. (1997). Rhythms of immunity. *Archivum Immunologiae et Therapiae Experimentalis, 45,* 157–162.

Plytycz, B., & Szarski, H. (1987). Inguinal bodies of some Bufo species. *Journal of Herpetology, 21,* 236–237.

Plytycz, B., Chadzinska, M., Józkowicz, A., Gruca, P., & Seljelid, R. (1996). Stressing fish before sacrificing affects the in vitro cell activity. *Central-European Journal of Immunology, 21,* 278–280.

Plytycz, B., Dulak, J., Bigai, J., & Janeczko, K. (1991). Annual cycle of mitotic activity in the thymus of the frog, *Rana temporaria. Herpetopathologia, 2,* 23–29.

Plytycz, B., Kusina, E., & Józkowicz, A. (1993). Effects of hydrocortisone on the lymphoid organs of *Rana temporaria. Folia Histochemica and Cytobiologica, 31,* 129–132.

Pulsford, A. L., Crampe, M., Langston, A., & Glynn, P. J. (1995). Modulatory effects of disease, stress, copper, TBT and vitamin E on the immune system of flatfish. *Fish and Shellfish Immunology, 5,* 631–643.

Pulsford, A. L., Lemaire-Gony, S., Tomlinson, M., Collingwood, N., & Glynn P. J. (1994). Effects of acute stress on the immune system of the dab, *Limanda limanda. Comparative Biochemistry and Physiology, 109C,* 129–139.

Ramirez-Amaya, V., & Bermudez-Rattoni, F. (1999). Conditioned enhancement of antibody production is disrupted by insular cortex and amygdala but not hippocampal lesions. *Brain, Behavior, and Immunity, 13,* 46–60.

Rollins-Smith, L. A. (1998). Metamorphosis and the amphibian immune system. *Immunological Reviews, 166,* 221–230.

Rollins, L. A., & Cohen, N. (1980). On tadpoles, transplantation, and tolerance. In J. D. Horton (Ed.), *Development and differentiation of vertebrate lymphocytes* (pp. 203–214). Amsterdam: Elsevier/ North-Holland.

Rollins-Smith, L. A., & Blair, P. J. (1990a). Expression of class II major histocompatibility complex antigens on adult T-cells in *Xenopus* is metamorphosis dependent. *Developmental Immunology, 1,* 97–104.

Rollins-Smith, L. A., & Blair, P. (1990b). Contribution of ventral blood island mesoderm to hematopoiesis in postmetamorphic and metamorphosis-inhibited *Xenopus laevis. Developmental Biology, 142,* 178–183.

Rollins-Smith, L. A., & Blair, P. J. (1993). The effects of corticosteroid hormones and thyroid hormones on lymphocyte viability and proliferation during development and metamorphosis of *Xenopus laevis. Differentiation, 54,* 155–160.

Rollins-Smith, L. A., & Cohen, N. (1995). Metamorphosis: An immunologically unique period in the life of the frog. In L. J. Gilbert, B. G. Atkinson, & J. Tata (Eds.), *Metamorphosis/postembryonic reprogramming of gene expression in amphibian and insect cells.* (pp. 626–646). London: Academic Press.

Rollins-Smith, L. A., & Cohen, N. (1982). Self-pituitary grafts are not rejected by frogs deprived of their pituitary anlagen as embryos. *Nature, 299,* 820–821.

Rollins-Smith, L. A., Barker, K. S., & Davis, A. T. (1997). Involvement of glucocorticoids in the reorganization of the amphibian immune system at metamorphosis. *Developmental Immunology, 5,* 145–152.

Rollins-Smith, L. A., Blair, P. J., & Davis, A. T. (1992). Thymus ontogeny in frogs T-cell renewal at metamorphosis. *Developmental Immunology, 2,* 207–213.

Rollins-Smith, L. A., Davis, A. T., & Blair, L. A (1993). Effects of thyroid hormone deprivation on immunity in postmetamorphic frogs. *Developmental and Comparative Immunology, 17,* 157–164.

Rollins-Smith, L. A., Flajnik, M. F., Blair, P., Davis, A. T., & Green, W. F. (1994). Expression of MHC class I antigens during ontogeny in *Xenopus* is metamorphosis-independent. *Developmental and Comparative Immunology, 18,* S95.

Rollins-Smith, L. A., Parsons, S., & Cohen, N. (1984). During frog ontogeny, PHA and Con A responsiveness of splenocytes precedes that of thymocytes. *Immunology, 52,* 491–500.

Romano, T. A., Felten, S. Y., Felten, D. L., & Olschowka, J. A. (1991). Neuropeptide-Y innervation of the rat spleen: Another potential immunomodulatory neuropeptide. *Brain, Behavior, and Immunity, 5,* 116–131.

Romano, T. A., Felten, S. Y., Olschowka, J. A., & Felten, D. L. (1994). Noradrenergic and peptidergic innervation of lymphoid organs in the beluga, *Delphinapterus leucas*: An anatomical link between the nervous and immune systems. *Journal of Morphology, 221,* 243–259.

Rome, A., & Bell, C. (1983). Catecholamines in the sympathetic nervous system of the domestic fowl. *Journal of the Autonomic Nervous System, 8,* 331–342.

Romero, L. M., & Wingfield, J. C. (1999). Alterations in hypothalamic-pituitary-adrenal function associated with captivity in Gambel's white-crowned sparrows (*Zonotrichia leucophrys gambelii*). *Comparative Biochemistry and Physiology, Part B, Biochemistry & Molecular Biology, 122,* 13–20.

Romero, L. M., Ramenofsky, M., & Wingfield J. C. (1997). Season and migration alters the corticosterone response to capture and handling in an Arctic migrant, the white-crowned sparrow (*Zonotrichia leucophrys* gambelii). *Comparative Biochemistry and*

Physiology, Part C, Pharmacology, Toxicology/Endocrinology, 116, 171–177.

Roszman, T. L., & Carlson, S. L. (1991). Neurotransmitters and molecular signaling in the immune response. In R. Ader, D L. Felten, & N, Cohen (Eds.), *Psychoneuroimmunology*, (2nd ed., pp. 311–335). San Diago: Academic Press.

Rothman, R. J., & Mech, L. D. (1979). Scent-marking in lone wolves and newly formed pairs. *Animal Behaviour, 27*, 750–760.

Ruben, L. N., Proochista, A., Johnson, R. O., Buchholz, D. R., Clothier, R. H., & Shiigi, S. (1994). Apoptosis in the thymus of developing *Xenopus laevis*. *Developmental and Comparative Immunology, 18*, 343–352.

Saad, A.-H. (1993). Neuroimmunomodulation in reptiles. I. Pathways of neuro-immune interactions in the turtle, *Mauremys caspica*. *Journal of the Egyptian General Society of Zoology, 10*, 81–103.

Saad, A.-H, & Ali, W. (1992). Seasonal changes in humoral immunity and blood thyroxine levels in the toad, *Bufo regularis*. *Zoological Science, 9*, 349–356.

Saad, A.-H., & Bassiouni, W. M. (1991). Ultrastructural changes in the thymus of the lizard, *Chalcides ocellatus* following hydrocortisone treatment. *Journal of the Egyptian General Society of Zoology, 6*, 39–44.

Saad, A.-H., & El Ridi, R. (1988). Endogenous corticosteroids mediate seasonal cyclic changes in immunity of the lizard. *Immunobiology, 177*, 390–403.

Saad, A.-H., & Plytycz, B. (1994). Hormonal and nervous regulation of amphibian and reptilian immunity. *Folia Biologica, 42*, 63–78.

Saad, A.-H., & Shoukrey, N (1988). Sexual dimorphism on the immune responses of the snake *Psammophis siblans*. *Immunobiology, 177*, 404–419.

Saad, A.-H., Abdel Khalek, N., & El Ridi, R. (1990). Blood testosterone level: A season-dependent factor regulating immune reactivity in lizards. *Immunobiology, 180*, 184–190.

Saad, A.-H, El Ridi, R., El Deeb, S., & Soliman, M. A. W (1986). Effects of hydrocortisone on the immune response of the lizard, *Chalcides ocellatus*. III. Effect on cellular and humoral immune responses. *Developmental and Comparative Immunology, 10*, 235–245

Saad, A.-H., El Ridi, R., Zada, S., & Badir, N. (1984a). Effects of hydrocortisone on the immune response of the lizard, *Chalcides ocellatus*. I. Response of lymphoid tissues and cells to in vivo and in vitro hydrocortisone. *Developmental and Comparative Immunology, 8*, 121–130.

Saad, A.-H., El Ridi, R., Zada, S., & Badir, N. (1984b). Effects of hydrocortisone on the immune response of the lizard, *Chalcides ocellatus*. II. Differential action on T and B lymphocytes. *Developmental and Comparative Immunology, 8*, 835–844.

Saad, A.-H., Mansour, H., El Yazji, M., & N. Badir. (1992). Endogenous testosterone controls humoral immunity in the lizard, *Chalcides ocellatus*. *Zoological Science, 9*, 1037–1045.

Saad, A.-H, Nabil, M., & Raheem, K. (1993). Neuroimmunomodulation in reptiles. II. Seasonal changes in immune response and brain monoamine levels in the lizard, *Eumeces schneideri*. *Journal of the Egyptian General Society of Zoology, 10*, 355–371.

Saad, A.-H., Torroba, M., Varas, A., & Zapata, A. (1991a). Testosterone induces lymphopenia in turtles. *Veterinary Immunology and Immunopathology, 28*, 173–180.

Saad, A.-H., Torroba, M., Varas, A., & Zapata, A. (1991b). Structural changes in the thymus gland of turtles following testosterone treatment. *Thymus, 17*, 129–132.

Salonius, K., & Iwama, G. K. (1993). Effect of early rearing environment on stress response, immune function, and disease resistance in juvenile coho (*Oncorhynchus kisutch*) and chinook salmon (*O. tshawytscha*). *Canadian Journal of Aquatic Science, 50*, 759–766.

Sanders, V. M., Baker, R. A., Ramer-Quinn, D. J., Kasprowicz, B. A., Fuchs, B. A., & Street, N. A. (1997), *Journal of Immunology, 158*, 4200–4210.

Sapolsky, R., Rivier, C., Yamamoto, G., Plotsky, P., & Vale, W. (1987). Interleukin-1 stimulates the secretion of hypothalamic corticotropin-releasing factor. *Science, 238*, 522–524.

Sassi D., Kletsas, D., & Ottaviani E. (1998). Interactions of signaling pathways in ACTH (1–24)-induced cell shape changes in invertebrate immunocytes. *Peptides, 19*, 1105–1110.

Schauenstein, K., Fässler, R., Dietrich, H., Schwartz, S., Krömer, G., & Wick, G. (1986). Disturbed immune-endocrine communication in autoimmune disease: Lack of corticosterone response to immune signals in obese chickens with spontaneous autoimmune thyroiditis. *Journal of Immunology, 139*, 1830–1833.

Secombes, C., Zou, J., Daniels, G., Cunningham, C., Koussounadis, A., & Kemp, G. (1998). Rainbow trout cytokine and cytokine receptors genes. *Immunological Reviews, 166*, 333–340.

Sharma, J. M. (1991). Overview of the avian immune system. *Veterinary Immunology and Immunopathology, 30*, 13–17.

Shimizu, N., Hori, T., & Nakane, H. (1994). An interleukin-1β-induced noradrenaline release in the spleen is mediated by brain corticotropin-releasing factor: An in vivo microdialysis study in conscious rats. *Brain, Behavior, and Immunity, 7*, 14–23.

Skwarlo-Sonta, K. (1992). Prolactin as an immunoregulatory hormone in mammals and birds. *Immunology Letters, 33*, 105–122.

Smith, E., Hughes, T., Leung, M., & Stefano, G. B. (1991). The production and action of ACTH-related peptides in invertebrate hemocytes. *Advances in Neuroimmunology, 1*, 7–16.

Sonetti D., Ottaviani, E., Bianchi, F., Rodriguez, M., Stefano, M. L., Scharrer, B., & Stefano G. B. (1994). Microglia in invertebrate ganglia. *Proceedings of the National Academy of Sciences of the United States of America, 91*, 180–184.

Sonetti, D., Ottaviani, E., & Stefano, G. B. (1997). Opiate signaling regulates microglia activities in the invertebrate nervous system. *General Pharmacology*, 29, 39–47.

Spangelo, B. L., Judd, A. M., Isakson, P. C., & MacLeod, R. M. (1991). Interleukin-1 stimulates interleukin-6 release from rat anterior pituitary cells in vitro. *Endocrinology, 128*, 2685–2692.

Spieler, R. E. (1979). Daily rhythms of circulating prolactin, cortisol, thyroxine, and triiodothyronine levels in fishes: A review. *Review of Canadian Biology, 38*, 301–315.

Spooner, C. E., & Winters, W. D. (1966). Distribution of monoamines and regional uptake of DL-norepinephrine-7-H^3 in the avian brain. *Pharmacologist, 8*, 189.

Stave, J. B., & Roberson, B. S. (1985). Hydrocortisone suppresses the chemiluminescent response of striped bass phagocytes. *Developmental and Comparative Immunology, 9*, 77–84.

Stefano, G. B., Cadet, P., & Scharrer, B. (1989). Stimulatory effects of opioid neuropeptides on locomotory activity and conformational changes in invertebrate and human immunocytes: Evidence for a subtype of ∂ receptor. *Proceedings of the National Academy of Science of the United States of America, 86*, 6307–6311.

Stefano, G. B., Digenis, A., Spector, S., Leung, M. K., Bilfinger, T. V., Makman, M. H., Scharrer, B., & Abumrad, N. N. (1993). Opiate-like substances in an invertebrate, an opiate receptor on invertebrate and human immunocytes, and a role in immunosuppression. *Proceedings of the National Academy of Science of the United States of America, 90*, 11099–11103.

Stefano, G. B., Leung, M., Zhao, X., & Scharrer, B. (1989). Evidence for the involvement of opioid neuropeptides in the adherence and migration of immunocompetent invertebrate hemocytes.

Proceedings of the National Academy of Science of the United States of America, 86, 626–630.

Stefano, G. B., Shipp, M., & Scharrer, B. (1991). A possible immunoregulatory function for [Met]-enkephalin-Arg6-Phe[7] involving human and invertebrate granulocytes. *Journal of Neuroimmunology, 31*, 97–103.

Stefano, G. B., Smith, E., & Hughes, T. (1991). Opioid induction of immunoreactive interleukin-1 in *Mytilus edulis* and human immunocytes: An interleukin-1-like substance in invertebrate neural tissue. *Journal of Neuroimmunology, 32*, 29–34.

Sumpter, J. P., Pottinger, T. G. Rand-Weaver, M., & Campbell, P. M. (1994). The wide-ranging effects of stress on fish. In K. G. Davey, R. E. Peter & S. S. Tobe (Eds.), *Perspectives in comparative endocrinology* (pp. 535–538). Ottawa: National Research Council of Canada.

Tripp, R. A., Maule, A. G., Schreck, C. B., & Kaattari, S. L. (1987). Cortisol mediated suppression of salmon lymphocyte responses in vitro. *Developmental and Comparative Immunology, 11*, 565–576.

Trout, J. M., & Mashaly, M. M., (1995). Effects of in vitro corticosterone on chicken T- and B-lymphocyte proliferation. *British Poultry Science, 36*, 813–820.

Turnbull, A. V., & Rivier, C. (1995). Regulation of the HPA axis by cytokines. *Brain, Behavior, and Immunity, 9*, 253–275.

Vacchio, M. S., Papadopoulos, V., & Ashwell, J. D. (1994). Steroid production in the thymus: Implications for thymocyte selection. *Journal of Experimental Medicine, 179*, 1835–1846.

Vankelecom, H., Matthys, P., van Damme, J., Heremans, H., Billiau, A., & Denef, C. (1993). Immunocytochemical evidence that S-100-positive cells of the mouse anterior pituitary contain interleukin-6 immunoreactivity. *Journal of Histochemistry and Cytochemistry, 41*, 151–156.

Varas A., Torroba M., & Zapata A. G. (1992). Changes in the thymus and spleen of the turtle *Mauremys caspica* after testosterone injection: A morphometric study. *Developmental and Comparative Immunology, 16*, 165–174.

Verburg-van Kemenade B. M. L., Nowak, B., Engelsma, M. Y., & Weyts F. A. A. (1999). Differential effects of cortisol on apoptosis and proliferation of carp B lymphocytes from head kidney, spleen and blood. *Fish and Shellfish Immunology, 9*, 405–415.

Verburg-van Kemenade, B. M. L., Weyts, F. A. A., Debets R., & Flik, G. (1995). Carp macrophages and neutrophilic granulocytes secrete an interleukin-1-like factor. *Developmental and Comparative Immunology, 19*, 59–70.

Wang, R., & Belosevic, M. (1995). The in vitro effects of estradiol and cortisol on the function of a long-term goldfish macrophage cell line. *Developmental and Comparative Immunology, 19*, 327–336.

Wechsler S. J., McAllister, P. E., Hetrick, F. M., & Anderson, D. P. (1986). Effect of exogenous corticoisteroids on circulating virus and neutralizing antibodies in striped bass (*Morone saxatilis*) infected with infectious pancreatic necrosis virus. *Veterinary Immunology and Immunopathology, 12*, 305–311.

Weller, R. O., Engelhardt, B., & Phillips, M. M. (1996). Lymphocyte targeting of the central nervous system: A review of afferent and efferent CNS-immune pathways. *Brain Pathology, 6*, 275–288.

Wendelaar Bonga, S. E. (1997). The stress response in fish. *Physiological Reviews, 77*, 591–625.

Weyts, F., Flik, G., Cohen, N., & L. Verburg-van Kemenade. (1999). Interactions between the immune system and hypothalamo-pituitary-interrenal axis in fish. *Fish and Shellfish Immunology, 9*, 1–20.

Weyts, F. A. A., Verburg-van Kemenade, B. M. L., & Flik, G. (1998a). Characterization of corticoid receptors in carp, *Cyprinus carpio L.*, peripheral blood leukocytes. *General and Comparative Endocrinology*, 111, 1–8.

Weyts, F. A. A., Flik, G., Rombout, J. H. W. M., & Verburg-van Kemenade, B. M. L. (1998b). Cortisol induces apoptosis in activated B cells, but not in thrombocytes or T cells of common carp, *Cyprinus carpio* L. *Developmental & Comparative Immunology, 22*, 551–562.

Weyts, F. A. A., Flik, G., & Verburg-van Kemenade, B. M. L. (1998c). Cortisol inhibits apoptosis in carp neutrophilic granulocytes. *Developmental and Comparative Immunology, 22*, 563–572.

Weyts, F. A. A., Verburg-van Kemenade, B. M. L., Flik, G., Lambert, J. G. D., & Wendelaar Bonga, S. E. (1997). Conservation of apoptosis as an immune regulatory mechanism: Effects of cortisol and cortisone on carp lymphocytes. *Brain, Behavior, and Immunity, 11*, 95–105.

White, B., & Nicoll, C. (1981). Hormonal control of amphibian metamorphosis. In L. Gilbert & E. Frieden (Eds.), *Metamorphosis:* A problem in developmental biology (pp. 363–395). New York: Plenum Press.

Wick, G., Brezinschek, H. P., Hala, K., Dietrich, H., Wolf, H., & Krömer, G. (1990). The obese strain of chickens: An animal model with spontaneous autoimmune thyroiditis. *Advances in Immunology, 47*, 433–500.

Wick, G., Hu, Y., Schwarz, S., & Krömer, G. (1993). Immunoendocrine communication via the hypothalamo-pituitary-adrenal axis in autoimmune diseases. *Endocrine Reviews, 14*, 539–563.

Wilder, R. L. (1995). Neuroendocrine-immune system interactions and autoimmunity. *Annual Review of Immunology, 13*, 307–338.

Wojtaszek, J. S. (1992). Seasonal changes of circulating blood parameters in the grass snake *Natrix natrix natrix* L. *Comparative Biochemistry and Physiology, 103A*, 461–471.

Wojtowicz, A., & Plytycz, B. (1997). Seasonal changes of the gut-associated lymphoid tissues in the common toad, *Bufo bufo*. *Journal of Nutritional Immunology, 52*, 57–65.

Worley, R. T. S., & Jurd, R. D. (1979). The effect of a laboratory environment on graft rejection in *Lacerta viridis*, the European green lizard. *Developmental and Comparative Immunology, 3*, 653–665.

Yamaguchi, A., Teshima, C., Kurashige, S., Saito, T., & Mitsuhasi, S. (1981). Seasonal modulation and antibody formation in rainbow trout (*Salmo gaidneri*). In J. B. Solomon (Ed.), *Aspects of developmental and comparative immunology* (pp. 483). Oxford: Pergamon Press.

Yin, Z., Lam, T. J., & Sin, Y. M. (1995). The effects of crowding stress on the non-specific immune response in fancy carp (*Cyprinus carpio L.*). *Fish and Shellfish Immunology, 5*, 519–529.

Zapata, A., Garrido, F., Laceta, J., & Gomariz, R. P. (1983). Relationships between neuroendocrine and immune systems in amphibians and reptiles. *Developmental and Comparative Immunology, 7*, 771–774.

Zapata, A., & Leceta, J. (1986). Seasonal variations in the immune response of the tortoise *Mauremys caspica*. *Immunology, 57*, 483–487.

Zapata, A., Varas, A., & Torroba, M. (1992). Seasonal variations in the immune system of lower vertebrates. *Immunology Today, 13*, 142–147.

Zapata, A., Villena, A., & Cooper, E. L. (1982). Direct contacts between nerve endings and lymphoid cells in the jugular body of *Rana pipiens*. *Experientia, 38*, 623–624.

Zentel, H. J., Nohr, D., Albrecht, R., Jeurissen, S. H. M., Vainio, O., & Weihe, E. (1991). Peptidergic innervation of the bursa fabric: Interrelation with T-lymphocyte subsets. *International Journal of Neuroscience, 59*, 177–188.

Zentel, H. J., & Weihe, E. (1991). The neuro-B cell link of peptidergic innervation of the bursa fabric. *Brain, Behavior, and Immunity, 5*, 132–147.

C H A P T E R

2

Innervation of Lymphoid Organs—Association of Nerves with Cells of the Immune System and Their Implications in Disease

DENISE L. BELLINGER, DIANNE LORTON, CHERI LUBAHN, DAVID L. FELTEN

I. INTRODUCTION

The term *neuroimmunomodulation* refers to the ability of neurotransmitters to regulate immune function via neurophysiologic signaling. This capacity for neural–immune signaling derives from several observations: (1) immunocytes reside in a microenvironment in which they can be exposed to specific neurotransmitters; (2) cells of the immune system contain the machinery to respond to specific neurotransmitters; and (3) manipulation of the nervous system can alter immune responses in predictable ways. Neurotransmitters may be present in the microenvironment of lymphoid cells through several routes or sources. Nerves innervate cellular compartments of lymphoid organs, and distribute to mucosal sites where cells of the immune system form diffuse and aggregated lymphoid tissue. To understand the precise communication channels, it is important to determine the phenotype of immunocytes that are targets for these nerves, the molecular pathways through which the specific neurotransmitters convey their messages, and how changes in important signaling pathways alter immune function over the life span of an individual, under different physiologic conditions, and in disease states.

Other routes of neurotransmitter delivery to immunocytes exist in addition to direct innervation. Neurotransmitters may be produced and secreted by cells of the immune system, and may act in both an autocrine and paracrine fashion. Furthermore, since nerves have autoreceptors specific for the neurotransmitters that they release, secretion of neurotransmitters from immunocytes that reside adjacent to nerves is likely to regulate neurotransmitter release from nerves in lymphoid organs. Signal molecules from the nervous system also may arrive in lymphoid tissue via the circulation, as hormones. Some neurotransmitters (e.g., norepinephrine [NE]) may impinge on cells of the immune system by several routes.

Substantial research from a variety of fields confirms the presence of specific receptors for neurotransmitters on cells of the immune system. Interaction of the neurotransmitter with these receptors influences critical cellular events in immune reactions in vivo. Neurotransmitters in lymphoid organs also may have nonlymphoid cellular targets, such as vascular smooth muscle and endothelial cells, lymphatic vessels, and reticular cells that provide the supportive framework of the organ. Innervation of these targets may influence immune function indirectly by altering vascular permeability and blood flow, chemotaxis, cellular migration, and release or signaling of other mediators from targets that effect lymphocyte function.

In this chapter we describe neurotransmitter-specific innervation of lymphoid tissue, and the anatomical relationship between nerves and cells of the immune system. Anatomical studies are capable of revealing spatial relationships between nerves and cells of the immune system, and provide evidence for potential immune targets of these nerves. The intracellular pathways that neurotransmitters act through, and the functional consequences of receptor interaction with specific neurotransmitters, are discussed in other chapters. Lastly, in both the peripheral nervous system (PNS) and the central nervous system (CNS), products from immunocytes can alter neural function, including neuronal activity, neurotransmitter synthesis and release, the neurotransmitter phenotype of some neurons, and nerve fiber density. There is substantial evidence that changes in immune function can influence nerves that distribute to lymphoid tissues as well. Nerves in lymphoid organs are not static; they respond to immune cell signals in a variety of ways. The response of these nerves can, in turn, influence the ability of the immune system to handle immunologic challenges and reestablish homeostasis. In some pathologic situations the inability of the immune system to deal effectively with a challenge may in part be determined by neural signaling at the site of antigen processing, such as a neurally driven or chronic inflammatory response that results in the release of immune mediators, which feed back to alter neural input at that site. In this chapter, we summarize how nerves in lymphoid tissue respond to changes in immune function under normal conditions and disease states. We also discuss the possible consequences of nerve plasticity in certain disease states.

II. NEUROCHEMICALLY-SPECIFIC NERVES IN LYMPHOID TISSUE

A. Noradrenergic Sympathetic Nerves

1. *Bone Marrow*

General histological staining methods (such as silver stains and methylene blue) and electron microscopy (Calvo, 1968; Calvo & Forteza-Vila, 1969; DePace & Webber, 1975; Lichtman, 1981) reveal nerve bundles that supply the periosteum and enter the interior of the bone via the nutrient foramena to the medulla. These medullary bundles, consisting of both myelinated and unmyelinated nerve fibers, then distribute in a fashion similar to the branching of the nutrient artery. Some nerve fibers enter the parenchyma to course among blood-forming cells in the marrow. Clearly, some, but not all, of these nerves are noradrenergic (NA) (DePace & Webber, 1975), because sympathectomy results in the degeneration of some of these fibers (Kawahara & Osada, 1962; Takase & Nomura, 1957).

Recently, NA innervation of the bone marrow has been examined with immunocytochemistry for localization of tyrosine hydroxylase (TH), the rate-limiting enzyme in the synthesis of NE (Tabarowski, Gibson-Berry, & Felten, 1996), and with glyoxylic acid-induced fluorescence histochemistry for localizing catecholamines (S. Y. Felten & Felten, 1991). In young adult rodents, NA postganglionic sympathetic innervation that distributes to long bones courses along branches of the appropriate spinal nerve supplying that region of the body. These NA nerves then form small nerve bundles that supply the bone through the nutrient foramena, along with the vasculature. Within the marrow, the majority of NA nerves (Figure 1) form dense plexuses along the vasculature (D. L. Felten,

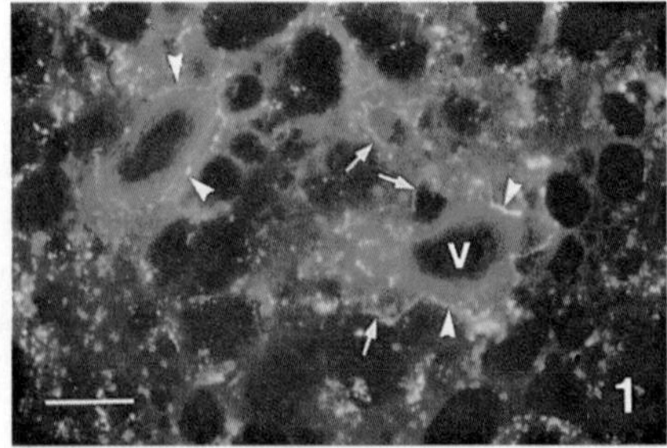

FIGURE 1 In the bone marrow of the rat femur, NA sympathetic nerves surround several blood vessels (v) (arrowheads), and course in the surrounding parenchyma (arrows). Glyoxylic acid-induced histofluorescence (HF) for catecholamines (CAs); X43. Calibration bar = 100 μm.

Felten, Carlson, Olschowka, & Livnat, 1985; S. Y. Felten & Felten, 1991; Tabarowski et al., 1996). From these vascular plexuses, numerous nerve fibers branch into the surrounding parenchyma among hemopoietic cells in the marrow. With functional and pharmacological studies, adrenoceptors have been demonstrated on granulocyte-macrophage progenitor cells and primitive progenitor cells (Maestroni & Conti, 1994; Setchenska, Bonanou-Tzedaki, & Arnstein, 1986). Neurochemical measurements of catecholamines in murine bone marrow reveal the presence of NE in the range of 1–3 ng per g bone marrow tissue (Maestroni et al., 1998; Marino et al., 1997), one to two orders of magnitude lower than is generally found in secondary lymphoid organs in rats (Besedovsky, del Rey, Sorkin, Da Prada, & Keller, 1979; Madden, Sanders, & Felten, 1995).

Interleukin (IL)-1-immunoreactive nerves were demonstrated in the marrow of developing heterotopic bone, induced by demineralized allogeneic bone matrix in the rat. These nerves closely resembled NA sympathetic innervation in their shape, density of nerve profiles, and compartmentation (Kreicbergs et al., 1995). Whether these IL-1^+ nerves are sympathetic, and whether IL-1 and NE are colocalized in nerves in the bone marrow in vivo, awaits further investigation.

The functional significance of sympathetic nerves in bone marrow is not yet clear. The presence of NA nerves adjacent to the vasculature suggests that NE may have vasomotor activity, controlling blood flow and volume within the bone marrow. An electron microscopic study (Yamazaki & Allen, 1990) demonstrated direct apposition between nerve terminals and a particular type of stromal cell, the periarterial adventitial cell, an important source of growth factors and adhesion molecules. Periarterial adventitial cells are characterized by a thin veil-like cytoplasm that concentrically surrounds both nerves and arterioles. Nonmyelinated and myelinated nerves distribute mainly between the layers of periarterial adventitial cells. Efferent nerves also appose sinus adventitial reticular cells and intersinusoidal reticular cells; all three cell types are connected by gap junctions. Some authors suggest that efferent nerves may regulate hematopoiesis via modulation of factors released by these stromal cells (Afan, Broome, Nicholls, Whetton, & Miyan, 1997; Yamazaki & Allen, 1990). Temporal development of innervation of the rat bone marrow correlates with the onset of hemopoietic activity (Calvo & Forteza-Vila, 1969; Garcia & van Dyke, 1961). Data from several studies are consistent with this hypothesis. NE and dopamine concentrations in mouse bone marrow exhibit diurnal rhythmicity, with peak values occurring at night (Maestroni et al., 1998). This phenomenon positively correlates with the G2/M and S phases of the cell cycle (Cosentino et al., 1998; Maestroni et al., 1998), suggesting a possible neural association.

Chemical sympathectomy with 6-hydroxydopamine (6-OHDA), or administration of the α_1-adrenergic antagonist, prazosin, enhances myelopoiesis and exerts an inhibitory effect on lymphopoiesis (Maestroni, Conti, & Pedrinis, 1992; Maestroni & Conti, 1994). Feldman and co-workers (Feldman, Rachmilewitz, & Izak, 1966) have shown that stimulation of the posterior hypothalamus causes a release of reticulocytes, via activation of descending sympathetic innervation to the bone marrow. However, it is not yet clear whether the release of reticulocytes is due to a direct action of NE on these cells or to an indirect action of NE on the vasculature. Within 24 hours after transection of the femoral nerve, or after chemical sympathectomy with 6-OHDA, bone marrow cellularity decreases, resulting from mobilization of mature cells; this phenomenon is attributed to the bolus release of NE from damaged nerves (Afan et al., 1997). Femoral nerve transection also releases progenitor cells from the bone marrow into the circulation. In contrast, following neonatal chemical sympathectomy, surgical denervation of the hind limb, or electrical stimulation of the hind limb, Benestad et al. (Benestad, Strom-Gundersen, Ole Iversen, Haug, & Nja, 1998) found no change in blood flow, bone marrow cellularity, or efflux of tibial marrow cells into the circulation. NE also mobilizes fat from the bone marrow (Tran, Dang, Lafontan, & Montastruc, 1985).

Wu and colleagues (D. L. Felten, Gibson-Berry, & Wu, 1996) have utilized a three-dimensional bone marrow culture system to test the effects of neurotransmitters on hematopoiesis. They found that isoproterenol treatment of murine bone marrow cultures greatly enhanced cell proliferation in the culture, and stimulated granulopoiesis in a dose-dependent fashion. In fact, isoproterenol was as effective as granulocyte colony stimulating factor in stimulating granulopoiesis, and synergized the stimulating effects of granulocyte colony stimulating factor.

2. *Thymus*

NA sympathetic innervation of the thymus originates from postganglionic cell bodies in the upper paravertebral ganglia of the sympathetic chain, primarily the superior cervical and stellate ganglia (Bulloch & Pomerantz, 1984; Nance, Hopkins, & Bieger, 1987; Tollefson & Bulloch, 1990). NA innervation of the thymus is well characterized in rodents (Al

Shawaf, Kendall, & Cowen, 1991; Bellinger, Felten, & Felten, 1988; Besedovsky et al., 1987; Bulloch & Pomerantz, 1984; D. L. Felten & Felten, 1989; D. L. Felten et al., 1985; S. Y. Felten, Felten et al., 1988; Kendall & Al-Shawaf, 1991; Kranz, Kendall, & von Gaudecker, 1997; Madden et al., 1997; reviewed in D. L. Felten & Felten, 1989; S. Y. Felten & Felten, 1991; Mitchell, Kendall, Adam, & Schumacher, 1997; Müller & Weihe, 1991; Nance et al., 1987; Sergeeva, 1974; Williams & Felten, 1981; Williams et al., 1981). Several reports briefly indicate sympathetic nerves in the chicken (Chan, 1992) and human (de Leeuw et al., 1992; Kranz et al., 1997) thymus. NA fibers enter the thymus adjacent to large blood vessels as dense vascular plexuses, and travel in the capsule (Figures 2 and 5) and interlobular septa (Figure 3), or continue with the vasculature into the cortex (Figure 4). From these plexuses, NA nerves appear to course along very fine septa into the cortical region, in close proximity to thymocytes (less than 1 μm). Cortical fibers often reside in close proximity to cells with yellow autofluorescence, a macrophage-like cell in the cortex in thymic tissue stained with fluorescence histochemistry for catecholamines.

In the capsule and interlobular septa, NA nerve fibers course adjacent to mast cells (Bellinger et al., 1990; Müller & Weihe, 1991), corticotropin releasing hormone (CRH)-immunoreactive cells (Figure 5) (Brouxhon, Prasad, Joseph, Bellinger, & Felten, 1994), and ED3$^+$ macrophages (Figure 2). At the corticomedullary junction, NA nerves are present along the medullary venous sinuses, which are continuous with the system of innervated vessels in the septa. NA fibers extend from these sinuses into the adjacent cortical region and occasionally into the medullary parenchyma. TH$^+$ nerves also course adjacent to ED1$^+$ corticomedullary macrophages (Müller & Weihe, 1991). Neurochemical analysis of catecholamines in the thymus indicates that virtually all the catecholamine-containing nerves are NA. It appears that not all of the NA nerve fibers are positive for PGP 9.5 (Al Shawaf et al., 1991), a general marker for nerve fibers regardless of the neurotransmitter phenotypes (Thompson, Doran, Jackson, Dhillon, & Rode, 1983).

Another potential target of NA nerves in the thymus appears to be thymic epithelial cells, which the NA nerve fibers closely appose (Kurz et al., 1997). Further, mRNA for β_1 and β_2-adrenoceptors have been detected in cultured thymic epithelial cells by reverse transcription-polymerase chain reaction using sequence-specific primers and surface expression

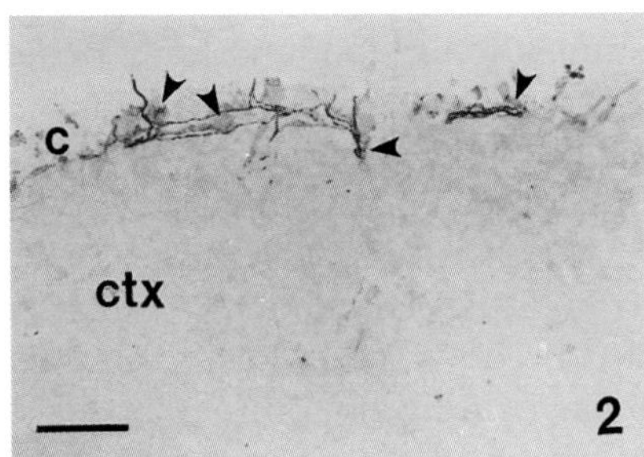

FIGURE 2 Tyrosene hydroxylase (TH)$^+$ nerves (black) course in the capsule (c) of the rat thymus among ED3$^+$ macrophages (brown) (arrowheads). ctx, thymic cortex. Double-label immunocytochemistry (ICC) for TH and ED3, a macrophage marker. X43. Calibration bar = 100 μm.

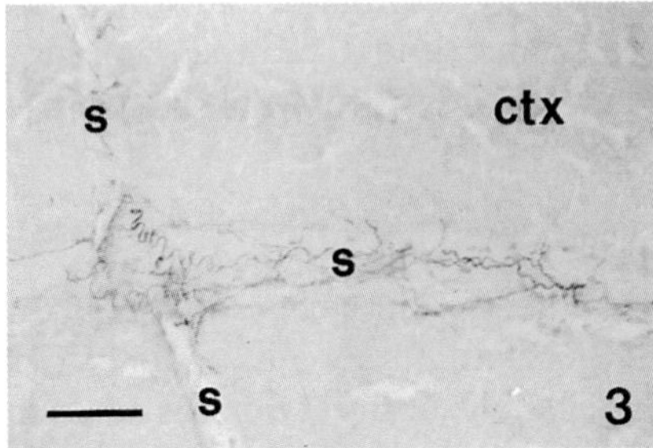

FIGURE 3 TH$^+$ nerve fibers (black) reside in the interlobular septum (s) of the rat thymus. ctx, thymic cortex. Single-label ICC for TH. X43. Calibration bar = 100 μm.

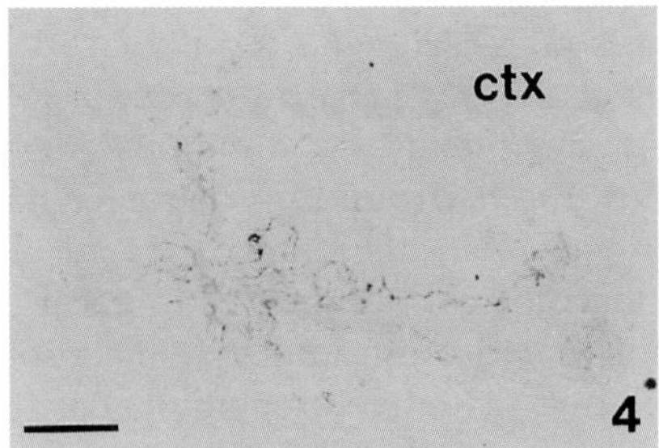

FIGURE 4 Linear varicose TH$^+$ nerve fibers form a plexus associated with a blood vessel in the rat thymic cortex (ctx) . Single-label ICC for TH. X43. Calibration bar = 100 μm.

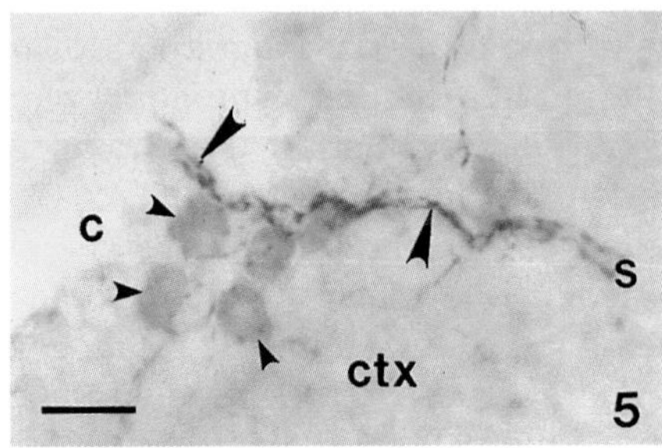

FIGURE 5 Beneath the capsule (c) and in the interlobular septum (s) of the rat thymus, TH$^+$ nerve fibers (black) (large arrowheads) reside in close proximity to corticotropin releasing hormone (CRH)$^+$ cells (brown) (small arrowheads). ctx, thymic cortex. Double-label ICC for TH and CRH. X85. Calibration bar = 50 μm.

confirmed by pharmacological means, including binding studies and adenosine 3′,5′-cyclic monophosphate (cAMP) generation by epithelial cells (Kurz et al., 1997). Close appositions between nonmyelinated nerves containing dense core vesicles and myoid cells and fibroblasts also have been reported in the chick thymus (Chan, 1992).

Without the presence of a diffusion barrier associated with the fine septa, it is likely that NE released from NA nerves can interact with thymocytes, particularly since extensive diffusion of NE from sympathetic postganglionic nerves is well documented in other peripheral target organs. The functional significance of NA innervation of the thymus is not clear. Experimental studies by Singh and Owen (Singh, 1979a, 1979b; 1985a, 1985b; Singh & Owen, 1975, 1976) suggest that NE exerts an effect on the maturation of thymocytes, since it inhibits proliferation and promotes differentiation of thymocytes in vitro. This effect is mediated through the activation of β-adrenergic receptors via cAMP as a second messenger (reviewed in Felten et al., 1987; Livnat, Felten, Carlson, Bellinger, & D. L. Felten, 1985).

3. *Spleen*

Innervation of the spleen has been studied more widely than innervation of other lymphoid organs. Both fluorescence histochemical localization of catecholamines and immunocytochemical staining for TH or NE demonstrate robust NA sympathetic innervation of the spleen in a variety of species, including humans (Kudoh, Hoshi, & Murakami, 1979), dogs (Dahlström & Zetterström, 1965), cats (Fillenz, 1966a, 1966b), beluga whales (Romano, Felten, Olschowka, & Felten, 1994), mice (Besedovsky et al., 1987; Carlson, Felten, Livnat, & Felten, 1987; Madden et al., 1997; F. D. Reilly, McCuskey, Miller, McCuskey, & Meineke, 1979; Williams & Felten, 1981), rats (Ackerman, Felten, Bellinger, & Felten, 1987; Ackerman, Felten, Bellinger, Livnat, & Felten, 1987; Ackerman, Felten, Dijkstra, Livnat, & Felten, 1989; Bellinger, Ackerman, Felten, & Felten, 1992; Bellinger, Felten, Collier, & Felten, 1987; Bellinger, Felten, Lorton, & Felten, 1989; S. Y. Felten & Olschowka, 1987; S. Y. Felten, Olschowka, Ackerman, & Felten, 1988; Fillenz & Pollard, 1976), African lungfish (Abrahamsson, Holmgren, Nilsson, & Pettersson, 1979), dogfish (Abrahamsson et al., 1979), cod (Nilsson & Grove, 1974; Winberg, Holmgren, & Nilsson, 1981), salamanders (Kinney, Cohen, & Felten, 1994), caecilians (Kinney et al., 1994), frogs (Kinney, Felten, & Cohen, 1991; Kinney et al., 1994), and cane toads (Nilsson, 1978). In salamanders and caecilians, NA nerves are scattered throughout the spleen, whereas in frogs, NA nerves are clearly defined in compartments of red pulp and white pulp much as it is in the mammalian spleen (Kinney et al., 1994). In addition to NE-containing nerves, neuropeptide Y $(NPY)^+$ and substance P $(SP)^+$ nerves were found in spleens from frogs (Kinney et al., 1994). In the South African clawed frog, NA innervation occurred late in larval life, and was sensitive to environmental conditions and to the rapidity at which development occurred. Prevention of overt metamorphosis by sodium perchlorate blockade prevented the development of NA splenic innervation in some of the tadpoles examined, but depletion of T lymphocytes by early larval thymectomy did not alter the kinetics or pattern of splenic NA innervation (Kinney et al., 1991).

NA nerves that distribute in the spleen in the rat derive from postganglionic cell bodies mainly in the superior mesenteric-celiac ganglionic complex (Bellinger, Felten, et al., 1989; D. L. Felten, Bellinger, Ackerman, & Felten, 1986; Nance & Burns, 1989; Trudrung, Furness, Pompolo, & Messenger, 1994), and to a lesser extent, the sympathetic trunk (Nance & Burns, 1989; Trudrung et al., 1994) that sends fibers through the superior mesenteric-celiac ganglion. A recent retrograde tracing study in the cat (Chen, Itoh, Sun, Miki, & Takenuchi, 1996) is consistent with similar studies in rodents, showing heavy labeling mainly in the celiac ganglia bilaterally and some labeled neurons in the superior mesenteric ganglion after injection of wheat germ agglutinin-horseradish peroxidase (WGA-HRP) into the spleen. With fluorescence histochemistry for catecholamines, NA nerves enter the spleen as a dense plexus associated with the splenic artery and branch beneath the capsule of the spleen. From this subcapsular plexus, NA fibers plunge into the depths of the spleen along the trabeculae and its associated vasculature. NA plexuses follow the central arterioles and their branches into the white pulp of the spleen (Figure 6). Many of these NA nerve fibers exit this central arteriolar vascular plexus and travel into the surrounding periarteriolar lymphatic sheaths (PALS), regions composed primarily of T lymphocytes.

In transgenic mice that overexpress nerve growth factor (NGF) in the skin and other epithelial structures, the marginal zone is hyperinnervated compared with control mice (Carlson et al., 1995). Further, concanavalin A (Con A)-induced proliferation is suppressed in splenocytes from NGF transgenic mice. These findings are consistent with NGF's neurotrophic role, and suggest that either an increase in NGF in the spleen and/or NGF-induced sympathetic

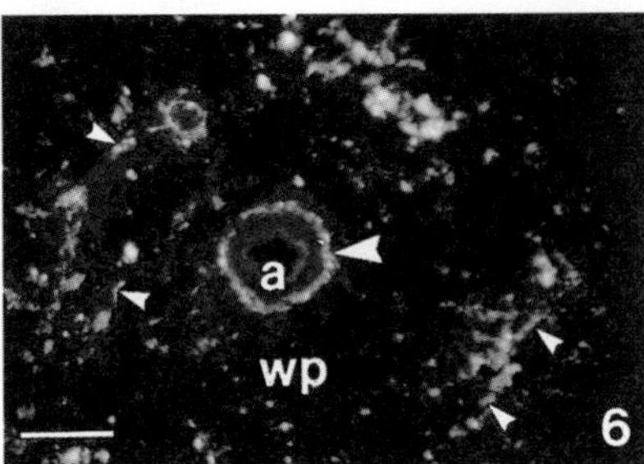

FIGURE 6 NA sympathetic nerve fibers (large arrowhead) travel along the central arteriole (a) in the white pulp (wp) of the rat spleen. Additional NA nerve fibers (small arrowheads) are present along blood vessels and as free fibers in the outer white pulp. HF. X43. Calibration bar = 100 μm.

hyperinnervation of the spleen and has functional consequences on immune response (Carlson et al., 1995).

Developmental studies by Ackerman et al. (Ackerman, 1989; Ackerman, Bellinger, Felten, & Felten, 1991; Ackerman et al., 1989) have found that NA nerve fibers enter the parenchymal lymphoid component of the 1-day-old rat spleen and form neuroeffector junctions with lymphocytes and macrophages at a time before smooth muscle even exists along the vasculature and before NA fibers are found along the vasculature. NA nerves also are present along the marginal sinus and in the marginal zone along blood vessels, in nerve bundles or as free fibers that course adjacent to B lymphocytes and macrophages. Occasionally, NA fibers are found in the follicles among B lymphocytes, but this is seen more frequently in neonatal development. In the red pulp, NA fibers are found along the trabeculae and venous sinuses that drain splenic blood. A few fibers can be seen exiting these plexuses to course through the parenchyma of the red pulp. The early presence of NA nerve fibers in the parenchyma of the white pulp prior to development of vascular nerve plexuses raises the possibility of separate origins for these two nerve components.

Immunocytochemical studies for the localization of TH confirm and extend observations with fluorescence histochemistry (Ackerman, Felten, Bellinger, Livnat, et al., 1987; Ackerman et al., 1989; Bellinger, Ackerman, et al., 1992; S. Y. Felten & Olschowka, 1987). Spleen sections stained with antibodies directed against TH and antibodies directed against surface antigens specific for different populations of immunocytes reveal the anatomical relationship of TH^+ nerves with specific populations of cells of the immune system. In the PALS, TH^+ nerves (Figure 7) reside in close proximity to T lymphocytes of both the T-helper and T-cytotoxic/suppressor subsets. TH^+

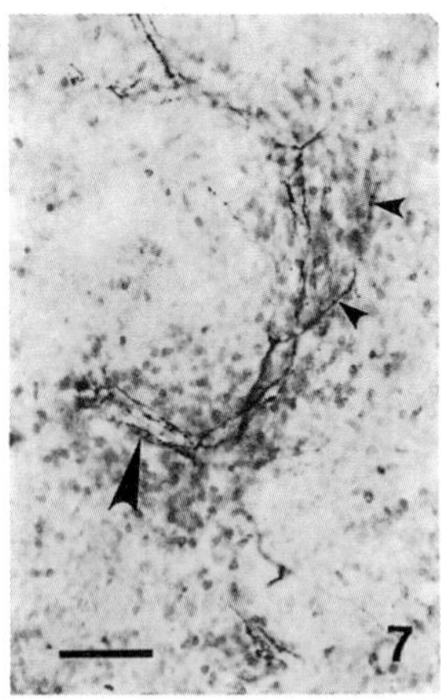

FIGURE 7 A dense plexus of TH^+ nerve fibers (black) (large arrowhead) closely appose the central arteriole in the white pulp of the rat spleen. TH^+ nerve fibers (small arrowheads) exit this vascular plexus and enter into the surrounding periarteriolar lymphatic sheath among fields of $OX19^+$ T lymphocytes (brown). Double-label ICC for TH and OX19, a pan T lymphocyte marker. X43. Calibration bar = 100 μm.

nerves also course along the marginal sinus adjacent to $ED3^+$ macrophages and in the marginal zone in close association with $ED3^+$ macrophages (Figure 8) and immunoglobulin $(Ig)M^+$ B lymphocytes (Figure 9). Only an occasional TH^+ nerve fiber is present among IgM^+ B lymphocytes in the follicle.

Electron microscopic examination of sections immunocytochemically stained for TH (S. Y. Felten & Olschowka, 1987) have revealed TH^+ nerve terminals adjacent to smooth muscle cells of the central arteriole. Similar to typical sympathetic neuroeffector junctions in other nonlymphoid target organs, TH^+ terminals are separated from these smooth muscle cells by a basement membrane and often by addi-

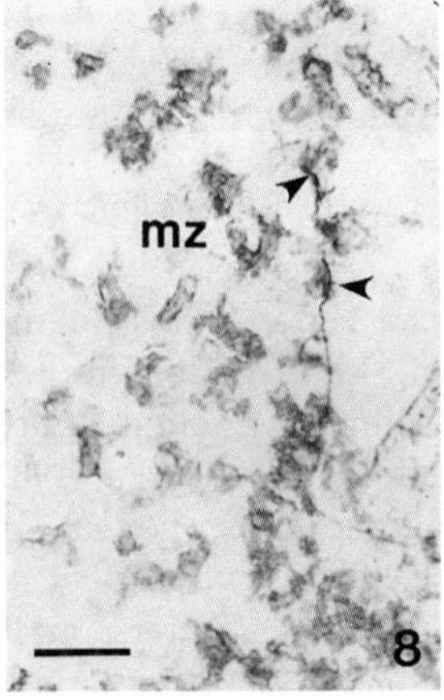

FIGURE 8 Linear TH^+ nerve fibers (black) (arrowheads) are present at the site of the marginal sinus and in the marginal zone (mz) adjacent to $ED3^+$ macrophages (brown). Double-label ICC for TH and ED3. X85. Calibration bar = 50 μm.

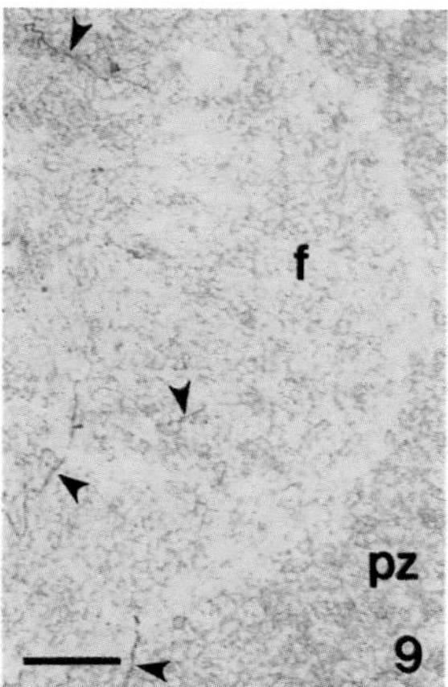

FIGURE 9 TH+ nerve fibers (black) course as free fibers (arrowheads) among IgM+ B lymphocytes (brown) in the parafollicular zone (pz), and sometimes extending into the follicle (f). Double-label ICC for TH and IgM, a marker for B lymphocytes. X43. Calibration bar = 100 μm.

tional cell processes. These neuroeffector junctions are in the range of 150 nm or more. Surprisingly, TH+ nerve terminals also are found in direct contact with lymphocytes in the PALS (Figure 10), at sites distant from the central arterioles. These terminals possess long, smooth zones of contact with lymphocyte plasma membranes, separated by as little as 6 nm. In many cases, the TH+ terminals indent along the lymphocyte membrane. Similar close appositions are present at the marginal sinus and in the marginal zone between TH+ nerve terminals and lymphocytes and macrophages. No postsynaptic specializations are apparent. However, such CNS-type synaptic specialization is rarely found at peripheral sympathetic neuroeffector junctions with other target cells. These TH+ profiles are not present in spleens denervated either by 6-OHDA, a neurotoxin that destroys nerve terminals, or by ganglionectomy, and they are not present in immunocytochemically stained tissue sections incubated with goat antirabbit IgG (the secondary antibody) alone.

An ultrastructural study in horses and pigs describes S-100 protein-immunoreactive nerve profiles that contain small and large dense core vesicles and terminate around the cytoplasmic processes of reticular cells in the red pulp of the spleen (Ueda, Abe, Takehana, Iwasa, & Hiraga, 1991). In the guinea pig splenic capsule, regions of unmyelinated axons devoid of a Schwann cell sheath appose spleen cells with variable intervals of extracellular space and interposed basal lamina material. Some nonmyelinated axons contact splenic cells with very little

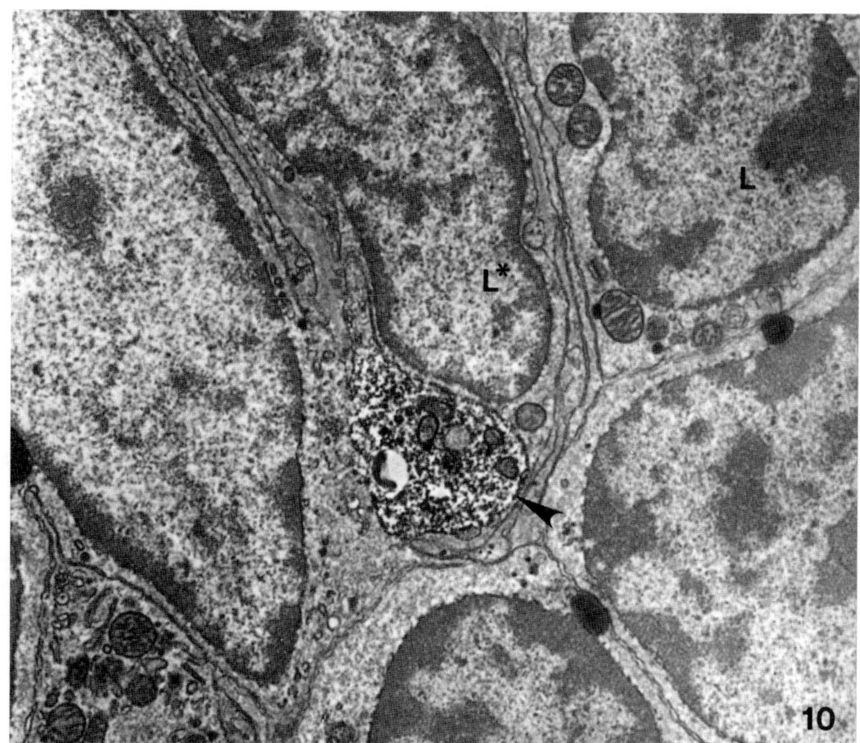

FIGURE 10 TH+ nerve terminal (large arrowhead) in direct contact with a lymphocyte (L*) in the periarteriolar lymphatic sheath of the rat spleen. L, lymphocyte. Single-label ICC for TH with TEM. X10,600.

intervening extracellular space and no basal lamina interposed (Elfvin, Johansson, Hoijer, & Aldskogius, 1994).

Strain differences have been used to explain differing results when studying neural–immune interactions in laboratory animals (Kelley, Grota, Felten, Madden, & Felten, 1996). This possibility was examined for NA innervation of the spleen using three mouse strains (BALB/cJ, C57Bl/6J, and DBA/2). Small but significant differences between these strains were demonstrated in total resting splenic NE content (BALB/cJ > C57Bl6J > DBA/2) and in resting NE concentration (C57Bl/6J > BALB/cJ > DBA/2). These findings may in part be due to differences in the size of the spleens from these murine strains (BALB/cJ > DBA/2 > C57Bl/6J). No diurnal differences were found in NE content or NE concentration of the spleen, but the expected diurnal pattern of plasma corticosterone (serving as a positive control) was observed in all strains.

4. *Lymph Nodes*

NA sympathetic innervation of lymph nodes in rats (Giron, Crutcher, & Davis, 1980) and several strains of mice (Ackerman, Felten, Bellinger, & Felten, 1987; Ackerman, Felten, Bellinger, Livnat, et al., 1987; Bellinger, Ackerman, Felten, Lorton, & Felten, 1989; Bellinger, Felten, & Felten, 1992; Felten et al., 1987; Felten, Livnat, Felten, Carlson, Bellinger, & Yeh, 1984) occurs as dense plexuses of NA nerves along blood vessels at the hilus, the presumed point of entry of NA nerves. In the lymph nodes, NA nerves travel in a subcapsular plexus (Figure 11), or continue in vascular plexuses and individual fibers in the medullary cords (Figure 11). In the medulla, NA fibers distribute adjacent to many lymphoid cell types and to both vascular and lymphatic channels. These

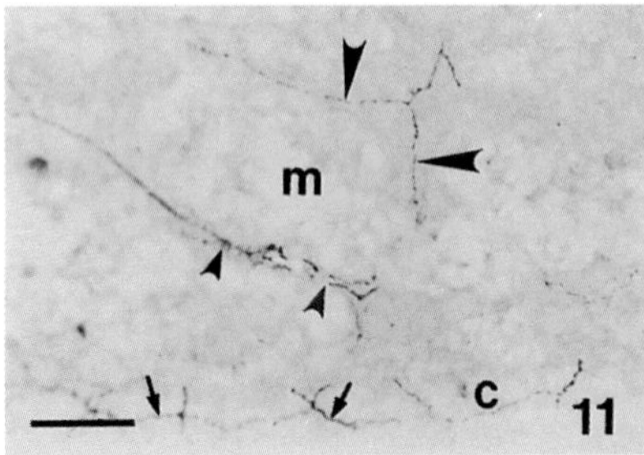

FIGURE 11 In the mesenteric lymph node of a rat, TH$^+$ nerve fibers (black) are seen coursing in the capsule (c) (arrows), along the medullary cords (small arrowheads) in the medulla (m), and in the parenchyma of the medulla (large arrowheads). Single-label ICC for TH. X43. Calibration bar = 100 μm.

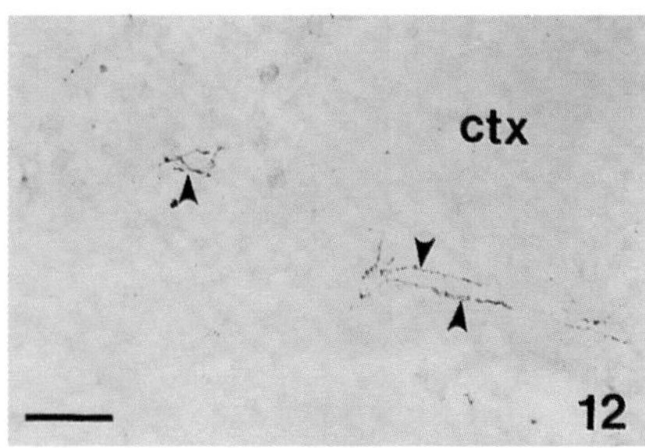

FIGURE 12 TH$^+$ nerve fibers (black) (arrowheads) are present in the cortex (ctx) of the rat mesenteric lymph nodes near the corticomedullary junction. Single-label ICC for TH. X43. Calibration bar = 100 μm.

fibers continue along small vessels that course from the medulla into the paracortical regions, which are rich in T lymphocytes. Single NA profiles exit these vascular plexuses and travel in the paracortical parenchyma (Figure 12). NA fibers that contribute to subcapsular plexuses also course along small vessels into the cortex and give off individual fibers that project into the cortical parenchyma. Linear fibers that enter into T lymphocyte compartments of the cortex and paracortex do not travel into the adjacent nodular regions and germinal centers where B lymphocytes predominate. Dopa-mine β-hydroxylase$^+$ (an enzyme that converts the precursor, dopamine, to NE) nerve fibers have been demonstrated in lymph nodes from rats, guinea pigs, mice, cats, pigs, and humans (Fink & Weihe, 1988).

In NGF transgenic mice where NGF is overexpressed by the skin, peripheral lymph nodes that drain the skin are more densely innervated compared with peripheral lymph nodes from control mice and compared with mesenteric lymph nodes from transgenic and control mice (Carlson et al., 1995). NGF concentration in peripheral lymph nodes from NGF transgenic mice is also elevated 13-fold over that found in control mice. These findings suggest that NGF provides trophic influence on sympathetic nerves in this genetic mouse model.

At the ultrastructural level, Novotny and Kliche (Novotny, 1988; Novotny & Kliche, 1986) have described axonal profiles with synaptic vesicles, presumed to be NA, in close proximity to vascular smooth muscle, reticular cells, plasma cells, and lymphocytes. They report at least three different vesicle populations and suggest that these populations result from colocalization of peptides. NA nerves also distribute along lymphatic vessels (Alessandrini et al., 1981) forming a loose network in the adventitia of the lymph vessel, where they are proposed to regulate vessel constriction.

The origin of NA innervation of lymph nodes has not been thoroughly investigated. Removal of the superior cervical ganglia decreases NA innervation of the cervical nodes in the rat (Giron et al., 1980). It is presumed that since lymph nodes are regional structures draining the areas with which they are associated, their innervation must also be regional.

The compartmentalization of NA nerves in lymph nodes displays many similarities with NA innervation of the spleen, suggesting a common functional role in both organs (reviewed in D. L. Felten et al., 1987). A role for NE in antigen processing, i.e., antigen capture and antigen presentation, is supported by studies showing reduced primary antibody responses in spleen and lymph nodes following sympathetic denervation (Livnat et al., 1985). Egress of activated lymphocytes into the circulation from spleen and lymph nodes occurs following the infusion of catecholamines (Ernström & Sandberg, 1974; Ernström & Söder, 1975; D. L. Felten et al., 1987) suggesting an additional role for NE at these secondary lymphoid organs in lymphocyte trafficking.

5. *Functional Significance*

The functional significance of NE in immunomodulation is highly complex, and depends on the organ, the cell type, the state of differentiation or activation, aging, and the presence of other signal molecules, including other neurotransmitters, hormones, and cytokines. This is discussed in a separate chapter in this volume.

B. Cholinergic Innervation of Lymphoid Organs

A variety of techniques can be used to demonstrate the presence of cholinergic innervation. With antibodies directed against choline acetyltransferase (ChAT), an enzyme necessary for the synthesis of acetylcholine (ACh), immunocytochemistry has been used successfully to demonstrate cholinergic neurons and their projections in the CNS, since other techniques used in conjunction with this method such as measurements of ACh content and ChAT activity can confirm the existence of cholinergic innervation in these sites. In the past, acetylcholinesterase (AChE) staining has been the method of choice for revealing putative cholinergic innervation in many peripheral organs. In lymphoid organs, however, interpretation of AChE staining is greatly complicated because many cellular elements stain positively for AChE, including thymocyte and lymphocyte membranes, reticular cells, dendritic cells, and smooth muscle of the vascular and connective tissue. Furthermore, noncholinergic nerves, including NA nerve fibers, appear to contain AChE. Thus, given the inherent problems with anatomical staining methods for cholinergic nerves, accurate neurochemical measurements of ACh and measurements of ChAT activity are necessary to even propose the existence of any putative cholinergic nerves in lymphoid organs. For most lymphoid organs, a thorough examination of putative cholinergic innervation is not available.

1. *Bone Marrow*

Few studies have examined the possibility of cholinergic innervation of bone marrow. DePace and Webber (1975) described $AChE^+$ staining in blood vessel walls of the bone marrow and interpreted these as $AChE^+$ nerve fibers that are sensory in function, although no further experimental evidence is given to support either the cholinergic nature of $AChE^+$ nerve fibers or any sensory function. They reported such nerve fibers within the parenchyma, but found no nerve endings, suggesting that these fibers pass through the area without specific association with hemopoietic cells.

2. *Thymus*

Several lines of evidence have been cited to infer cholinergic innervation in the thymus. Studies using retrograde tracing with horseradish peroxidase (HRP) injected into the mouse and rat thymus to determine the cells of origin of the nerve fibers have been performed by Bulloch and colleague (Bulloch & Moore, 1981). They described labeled neurons in three areas of the brain stem (the retrofacial nucleus, nucleus ambiguus, and the dorsal medullary tegmentum adjacent to the dorsal motor nucleus of the vagus) and three areas of the spinal cord (C_2-C_4 lateral ventral horn, C_2-C_4 medial ventral horn, and a group of large motoneurons in the medial ventral horn from the decussation of the pyramids through the C_1 segment).

Later, work by Bulloch and Pomerantz (1984) combined gross anatomical observations with AChE staining to identify $AChE^+$ nerves in the thymus. They reported that the mouse thymus receives $AChE^+$ nerves from the vagus nerve, the phrenic nerve, and the recurrent laryngeal nerve. They further reported that the latter two sources, along with fibers from the sympathetic chain, provide innervation in the subcapsular region, but did not provide supporting experimental evidence.

In similar studies in the 1-day-old chick, using retrograde tracing from the thymus, positive-labeled neurons were found in the cervical spinal cord and in the IX and X nerve nuclei of the brain stem contain retrogradely traced dye from the thymus (Bulloch, 1988). More recently, a double-label retrograde tracing study by Tollefson and Bulloch (1990) reported that tracers injected into the thymus and the esophagus adjacent to the thymus label separate cell populations in both the spinal cord and brain stem. However, as many as 30% of cells in the nucleus ambiguus and 20% of cells in the nucleus retrofacial and spinal cord are labeled with both tracers. Double-labeling of these cells were interpreted to indicate that either the tracer diffused directly onto adjacent tissue or into the lymphatics, or that collaterals of vagus nerve fibers innervate these areas.

In support of these findings, Dovas et al. (1998) performed a retrotrade tracing study where one tracer was injected into the cranial portion of the right lobe of the thymus, a second dye applied around the cut end of the right recurrent laryngeal nerve, and a third dye applied to the central stump of this nerve. Vagal efferent fibers of the recurrent laryngeal nerve arise from the nucleus retroambigualis, nucleus ambiguus, and to a lesser extent, the nucleus retrofacialis. Dye injected into the thymus retrogradely traced to cells in these nuclei. This study suggests that thymic vagal fibers originate from neurons of the dorsal motor nucleus of the vagus. Whether these are neurons are cholinergic was not investigated.

Nance and co-workers (1987) carefully reinvestigated innervation of the thymus, using injections of HRP conjugated to WGA-HRP into the thymus, but using small injection volumes followed by application of wound sealants to eliminate diffusion of the dye from the thymus. They confirmed Bulloch and co-workers' findings of sympathetic innervation (Bulloch & Moore, 1981; Bulloch & Pomerantz, 1984), but were unable to verify any labeled cells in the spinal cord and brain stem. Control injections into the esophagus and the longus colli muscles produced extensive labeling of nucleus ambiguus and the cervical spinal cord, respectively. They have suggested that the CNS-derived innervation from the dorsal motor nucleus of the vagus to the thymus (Tollefson & Bulloch, 1990) is an artifact caused by the diffusion of tracer from the thymus onto these adjacent structures.

The problem of the diffusion of tracer from peripherally innervated organs is not a new one. Early reports of direct CNS innervation of the pancreas (Laughton & Powley, 1979) have been shown to result from diffusion of the tracer from the organ (Fox & Powley, 1986). In fact, the gradual diffusion of the label from an injected organ can produce even denser CNS labeling than direct injection of the tracer into the peritoneum, possibly because slowly diffusing tracers escape phagocytosis by macrophages. In our laboratory we were unable to show anterograde tracing from the brain stem to the thymus (D. L. Bellinger, unpublished results) using either WGA-HRP or fluorogold, although these labels were transported in an anterograde fashion to the esophagus.

The second line of evidence for cholinergic innervation of the thymus comes from AChE staining. There are many reports in the literature of AChE$^+$ nerve fibers distributing to the thymus (Bulloch, 1988; Bulloch, Cullen, Schwartz, & Longo, 1987; Bulloch & Pomerantz, 1984; Fatani, Qayyum, Mehta, & Singh, 1986). It has been inferred that these nerves derive from branches of the vagus nerve on its course through the diaphragm to innervate other visceral organs. However, AChE staining is not diminished by experimental vagotomy in the rat (Nance et al., 1987), suggesting that even if some nerve fibers from the vagus do supply the thymus, they most likely are not AChE$^+$ and are therefore not likely to be cholinergic, or that the AChE$^+$ component is so minute that vagotomy has little effect on AChE staining.

We have performed AChE staining in the thymus and indeed, at both the light and ultrastructural level, and found nerve profiles that are positively stained for AChE, particularly around the vasculature (Bellinger, Ackerman, et al., 1989; Bellinger, Lorton, Hamill, Felten, & Felten, 1993). Despite this staining, we are not sure that these nerve profiles are cholinergic, since noncholinergic nerve fibers also can stain for AChE. Clearly, at least some of the AChE is colocalized within NA nerves, because chemical sympathectomy with 6-OHDA also diminishes AChE staining in neural profiles in these sites of the thymus. In our AChE-stained sections of the thymus, the AChE$^+$ cellular elements, which comprise most of the AChE staining, are the more prominent features. These cellular elements include thymocyte membranes and endoplasmic reticulum of epithelial reticular cells. Similar staining is reported in the human thymus (Topilko & Caillou, 1985).

The presence of such large amounts of AChE may be important for neurotransmission with neuropeptides. Besides hydrolyzing ACh, AChE also hydrolyzes and inactivates SP (Chubb, Hodgson, & White, 1980) and perhaps other peptides (Chubb, Ranieri, White, & Hodgson, 1983; Dowton & Boelen, 1988; Ismael, Millar, Small, & Chubb, 1986). Therefore, the presence of AChE$^+$-stained profiles, even if they are shown to be nerves, is not evidence for cholinergic innervation.

An alternative to staining for AChE is to use immunocytochemistry for ChAT. There are no convincing data indicating cholinergic innervation of the thymus using this technique. Fatani and colleagues (1986) reported a rather modest density of stained profiles that were presumed to be nerves, largely associated with the vasculature, with only a few fibers extending into the parenchyma. They did not report extensive subcapsular plexuses, and contrary to studies using AChE staining that report staining early in ontogeny, these ChAT$^+$ profiles were not seen until day 17 or 18 of gestation. If these are nerve fibers, the discrepancy could result from differential expression of genes that code for these two enzymes that are turned on at different time periods during development.

Interpretation of immunocytochemistry for ChAT must be done with utmost caution. The enzyme appears to be processed posttranslationally, is notoriously unreliable for demonstrating even the most robust peripheral cholinergic nerve fibers, and is problematic for false-positive staining. In a collaborative study between our laboratory and Robert Hamill we have measured ChAT activity and total acetyltransferase activity in lymphoid organs (Bellinger et al., 1988, 1993). In the rat thymus, only a very low level of total activity is measurable, less than the 2X background activity that is needed to claim that activity is present. This low level of ChAT activity is not consistent with a large cholinergic nerve supply, and is substantially below the levels detected in other peripheral organs, such as the heart, salivary glands, and penile corpora, that are known to be innervated by parasympathetic cholinergic nerve fibers.

The third line of evidence cited in support of cholinergic innervation of lymphoid organs, the presence of muscarinic receptors on lymphocytes (Gordon, Cohen, & Wilson, 1978; Hadden, 1977; Maslinski, Kullberg, Nordström, & Bartfai, 1988; Strom, Lundin, & Carpenter, 1977), is the best established component of a possible cholinergic link for cells of the immune system. Of course, the presence of muscarinic receptors on cells of the immune system does not provide any clues about a possible ligand, if one exists. Mismatches between localization of presynaptic neurotransmitters and their receptors on the responding cells are commonplace both centrally and peripherally. This is not to say that thymocytes that possess muscarinic receptors will never be in a microenvironment where there is ligand to bind to muscarinic receptors. It is possible that muscarinic receptors will become activated on cells that migrate from the thymus into a site (i.e., skin, gut, or lung) where cholinergic nerves are present and can secrete the ligand, ACh. It also is possible that the endogenous ligand for muscarinic receptors on cells of the immune system is a peptide.

In summary, at the present time the evidence for cholinergic innervation of the thymus is weak. If cholinergic innervation is present, it is most probably minimal when contrasted with NA innervation of the thymus and with cholinergic innervation of other target tissues. Niijima (1995) has examined vagal innervation of the rat thymus using electrophysiological techniques under general anesthesia, and reports that the majority of vagal fibers in the thymic branch of the vagus nerve are nonmyelinated C fibers, and these fibers innervate the thymus bilaterally. The neurotransmitter content of the these nerve fibers was not determined, but SP and/or calcitonin gene-related peptide (CGRP) are likely candidates.

3. *Spleen*

In the spleen, histochemical staining for AChE has been demonstrated by numerous investigators (Figures 13–15) (Bellinger et al., 1993; Fillenz, 1966a; Kudoh et al., 1979; F. D. Reilly et al., 1979). These studies describe the largest compartment of AChE staining to be in cellular elements. These authors are generally cautious in their statements of AChE staining in nerve profiles in the spleen. Kudoh et al. (1979) reported AChE$^+$ nerve fibers associated with trabecular arteries, presuming them to be cholinergic, a contention unsubstantiated by other evidence. We have found extensive AChE staining associated with lymphoid and reticular elements of the spleen (Figures 14–15) (Bellinger et al., 1993), some of which resemble nerve-like profiles but are not nerves; this supports findings in the earlier literature (Fillenz, 1966a; Kudoh et al., 1979; F. D. Reilly et al., 1979). In addition, we have found AChE staining in nerve-like profiles in the splenic nerve (Figure 13) and along the central arterioles (Figure 14), in the white pulp, and along the trabeculae (Figure 15); however, bilateral subdiaphragmatic vagotomy did not alter this staining pattern. Instead, surgical removal of the superior mesenteric-celiac ganglion totally eliminated all neural and nonneural AChE staining. Chemical sympathectomy with 6-OHDA eliminated some, but not all, of the AChE staining. Collectively, these studies indicate that the majority of AChE staining in the rat spleen is nonneural, and that AChE staining present in nerves derives from sympathetic NA nerves as well as from non-NA, nonvagal nerves. The presence of AChE staining in nonneural cellular

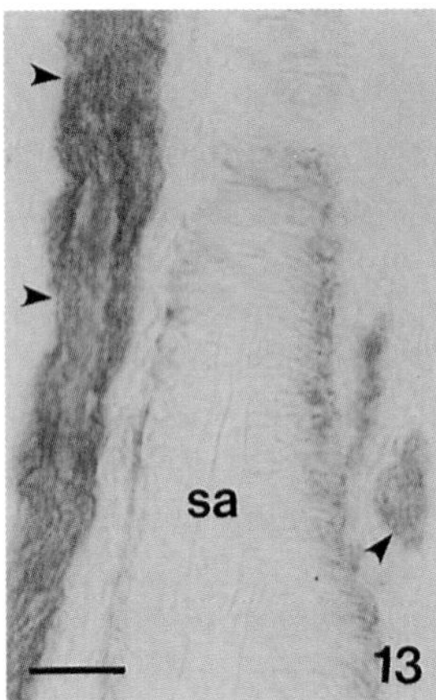

FIGURE 13 AChE$^+$ nerve bundle (black) (arrowheads) travels adjacent to the splenic artery (sa) close to the entry site into the rat spleen. AChE staining with nickel enhancement. X64. Calibration bar = 75 μm.

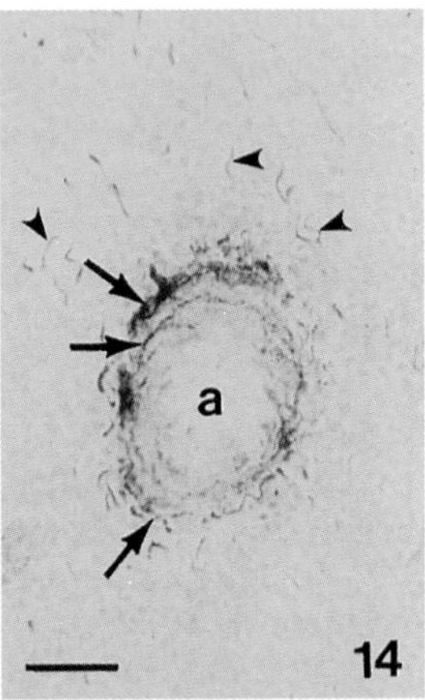

FIGURE 14 AChE staining in the rat spleen reveals short non-neural connective tissue fibers that lightly stain AChE$^+$ in the periarteriolar lymphatic sheath (small arrowheads), and more densely stained, varicose, linear profiles that resemble nerve profiles (arrows) in close association with the central arteriole (a). AChE staining with nickel enhancement. X64. Calibration bar = 75 μm.

elements of the spleen may function in detoxification of bacterial toxins (Ballantyne, 1968) or hydrolysis of peptides (Chubb et al., 1980, 1983; Dowton & Boelen, 1988; Ismael et al., 1986). After injection of WGA-HRP into the cat spleen (Chen et al., 1996), labeled neurons were found throughout the rostrocaudal extent of the dorsal motor nucleus of the vagus nerve bilaterally, with the highest concentration found at the level of the obex.

4. *Lymph Nodes*

There are a few preliminary reports of AChE staining in nerve profiles that innervate lymph nodes

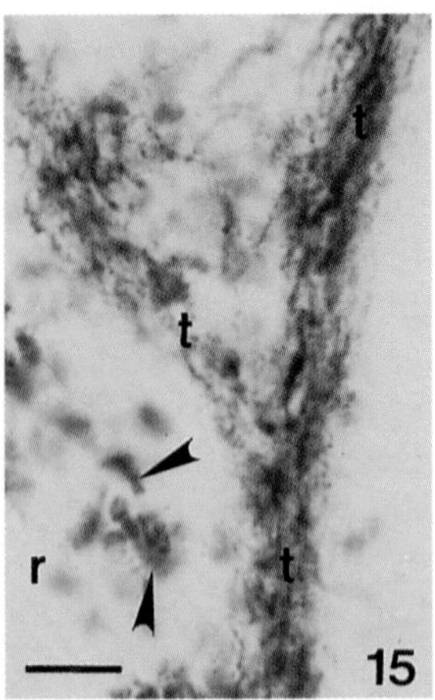

FIGURE 15 In the trabeculae (t), AChE$^+$ staining is present in connective tissue fibers and in linear, varicose, nerve-like profiles. AChE$^+$ cells (arrowheads) also are seen in the red pulp (r) of the rat spleen. AChE staining with nickel enhancement. X64. Calibration bar = 75 μm.

(Bellinger, Felten, Coleman, Yeh, & Felten, 1985), but no definitive evidence that these nerves are cholinergic. Clearly, there are non-NA nerve fibers in lymph nodes as seen with electron microscopy (Novotny, 1988; Novotny & Kliche, 1986) and immunocytochemical studies (Fink & Weihe, 1988). The possibility that some of these fibers are cholinergic remains to be demonstrated.

C. Neuropeptidergic Nerves—NPY

1. *Bone Marrow*

The identification of neurotransmitter-specific nerves other than NA sympathetic nerves innervating the bone marrow is not clearly established. The localization of peptidergic nerves with immunocytochemistry in the bone marrow has been hampered by the difficulty in preserving antigenicity with standard decalcification methods used in the tissue preparation of bone. Recently, immunocytochemistry for PGP 9.5, TH, and NPY (Tabarowski et al., 1996) has been performed in rat bone marrow (Tabarowski et al., 1996). NPY$^+$ profiles have a distribution similar to that of TH$^+$ nerves, traveling adjacent to the vasculature and in the parenchyma among hemopoietic and lymphopoietic cells in the marrow (Tabarowski et al., 1996). The overlapping distribution of NA- and NPY-containing nerves suggests that these neurotransmitters are colocalized in nerves that innervate bone marrow. With a radioimmunoassay (RIA), NPY content in bone, periosteum, and bone marrow of male Lewis rats has been measured as a combined mean in picomoles per gram wet weight (Ahmed, Srinivasan, Theodorsson, Bjurholm, & Kreicbergs, 1994). NPY content in these sites is higher than SP, CGRP, and vasoactive intestinal polypeptide (VIP), consistent with findings in other lymphoid organs. Compared with bone (1.47 ± 0.33), the concentrations in the periosteum (2.04 ± 0.39) and bone marrow (5.09 ± 0.17) were 1.4 and 3.5 times higher. At least some of the NPY in the bone marrow is nonneural, occurring in resident megakaryocytes and platelets (Ericsson et al., 1987).

2. *Thymus*

NPY^+ nerves (Bellinger et al., 1990; Kendall & Al-Shawaf, 1991; Kranz et al., 1997; Weihe, Müller, Fink, & Zentel, 1989) provide the most extensive peptidergic innervation of the rodent thymus identified to date. The distribution of NPY^+ nerves overlaps with the NA innervation of the thymus, and chemical sympathectomy by administration of the neurotoxin, 6-OHDA destroys NPY-immunoreactive nerves in the rat thymus (Kendall & Al-Shawaf, 1991). NPY^+ fibers travel in bundles that enter the thymus through the capsule or with surface arteries that extend along the thymic capsule and traverse the interlobular septa. In the septa these fibers course adjacent to mast cells and macrophages (Müller & Weihe, 1991; Weihe et al., 1989). From these subcapsular and septal plexuses, NPY^+ nerves extend into superficial and deep cortical regions in association with blood vessels (Figure 16), or as individual fibers (Figure 17), arborizing among thymocytes and other supportive cells of the thymus. The densest innervation occurs at the corticomedullary junction. NPY^+ profiles are also found in the medulla along the vasculature adjacent to the corticomedullary junction. A similar distribution of NPY^+ nerves recently has been described in the chicken thymus, but NPY^+ fibers are not as numerous as VIP^+ fibers (Gulati, Tay, & Leong, 1997). Close associations of NPY^+ nerves with macrophages and mast cells similar to that described for NA nerves have been reported (Bellinger et al., 1990; Müller & Weihe, 1991).

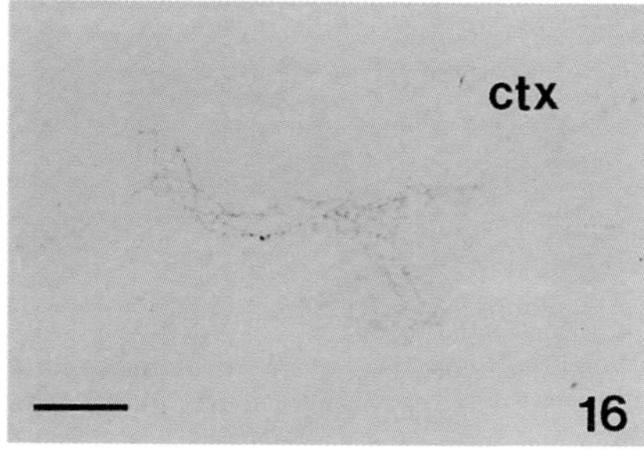

FIGURE 16 NPY^+ nerve fibers (black) course along a blood vessel in the cortex (ctx) of the rat thymus. Single-label ICC for NPY. X43. Calibration bar = 100 μm.

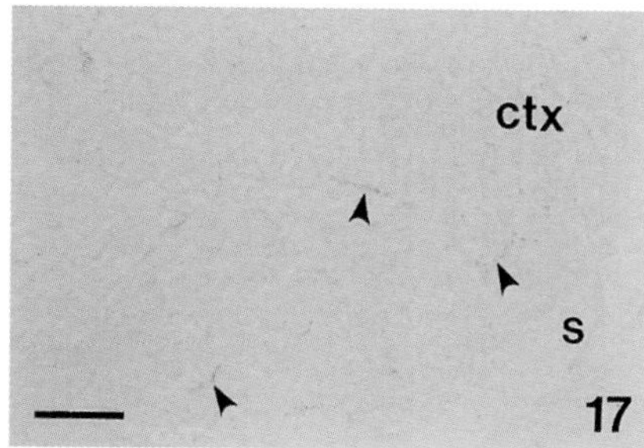

FIGURE 17 In the cortex (ctx) of the rat thymus, very fine, varicose, NPY-immunoreactive nerve fibers (black) (arrowheads) are present among thymocytes and stromal cells. s, interlobular septum. Single-label ICC for NPY. X43. Calibration bar = 100 μm.

3. *Spleen*

Early observations from our laboratories using immunofluorescent techniques identified the presence of NPY-immunoreactive profiles along the central arteriole of the white pulp and its smaller branches, with only sparse numbers of fibers entering the parenchyma (D. L. Felten et al., 1985). Lundberg et al. (Lundberg, Rudehill, Sollevi, Theodorsson-Norhein, & Hamberger, 1986) reported NPY innervation of the splenic vasculature, indicating that these nerves mediate vascular and volume control. These investigators did not further describe the distribution of NPY^+ nerves in specific compartments of the spleen.

With light microscopic immunocytochemical methods, NPY^+ nerves have been found along the vasculature and in lymphoid compartments of the spleen (Bellinger et al., 1990; Olschowka, Felten, Bellinger, Lorton, & Felten, 1988; Romano, Felten, Felten, & Olschowka, 1991; Romano et al., 1994). The distribution of NPY^+ nerves (Romano et al., 1991, 1994; Bellinger et al., 1990; Olschowka et al., 1988) closely parallels NA innervation of the spleen. NPY^+ nerves travel along the capsular, trabecular (Figure 18), and venous systems, and along the arterial systems, including prominent innervation of the central arterioles in the white pulp (Figure 19). NPY^+ nerves in the trabecular plexuses course near $OX8^+$ T cells in the surrounding red pulp (Figure 18). In the white pulp, NPY^+ nerves arborize in the PALS away from the central arteriolar plexuses; these fibers end among T lymphocytes (Figure 19). Additional NPY^+ fibers extend along the marginal sinus and are scattered in the marginal zone (Figures 19–22), where they branch among IgM^+ B lymphocytes (Figure 20),

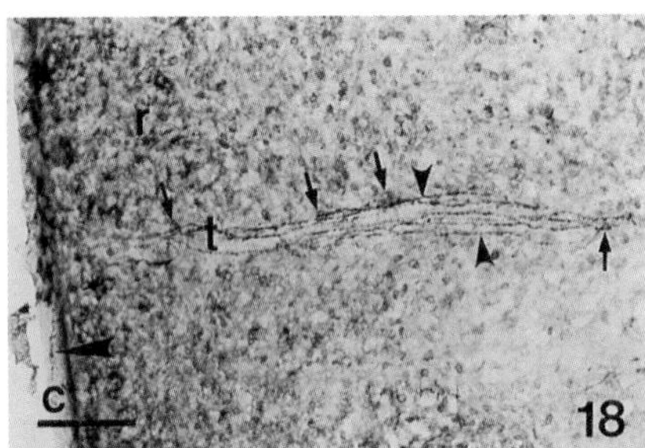

FIGURE 18 In the rat spleen, NPY$^+$ nerve fibers are present in the capsule (c) (large arrowhead), and associated with the trabeculae (t) (small arrowheads) in the red pulp (r). OX8$^+$ T suppressor/cytotoxic cells (brown) reside in close proximity to NPY$^+$ nerve fibers near the trabecular nerve plexus (arrows). Double-label ICC for NPY and OX8, a T suppressor/cytotoxic cell marker. X43. Calibration bar = 100 μm.

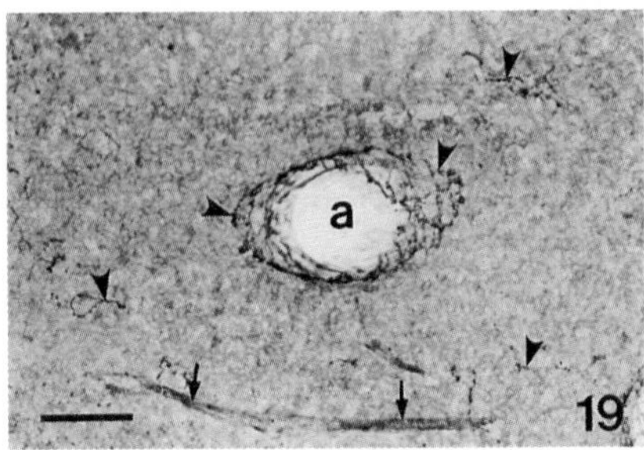

FIGURE 19 NPY-immunoreactive nerve fibers (black) form a dense vascular plexus around the central arteriole (a) of the rat spleen. Additional NPY$^+$ nerves (small arrowheads) exit this plexus to course among OX8$^+$ T lymphocytes in the PALS. Large NPY$^+$ nerve bundles (arrows) also course in the outer periarteriolar lymphatic sheath. Double-label ICC for NPY and OX8. X43. Calibration bar = 100 μm.

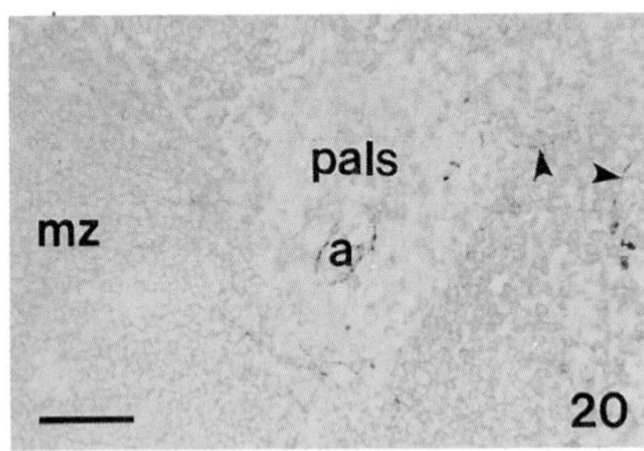

FIGURE 20 NPY$^+$ nerve fibers are seen coursing along a small central arteriole (a). In the marginal zone (mz), NPY$^+$ nerve fibers (black) (arrowheads) are present in close association with IgM$^+$ B lymphocytes (brown). pals, perarteriolar lymphatic sheath. Double-label ICC for NPY and IgM. X43. Calibration bar = 100 μm.

ED1$^+$ macrophages (Meltzer, Grimm, Greenberg, & Nance, 1997), and ED3$^+$ macrophages (Figure 21). Ultrastructural analysis of immunocytochemically stained spleen sections revealed direct contacts between NPY$^+$ terminals and lymphocytes, similar to those seen

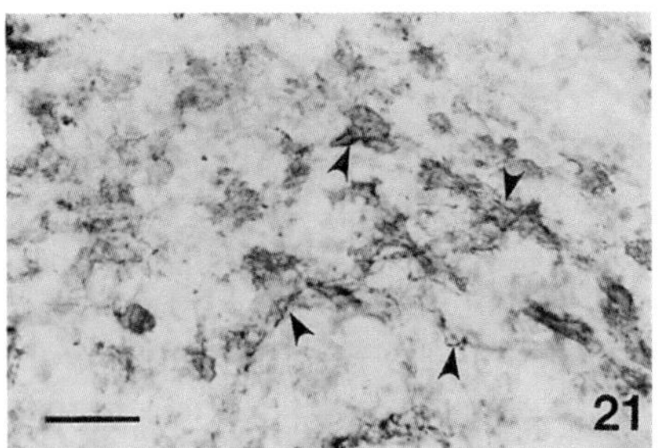

FIGURE 21 NPY$^+$ nerve fibers (black) (arrowheads) course in close proximity to ED3$^+$ macrophages (brown) in the marginal zone of the rat spleen. Double-label ICC for NPY and ED3. Double-label ICC for NPY and ED3. X170. Calibration bar = 50 μm.

for TH$^+$ terminals (Olschowka et al., 1988; Romano et al., 1991).

Romano and colleagues (1991) have shown that destruction of sympathetic NA nerves with 6-OHDA depletes NPY and eliminates NPY$^+$ profiles in immunocytochemically stained sections, even though NPY concentration as measured with an RIA is not significantly reduced in spleens from sympathectomized animals (D. L. Bellinger, unpublished observations; personal communications with Dwight Nance and Arnold Greenberg). This could result from the binding and internalization of released NPY from damaged sympathetic nerve terminals into cells in the spleen, and/or from the high concentration of NPY in megakaryocytes, platelets, or other cells in the spleen (Ericsson et al., 1987), obscuring small changes in splenic NPY concentration. By differential staining of consecutive tissue sections, they also showed direct colocalization of TH and NPY in some nerve fibers in the rat spleen. Studies of the bovine splenic nerve (Fried et al., 1986) demonstrated NE and NPY colocalized in large, dense core vesicles with enkephalins. Immunofluorescence staining also supports

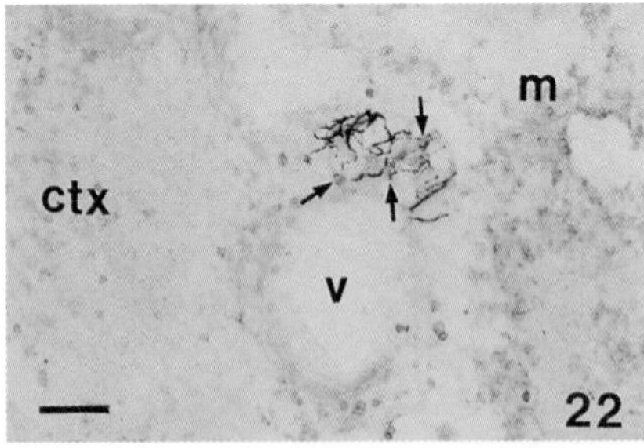

FIGURE 22 A loose bundle of NPY$^+$ nerve fibers (black) is present next to a blood vessel (v) at the corticomedullary junction in the mesenteric lymph node from a rat. Double labeling reveals a close association between NPY$^+$ nerve fibers and W3/13 T helper lymphocytes (brown) (arrows). m, medulla; ctx, cortex. X43. Double-label ICC for NPY and W3/13, a T helper lymphocyte marker. Calibration bar = 100 μm.

colocalization of these neurotransmitters in some nerves along the large blood vessels near their entry into the bovine spleen. NE and NPY colocalize in vascular and trabecular nerves of spleens from cats (Rosenstein & Brightman, 1983) and pigs (Lundberg, Änggård, Pernow, & Hökfelt, 1985), where NPY is believed to mediate vasoconstriction and possibly play a neuromodulatory role, enhancing the action of NE on the vasculature.

4. *Lymph Nodes*

Immunoreactivity for NPY in nerves have been described in lymph nodes in a variety of mammalian species including the rat (Bellinger et al., 1990; S. Y. Felten & Felten, 1991; Fink & Weihe, 1988; Romeo, Fink, Yanaihara, & Weihe, 1994), mouse (Enzmann & Drossler, 1994; Fink & Weihe, 1988), guinea-pig (Enzmann & Drossler, 1994; Fink & Weihe, 1988), cat (Fink & Weihe, 1988; Popper, Mantyh, Vigna, Magioos, & Mantyh, 1988), pig (Fink & Weihe, 1988), beluga whale (Romano et al., 1994), and human (Fink & Weihe, 1988). Retrograde tracing studies in Wistar rats indicate that NPY-containing neurons of the superior cervical ganglia project to the submaxillary lymph nodes (Romeo et al., 1994), and do not colocalize proenkephalin in fibers that distribute to these lymph nodes.

Studies from our laboratories have demonstrated NPY-immunoreactive nerve fibers in mesenteric, popliteal, and inguinal lymph nodes of the rat (Bellinger et al., 1990; S. Y. Felten & Felten, 1991). The distribution of NPY^+ nerves again appears to overlap NA innervation. NPY^+ nerve fibers course along blood vessels in the hilar, corticomedullary (Figure 22), and interfollicular regions of lymph nodes. Individual NPY^+ fibers are present as linear varicose profiles in the capsule among ED3+ macrophages (Figure 23), and in the parenchyma of the medulla (Figures 24 and 25), paracortex, and cortex, where they end among fields of lymphocytes.

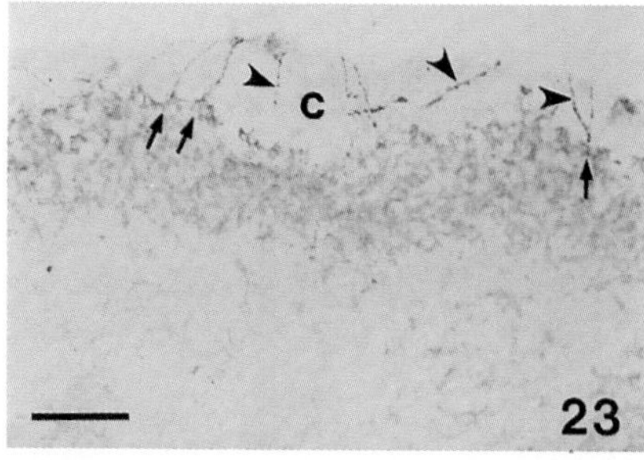

FIGURE 23 NPY^+ nerve fibers (black) (arrowheads) course in the capsule (c) of the rat mesenteric lymph nodes, and appear to end on $ED3^+$ macrophages (brown) (arrows) at the base of the capsule in the cortex of the node. Double-label ICC for NPY and ED3. X43. Calibration bar = 100 μm.

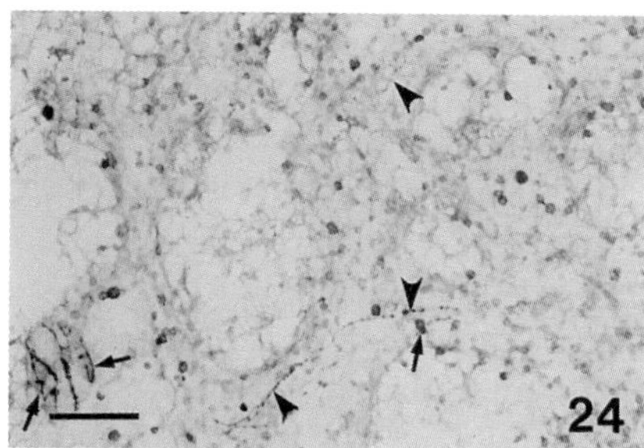

FIGURE 24 In the medulla of a rat mesenteric lymph node, NPY^+ nerve fibers (black) (arrowheads) travel as free fibers along the medullary cords. Frequently, these nerve fibers reside in close proximity to $OX19^+$ T lymphocytes (brown) (arrows). Double-label ICC for NPY and OX19, a pan T lymphocyte marker. X43. Calibration bar = 100 μm.

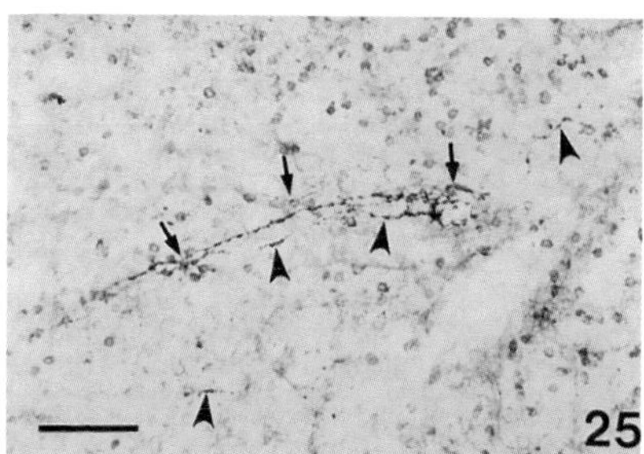

FIGURE 25 Individual, varicose NPY^+ nerve fibers (black) (arrowheads) in the medulla of the rat mesenteric lymph node are found along the medullary cords, and closely apposed to $W3/13^+$ T helper lymphocytes (brown) (arrows). Double-label ICC for NPY and W3/13. X43. Calibration bar = 100 μm.

5. *Functional Significance*

NPY potently inhibits spontaneous activation of human granulocytes and macrophages as well as mytilus edulis immunocytes in a concentration-dependent manner (Dureus, Louis, Grant, Bilfinger, & Stefano, 1993). NPY also inhibit the chemotaxic response of these immunocytes to the chemoattractant formyl-methionyl-leucyl-phenylalanine (fMLP). Incubation of both human and invertebrate immunocytes in fMLP (10^{-9} M) causes "activation" as noted by random locomotion (chemokinesis), an effect blocked by NPY. NPY at 10^{-9} to 10^{-12} M produces a significant dose-dependent suppression of natural killer (NK) cell activity against K 562 target cells (Nair, Schwartz, Wu, & Kronfol, 1993), an effect inhibited by rabbit anti-NPY antisera at 1:800 and 1:1600 dilutions. NPY (in the same range of concentrations) also inhibits, in a dose-dependent fashion, NK cell activities of NK cell-enriched large granular lymphocytes against lymphadenopathy-associated virus (LAV)-infected 8E5/LAV target cells. This effect is not due to direct toxicity of NPY on effector cells, since lymphocytes treated with NPY show normal levels of ^{51}Cr release and their viability is comparable to that of untreated control cells.

NPY and peptide YY (10^{-12} to 10^{-8} M) stimulate several functions of resting peritoneal macrophages from BALB/c mice in vitro, including adherence to substrate, chemotaxis, ingestion of inert particles (latex beads) and foreign cells (*Candida albicans*), and production of superoxide anion measured by nitroblue tetrazolium reduction. This latter effect is dose-dependent, with maximal stimulation of functions at 10^{-10} M (De La Fuente, Bernaez, Del Rio, & Hernanz, 1993). These effects seem to be mediated via simulation of protein kinase C. NPY upregulates the adhesiveness of human umbilical vein endothelial cells for ^{51}Cr-labeled human neutrophils or human monocytic U937 cell line leukocytes (0.01–1 μM) in a dose- and time-dependent manner (Sung, Arleth, & Feuerstein, 1991). NPY also primes polymorphonuclear neutrophil oxidative metabolism, and causes a direct and dose-related increase in cytosolic calcium concentrations in these cells (Hafstrom, Ringertz, Lundeberg, & Palmblad, 1993).

D. Neuropeptidergic Nerves—SP and CGRP

1. *Bone Marrow*

PGP 9.5 staining reveals a greater density of nerve profiles associated with the vasculature and parenchyma in the marrow than is seen with TH- or NPY-staining, indicating the presence of non-NA sympathetic nerve fibers (Tabarowski et al., 1996). In support of these findings, several investigators (Bjurholm, Kreicbergs, Broden, & Schultzberg, 1989; Imai, Tokunaga, Maeda, Kikkawa, & Hukuda, 1997; Iwasaki, Inoue, & Hukuda, 1995) have reported SP^+ and $CGRP^+$ nerves in the bone marrow. The distribution of these two types of nerves is similar, although $CGRP^+$ fibers are more numerous suggesting a colocalization of SP with some but not all $CGRP^+$ nerves (Bjurholm et al., 1989). Varicose arrays of winding fibers are present among hemopoietic cells of the bone marrow and generally do not course along the vasculature. Long, nonvaricose fibers course along the bone trabeculae and in close relation to blood vessels in the marrow. In male Lewis rats, Ahmed et al. (1994) have measured SP and CGRP content, expressed as mean concentrations in picomoles per gram, in bone (0.06 ± 0.02 and 0.15 ± 0.02, respectively), periosteum (0.57 ± 0.15 and 0.99 ± 0.13, respectively), and bone marrow (2.39 ± 0.6 and 0.93 ± 0.18, respectively).

Although the function of these nerves in bone marrow is not clear, some studies report that SP is involved in the regulation of hematopoiesis either by direct interaction with primitive bone marrow stem cells and/or by modulation of cytokines that in turn regulate this process (Maestroni, 1998; Manske, Sullivan, & Andersen, 1995; Rameshwar, Ganea, & Gascon, 1993, 1994; Rameshwar & Gascon, 1996, Rameshwar, Poddar, & Gascon, 1997). Similarly, CGRP appears to modulate early B lymphocyte differentiation of bone marrow cells (McGillis, Rangnekar, & Ciallella, 1995).

2. *Thymus*

The thymus also receives innervation from SP/tachykinin- and CGRP-containing nerve fibers (Bellinger, Felten, & Felten, 1992a; Bellinger et al., 1990; Bulloch, Hausman, Radojcic, & Short, 1991; Bulloch et al., 1991; Jurjus, More, & Walsh, 1998; Kranz et al., 1997; Lorton, Bellinger, Felten, & Felten, 1990; Müller & Weihe, 1991; Weihe et al., 1989). SP/tachykinin$^+$ and $CGRP^+$ nerves enter the thymus along the capsule and travel along the interlobular septa, where they frequently reside adjacent to mast cells (Figure 26). An occasional nerve fiber exits from the interlobular septa to pass among immature thymocytes in the parenchyma of the cortex or to enter the medulla. SP^+ and $CGRP^+$ fibers also course along blood vessels, particularly those of the corticomedullary boundary, and are found in close association with the large number of mast cells also present along these vessels (Lorton et al., 1990; Müller & Weihe, 1991). SP/CGRP-containing nerves reside adjacent to mast cells in the capsule, interlobular septum, and at the corticomedullary junction (Bulloch et al., 1991; Lorton et al., 1990; Müller & Weihe, 1991). Free SP fibers are especially prominent at the

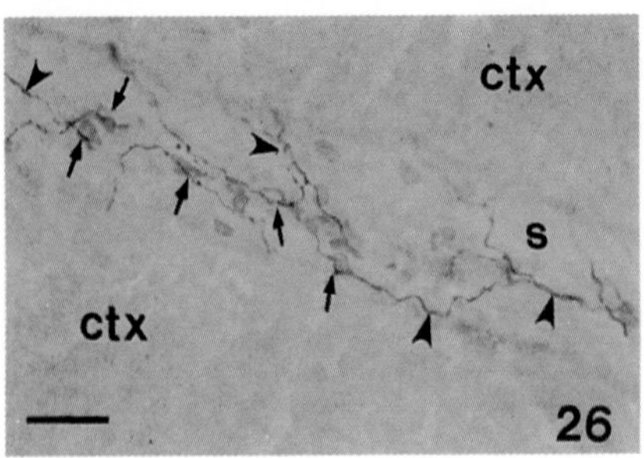

FIGURE 26 In the rat thymus, SP^+ nerve fibers (black) (arrowheads) traverse the interlobular septum (s) adjacent to mast cells (arrows). ctx, thymic cortex. Single-label ICC for SP. X43. Calibration bar = 100 μm.

corticomedullary junction, and form close associations with SP-positive cells in this region (Jurjus et al., 1998). They also closely appose $ED1^+$ and $ED3^+$ macrophages in the capsule, interlobular septum, cortex, and corticomedullary junction (Lorton et al., 1990; Müller & Weihe, 1991).

Weihe et al. (1989) have suggested that tachykinins, including SP, and CGRP serve a sensory function. Treatment with capsaicin, a neurotoxin specific for small nonmyelinated afferent nerves when administered in low concentrations, depletes SP in the thymus (Geppetti et al., 1987), indicating that SP resides in neural compartments. These findings support a sensory origin for SP. The distribution of $CGRP^+$ nerves in the thymus closely overlaps the distribution of SP^+ staining. Based on neurochemical measurements of SP and CGRP using an RIA following capsaicin treatment, these two peptides do not appear to be colocalized in the thymus (Geppetti et al., 1988). However, results from anterograde tracing methods from the C_2–C_4 dorsal root ganglia of the guinea pig demonstrate nerve fibers positive for both the tracer and for SP or CGRP, mainly in the ipsilateral thymus, suggesting that, at least in part, these nerves are primary sensory afferents arising from cervical dorsal root ganglia (Elfvin, Aldskogius, & Johansson, 1993).

3. *Spleen*

SP-immunoreactive nerves innervate the vasculature of the pig and cat spleens, and modulate vascular tone and blood volume (Lundberg et al., 1985, 1986). In rodents, SP^+, and $CGRP^+$ nerves have been described along the vasculature and in lymphoid compartments of the spleen (Bellinger et al., 1990; Lorton, Bellinger, Felten, & Felten, 1991; Olschowka et al., 1988; Romano et al., 1991, 1994). SP^+ and $CGRP^+$ nerves (Bellinger et al., 1992a; Bellinger et al., 1990; Lorton et al., 1991) also appear to have overlapping distributions in the rat spleen, but different from TH^+, NPY^+, or VIP^+ nerve fibers. Overall, the spleen is more densely innervated by $CGRP^+$ nerves than SP^+ nerves. SP^+ and $CGRP^+$ nerves travel along the large venous sinuses (Figure 27) and extend from these sinuses along the trabeculae. Numerous linear SP^+ and $CGRP^+$ nerves extend from the venous plexuses and trabeculae into the surrounding red pulp (Figure 28). Long, linear, SP^+ and $CGRP^+$ profiles, or vascular plexuses of SP^+/$CRGP^+$ nerves, occasionally travel through the marginal zone, and to a lesser extent, the PALS (Figure 29). SP^+ fibers are present adjacent to large arteries near the hilus of the spleen, which is presumably their site of entry into the spleen.

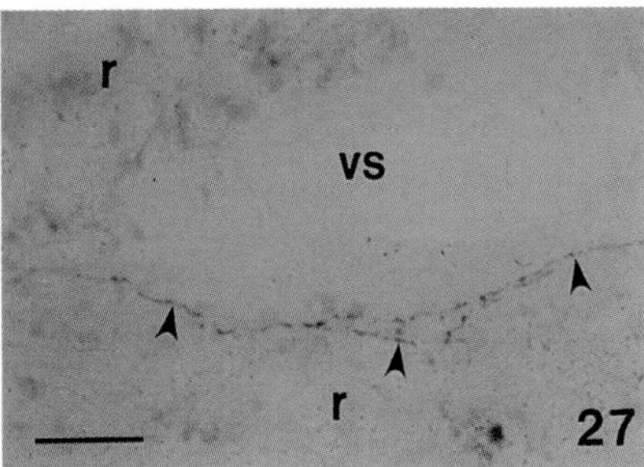

FIGURE 27 $CGRP^+$ nerve fibers (black) (arrowheads) travel along a venous sinus (vs) in the red pulp (r) of the rat spleen. Single-label ICC for CGRP. X43. Calibration bar = 100 μm.

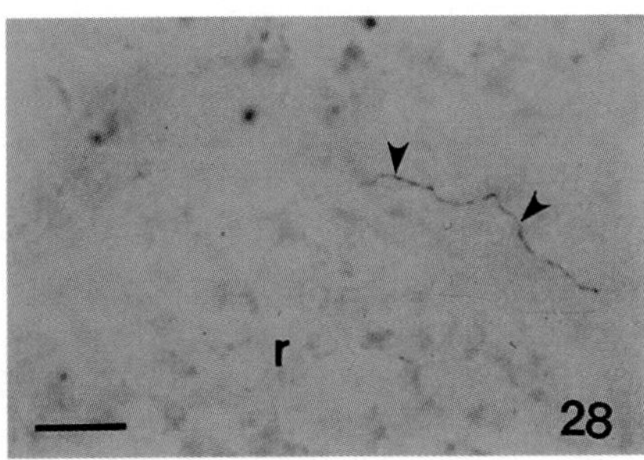

FIGURE 28 An individual SP^+ nerve fiber (black) (arrowheads) present in the red pulp (r) of the rat spleen. Single-label ICC for SP. X43. Calibration bar = 100 μm.

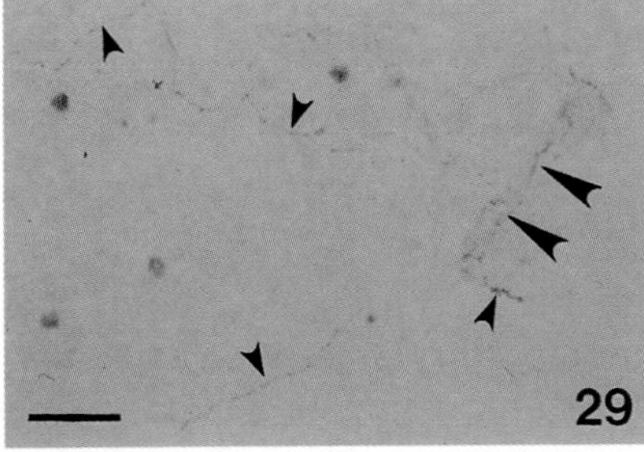

FIGURE 29 SP^+ nerve fibers (black) form a vascular plexus (large arrowheads) along a blood vessel, or course as free fibers (small arrowheads) in the periarteriolar lymphatic sheath of the rat spleen. Single-label ICC for SP. X85. Calibration bar = 50 μm.

Whether SP^+ and $CGRP^+$ nerves in the spleen represent sensory innervation is not clear. Very few myelinated fibers are reported in the splenic nerve (Baron & Jänig, 1988; Fillenz, 1970), and none has been described within the spleen itself. Tracing studies reveal very few labeled cells in sensory ganglia (Bellinger, Felten, Lorton, & Felten, 1989; Nance & Burns, 1989). In a careful tracing study by Baron and Jänig (1988), only 5% of the fibers in the splenic nerve of the cat were sensory. Anterograde tracing of primary sensory afferents from thoracic dorsal root ganglia (T_7–T_{12}) also indicates the existence of sensory nerve fibers that contain SP and CGRP in the guinea-pig spleen (Elfvin, Aldskogius, & Johansson, 1992). Physiological evidence indicates that some nerve fibers are able to evoke reflex responses between the spleen and kidney (reviewed in S. Y. Felten & Felten, 1991).

4. *Lymph Nodes*

Immunoreactivity for SP and CGRP in nerves have been described in a variety of lymph nodes from many mammalian species, including the rat (Bellinger et al., 1990; S. Y. Felten & Felten, 1991; Fink & Weihe, 1988; Romeo et al., 1994), mouse (Enzmann & Drossler, 1994; Fink & Weihe, 1988), guinea-pig (Enzmann & Drossler, 1994; Fink & Weihe, 1988), cat (Fink & Weihe, 1988; Popper et al., 1988), pig (Fink & Weihe, 1988), beluga whale (Romano et al., 1994), and human (Fink & Weihe, 1988). In mesenteric, popliteal, and inguinal lymph nodes from the rat (Bellinger et al., 1990; S. Y. Felten & Felten, 1991), SP^+ and $CGRP^+$ nerves closely overlap in their distribution. These nerves are found in the hilus, beneath the capsule, at the corticomedullary junction (Figure 30), in medullary regions (Figure 31), and in internodal regions of the lymph nodes. SP^+ and $CGRP^+$ nerve fibers often course as individual fibers in the parenchyma of the cortex and medulla among lymphocytes (Figure 31) and accessory cells.

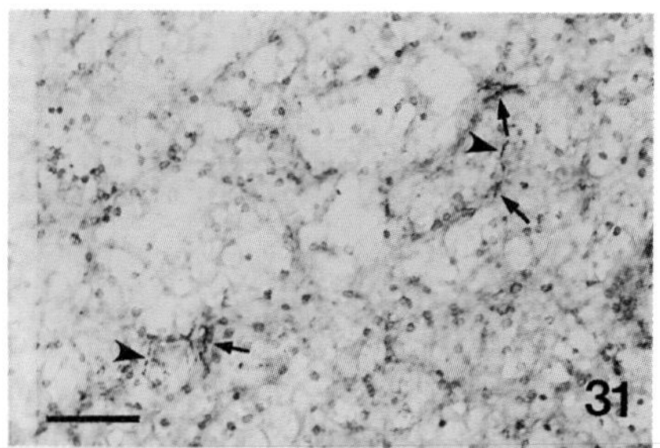

FIGURE 31 Individual SP^+ nerve fibers (black) (arrowheads) travel in the medulla of the rat mesenteric lymph node. These SP^+ nerve fibers (arrows) often closely appose $OX19^+$ T lymphocytes (brown). Double-label ICC for SP and OX19. X43. Calibration bar = 100 μm.

E. Neuropeptidergic Nerves—VIP

1. *Bone Marrow*

Although VIP nerve fibers have not been demonstrated immunocytochemically in bone marrow, VIP has been measured using an RIA in the periosteum, bone, and bone marrow of the Lewis rat (Ahmed et al., 1994). VIP concentrations in the periosteum (1.42 ± 0.31 pmol per gm) and bone marrow (0.47 ± 0.17 pmol per gm) are approximately 9 and 3 times higher than in bone (0.16 ± 0.04 pmol per gm), respectively. VIP in these bone sites could be localized in resident cells, nerves, or both.

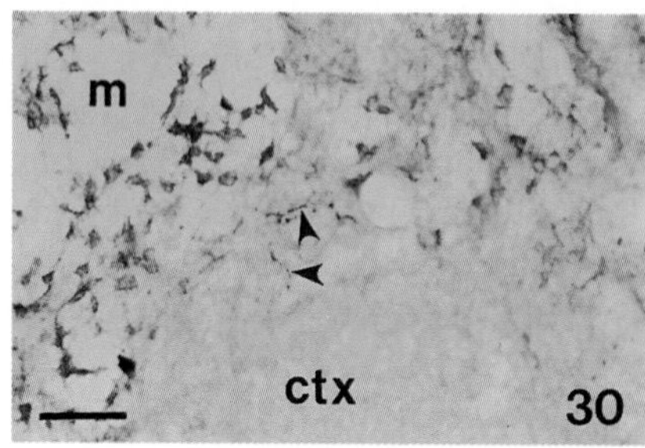

FIGURE 30 At the junction between the medulla (m) and the cortex (ctx) of the rat mesenteric lymph node, delicate, varicose $CGRP^+$ nerve fibers (black) (arrowheads) are present near $ED3^+$ macrophages (brown) in the medulla. Double-label ICC for CGRP and ED3. X43. Calibration bar = 100 μm.

2. *Thymus*

VIP^+ nerves have been demonstrated in primary lymphoid organs, including the thymus in rodents (Bellinger, Lorton, Brouxhon, Felten, & Felten, 1996; Bellinger, Lorton, Horn, Felten, & Felten, 1997; Bellinger et al., 1990; D. L. Felten et al., 1985; Kendall & Al-Shawaf, 1991) and chickens (Gulati et al., 1997), and the bursa fabricii of birds (Inoue, 1973). VIP^+ nerves have a different pattern of innervation than SP^+ and $CGRP^+$ nerves. Most VIP^+ fibers are present in the capsule and interlobular septa, often residing close to mast cells (Figure 32). Some VIP^+ nerves also are seen along blood vessels at the corticomedullary junction and adjacent to perivascular mast cells (Figure 33) and macrophages (Bellinger et al., 1997; Müller & Weihe, 1991), and

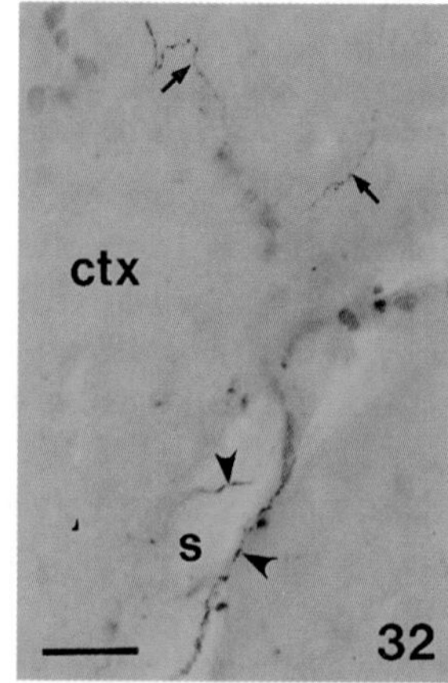

FIGURE 32 VIP^+ nerve fibers (black) (arrowheads) reside in the interlobular septum (s) of the rat thymus, and extend (arrows) from this compartment into the adjacent thymic cortex (ctx). Single-label ICC for VIP. X43. Calibration bar = 100 μm.

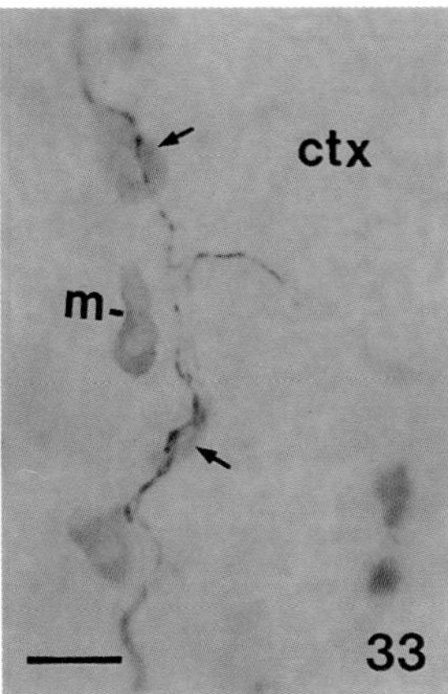

FIGURE 33 VIP$^+$ nerves (black) (arrows) are present in close proximity to mast cells (m) in the interlobular septum of the rat thymus. Single-label ICC for VIP. X85. Calibration bar = 50 μm.

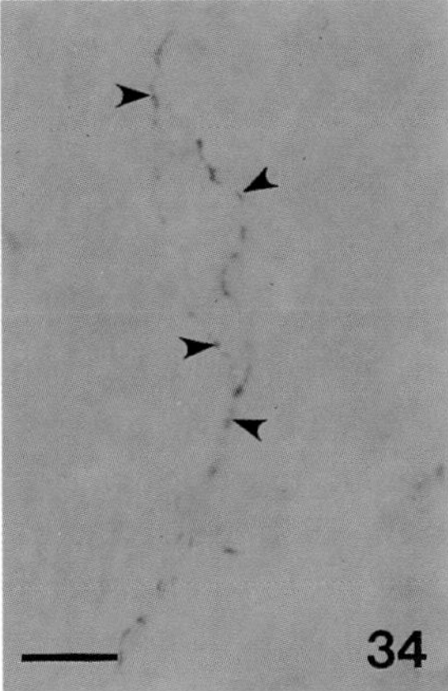

FIGURE 34 Long, linear, and varicose VIP$^+$ nerve fibers (black) (arrowheads) course deep into the cortex of the rat thymus medulla. Single-label ICC for VIP. X85. Calibration bar = 50 μm.

also exist as free fibers in the capsule, cortex (Figure 34), and medulla (Figure 35). In the medulla, VIP+ nerve fibers have close associations with a heterogeneous mix of VIP-immunoreactive cells (Figure 35). The association of peptide-containing nerves with mast cells is similar to that described in the mucosa of the gut (Stead et al., 1987), and may be a source of neuropeptide signals for regulation of mast cell secretion. In the chicken, VIP fibers are more abundant than NPY$^+$, SP$^+$ or CGRP$^+$ nerves (Gulati et al., 1997).

3. Spleen

Lundberg et al. (1986) report VIP innervation of the splenic vasculature that mediates vascular and volume responses. These investigators do not further describe the distribution of these nerves in specific compartments of the spleen. Fried and colleagues

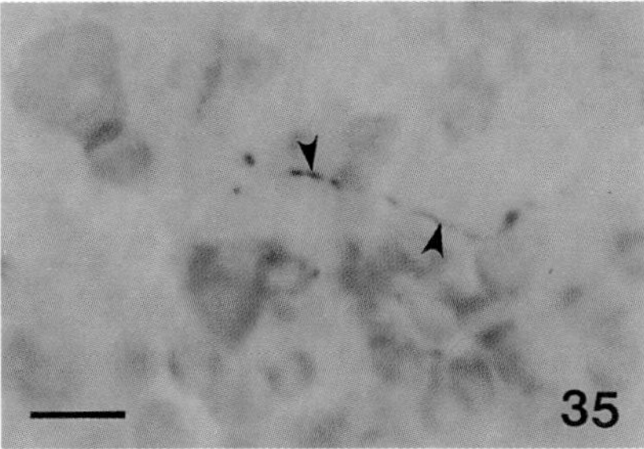

FIGURE 35 In the medulla of the rat thymus, a VIP$^+$ nerve fiber (black) (arrowheads) present among a cluster of VIP-immunoreactive cells (black). Single-label ICC for VIP. X85. Calibration bar = 50 μm.

(1986) report the presence of SP$^+$, somatostatin (SOM)$^+$, and VIP$^+$ nerve profiles in the bovine splenic nerve that are not colocalized with NE. VIP also is described along the vasculature in the cat spleen (Lundberg et al., 1986). In the rat spleen, VIP$^+$ nerves travel with the splenic artery into the spleen often in close proximity with clusters of T lymphocytes (Figure 36). VIP$^+$ nerves course along large arteries and central arterioles (Figure 37), and in the white pulp (Figures 38 and 39), venous/trabecular system (Figure 40), and red pulp (Bellinger et al., 1997). VIP innervation is more robust in Long-Evans hooded rats (Figure 38) than in Fischer 344 (F344) rats (Figure 39) (Bellinger et al., 1997). Surgical sympathectomy of the superior mesenteric-celiac ganglionic complex, the major source of sympathetic fibers to the spleen, does not alter splenic VIP content or the density of VIP$^+$ nerves in the spleen (Bellinger et al., 1997).

Infusion of VIP results in vasodilation and increased splenic volume, suggesting that VIP may exert at least some of its effects directly on the vasculature. We have found a sparse VIP innervation of the splenic vasculature (Bellinger et al., 1990; D. L. Felten et al., 1985) and adjacent PALS, and a relatively low VIP concentration in the rat spleen (Bellinger,

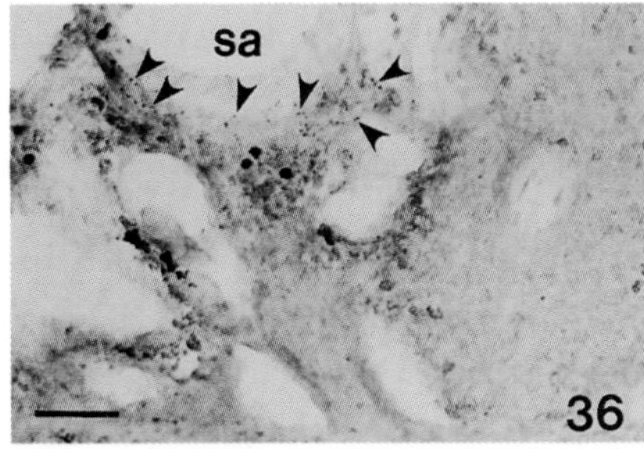

FIGURE 36 VIP$^+$ nerve fibers (black) (arrowheads) travel along the splenic artery (sa) and its branches as they enter the Fischer 344 (F344) rat spleen. These VIP$^+$ nerve fibers often reside near OX19$^+$ T lymphocytes (brown) at this vascular entry zone. Double-label ICC for VIP and OX19. X43. Calibration bar = 100 μm.

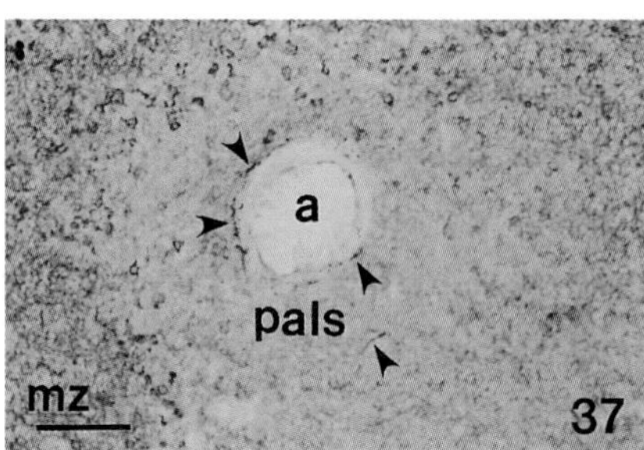

FIGURE 37 VIP+ fibers (black) (arrowheads) are present around the large central arteriole (a) and in the adjacent periarteriolar lymphatic sheath (pals) of the F344 rat splenic white pulp. mz, marginal zone. Double-label ICC for VIP and OX8. X43. Calibration bar = 100 μm.

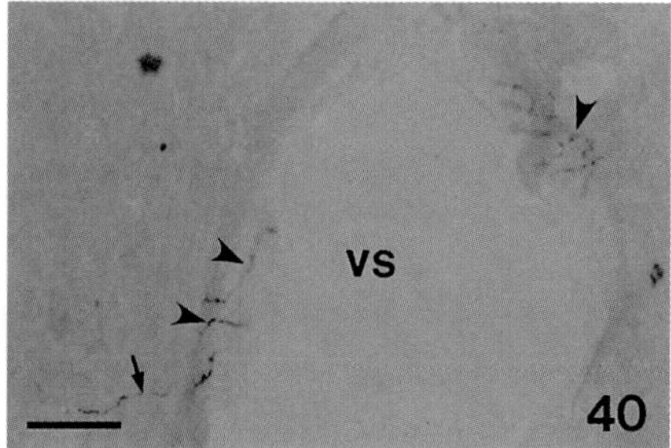

FIGURE 40 VIP+ nerve fibers (black) (arrowheads) travel along the venous sinus (vs) of the F344 rat spleen, and occasionally exit this plexus (arrow) into the surrounding red pulp. Single-label ICC for VIP. X43. Calibration bar = 100 μm.

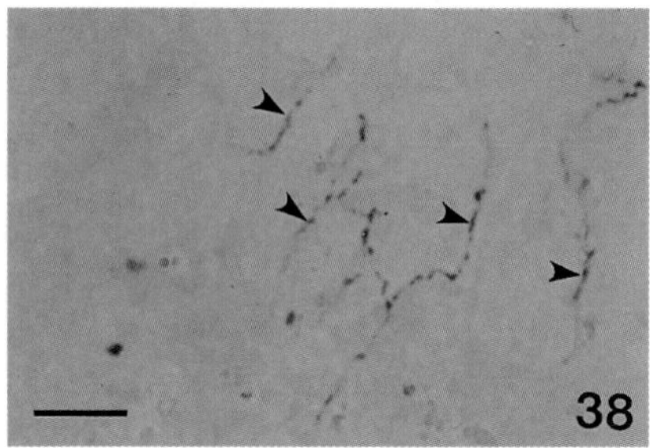

FIGURE 38 Spleens from Long-Evans hooded rats are more densely innervated than that seen in F344 rats as demonstrated in this photomicrograph of VIP+ nerve fibers (black) (arrowheads) coursing in the periarteriolar lymphatic sheath near a central arteriole (not shown in the picture) (see Fig. 39 for comparison). Single-label ICC for VIP. X85. Calibration bar = 50 μm.

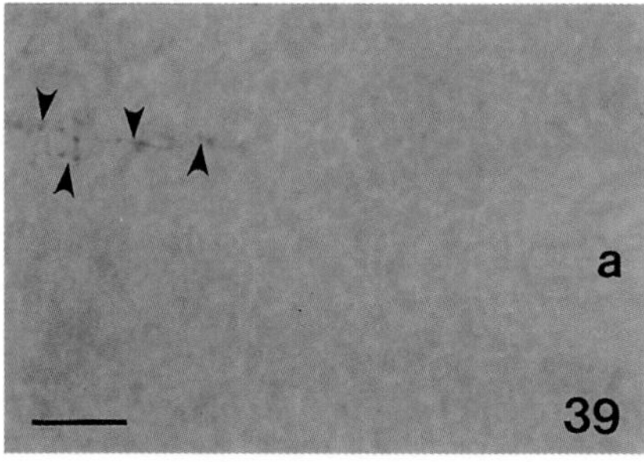

FIGURE 39 VIP+ nerve fibers (black) (arrowheads) in the periarteriolar lymphatic sheath of the F344 rat spleen coursing radially a short distance away from the central arteriole (a). Single-label ICC for VIP. X85. Calibration bar = 50 μm.

Earnest, Gallagher, & Felten, 1992). VIP+ nerves course along the venous sinuses and trabeculae, in the red pulp, in the marginal zone, and along the central artery and in the adjacent PALS (Figure 17). The paucity of VIP+ nerve fibers in the spleen is supported by the findings of Chevendra and Weaver (1992), reporting that less than 1% of the mesenteric neurons that innervate the spleen are VIP-immunoreactive. They also reported that no SOM+ neurons innervate the spleen, consistent with negative results following our efforts to stain for SOM in the spleen. VIP immunoreactivity is also present in cells of the immune system, suggesting an additional source of VIP in the spleen (reviewed in Bellinger, Lorton, et al., 1996).

4. *Lymph Nodes*

Immunoreactivity for VIP in nerves is found along the vasculature in internodal regions of the cortex and along medullary cords, with meager innervation of surrounding parenchyma (Figure 22) (Fink & Weihe, 1988; Popper et al., 1988). VIP and peptide histidine isoleucine (PHI) staining overlap in their distribution and may be colocalized. These fibers generally are found in association with the vasculature. In the rat, VIP+ nerves were found in mesenteric lymph nodes but not in popliteal lymph nodes (Bellinger et al., 1997). These findings suggest differences in peptide innervation depending on regional location, i.e., whether the lymph nodes drain peripheral sites or they drain the viscera.

F. Neuropeptidergic—Other Neurotransmitter-Specific Nerves

1. *Bone Marrow*

With immunoelectron microscopy, Elhassan and co-workers (Elhassan, Adem, Hultenby, & Lindgren, 1998) have demonstrated SOM labeling in myelinated nerves of the periosteum and in cells of the bone marrow. Measurements of SOM content using an RIA indicate the highest concentrations of SOM in bone marrow, followed by periosteum and cortical bone (approximately 8–11, 4, and 2 pmol per gm tissue, respectively). Involvement of SOM in nociception and in bone growth in the periosteum has been suggested since SOM inhibits cell growth in vitro. SOM+ nerves in the bone marrow, however, have not been demonstrated.

2. Thymus

Measurable levels of SOM (78.1 ± 7.9 pg per mg protein in the rat), as well as mRNA for SOM, exist in the thymus (Aguila, Dees, Haensely, & McCann, 1991; Sundler, Carraway, Hakanson, Alumets, & Dubois, 1978). With immunofluorescent staining, SOM$^+$ cells are present in the medulla and at the corticomedullary junction. At least some of the SOM$^+$ cells are thymocytes (Aguila et al., 1991). Immunocytochemistry for SOM has not provided convincing evidence for SOM$^+$ nerves in the thymus. In support of nonneural sources of SOM in the thymus, Geppetti and co-workers (Geppetti et al., 1987) found that SOM-like immunoreactivity was not affected by either capsaicin or 6-OHDA treatment.

Similarly, immunoreactivity for oxytocin, vasopressin, and associated neurophysins are present in epithelial cells, nurse cells, and other nonneural elements in the human thymus (Clements & Funder, 1986; Geenen et al., 1986; Geenen et al., 1987; Markwick, Lolait, & Funder, 1986) but has not been reported in nerves. Nicotinamide adenine dinucleotide phosphate-diaphorase (NADPH-d) histochemistry demonstrates the presence of nitric oxide in nerves of the chick thymus (Gulati, Leong, & Chan, 1998), where it colocalizes with nitric oxide synthetase (Gulati et al., 1997). NADPH-d$^+$ nerves occasionally were seen in the interlobular septa by embryonic day 18/19 in the chick thymus (Gulati et al., 1998). By day 21, these nerves formed perivascular plexuses, and occasional fibers were present in the medullary parenchyma.

3. Spleen

SOM also is present in cells of the spleen, and measurements by RIA indicate approximately 34.44 ± 6.6 pg per mg of protein of SOM is present in the spleen (Aguila et al., 1991). SOM mRNA$^+$ and SOM$^+$ cells occur in clusters in the white pulp, and are dispersed in the red pulp of the rat and chicken spleen. At least a subset of these cells are B lymphocytes. Again, SOM in nerves has not been revealed in the spleen.

A report by Schultzberg and colleagues (Schultzberg, Svenson, Unden, & Bartfai, 1987) described IL-1-containing nerve fibers in the spleen, perhaps colocalized in sympathetic NA nerves. An early report by D. L. Felten et al. (1985) noted met-enkephalin-containing nerves in the rodent spleen. Nohr et al. (Nohr, Michel, Fink, & Weihe, 1995) recently have demonstrated proenkephalin opioid peptides in the porcine and bovine splenic nerves, but were unable to find them in splenic nerves from rats, mice, hamsters, and guinea pigs. This study confirms earlier work by Fried and co-workers (1986), who reported enkephalin-immunoreactive nerves in bovine spleen. In addition, Fried et al. (1986) have provided evidence that enkephalin is coexpressed with NA and NPY in the splenic nerve. Nohr et al. (1995) did not confirm the report by D. L. Felten et al. (1985) of enkephalin-containing nerves in the rat spleen. This discrepancy may be due to the use of antibodies with different specificities, or to strain differences. Enkephalin-containing nerves form a dense plexus along blood vessels in the spleen suggesting a functional role of opioid peptides in modulating vascular effector functions similar to that described for NPY and NE (Nohr et al., 1995). In the PALS, numerous peri- and paravascular proenkephalin-immunoreactive fibers course in close apposition to lymphocytes and reticular cells. Proenkephalin-immunoreactive fibers also reside in the red pulp.

4. Lymph Nodes

Immunoreactivity for PHI, dynorphin A, enkephalin, and cholecystokinin (CCK) in nerves have been described in lymph nodes. Dynorphin A$^+$ and CCK$^+$ profiles travel in the medulla of lymph nodes from guinea pigs (Kurkowski, Kummer, & Heym, 1990). In contrast to the spleen and thymus, SOM-immunoreactive cells are apparently not found in lymph nodes (Aguila et al., 1991), even though SOM receptors may be present in human peripheral lymph nodes in some sites (Reubi, Horisberger, Dappeler, & Laissue, 1998). Popper, however, could not detect SOM binding sites in mesenteric lymph nodes from cats (Popper et al., 1988), suggesting regional differences in the cell composition and receptor expression in lymph nodes, or species differences. Retrograde tracing studies in Wistar rats indicate proenkephalin-containing neurons of the superior cervical ganglia project to the submaxillary lymph nodes (Romeo et al., 1994).

G. Nerves in Gut-Associated Lymphoid Tissue

The epithelium of the gastrointestinal tract is continuously exposed to an external environment containing food antigens, microbes, and other pathogens. Immunologic and nonimmunologic mechanisms contribute to the neutralization and elimination of these foreign antigens. The immune system of the intestine is the most extensive in mammals and involves diffuse populations of immune cells, lymphoid aggregates, and intraepithelial lymphocytes.

The more diffuse accumulations of lymphoid tissue in the mucosa of the gastrointestinal and respiratory systems make interpretation of innervation more difficult. It is not clear whether the nerve fibers that are present signal lymphoid cells as an important physiologic function, or whether other nonlymphoid components are targets with the lymphoid cells associated with nerve profiles as a coincidental epiphenomenon. However, if a transmitter released from nerves binds to the appropriate receptor on lymphoid cells in these sites, and the lymphoid cell is altered intracellularly by this ligand-receptor interaction, then important classic criteria for neurotransmission are met.

In vitro studies show that transient exposure of lymphocytes or other immunocytes to a variety of neurotransmitters can result in profound functional alterations (reviewed in Bellinger et al., 1990). It does not matter if the association with the target cell is transient; this may be the case for some cells in other lymphoid organs as well, such as the spleen and thymus. The presence of the target cell may in fact have resulted from a previous interaction of receptors with transmitter substances, such as VIP, that determines the migration of the cell to that location, as shown in elegant studies by Ottaway (Ottaway, 1984; Ottaway, 1985; Ottaway & Greenberg, 1984; Ottaway, Lewis, & Asa, 1987). He and his colleagues have demonstrated that the expression of VIP receptors on murine T lymphocytes mediates cell homing to Peyer's patches and mesenteric lymph nodes. Very high concentrations of VIP in mesenteric lymph nodes in the rat, compared with levels in spleen, thymus, or lymph nodes from other sites in the body, are consistent with their findings (Bellinger, Lorton, et al., 1996).

1. *Lamina Propria*

The lamina propria of the intestines receives an extensive plexus of nerves that arise from the enteric nervous system, and from sympathetic, parasympathetic, and dorsal root ganglia. Nerves in the lamina propria reside in specific compartments of the gut mucosa, depending on the neurotransmitter phenotype. These nerve fibers contain a variety of neuropeptides, including SP, SOM, VIP, CCK, and CGRP (Cooke, 1986; Lundbert, Saria, Brodin, Rosell, & Folkars, 1983; Probert, de Mey, & Polak, 1981). Several neuropeptides may be present in the same nerve fiber. For example, NPY is colocalized with VIP in submucosal nerves of the rat jejunum, and with ChAT and SOM in the guinea pig ileum (Lomax, Bertrand, & Furness, 1998), but NPY staining is not colocalized in NA nerves associated with blood vessels (Cox, Rudolph, & Gschmeissner, 1994).

TH^+ (Figure 41), NPY^+ (Figure 42), SP^+ (Figure 43), $CGRP^+$, VIP^+ (Figures 44 and 45), SOM^+, and CRH^+ (Figure 46) nerves extend throughout the lamina propria and form a dense network of fibers around the epithelial crypts. These nerves also ramify throughout the villi. Some of these fibers, depending on their neurotransmitter content, extend beneath the basement membrane of the epithelium, especially nerves that contain VIP, TH, and NPY. VIP^+ nerves appear to form the densest nerve plexus, followed by TH^+/NPY^+ nerves. There are fewer SP^+, SOM^+, and CRH^+ nerves in the lamina propria. SOM^+ nerves are present in pericryptal networks, but are infrequently found in the villi of the mucosa.

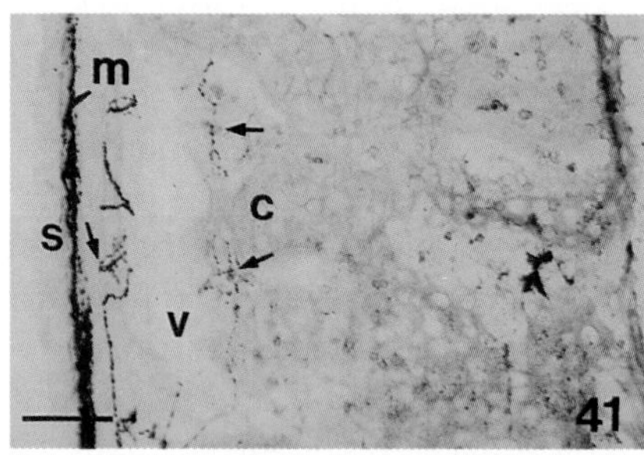

FIGURE 41 TH^+ neurons and nerve fibers (black) are present in the myenteric plexus (m) just beneath the serosa (s) in the rat ileum. TH^+ nerve fibers (arrows) also are found adjacent to $OX8^+$ T lymphocytes (brown) near large diameter postcapillary venules (v) at the base of the epithelial crypts (c). Double-label ICC for TH and OX8. X43. Calibration bar = 100 μm.

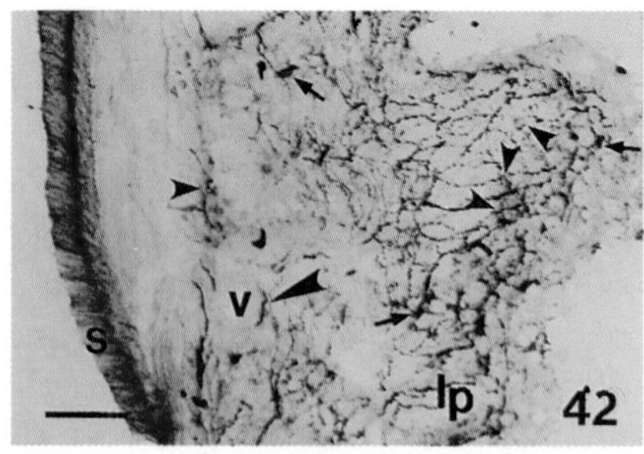

FIGURE 42 NPY^+ nerve fibers (black) abundantly innervate the lamina propria (lp) of the rat ileum. These fibers extend to the epithelium, and can sometimes be seen adjacent to $OX8^+$ intraepithelial cells. NPY^+ nerve fibers also are present near postcapillary venules (v) (large arrowhead). In the lamina propria, NPY^+ nerve fibers often closely appose $OX8^+$ T lymphocytes (brown) (small arrowheads) and NPY-immnoreactive cells (black) (arrows). Double-label ICC for NPY and OX8. X43. Calibation bar = 100 μm.

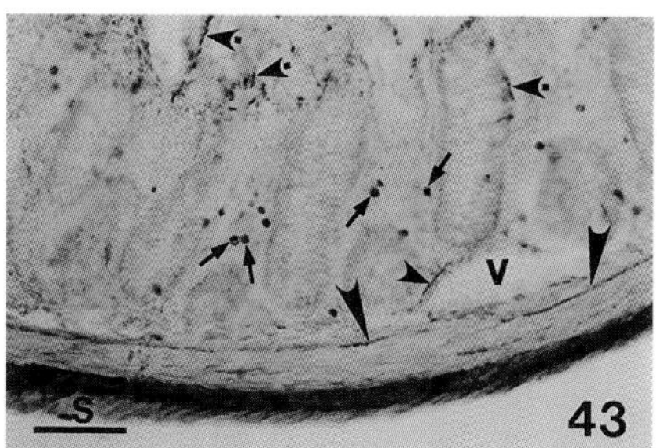

FIGURE 43 In the rat ileum, SP-immunoreactivity is present in nerve fibers (black) in the outer muscle layers (large arrowheads), and near the postcapillary venules (v) (small arrowhead). SP immunoreactivity also is present in cells (black) that reside in the lamina propria and epithelium. A close look at the SP-immunoreactive cells reveals that many of these cells stain positive for OX8 (arrows). SP^+ nerve fibers can be seen coursing adjacent to SP^+, and $SP^+/OX8^+$ cells (dot-small arrowheads). s, serosa. X43. Calibration bar = 100 μm.

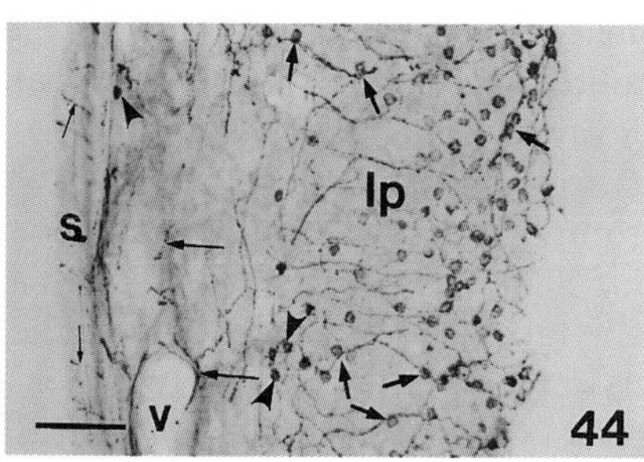

FIGURE 44 Photomicrograph from the rat ileum stained immunocytochemically for VIP reveals VIP^+ nerve fibers (black) in the serosa (s) (long, thin arrows), along the postcapillary venules (v) (large, thin arrows), in the muscle layers of the gut, and in the lamina propria (lp). Additionally, VIP immunoreactivity (black) is present in lymphoid cells of the lamina propria. Many of these VIP^+ cells are also positive for OX8 (brown) (small arrowheads). VIP^+ nerve fibers course in close proximity with VIP^+, $OX8^+$, and $VIP^+/OX8^+$ cells in the laminal propria (short, thick arrows). Double-label ICC for VIP and OX8. X43. Calibration bar = 100 μm.

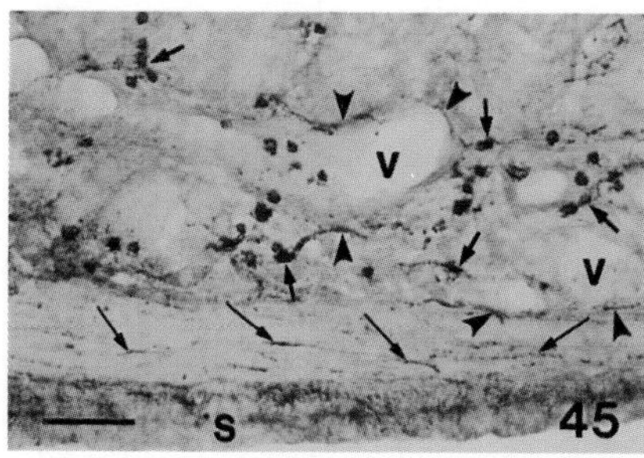

FIGURE 45 VIP^+ nerve fibers (black) course along the large postcapillary venules (v) at the base of the crypts (arrowheads), in the muscle layers next to the serosa (s) (long, thin arrows), and adjacent to VIP^+, $VIP^+/OX8^+$ (brown), and $OX8^+$ cells (short, thick arrow). Double-label ICC for VIP and OX8. X43. Calibration bar = 100 μm.

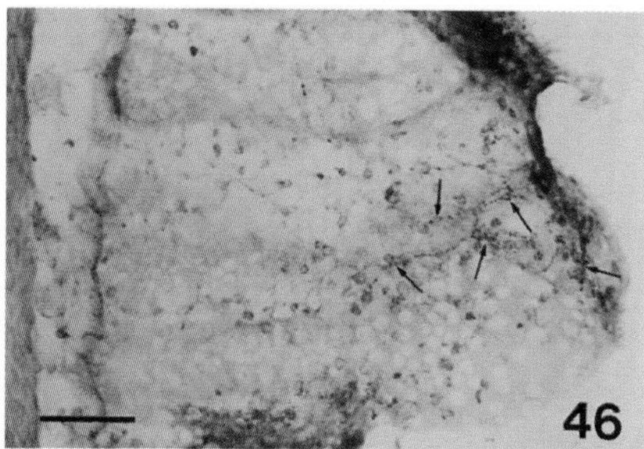

FIGURE 46 In the rat ileum, very fine CRH^+ nerve fibers (black) are present in the lamina propria and along the crypts, often adjacent to $OX8^+$ T lymphocytes (brown) (arrows). Double-label ICC for CRH and OX8. X43. Calibration bar = 100 μm.

These nerves also are present in the area surrounding the bases of the crypts, a region where capillaries serving the villus coalesce to form larger-diameter postcapillary venules (Figures 41–45). Close association of NA and peptidergic nerves with postcapillary venules suggest a role for these nerves in regulating trafficking of activated effector blast cells, and unactivated effector cells from the blood stream into the mucosa (Bienenstock, Befus, & McDermott, 1983; Husband, 1982; Jeurissen, Duijvestijn, & Sontag, 1987).

Keast and colleagues (Keast, Furness, & Costa, 1984) have investigated the origin of many neurotransmitter-specific nerves in the mucosa of the guinea pig small intestine. They report that nerve fibers in the mucosa with immunoreactivity for VIP, SOM, CCK, and NPY arise from cell bodies in the overlying submucous plexus. SP fibers arise in part from the overlying submucous plexus and in part from the myenteric plexus. Mucosal NE fibers arise from extrinsic sympathetic ganglia. Enkephalin, gastrin-releasing peptide, and serotonin, which are in some enteric nerves, are not found in submucous nerve cells and few, if any, fibers containing these substances supply the mucosa.

In the rat ileum, double-label immunocytochemical staining for a variety of neurotransmitters and specific markers for lymphoid cells has been performed in our laboratory. $OX19^+$ (pan T cell marker) and $OX8^+$ (suppressor/cytotoxic T cell marker) T cells are scattered throughout the lamina propria; sometimes they form small aggregates predominantly seen at the base of the crypts. OX8 staining also reveals intraepithelial lymphocytes in the epithelium of the luminal surface of the gut (Figures 41–46). Nerves in the lamina propria that are immunoreactive for TH, NPY, VIP, SP, CGRP, and CRH form close associations with T cells positive for OX19, a pan T cell marker. Immunocytochemical staining with antibodies for $OX8^+$, a CD8 T cell marker, further indicates that many of these cells are CD8 T lymphocytes

(Figures 41–46). Some of these T cells double-label for CRH (Figure 46), SP (Figure 43), and VIP (Figures 44–45). VIP (Figure 44), TH (Figure 41), and NPY (Figure 42) nerves also course adjacent to the basement membrane of the epithelium, in close proximity to $CD8^+$ intraepithelial lymphocytes. Close appositions between $ED3^+$ macrophages and TH, NPY, VIP, SP, CGRP, and CRH nerves also occurred in the lamina propria.

Although it is clear that these nerves course among lymphocytes, plasma cells, mast cells, and macrophages in the lamina propria, descriptions of interactions between nerves and lymphoid cells in the gut mucosa are limited. Intestinal mucosal mast cells from normal and nematode-infected rats (nematode infection causes mast cell hyperplasia) have contacts with nerves (Stead, Tomioka, Quinonez, et al., 1987) that contain SP and CGRP (Stead, Tomioka, Riddell, & Bienenstock, 1988). Similarly, in the human intestinal mucosa, mast cells also are apposed to PGP 9.5^+ nerves (Stead, Dixon, Bramwell, Riddell, & Bienenstock, 1989). Other investigators have noted the close proximity of mast cells and nerves in the duodenal mucosa (Stach, 1973), rat colon (Yonei et al., 1985), and the gastric glands of the opossum (Seelig, Schlusselberg, Smith, & Woodward, 1985). Yonei (1987) reported degranulated mast cells closely associated with cholinergic nerves in ulcerative colitis.

AChE staining has been reported in nerve-like fibers in the lamina propria (D. L. Felten, Overhage, Felten, & Schmedtje, 1981; Inoue, 1973; Yamashita, Kumazawa, Kozuki, Amano, Tomoda, & Kumazawa, 1984). ChAT/NPY/SOM-immunoreactive and ChAT/calbindin-immunoreactive neurons are present in the myenteric plexus, and $ChAT^+$/$tachykinin^+$ neurons are present in the submucous plexus (Lomax et al., 1998). Vagal afferent nerves have been described penetrating the jejunal mucosa and contacting intestinal mucosal mast cells (IMMCs) (Gottwald, Lhotak, & Stead, 1997). Further, electrical stimulation of the vagus nerve results in increased IMMC histamine content. Three weeks after truncal vagotomy, 25% fewer IMMCs were seen in vagotomized animals than in controls (Gottwald et al., 1997). Three months after neonatal capsaicin treatment 28% fewer IMMCs were found in treated rat jejunum. Three weeks after vagotomy, IgA^+ plasma cell densities were increased, whereas the proportion of lamina propria areas remained stable. Growth-associated protein-43 (GAP-43)-immunoreactive indicated no change in nerve density 3 weeks after vagotomy.

Eosinophils form close associations with nerves in the rat and human gastrointestinal mucosa, but to a lesser extent than found for mast cells (Bramwell, Ridell, Colley, & Stead, 1989; Quinonez et al., 1989). Stach (1973) noted plasma cell-nerve associations in the gastrointestinal tract. A light and electron microscopic study in the mouse small bowel confirms and extends this observation, demonstrating enteric nerves in contact with plasma cells or B immunoblasts in the mucosa and submucosa (Crivellato, Soldano, Travan, Fusaroli, & Mallardi, 1998) at an incidence level that is 3–4 times greater than would be expected by chance alone.

2. *Aggregated Lymphoid Tissue*

In some regions of the gut, lymphoid tissue forms discrete compartments, including tonsils, Peyer's patches, and the appendix, that are integral, large, important compartments in the gut-associated immune system. A variety of neurotransmitter-specific nerves have been described in these lymphoid compartments. Sympathetic NA innervation is present in the human palatine tonsils and paratonsillar glands (Ueyama et al., 1990; Yamashita et al., 1984), the rabbit appendix (D. L. Felten et al., 1981), the sacculus rotundus and Peyer's patches of the rabbit (Jesseph & Felten, 1984), and the bursa of Fabricius of the chicken (Inoue, 1973). Even though the bursa of Fabricius is considered a primary lymphoid organ in birds, it is associated with, and anatomically similar to, other gut-associated lymphoid tissue (GALT), so it will be included in this section.

In the tonsil (Ueyama et al., 1990; Yamashita et al., 1984), NA nerves distribute in dense perivascular plexuses, particularly along the arteries. Individual fluorescent profiles enter parafollicular regions of the tonsil, but no fibers travel into the epithelium or the germinal centers. In the human appendix, a significant relationship exists between the density of PGP 9.5^+ nerves and mast cells in the lamina propria (Stead, Franks, Goldsmith, Bienenstock, & Dixon, 1990). Neurotransmitter phenotypes were not characterized in these nerves. In the rabbit appendix (D. L. Felten et al., 1981), NA nerves enter lymphoid tissue with the vasculature and muscularis interna. NA fibers travel longitudinally inside the muscularis interna for short distances until they reached a zone between lymphoid nodules. These NA plexuses turn radially to course perpendicular to the long axis of the lumen and continue toward the lumen between the large lymphoid nodules. As in the tonsil, no fibers enter into the lymphoid nodules. NA nerves traverse through interdomal zones of T lymphocytes between lymphoid nodules at the entrance to the lamina propria. NA fibers then enter the lamina propria, traveling along small blood vessels and arborizing into the surrounding parenchyma to end among lymphocytes, enterochromaffin cells (some of which may contain serotonin), and other accessory cells. They also form delicate arborizations in the subepithelial region adjacent to plasma cells.

The general pattern of NA innervation in the sacculus rotundus and Peyer's patches (Jesseph & Felten, 1984) is similar to that in the appendix. However, the enterochromaffin cells that are juxtaposed with NA terminals are more abundant in the appendix. A similar pattern of innervation is present in the bursa of Fabricius. NA nerves form perivascular plexuses in the perimuscular connective tissue, muscle, and mucosa, often in close proximity to autofluorescent cells. Fine linear fibers travel between the lymphoid nodules, but do not enter the nodules. NA fibers also are not found in the epithelium. NPY fibers in the submucosa are a conspicuous feature of the duodenum, caecum, transverse colon, descending colon, and rectum, but not of the ileum, ascending colon, or distal spiral (Hsieh et al., 1996). In the rat ileum, an occasional NPY^+ nerve fiber can be seen in the periphery of Peyer's patches (Figure 47).

AChE staining has been reported in GALT (D. L. Felten et al., 1981; Inoue, 1973; Yamashita et al., 1984) in nerve-like fibers in the lamina propria and between lymphoid nodules of the rabbit appendix, and lymphoid nodules of the human tonsil. There is no evidence that these nerves represent cholinergic fibers; some of these fibers may be sympathetic. This is probably the case for some of the nerve-like $AChE^+$ staining in the rabbit appendix (D. L. Felten et al., 1981). It is probable that at least some of the $AChE^+$ staining in GALT represent cholinergic nerve fibers, because parasympathetic ganglia are present within the enteric nervous system, and vagal afferents innervate the gastrointestinal tract. However, no definitive studies have demonstrated that $AChE^+$ nerve fibers in GALT are truly cholinergic. In addition, there is a more diffuse nonneural AChE staining associated with the lymphoid nodules. In the rabbit appendix (D. L. Felten et al., 1981), this staining forms a dense network surrounding the B lymphocytes deep within the nodules and at the crown of the domes. Similar staining is seen in the germinal centers in the tonsil (Yamashita et al., 1984).

Direct demonstration of peptidergic nerves innervating lymphoid components of the gut is incomplete (reviewed in Stead, Bienenstock, & Stanisz, 1987). Early studies using silver stains of the bursa of Fabricius indicate nerves within the nodules (Cordier, 1969; Inoue, 1971). These are not likely to be NA nerves, since fluorescence histochemistry fails to reveal NA nerves in lymphoid nodules. An ultrastructural study of Peyer's patches from the Syrian hamster demonstrated nonmyelinated nerve bundles traversing the lymphoid follicles (Pfoch & Unsicker, 1972). Within the lymphoid nodule, free nerve fibers containing synaptic vesicle aggregates reside within 20 nm of reticular cells and lymphocytes. Similar direct contacts were reported between catecholaminergic nerve terminals and plasma cells in the lacrimal gland of the pigeon (Walcott & McLean, 1985) and between nonmyelinated nerve endings and small lymphocytes in the jugular body, a lymphomyeloid organ, of the leopard frog (Zapata, Villena, & Cooper, 1982). In the human tonsil (Ueyama et al., 1990), VIP^+ nerve fibers have been reported along the tonsillar blood vessels, in extranodular lymphoid tissue, and in the marginal zone of the lymph nodules, but not in the germinal centers.

VIP^+ nerve fibers are present in murine (Ottaway, Lewis, & Asa, 1987) and cat (Ichikawa, Sreedharan, Goetzl, & Owen, 1994) Peyer's patches, coursing predominantly along small-caliber blood vessels. In the rat ileum, VIP^+ nerve fibers course along the edge of Peyer's patches, and sometimes into a short distance into the patch (Figure 48). In the human colon, SP^+ nerves are in close apposition with both T_4-

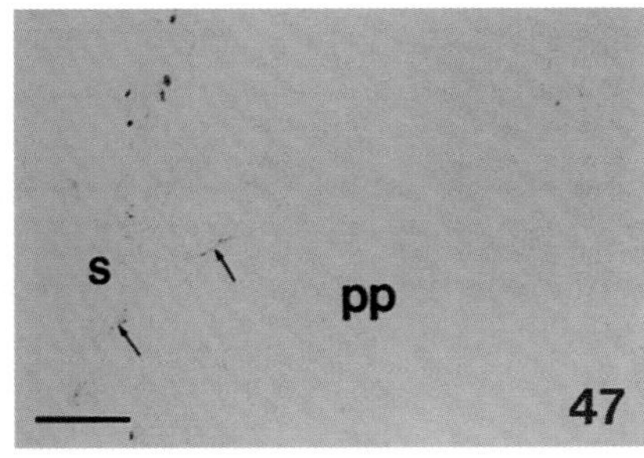

FIGURE 47 A VIP^+ nerve fiber (black) (arrows) course under the serosa (s) and extends into a Peyer's patch (pp) in the rat ileum. Single-label ICC for VIP. X43. Calibration bar = 100 μm.

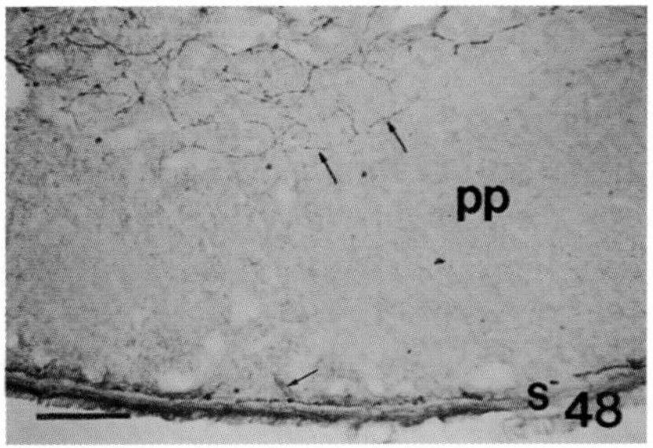

FIGURE 48 NPY^+ nerve fibers (black) are present under the serosa (s), and in the parenchyma adjacent to the Peyer's patch (pp) in the rat ileum. Occasionally, NPY^+ nerve fibers extend from these compartments into the periphery of the patch (arrows). Double-label ICC for NPY and OX8. X43. Calibration bar = 100 μm.

cells and IgA-bearing B cells (Weisz-Carrington et al., 1991). SOM-immunoreactive nerves also have been described in the Peyer's patches from cats (Feher, Foror, & Burnstock, 1992). SOM^+ nerves and SOM^+ cell bodies of enteric neurons are present in the tela submucosa very close to the Peyer's patches. SOM^+ (Feher et al., 1992) and VIP^+ (Ottaway et al., 1987; Ichikawa et al., 1994) fibers course along the margin of the follicle and few fibers are found in the follicle.

With electron microscopic analysis, very close contacts of SOM-immunoreactive nerves with lymphocytes and plasma cells (gap junction of 20–200 nm) with no Schwann cell sheath interposed have been observed (Feher et al., 1992). The source of SOM innervation of Peyer's patches is not clear. SOM and NE colocalize in neurons from the mesenteric-celiac ganglia that innervate the intestines (Chevendra & Weaver, 1992). Using retrograde tracing after injection of tracer into the intestines, Chevendra and Weaver (1992) have identified mesenteric postganglionic neurons in rat sympathetic ganglia double-labeled for tracer and SOM. An alternative source of these nerves may be the submucous plexus of the enteric nervous system (Keast et al., 1984).

Four different peptides in nerve compartments have been found in the bursa fabricius, tachykinins, VIP, galanin, and CGRP; they are distributed throughout the different bursal compartments, except for the medulla of the bursal follicles, where the early stages of lymphocyte maturation occur (Zentel & Weihe, 1991). Double labeling reveals three populations of fibers, VIP/galanin double-positive nerves, tachykinin and CGRP double-positive nerves, and tachykinin single-positive nerves. Some of the tachykinin$^+$ fibers also may contain VIP. These nerves are found adjacent to B cells in the follicle cortex. VIP fibers also are seen close apposed to macrophages.

H. Nerves in Mucosa-Associated Lymphoid Tissue

1. *Bronchus-Associated Lymphoid Tissue*

The respiratory tract of mammals contains aggregations of various lymphoid cells in its mucosal layer, referred to as bronchus-associated lymphoid tissue (BALT). This lymphoid tissue randomly distributes along the bronchial tract and at bifurcations (reviewed by Nohr & Weihe, 1991). Individual aggregates are referred to as bronchus-associated lymphoid units (BALUs), which are located beneath the bronchial epithelium, crossing the muscularis mucosa, and extending into the submucosa. BALUs contain primary as well as secondary follicles, high endothelial venules, and efferent lymph vessels, and in principle are accompanied by an artery and a nerve. They possess all cells typical of peripheral lymphoid organs, but have no bordering capsule.

NA and peptidergic nerve fibers in the BALT of the rat (Inoue, Magari, & Sakanaka, 1990; Nohr & Weihe, 1991) and cat (Nohr & Weihe, 1991) have been examined using immunocytochemistry. The rat BALT receives NPY, SP, CGRP, and VIP innervation (Inoue et al., 1990). PGP 9.5 stained all nerve fibers except some smaller $CGRP^+$ nerves. Immunoreactivity for SP, CGRP, NPY, leu-enkephalin, met-enkephalin, and TH in nerves are distributed throughout the different compartments of the BALT. Nerve fibers are found under the epithelium, in the smooth muscle layer, along the vasculature, and among immune cells of the BALT parenchyma. Peptidergic and NA nerve fibers form close contacts with mast cells, $ED1^+$ macrophages, and other lymphoid cells with varying frequencies. Although there do not appear to be differences in the specific compartments innervated by the different neurotransmitters, differences are present in the density of the different peptidergic and adrenergic fibers that innervated different regions and targets.

TH and NPY fibers preferentially supply blood vessels, often forming dense perivascular plexuses (Nohr & Weihe, 1991). These fibers enter the BALT together with pulmonary arterial branches, and frequently reach the central zone of the BALT to give rise to fine, tortuous fibers (Inoue et al., 1990). A few TH or NPY fibers are seen between lymphoid cells in the parenchyma of the BALU (Nohr & Weihe, 1991). NPY and TH^+ fibers are more numerous in association with perivascular plexuses than nerves containing both SP and CGRP.

In contrast, SP^+ and $CGRP^+$ nerve fibers enter the BALT as fibers branching from the walls of the bronchi and then distribute primarily in the subepithelial zones of the BALT. SP^+ and $CGRP^+$ nerves are located in the area under the epithelium, in the smooth muscle layer of and in the BALUs. These fibers seem to distribute predominantly in the subepithelial zone of the BALT after dissociating from the fiber networks in the walls of the bronchi, although small numbers of SP^+ and $CGRP^+$ nerves are seen in the BALT central zone. Within the BALUs, SP and CGRP-immunoreactive fibers reside in peri- and paravascular locations and intermingle with lymphoid cells in the parenchyma of the BALU (Inoue et al., 1990; Nohr & Weihe, 1991). Although $CGRP^+$ nerves have a similar distribution, they outnumber the SP^+ nerve fibers (Inoue et al., 1990; Nohr & Weihe, 1991). SP coexists with CGRP in most nerves (Nohr &

Weihe, 1991). Similarly, Nilsson and co-workers (G. Nilsson, Alving, Ahlstedt, Hokfelt, & Lundberg, 1990) demonstrated the presence neurokinin A in the lining respiratory epithelium, bronchial smooth muscle, around blood vessels and close to lymphoid aggregates using immunocytochemistry. These nerve fibers are markedly decreased following capsaicin treatment, suggesting a sensory origin.

VIP^+/PHI^+ nerves appear under the epithelium, in peri- and paravascular regions, in smooth muscle layer, and between lymphocytes (Inoue et al., 1990; Nohr & Weihe, 1991). VIP inhibits antigen-induced histamine release (Undem, Dick, & Buckner, 1983). Nerves staining for opioid peptides leu-enkephalin and met-enkephalyl-Arg-Gly-Leu and for the opioid sequence Tyr-Gly-Gly-Phe, are found mainly beneath the epithelium (Nohr & Weihe, 1991), but also occur in the smooth muscle layer, in peri- and paravascular regions, and between lymphocytes. Nerves are not detected in the lymphoid epithelium of the BALU. $ED1^+$ macrophages and mast cells were found mainly in peripheral regions of BALUs. $CGRP^+$, met-enkephalyl-Arg-Gly-Leu^+, and SP^+ fibers contact $ED1^+$ macrophages, and to a lesser extent mast cells (Inoue et al., 1990; Nohr & Weihe, 1991). $Tachykinin^+$ and $CGRP^+$ nerve fibers travel in close association with $serotonin^+$ mast cells in the bronchi of the lung (G. Nilsson et al., 1990). Very few associations occur between VIP^+/PHI^+, NPY^+ dopamine β-$hydroxylase^+$ and TH^+ nerve fibers and either $ED1^+$ macrophages or mast cells. These findings support a role for these four neuropeptides in control of mucosal immunity, lymphocyte migration, and proliferation within the BALT.

2. *Nerves Associated with the Cutaneous Immune System*

As a first line of defense, the skin is poised to respond to external challenges for the protection and preservation of the organism. The skin contains a complex and interactive neural network that detects irritants and maintains homeostasis. Sensory nerves that innervate the skin and release neuropeptides have been demonstrated to modulate functions of keratinocytes, Langerhans cells, mast cells, dermal microvascular endothelial cells, and infiltrating immune cells, influencing such functions as cell proliferation, cytokine production, and antigen presentation under normal or disease conditions. Changes in nerve-cutaneous immune cell interactions play an important role in certain skin disorders, such as psoriasis and atopic dermatitis. There is a growing body of evidence indicating that stress can influence immune competence in the skin. For example, psoriasis and atopic dermatitis may be exacerbated by psychic stress. Similarly, immobilization stress just before sensitization can reduce a delayed-type hypersensitivity (DTH) response in a time-dependant manner, and cause marked alterations in Langerhans cell morphology in the sensitized area in stressed mice (Kawaguchi et al., 1997). This stress effect has been associated with an increase in the activity of $CGRP^+$ nerves (Kawaguchi et al., 1997).

Nerves that innervate the skin express a variety of neurotransmitters, including SP, VIP, SOM, CGRP, gastrin-releasing peptide, calretinin, NPY, PHI, neurotensin, neurokinin A and B, bradykinin, ACh, catecholamines, histamine, pituitary adenylate cyclase activating polypeptide, endorphins, and enkephalins (Al'Abadie, Senior, Bleehen, & Gawkrodger, 1994; Dalsgaard et al., 1989; Hardebo, Suzuki, & Ekman, 1992; Gibbins, Wattchow, & Coventry, 1987; Johansson, 1986; Johansson, Virtanen, & Hilliges, 1995; Moller et al., 1993; Odum, Petersen, Skov, & Ebskov, 1998; Ositelu, Morris, & Vaillant, 1987; D. M. Reilly et al., 1997; Schulze, Witt, Fink, Hofer, & Funk, 1997; Wallengren, Ekman, & Sundler, 1987; reviewed by Misery, 1997; Wallengren, Moller, & Ekman, 1987). Neurotransmitter-specific nerves distribute to specific compartments in the skin. SP^+, neurokinin A^+, and $CGRP^+$ nerves are present in the epidermis. $CGRP^+$ nerves are located close to the epidermal basement membrane. Nerves that contain SP, calretinin, VIP, CGRP, and neurokinin A reside in the dermis.

In the dermis of skin, $CGRP^+$ nerves leave large nerve bundles to distribute to blood vessels, eccrine sweat glands, and to enter the epidermis directly or in association with Meissner's corpuscles in the dermal papillae (Ishida-Yamamoto, Senba, & Tohyama, 1989). In the epidermis, $CGRP^+$ nerves distribute widely. Some $CGRP^+$ fibers are associated with Merkel cells and keratinocytes (Ishida-Yamamoto et al., 1989). Depletion of SP^+ and $CGRP^+$ nerves follows capsaicin treatment, suggesting a sensory origin for these nerves (D. M. Reilly et al., 1997). Morphologic studies indicate that Langerhans cells are frequently apposed to epidermal nerves that are $CGRP^+$, and Langerhans cells are responsive to changes in CGRP concentrations in the skin (Kawaguchi et al., 1997).

Calretinin is particularly prominent in large myelinated cutaneous nerve fibers. NPY and TH predominate along the wall of arteries, arterioles, and veins, while neurokinin A^+ and SP^+ nerves are less commonly seen adjacent to blood vessels, usually observed in deeper dermal layers (D. M. Reilly et al., 1997). The density of these nerves varies depending on the region of skin. For example, VIP^+ nerves are more common in face skin than in the forearm, whereas in forearm there are more NPY^{+}, $CGRP^{+}$, neurokinin A^{+}, and SP^{+} nerve fibers than in face skin.

Receptors for these neuropeptides, and the presence of neuropeptide-specific peptidases in target cells or tissues of the skin, have been documented (Kemeny, von Restorff, Michel, & Ruzicka, 1994; Staniek, Doutremepuich, Schmitt, Claudy, & Misery, 1999; Staniek et al., 1997). VIP stimulates cell proliferation of cultured keratinocytes (Haegerstrand, Jonzon, Dalsgaard, & Nilsson, 1989). SP modulates IL-1 and IL-8 production in keratinocytes (Viac et al., 1996) and tumor necrosis factor-alpha (TNF_{α}) release from skin mast cells (Okayama, Ono, Nakazawa, Church, & Mori, 1998). SP also stimulates the expression of high levels of vascular cellular adhesion molecule-1 by dermal microvascular endothelial cells (Scholzen et al., 1998). Both SP and CGRP have been demonstrated to modulate leukocyte infiltration into skin during allergic contact dermatitis (Goebeler, Henseleit, Roth, & Sorg, 1994). CGRP is capable of stimulating dermal microvascular endothelial cells to secrete IL-8 (Scholzen et al., 1998) and inhibits the antigen-presenting capacity of Langerhans cells and macrophages (Hosoi et al., 1993; Scholzen et al., 1998; Torii, Hosoi, Asahina, & Granstein, 1997).

The effects of CGRP on Langerhans cells function have been examined using (1) in vitro alloantigen presentation; (2) specific protein presentation to a responsive T cell line; and (3) ability of enriched Langerhans cells to present tumor-associated antigens for induction and elicitation of DTH response in tumor-immune mice (Hosoi et al., 1993; Torii et al., 1997a). CGRP inhibits antigen presentation by Langerhans cells in all three assays. Intradermally administered CGRP suppresses the induction of contact hypersensitivity to a hapten applied to the injection site, whereas systemic treatment with capsaicin increases contact and DTH reactions (Girolomoni & Tigelaar, 1990; G. Nilsson & Ahlstedt, 1989; Wallengren, Ekman, & Möller, 1991). These studies support the concept that CGRP is an endogenous modulator of immune function in the skin and suggest that CGRP or analogs/inhibitors might have therapeutic value in skin disorders and in inflammation.

Mechanisms through which CGRP suppresses DTH responses have been investigated. Intracellular cAMP is significantly increased in freshly prepared Langerhans cells after exposure to CGRP, an effect that is prevented by a specific CGRP receptor antagonist. In the Langerhans cell-like line, XS52, lipopolysaccharide (LPS)- and granulocyte-macrophage colony-stimulating factor (GM-CSF)-induced B7-2 expression is suppressed by CGRP (Asahina, Hosoi, Grabbe, & Granstein, 1995). Similar effects of CGRP on GM-CSF-induced B7-2 expression occur in LPS-stimulated peritoneal macrophages, perhaps accounting for, at least in part, the inhibitory effects of CGRP. CGRP also modulates synthesis and release of cytokines by Langerhans cells (Asahina et al., 1995). CGRP potentiates LPS- and GM-CSF-induced expression of IL-10 but suppresses the expression of IL-1β by Langerhans cells (Torii, Hosoi, Beissert, et al., 1997). The suppressive effect of CGRP on B7-2 expression by Langerhans cells is blocked by neutralizing antibodies to IL-10. IL-10 also prevents CGRP-induced suppression of epidermal cell presentation of tumor-associated antigens (from the S1509a spindle cell carcinoma) for elicitation of DTH in S1509a-immune mice. Collectively, these findings suggests that suppression of the antigen-presenting function by CGRP is mediated, at least in part, by changes in cytokine expression that favor less robust antigen presentation for cell-mediated immunity.

Intraepidermal nerve endings also contact melanocytes in human skin (Hara et al., 1996). Nerves that are not cholinergic or sympathetic also have been reported to contact melanocytes in the rabbit choroid (Sugita, Yoshioka, & Okita, 1983). At the ultrastructural level, thickenings of apposing plasma membranes between melanocytes and nerve fibers are present, similar to synaptic contacts seen in nervous tissue. In functional studies CGRP stimulates an increase in the rate of DNA synthesis of cultured melanocytes that is both time- and dose-dependent. By day 5 after CGRP addition to the cultures, cell yields are increased 25% over control cultures maintained in an otherwise optimized medium. Stimulation by CGRP induces rapid and dose-dependent accumulation of intracellular cAMP, suggesting that the mitogenic stimulatory effect is mediated by the cAMP pathway.

Similarly, CGRP, VIP, peptide histidine methionine, and growth hormone releasing hormone stimulate a rapid and marked formation of intracellular cAMP in cultured human keratinocytes in a dose-dependent manner, associated with stimulation of adenylate cyclase and the presence of guanosine 5′-triphosphate (GTP) (Takahashi, Nakanishi, & Imamura, 1993) Furthermore, these peptides stimulate DNA synthesis and proliferation in a human keratinocyte cell line in a dose-dependent manner. NPY inhibits forskolin-induced cAMP accumulation in keratinocytes, an effect that is completely eliminated by pretreating cultured keratinocytes with glucocorticoid.

3. *Other Mucosal Lymphoid Tissues*

The nerve distribution in mucosal-associated tissue is similar to that found in other lymphoid organs. In the conjunctival lymph follicles from cynomolgus monkeys (Ruskell & VanderWerf, 1997), fine nerve branches enter the follicle parenchyma. Sensory nerve endings branch into fine reticular fibers. Many of these fibers have been identified as autonomic based on their morphology. Few terminals directly contact lymphocytes, and none are found in germinal centers. Some fibers in the follicles associate with the epithelium. With lesions of the conjunctiva, nerves in the follicles display degenerative changes, and lose their association with the epithelium.

Confocal laser scanning microscopy from single focal planes reveals apparent contacts between thin, varicose nerves and immunocompetent cell in dental pulp from rats (Okiji et al., 1997). Close associations are most frequently seen in the para-odontoblastic region of the coronal pulp, where more than 70% and 50% of class II antigen-presenting $OX6^{+}$ cells show proximity to $CGRP^{+}$ and SP nerves, respectively. $ED2^{+}$ macrophages less frequently associate closely with nerves.

III. RELATIONSHIP OF NERVES WITH MAST CELLS

Mast cells reside in tissues throughout the body, particularly in connective tissue associated with blood vessels and nerves, and along surfaces that interface the external environment. Mast cells are bone marrow-derived and depend on stem cell factor for survival. Biological functions of mast cells are thought to include a role in innate immunity, involvement in host defense mechanisms against parasitic infestations, modulation of the immune system, and tissue repair and angiogenesis (reviewed by Metcalfe, Baram, & Mekori, 1997).

Investigators using immunocytochemisty have reported transmitter-specific nerve fibers in close contact with mast cells in a variety of tissues (Bellinger et al., 1990; Crivellato, Damiani, Mallardi, & Travan, 1991; Dimitriadou et al., 1994; Egan et al., 1998; Elitsur, Luk, Colberg, Gesell, Dosescu, & Moshier, 1994; Lorton et al., 1990; Stead, Tomioka, et al., 1987, 1989; Sung et al., 1991). This has been confirmed at the ultrastructural level. Unmyelinated SP^{+} and $CGRP^{+}$ nerve fibers are contacted by mast cells that possess lamellipodia that wrap around and enclose the fibers (Keith, Jin, & Saban, 1995). Numerous studies provide support not only for close contacts between nerve fibers and mast cells, but also suggest coordinated changes in mast cell number and nerve densities with development of inflammatory responses. Stead and co-workers (Stead, Tomioka, et al., 1987) have reported that changes in mast cell numbers in the lamina propria correlate with changes in nerve fiber densities that occur during the course of the infection. In lamina propria of the jejunal intestinal mucosa from uninfected mice, $47 \pm 4\%$ of the IMMC directly appose neuron-specific enolase-containing nerve fibers (Stead, Tomioka, et al., 1987). In contrast, there is a significantly greater number of IMMCs apposed to the nerves in the lamina propria ($67 \pm 4\%$) from animals sacrificed 35 days after nematode infection (Stead, Tomioka, et al., 1987).

Similarly, in "normal" human intestinal specimens, 40 to 77% of mucosal mast cells are apposed to PGP 9.5-immunoreactive nerves (Stead et al., 1989). In the dog colon, $70.77 \pm 3.43\%$ and $13.51 \pm 2.36\%$ of the IMMCs are closely associated with nerves in the luminal and basal regions of the mucosa, respectively. Electron microscopic evaluation of rodent and human intestinal specimens reveal frequent degenerating axonal profiles adjacent to mast cells that appear to be degranulating or regranulating (Stead et al., 1989), a phenomenon that becomes more pronounced in rats during acute infection.

In the rat lung and spleen, nerve fibers closely associated with mast cells appear to be nonmyelinated C fibers, since they are destroyed by neonatal treatment with capsaicin (Dimitriadou et al., 1994). Capsaicin treatment markedly increases the number of mast cells in the lung and spleen (Dimitriadou et al., 1994). Similarly, the number of mast cells present among SP, CGRP, VIP, and NPY nerve fibers in the lacrimal gland appears to depend on the density of these nerve fibers (Sung et al., 1991). With aging, a large increase in mast cells has been observed in 24-month-old compared with 3–5- month-old rats in lacrimal glands that is associated with a decrease in innervation. The loss of innervation is particularly associated with damage to the gland (chronic inflammation), and may contribute to reduced tear output in aging (Sung et al., 1991).

One explanation for the apparent correlation between numbers of tissue mast cells and density of innervation may be the increase in NGF that occurs within tissues at sites of inflammation (G. Nilsson et al., 1997). During an inflammatory response, nerve fibers are damaged and degenerate. This loss of innervation is coupled with an increased production of tissue NGF. Rodent mast cells proliferate in the presence of NGF. Mast cells express functional TrkA and synthesize NGF, suggesting a mechanism by which NGF may act in an autocrine fashion in mast cells, and by which mast cells and nerves may interact (G. Nilsson et al., 1997).

Studies have indicated that coordinated changes in mast cell and nerve densities may play a role in disease processes. In the dermal lesions of prurigo nodularis, increases in histamine-containing mast cell number and the number of NGF receptor$^+$ nerve fibers have been reported (Liang, Marcusson, Jacobi, Haak-Frendscho, & Johansson, 1998). Mast cell size also increases and the shape is more dendritic. Mast cells are in close proximity to NGF receptor$^+$ nerves. Similarly, a 130% increase in mast cell density in the superficial oral buccal mucosa in patients with oral lichen planus compared with normal oral buccal mucosa is accompanied by an approximate twofold increase in nerve-mast cell associations (Zhao, Savage, Pujic, & Walsh, 1997). These studies suggest that increases in mast cell numbers and their association with nerve fibers regulate lesional cell populations, and subsequently play a secondary role in immune responses once this becomes established.

Mast cells have received a great deal of attention as potential targets for neural signals. Functional studies indicate that SP can induce release of histamine from mast cells (Skofitsch, Savitt, & Jacobowitz, 1985). Neonatal capsaicin treatment also suppresses the ability of a histamine H_3 receptor antagonist to enhance histamine synthesis in mast cells from infected organs. These findings suggest that neuropeptide-containing nerves are involved in histamine metabolism in mast cells. This local neuron-mast cell feedback loop is likely to play a significant role in processes such as neurogenic inflammation, since this loop still functions when mast cells proliferate in an inflammatory condition.

IV. NERVE REMODELING AND PLASTICITY IN LYMPHOID TISSUE

Nerves in peripheral tissues are generally thought to be stable unless they receive a direct insult; however, it is clear that neurons depend on trophic factors produced by their targets to maintain innervation. Disturbances in homeostasis in lymphoid tissues often result in changes in neurotransmitter turnover, or a more dramatic remodeling of nerves that distribute to them. The integrity of nerves in lymphoid organs change over the life span of an individual (Ackerman, Felten, Bellinger, & Felten, 1987; Ackerman et al., 1991; Bellinger et al., 1987, 1988; Bellinger, Ackerman, et al., 1989, 1992; Felten, Bellinger, Collier, Coleman, & Felten, 1987), with normal physiological events (Kendall et al., 1994), following immune activation (Novotny & Hsu, 1993; Novotny, Heuer, Schottelndreier, & Fleisgarten, 1994; Yang, Wang, & Huang, 1998), in response to disease states (Bellinger, Lorton, Felten, & Felten, 1992; Bracci-Laudiero, Aloe, Stenfors, Theodorsson, & Lundeberg, 1998; S.Y. Felten, Felten, Bellinger, & Olschowka, 1992; Levine, Dardick, Roizen, Helms, & Basbaum, 1986; Levine, Goetzl, & Basbaum, 1991; Lorton, Lubahn, Felten, & Bellinger, 1997; Lubahn, Almond, Zhu, Hoffman, & Lorton, 1997, 1999; Lubahn & Lorton, 1998; Mitchell et al., 1997; Stead, Kosecka-Janiszewska, Oestreicher, Dixon, & Bienenstock, 1991), and with injury, inflammatory, and reparative processes. Given the vast literature demonstrating neural-immune signaling, changes in nerve density and state of activity has consequences for the vigor of immune responses, recovery from injury, and disease outcome.

Mechanisms for changes in neurotransmitter content in lymphoid organs have not been thoroughly investigated at present. Decreased NA or peptidergic innervation could result from an increase in target tissue volume, decreased production of neurotransmitter via regulation of TH or neuropeptide mRNA expression, decreased turnover, or destruction of nerve terminals due to loss of trophic factors, production of toxic products by immune cells, or reactive oxygen intermediates from breakdown products of catecholamines. Few studies have examined the mechanisms for decreases in innervation of lymphoid organs in the conditions indicated above; however, there is some indication that each of the above proposed mechanisms does occur in at least some cases. An increase in the volume of lymphoid organs results in decreased availability of neurotransmitters in the absence of nerve fiber sprouting, whereas a decrease in the volume of lymphoid organs causes an increase in the density of nerve terminals and availability of NE. These conditions have been described for primary and secondary lymphoid organs with aging, and during the onset of some autoimmune diseases (Bellinger et al., 1988; Breneman, Moynihan, Grota, Felten, & Felten, 1993; Lorton et al., 1997). In support of the theory that activation of the immune system can alter neurotransmitter synthesis by altering expression of machinery for its synthesis, Friedman and co-workers (Barbany, Friedman, & Persson, 1991) have found that coculture of splenocytes with superior cervical ganglion neurons in vitro leads to a significant decrease in the expression of mRNA for TH.

A. Genetic Models

In severe combined immunodeficient (SCID) mice that are deficient in both B and T lymphocytes

(Bosma, 1992), the thymus consists of an encapsulated, uniform collection of epithelial cells (Mitchell et al., 1997). There is no distinction between the cortex and medulla, and a small number of cystic areas are apparent. At the ultrastructural level, nerve bundles consist typically of 15–30 nonmyelinated fibers and reside close to blood vessels and mast cells in the thymus from SCID mice. Immunocytochemistry for TH demonstrate that the perithymic fat is densely innervated with TH^+ nerves. The thymus is innervated with a higher density of NA fibers compared with normal sympathetic innervation of the thymus in BALB/c mice (Mitchell et al., 1997), from which SCID mice are derived. This apparent increase in TH^+ nerve density may reflect the diminished size of the thymus in SCID mice compared with their normal counterpart BALB/c mice. TH^+ nerves distribute in the capsular region, adjacent to the vasculature, in the thymic septa, and among the epithelial cells in the parenchyma of the thymus.

In SCID mice NPY innervation of the thymus is less dense than NA innervation but is overlapping with it. NPY^+ nerves are located in the parenchymal, capsular, septal, and perivascular compartments, similar to that seen for TH staining (Mitchell et al., 1997). VIP^+ nerves in the thymus from SCID mice are similar in density and distribution to VIP innervation of normal thymus from BALB/c mice (Mitchell et al., 1997). No SP^+ or leu-enkephalin$^+$ nerve fibers are present in the thymus of SCID mice (Mitchell et al., 1997).

In SCID mice 10 weeks following transplantation of bone marrow cells from BALB/c mice, normal morphologic features of the thymus were restored, but nerve fibers were undetectable with immunocytochemistry for PGP 9.5 or neurotransmitter markers in the thymus (Purcell & Gattone, 1992). However, 6 months after the bone marrow transplant TH^+ and PGP 9.5^+ nerves were restored to the capsular region of the thymus. Kendall et al. (Mitchell et al., 1997) have suggested that innervation of the thymus is regulated independently from its lymphocytic population. They suggest that the microenvironment of the thymus relevant to innervation is not altered by the deficit in lymphocytes.

Increases in the density of NA innervation of the thymus also have been reported in a genetic model for hypertension. Purcell and Gattone (1992) have reported that the density of sympathetic nerves in the thymus of the spontaneously hypertensive rat (SHR) at 2 and 12 weeks of age is significantly greater compared with the Wistar-Kyoto, F344, and Long-Evans strains. In the spleen from SHR rats, NA innervation is delayed until 2 weeks after birth, but thereafter rapidly increases in density to a greater extent than seen in the other strains by 12 weeks of age. By 24 weeks of age NA nerves regress to a level comparable with densities in the spleen and thymus of other rat strains.

Similarly, higher splenic NA levels are present in 7-, 11-, and 21-day old athymic nude mice (nu/nu) compared with normal thymus-bearing littermates (nu/+) (Besedovsky et al., 1987). Thymus transplantation or thymocyte injection into newborn nude mice results in splenic NA levels comparable with normal nu/+ mice. Collectively, these data suggests that cells of the immune system or their products can influence the density of neurotransmitter-specific nerve fibers that innervate primary and secondary lymphoid tissues, and that alterations in the cellular makeup of these tissues can result in altered innervation and neurotransmitter content in lymphoid organs.

The mechanisms by which immunocytes direct remodeling of nerve fibers is not entirely clear at present; however, lymphocytes and macrophages do produce trophic factors that are likely to play a role in the restructuring of innervation under different physiological conditions. This notion is supported by studies of NGF-transgenic mice in which secondary lymphoid tissues are hyperinnervated by NA nerve fibers (Carlson, Fox, & Abell, 1997). The extent of NA innervation corresponds to levels of NGF present in the tissue. Splenic innervation in NGF transgenics gradually diverges from controls during the first 2 postnatal weeks, with the greatest change occurring between postnatal days 13 and 16, when the splenic organization is reaching the adult pattern (Carlson, Johnson, Parrish, & Cass, 1998). In contrast, peripheral lymph nodes are hyperinnervated at an earlier age. Sympathetic innervation of mesenteric lymph nodes never diverge from the normal pattern. NGF levels in transgenic spleens were much higher than controls at postnatal days 1 and 2, when little innervation was present, and declined as the tissue matured, possibly because of NGF uptake by the ingrowing sympathetic nerves. Thus, it appears that immune tissues are capable of concentrating NGF, which in turn modulates the pattern of innervation by the sympathetic nervous system.

Trophic factors also play a regulatory role in maintenance of innervation of the cutaneous immune system. In transgenic mice that overexpress insulin-like growth factor II using the keratin promoter, immunocytochemical staining for PGP 9.5 at postnatal days 0 and 21 reveals markedly reduced innervation by cutaneous nerves of the hind limb to the skin, particularly in superficial dermis and epidermis; in some areas innervation is completely absent (Reynolds, Ward, Graham, Coggeshall, & Fitzgerald,

1997). The effect is greatest in the distal skin and increases with age. This effect is not due to a loss of dorsal root ganglion cells that innervate the hind limb. Insulin-like growth factor II is reported to be a sensory neurotrophic factor and is thought to inhibit terminal axon growth directly via receptors on sensory neurons of peripheral glia.

B. Physiological Events and Aging

Changes in neurotransmitter content and in the density of innervation in lymphoid tissues also occurs with normal physiologic changes and with aging. These changes are likely due to increases or decreases in tissue volume, altered turnover of the transmitter, and/or remodeling of nerve fibers supplying the lymphoid tissue. NA innervation of the rat thymus during pregnancy and the postpartum period has been examined by a sucrose glyoxylic acid method for localizing catecholamines and by high performance liquid chromatography (HPLC) with electrochemical detection. Fluorescent nerves decrease in number throughout pregnancy when there is an overall loss in thymic weight due to cortical involution. These changes are maximal by parturition. There is a dramatic increase in nerves between day 21 of pregnancy and day 1 after parturition, especially in the capsule and around blood vessels in the connective tissue septa. When the neonates are removed at parturition, thymic weight is rapidly regained. The increased number of nerves remains throughout pregnancy and the postpartum period, but does not parallel thymic weight changes. The mean concentration of NE in the virgin thymus is approximately $1063 \pm 107\,pg/mg$ protein. Levels remain similar during early pregnancy and increase significantly at day 16. Virgin levels are regained by day 21. Values peak after parturition but rapidly decrease over the next 3 days, and remain at or below virgin levels until day 28 except for a transient rise at day 10 postpartum. This study demonstrates that there are variations in both density of nerves, and in neurotransmitter content in the thymus during the course of pregnancy and the postpartum period. Changes in density of nerves and neurotransmitter content could influence thymic function during pregnancy and parturition.

A study in our laboratory has examined the NA innervation of the splenic white pulp in postpartum female rats. For 3 weeks following delivery, the splenic white pulp is reduced in cellularity and demonstrates a marked increase in the density of NA innervation. This increased density disappears following weaning of the pups, as cellularity is restored to the spleen. We consider this change in innervation density to be a remodeling of existing nerves to maintain compartmentation in the shrinking white pulp (D. Felten and R. Christie, unpublished observations).

Our laboratories have been interested in understanding the relationship between the sympathetic nervous system and the immune system with age. We have shown a loss of NA sympathetic innervation in spleen and lymph nodes (Ackerman et al., 1991; Bellinger et al., 1987; Bellinger, Ackerman, et al., 1989, 1992; Bellinger, Ackerman, et al., 1992), but not in primary lymphoid organs (Ackerman et al., 1991; Bellinger et al., 1988; Bellinger et al., 1992b) with increasing age. NE content in the 17-month-old F344 (F344) rat spleen was reduced by 25%, and by 50 to 70% between 24 and 27 months of age (S. Y. Felten et al., 1987). Morphometric analysis of histofluorescent-stained spleen sections revealed about a 70% loss in innervation by 21 months of age (Bellinger et al., 1987). Corresponding to this change, splenocyte β-AR expression was increased in rats between 17 and 27 months of age compared with 3-month-old rats, possibly reflecting a compensatory mechanism to increase cell sensitivity to the decrease in concentration of NE (Ackerman et al., 1991). These age-related changes in NA innervation parallel diminished cell-mediated immunity in the rat. Changes in innervation of lymphoid tissue with aging are summarized more extensively in chapter 8, in this volume.

In contrast to the decline in NA innervation of secondary lymphoid organs, the innervation of the thymus is maintained with increasing age (Bellinger et al., 1988). The thymus is one of the first organs to involute with the normal aging process (Boyd, 1932). This primary lymphoid organ reaches its greatest weight at puberty. Following puberty the thymus begins to involute early in adulthood. Thymic involution is associated with a decline in thymic hormone secretion that begins prior to the observed loss in thymic mass. The decline in the size and cellularity of the rat thymus also is associated with an increase in the density of NA nerve fibers in all compartments (Bellinger et al., 1988). NE content per whole thymus remains relatively stable from 3 to 17 months of age. When thymic NE concentration is expressed as NE per milligram wet weight, there is a progressive increase in NE concentration from 3 to 17 months of age, followed by a decline to a second plateau from 21 to 27 months of age. These findings are consistent with a maintenance of NA fibers within a collapsing thymic parenchyma. As the thymic parenchyma recedes, the remaining fibers are packed into a smaller volume, yielding increased

NE concentration in the remaining tissue. The decreased concentration of NE per milligram wet weight of thymus at 21 to 27 months of age may reflect an infiltration of fat, which is not innervated as abundantly as the remaining tissue.

C. Immune Activation

Some reports suggest that immune activation can induce changes in nerve fibers that innervate lymphoid organs, such as altered neurotransmitter metabolism, induction of the expression of neurotransmitters in the nerves, and promotion of axonal sprouting or neuronal degeneration. These findings support the hypothesis that nerve fibers supplying lymphoid tissues are not stable anatomical entities, but rather dynamic components of the lymphoid organs that are responsive to changes in immune function. Novotny and Hsu (1993) found reduced numbers of mitotic cells in the thymic cortex after antigenic stimulation that corresponded with an increase in the density of innervation along blood vessels and nonvascular innervation in the septa. Similarly, differences in nerve density in the medulla of draining lymph nodes are demonstrated in rats after antigen challenge with bovine albumin (Novotny et al., 1994). These differences are most pronounced 4 months after antigen challenge. At the ultrastructural level, the density of incompletely ensheathed axonal profiles in the parenchyma of the medulla increases, while the number of nerves associated with blood vessels do not change.

Yang and co-workers (1998) describe a significant increase in the density and distribution of GAP-43$^+$ nerve fibers, a marker for synaptogenesis, in spleens from mice immunized with a purified protein derivative of tuberculin, compared with control mice. In control animals, GAP-43$^+$ nerve fibers reside mainly in vascular plexuses, with minor extensions into the parenchyma of the inner zone of the PALS. In the immunized animals, in addition to denser vascular plexuses, more fibers appear in the outer zone of the PALS, the marginal zone, and the red pulp, sites where lymphoid cells reside. These results suggest that active nerve remodeling takes place in the primary and secondary lymphoid organs during an immune response. These studies also suggest that immunostimulation leads to functional activation of the autonomic nervous system through the immune system.

Neural remodeling may serve as a mechanism through which the nervous system regulates immune responses. Activation of the immune system can increase neurotransmitter synthesis/turnover of existing nerve terminals. The basal NE concentration in the spleen is inversely related to immunological activity (del Rey, Besedovsky, Sorkin, Da Prada, & Arrenbrecht, 1981). Following immunologic challenge, NE levels decrease (Besedovsky et al., 1979; Engels, Folkerts, van Heuven-Nolsen, & Nijkamp, 1987), which has been attributed to an increase in NE turnover. Besedovsky et al. (1979) also find that the magnitude of the reduction in NE levels is proportional to the magnitude of the immune response. In support of these findings, an increase in sympathetic nerve activity occurs after immunostimulation by intravenous treatment with LPS or IL-1β (Carlson, Brooks, & Roszman, 1989; MacNeil, Jansen, Greenberg, & Nance, 1996; Niijima, 1998; Saito, Akiyoshi, & Shimizu, 1991). Together, these studies indicate that activation of the immune system can alter neural outflow that, in turn, modulates immune functions.

TNF$_\alpha$ (Soliven & Albert, 1992), IL-1 (Hurst & Collins, 1994; Saito et al., 1991), IL-2 (Barbany et al., 1991; Zalcman et al., 1994), and IL-6 (Hurst & Collins, 1993) may mediate these changes in splenic NE concentrations after immunization, since these cytokines have been demonstrated to alter NE synthesis/release. Barbany et al. (1991) reported that splenocytes cocultured with dissociated sympathetic neurons can differentially regulate neurotransmitter gene expression (TH and NPY). IL-2 receptors are present on cultured rat superior cervical ganglion neurons (Barbany et al., 1991) and on dissociated rat and chick sympathetic neurons (Haugen & Letoumeau, 1989). IL-2 receptor mRNA and IL-2 protein are present in superior mesenteric-celiac neurons, and their expression can be enhanced by immune activation (Bellinger, Brouxhon, Henderson, Felten, & Felten, 1996; Brouxhon, Bellinger, Mukheraji, & Felten, 1996). Administration of i.p. IL-2 alters splenic NE concentrations (Bellinger, Brouxhon et al., 1996), and both IL-1 and IL-2 can alter NE release from the spleen (Bognar et al., 1994) (Dave Snyder, Medical College of Pennsylvania, personal communications). IL-1β administration given i.p. (Akiyoshi, Shimizu, & Saito, 1990; Shimizu, Hori, & Nakane, 1994) or centrally (Vriend, Zuo, Dyck, Nance, & Greenberg, 1993) facilitates release in the spleen by activating sympathetic nerves, and increasing sympathetic activity, an effect that is partly mediated by the activation of hypothalamic CRH neurons (Shimizu et al., 1994; Terao, Oikawa, & Saito, 1994; Vriend et al., 1993).

TNF$_\alpha$ can suppress catecholamine release from cultured sympathetic neurons (Soliven & Albert, 1992), and in vivo in the rat myenteric plexus (Hurst & Collins, 1994). TNF$_\alpha$ also can induce the expression of SP in sympathetic neurons (Ding, Hart, & Jonakait, 1995; Kessler, Freidin, Kalberg, & Chandross, 1993; Shadlack, Hart, Carlson, & Jonakait, 1993), an effect that is mediated via IL-1 (Ding et al., 1995) and leukemia inhibitory factor (Ding et al., 1995; Shadlack et al., 1993). Hurst and Collins (1993) have shown that IL-1β can modulate NE release from rat myenteric nerves, causing a biphasic, time-dependent suppression of evoked NE release that is delayed in onset and blocked by applying a neutralizing anti-IL-1β antibody or by preincubation of the tissue with an IL-1 receptor antagonist. Further, exogenously applied IL-6 alters NE release from the rat jejunal myenteric plexus in a dose-dependent dual manner, with lower concentrations increasing release and higher concentrations suppressing release (Ruhl, Hurst, & Collins, 1994).

Lastly, Watkins and colleagues (Watkins, Goehler, Relton, Brewer, & Maier, 1995; Watkins et al., 1994) have reported IL-1 receptors on a subpopulation of paraganglion cells embedded in the hepatic branch of the vagus nerve that mediate LPS-, IL-1β-, or TNF$_{\alpha}$-induced hyperalgesia. IL-1β-induced corticosterone elevation and hypothalamic NE depletion (Fleshner et al., 1995), IL-1β-induced conditioned taste aversion (Goehler et al., 1995), and IL-1β suppression of feeding behavior (Bret-Dibat, Bluthe, Kent, Kelley, & Dantzer, 1995) are also vagally mediated. These data suggest that paraganglionic cells are sensitive to circulating cytokines associated with immune activation and convey this information to the brain via the vagus nerve. Indeed, peripheral administration of LPS (which causes IL-1β release) induces intense c-fos activation in the nucleus tractus solitarius (Ericsson, Kovacs, & Sawchenko, 1994), where the majority of vagal afferents terminate (Cohen et al., 1992; Leslie, Reynolds, & Lawes, 1992).

In some cases neurotransmitters that are not normally observed under homeostatic conditions of the animal are observed in nerve fibers after an antigen challenge. Enzman and Drossler (1994) find that they can only identify SP and VIP in nerves in auricular lymph nodes from immunized mice (SP, VIP) and guinea pigs (SP). Recently, we found CRH and arginine-vasopressin-containing nerves in the thymus and spleen 12 and 24 hours after i.p. injection of human recombinant IL-2 into F344 rats (Brouxhon, Bellinger, & Felten, 1996). In vehicle-treated and untreated F344 rats, we were unable to detect CRH-immunoreactive fibers in the thymus or spleen. After treatment with human recombinant IL-2 (50–200 ng/rat, i.p.), CRH-immunoreactive nerves are transiently expressed in the spleen and thymus. In the thymus they appear in the interlobular septa (Figure 49), in

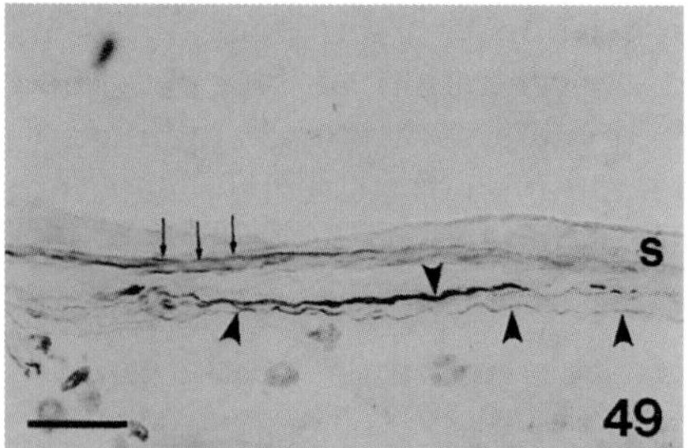

FIGURE 49 CRH immunoreactivity is present in nerve fibers (black) (arrowheads) in the interlobular septum (s) of the rat thymus 12 hours after i.p. administration of 100 ng of human recombinant (hr) IL-2, i.p. Several CRH$^+$ nerve fibers are closely apposed with mast cells (arrows). Single-label ICC for CRH. X43. Calibration bar = 100 μm.

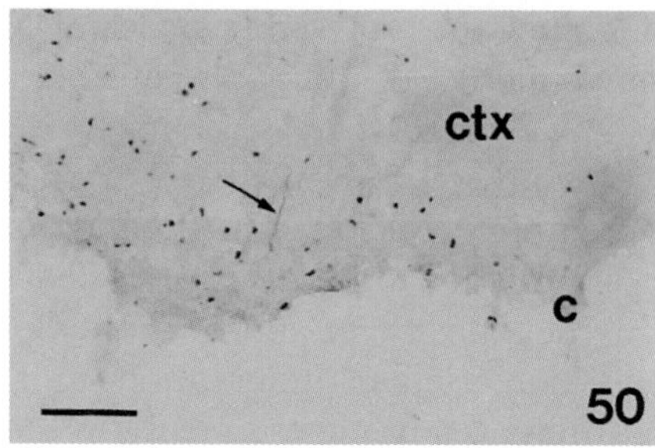

FIGURE 50 Twenty-four hours after IL-2 treatment (200 ng of hrIL-2/rat, i.p.), CRH$^+$ nerve fibers (black) (arrow) can been found in the outer cortex (ctx) of the thymus. CRH-immunoreactive cells also are present in the outer cortex. c, capsule. Single-label ICC for CRH. X43. Calibration bar = 100 μm.

the capsule, along the vasculature at the corticomedullary junction (Figure 50), and in cortical regions (Figure 51). In the spleen they are present in the hilus, and along the trabeculae (Figure 52) and venous sinuses (Figure 53) of the splenic red pulp. After administration of higher doses of IL-2 (2400 ng/rat, i.p.) CRF$^+$ nerve fibers can be found in the outer white pulp of the spleen (Figure 54). IL-2 treatment also induces the expresses of arginine-vasopressin$^+$ nerves along blood vessels near the hilus of the spleen (Figure 55), and overlaps the distribution of CRH$^+$

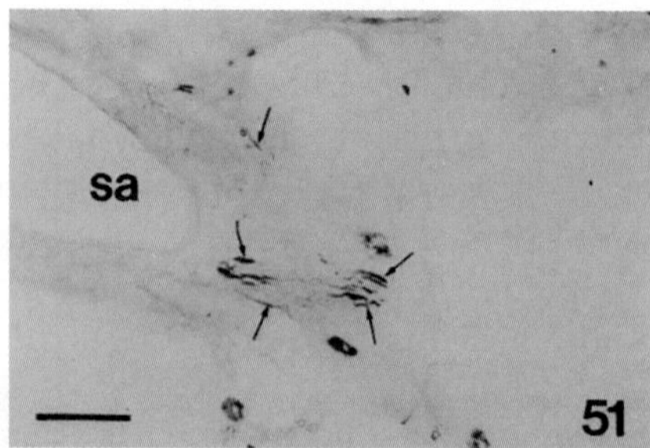

FIGURE 51 CRH$^+$ nerve fibers (black) (arrows) are apparent in the hilus of the rat spleen near the splenic artery (sa) by 4 hours after i.p. injection of 100 ng of hrIL-2. X43. Calibration bar = 100 μm.

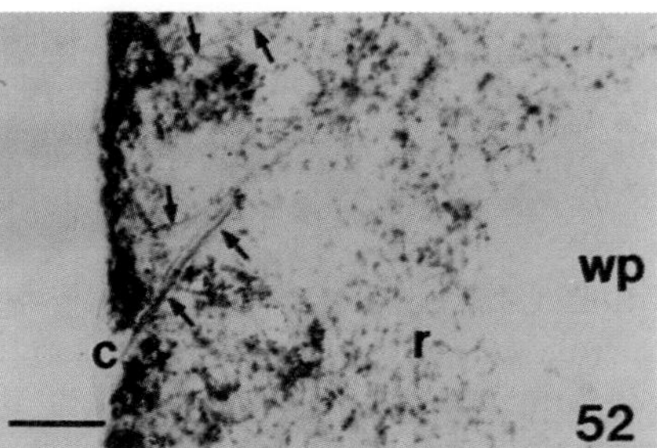

FIGURE 52 In the rat spleen, CRH$^+$ nerve fibers (black) (arrrows) are present along the trabeculae near the capsule (c) of the spleen 24 hours after i.p. administration of 50 ng hrIL-2. r, red pulp; wp, white pulp. Single-label ICC for CRH. X43. Calibration bar = 100 μm.

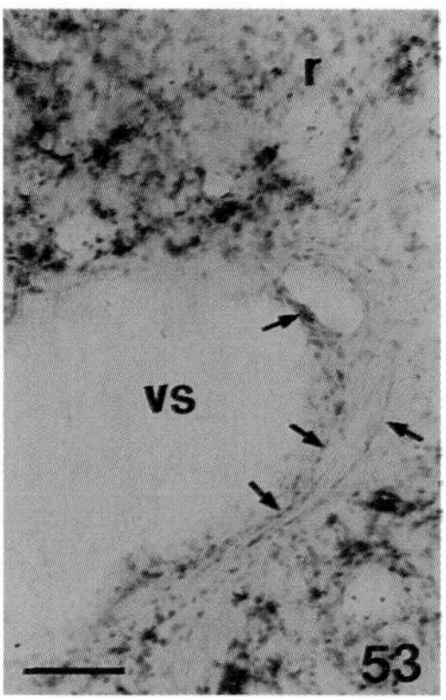

FIGURE 53 Treatment with hrIL-2 (50 ng/rat, i.p., 24 hours later) reveals CRH$^+$ nerve fibers (black) (arrows) along the venus sinuses (vs) of the spleen. r, red pulp. Single-label ICC for CRH. X43. Calibration bar = 100 μm.

FIGURE 54 At high doses of hrIL-2 (2400 ng/rat, i.p.) individual CRH$^+$ nerve fibers (black) (arrow) are occasionally found in the white pulp of the rat spleen. Single-label ICC for CRH. X43. Calibration bar = 100 μm.

fibers within the spleen. These fibers are likely to be sympathetic in nature, since we also found an increase in CRH immunoreactivity in the superior mesenteric-celiac and superior cervical ganglia at 12

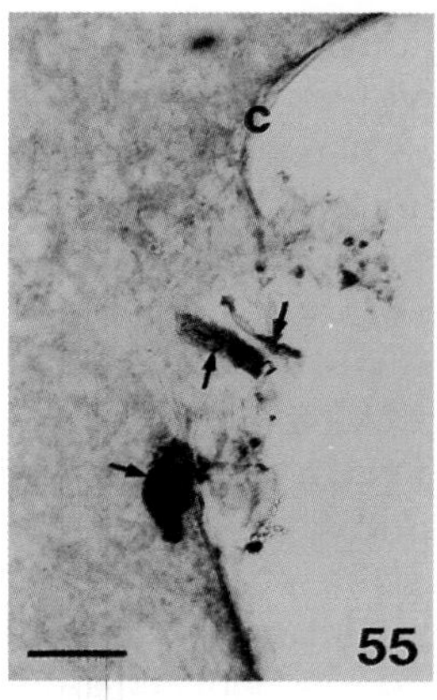

FIGURE 55 AVP$^+$ nerve fibers (black) (arrows) are present in large nerve bundles at the hilus of the rat spleen examined 24 hours after treatment with 50 ng of hrIL-2 (i.p.). c, capsule. Single-label ICC for CRH. X43. Calibration bar = 100 μm.

and 24 hours after IL-2 treatment, sources of sympathetic innervation of spleen and thymus, respectively.

D. Injury, Inflammation, and Reparative Processes

Changes in nerve fiber remodeling also occur at sites of inflammation and tissue damage. The restructuring of nerve fibers at inflammatory sites may be due to changes in distribution of their target cells. Studies have indicated that coordinated changes in mast cell and nerve densities occur in the gut mucosa, during progressive fibrosis; however, until recently there has been no experimental evidence to support remodeling of intestinal nerve fibers as a part of the disease process. In rats infected with the nematode *Nippostrongylus brasiliensis*, an initial loss of stainable intestinal mucosal mast cells occurs during an acute inflammatory phase (Stead et al., 1991). Following the acute inflammatory phase, mast cell hyperplasia occurs.

Using immunocytochemical staining for GAP-43, Stead and co-workers observed an initial small decrease in the numbers of GAP-43$^+$ nerve fibers per intestinal villus at day 7 postinfection followed by an increased number of GAP-43$^+$ nerve fibers per villus by day 49 compared with control rats (30% increase). Electron microscopic examination reveals GAP-43-labeled neurons with axonal dilation and degeneration. The early degenerative and later regenerative phases correlate with changes in mast cell densities that occur throughout the course of infection. Reported increases in expression of GAP-43 in the terminal fields of pancreatic nerves in chronic alcohol-induced pancreatitis also suggest that the innervation of human pancreases undergoes continual toposelective remodeling (Fink, Sebastiano, Buchler, Beger, & Weihe, 1994). An increased density of GAP-43-immunoreactive nerve fibers in enlarged nerve trunks of the pancreatic nerve parallels an augmentation in the expression of GAP-43 in intrinsic neurons and a reduction in parenchymal GAP-43^+ nerve fiber innervation.

Under conditions in which there is inflammation of the intestinal mucosa, the density of sensory and autonomic nerve fibers are altered. A few examples are presented here. In an experimental model of colitis in rats, hyperplasia of both mucosal SP^+ and NPY^+ nerves in regions with crypt abnormalities occurs, associated with an increase in the permeability of Evans blue from the lumen into the wall (Bjorck, Jennische, Dahlsrom, & Ahlman, 1997). In rectal biopsy specimens from patients with ulcerative proctitis/proctosigmoiditis, NPY^+ and TH^+ nerves markedly increase in number, and in a few patients there also is hyperinnervation of VIP^+ and SP^+ nerve (Bjorck, Dahlstrom, & Ahlman, 1989). Similarly, patients with celiac disease have an increased number of NPY^+ nerve fibers and significantly elevated tissue concentrations of NPY compared with controls (Sjolund & Elman, 1988). Lastly, Akesson, Ekman, Prytz, and Sundler (1998) examined esophageal hypomotility and abnormalities of the intestinal mucosa in systemic sclerosis patients. They found that CRH increases twofold, while tissue concentration of motilin, NPY, and peptide YY decreased by approximately 50% among patients with dysfunction compared with patients with impaired esophageal motility alone. HPLC characterization of motilin, NPY, and peptide YY revealed a different pattern of fragments among patients from these two groups. No change in NPY nerve frequency occurred in the intestinal mucosa in systemic sclerosis patients. Peptide YY, SOM, and motilin was present in cells of the mucosa, while the NPY immunoreactivity was present in neural compartments (Akesson et al., 1998).

Immunoreactivity of GAP-43 in the urinary bladder from rats with cyclophosphamide-induced acute cystitis was significantly increased in the muscle layer (Wakabayashi, Maeda, Aimi, & Kwok, 1998; Wakabayashi, Maeda, Tomoyoshi, & Kwok, 1998). PGP 9.5 was not augmented following this treatment. Double-label immunocytochemistry revealed that SP immunoreactivity was present in most GAP-43^+ fibers (90.2%) in the inflamed bladder. Some GAP-43^+ axons showed degeneration with electron microscopy. These data provide evidence for dramatic plasticity of nerve fiber innervation at sites of inflammation. These changes in innervation may occur in response to changes in the density of target cells with development of an inflammatory response. Further, neurotransmitter-specific changes also may occur within tissue undergoing an acute inflammatory response.

Interstitial cystitis is a bladder condition characterized by urinary frequency, urgency, nocturia, and suprapubic pain, occurs almost exclusively in women, and is associated with bladder mastocytosis (Sant & Theoharides, 1994). Almost 40% of these patients have irritable bowel syndrome (Koziol, Clark, Gittes, & Tan, 1993). Irritable bowel syndrome refers to a symptom complex with pain, bloating, and abnormal defecation (Farthing, 1995). In interstitial cystitis, there is an increase in the number (Larson et al., 1982; Theoharides et al., 1995) and activation (Theoharides et al., 1995) of bladder mast cells, and an elevation of methyl-histamine (a major metabolite of mast cell mediator histamine) (El-Mansoury, Boucher, Sant, & Theoharides, 1994) and mast cell enzyme tryptase (Boucher, El-Mansoury, Pang, Sant, & Theoharides, 1995). Further, there is an increase in bladder nerve fiber density in untreated patients with interstitial cystitis, specifically nerves that contain SP (Christmas, Rode, Chapple, Milroy, & Turner-Warwick, 1990; Pang, Marchand, Sant, Kream, & Theoharides, 1995). Accumulation of mast cells and increased density of SP^+ in bowel and bladders of patients with irritable bowel syndrome also has been reported (Weston, Biddle, Bhatia, & Miner, 1993; Pang, Boucher, Triadafilopoulos, Sant, & Theoharides, 1996). SP triggers mast cell secretion, and this action is augmented by estradiol (Sant & Theoharides, 1994). Bladder mast cells express estrogen receptors (Sant & Theoharides, 1994). Both syndromes (interstitial cystitis and irritable bowel syndrome) may have a common neuroimmunoendocrine bases, which may also explain why their symptoms are readily exacerbated by stress and during specific phases of the menstrual cycle.

IL-6-like immunoreactivity is present in the dermis and epidermis of normal skin, and in skin from patients with atopic dermatitis, prurigo nodularis, and positive epicutaneous patch-test reactions to nickel sulfate (Nordlind, Libing, Ahmed, Ljungberg, & Liden, 1995). In patch test skin, there is an increase in the density of IL-6 reactive nerves in the epidermis compared with normal skin, but no difference in the density of these fibers in the papillary dermis. There are clusters of IL-6^+ fibers in the dermis of prurigo nodularis lesions. IL-6 nerves colocalize with CGRP, and their presence surrounding the eccrine sweat glands suggests that IL-6 is present in autonomic as well as sensory nerves. SOM^+ nerves are not found in the skin of atopic dermatitis, whereas a normal pattern of immunoreactivity is detectable in most healthy subjects (Pincelli et al., 1990). SP^+ nerves are present in skin in most cases of atopic dermatitis, but not in normal controls (Pincelli et al., 1990).

The microenvironment is important is determining the extent of reinnervation into a target tissue. Korsgren, Jansson, Anderssons, and Sundler (1993) have shown marked differences in the extent and pattern of reinnervation of sympathetic, peptidergic, and $AChE^+$ nerves in transplanted pancreatic islets depending on the site of implantation (spleen, liver, or kidney). Sympathetic fibers sprout best into transplants in the spleen, whereas peptidergic (VIP, CGRP, SP) and AChE do not enter islet transplants in spleen or liver.

Growth factors and neurotrophic factors play a significant role in the response of the nervous system to injury and at sites of inflammation. NGF is necessary for the normal development of peripheral sensory and sympathetic neurons. Sympathetic and sensory neurons are responsive to NGF throughout their life spans. Drastic changes, including the loss of sympathetic cell bodies, are seen in adult animals autoimmunized against NGF, indicating that the maintenance of the functional and structural integrity of adult sympathetic neurons requires the presence of NGF.

Factors involved in the regulation of immune and inflammatory responses are able to influence nerve growth. IL-1 induces neurite outgrowth from murine superior cervical ganglia in vitro (Kannan, Bienenstock, Ohta, Stanisz, & Stead, 1996), and is important in peripheral nerve regeneration (Brenneman, Schultzberg, Bartfai, & Gozes, 1992). Application of granulation tissue, rich in $ED1^+$ and $ED2^+$ macrophages, to a peripheral nerve induces a conditioning effect; it enhances the regeneration capability of peripheral nerves after a test crush lesion (Miyauchi, Kanje, Danielsen, & Dahlin, 1997). This response may involve IL-1 production and release from macrophages; following peripheral nerve injury, the local synthesis of NGF is stimulated by IL-1 produced from infiltrating macrophages (Heumann, 1987). Other interleukins (Araujo & Cotman, 1993; Awatsuji, Furukawa, Nakajima, Furukawa, & Hayashi, 1993; Kashima, Hama, & Hatanaka, 1992; Keely Haugen & Letourneau, 1990; Mehler, Rozental, Dougherty, Spray, & Kessler, 1993; van Coelln, Unsicker, & Krieglstein, 1995), as well as GM-CSF (van Coelln et al., 1995), transforming growth factor-β (Poulsen et al., 1994), stem cell factor (Carnahan, Patel, & Miller, 1994), and leukemia inhibitor factor (Murphy, Reid, Brown, & Bartlett, 1993) have been reported to enhance nerve growth. Rat lymphoid tissue explants have neurostimulatory action when cocultured with rat superior cervical ganglion neurons (Kannan, Stead, Goldsmith, & Bienenstock, 1994).

Senapati et al. (1986) have reported significant depletion of the neuropeptides, SP, CGRP, and SOM, in regions of the skin undergoing wound healing, evident by 2 days after injury, and persisting for 2 weeks, possibly due to a loss of neurotrophic factors from immune cells in the skin. In support of this hypothesis, supernatants conditioned by LPS-stimulated XS52 Langerhans-like cells, and enriched murine Langerhans cells, can induce the differentiation of the pheochromocytoma line PC12 into sympathetic neuron-like cells (Torii, Yan, Hosoi, & Granstein, 1997). Most of this effect is due to IL-6 and a small amount is due to NGF and basic fibroblast growth factor, all of which are expressed in the XS52-4D cell line, and enriched Langerhans cells.

Many investigators have reported proliferation of terminal cutaneous nerves and the upregulation of various neuropeptides (SP, VIP, CGRP) in psoriatic lesions. NGF promotes growth of nerves and causes upregulation of neuropeptides such as SP and CGRP. NGF is detected only in keratinocytes in skin (Raychaudhuri, Jiang, & Farber, 1998). In psoriatic tissue the number of keratinocytes per square millimeter of epidermis positive for NGF is 84.7 ± 46.3 compared with 44.8 ± 29.9, 18.9 ± 11.8, and 7.5 ± 16.9, respectively, in nonlesional psoriatic skin, normal skin, and lichen planus (Raychaudhuri et al., 1998). Increased expression of NGF mechanistically explains the larger numbers of terminal cutaneous nerves and upregulation of SP and CGRP in psoriatic lesions. NGF is mitogenic to keratinocytes, activates T lymphocytes, and can induce migration of inflammatory cellular infiltrates, histological features that are characteristic of psoriasis. Recently, Staniek et al. (1999) reported overexpression of SP (NK_1) receptors on keratinocytes, suggesting a role for SP in the pathology of psoriasis.

Collectively, these findings support the view that use of growth factor mechanisms may counteract neurodegeneration. In animal models, the administration of neurotrophic factors can attenuate age-related and experimentally induced degeneration and behavioral deficits. NGF treatment may be useful in preserving and/or restoring sympathetic innervation in lymphoid organs in a variety of diseases and harmful conditions. For example, prenatal alcohol exposure selectively delays development of sympathetic innervation in lymphoid organs (Gottesfeld, Simpson, Yuwiler, & Perez-Polo, 1996). Chronic, but not acute, NGF treatment reverses the prenatal alcohol exposure-related deficits in splenic NE concentrations in a time- and age-dependent manner. Altered NE may play a role in immune deficits associated with exposure to alcohol in utero.

Pharmacological strategies in pursuit of therapeutic treatments may exploit the role of NGF on the immune system (Matsuda, Coughlin, Bienenstock, & Denburg, 1988). For example, NGF stimulates production of NPY in human lymphocytes from the human tonsil (Bracci-Laudiero, Aloe, et al., 1996); NPY is not detectable by RIA in unstimulated lymphocytes, but is induced after cell activation. Addition of NGF to the culture has a similar effect to that of mitogens, leading to the production of NPY. Only unstimulated T cells respond to NGF by synthesizing NPY. NPY synthesis is not seen in purified B cells treated with NGF.

Initially, most of the characterized actions of growth and neurotrophic factors on neurons have been related to developmental processes. However, it has become clear that growth factors also are important in the function of the adult nervous system and for maintenance of structural integrity and regulation of synaptic plasticity. These processes are altered in degenerative events following acute injury to the nervous system, prompting the speculation that growth factors are involved in the cascade of structural alterations in response to injury and disease. Insufficient neurotrophic factor functions could diminish the plastic capabilities of a neuronal system and reduce its functional adaptation to disease-related structural alterations. Alternatively, hyperfunction of growth factor mechanisms may induce synaptic malfunction or aberrant growth. In traumatic injury or loss of innervation related to inflammation or immune activation, changes in synthesis or release of growth factors may protect vulnerable neurons or alternatively may enhance the detrimental effects of the injury. Although many speculations have been put forward, at present only minimal data are available on the status of growth factors in nerve degeneration.

E. Autoimmunity

Changes in innervation patterns also occur with development of autoimmune diseases. In mice that develop lupus-like syndromes, NE content and the density of sympathetic nerves in the spleen and lymph nodes decline just prior to the onset of disease, a process that continues as the disease progresses (Bellinger, Ackerman et al., 1989; Breneman et al., 1993). Similarly, NE concentrations and nerve density in secondary lymphoid organs of adjuvant-induced arthritic (AA) rats also are reduced significantly compared with non-AA controls (Lorton et al., 1997). The innervation pattern of NA fibers of spleens obtained from AA rats 28 days after CFA challenge is similar to previous reports from our laboratories (D. L. Felten et al., 1985, 1987; Bellinger et al., 1987); however, there are differences in the numbers of these nerve fibers present in spleens from the different treatment groups. In AA rats (Figures 57, 59, and 63), there are fewer TH$^+$ fibers in regions of the spleen more distal to the hilus compared with non-AA rats (Figures 56, 58, and 62). In contrast, white pulp near the hilus of spleens from AA rats, the point of NA fiber entry into the spleens, appears to be hyperinnervated (Figures 60 and 61). Morphometric, biochemical, and immunocytochemical studies are underway to confirm whether there is a loss of NA nerve terminals distal to sites of nerve entry into the spleen with a compensatory sprouting response occurring at the nerve entry site with development of AA.

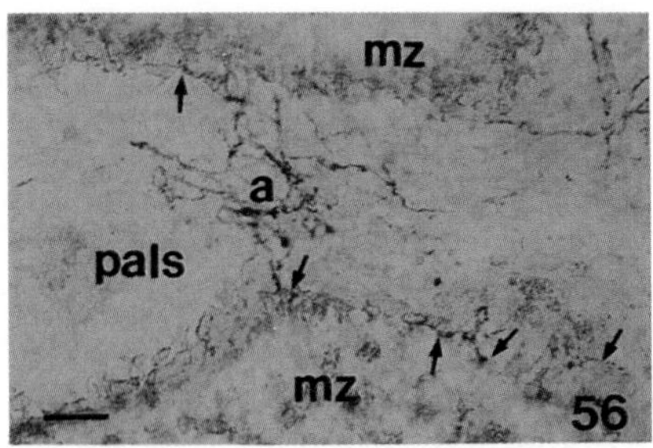

FIGURE 56 TH$^+$ nerve fibers (black) (arrowheads) course in the inner and outer marginal zones (mz) adjacent to ED3$^+$ macrophages (brown) (arrows) in vehicle-treated Lewis rats. a, central arteriole; pals, periarteriolar lymphatic sheath. Double-label ICC for TH and ED3. X54. Calibration bar = 100 μm.

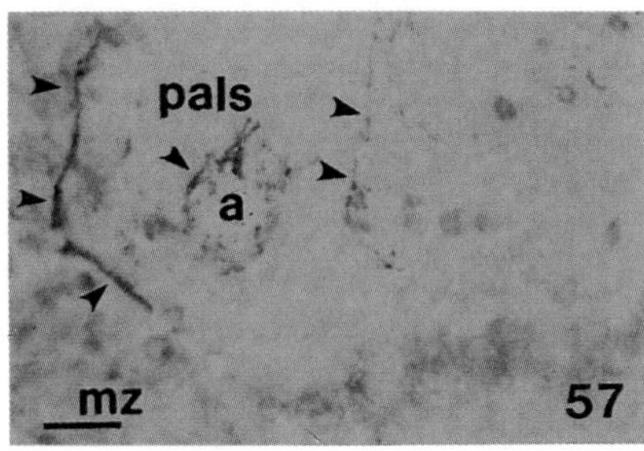

FIGURE 57 A region of the spleen distal to the hilus from a Lewis rat treated with CFA and sacrificed 28 days later reveals a decrease in the density of TH$^+$ nerve fibers (black) associated with the central arteriole (a), and coursing in the periarteriolar lymphatic sheath (pals) and marginal zone (mz). Double staining techniques also reveal a corresponding loss in ED3$^+$ macrophages (brown) in the marginal zone. Double-label ICC for TH and ED3. X78.5. Calibration bar = 100 μm.

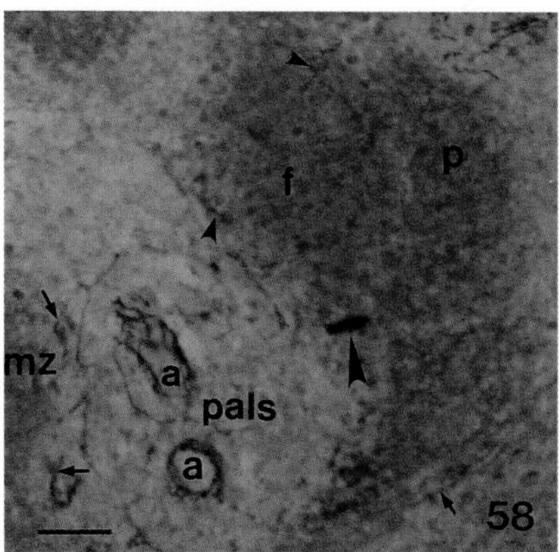

FIGURE 58 A region near the hilus of the spleen taken from a vehicle-treated Lewis rat demonstrates relatively robust density of TH^+ nerve fibers along the central arteriole (a) and in the surrounding periarteriolar lymphatic sheath (pals). In the marginal zone (mz) and the parafollicular zone (p), TH^+ nerves (arrows) are commonly seen in close proximity with IgM^+ B lymphocytes (brown). Occasionally TH^+ nerve fibers, in bundles (large arrowhead) or as free fibers (small arrowheads) are present in the follicle (f). Double-label ICC for TH and IgM. X82.5. Calibration bar = 100 μm.

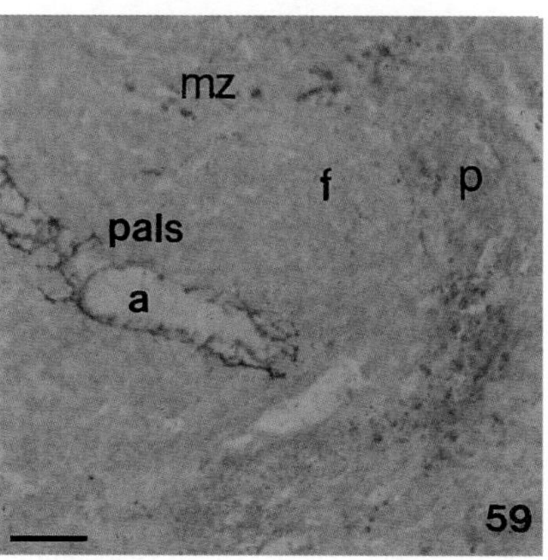

FIGURE 59 Slightly diminished density of TH^+ nerve fibers in the white pulp midway from the hilus and the distal regions of a spleen from arthritic rats is apparent compared with that seen in Figure 58. There is a dramatic decline in the density of IgM^+ B lymphocytes (brown) in the marginal zone (mz), parafollicular zone (p), and follicle (f) that occurs uniformly throughout the spleen in arthritic rats. a, central arteriole; pals, periarteriolar lymphatic sheath. Double-label ICC for TH and IgM. X82.5. Calibration bar = 100 μm.

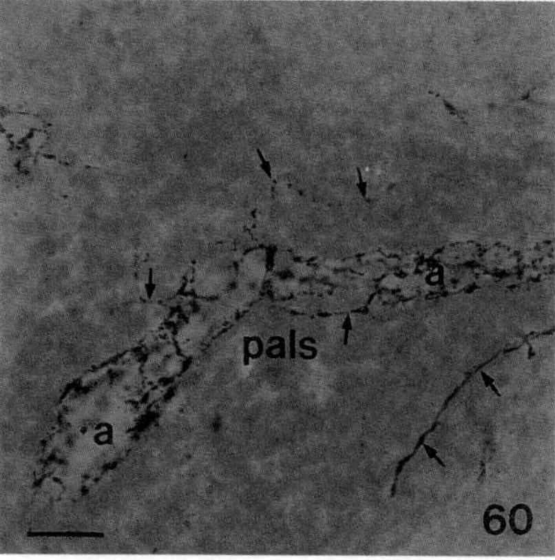

FIGURE 60 In a region near the hilus of the spleen from a vehicle-treated Lewis rat, a longitudinally sectioned central arteriole (a) is present associated with a robust TH^+ nerve plexus (black). $CD4^+$ T lymphocytes (brown) cluster around the central arteriole to form the periarteriolar lymphatic sheath (pals). TH^+ nerve fibers closely appose CD^+ T lymphocytes (arrows). Double-label ICC for TH and W3/25, a CD4 T lymphocyte marker. X82.5. Calibration bar = 100 μm.

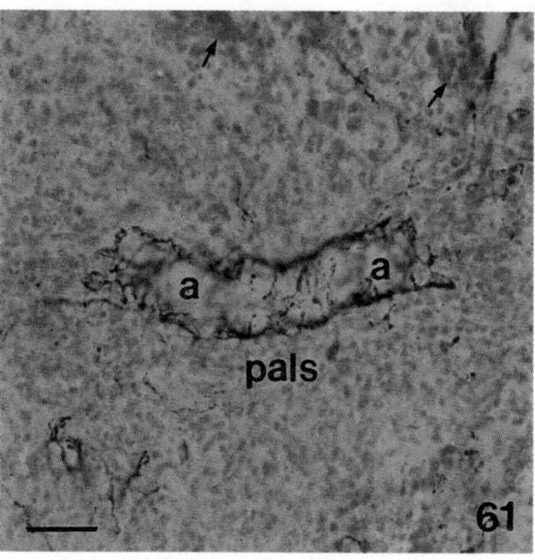

FIGURE 61 In the hilar region of arthritic rat spleens TH^+ nerve fibers (black) travel along the central arteriole (a), and are present in the adjacent periartiolar lymphatic sheath (pals). In arthritic rats there is a marked decrease in the density of $CD4^+$ T lymphocytes (brown) in the white pulp of the spleen, with prominent clusters of these cells in the marginal zone (arrows) and in the red pulp. This change in $CD4^+$ T cell density occurs uniformly throughout the spleen, and apparently is independent of the proximal-to-distal loss in NA innervation. Double-label ICC for TH and W3/25. X82.5. Calibration bar = 100 μm.

Double-label immunocytochemical staining in spleens from AA rats 28 days after antigen challenge reveals a dramatic loss in the density of $ED3^+$ cells in the marginal and parafollicular zones (Figure 57) compared with vehicle-treated animals (Figure 56). Similarly, a decline in the density of IgM^+ B cells occurs in the follicles and the marginal and parafollicular zones from AA treated rats (Figure 58) over that seen in control animals (Figure 59). $ED3^+$ and IgM^+ cell loss is most severe in white pulp where there also is a decline in the density of TH^+ nerves. CD4+ T cells also are depleted in the periarteriolar lymphatic sheaths in adjuvant-treated rats (Figures 60 and 61), but loss of the cell type occurs throughout the splenic white pulp regardless of whether NA sympathetic nerves are lost. $CD4^+$ T cells are most prevalent groups in small aggregates in the red pulp. In contrast, $CD8^+$ T cells are densely packed in the

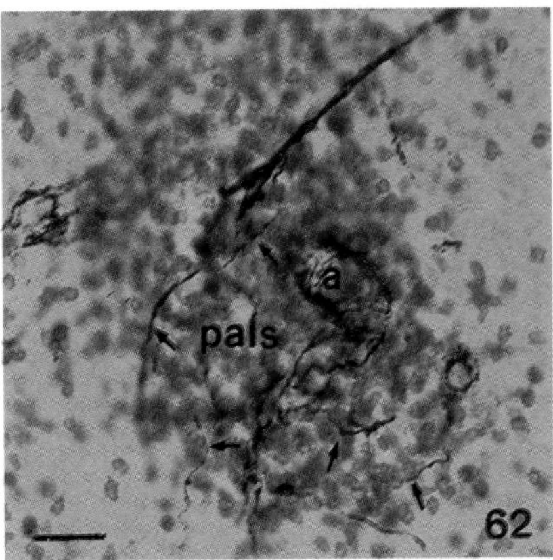

FIGURE 62 In the region of the vehicle-treated rat spleen that is distal to the hilus, TH^+ nerve fibers (black) form a dense vascular plexus along the central arteriole (a). Frequently, TH^+ nerve fibers exit this vascular plexus to end among fields of $CD8^+$ T lymphocytes (brown) in the periarteriolar lymphatic sheath (pals) (arrows). Double-label ICC for TH and W3/13, a CD8 T lymphocyte marker. X82.5. Calibration bar = 100 μm.

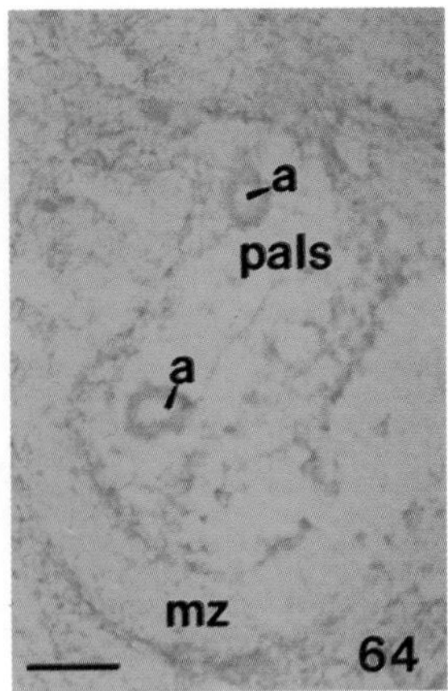

FIGURE 64 Nerve growth factor immunoreactivity (brown) is present in the central arteriole (a), in a reticular-like pattern in the outer region of the periarteriolar lymphatic sheath (pals), and in the inner and outer marginal zone (mz) in spleens from vehicle-treated rats. X43. Calibration bar = 100 μm.

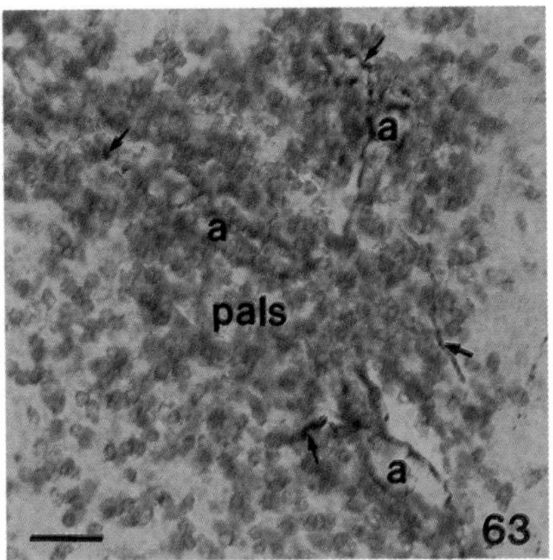

FIGURE 63 In arthritic rats the density of $CD8^+$ T lymphocytes (brown) in the white pulp of the spleen is similar to that shown in Figure 62. The loss of TH^+ nerve fibers (black) in the vascular plexuses and in the periarteriolar lymphatic sheath (pals) is apparent in this photomicrograph of a white pulp that is distal to the hilus. a, central arteriole. The disease-resistant TH+ nerve fibers maintain their close proxmity to CD8+ T lymphocytes (arrow). Double-label ICC for TH and W3/13. X82.5. Calibration bar = 100 μm.

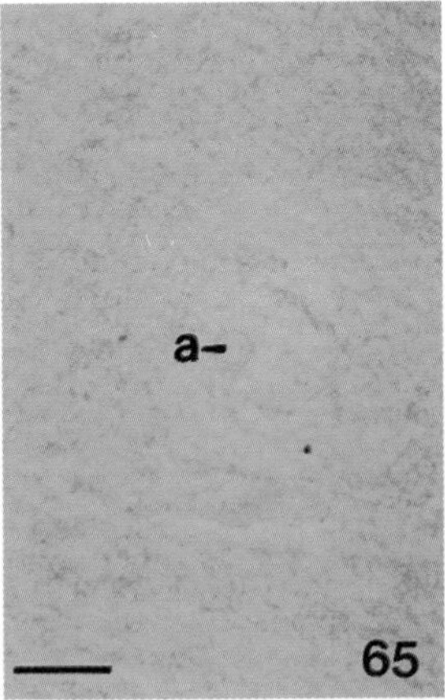

FIGURE 65 In the white pulp of spleens from arthritic rats (30 days after CFA treatment), nerve growth factor immunoreactivity (brown) is greatly reduced in the central arteriole (a) and in the compartments in which staining is seen in control animals. Additionally, staining in the white pulp is less clearly defined, with a loss of the reticular pattern of staining in the outer periarteriolar lymphatic sheath and macrophage-like staining in the marginal zone. X43. Calibration bar = 100 μm.

PALS, and their density is not affected by the development and progression of AA (Figures 62 and 63).

We have used immunocytochemistry for NGF to explore possible mechanisms for loss of NA nerve fibers with development of AA (Figures 64–66). Animals were challenged with CFA at the base of the tail to induce arthritis. Control rats were given a vehicle injection of the same volume. At 30 days after the CFA challenge spleens were harvested and prepared for immunocytochemical staining for NGF. In spleens from control rats, cells in the marginal zone, presumably macrophages, stained positive for NGF (Figure 64). NGF immunoreactivity also was present in a reticular-like pattern in the outer region of the periarteriolar lymphatic sheath, and in the inner and outer marginal zone (mz) in spleens when compared with negative control tissue (Figure 66). In contrast, although NGF immunoreactivity was observed compared with negative control tissue (Figure 66), most of the cellular staining in the marginal zone and outer periarteriolar lymphatic sheath was absent in spleens obtained from rats with AA (Figure 65). These findings suggest that NA nerve fibers that innervate the PALS may lose the

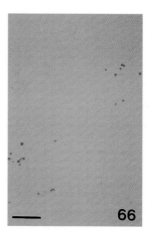

FIGURE 66 This photomicrograph demonstrates the lack of immunoreactivity in a spleen section used as a negative control for nerve growth factor staining (incubation with the primary antibody is not performed in these sections). X43. Calibration bar = 100 μm.

trophic support of NGF-producing macrophages that reside in the marginal zone as their density declines with the development of AA. Whether the NGF$^+$ macrophages migrate out of the spleen or undergo apoptosis with disease onset is currently under investigation.

Similarly, reports of altered neuropeptide-containing nerve fibers that innervate lymphoid organs of autoimmune prone mice have been reported (Lubahn et al., 1997, 1999; Bracci-Laudiero et al., 1998). Bracci-Laudiero and co-workers (1998) observed a significant decrease in SP, CGRP, VIP, and NPY content in the thymus of New Zealand Black/White (NZBW) mice with lupus-like syndrome at 8 months compared with New Zealand Black (NZB) and New Zealand White (NZW) control mice. They also found reduced SP and CGRP concentrations in the spleens of lupus mice compared with concentrations observed in the parental strains at 8 months. Despite decreased NA innervation in NZBW lupus-prone mice and the fact that NPY is colocalized with NE nerve terminals, an increase was found in the levels of NPY during the course of the disease for lupus mice compared with the NZW parental strain. The authors attributed the increased NPY concentrations in the lupus mouse spleens to increased synthesis of NPY by activated B and T lymphocyte (Schwarz, Villiger, von Kempis, & Lotz, 1994) in lymphoid tissue undergoing extensive lymphoproliferation. These authors further suggest that elevated NPY levels may be due to overexpression of NGF, which stimulates enhanced production of NPY by activated lymphocytes (Bracci-Laudiero, Lundeberg, et al., 1996b).

Our laboratories also have found changes in SP concentrations in primary and secondary lymphoid tissue from MRL-lpr/lpr mice compared with MRL-mp and BALB/c mice. Shortly after the onset of autoimmune disease (16 weeks) in the MRL-lpr/lpr mice, a significant decline in SP concentrations (expressed as micrograms SP per gram wet weight) occurred in spleen (Figure 73A). This decline likely results from the greater than four fold increase in spleen weight from 4 to 16 weeks of age. However, when splenic SP content is expressed in micrograms SP per whole organ, we find a striking increase in the amount of SP in the MRL-lpr/lpr mice compared with both the MRL-mp and BALB/c mice at 16 weeks (Figure 73C). At 16 weeks of age, SP concentration in the thymus from the lupus mice also increases significantly (Figure 73B, expressed as micrograms/wet weight). The enhanced SP concentration in the thymus appears to result from a 13% decrease in tissue volume between 4 and 16 weeks with disease development, since no differences were detected in SP content per whole thymus in lupus mice compared with MRL-mp or BALB/c mice (Figure 73D).

The large increase in total SP content in whole spleens from MRL-lpr/lpr mice at the onset of autoimmunity may be accounted for by (1) an increase in SP synthesis/turnover of existing nerve terminals; (2) sprouting by SP-containing nerve fibers in response to changes in the splenic architecture that occurs with disease progression; (3) induction of SP by cellular constituents of the spleen; (4) an increase in the synthesis of SP by cellular components of the spleen; and/or (5) an infiltration of SP$^+$ cells into the spleen. Immunocytochemical staining of spleen sections obtained from MRL-lpr/lpr, MRL-mp, and BALB/c do not provide supportive evidence for a change in the density of SP$^+$ nerves or SP$^+$ synthesis in nerves (Figures 67–72). The density of SP$^+$ nerves, and their staining intensity, is similar in spleens

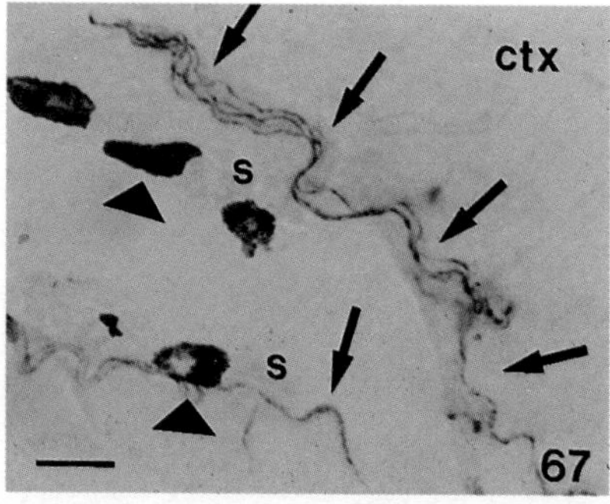

FIGURE 67 SP$^+$ nerve fibers (black) (arrows) reside in the interlobular septum (s) of the thymus from an 8-week-old MRL/mp mouse. Cells with the appearance of mast cells (black) (arrowheads) also are immunoreactive for SP. ctx, thymic cortex. Single-label ICC for SP. X82.5. Calibration bar = 100 μm.

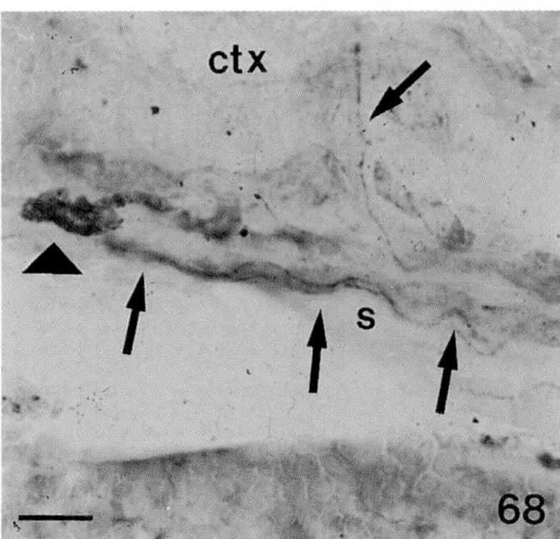

FIGURE 68 SP+ nerve fibers (black) (arrows) course in the interlobular septum (s) of the MRL/lpr mouse thymus at 8 weeks of age, often in close proximity with SP-immunoreactive (black) mast cells (arrowheads). The density of SP+ nerves, and the intensity of staining is similar compared with MRL/mp mice (see Fig. 67). ctx, thymic cortex. Single-label ICC for SP. X82.5. Calibration bar = 100 μm.

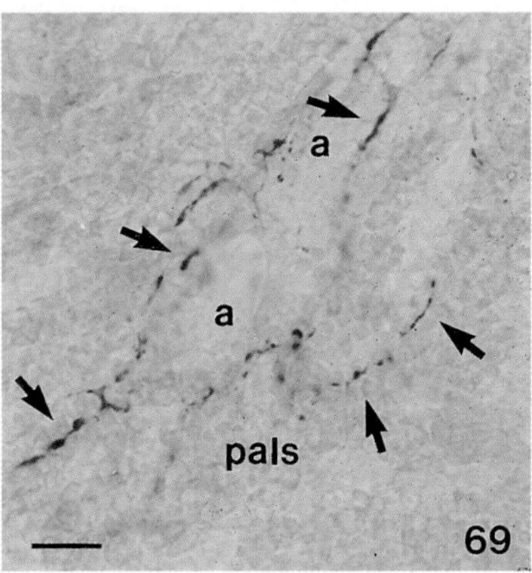

FIGURE 69 Along the central arteriole (a) in the white pulp of the MRL/mp mouse spleen at 8 weeks of age, a relatively dense plexus of SP+ nerves (black) (arrows) can be found. From this vascular plexus, SP+ nerve fibers (arrows) course into the surrounding perarteriolar lymphatic sheath (pals). Single-label ICC for SP. X82.5. Calibration bar = 100 μm.

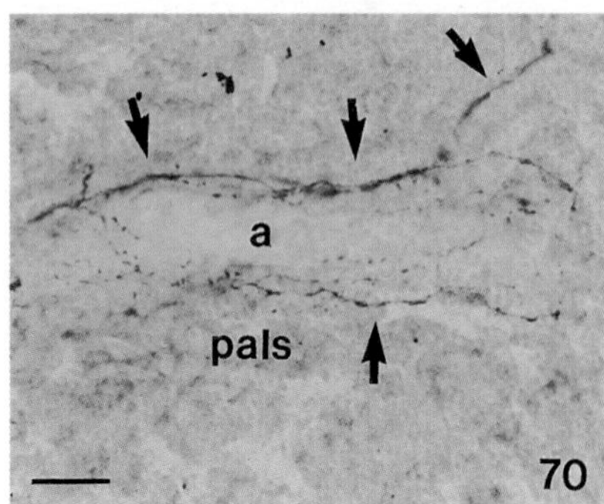

FIGURE 70 A similar density and distribution of SP+ nerve fibers is present in the white pulp of spleens from MRL/lpr mice compared with neural staining in the MRL/mp mice (see Figure 69). Single-label ICC for SP. X82.5. Calibration bar = 100 μm.

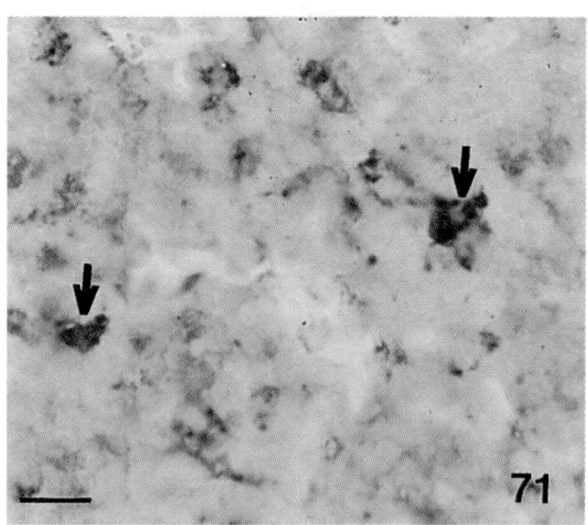

FIGURE 71 SP-immunoreactive cells (black) (arrows) are commonly seen throughout the red pulp of spleens from 8-week-old MRL/mp mice. Single-label ICC for SP. X82.5. Calibration bar = 100 μm.

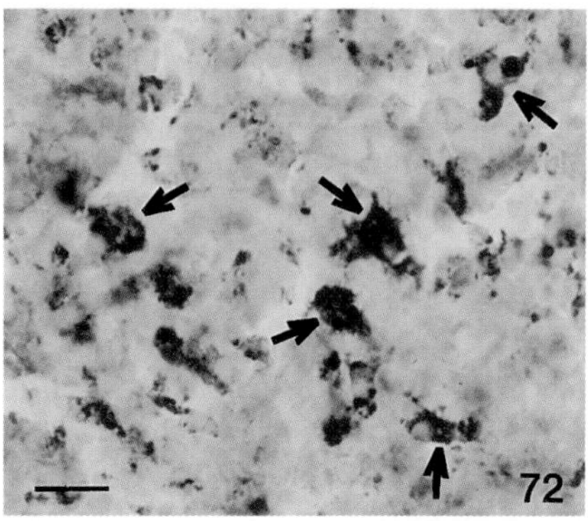

FIGURE 72 The density of SP-immunoreactive cells (black) (arrows) in the red pulp of spleens from 8-week-old MRL/lpr mice increase dramatically as the autoimmune disease progresses. Single-label ICC for SP. X82.5. Calibration bar = 100 μm.

(Figures 69 and 70) and thymuses (Figures 67 and 68) in MRL+/+ (Figures 67 and 69), MRL lpr/lpr (Figures 68 and 70), and BALB/c mice. Additionally we find a striking increase in the number of cellular components in the MRL-lpr/lpr spleens that immunoreact with SP. These cells are especially prominent in trabeculae and capsule, and in the red pulp and PALS of spleens from lupus mice (Figure 71) compared with MRL-mp mice (Figure 72). Collectively, these findings suggest that the increase in total SP content in spleens from MRL-lpr/lpr mice at the time of disease onset results primarily from changes in the cellular compartment of the spleen, and not from changes in SP innervation.

Nerve fiber remodeling contributes to the pathogenesis at sites of inflammation in several autoimmune diseases. In the inflamed kidneys of lupus-prone NZBW mice, the content of SP and CGRP is elevated at 5 months and NPY at 5 and 8 months. Studies with patients suffering from rheumatoid arthritis (Gronblad et al., 1988; Menkes et al., 1993; Pereira

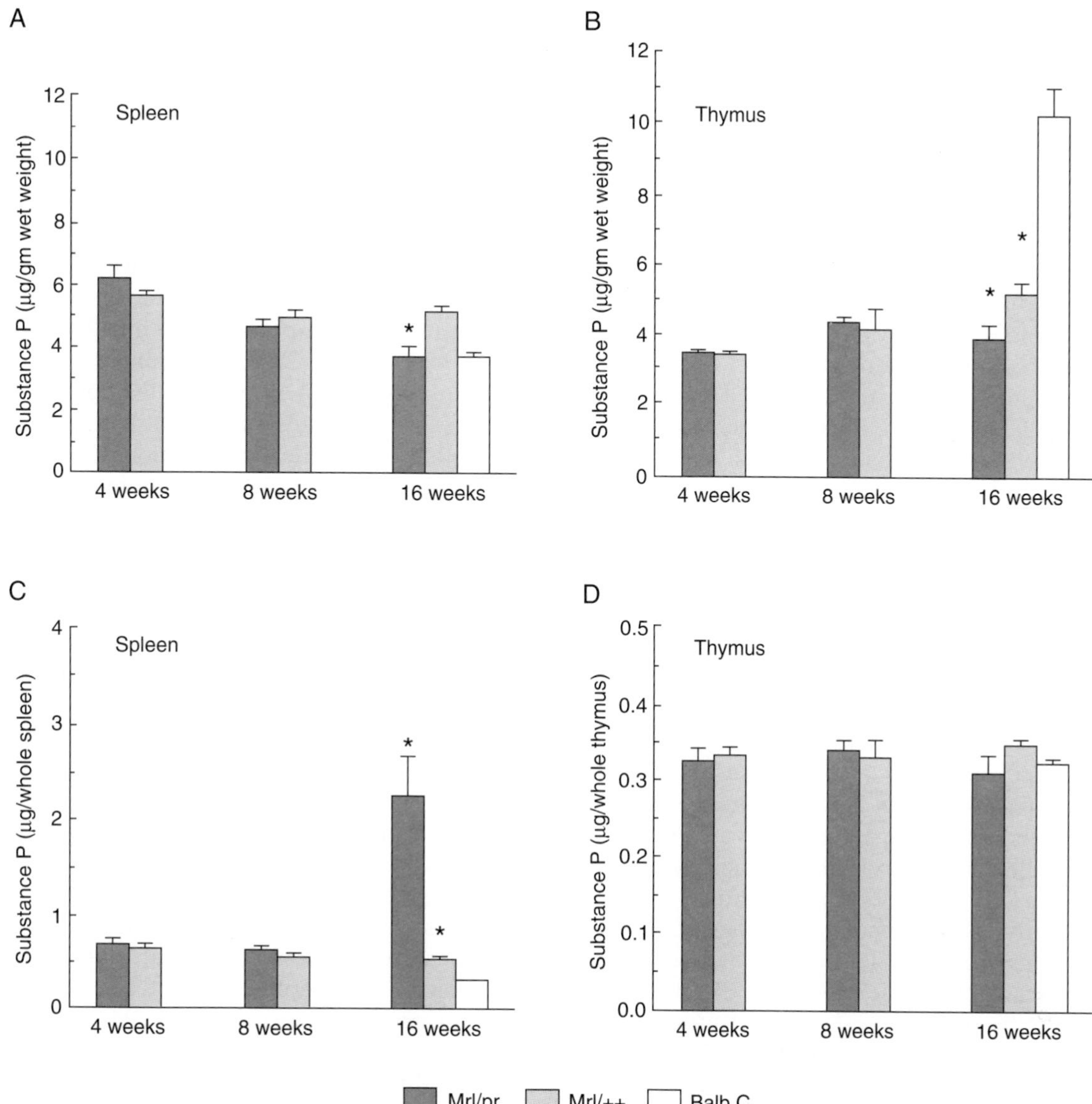

FIGURE 73 Substance P content in spleen (A and C) and thymus (B and D) from MRL-lpr/lpr, MRL-mp, and BALB/c mice measured at 4, 8, and 16 weeks of age demonstrates a significant decrease in SP concentration (A, expressed as μg/gm wet weight) in spleens from MRL-lpr/lpr by 16 weeks of age, the time of onset of lupus in these mice. In contrast, a significant increase in total SP content in spleens from MRL-lpr/lpr mice (C, expressed as μg/whole spleen) occurs between 8 and 16 weeks of age. These findings are attributed to an increase in spleen weight with disease onset, and changes in SP content in cellular compartments of the spleen. There also is a slight but significant decrease in total SP content in spleens of MRL-mp mice between 4 and 16 weeks of age. In the thymus, SP concentation (B, expressed as μg/gm wet weight) significantly increases in both MRL-lpr/lpr and MRL-mp mice between 8 and 16 weeks of age. This increase is attributed to a loss in thymic weight, since there is no difference in total SP content in the thymus (D, expressed as SP/whole thymus) during this time period. $n = 6$ to 7 animals per group. Analysis of variance (ANOVA) and subsequent Neuman-Keuls posthoc test performed when the ANOVA revealed significant differences ($p < 0.05$). RIA for SP.

da Silva, & Carmo-Fonseca, 1990) and experimental models of rheumatoid arthritis (Konttinen et al., 1990) demonstrate similar modifications in neuropeptide concentrations and neuropeptide-containing nerve density in the synovium of inflamed joints. NGF content within sites of inflammation are elevated (Bracci-Laudiero Lundeberg, et al., 1996), and may indicate a plasticity response by sensory and/or sympathetic nerve fibers at these sites. Collectively, these findings support a role for these sensory neuropeptides in the inflammatory processes in these autoimmune diseases. The changes in neuropeptide concentrations observed at sites of inflammation in autoimmune diseases as well as in the immunoregulatory organs strongly support a close interaction between the nervous and immune systems. The altered pattern of peptide synthesis and perhaps innervation could play a crucial role in the development of autoimmune disease.

The altered neurotransmitter concentrations observed in lymphoid organs from subjects with autoimmune diseases may be partly responsible for altered immune responses, and may contribute to the development of autoimmune diseases. This is supported by animal research (Colpaert, Donnerer, & Lembeck, 1983; Levine et al., 1984; Levine, Moskowitz, & Basbaum, 1985, 1988; Levine, Dardick, Basbaum, & Scipio, 1985) and clinical studies (Kaplan, Robinson, Scavulli, & Vaughan, 1980; Levine, Fye, Heller, Basbaum, & Whiting-O'Keefe, 1986; Vyden, Groseth-Dittrich, Callis, Lars, & Weinberger, 1971), which point toward involvement of the nervous system in autoimmune disease pathology. Denervation studies utilizing a variety of animal models for autoimmune disorders, including AA, New Zealand, and MRL mice strains as models for hemolytic anemia and lupus-like syndrome, and experimental allergic encephalomyelitis, a model for multiple sclerosis, support this notion. Sympathectomy with 6-OHDA in newborn Lewis rats exacerbates the severity of experimental allergic encephalomyelitis, whereas treatment with isoproterenol, a β-agonist, protects susceptible rats from developing this induced autoimmune disease (Chelmicka-Schorr, Checinski, & Arnason, 1988; Chelmicka-Schorr, Kwasniewski, Thomas, & Arnason, 1989). However, Colburn et al. (1990) have reported that administration of isoproterenol is associated with increased anti-DNA antibody titers in MRL-lpr/lpr mice, a measure often used as an index of disease severity. Similarly, chemical sympathectomy with 6-OHDA augments the severity of an animal model for myasthenia gravis (Agius, Checinski, Richman, & Chelmicka-Shorr, 1987). These studies suggest that peptidergic and NA activity in secondary lymphoid organs plays a role autoimmune disease pathology in susceptible animals.

Based on extensive studies by Levine and colleagues (Levine et al., 1984 1988, 1991; Levine, Collier, Basbaum, Moskowitz, & Helms, 1985; Levine, Dardick, et al., 1985, 1986; Levine, Fye, et al., 1986; Levine, Moskowitz, et al., 1985; Levine, Taiwo, Collins, & Tam, 1986), both SP and NE have been implicated in the expression of AA in Lewis rats. SP injected directly into the arthritic joint increases inflammation and joint destruction. Systemic denervation of primary sensory SP nerves protects the joint from inflammatory responses (Levine et al., 1988). Similarly, systemic depletion of NE by guanethidine or reserpine treatment diminishes the inflammatory response and arthritic changes in Lewis rats (Levine, Dardick, et al., 1986). In the collagen type II arthritic DBA/1 mouse model, Josefsson et al. (Josefsson, Mansson, Blennow, & Tarkowski, 1994) also found that systemic depletion of NE with 6-OHDA treatment suppressed the inflammatory response at the time of disease onset. We found a similar attenuation of inflammatory response at the time of disease onset with systemic 6-OHDA administration prior to immunization in AA Lewis rats (Lorton, Bellinger, Duclos, Felten, & Felten, 1996). These findings are consistent with clinical observations that propranolol, a β-antagonist, diminishes inflammation in patients with rheumatoid arthritis (Kaplan et al., 1980), and that regional sympathetic blockade with guanethidine reduces pain and enhances performance in patients with rheumatoid arthritis (Levine, Fye, et al., 1986). All of these experimental studies of rheumatoid arthritis and therapies in rheumatoid arthritic patients manipulate catecholamines or SP systemically or in the arthritic joints. Clearly, the tissue affected by rheumatoid arthritis, joint tissue, is innervated by SP and NA nerves, and would be expected to respond to these pharmacological manipulations as the end-point mechanism.

We have hypothesized that NA nerve fibers in secondary lymphoid organs where relevant adjuvant antigens are processed also contribute to the pathophysiology of experimental AA. To test this hypothesis, we examined the effect of 6-OHDA injections (0.5 mg total with $2 \times 4\,\mu L$ injections) into the fat pads surrounding draining lymph nodes prior to CFA challenge to induce AA. This procedure denervates NA nerves from draining lymph nodes and spleen, while leaving NA innervation of the joints and vasculature intact (Lorton et al., 1996). Rats receiving this treatment 1 day prior to CFA challenge displayed an earlier onset of inflammatory changes in hind limb joints and more severe inflammation and joint destruction at 27 days after CFA administration compared with changes in control CFA-treated animals (Lorton et al., 1996). These findings are consistent with the work of Chelmicka-Schorr et al. (1988, 1989) indicating that systemic sympathectomy prior to induction of autoimmune disease exacerbates the severity of the response. These findings are in contrast to the results of systemic manipulation (Levine, Collier, et al., 1985; Levine, Dardick, et al., 1985; Levine, Frye, et al., 1986; Levine, Moskowitz, et al., 1986) of NE in AA Lewis rats, and suggest that manipulation of NA nerves in relevant secondary lymphoid organs and joints may have directionally opposite effects.

During the course of autoimmune-related skin disorders, the neuroimmunocutaneous system destablizes, i.e., especially in psoriasis. Whether destabilization of the neuroimmunocutaneous interactions are secondary or are responsible for the induction and maintenance of the inflammatory process is unclear at present (reviewed by Misery, 1997). Analysis of neuropeptide-containing nerve fibers in such disorders reveals altered density of neuropeptide-containing nerves and concentrations of sensory neuropeptides within the skin. Ultrastructural analysis of skin with atopic dermatitis reveals a significant increase in the density of nerve fibers compared with uninvolved skin from these patients (Sugiura, Omoto, Hirota, Danno, & Uehara, 1997). The bulging of axons with many mitochondria and a loss of their surrounding sheath of Schwann cells suggest an active state of excitation. Additionally, pinocytotic vesicles in the periphery of basal keratinocytes facing nerve endings suggests a potential for reciprocal interaction between these entities.

The number of SP^+ nerves in the epidermis in biopsies from lesional skin of psoriasis and spongiotic dermatitis increases compared with nonlesional psoriatic skin and normal skin (Chan, Smoller, Raychauduri, Jiang, & Farber, 1997). But no difference in VIP^+ and $CGRP^+$ intraepidermal nerves in lesional psoriatic skin was noted, except in 5 of 36 patients (Chan et al., 1997). There is a report that denervation of a patient with psoriasis resulted in clearing of the psoriasis from the denervated area (Dewing, 1971).

In affected skin from vitiligo vulgaris patients, there was a reduction in the number and intensity of low affinity (p75) NGF receptor-immunoreactive basal keratinocytes, and an increase in the number of NGF receptor-immunoreactive nerve fibers (Liu, Bondesson, Lontz, & Johansson, 1996). The number of $CGRP^+$ nerves in the epidermis and papillary dermis dramatically increased in involved skin compared with uninvolved and control skin. No clear difference was found in the distribution of VIP^+ and NPY^+ nerve fibers. Collectively, these studies suggest that changes in the balance of neuropeptides innervating the epidermis play a critical role in the pathogenesis in autoimmune diseases that affect the skin.

V. SUMMARY

Lymphoid organs and tissues are comprised of a heterogeneous mix of lymphoid and myeloid cells residing in a reticular stroma that provides a supporting framework. NA, cholinergic, and peptidergic nerve fibers distribute to both primary and secondary lymphoid organs among cells of the immune system. Studies to determine the cellular targets of these nerves are currently in progress in several laboratories. This is a complex issue, since cells of the immune system may be targets only under certain conditions. Many of the cells in lymphoid organs are mobile, and may become targets of a set of nerves only when they have been activated or subsequently migrate into a site of immunological activity. Further, under certain conditions, nerves may be induced to express and release a neurotransmitter for which immunocytes express receptors.

In spite of these complexities, it is clear from previous extensive research that (1) specific compartments exist within lymphoid organs that subserve specific functions; (2) NA, cholinergic, and peptidergic nerves selectively innervate many of these compartments, and (3) neurotransmitters released from these nerves can influence specific functions of specific subsets of cells at these sites. Secondary lymphoid organs and aggregates of lymphoid tissue have T-dependent zones and B-dependent regions (generally nodules or follicles). Generally, there is a greater density of NA and peptidergic innervation of T-dependent areas, and only occasionally are nerve fibers found in B-dependent areas. There also are regions in lymphoid tissue, generally associated with blood or lymph sinus, that contain a mix of macrophages, B and T lymphocytes, and other cell types. These areas are often sites where antigen presentation occurs, and often are innervated densely, especially by NA/NPY-containing nerves.

A summary of the literature and new data from our laboratory showing anatomical associations between nerves and immunocytes in lymphoid tissue is described in this chapter. We assume that these associations form an anatomical substrate for direct neural modulation of the immune system, since many of these cells possess receptors for a variety of neurotransmitters that also are present in nerves in the lymphoid organ. We also have discussed evidence from the literature that is consistent with the concept that immune cell products, such as cytokines, lymphokines, lymphotoxins, and chemokines, can be released from lymphoid cells and modulate nerve terminal activity, viability, and neurotransmitter release. Additionally, these products can enter the circulation to provide feedback to the CNS. In fact, the distinction of what is a neurotransmitter versus. a cytokine has become less clear, since nerves can synthesize and release cytokines such as histamine, IL-1, and IL-6, and cells of the immune system can synthesize and secrete neurotransmitters or neurohormones, such as CRH, adrenocorticotropic hormone, beta-endorphin, VIP, SP, NPY, and NE. Some neurotransmitters have been found to have minimal effect on a particular immune parameter alone, but when administered in the presence of a cytokine were found to potentiate the cytokine influence on the immune response (Carlson et al., 1989). Thus, synergistic as well as countersynergistic modulation are likely to occur between neurotransmitters and cytokines, or between two neurotransmitters.

The neurotransmitters thus far described in nerves in lymphoid tissues all have vasoactive capability to some extent, and can modulate blood flow, perfusion pressure, blood volume, and cell trafficking. Changes in vasculature alone can influence cell traffic to and from the lymphoid organ. Additionally, specific neurotransmitters could directly interact with lymphoid cells to direct trafficking, as is the case for VIP in the GALT.

Neurotransmitter-specific nerves transmit signals to the immune system that are capable of altering immune reactivity. Dynamic changes can occur in sympathetic and peptidergic innervation in lymphoid compartments over the life span of an individual and under a variety of physiological conditions, with possible functional implications for lymphoid development and age-related senescence of the immune system. Studies described in this chapter indicate that the development of disease states, especially autoimmune disorders, depend on highly complex interactions between the nervous and immune systems at multiple sites (i.e., at effector tissues, at sites of antigen presentation and processing, and in the PNS and CNS). How nerves in lymphoid tissues respond to ongoing immune responses is important in determining whether the immune system can successfully eliminate the immunogen and return to homeostatic levels of activity. Aberrant nerve-immune interactions may precipitate and/or determine the severity of neurogenic inflammation and chronic inflammatory diseases.

Studies examining the mechanisms of action, routes of communication, and the neural and immune mediators involved in disease processes are currently under way. Anatomical studies will be important in this regard, since they provide important clues to neural and immune players in the disease pathology. The development of antibodies directed to signal molecules of nerves and immune cells has been an important tool, allowing investigators to examine the relationships of important mediators of immune responses in anatomically defined compartments during disease progression. These studies will provide critical information for a better understanding of neural–immune interactions in vivo. Ultimately, this line of research is likely to advance the development of unique pharmacologic interventions aimed at neural mechanisms important in immune-mediated disease processes.

References

Abrahamsson, T., Holmgren, S., Nilsson, S., & Pettersson, K. (1979). Adrenergic and cholinergic effects on the heart, the lung and the spleen of the African lungfish, *Protopterus aethiopicus. Acta Physiologica Scandinavica, 107*, 141–147.

Ackerman, K. D. 1989. *Noradrenergic sympathetic neurotransmission in the adult and neonatal rat spleen.* Unpublished doctoral dissertation. University of Rochester, Rochester, New York.

Ackerman, K. D., Bellinger, D. L., Felten, S. Y., & Felten, D. L. (1991). Ontogeny and senescence of noradrenergic innervation of the rodent thymus and spleen. In Ader, R., Felten, D. L. & Cohen, N. (Eds.), *Psychoneuroimmunology* (2nd ed.; pp. 71–125). New York: Academic Press.

Ackerman, K. D., Felten, S. Y., Bellinger, D. L., & Felten, D. L. (1987). Noradrenergic sympathetic innervation of the spleen: III. Development of innervation in the rat spleen. *Journal of Neuroscience Research, 18*, 49–54.

Ackerman, K. D., Felten, S. Y., Bellinger, D. L., Livnat, S., & Felten, D. L. (1987). Noradrenergic sympathetic innervation of spleen and lymph nodes in relation to specific cellular compartments. *Progress in Immunology, 6*, 588–600.

Ackerman, K. D., Felten, S. Y., Dijkstra, C. D., Livnat, S., & Felten, D. L. (1989). Parallel development of noradrenergic innervation and cellular compartmentation in the rat spleen. *Experimental Neurology, 103*, 239–255.

Afan, A. M., Broome, C. S., Nicholls, S. E., Whetton, A. D., & Miyan, J. A. (1997). Bone marrow innervation regulates cellular retention in the murine haemopoietic system. *British Journal of Haematology, 98*, 569–577.

Agius, M. A., Checinski, M. E., Richman, D. P., & Chelmicka-Shorr, E. (1987). Sympathectomy enhances the severity of experimental autoimmune myasthenia gravis (EAMG). *Journal of Neuroimmunology, 16*, 11–12.

Aguila, M. C., Dees, W. L., Haensely, W. E., & McCann, S. M. (1991). Evidence that somatostatin is localized and synthesized in lymphoid organs. *Proceedings of the National Academy of Science of the United States of America, 88*, 11485–11489.

Ahmed, M., Srinivasan, G. R., Theodorsson, E., Bjurholm, A., & Kreicbergs, A. (1994). Extraction and quantitation of neuropeptides in bone by radioimmunoassay. *Regulatory Peptides, 51*, 179–188.

Akesson, A., Ekman, R., Prytz, H., & Sundler, F. (1998). Tissue concentrations of gastrointestinal regulatory peptides in the duodenal mucosa in systemic sclerosis. *Clinical Experimental Rheumatology, 16*, 141–148.

Akiyoshi, M., Shimizu, Y., & Saito, M. (1990). Interleukin-1 increases norepinephrine turnover in the spleen and lung in rats. *Biochemical Biophysical Research Communications, 173*, 1266–1270.

Al'Abadie, M. S., Senior, H. J., Bleehen, S. S., & Gawkrodger, D. J. (1994). Neuropeptide and neuronal marker studies in vitiligo. *British Journal of Dermatology, 131*, 160–165.

Al Shawaf, A. A., Kendall, M. D., & Cowen, T. (1991). Identification of neural profiles containing vasoactive intestinal polypeptide, acetylcholinesterase and catecholamines in the rat thymus. *Journal of Anatomy, 174*, 131–143.

Alessandrini, C., Gerli, R., Sacchi, G., Ibba, L., Pucci, A. M., & Fruschelli, C. (1981). Cholinergic and adrenergic innervation of mesenterial lymph vessels in guinea pig. *Lymphology, 14*, 1–6.

Araujo, D. M., & Cotman, C. W. (1993). Trophic effects of interleukin-4, -7, and 8 on hippocampal neuronal cultures: Potential involvement of glial-derived factors. *Brain Research, 600*, 49–55.

Asahina, A., Hosoi, J., Grabbe, S., & Granstein, R. D. (1995). Modulation of Langerhans cell function by epidermal nerves. *Journal of Allergy & Clinical Immunology, 96*, 1178–1182.

Awatsuji, H., Furukawa, M., Nakajima, M., Furukawa, S., & Hayashi, K. (1993). Interleukin-2 as a neurotrophic factor for supporting the survival of neurons cultured from various regions of fetal rat brain. *Journal of Neuroscience Research, 35*, 305–311.

Ballantyne, B. (1968). The reticuloendothelial localization of splenic esterases. *Journal of the Reticuloendothelial Society, 5*, 399–411.

Barbany, G., Friedman, W. J., & Persson, H. (1991). Lymphocyte-mediated regulation of neurotransmitter gene expression in rat sympathetic ganglia. *Journal of Neuroimmunology, 32*, 97–104.

Baron, R., & Jänig, W. (1988). Sympathetic and afferent neurons projecting in the splenic nerve of the cat. *Neuroscience Letters, 94*, 109–113.

Bellinger, D. L., Ackerman, K. D., Felten, S. Y., & Felten, D. L. (1992). A longitudinal study of age-related loss of noradrenergic nerves and lymphoid cells in the aged rat spleen. *Experimental Neurology, 116*, 295–311.

Bellinger, D. L., Earnest, D. J., Gallagher, M., & Felten, D. L. (1992). Presence and availability of VIP in primary and secondary lymphoid organs [Abstract]. *Society for Neuroscience, 18*, 1009.

Bellinger, D. L., Lorton, D., Felten, S. Y., & Felten, D. L. (1992). Innervation of lymphoid organs and implications in development, aging, and autoimmunity. *International Journal of Immunopharmacology, 14*, 329–344.

Bellinger, D. L., Ackerman, K. D., Felten, S. Y., Lorton, D., & Felten, D. L. (1989). Noradrenergic sympathetic innervation of thymus, spleen and lymph nodes: Aspects of development, aging and plasticity in neural-immune interactions. In Nistico, G. (Ed.), *Proceedings of a Symposium on Interactions Between the Neuroendocrine and Immune Systems* (pp. 35–66). Rome: Pythogora Press.

Bellinger, D. L., Felten, S. Y., Lorton, D., & Felten, D. L. (1989). Origin of noradrenergic innervation of the spleen in rats. *Brain, Behavior, and Immunity, 3*, 291–311.

Bellinger, D. L., Felten, S. Y., Coleman, P. D., Yeh, P., & Felten, D. L. (1985). Noradrenergic innervation and acetylcholinesterase activity of lymph nodes in young adult and aging mice [Abstract]. *Society for Neuroscience, 11*, 663.

Bellinger, D. L., Felten, S. Y., Collier, T. J., & Felten, D. L. (1987). Noradrenergic sympathetic innervation of the spleen: IV. Morphometric analysis in adult and aged F344 rats. *Journal of Neuroscience Research, 18*, 55–63.

Bellinger, D. L., Felten, S. Y., & Felten, D. L. (1988). Maintenance of noradrenergic sympathetic innervation in the involuted thymus of the aged Fischer 344 rat. *Brain, Behavior, and Immunity, 2*, 133–150.

Bellinger, D. L., Felten, S. Y., & Felten, D. L. (1992a). Neural-immune interactions: Neurotransmitter signaling of cells of the immune system. *Annual Review of Psychiatry, 11*, 127–144.

Bellinger, D. L., Felten, S. Y., & Felten, D. L. (1992b). Noradrenergic sympathetic innervation of lymphoid organs during development, aging, and autoimmunity. In Amenta, F. (Ed.), *Aging of the Autonomic Nervous System* (pp. 243–284). Boca Raton, Florida: CRC Press.

Bellinger, D. L., Lorton, D., Brouxhon, S., Felten, S. Y., & Felten, D. L. (1996). The significance of vasoactive intestinal polypeptide (VIP) in immunomodulation. *Advances in Neuroimmunology, 6*, 5–27.

Bellinger, D. L., Brouxhon, S., Henderson, D., Felten, D. L., & Felten, S. Y. (1996). IL-2 increases IL-2R expression in superior mesenteric-celiac ganglion and alters splenic norepinephrine concentration [Abstract]. *Society for Neuroscience, 22*, 1353.

Bellinger, D. L., Lorton, D., Hamill, R., Felten, S. Y., & Felten, D. L. (1993). Acetylcholinesterase staining and choline acetyltransferase activity in the young adult rat spleen: Lack of evidence for cholinergic innervation. *Brain, Behavior, and Immunity, 7*, 191–204.

Bellinger, D. L., Lorton, D., Horn, L., Felten, S. Y., & Felten, D. L. (1997). Vasoactive intestinal polypeptide (VIP) innervation of rat spleen, thymus, and lymph nodes. *Peptides, 18*, 1139–1149.

Bellinger, D. L., Lorton, D., Romano, T., Olschowka, J. A., Felten, S. Y., & Felten, D. L. (1990). Neuropeptide innervation of lymphoid organs. *Annals of the New York Academy of Science, 594*, 17–33.

Benestad, H. B., Strom-Gundersen, I., Ole Iversen, P., Haug, E., & Nja, A. (1998). No neuronal regulation of murine bone marrow function. *Blood, 91*, 1280–1287.

Besedovsky, H. O., del Rey, A. E., Sorkin, E., Burri, R., Honegger, C. G., Schlumpf, M., & Lichtensteiger, W. (1987). T lymphocytes affect the development of sympathetic innervation of mouse spleen. *Brain, Behavior, and Immunity, 1*, 185–193.

Besedovsky, H. O., del Rey, A., Sorkin, E., Da Prada, M., & Keller, H. H. (1979). Immunoregulation mediated by the sympathetic nervous system. *Cellular Immunology, 48*, 346–355.

Bienenstock, J., Befus, A., & McDermott, M. (1983). Regulation of lymphoblast traffic in mucosal tissue with emphasis of IgA. *Federation Proceedings, 42*, 3213–3217.

Bjorck, S., Dahlstrom, S., & Ahlman, H. (1989). Topical treatment of ulcerative proctitis with lidocaine. *Scandinavian Journal of Gastroenterology, 24*, 1061–1072.

Bjorck, S., Jennische, E., Dahlsrom, A., & Ahlman, H. (1997). Influence of topical rectal application of drugs on dextran sulfate-induced colitis in rats. *Digestive Diseases and Sciences, 42*, 824–832.

Bjurholm, A., Kreicbergs, A., Broden, E., & Schultzberg, M. (1989). Substance P- and CGRP-immunoreactive nerves in bone. *Peptides, 9*, 165–171.

Bognar, I. T., Albrecht, S. A., Farasaty, M., Schmitt, E., Seidel, G., & Fuder, H. (1994). Effects of human recombinant interleukins on stimulation-evoked noradrenaline overflow from the rat perfused spleen. *Naunyn-Schmeideberg's Archives of Pharmacology, 349*, 497–502.

Bosma, M. J. (1992). B and T cell leakiness in the scid mouse mutant. *Immunodeficiency Reviews, 3*, 261–276.

Boucher, W., El-Mansoury, M., Pang, X., Sant, G. R., & Theoharides, T. C. (1995). Elevated mast cell tryptase in the urine of patients with interstitial cystitis. *British Journal of Urology, 76*, 94–100.

Boyd, E. (1932). The weight of the thymus gland in health and in disease. *American Journal of Diseases in Children, 43*, 1162–1214.

Bracci-Laudiero, L., Aloe, L., Stenfors, C., Theodorsson, E., & Lundeberg, T. (1998). Development of systemic lupus erythematosus in mice is associated with alteration of neuropeptide concentrations in inflamed kidneys and immunoregulatory organs. *Neuroscience Letters*, 97, 100.

Bracci-Laudiero, L., Aloe, L., Stenfors, C., Tirassa, P., Theodorsson, E., & Lundberg, T. (1996). Nerve growth factor stimulates production of neuropeptide Y in human lymphocytes. *Neuroreport, 7*, 485–488.

Bracci-Laudiero, L., Lundeberg, T., Stenfors, C., Theodorsson, E., Tirassa, P., & Aloe, L. (1996). Modification of lymphoid and brain nerve growth factor levels in systemic lupus erythematosus mice. *Neuroscience Letters, 204*, 13–16.

Bramwell, N. H., Ridell, R. H., Colley, E. C. C., & Stead, R. H. (1989). Eosinophils are in intimate contact with nerve fibers in the human gastrointestinal tract. *Gastroenterology, 96*, A961.

Breneman, S. M., Moynihan, J. A., Grota, L. J., Felten, D. L., & Felten, S. Y. (1993). Splenic norepinephrine is decreased in MRL-lpr/lpr mice. *Brain, Behavior, and Immunity, 7*, 135–143.

Brenneman, D. E., Schultzberg, M., Bartfai, T., & Gozes, I. (1992). Cytokine regulation of neuronal survival. *Journal of Neurochemistry 58*, 454–460.

Bret-Dibat, J.-L., Bluthe, R.-M., Kent, S., Kelley, K. W., & Dantzer, R. (1995). Lipopolysaccharide and interleukin-1 depress food-motivated behavior in mice by a vagal-mediated mechanism. *Brain, Behavior, and Immunity, 9*, 242–246.

Brouxhon, S. M., Bellinger, D. L., & Felten, D. L. (1996). Corticotropin-releasing factor (CRF) expression in the immune system following IL-2 administration [Abstract]. *Society for Neuroscience, 22*, 1353.

Brouxhon, S. M., Bellinger, D. L., Mukheraji, P., & Felten, D. L. (1996). Interleukin-2 (IL-2) regulation of CRF expression in the rat superior cervical ganglion [Abstract]. *Society for Neuroscience, 22*, 1353.

Brouxhon, S. M., Prasad, A. V., Joseph, S. A., Bellinger, D. L., & Felten, D. L. (1994). Localization of CRF in the primary and secondary lymphoid organs of the rat [Abstract]. *Society for Neuroscience, 20*, 950.

Bulloch, K. (1988). A comparative study of the autonomic nervous system innervation of the thymus in the mouse and chicken. *Internal Journal of Neurosciences, 40*, 129–140.

Bulloch, K., Cullen, M. R., Schwartz, R. H., & Longo, D. L. (1987). Development of innervation within syngeneic thymus tissue transplanted under the kidney capsule of the nude mouse: A light and ultrastructural microscope study. *Journal of Neuroscience Research, 18*, 16–27.

Bulloch, K., Hausman, J., Radojcic, T., & Short, S. (1991). Calcitonin gene-related peptide in the developing and aging thymus. An immunocytochemical study. *Annals New York Academy of Sciences, 621*, 218–228.

Bulloch, K., & Moore, R. Y. (1981). Innervation of the thymus gland by brain stem and spinal cord in mouse and rat. *American Journal of Anatomy, 162*, 157–166.

Bulloch, K., & Pomerantz, W. (1984). Autonomic nervous system innervation of thymic related lymphoid tissue in wild-type and nude mice. *Journal of Comparative Neurology, 228*, 57–68.

Bulloch, K., Radojcic, T., Yu, R., Hausman, J., Lenhard, L., & Baird, S. (1991). The distribution and function of calcitonin gene-related peptide in the mouse thymus and spleen. *Progress in NeuroEndocrinImmunology, 4*, 186–194.

Calvo, W. (1968). The innervation of the bone marrow in laboratory animals. *American Journal of Anatomy, 123*, 315–328.

Calvo, W., & Forteza-Vila, J. (1969). On the development of bone marrow innervation in new-born rats as studied with silver impregnation and electron microscopy. *American Journal of Anatomy, 126*, 355–359.

Carlson, S. L., Albers, K. M., Beiting, D. J., Parish, M., Conner, J. M., & Davis, B. M. (1995). NGF modulates sympathetic innervation of lymphoid tissues. *Journal of Neuroscience, 15*, 5892–5899.

Carlson, S. L., Brooks, W. H., & Roszman, T. L. (1989). Neurotransmitter-lymphocyte interactions: Dual receptor modulation of lymphocyte proliferation and cAMP production. *Journal of Neuroimmunology, 24*, 155–162.

Carlson, S. L., Felten, D. L., Livnat, S., & Felten, S. Y. (1987). Noradrenergic sympathetic innervation of the spleen: V. Acute drug-induced depletion of lymphocytes in the target fields of innervation results in redistribution of noradrenergic fibers but maintenance of compartmentation. *Journal of Neuroscience Research, 18*, 64–69.

Carlson, S. L., Fox, S., & Abell, K. M. (1997). Catecholamine modulation of lymphocyte homing to lymphoid tissues. *Brain, Behavior, and Immunity, 11*, 307–320.

Carlson, S. L., Johnson, S., Parrish, M. E., & Cass, W. A. (1998). Development of immune hyperinnervation in NGF-transgenic mice. *Experimental Neurology, 149*, 209–220.

Carnahan, J. F., Patel, D. R., & Miller, J. A. (1994). Stem cell factor is a neurotrophic factor for neural crest-derived chick sensory neurons. *Journal of Neurosciences, 14*, 1433–1440.

Chan, A. S. (1992). Association of nerve fibres with myoid cells in the chick thymus. *Journal of Anatomy, 181*, 509–512.

Chan, J., Smoller, B. R., Raychauduri, S. P., Jiang, W. Y., & Farber, E. M. (1997). Intraepidermal nerve fiber expression of calcitonin gene-related peptide, vasoactive intestinal peptide and substance P in psoriasis. *Archives of Dermatology Research, 289*, 611–616.

Chelmicka-Schorr, E., Checinski, M., & Arnason, B. G. W. (1988). Chemical sympathectomy augments the severity of experimental allergic encephalomyelitis. *Journal of Neuroimmunology, 17*, 347–350.

Chelmicka-Schorr, E., Kwasniewski, M. N., Thomas, B. E., & Arnason, B. G. W. (1989). The β-adrenergic agonist isoproterenol suppresses experimental allergic encephalomyelitis in Lewis rats. *Journal of Neuroimmunology, 25*, 203–207.

Chen, S. H., Itoh, M., Sun, W., Miki, T., & Takenuchi, Y. (1996). Localization of sympathetic and parasympathetic neurons innervating pancreas and spleen in the cat. *Journal of the Autonomic Nervous System, 59*, 12–16.

Chevendra, V., & Weaver, L. C. (1992). Distribution of neuropeptide Y, vasoactive intestinal peptide and somatostatin in populations of postganglionic neurons innervating the rat kidney, spleen and intestine. *Neuroscience, 50*, 727–743.

Christmas, T. J., Rode, J., Chapple, C. R., Milroy, E. J., & Turner-Warwick, R. T. (1990). Nerve fibre proliferation in interstitial cystitis. *Virchows Archives of Pathology, Anatomy, & Histopathology, 416*, 447–451.

Chubb, I. W., Hodgson, A. J., & White, G. H. (1980). Acetylcholinesterase hydrolyzes substance P. *Neuroscience, 5*, 2065–2072.

Chubb, I. W., Ranieri, R., White, G. H., & Hodgson, A. J. (1983). The enkephalins are amongst the peptides hydrolyzed by purified acetylcholinesterase. *Neuroscience, 10*, 1369–1377.

Clements, J. A., & Funder, J. W. (1986). Arginine vasopressin (AVP) and AVP-like immunoreactivity in peripheral tissues. *Endocrine Review, 7*, 449–460.

Cohen, J., Arai, M., Prak, E. L., Brooks, S. A., Young, L. H., & Prystowsky, M. B. (1992). Characterization of a novel mRNA expressed by neurons in mature brain. *Journal of Neuroscience Research, 31*, 273–284.

Colburn, K., Boucek, R., Gusewitch, G., Wong, A., Wat, P., & Weeks, D. (1990). β-adrenergic receptor stimulation increases anti-DNA antibody production in MRL/1pr mice. *Journal of Rheumatology, 17*, 138–141.

Colpaert, F. C., Donnerer, J., & Lembeck, F. (1983). Effects of capsaicin on inflammation and on the substance P content of nervous tissue in rats with adjuvant arthritis. *Life Sciences, 32*, 1827–1834.

Cooke, H. J. (1986). Neurobiology of the intestinal mucosa. *Gastroenterology, 90*, 1057–1081.

Cordier, A. (1969). L'innervation de la bourse de fabricius durant l'embryogenese et la vie adulte. *Acta Anatomy, 73*, 38–47.

Cosentino, M., Marino, F., Bombelli, R., Ferrari, M., Maestroni, G. J., Conti, A., Rasini, E., Lecchini, S., & Frigo, G. (1998). Association between the circadian course of endogenous noradrenaline and the hematopoietic cell cycle in mouse bone marrow. *Journal of Chemotherapy, 10*, 179–181.

Cox, H. M., Rudolph, A., & Gschmeissner, S. (1994). Ultrastructural co-localization of neuropeptide Y and vasoactive intestinal polypeptide in neurosecretory vesicles of submucous neurons in the rat jejunum. *Neuroscience, 59*, 469–476.

Crivellato, E., Damiani, D., Mallardi, F., & Travan, L. (1991). Suggestive evidence for a microanatomical relationship between mast cells and nerve fibers containing substance P, calcitonin gene-related peptide, vasoactive intestinal polypeptide, and somatostatin in the rat mesentery. *Acta Anatomy, 141*, 127–131.

Crivellato, E., Soldano, R., Travan, L., Fusaroli, P., & Mallardi, F. (1998). Apposition of enteric nerve fibers to plasma cells and immunoblasts in the mouse small bowel. *Neuroscience Letters, 241*, 123–126.

Dahlström, A. B., & Zetterström, B. E. M. (1965). Noradrenaline stores in nerve terminals of the spleen: Changes during hemorrhagic shock. *Science, 147*, 1583–1585.

Dalsgaard, C. J., Jernbeck, J., Stains, W., Kjartansson, J., Haegerstrand, A., Hokfelt, T., Brodin, E., Cuello, A. C., & Brown, J. C. (1989). Calcitonin gene-related peptide-like immunoreactivity in nerve fibers in the human skin. Relation to fibers containing substance P-, somatostatin- and vasoactive intestinal polypeptide-like immunoreactivity. *Histochemistry, 91*, 35–38.

De La Fuente, M., Bernaez, I., Del Rio, M., & Hernanz, A. (1993). Stimulation of murine peritoneal macrophage functions by neurpeptide Y and peptide YY. Involvement of protein kinase C. *Immunology, 80*, 259–265.

de Leeuw, F. E., Jansen, G. H., Batanero, E., van Wichen, D. F., Huber, J., & Schuurman, H. J. (1992). The neural and neuroendocrine component of the human thymus. I. Nerve-like structures. *Brain, Behavior, and Immunity, 6*, 234–248.

del Rey, A., Besedovsky, H. O., Sorkin, E., Da Prada, M., & Arrenbrecht, S. (1981). Immunoregulation mediated by the sympathetic nervous system. *Cellular Immunology, 63*, 329–334.

DePace, D. M., & Webber, R. H. (1975). Electrostimulation and morphologic study of the nerves to the bone marrow of the albino rat. *Acta Anatomy, 93*, 1–18.

Dewing, S. B. (1971). Remission of psoriasis associated with cutaneous nerve section. *Archives of Dermatology, 104*, 220–221.

Dimitriadou, V., Rouleau, A., Dam Trung Tuong, M., Newlands, G. J., Miller, H. R., Luffau, G., Schwartz, J. C., & Garbarg, M. (1994). Functional relationship between mast cells and C-sensitive nerve fibres evidenced by histamine H_3-receptor modulation in rat lung and spleen. *Clinical Sciences, 87*, 151–163.

Ding, M., Hart, R. P., & Jonakait, G. M. (1995). Tumor necrosis factor-a induces substance P in sympathetic ganglia through sequential induction of interleukin-1 and leukemia inhibitory factor. *Journal of Neurobiology, 28*, 445–454.

Dovas, A., Lucchi, M. L., Bortolami, R., Grandis, A., Palladino, A. R., Banelli, E., Carreta, M., Magni, F., & Paolocci, N. (1998). Collaterals of recurrent laryngeal nerve fibres innervate the thymus: A fluorescent tracer and HRP investigation of efferent vagal neurons in the rat brainstem. *Brain Research, 809*, 141–148.

Dowton, M., & Boelen, M. (1988). Acetylcholinesterase converts Met_5-enkephalin-containing peptides to Met_5-enkephalin. *Neuroscience Letters, 94*, 151–155.

Dureus, P., Louis, D., Grant, A. V., Bilfinger, T. V., & Stefano, G. B. (1993). Neuropeptide Y inhibits human and invertebrate immunocyte chemotaxis, chemokinesis, and spontaneous activation. *Cellular and Molecular Neurobiology, 13*, 541–546.

Egan, C. L., Viglione-Schneck, M. J., Walsh, L. J., Green, B., Trojanowski, J. W., Whitaker-Menezes, D., & Murphy, G. F. (1998). Characterization of unmyelinated axons uniting epidermal and dermal immune cells in primate and murine skin. *Journal of Cutaneous Pathology, 25*, 20–29.

Elfvin, L.-G., Aldskogius, H., & Johansson, J. (1992). Splenic primary sensory afferents in the guinea pig demonstrated with anterogradely transported wheat-germ agglutinin conjugated to horseradish peroxidase. *Cell and Tissue Research, 269*, 229–234.

Elfvin, L. G., Aldskogius, H., & Johansson, J. (1993). Primary sensory afferents in the thymus of the guinea pig demonstrated with anterogradely transported horseradish peroxidase conjugates. *Neuroscience Letters, 150*, 35–38.

Elfvin, L. G., Johansson, J., Hoijer, A. S., & Aldskogius, H. (1994). The innervation of the splenic capsule in the guinea pig: An immunohistochemical and ultrastructural study. *Journal of Anatomy, 185*, 267–278.

Elhassan, A. M., Adem, A., Hultenby, K., & Lindgren, J. U. (1998). Somatostatin immunoreactivity in bone and joint tissues. *Neuroreport, 9*, 2573–2575.

Elitsur, Y., Luk, G. D., Colberg, M., Gesell, M. S., Dosescu, J., & Moshier, J. A. (1994). Neuropeptide Y (NPY) enhances proliferation of human colonic lamina propria lymphocytes. *Neuropeptides, 26*, 289–295.

El-Mansoury, M., Boucher, W., Sant, G. R., & Theoharides, T. C. (1994). Increased urine histamine and methylhistamine in interstitial cystitis. *Journal of Urology, 152*, 350–353.

Engels, F., Folkerts, G., van Heuven-Nolsen, D., & Nijkamp, F. P. (1987). Haemophilus influenzae-induced decreases in lung beta-adrenoceptor function and number coincide with decreases in spleen noradrenaline. *Naunyn-Schmeideberg's Archives of Pharmacology, 336*, 274–279.

Enzmann, V., & Drossler, K. (1994). Immunohistochemical detection of substance P and vasoactive intestinal peptide fibres in the auricular lymph nodes of sensitized guinea-pigs and mice. *Acta Histochemica Jena, 96*, 15–18.

Ericsson, A., Kovacs, K. J., & Sawchenko, P. E. (1994). A functional anatomical analysis of central pathways subserving the effects of interleukin-1 on stress-related neuroendocrine neurons. *Journal of Neuroscience, 14*, 897–913.

Ericsson, A., Schalling, M., McIntyre, K. R., Lundberg, J. M., Larhammar, D., Seroogy, K., Hokfelt, T., & Persson, H. (1987). Detection of neuropeptide Y and its mRNA in megakaryocytes: Enhanced levels in certain autoimmune mice. *Proceedings of the National Academy of Sciences of the United States of America, 84*, 5585–5589.

Ernström, U., & Sandberg, G. (1974). Stimulation of lymphocyte release from the spleen by theophylline and isoproterenol. *Acta Physiologica Scandinavica, 90*, 202–209.

Ernström, U., & Söder, O. (1975). Influence of adrenaline on the dissemination of antibody-producing cells from the spleen. *Clinical and Experimental Immunology, 21*, 131–140.

Farthing, M. J. (1995). Irritable bowel, irritable body, or irritable brain? *British Medical Journal, 310*, 171–175.

Fatani, J. A., Qayyum, M. A., Mehta, L., & Singh, U. (1986). Parasympathetic innervation of the thymus: A histochemical and immunocytochemical study. *Journal of Anatomy, 147*, 115–119.

Feher, E., Foror, M., & Burnstock, G. (1992). Distribution of somatostatin-immunoreactive nerve fibres in Peyer's patches. *Gut, 33*, 1195–1198.

Feldman, S., Rachmilewitz, E. A., & Izak, G. (1966). The effect of central nervous system stimulation on erythropoiesis in rat with chronically implanted electrodes. *Journal of Laboratory and Clinical Medicine, 67*, 713–725.

Felten, D. L., Bellinger, D. L., Ackerman, K. D., & Felten, S. Y. (1986). Denervation of splenic sympathetic fibers in the young adult rat [Abstract]. *Society for Neuroscience, 12*, 1064.

Felten, D. L., & Felten, S. Y. (1989). Innervation of the thymus. In Kendall, M. D. & Ritter, M. A. (Eds.), *Thymus update* (pp. 73–88). London: Harwood Academic Publishers.

Felten, D. L., Felten, S. Y., Bellinger, D. L., Carlson, S. L., Ackerman, K. D., Madden, K. S., Olschowka, J. A., & Livnat, S. (1987). Noradrenergic sympathetic neural interactions with the immune system: Structure and function. *Immunological Reviews, 100*, 225–260.

Felten, D. L., Felten, S. Y., Carlson, S. L., Olschowka, J. A., & Livnat, S. (1985). Noradrenergic and peptidergic innervation of lymphoid tissue. *Journal of Immunology, 135*, 755s–765s.

Felten, D. L., Gibson-Berry, K., & Wu, J. H. D. (1996). Innervation of bone marrow by tyrosine hydroxylase-immunoreactive nerve fibers and hemopoiesis-modulating activity of a β-adrenergic agonist in mouse. *Molecular Biology of Hematopoiesis, 5*, 627–636.

Felten, D. L., Livnat, S., Felten, S. Y., Carlson, S. L., Bellinger, D. L., & Yeh, P. (1984). Sympathetic innervation of lymph nodes in mice. *Brain Research Bulletin, 13*, 693–699.

Felten, D. L., Overhage, J. M., Felten, S. Y., & Schmedtje, J. F. (1981). Noradrenergic sympathetic innervation of lymphoid tissue in the rabbit appendix: Further evidence for a link between the nervous and immune systems. *Brain Research Bulletin, 7*, 595–612.

Felten, S. Y., Bellinger, D. L., Collier, T. J., Coleman, P. D., & Felten, D. L. (1987). Decreased sympathetic innervation of spleen in aged Fischer 344 rats. *Neurobiology of Aging, 8*, 159–165.

Felten, S. Y., & Felten, D. L. (1991). The innervation of lymphoid tissue. In Ader, R., Felten, D. L. & Cohen, N. (Eds.), *Psychoneuroimmunology* (2nd ed.; pp. 27–69). New York: Academic Press.

Felten, S. Y., Felten, D. L., Bellinger, D. L., Carlson, S. L., Ackerman, K. D., Madden, K. S., Olschowka, J. A., & Livnat, S. (1988). Noradrenergic sympathetic innervation of lymphoid organs. *Progress in Allergy, 43*, 14–36.

Felten, S. Y., Felten, D. L., Bellinger, D. L., & Olschowka, J. A. (1992). Noradrenergic and peptidergic innervation of lymphoid organs. In Blalock, J. E. (Ed.), *Chemical immunology: neuroimmunoendocrinology* (pp. 25–48). Basel: S. Karger.

Felten, S. Y., & Olschowka, J. A. (1987). Noradrenergic sympathetic innervation of the spleen: II. Tyrosine hydroxylase (TH)-positive nerve terminals form synaptic-like contacts on lymphocytes in the splenic white pulp. *Journal of Neuroscience Research, 18*, 37–48.

Felten, S. Y., Olschowka, J. A., Ackerman, K. D., & Felten, D. L. (1988). Catecholaminergic innervation of the spleen: Are lymphocytes targets of noradrenergic nerves? In Dahlström, A., Belmaker, R. H. & Sandler, M. (Eds.), *Progress in catecholamine research, part A: Basic aspects and peripheral mechanisms* (pp. 525–531). New York : Alan R. Liss.

Fillenz, M. (1966a). Innervation of the cat spleen. *Proceedings of the Physiological Society, 25–26*, 2P–3P.

Fillenz, M. (1966b). Innervation of blood vessels of lung and spleen. In Karger, B. (Ed.), *Sympathetic electric activation and innervation of blood vessels* (pp. 56–59). London: Cambridge.

Fillenz, M. (1970). The innervation of the cat spleen. *Proceedings of the Royal Society of London, 174*, 459–468.

Fillenz, M., & Pollard, R. M. (1976). Quantitative differences between sympathetic nerve terminals. *Brain Research, 109*, 443–454.

Fink, T., Sebastiano, P. D., Buchler, M., Beger, H. G., & Weihe, E. (1994). Growth-associated protein 43 and protein gene-product 9.5 innervation in human pancreas: Changes in chronic pancreatitis. *Neuroscience, 63*, 249–266.

Fink, T., & Weihe, E. (1988). Multiple neuropeptides in nerves supplying mammalian lymph nodes: Messenger candidates for sensory and autonomic neuroimmunomodulation? *Neuroscience Letters, 90*, 39–44.

Fleshner, M., Goehler, L. E., Hermann, J., Relton, J. K., Maier, S. F., & Watkins, L. R. (1995). Interleukin-1β induced corticosterone elevation and hypothalamic NE depletion is vagally mediated. *Brain Research Bulletin, 37*, 605–610.

Fox, E. A., & Powley, T. L. (1986). Tracer diffusion has exaggerated CNS maps of direct preganglionic innervation of pancreas. *Journal of the Autonomic Nervous System, 15*, 55–69.

Fried, G., Terenius, L., Brodin, E., Efendic, S., Dockray, G., Fahrenkrug, J., Goldstein, M., & Hökfelt, T. (1986). Neuropeptide Y, enkephalin and noradrenaline coexist in sympathetic neurons innervating the bovine spleen. Biochemical and immunohistchemical evidence. *Cell & Tissue Research, 243*, 495–508.

Garcia, J. F., & van Dyke, D. C. (1961). Response of rats of various ages to erythropoietin. *Proceedings of the Society of Experimental Biology and Medicine, 106*, 585–588.

Geenen, V., Legros, J.-J., Franchimont, P., Baudrihaye, M., Defresne, M. P., & Boniver, J. (1986). The neuroendocrine thymus: Coexistence of oxytocin and neurophysin in the human thymus. *Science, 232*, 508–510.

Geenen, V., Legros, J.-J., Franchimont, P., Defresne, M. P., Boniver, J., Ivell, R., & Richter, D. (1987). The thymus as a neuroendocrine organ: Synthesis of vasopressin and oxytocin in human thymic epithelium. *Annals of the New York Academy of Science, 496*, 56–66.

Geppetti, P., Frilli, S., Renzi, d., Santicioli, P., Maggi, C. A., Theodorsson, E., & Fanciullacci, M. (1988). Distribution of calcitonin gene-related peptide-like immunoreactivity in various rat tissues: Correlation with substance P and other tachykinins and sensitivity to capsaicin. *Regulatory Peptides, 23*, 289–298.

Geppetti, P., Maggi, C. A., Zecchi-Orlandini, S., Santicioli, P., Meli, A., Frilli, S., Spillantini, M. G., & Amenta, F. (1987). Substance P-like immunoreactivity in capsaicin-sensitive structures of the rat thymus. *Regulatory Peptides, 18*, 321–329.

Gibbins, I. L., Wattchow, D., & Coventry, B. (1987). Two immunohistochemically identified populations of calcitonin gene-related peptide (CGRP)-immunoreactive axons in human skin. *Brain Research, 414*, 143–148.

Girolomoni, G., & Tigelaar, R. E. (1990). Capsaicin-sensitive primary sensory neurons are potent modulators of murine delayed-type hypersensitivity reactions. *Journal of Immunology, 145*, 1105–1112.

Giron, L. T., Crutcher, K. A., & Davis, J. N. (1980). Lymph nodes — a possible site for sympathetic neuronal regulation of immune responses. *Annals of Neurology, 8*, 520–525.

Goebeler, M., Henseleit, U., Roth, J., & Sorg, C. (1994). Substance P and calcitonin gene-related peptide modulate leukocyte infiltration to mouse skin during allergic contact dermatitis. *Archives of Dermatology Research, 286*, 341–346.

Goehler, L. E., Busch, C. R., Tartaglia, N., Relton, J., Sisk, D., Maier, S. F., & Watkins, L. R. (1995). Blockade of cytokine induced conditioned taste aversion by subdiaphragmatic vagatomy: Further evidence for vagal mediation of immune-brain communication. *Neuroscience Letters, 185*, 163–166.

Gordon, M. A., Cohen, J. J., & Wilson, I. B. (1978). Muscarinic cholinergic receptors in murine lymphocytes: Demonstration by direct binding. *Proceedings of the National Academy of Science of the United States of America, 75*, 2902–2904.

Gottesfeld, Z., Simpson, S., Yuwiler, A., & Perez-Polo, J. R (1996). Effect of nerve growth factor on splenic norepinephrine and pineal N-acetyl-transferase in neonate rats exposed to alcohol *in utero*: Neuroimmune correlates. *International Journal of Developmental Neurosciences, 14*, 655–622.

Gottwald, T., Lhotak, S., & Stead, R. H. (1997). Effect of truncal vagotomy and capsaicin on mast cells and IgA-positive plasma cells in rat jejunal mucosa. *Neurogastroenterology & Motility, 158*, 5178–5184.

Gronblad, M., Konttinen, Y. T., Korkala, O., Liesi, P., Hukkanen, M., & Polak, J. M. (1988). Neuropeptides in synovium of patients with rheumatoid arthritis and osteoarthritis. *Journal of Rheumatology, 15*, 1807–1810.

Gulati, P., Leong, S., & Chan, A. S. (1998). Ontogeny of NADPH-d expression in the thymic microenvironment of the chick embryo. *Cell and Tissue Research, 294*, 335–343.

Gulati, P., Tay, S. S., & Leong, S. K. (1997). Nitrergic, peptidergic and substance P innervation of the chick thymus. *Journal für Hirnforschung, 38*, 553–564.

Hadden, J. W. (1977). Cyclic nucleotides in lymphocyte proliferation and differentiation. In Hadden, J. W., Coffey, R. G. & Spreafico, F. (Eds.), *Immunopharmacology* (pp. 1–28). New York: Plenum Press.

Haegerstrand, A., Jonzon, B., Dalsgaard, D. J., & Nilsson, J. (1989). Vasoactive intestinal polypeptide stimulates cell proliferation and adenylate cyclase activity of cultured human keratinocytes. *Proceedings of the National Academy of Science of the United States of America, 86*, 5993–5996.

Hafstrom, I., Ringertz, B., Lundeberg, T., & Palmblad, J. (1993). The effect of endothelin, neuropeptide Y, calcitonin gene-related peptide and substance P. *Acta Physiologica Scandinavica, 148*, 341–346.

Hara, M., Toyoda, M., Yaar, M., Bhawan, J., Avila, E. M., Penner, I. R., & Gilchrest, B. A. (1996). Innervation of melanocytes in human skin. *Journal of Experimental Medicine, 184*, 1385–1395.

Hardebo, J. E., Suzuki, N., & Ekman, R. (1992). Presence of gastrin-releasing peptide in neurons of the geniculate ganglion in rat and man. *Neuroscience Letters, 139*, 239–242.

Haugen, P.K, & Letoumeau, P. C. (1990). Interleukin-2 enhances chick and rat sympathetic, but not sensory, neurite outgrowth *Journal of Neuroscience Research, 25*, 443–452.

Heumann, R. (1987). Regulation of synthesis of nerve growth factor. *Journal of Experimental Biology, 132*, 133–150.

Hosoi, J., Murphy, G. F., Egan, C. L., Lerner, E. A., Grabbe, S., Asahina, A., & Granstein, R. D. (1993). Regulation of Langerhans cell function by nerves containing calcitonin gene-related peptide. *Nature, 363*, 159–163.

Hsieh, S. T., Choi, S., Lin, W. M., Chang, Y. C., Mcarthur, J. C., & Griffin, J. W. (1996). Epidermal denervation and its effects on keratinocytes and Langerhans cells. *Journal of Neurocytology, 25*, 513–524.

Hurst, S., & Collins, S. M. (1993). Interleukin-1β modulation of norepinephrine release from rat myenteric nerves. *American Journal of Physiology, 264*, G30–G35.

Hurst, S. M., & Collins, S. M. (1994). Mechanism underlying tumor necrosis factor-α suppression of norepinephrine release from rat myenteric plexus. *American Journal of Physiology, 266*, G1123–G1129.

Husband, A. J. (1982). Kinetics of extravasation and redistribution of IgA-specific antibody containing cells in the intestine. *Journal of Immunology, 128*, 1355–1359.

Ichikawa, S., Sreedharan, S. P., Goetzl, E. J., & Owen, R. L. (1994). Immunohistochemical localization of peptidergic nerve fibers and neuropeptide receptors in Peyer's patches of the cat ileum. *Regulatory Peptides, 54*, 385–395.

Imai, S., Tokunaga, Y., Maeda, T., Kikkawa, M., & Hukuda, S. (1997). Calcitonin gene-related peptide, substance P, and tyrosine hydroxylase-immunoreactive innervation of the rat bone marrow: An immunohistochemical and ultrastructural investigation on possible efferent and afferent mechanisms. *Journal Orthopedic Research, 15*, 133–140.

Inoue, K. (1973). Distribution of adrenergic and cholinergic nerve cells and fibers in the bursa of fabricius of chicken. *Okajimas Folia Anatomica Japonica, 50*, 317–325.

Inoue, K. (1971). Innervation of the bursa of Fabricius in the domestic fowl. *Acta Anatomica Nippon, 46*, 403–415.

Inoue, N., Magari, S., & Sakanaka, M. (1990). Distribution of peptidergic nerve fibers in rat bronchus-associated lymphoid tissue: Light microscopic observations. *Lymphology, 23*, 155–160.

Ishida-Yamamoto, A., Senba, E., & Tohyama, M. (1989). Distribution and fine structure of calcitonin gene-related peptide-like immunoreactive nerve fibers in the rat skin. *Brain Research, 491*, 93–101.

Ismael, Z., Millar, T. J., Small, D. H., & Chubb, I. W. (1986). Acetylcholinesterase generates enkephalin-like immunoreactivity when it degrades the soluble proteins (chromogranins) from adrenal chromaffin granules. *Brain Research, 376*, 230–238.

Iwasaki, A., Inoue, K., & Hukuda, S. (1995). Distribution of neuropeptide-containing nerve fibers in the synovium and adjacent bone of the rat knee joint. *Clinical and Experimental Rheumatology, 13*, 173–178.

Jesseph, J. M., & Felten, D. L. (1984). Noradrenergic innervation of the gut-associated lymphoid tissues (GALT) in the rabbit [Abstract]. *Anatomical Records, 208*, 81A.

Jeurissen, S. H., Duijvestijn, A. M., Sontag, Y., & Kraal, G. (1987). Lymphocyte migration into lamina propria of the gut is mediated by specialized HEV-like blood vessels. *Immunology, 62*, 273–277.

Johansson, O. (1986). A detailed account of NPY-immunoreactive nerves and cells of the human skin. Comparison with VIP-, substance P- and PHI-containing structures. *Acta Physiologica Scandinavica, 128*, 147–153.

Johansson, O., Virtanen, M., & Hilliges, M. (1995). Histaminergic nerves demonstrated in the skin. A new direct mode of neurogenic inflammation? *Experimental Dermatology 4*, 93–96.

Josefsson, E., Mansson, J.-E., Blennow, K., & Tarkowski, A. (1994). Immunomodulating and anti-inflammatory properties of the sympatholytic compound 6-hydroxydopamine. *Journal of Neuroimmunology, 55*, 161–169.

Jurjus, A. R., More, N., & Walsh, R. J. (1998). Distribution of substance P positive cells and nerve fibers in the rat thymus. *Journal of Neuroimmunology, 90*, 143–148.

Kannan, Y., Bienenstock, J., Ohta, M., Stanisz, A. M., & Stead, R. H. (1996). Nerve growth factor and cytokines mediate lymphoid tissue-induced neurite outgrowth from mouse superior cervical ganglia in vitro. *Journal of Immunology, 156*, 313–320.

Kannan, Y., Stead, R. H., Goldsmith, C. H., & Bienenstock, J. (1994). Lymphoid tissues induce NGF-dependent and NGF-independent neurite outgrowth from rat superior cervical ganglia explants in culture. *Journal of Neuroscience Research, 37*, 374–383.

Kaplan, R., Robinson, C. A., Scavulli, J. F., & Vaughan, J. H. (1980). Propranolol and the treatment of rheumatoid arthritis. *Arthritis and Rheumatism, 23*, 253–255.

Kashima, Y., Hama, T., & Hatanaka, H. (1992). Interleukin-6 as a neurotrophic factor for promoting the survival of cultured catecholaminergic neurons in a chemically defined medium from fetal and postnatal rat midbrains. *Journal of Neuroscience Research, 13,* 267–280.

Kawaguchi, Y., Okada, T., Konishi, H., Fujino, M., Asai, J., & Ito, M. (1997). Reduction of the DTH response is related to morphological changes of Langerhans cells in mice exposed to acute immobilization stress. *Clinical and Experimental Immunology, 109,* 397–401.

Kawahara, G., & Osada, N. (1962). Studies on the innervation of bone marrow with special reference to the intramedullary fibers in the dog and goat. *Archivum Histologicum Japanicum, 24,* 471–487.

Keast, J. R., Furness, J. B., & Costa, M. (1984). Origins of peptide and norepinephrine nerves in the mucosa of the guinea pig small intestine. *Gastroenterology, 86,* 637–644.

Keith, J. M., Jin, J., & Saban, R. (1995). Nerve-mast cell interaction in normal guinea pig urinary bladder. *Journal of Comparative Neurology, 363,* 28–36.

Kelley, S. P., Grota, L. J., Felten, S. Y., Madden, K. S., & Felten, D. L. (1996). Norepinephrine in mouse spleen shows minor strain differences and no diurnal variation. *Pharmacological and Biochemical Behavior, 53,* 141–146.

Kemeny, L., von Restorff, B., Michel, G., & Ruzicka, T. (1994). Specific binding and lack of growth-promoting activity of substance P in cultured keratinocytes. *Journal of Investigative Dermatology, 103,* 605–606.

Kendall, M. D., & Al-Shawaf, A. A. (1991). Innervation of the rat thymus gland. *Brain, Behavior, and Immunity, 5,* 9–28.

Kendall, M. D., Atkinson, B. A., Munoz, F. J., De La Riva, C., Clarke, A. G., & von Gaudecker, B. (1994). The noradrenergic innervation of the rat thymus during pregnancy and in the post-partum period. *Journal of Anatomy, 185,* 617–625.

Kessler, J. A., Freidin, M. M., Kalberg, C., & Chandross, K. J. (1993). Cytokines regulate substance P expression in sympathetic neurons. *Regulatory Peptides, 46,* 70–75.

Kinney, K. S., Cohen, N., & Felten, S. Y. (1994). Noradrenergic and peptidergic innervation of the amphibian spleen: Comparative studies. *Developmental and Comparative Immunology, 18,* 511–521.

Kinney, K. S., Felten, S. Y., & Cohen, N. (1991). Sympathetic innervation of the amphibian spleen. *Fifth ISDCI Congress.*

Konttinen, Y. T., Rees, R., Hukkanen, M., Gronblad, M., Tolvanen, E., Gibson, S. J., Polak, J. M., & Brewerton, D. A. (1990). Nerves in inflammatory synovium: Immunohistochemical observations on the adjuvant arthritis rat model. *Journal of Rheumatology, 17,* 1586–1591.

Korsgren, O., Jansson, L., Andersson, A., & Sundler, F. (1993). Reinnervation of transplanted pancreatic islets. A comparison among islets implanted into the kidney, spleen, and liver. *Transplantation, 56,* 138–143.

Koziol, J. A., Clark, D. C., Gittes, R. F., & Tan, E. M. (1993). The natural history of interstitial cystitis: A survey of 374 patients. *Journal of Urology, 149,* 465–469.

Kranz, A., Kendall, M. D., & von Gaudecker, B. (1997). Studies on rat and human thymus to demonstrate immunoreactivity of calcitonin gene-related peptide, tyrosine hydroxylase and neuropeptide Y. *Journal of Anatomy, 191,* 441–450.

Kreicbergs, A., Ahmed, M., Ehrnberg, A., Schultzberg, M., Svenson, S. B., & Bjurholm, A. (1995). Interleukin-1 immunoreactive nerves in heterotopic bone induced by DBM. *Bone, 17,* 341–345.

Kudoh, G., Hoshi, K., & Murakami, T. (1979). Fluorescence microscopic and enzyme histochemical studies of the innervation of the human spleen. *Archivum Histologicum Japanicum, 42,* 169–180.

Kurkowski, R., Kummer, W., & Heym, C. (1990). Substance P-immunoreactive nerve fibers in tracheobronchial lymph nodes of the guinea pig: Origin, ultrastructure and coexistence with other peptides. *Peptides, 11,* 13–20.

Kurz, B., Feindt, J., von Gaudecker, B., Kranz, A., Loppnow, H., & Mentlein, R. (1997). Beta-adrenoceptor-mediated effects in rat cultured thymic epithelial cells. *British Journal of Pharmacology, 120,* 1401–1408.

Larson, S., Thompson, S. A., Hald, T., Barnard, R. J., Gilpin, C. J., Dixon, J. S., & Gosling, J. A. (1982). Mast cells in interstitial cystitis. *British Journal of Urology, 54,* 283–286.

Laughton, W., & Powley, T. L. (1979). Four central nervous system sites project to the pancreas [Abstract]. *Society for Neuroscience, 5,* 46.

Leslie, R. A., Reynolds, J. M., & Lawes, I. N. C. (1992). Central connections of the nuclei of the vagus nerve. In Ritter, R., Ritter, S. C. & Barnes, C. D. (Eds.), *Neuroanatomy and physiology of abdominal vagal afferents* (pp. 81–98). Ann Arbor: CRC Press.

Levine, J. D., Clark, R., Devor, M., Helms, C., Moskowitz, M. A., & Basbaum, A. I. (1984). Intraneuronal substance P contributes to the severity of experimental arthritis. *Science, 226,* 547–549.

Levine, J. D., Collier, D. H., Basbaum, A. I., Moskowitz, M. A., & Helms, C. A. (1985). Hypothesis: The nervous system may contribute to the pathophysiology of rheumatoid arthritis. *Journal of Rheumatology, 12,* 406–411.

Levine, J. D., Dardick, S. J., Basbaum, A. I., & Scipio, E. (1985). Reflex neurogenic inflammation. I. Contribution of the peripheral nervous system to spatially remote inflammatory responses that follow injury. *Journal of Neuroscience, 5,* 1380–1386.

Levine, J. D., Moskowitz, M. A., & Basbaum, A. I. (1985). The contribution of neurogenic inflammation in experimental arthritis. *Journal of Immunology, 135,* 843s–847s.

Levine, J. D., Dardick, S. J., Roizen, M. F., Helms, C., & Basbaum, A. L. (1986). Contribution of sensory afferents and sympathetic efferents to joint injury in experimental arthritis. *Journal of Neuroscience, 6,* 3423–3429.

Levine, J. D., Fye, K., Heller, P., Basbaum, A. I. & Whiting-O'Keefe, Q. (1986). Clinical response to regional intravenous guanethidine in patients with rheumatoid arthritis. *Journal of Rheumatology, 13,* 1040–1043.

Levine, J. D., Taiwo, Y. O., Collins, S. D., & Tam, J. K. (1986). Noradrenaline hyperalgesia is mediated through interaction with sympathetic postganglionic neuron terminals rather than activation of primary afferent nociceptors. *Nature, 323,* 158–160.

Levine, J. D., Goetzl, E. J., & Basbaum, A. I. (1991). Contribution of the nervous system to the pathophysiology of rheumatoid arthritis and other polyarthritides. *Rheumatic Disease Clinics of North America, 13,* 369–383.

Levine, J. D., Moskowitz, M. A., & Basbaum, A. I. (1988). The effect of gold, an antirheumatic therapy, on substance P levels in rat peripheral nerve. *Neuroscience Letters, 87,* 200–202.

Liang, Y., Marcusson, J. A., Jacobi, H. H., Haak-Frendscho, M., & Johansson, O. (1998). Histamine-containing mast cells and their relationship to NGFr-immunoreactive nerves in prurigo nodularis: A reappraisal. *Journal of Cutaneous Pathology, 25,* 189–198.

Lichtman, M. A. (1981). The ultrastructure of the hemopoietic environment of the marrow: A review. *Experimental Hematology, 9,* 391–410.

Liu, P. Y., Bondesson, L., Lontz, W., & Johansson, O. (1996). The occurrence of cutaneous nerve endings and neuropeptides in vitiligo vulgaris: A case-control study. *Archives of Dermatology Research, 288,* 670–675.

Livnat, S., Felten, S. Y., Carlson, S. L., Bellinger, D. L., & Felten, D. L. (1985). Involvement of peripheral and central catecholamine systems in neural-immune interactions. *Journal of Neuroimmunology, 10*, 5–30.

Lomax, A. E., Bertrand, P. P., & Furness, J. B. (1998). Identification of the populations of enteric neurons that have NK_1 receptors in the guinea-pig small intestine. *Cell and Tissue Research, 294*, 27–33.

Lorton, D., Bellinger, D. L., Duclos, M., Felten, S. Y., & Felten, D. L. (1996). Application of 6-hydroxydopamine into the fatpads surrounding the draining lymph nodes exacerbates adjuvant-induced arthritis. *Journal of Neuroimmunology, 64*, 103–113.

Lorton, D., Bellinger, D. L., Felten, S. Y., & Felten, D. L. (1991). Substance P innervation of spleen in rats: Nerve fibers associate with lymphocytes and macrophages in specific compartments of the spleen. *Brain, Behavior, and Immunity, 5*, 29–40.

Lorton, D., Bellinger, D. L., Felten, S. Y., & Felten, D. L. (1990). Substance P innervation of the rat thymus. *Peptides, 11*, 1269–1275.

Lorton, D., Lubahn, C., Felten, S. Y., & Bellinger, D. L. (1997). Norepinephrine content in primary and secondary lymphoid organs is altered in rats with adjuvant-induced arthritis. *Mechanisms of Ageing and Development, 94*, 145–63.

Lubahn, C., Almond, S., Zhu, Y., Hoffman, S., & Lorton, D. (1997). Substance P innervation of lymphoid organs in autoimmune prone mice [Abstract]. *Society for Neuroscience, 23*, 1512.

Lubahn, C., Almond, S., Zhu, Y., Hoffman, S., & Lorton, D. (1999). Substance P levels are altered in lymphoid organs of lymphoid organs of autoimmune mice [Abstract]. *Society for Neuroscience, 25*, 942.

Lubahn, C., & Lorton, D. (1998). Parallel loss of noradrenergic nerves (NA) and lymphoid cells in spleens from rats with adjuvant arthritis [Abstract]. *Society for Neuroscience, 24*, 1855.

Lundberg, J. M., Rudehill, A., Sollevi, A., Theodorsson-Norhein, E., & Hamberger, B. (1986). Frequency- and reserpine-dependent chemical coding of sympathetic transmission: differential release of noradrenaline and neuropeptide Y from pig spleen. *Neuroscience Letters, 63*, 96–100.

Lundberg, J. M., Änggård, A., Pernow, J., & Hökfelt, T. (1985). Neuropeptide Y-, substance P- and VIP-immunoreactive nerves in cat spleen in relation to autonomic vascular and volume control. *Cell & Tissue Research, 239*, 9–18.

Lundbert, J. M., Saria, A., Brodin, E., Rosell, S., & Folkars, K. (1983). A substance P antagonist inhibits vagally-induced increase in vascular permeability and bronchial smooth muscle contraction in the guinea pig. *Proceedings of the National Academy of Science of the United States of America, 80*, 1120–1124.

MacNeil, B. J., Jansen, A. H., Greenberg, A. H., & Nance, D. M. (1996). Activation and selectivity of splenic sympathetic nerve electrical activity response to bacterial endotoxin. *American Journal of Physiology, 270*, R264–R270.

Madden, K. S., Bellinger, D. L., Felten, S. Y., Synder, E., Maida, M. E., & Felten, D. L. (1997). Alterations in sympathetic innervation of thymus and spleen in aged mice. *Mechanisms of Ageing and Development, 94*, 165–175.

Madden, K. S., Sanders, V. M., & Felten, D. L. (1995). Catecholamine influences and sympathetic neural modulation of immune responsiveness. *Annals Review of Pharmacology and Toxicology, 35*, 417–448.

Maestroni, G. J. (1998). Is hematopoiesis under the influence of neural and neuroendocrine mechanisms? *Histology and Histopathology, 13*, 271–274.

Maestroni, G. J., & Conti, A. (1994). Modulation of hematopoiesis via alpha 1-adrenergic receptors on bone marrow cells. *Experimental Hematology, 22*, 313–320.

Maestroni, G. J. M., Conti, A., & Pedrinis, E. (1992). Effect of adrenergic agents on hematopoiesis after syngeneic bone marrow transplantation in mice. *Blood, 80*, 1178–1182.

Maestroni, G. J. M., Cosentino, M., Marino, F., Togni, M., Conti, A., Lecchini, S., & Frigo, G. (1998). Neural and endogenous catecholamines in the bone marrow. Circadian association of norepinephrine with hematopoiesis. *Experimental Hematology, 26*, 1172–1177.

Manske, J. M., Sullivan, E. L., & Andersen, S. M. (1995). Substance P mediated stimulation of cytokine levels in cultured murine bone marrow stromal cells. *Advances in Experimental and Medical Biology, 383*, 53–64.

Marino, F., Cosentino, M., Bombelli, R., Ferrari, M., Maestroni, G. J., Conti, A., Lecchini, S., & Frigo, G. (1997). Measurement of catecholamines in mouse bone marrow by means of HPLC with electrochemical detection. *Haematologica, 82*, 392–394.

Markwick, A. J., Lolait, S. J., & Funder, J. W. (1986). Immunoreactive arginine vasopressin in the rat thymus. *Endocrinology, 119*, 1690–1696.

Maslinski, W., Kullberg, M., Nordström, O., & Bartfai, T. (1988). Muscarinic receptors and receptor-mediated actions on rat thymocytes. *Journal of Neuroimmunology, 17*, 265–274.

Matsuda, H., Coughlin, M. D., Bienenstock, J., & Denburg, J. A. (1988). Nerve growth factor promotes human hemopoietic colony growth and differentiation. *Proceedings of the National Academy of Science of the United States America, 85*, 6508–6512.

McGillis, J. P., Rangnekar, V., & Ciallella, J. R. (1995). A role for calcitonin gene-related peptide (CGRP) in the regulation of early B lymphocyte differentiation. *Canadian Journal of Physiology and Pharmacology, 73*, 1057–1064.

Mehler, M. F., Rozental, R., Dougherty, M., Spray, D. C., & Kessler, J. A. (1993). Cytokine regulation of neuronal differentiation of hippocampal progenitor cells. *Nature, 362*, 62–65.

Meltzer, J. C., Grimm, P. C., Greenberg, A. H., & Nance, D. M. (1997). Enhanced immunohistochemical detection of autonomic nerve fibers, cytokines and inducible nitric oxide synthase by light and fluorescent microscopy in rat spleen. *Journal of Histochemistry and Cytochemistry, 45*, 599–610.

Menkes, C. J., Renoux, M., Laoussadi, S., Mauborgne, A., Bruxelle, J., & Cesselin, F. (1993). Substance P levels in the synovium and synovial fluid from patients with rheumatoid arthritis and osteoarthritis. *Journal of Rheumatology 20*, 714–717.

Metcalfe, D. D., Baram, D., & Mekori, Y. A. (1997). Mast cells. *Physiological Reviews, 77*, 1033–1079.

Misery, L. (1997). Skin, immunity and the nervous system. *British Journal of Dermatology, 137*, 843–850.

Mitchell, B., Kendall, M., Adam, E., & Schumacher, U. (1997). Innervation of the thymus in normal and bone marrow reconstituted severe combined immunodeficient (SCID) mice. *Journal of Neuroimmunology, 75*, 19–27.

Miyauchi, A., Kanje, M., Danielsen, N., & Dahlin, L. B. (1997). Role of macrophages in the stimulation and regeneration of sensory nerves by transposed granulation tissue and temporal aspects of the response. *Scandinavian Journal of Plastic & Reconstructive Surgery & Hand Surgery, 31*, 17–23.

Moller, K., Zhang, Y. Z., Hakanson, R., Luts, A., Sjolund, B., Uddman, R., & Sundler, F. (1993). Pituitary adenylate cyclase activating peptide is a sensory neuropeptide: immunocytochemical and immunochemical evidence. *Neuroscience, 57*, 725–732.

Murphy, M., Reid, K., Brown, M. A., & Bartlett, P. F. (1993). Involvement of leukaemia inhibitory factor and nerve growth factor in the development of dorsal root ganglion neurons. *Development, 117*, 1173–1182.

Müller, S., & Weihe, E. (1991). Interrelation of peptidergic innervation with mast cells and ED1-positive cells in rat thymus. *Brain, Behavior, and Immunity, 5*, 55–72.

Nair, M. P., Schwartz, S. A., Wu, K., & Kronfol, Z. (1993). Effect of neuropeptide Y on natural killer activity of normal human lymphocytes. *Brain, Behavior, and Immunity, 7*, 70–78.

Nance, D. M., & Burns, J. (1989). Innervation of the spleen in the rat: Evidence for absence of afferent innervation. *Brain, Behavior, and Immunity, 3*, 281–290.

Nance, D. M., Hopkins, D. A., & Bieger, D. (1987). Re-investigation of the innervation of the thymus gland in mice and rats. *Brain, Behavior, and Immunity, 1*, 134–147.

Niijima, A. (1998). An electrophysiological study on the autonomic innervation of the mesenteric lymph node in the rat. *Neuroscience Letters, 243*, 144–146.

Niijima, A. (1995). An electrophysiological study on the vagal innervation of the thymus in the rat. *Brain Research Bulletin, 38*, 319–323.

Nilsson, G., & Ahlstedt, S. (1989). Increased delayed-type hypersensitivity reaction in rats neuromanipulated with capsaicin. *International Archives of Allergy and Applied Immunology, 90*, 256–260.

Nilsson, G., Alving, K., Ahlstedt, S., Hokfelt, T., & Lundberg, J. M. (1990). Peptidergic innervation of rat lymphoid tissue and lung: relation to mast cells and sensitivity to capsaicin and immunization. *Cell and Tissue Research, 262*, 125–133.

Nilsson, G., Forsberg-Nilsson, K., Xiang, Z., Hallbook, F., Nilsson, K., & Metcalfe, D. D. (1997). Human mast cells express functional TrkA and are a source of nerve growth factor. *European Journal of Immunology, 27*, 2295–2301.

Nilsson, S. (1978). Sympathetic innervation of the spleen of the cane toad, *Bufo marinus. Comparative Biochemistry and Physiology, C: Comparative Pharmacology, 61C*, 133–139.

Nilsson, S., & Grove, D. J. (1974). Adrenergic and cholinergic innervation of the spleen of the cod: *Gadus morhua. European Journal of Pharmacology, 28*, 135–143.

Nohr, D., Michel, S., Fink, T., & Weihe, E. (1995). Pro-enkephalin opioid peptides are abundant in porcine and bovine splenic nerves, but absent from nerves of rat, mouse, hamster, and guinea-pig spleen. *Cell and Tissue Research, 281*, 215–219.

Nohr, D., & Weihe, E. (1991). The neuroimmune link in the bronchus-associated lymphoid tissue (BALT) of cat and rat: Peptides and neural markers. *Brain, Behavior, and Immunity, 5*, 84–101.

Nordlind, K., Libing, C., Ahmed, A. A., Ljungberg, A., & Liden, S. (1995). Immunohistochemical localization of interleukin-6 like immunoreactivity to peripheral nerve-like structures in normal and inflamed human skin. *Annals of the New York Academy of Science, 762*, 450–451.

Novotny, G. E., Heuer, T., Schottelndreier, A., & Fleisgarten, C. (1994). Plasticity of innervation of the medulla of axillary lymph nodes in the rat after antigenic stimulation. *Anatomical Records, 238*, 213–224.

Novotny, G. E., & Hsu, Y. (1993). The effect of immunostimulation on thymic innervation in the rat. *Journal fur Hirnforschung 34*, 155–163.

Novotny, G. E. K. (1988). Ultrastructural analysis of lymph node innervation in the rat. *Acta Anatomica, 133*, 57–61.

Novotny, G. E. K., & Kliche, K. O. (1986). Innervation of lymph nodes: A combined silver impregnation and electron-microscopic study. *Acta Anatomica, 127*, 243–248.

Odum, L., Petersen, L. J., Skov, P. S., & Ebskov, L. B. (1998). Pituitary adenylate cyclase activating polypeptide (PACAP) is localized in human dermal neurons and causes histamine release from skin mast cells. *Inflammation Research, 47*, 488–492.

Okayama, Y., Ono, Y., Nakazawa, T., Church, M. K, & Mori, M. (1998). Human skin mast cells produce TNF-alpha by substance P. *International Archives of Allergy and Applied Immunology, 117*(Suppl. 1), 48–51.

Okiji, T., Jontell, M., Belichenko, P., Dahlgren, U., Bergenholtz, G., & Dahlstrom, A. (1997). Structural and functional association between substance P- and calcitonin gene-related peptide-immunoreactive nerves and accessory cells in the rat dental pulp. *Journal of Dental Research 76*, 1818–1824.

Olschowka, J. A., Felten, S. Y., Bellinger, D. L., Lorton, D., & Felten, D. L. (1988). NPY-positive nerve terminals contact lymphocytes in the periarteriolar lymphatic sheath of the rat splenic white pulp. *Society for Neuroscience, Abstract, 14*, 1280.

Ositelu, D. O., Morris, R., & Vaillant, C. (1987). Innervation of facial skin but not masticatory muscles or the tongue by trigeminal primary afferents containing somatostatin in the rat. *Neuroscience Letters, 78*, 271–276.

Ottaway, C. A. (1985). Evidence for local neuromodulation of T cell migration in vivo. *Advances in Experimental Medicine, 186*, 637–645.

Ottaway, C. A. (1984). In vitro alteration of receptors for vasoactive intestinal peptide changes the in vivo localization of mouse T cells. *Journal of Experimental Medicine, 160*, 1054–1069.

Ottaway, C. A., & Greenberg, G. R. (1984). Interaction of vasoactive intestinal peptide with mouse lymphocytes: Specific binding and the modulation of mitogen responses. *Journal of Immunology, 132*, 417–423.

Ottaway, C. A., Lewis, D. L., & Asa, S. L. (1987). Vasoactive intestinal peptide-containing nerves in Peyer's patches. *Brain, Behavior, and Immunity, 1*, 148–158.

Pang, X., Boucher, W., Triadafilopoulos, G., Sant, G. R., & Theoharides, T. C. (1996). Mast cell and substance P-positive nerve involvement in a patient with both irritable bowel syndrome and interstitial cystitis. *Urology, 47*, 436–438.

Pang, X., Marchand, J., Sant, G. R., Kream, R. M., & Theoharides, T. C. (1995). Increased number of substance P positive nerve fibers in interstitial cystitis. *British Journal of Urology, 75*, 744–750.

Pereira da Silva, J. A., & Carmo-Fonseca, M. (1990). Peptide containing nerves in human synovium: immunohistochemical evidence for decreased innervation in rheumatoid arthritis. *Journal of Rheumatology, 17*, 1592–1599.

Pfoch, M., & Unsicker, K. (1972). Electron microscopic study on the innervation of Peyer's patches of Syrian hamster. *Zeitschrift fur Zellforsch und Mikoscopische Anatomie, 123*, 425–429.

Pincelli, C., Fantini, F., Massimi, P., Girolomoni, G., Seidenari, S., & Giannetti, A. (1990). Neuropeptides in skin from patients with atopic dermatitis: An immunohistochemical study. *British Journal of Dermatology, 122*, 745–750.

Popper, P., Mantyh, C. R., Vigna, S. R., Magioos, J. E., & Mantyh, P. W. (1988). The localization of sensory nerve fibers and receptor binding sites for sensory neuropeptides in canine mesenteric lymph nodes. *Peptides, 9*, 257–267.

Poulsen, K. T., Armanini, M. P., Klein, R. D., Hynes, M. A., Phillips, H. S., & Rosenthal, A. (1994). $TGF_{\beta2}$ and $TGF_{\beta3}$ are potent survival factors for midbrain dopaminergic neurons. *Neuron, 13*, 1245–1252.

Probert, L., de Mey, J., & Polak, J. M. (1981). Distinct subpopulations of enteric p-type neurones contain substance P and vasoactive intestinal polypeptide. *Nature, 294*, 470–471.

Purcell, E. S., & Gattone, V. H. (1992). Immune system of the spontaneously hypertensive rat. I. Sympathetic innervation. *Experimental Neurology, 117*, 44–50.

Quinonez, G., Bramwell, N. H., Colley, E. C. C., Simon, G. T., Bienenstock, J., & Stead, R. H. (1989). Eosinophils in normal nematode-infected rat intestine are in direct contact with "p-type" post-ganglionic axons. *Laboratory Investigation, 60*, 75A.

Rameshwar, P. & Gascon, P. (1997). Hematopoietic modulation by the tachykinins. *Acta Haematologica, 98*, 59–64.

Rameshwar, P., & Gascon, P. (1996). Induction of negative hematopoietic regulators by neurokinin-A in bone marrow stroma. *Blood, 88*, 98–106.

Rameshwar, P., Ganea, D., & Gascon, P. (1994). Induction of IL-3 and granulocyte-macrophage colony-stimulating factor by substance P in bone marrow cells is partially mediated through the release of IL-1 and IL-6. *Journal of Immunology, 152*, 4044–4054.

Rameshwar, P., Ganea, D., & Gascon, P. (1993). *In vitro* stimulatory effect of substance P on hematopoiesis. *Blood, 81*, 391–398.

Rameshwar, P., Poddar, A., & Gascon, P. (1997). Hematopoietic regulation mediated by interactions among the neurokinins and cytokines. *Leukocytes and Lymphomas, 28*, 1–10.

Raychaudhuri, S. P., Jiang, W. Y., & Farber, E. M. (1998). Psoriatic keratinocytes express high levels of nerve growth factor. *Acta Dermatovenerealogica, 78*, 84–86.

Reilly, D. M., Ferdinando, D., Johnston, C., Shaw, C., Buchanan, K. D., & Green, M. R. (1997). The epidermal nerve fibre network: Characterization of nerve fibres in human skin by confocal microscopy and assessment of racial variations. *British Journal of Dermatology, 137*, 163–170.

Reilly, F. D., McCuskey, P. A., Miller, M. L., McCuskey, R. S., & Meineke, H. A. (1979). Innervation of the periarteriolar lymphatic sheath of the spleen. *Tissue and Cell, 11*, 121–126.

Reubi, J. C., Horisberger, U., Dappeler, A., & Laissue, J. A. (1998). Localization of receptors for vasoactive intestinal peptide, somatostatin, and substance P in distinct compartments of human lymphoid organs. *Blood, 92*, 191–197.

Reynolds, M. L., Ward, A., Graham, C. F., Coggeshall, R., & Fitzgerald, M. (1997). Decreased skin sensory innervation in transgenic mice overexpressing insulin-like growth factor-II. *Neuroscience, 79*, 789–797.

Romano, T. A., Felten, S. Y., Felten, D. L., & Olschowka, J. A. (1991). Neuropeptide-Y innervation of the rat spleen: Another potential immunomodulatory neuropeptide. *Brain, Behavior, and Immunity, 5*, 116–131.

Romano, T., Felten, S. Y., Olschowka, J. A., & Felten, D. L. (1994). Noradrenergic and peptidergic innervation of lymphoid organs in the beluga, *Delphinapterus leucas*: an anatomical link between the nervous and immune systems. *Journal of Morphology, 221*, 243–259.

Romeo, H. E., Fink, T., Yanaihara, N., & Weihe, E. (1994). Distribution and relative proportions of neuropeptide Y- and proenkephalin-containing noradrenergic neurones in rat superior cervical ganglion: Separate projections to submaxillary lymph nodes. *Peptides, 15*, 1479–1487.

Rosenstein, J. M., & Brightman, M. W. (1983). Circumventing the blood-brain barrier with autonomic ganglion transplants. *Science, 221*, 879–881.

Ruhl, A., Hurst, S., & Collins, S. M. (1994). Synergism between interleukins 1β and 6 on noradrenergic nerves in rat myenteric plexus. *Gastroenterology, 107*, 993–1001.

Ruskell, G. L., & VanderWerf, F. (1997). Sensory innervation of conjunctival lymph follicles in cynomolgus monkeys. *Investigative Ophthalmology and Visual Science, 38*, 884–892.

Saito, M., Akiyoshi, M., & Shimizu, Y. (1991). Possible role of the sympathetic nervous system in responses to interleukin-1. *Brain Research Bulletin, 27*, 305–308.

Sant, G. R., & Theoharides, T. C. (1994). The role of the mast cell in interstitial cystitis. *Urology Clinics of North America, 21*, 41–53.

Scholzen, T., Armstrong, C. A., Bunnett, W., Luger, T. A., Olerud, J. E., & Ansel, J. C. (1998). Neuropeptides in the skin: interactions between the neuroendocrine and the skin immune systems. *Experimental Dermatology, 7*, 81–96.

Schultzberg, M., Svenson, S. B., Unden, A., & Bartfai, T. (1987). Interleukin-1-like immunoreactivity in peripheral tissues. *Journal of Neuroscience Research, 18*, 184–189.

Schulze, E., Witt, M., Fink, T., Hofer, A., & Funk, R. H. (1997). Immunohistochemical detection of human skin nerve fibers. *Acta Histochemica, 99*, 301–309.

Schwarz, H., Villiger, P. M., von Kempis, J., & Lotz, M. (1994). Neuropeptide Y is an inducible gene in the human immune system. *Journal of Neuroimmunology, 51*, 53–61.

Seelig, L. L., Jr., Schlusselberg, D. S., Smith, W. K., & Woodward, D. J. (1985). Mucosal nerves and smooth muscle relationships with gastric glands of the opossum: An ultrastructural and three-dimensional reconstruction study. *American Journal of Anatomy, 174*, 15–26.

Senapati, A., Anand, P., McGregor, G. P., Ghatei, M. A., Thompson, R. P., & Bloom, S. R. (1986). Depletion of neuropeptides during wound healing in rat skin. *Neuroscience Letters, 71*, 101–105.

Sergeeva, V. E. (1974). Histotopography of catecholamines in the mammalian thymus. *Bulletin of Experimental Biology and Medicine, 77*, 456–458.

Setchenska, M. S., Bonanou-Tzedaki, S. A., & Arnstein, H. R. (1986). Classification of beta-adrenergic subtypes in immature rabbit bone marrow erythroblasts. *Biochemical Pharmacology, 35*, 3679–3684.

Shadlack, A. M., Hart, R. P., Carlson, C. D., & Jonakait, G. M. (1993). Interleukin-1 induces substance P in sympathetic ganglia through the induction of leukemia inhibitory factor (LIF). *Journal of Neuroscience, 13*, 2601–2609.

Shimizu, N., Hori, T., & Nakane, H. (1994). An interleukin-1β-induced noradrenaline release in the spleen is mediated by brain corticotropin-releasing factor: an in vivo microdialysis study in conscious rats. *Brain, Behavior, and Immunity, 7*, 14–23.

Singh, U. (1979a). Effect of catecholamines on lymphopoiesis in fetal mouse thymic explants. *European Journal of Immunology, 14*, 757–759.

Singh, U. (1979b). Effect of catecholamines on lymphopoiesis in fetal mouse thymic explants. *Journal of Anatomy, 129*, 279–292.

Singh, U. (1985a). Lymphopoiesis in the nude fetal mouse thymus following sympathectomy. *Cellular Immunology, 93*, 222–228.

Singh, U. (1985b). Effect of sympathectomy on the maturation of fetal thymocytes grown within the anterior eye chambers in mice. *Advances in Experimental Biology and Medicine, 186*, 349–356.

Singh, U., & Owen, J. J. T. (1975). Studies on the effect of various agents on the maturation of thymus stem cells. *European Journal of Immunology, 5*, 286–288.

Singh, U., & Owen, J. J. T. (1976). Studies on the maturation of thymus stem cells. The effects of catecholamines, histamine, and peptide hormones on the expression of T alloantigens. *European Journal of Immunology, 6*, 59–62.

Sjolund, K., & Elman, R. (1988). Increased tissue concentration of neuropeptide Y in the duodenal mucosa in coeliac disease. *Scandinavian Journal of Gastroenterology, 24*, 607–612.

Skofitsch, G., Savitt, J. M., & Jacobowitz, D. M. (1985). Suggestive evidence for a functional unit between mast cells and substance P fibers in the rat diaphragm and mesentery. *Histochemistry, 82*, 5–8.

Soliven, B., & Albert, J. (1992). Tumour necrosis factor modulates the inactivation of catecholamine secretion in cultured sympathetic neurons. *Journal of Neurochemistry, 58*, 1073–1078.

Stach, W. (1973). Uber die Nervengeflechte der Duodenalzotten: licht- und elektronen-mikroskopische untersuchungen. *Acta Anatomica, 85*, 216–231.

Staniek, V., Doutremepuich, J., Schmitt, D., Claudy, A., & Misery, L. (1999). Expression of substance P receptors in normal and psoriatic skin. *Pathobiology, 67*, 51–54.

Staniek, V., Misery, L., Peguet-Navarro, J., Abello, J., Doutremepuich, J. D., Claudy, A., & Schmitt, D. (1997). Binding and in vitro modulation of human epidermal Langerhans cell functions by substance P. *Archives of Dermatological Research, 289*, 285–291.

Stead, R. H., Bienenstock, J., & Stanisz, A. M. (1987). Neuropeptide regulation of mucosal immunity. *Immunological Reviews, 100*, 333–359.

Stead, R. H., Tomioka, M., Quinonez, G., Simon, G., Felten, S. Y., & Bienenstock, J. (1987). Intestinal mucosal mast cells in normal and nematode-infected rat intestines are in intimate contact with peptidergic nerves. *Proceedings of the National Academy of Science of the United States of America, 84*, 2975–2979.

Stead, R. H., Dixon, M. F., Bramwell, N. H., Riddell, R. H., & Bienenstock, J. (1989). Mast cells are closely apposed to nerves in the human gastrointestinal mucosa. *Gastroenterology, 97*, 575–585.

Stead, R. H., Franks, A. J., Goldsmith, C. H., Bienenstock, J., & Dixon, M. F. (1990). Mast cells are closely apposed to nerves in the human gastrointestinal mucosa. *Gastroenterology, 97*, 575–585.

Stead, R. H., Kosecka-Janiszewska, U., Oestreicher, A. B., Dixon, M. F., & Bienenstock, J. (1991). Remodeling of B-50 (GAP-43)- and NSE-immunoreactive mucosal nerves in the intestines of rats infected with *Nippostrongylus brasiliensis*. *Journal of Neuroscience, 11*, 3809–3821.

Stead, R. H., Tomioka, M., Riddell, R. H., & Bienenstock, J. (1988). Substance P and/or calcitonin gene-related peptide are present in sub-epithelial enteric nerves apposed to intestinal mucosal mast cells. In MacDermott, R. P. (Ed.), *Inflammatory bowel disease: current status and future approach* (pp. 43–48). Amsterdam: Elsevier Press.

Strom, T. B., Lundin, A. P., & Carpenter, C. B. (1977). The role of cyclic nucleotides in lymphocyte activation and function. *Progress in Clinical Immunology, 3*, 115–153.

Sugita, A., Yoshioka, H., & Okita, T. (1983). Innervation of melanocytes in choroid. *Japanese Journal of Ophthalmology, 27*, 609–615.

Sugiura, H., Omoto, M., Hirota, Y., Danno, K., & Uehara, M. (1997). Density and fine structure of peripheral nerves in various skin lesions of atopic dermatitis. *Archives of Dermatological Research, 289*, 125–131.

Sundler, F., Carraway, R. E., Hakanson, R., Alumets, J., & Dubois, M. P. (1978). Immunoreactive neurotensin and somatostatin in the chicken thymus. *Cell and Tissue Research, 194*, 367–376.

Sung, C. P., Arleth, A. J., & Feuerstein, G. Z. (1991). Neuropeptide Y upregulates the adhesiveness of human endothelial cells for leukocytes. *Circulation Research, 68*, 314–318.

Tabarowski, Z., Gibson-Berry, K., & Felten, S. Y. (1996). Noradrenergic and peptidergic innervation of the mouse femur. *Acta Histochemica, 98*, 453–457.

Takahashi, K., Nakanishi, S., & Imamura, S. (1993). Direct effects of cutaneous neuropeptides on adenylyl cyclase activity and proliferation in a keratinocyte cell line: Stimulation of cyclic AMP formation by CGRP and VIP/PHM, and inhibition by NPY through G protein-coupled receptors. *Journal of Investigative Dermatology, 101*, 646–651.

Takase, B., & Nomura, S. (1957). Studies on the innervation of the bone marrow. *Journal of Comparative Neurology, 108*, 421–443.

Terao, A., Oikawa, M., & Saito, M. (1994). Tissue-specific increase in norepinephrine turnover by central interleukin-1, but not by interleukin-6, in rats. *American Journal of Physiology, 266*, R400–R404.

Theoharides, T. C., Sant, G. R., El-Mansoury, M., Letourneau, R. J., Ucci, A. A. Jr., & Meares, E. M. Jr. (1995). Activation of bladder mast cells in interstitial cystitis: A light and electron microscopic study. *Journal of Urology, 153*, 629–636.

Thompson, R. J., Doran, J. F., Jackson, P., Dhillon, A. P., & Rode, J. (1983). PGP 9.5: A new marker for vertebrate neurons and neuroendocrine cells. *Brain Research, 278*, 224–228.

Tollefson, L., & Bulloch, K. (1990). Dual-label retrograde transport: CNS innervation of the mouse thymus distinct from other mediastinum viscera. *Journal of Neuroscience Research, 25*, 20–28.

Topilko, A., & Caillou, B. (1985). Fine structural localization of acetylcholinesterase activity in rat submandibular gland. *Journal of Histochemistry and Cytochemistry, 33*, 439–445.

Torii, H., Hosoi, J., Asahina, A., & Granstein, R. D. (1997). Calcitonin gene-related peptide and Langerhans cell function. *Journal of Investigative Dermatology Symposium Proceeding, 2*, 82–86.

Torii, H., Hosoi, J., Beissert, S., Xu, S., Fox, F. E., Asahina, A., Takashima, A., Rook, A. H., & Granstein, R. D. (1997). Regulation of cytokine expression in macrophages and the Langerhans cell-like XS-52 by calcitonin gene-related peptide. *Journal of Leukocyte Biology, 61*, 216–223.

Torii, H., Yan, Z., Hosoi, J., & Granstein, R. D. (1997). Expression of neurotrophic factors and neuropeptide receptors by Langerhans cells and the Langerhans cell-like cell line XS52: Further support for a functional relationship between Langerhans cells and epidermal nerves. *Journal of Investigative Dermatology, 109*, 586–591.

Tran, M. A., Dang, T. L., Lafontan, M. S., & Montastruc, P. (1985). Adrenergic neurohumoral influences of FFA release from bone marrow adipose tissue. *Journal de Pharmacologie, 16*, 171–179.

Trudrung, P., Furness, J. B., Pompolo, S., & Messenger, J. P. (1994). Locations and chemistries of sympathetic nerve cells that project to the gastrointestinal tract and spleen. *Archives of Histology & Cytology, 57*, 139–150.

Ueda, H., Abe, M., Takehana, K., Iwasa, K., & Hiraga, T. (1991). Ultrastructure of the red pulp in spleen innervation in horse and pig. *Acta Anatomica, 141*, 151–158.

Ueyama, T., Kozuki, K., Houtani, T., Ikeda, M., Kitajiri, M., Tamashita, T., Kumazawa, T., Nagatsu, I., & Sugimoto, T. (1990). Immunolocalization of tyrosine hydroxylase and vasoactive intestinal polypeptide in nerve fibers innervating human palatine tonsil and paratonsillar glands. *Neuroscience Letters, 116*, 70–74.

Undem, B. J., Dick, E. C., & Buckner, C. K. (1983). Inhibition by vasoactive intestinal peptide of antigen-induced histamine release from guinea-pig minced lung. *European Journal of Pharmacology, 88*, 247–249.

van Coelln, R., Unsicker, K., & Krieglstein, K. (1995). Screening of interleukins for survival-promoting effects on cultured mesencephalic dopaminergic neurons from embryonic rat brain. *Developmental Brain Research, 89*, 150–154.

Viac, J., Gueniche, A., Doutremepuich, J. D., Reichert, U., Claudy, A., & Schmitt, D. (1996). Substance P and keratinocyte activation markers: An in vitro approach. *Archives of Dermatological Research, 288*, 85–90.

Vriend, C. Y., Zuo, L., Dyck, D. G., Nance, D. M., & Greenberg, A. H. (1993). Central administration of interleukin-1β increases norepinephrine turnover in the spleen. *Brain Research Bulletin, 31*, 39–42.

Vyden, J. K., Groseth-Dittrich, M. F., Callis, G., Lars, M. M., & Weinberger, H. (1971). The effect of propranolol on peripheral hemodynamics in rheumatoid arthritis. *Arthritis and Rheumatism, 14*, 420.

Wakabayashi, Y., Maeda, T., Aimi, Y., & Kwok, Y. N. (1998). Increase of low-affinity neurotrophin receptor p75 and growth-associated protein-43 immunoreactivities in the rat urinary bladder during experimentally induced nerve regeneration. *Journal of Urology, 160*, 1513–1517.

Wakabayashi, Y., Maeda, T., Tomoyoshi, T., & Kwok, Y. N. (1998). Increase of growth protein-43 immunoreactivity following cyclophosphamide-induced cystitis in rats. *Neuroscience Letters, 240*, 89–92.

Walcott, B., & McLean, J. R. (1985). Catecholamine-containing neurons and lymphoid cells in a lacrimal gland of the pigeon. *Brain Research, 328*, 129–137.

Wallengren, J., Ekman, R., & Möller, H. (1991). Capsaicin enhances allergic contact dermatitis in the guinea pig. *Contact Dermatitis, 24*, 30–34.

Wallengren, J., Ekman, R., & Sundler, F. (1987). Occurrence and distribution of neuropeptides in the human skin. An immunocytochemical and immunochemical study on normal skin and blister fluid from inflamed skin. *Acta Dermatologica Venereologica, 67*, 185–192.

Wallengren, J., Moller, H., & Ekman, R. (1987). Occurrence of substance P, vasoactive intestinal peptide, and calcitonin gene-related peptide in dermographism and cold urticaria. *Archives Dermatology, 279*, 512–515.

Watkins, L. R., Goehler, L. E., Relton, J., Brewer, M. T., & Maier, S. F. (1995). Mechanisms of tumor necrosis factor-α (TNF-α) hyperalgesia. *Brain Research, 692*, 244–250.

Watkins, L. R., Wiertelak, E. P., Goehler, L. E., Smith, K. P., Martin, D., & Maier, S. F. (1994). Characterization of cytokine-induced hyperalgesia. *Brain Research, 654*, 15–26.

Weihe, E., Müller, S., Fink, T., & Zentel, H. J. (1989). Tachykinins, calcitonin gene-related peptide and neuropeptide Y in nerves of the mammalian thymus: Interactions with mast cells in autonomic and sensory neuroimmunomodulation. *Neuroscience Letters, 100*, 77–82.

Weisz-Carrington, P., Nagomoto, N., Farraj, M., Buschmann, R., Rypins, E. B., & Stanisz, A. M. (1991). Analysis of SP/VIP fiber association with T_4 and T_8 lymphocytes in normal human colon. In Mestechky, J. (Ed.), *Advances in mucosal immunology* (pp. 559–561). New York: Plenum Press.

Weston, A. P., Biddle, W. L., Bhatia, P. S., & Miner, P. B. Jr. (1993). Terminal ileal mucosal mast cells in irritable bowel syndrome. *Digestive Diseases and Sciences, 38*, 1590–1595.

Williams, J. M., & Felten, D. L. (1981). Sympathetic innervation of murine thymus and spleen: A comparative histofluorescence study. *Anatomical Records, 199*, 531–542.

Williams, J. M., Peterson, R. G., Shea, P. A., Schmedtje, J. F., Bauer, D. C., & Felten, D. L. (1981). Sympathetic innervation of murine thymus and spleen: Evidence for a functional link between the nervous and immune systems. *Brain Research Bulletin, 6*, 83–94.

Winberg, M., Holmgren, S., & Nilsson, S. (1981). Effects of denervation of 6-hydroxydopamine on the activity of choline acetyltransferase in the spleen of the cod, *Gadus morhua*. *Comparative Biochemical Physiology, 69C*, 141–143.

Yamashita, T., Kumazawa, H., Kozuki, K., Amano, H., Tomoda, K., & Kumazawa, T. (1984). Autonomic nervous system in human palatine tonsil. *Acta Otolaryngology, 416*, 63–71.

Yamazaki, K., & Allen, T. D. (1990). Ultrastructural morphometric study of efferent nerve terminals on murine bone marrow stromal cells, and the recognition of a novel anatomical unit: The "neuro-reticular complex." *American Journal of Anatomy, 187*, 261–276.

Yang, H., Wang, L., & Huang, C. S. (1998). Plasticity of GAP-43 innervation of the spleen during immune response in the mouse. Evidence for axonal sprouting and redistribution of the nerve fibers. *Neuroimmunomodulation, 5*, 53–60.

Yonei, Y. (1987). Autonomic nervous alterations and mast cell degranulation in the exacerbation of ulcerative colitis. *Japanese Journal of Gastroenterology, 84*, 1045–1056.

Yonei, Y., Oda, M., Nakamura, M., Watanabe, N. H., Tsuskada, N., Komatsu, H. K., Akaiwa, Y., Ichikawa, E., Kaneko, K., Asakura, H., Fujiwara, T., & Tsuchiya, M. (1985). Evidence for direct interaction between the cholinergic nerve and mast cells in rat colonic mucosa. An electron microscopic cytochemical and autoradiographic study. *Journal of Clinical Electron Microscopy, 18*, 560–561.

Zalcman, S., Green-Johnson, J. M., Murray, L., Wan, W., Nance, D. M., & Greenberg, A. H. (1994). Interleukin-2-induced enhancement of an antigen-specific IgM plaque-forming cell response is mediated by the sympathetic nervous system. *Journal of Pharmacology and Experimental Therapeutics, 271*, 977–982.

Zapata, A., Villena, A., & Cooper, E. L. (1982). Direct contacts between nerve endings and lymphoid cells in the jugular body of *Rana pipiens*. *Experientia, 38*, 623–624.

Zentel, H. J., & Weihe, E. (1991). The neuro-B cell link of peptidergic innervation in the bursa Fabricii. *Brain, Behavior, and Immunity, 5*, 132–147.

Zhao, Z. Z., Savage, N. W., Pujic, Z., & Walsh, L. J. (1997). Immunohistochemical localization of mast cells and mast cell-nerve interaction in oral lichen planus. *Oral Diseases, 3*, 71–76.

CHAPTER

3

Introduction to Biological Signaling in Psychoneuroimmunology

DIANNE LORTON, CHERI LUBAHN, DENISE BELLINGER

I. INTRODUCTION

As more powerful anatomic, immunologic, cellular, and molecular techniques become available to study cells and the mechanisms they use to communicate with one another, the intricacies of signaling processes used by cells of the immune system are slowly being delineated. Cells of the immune system possess elaborate systems of proteins that enable them to respond to signals that are (1) self generated, (2) derived from other immunocytes, (3) conveyed by the neuroendocrine and autonomic nervous systems, or (4) generated in response to foreign substances in their microenvironment. Most of these signals are generated via the release of signaling molecules into extracellular compartments, and on reaching their target cells these signaling molecules interact with specific receptors in the plasma membrane or inside the target cell. Binding of the signaling molecules activates a cascade of protein systems. These systems of proteins include cell-surface and intracellular receptor proteins, protein kinases, protein phosphatases, guanosine triphosphate (GTP)-binding proteins, and many intracellular proteins with which these signaling proteins interact. In this chapter we will first discuss the general principles of intercellular signaling, with specific focus on the interaction between cells of the immune system, between neural mediators and immunocytes, and the signaling molecules that are important for these interactions to occur. Next, we will describe the families of cell-surface receptor proteins, and how they generate intracellular signals. Lastly, we will examine how cells of the immune system continuously adapt to respond sensitively to small changes in the concentration of an extracellular signaling molecule.

II. GENERAL PRINCIPLES OF CELL SIGNALING

Cells of the immune system communicate by means of hundreds of kinds of signaling molecules that are (1) secreted by exocytosis, (2) diffuse through the plasma membrane to be released into the extracellular fluids, or (3) remain tightly bound to the cell surface and influence only cells that contact the signaling cell. The nervous system also communicates with cells of the immune system through the evoked release of neurotransmitters, neuromodulators, and hormones. Secreted signaling molecules from these two interactive systems include a variety of structurally different substances, including proteins, small peptides, amino acids, nucleotides, steroids, retinoids, fatty acid derivatives, and even dissolved gases (reviewed in Hardie, 1999; Kahn, 1976; Snyder, 1985).

Regardless of the nature of the signal, cells of the immune system respond by means of specific proteins, called receptors. Binding of a signaling molecule to a specific receptor results in the initiation of a response by the target immune cells. As a rule, extracellular signaling molecules act at very low concentrations (generally $\leq 10^{-8}$ M), and the receptors that recognize them usually bind with high affinity ($K_a \geq 10^8$ L/mole) (Hardie, 1999; Kahn, 1976; Snyder, 1985). In most cases, receptors that bind extracellular signaling molecules are transmembrane proteins on the cell surface of the target cell, and when the extracellular signaling molecule, referred to as a ligand, binds to the receptor, the target cell becomes activated and subsequently generates a cascade of intracellular signals that alters the behavior of the target cell.

In some cases, the receptors for extracellular signaling molecules reside inside the target cell and the ligand must enter the cell to bind to them either in the cytosol or in the nucleus. For example, receptors for glucocorticoids (GC), estrogen, progesterone, and testosterone are not bound to the plasma membrane of cells of the immune system; rather, they are present in the cytosol or within the nucleus of these cells. Many of these ligands must be bound to carrier proteins and transported in the blood stream and other extracellular fluids, because their hydrophobic nature makes them nearly insoluble in aqueous solutions. Once they reach their target cell, they dissociate from their specific carrier proteins and diffuse into the target cell. One example of a signaling molecule that diffuses through the plasma membrane to directly regulate the activity of specific intracellular proteins is nitric oxide, which is produced as a local mediator by activated macrophages and neutrophils to help kill invading microorganisms, as well as by many types of neurons to signal neighboring cells, and is especially involved in neural regulation of blood flow by autonomic nerves (Bredt & Snyder, 1992; Lowenstein & Snyder, 1992; Moncada, Palmer, & Higgs, 1991; Stevens, 1992). Recent evidence supports a similar mechanism of action and signaling for carbon monoxide.

Other small, nongaseous, hydrophobic signaling molecules can diffuse across the plasma membrane, but instead of binding to enzymes as nitric oxide (NO) and carbon monoxide (CO) do, they bind to intracellular receptor proteins that directly regulate gene transcription. Included in this type of signaling molecule are the steroid hormones, thyroid hormones, retinoids, and vitamin D (Evans, 1988; Parker, 1991; Yamamoto, 1985). Once they have diffused across the plasma membrane they bind to intracellular receptor proteins in the steroid-hormone receptor superfamily, which in turn directly regulate the transcription of specific genes. Because of their hydrophobic nature, these signaling molecules resist degradation, persisting in the blood for hours to days, and thus they tend to mediate longer-lasting responses. After ligand binding to the intracellular receptor protein, in many cases there is first induction of the transcription of a small number of specific genes (within about 30 min), known as the primary response. The products of these genes, in turn, activate other genes and produce a delayed secondary response. In different types of cells the set of genes that these hydrophobic signaling molecules regulate can be very different, even when the intracellular receptor protein is identical. This occurs because more than one type of gene regulatory protein must bind to a gene to activate its transcription. This means that an intracellular receptor can activate a gene only if the right combination of other gene regulatory proteins is also present, and some of these are cell-type specific.

Signaling molecules that a cell secretes may act on distant targets or may act as local mediators affecting only cells in the immediate environment of the signaling cell. The latter process is called *paracrine signaling*. Paracrine signaling occurs between cells of the immune system, and with nerve-immune cell interactions. For example, norepinephrine (NE) released from sympathetic nerves that distribute to primary and secondary lymphoid tissue diffuses a short distance from the nerve terminal among nearby fields of immunocytes. Cells of the immune system that possess specific adrenergic receptors on their cell surface have the machinery to interact with this ligand, and respond to this neural signal. Similarly, cytokines released by cells of the immune system typically exert their effects on other immune cells through paracrine signaling. An important feature of this method of signaling is that the secreted signaling molecule must not be allowed to diffuse too far, so they are often rapidly taken up by neighboring target cells, destroyed by extracellular enzymes, or immobilized by the extracellular matrix.

Both the nervous and immune systems secrete signaling molecules that act on target sites distant from where the signaling molecule originates. Neurons can extend long processes, called axons, a great distance to contact target cells; this point of contact is specialized to receive signals from the nerve terminal and is called a *chemical synapse*. When an electrical impulse travels along its axon and reaches the nerve terminals, it stimulates the terminal to secrete a chemical signal, a neurotransmitter. This type of communication is designed to deliver the neurotransmitter signal rapidly and specifically. Chapter 2 of this volume describes the distribution of neurotransmitter-specific nerve fibers in primary and secondary lymphoid tissue and their potential lymphoid and myeloid cell targets. Although NE released from sympathetic nerves in lymphoid organs is thought to act in a paracrine fashion, neuropeptides released from nerves in these organs are probably more limited in their ability to diffuse, and act on target cells in the immediate vicinity of the nerve fiber.

Another way the nervous system signals the immune system is through specialized cells that generally control the behavior of the organism as a whole, referred to as neuroendocrine and/or endocrine cells. These cells secrete their signaling molecules, referred to as hormones, into the bloodstream, which then carries the signal to target cells distributed widely throughout the body. Similarly, products from activated immune cells can travel in the bloodstream to interact with peripheral nerves and/or neurons/glia in the central nervous system. Because this type of signaling relies on blood flow and diffusion, it is relatively slow, and local concentrations of hormones can be very high compared with the concentration of signaling molecules that use other delivery methods.

The forms of signaling discussed thus far allow one cell type to influence another; however, by the same mechanisms, cells also can send signals to other cells of the same type, and to themselves; this type of communication is called *autocrine signaling*. This is an important form of communication in cells of the immune system during their development and activation. Once an immune cell has been directed into a particular path of differentiation, it begins to secrete autocrine signals that reinforce this developmental decision. This is an effective way for simultaneously signaling neighboring cells of identical type to make the same developmental decisions. When immune cells are activated by tissue damage, or by some types of chemical signals, the rate of synthesis and release of certain signaling molecules, like eicosanoids and other inflammatory mediators that are both neural and immune cell derived, increase dramatically. This results in an increase in local levels of these signaling molecules, that in turn influences both the cells that made them and their immediate neighbors. Autocrine signaling also occurs when neurotransmitters released from a nerve terminal interact with specific receptors (autocrine receptors) on the same nerve terminal to regulate neurotransmitter metabolism and/or nerve impulse activity.

Lastly, neighboring cells can interact through gap junctions, a specialized cell–cell junction that can form between closely apposed plasma membranes. This allows for the exchange of small intracellular signaling molecules [intracellular mediators such as Ca^{2+} and cyclic adenosine 3′,5′-phosphate (cAMP)] across narrow water-filled channels that directly connect the cytoplasms of two neighboring cells. Like autocrine signaling, it is believed that gap junction communication helps adjacent cells of a similar type to coordinate their behavior (Caveney, 1985). This is a common mechanism of interaction between groups of similar neurons in the central nervous system.

III. CELLULAR RESPONSES TO SIGNALS

Cells of the immune system and neurons are both programmed to respond to specific combinations of signaling molecules in precise ways, whether it be to differentiate, proliferate, carry out some specialized functions, or undergo cell death (Raff, 1992). Cells of the immune system, as well as neurons, are programmed to depend on a specific set of signals simply for survival, and when they are deprived of the appropriate signals, they will activate a "suicide" program, apoptosis, designed to destroy itself. Depending on the cell type, there are different sets of survival signals. GC are well known for their ability to induce apoptosis in lymphocytes, and it also is clear that activation and survival of lymphocytes during an immune response depends of dual activation of receptor proteins that reside on their cell surfaces.

Two things determine how a cell responds to its environment: (1) the set of receptor proteins that a cell possesses, which in turn detects a particular set of available signaling molecules; and (2) the intracellular machinery by which the cell integrates and interprets the information that it receives from its receptors. This means that a single signaling molecule can have different effects on different target cells. Sometimes this can be explained by the receptor subtype that the cell possesses, but in many cases the same signaling molecule can bind to the same receptor subtype and yet produce very different responses in different types of target cells. This reflects differences in the intracellular machinery to which the receptors are coupled.

Cell surface receptor proteins act as signal transducers, that is, they bind the signaling ligand with high affinity and convert this extracellular event into one or more intracellular signals that alter the behavior of the target cell (Schimke, 1969). Most cell surface receptors belong to one of three classes that are defined by the transduction mechanism they use: (1) ion-channel-linked receptors or transmitter gated ion channels; (2) G protein-linked receptors; and (3) enzyme-linked receptors (Nishizuka, 1985). Ion channel-linked receptors are involved in rapid synaptic signaling between electrically excitable cells. This type of signaling is important for the propagation of an action potential along the axons of neurons, for contraction of muscle cells, and for postsynaptic neurotransmission between two or more neurons. Postsynaptic neurotransmission is mediated by a small number of neurotransmitters that transiently open or close the ion channel formed by the protein to which they bind, briefly changing the ion permeability of the plasma membrane, and subsequently the excitability of the postsynaptic cell.

All G protein-linked receptors belong to a large superfamily of homologous, seven-pass transmembrane proteins (Nishizuka, 1985). G protein-linked receptors indirectly regulate the activity of a plasma membrane-bound target protein, that can be either an enzyme or an ion channel. Trimeric GTP-regulatory proteins, or G proteins, mediate the interaction between the receptor and the target protein. The activation of the target protein either alters the concentration of one or more intracellular mediators if the target protein is an enzyme, or alters the ion permeability of the plasma membrane if the target protein is an ion channel. Activation of the target protein, in turn, alters the activity of other proteins in the cell.

Enzyme-linked receptors are generally a heterogeneous group of single-pass transmembrane proteins that either function directly as enzymes or are associated with enzymes (Nishizuka, 1985). Their ligand-binding site is outside the cell, and their catalytic site (generally either a protein kinase or associated with a protein kinase) is inside the cell. Signals received by these classes of receptors are often relayed to the nucleus, where they alter specific gene expression. This is accomplished by sequential activation of an elaborate set of intracellular signaling proteins. Generally, intracellular signaling proteins either become phosphorylated by protein kinases, dephosphorylated by protein phosphatases, or they are induced to bind triphosphate nucleotides producing proteins in an activated state (reviewed in Pelech, 1993; Posada & Cooper, 1992). They also tend to cause the phosphorylation of downstream proteins as part of a phosphorylation cascade.

Two main types of protein kinases mediate phosphorylation cascades: (1) serine/threonine kinases (phosphorylate proteins on serines and to a lesser extent, threonines); and (2) tyrosine kinases (phosphorylate proteins on tyrosines) (reviewed in Pelech, 1993; Posada & Cooper, 1992). Some protein kinases can do both. Cellular responses to signaling molecules are mediated by specific combinations of intracellular signals rather than by a single signal acting alone; therefore, the target cell must integrate the information coming from separate signals to make the proper response. This integration depends on the interactions between the various protein phosphorylation cascades that are activated by different extracellular signals (reviewed in Bourne & Nicoll, 1993; Cohen, 1992). Some of the intracellular signaling proteins in the cascades serve as integrating devices, that is, in response to multiple signal inputs they produce an output that is calibrated to cause the desired biological effect. A good example of the complexities of signal integration and diversity of responses is seen with antigen binding to appropriate receptors on cells of the immune system, and the T cell responses to activation of the T cell receptor (TCR). The specific details of integration and diversity of responsiveness in these signaling pathways are discussed later in the chapter.

IV. SIGNALING VIA G PROTEIN-LINKED RECEPTORS

G protein-linked receptors mediate cellular responses to a wide diversity of signaling molecules, including hormones, neurotransmitters, and cytokines, and the same ligand can activate many different families of trimeric GTP-binding proteins or G proteins (reviewed in Birnbaumer, 1990; Linder & Gilman, 1992). For example, NE can activate at least 9, acetylcholine acts via 5 or more, and serotonin interacts with at least 15 distinct G protein-linked receptors. Despite this diversity in G proteins, all G proteins have a similar structure, consisting of a single polypeptide chain that threads back and forth across the plasma membrane seven times. G protein-linked receptors that bind protein ligands have large extracellular ligand-binding domains formed by part of the polypeptide chain. Receptors for small ligands, like NE, have small extracellular domains, and the binding site is usually deep within the plane of the membrane and formed by several of the transmembrane segments. The intracellular domains have components that are responsible for binding to trimeric G proteins and components that become phosphorylated during receptor desensitization.

The function of G proteins is to couple the receptor to their target enzymes or ion channels in the plasma membrane (reviewed in Birnbaumer, 1990; Bourne, Sanders & McCormick, 1991; Hepler & Gilman, 1992; Linder & Gilman, 1992). These proteins are structurally distinct from the single-chain GTP-binding proteins called monomeric GTP-binding proteins, which help relay intracellular signals and regulate vascular traffic and other processes in the cell. GTP-binding proteins are GTPases that function as molecular switches, turning on and off between two states: an active state when GTP is bound, and an inactive state when guanosine diphosphate (GDP) is bound. In this process, the following occurs: (1) an intracellular ligand binds to a G protein-linked receptor; (2) the receptor changes its conformation and switches on the trimeric G proteins that associate with it by causing them to eject their GDP and replace it with GTP; (3) the G protein is inactivated when the G protein hydrolyzes its own bound GTP, converting it back to GDP; and (4) during this process the active protein, generated by the activation of an enzyme that is coupled to the G protein, diffuses away from the receptor and delivers its message to its downstream target.

G protein-linked receptors generally activate a chain of events that alters the concentration of one or more small intracellular signaling molecules, referred to as intracellular mediators or second messengers (reviewed in Birnbaumer, 1990; Bourne et al., 1991; Hepler & Gilman, 1992 Linder & Gilman, 1992). The most widely used second messengers are cAMP and Ca^{2+}. On receptor stimulation, cAMP concentrations can change fivefold in a matter of seconds, a response that requires the rapid synthesis of this molecule, with subsequent rapid breakdown or removal making it an effective signaling molecule. cAMP is synthesized from adenosine 5′-triphosphate (ATP) by a plasma membrane-bound enzyme, adenylyl cyclase, and it is rapidly and continuously destroyed by one or more cAMP phosphodiesterases, which hydrolyses cAMP to adenosine 5′-monophosphate (5′-AMP). Extracellular signaling molecules, such as vasoactive intestine polypeptide (VIP), NE, corticotropin releasing hormone (CRH), luteinizing hormone, and somatostatin, which act through this pathway, do so by altering the activity of adenylyl cyclase. Within a particular type of cells, it is generally found that all ligands that activate adenylyl cyclase usually produce the same effect, and the different receptors for these ligands activate a common pool of adenylyl cyclase molecules to which they are coupled by a trimeric G protein. Because this protein is involved in enzyme activation, it is referred to as a stimulatory G protein or G_s.

The best studied examples of G_s-linked receptors coupled to the activation of adenylyl cyclase are β_2-adrenergic receptors (β_2-AR) (Feder et al., 1986). β-AR are present on a wide variety of immunocytes (Bidart, Motte, Assicot, Bohuon, & Bellett, 1983; Bishopric, Cohen, & Lefkowitz, 1980; Hadden, Hadden & Middleton, 1970; Landmann, Bittiger, & Bühler, 1981; Landmann, Burgisser, West, & Buhler, 1985; Loveland, Jarrott, & McKenzie, 1981; Miles, Atweh, Otten, Arnason, & Chelmicka-Schorr, 1984; Motulsky, Cunningham, Deblasi, & Insel, 1986; Pochet & Delespesse, 1983; Pochet, Delespesse, Gausset, & Collet, 1979; Singh, 1984; Williams, Snyderman, & Lefkowitz, 1976). Agonist binding to β-AR on cells of the immune system, including B cells, T cells, and macrophages, stimulate an increase in cAMP (Bach, 1975; Bishopric et al., 1980; Geenen et al., 1986; Koff & Dunegan, 1986; Niaudet, Beaurain, & Bach, 1976; Stachelin, Müller, Portenier, & Harris, 1985), and result in subsequent changes in immune responses (Ernström & Sandberg, 1973, 1974; Ernström & Söder, 1975; D. L. Felten et al., 1987; D. L. Felten, Felten, Carlson, Olschowka, & Livnat, 1985; Livnat, Madden, Felten, & Felten, 1987; Madden et al., 1997; Madden,

Felten, Felten, Sundaresan, & Livnat, 1989; Madden et al., 1994; Madden, Sanders, & Felten, 1995; Singh, 1979; Yeh et al., 1985; Webber, DeFelice, Ferguson & Powell, 1970). The concentration of cAMP attained after β-AR stimulation depends on a number of variables, such as receptor density on the target cells (Khan, Sansoni, Silverman, & Engleman, 1986), and the activation state of the lymphocyte (Carlson, Brooks & Roszman, 1989; Roszman & Carlson, 1991). Signaling molecules that promote cAMP production must in some way integrate with signals that regulate cell division in lymphocytes, differentiation, and other cellular functions (Boynton & Whitfield, 1983; Carlson et al., 1989; Roszman & Carlson, 1991) known to be influenced by NE and other signaling molecules that increase intracellular cAMP in immunocytes. The intracellular mechanisms through which adrenergic receptor stimulation modulates lymphocyte and macrophage function, and how these pathways integrate with intracellular pathways that regulate cytokine production, proliferation, and differentiation are described in detail later in this chapter.

A trimeric G protein has three different polypeptide chains, an α, a β, and a γ chain. The G_s α chain, α_s, binds and hydrolyses GTP, which activates adenylyl cyclase (reviewed in Bourne et al., 1991; Hepler & Gilman, 1992; Linder & Gilman, 1992). The G_s β and γ chains form a tight complex, $\beta\gamma$, important for anchoring G_s to the cytoplasmic face of the plasma membrane. G_s, in its inactive form, exists as a trimer with GDP bound to an α_s subunit. When stimulated by binding to a ligand-activated receptor, α_s exchanges its GDP for GTP, causing α_s to dissociate from $\beta\gamma$, allowing α_s to bind instead to an adenylyl cyclase molecule, which it activates to produce cAMP from the hydrolysis of ATP. The GTPase activity of α_s is stimulated when α_s binds to adenylyl cyclase, which in turn causes hydrolysis of the bound GTP to GDP. This renders both α_s and adenylyl cyclase inactive. The α_s then reassociates with the $\beta\gamma$ complex to re-form an inactive G_s molecule. The bacterial toxin, cholera toxin, is an enzyme that acts by blocking the ability of α_s to hydrolyze its bound GTP in infected cells (Lai, 1980).

Some receptors, like α_2-AR, decrease cAMP production through its coupling to adenylyl cyclase via an inhibitory trimeric G protein, G_i (reviewed in Birnbaumer, 1990, 1992; Hepler & Gilman, 1992; Iniguez-Lluhi, Kleuss, & Gilman, 1993; Linder & Gilman, 1992). G_i can have the same $\beta\gamma$ subunit, but it has a different α subunit, α_i. When activated α_2-AR bind to G_i, causing α_i to bind to GTP and dissociate from the $\beta\gamma$ complex. Both the released α_i and $\beta\gamma$ subunits contribute to the inhibition of adenylyl cyclase. The α_i subunit inhibits adenylyl cyclase, and the $\beta\gamma$ subunit blocks cAMP synthesis in 2 ways: (1) by binding to adenylyl cyclase, and (2) by binding to any free α_s subunits and thus preventing them from activating adenylyl cyclase molecules. Activation of G_i proteins also can open K^+ channels. The bacterial-derived pertussis toxin acts by preventing the G_i complex from interacting with receptors, and so the complex remains bound to GDP and is unable to inhibit adenylyl cyclase or open K^+ channels. Because α_2-AR are present on cells of the immune system, a more detailed description of the downstream intracellular pathways is presented later in this chapter.

Trimeric G proteins are versatile intracellular signaling molecules (reviewed in Birnbaumer, 1993; Iniguez-Lluhi et al., 1993). From the above discussion, we have shown that either the α subunit, or both the α and the $\beta\gamma$ subunits, are active components in transducing extracellular signals. In other cases, receptors are coupled to their target proteins only by the released $\beta\gamma$ subunits. $\beta\gamma$ complexes also can act as conditional regulators of effector proteins, i.e., they can enhance the activation of some forms of adenylyl cyclase, but only if adenylyl cyclase has been activated by α_s.

cAMP exerts its effect in lymphocytes and other cells of the immune system mainly by activating cAMP-dependent protein kinase A (PKA), which catalyzes the transfer of the terminal phosphate group from ATP to specific serines or threonines of selected proteins (reviewed in Krebs, 1989; Taylor, Buechler & Yonemoto, 1990). Covalent phosphorylation of appropriate amino acids on these proteins, in turn, regulates their activity. PKA is found in all animal cells, and is believed to mediate all of the effects of cAMP in most cells. The substrates for PKA differ in different cell types, explaining why cAMP effects vary depending on the target cell. The inactive state of PKA consists of a complex of two catalytic subunits and two regulatory units that bind cAMP. The binding of cAMP alters the conformation of the regulatory subunits, causing them to dissociate from the complex. The released active catalytic subunits can subsequently phosphorylate specific substrate protein molecules.

In some cells, an increase in cAMP activates the transcription of specific genes. For example, in cells that secrete somatostatin cAMP turns on the gene that encodes this hormone. Cells of the immune system have been reported to synthesize somatostatin; however, the intracellular mechanisms that mediate somatostatin production in these cells has not been described. In these cases, there is a short DNA sequence, called the cAMP response element (CRE), that is present in the regulatory region of genes that can be turned on by cAMP. This sequence is recognized by a specific gene regulatory protein called CRE-binding (CREB) protein, and when CREB protein is phosphorylated by PKA on a single serine residue, it is activated to turn on the transcription of these genes (reviewed in Brindle & Montminy, 1992).

Dephosphorylation of PKA-induced phosphorylated serines and threonines inactivates the effects of cAMP (reviewed in Cohen, 1989). This reaction is catalyzed by four groups of serine/threonine phosphoprotein phosphatases, indicated as protein phosphatases I, IIA, IIB, and IIC. Protein phosphatase IIC is a minor phosphatase, unrelated to the others. The rest of these phosphatases are composed of a homologous catalytic subunit complexed with one or more regulatory subunits. Protein phosphatase I plays an important role in the response of cAMP, since it is responsible for dephosphorylating many of the proteins phosphorylated by PKA, including CREB. This enzyme can be bound and inactivated by another target of PKA, a specific phosphatase inhibitor protein under certain conditions, ultimately boosting the response of cAMP. Protein phosphatase IIA has a broad specificity and seems to be the main phosphatase responsible for reversing many of the phosphorylations catalyzed by serine/threonin kinases; it plays an important role in regulating the cell cycle. Protein phosphatase IIB, or calcineurin, is activated by Ca^{2+}.

Trimeric G proteins also couple receptors to another important enzyme, phospholipase C (PLC). The activation of this enzyme leads to an increase in Ca^{2+} concentration in the cytosol, a more widely used intracellular mediator than cAMP (reviewed in Carafoli, 1987). Generally, the intracellular concentration of Ca^{2+} is extremely low ($\leq 10^{-7}$ M), since it is concentrated in the endoplasmic reticulum (ER) (Koch, 1990), while the extracellular fluid contains relatively high Ca^{2+} levels (about 10^{-3} M). This sets up a large gradient that tends to drive Ca^{2+} into the cytosol across both the plasma membrane, and the ER membrane. Signaling molecules can transiently open Ca^{2+} channels in either of these membranes, allowing Ca^{2+} into the cytosol, and increasing local Ca^{2+} concentrations, which in turn activates Ca^{2+}-responsive proteins in the target cell.

Two pathways of Ca^{2+} signaling are well defined, one used mainly by electrically active or excitable cells (important for depolarization of their plasma membrane), and the other used by almost all other eucaryotic cells (reviewed in Carafoli, 1987; Koch, 1990). The first pathway is important for propagation of action potentials along the axons of nerve cells and for the release of neurotransmitters from nerve terminals. In the second Ca^{2+} pathway, binding of extracellular signaling molecules to cell surface receptors causes the release of Ca^{2+} from the ER. This occurs through the coupling of cell surface receptors to Ca^{2+} channels in the ER, via the second messenger, inositol triphosphate (IP_3). More than 25 different cell surface neurotransmitter receptors use this signal transduction pathway, including receptors for vasopression, acetylcholine, thrombin, and antigen.

The two phosphorylated derivatives of phosphatidylinositol (PI) most important in signal transduction are PI bisphosphate (PIP_2) and to a lesser extent, PI phosphate (PIP), which are located mainly in the inner half of the plasma membrane lipid bilayer (reviewed in Bansal & Majerus, 1990; Harden, 1992; Michell, 1992; Sekar & Hokin, 1986). Binding of the signaling molecule to a G protein-linked receptor in the plasma membrane, in this case a trimeric G_q protein, activates a PI-specific PLC called PLC-β, which in turn cleaves PIP_2 to generate two products, IP_3 and diacylglycerol (DAG). At this point, the signaling pathway diverges into two branches mediated by IP_3 and DAG. These two pathways often collaborate to produce a full cellular response. For example, stimulation of some cells to proliferate in culture requires activation of both pathways.

IP_3 diffuses away from the plasma membrane into the cytosol, where it releases Ca^{2+} from ER by binding to IP_3-gated Ca^{2+}-release channels in the ER membrane (reviewed in Berridge, 1993; Ferris & Snyder, 1992; Taylor & Marshal, 1992). Ca^{2+} can bind back to these channels, further increasing Ca^{2+} release, which tends to make release occur rapidly, in an all-or-none fashion. This response is terminated by two mechanisms: (1) IP_3 is rapidly dephosphorylated by specific phosphatases; and (2) Ca^{2+} that enters the cytosol is rapidly pumped largely into the extracellular fluid. However, not all of the IP_3 is dephosphorylated; instead, some can be further phosphorylated to form inositol 1,3,4,5-tetracisphosphate (IP_4), which may mediate slower and more prolonged responses in the cell or promote the refilling of the intracellular Ca^{2+} stores from the extracellular fluid, or both. The enzyme responsible for converting IP_3 to IP_4 is activated by the increase in cytosolic Ca^{2+} induced by IP_3. This provides a negative feedback mechanism for IP_3 concentrations. The IP_3 pathway can be mimicked by Ca^{2+} ionophores, such as A23187 or ionomycin, which allows Ca^{2+} to move into the cytosol from the extracellular fluid.

DAG exerts different effects in target cells; it has two potential signaling roles (reviewed in Asaoka,

Nakamura, Yoshida, & Nishizuka, 1992; Nishizuka, 1992; Sternweis & Smrcha, 1992). First, it can be cleaved to release arachidonic acid, which acts either as a messenger in its own right, or more importantly, can be used in the synthesis of eicosanoids. Synthesis of eicosanoids activates a crucial serine/threonine protein kinase that phosphorylates selected proteins in the target cell. This protein kinase is called protein kinase C (PKC) because it is Ca^{2+}-dependent. The IP_3-induced rise in cytosolic Ca^{2+} is believed to translocate PKC from the cytosol to the cytoplasmic surface of the plasma membrane where it is activated by the combination of Ca^{2+}, DAG, and a negatively charged membrane phospholipid, phosphatidylserine. DAG is rapidly metabolized and therefore cannot sustain the activity of PKC, so prolonged activation of PKC depends on a second wave of DAG production, catalyzed by phospholipases that cleave the major membrane phospholipid, phosphatidylcholine. The mechanisms for activating these later phospholipases are not clear.

Activated PKC phosphorylates specific serine or threonine residues on target proteins that vary depending on the cell type. In many cells, PKC activation increases the transcription of specific genes via at least two known pathways. PKC can activate a protein kinase cascade that leads to the phosphorylation and activation of a DNA-bound gene regulatory protein in one of the signaling pathways. In the other, PKC activation leads to the phosphorylation of an inhibitor protein, resulting in the release of a cytoplasmic gene regulatory protein that then migrates into the nucleus and stimulates the transcription of specific genes. The actions of DAG can be mimicked by phorbol esters, which bind to PKC and activate it directly.

Ca^{2+} concentrations inside cells are regulated by Ca^{2+}-binding proteins, such as troponin C in skeletal muscle cells and calmodulin found in all eucaryotic cells that have been examined (reviewed in Head, 1992; O'Neil & DeGrado, 1990). Calmodulin is a single polypeptide chain of about 150 amino acids with four high-affinity Ca^{2+}-binding sites, and it functions as a multipurpose intracellular Ca^{2+} receptor that mediates many Ca^{2+}-regulated processes. Ca^{2+} binding to calmodulin causes a conformational change in calmodulin, but this protein does not have enzyme activity; instead, the allosteric activation of calmodulin allows it to bind to other proteins and alter their activity. When Ca^{2+}-calmodulin binds to its target protein, it can undergo an additional, more dramatic conformational change. Target proteins of Ca^{2+}-calmodulin include a variety of enzymes and membrane transport proteins, for example, the Ca^{2+}-ATPase that pumps Ca^{2+} out of the cell. Most effects of Ca^{2+}-calmodulin, however, are more indirect and are mediated by binding to protein kinases.

The majority of Ca^{2+} effects in a cell are mediated by protein phosphorylations catalyzed by a family of Ca^{2+}-calmodulin-dependent protein kinases (CaM-kinases) (reviewed in Hanson & Schulman, 1992; Schulman, 1993). These kinases phosphorylate serines/threonines in proteins, and the response of the target cell to elevated Ca^{2+} depends on which CaM-kinases are present in the cell. Some CaM-kinases have narrow substrate specificities, but a number of CaM-kinases have been identified that have much broader specificities, and it is these kinases that seem to be responsible for mediating many of the actions of Ca^{2+} in animal cells. One such example is CaM-kinase II, which is present in all animal cells and is especially abundant in the nervous system. In activated catecholaminergic neurons, the influx of Ca^{2+} through voltage-gated Ca^{2+} channels in the plasma membrane stimulates these neurons to secrete their neurotransmitter, but also activates CaM-kinase II to phosphorylate tyrosine kinase, activating the rate-limiting enzyme in the synthesis of catecholamines. CaM-kinase can remain active even when Ca^{2+} is withdrawn, because this kinase can phosphorylate itself, as well as other proteins, when it is activated by Ca^{2+}-calmodulin. This signal is turned off when phosphatases overwhelm the autophosphorylating activity of the enzyme.

cAMP and Ca^{2+} intracellular signaling pathways can interact at several levels in the hierarchy of control (reviewed in Cohen, 1988). Cytosolic Ca^{2+} and cAMP concentrations can influence each other. The enzymes that make (adenylyl cyclase) and degrade (cAMP phosphodiesterase) cAMP are regulated by Ca^{2+}-calmodulin complexes. Conversely, PKA can phosphorylate some Ca^{2+} channels and pumps, altering their activity. PKA phosphorylates the IP_3 receptor in the ER, which can either inhibit or promote IP_3-induced Ca^{2+} release, depending the cell type. Enzymes directly regulated by Ca^{2+} and cAMP can influence each other. Some CaM-kinases are phosphorylated by PKA. Lastly, these enzymes can have interacting effects on shared downstream target molecules. PKA and CaM-kinases can phosphorylate different sites on the same protein (i.e., CREB), indicating regulation by both cAMP and Ca^{2+}.

Some trimeric G proteins regulate ion channels, and alter ion permeability and the excitability of the plasma membrane (reviewed in Brown & Birnbaumer, 1990; Hille, 1992). Muscarinic acetylcholine receptors are linked to G proteins that alter ion channels, called G_i proteins. Once activated, the α

subunit of G_i inhibits adenylyl cyclase, while the $\beta\gamma$ complex directly opens K^+ channels, this making the cell harder to depolarize. Other trimeric G proteins regulate the activity of ion channels indirectly, by regulating channel phosphorylation via enzymes like PKA, PKC, or CaM-kinase, or by causing the production or destruction of cyclic nucleotides that directly activate or inactivate ion channels.

V. FEATURES OF TRANSDUCING EXTRACELLULAR SIGNALING

All signaling systems that are triggered by G protein-linked receptors share certain features and are governed by similar general principles. (1) Most depend on complex cascades, or relay chains, of intracellular mediators. This is in contrast to the more direct signaling pathways used by intracellular receptors, and by ion channel-linked receptors. (2) Use of catalytic cascades of intracellular mediators allows for the amplification of the responses to extracellular signals (reviewed in Lamb & Pugh, 1992). For example, binding of NE to a β_2-AR may activate many molecules of G_s protein, each of which can activate an adenylyl cyclase molecule. G_s bound to adenylyl cyclase can keep adenylyl cyclase activated for seconds, time enough for adenylyl cyclase to catalyze the conversion of a large number of ATP molecules to cAMP molecules. (3) Cells contain counterbalancing mechanisms to keep these amplifying cascades of stimulatory signals in check at every step of the cascade, so that the system can be restored to its resting state when stimulation is terminated. (4) The time course for transducing extracellular signaling molecules depends on the intracellular mechanisms that are employed. Some cellular responses to signaling molecules are smoothly graded in simple proportion to the ligand concentration. For example, primary responses to steroid hormones often follow this pattern of activation (Mulvihill & Palmiter, 1997). This pattern of activation is thought to occur because each intracellular hormone receptor protein binds a single molecule of hormone, and each specific DNA recognition sequence in a steroid-hormone-responsive gene acts independently. Some responses to signaling ligands can begin abruptly as ligand concentration increases, even to the point of occurring in an all-or-none manner. The response is undetectable below a threshold concentration, and then reaches a maximal response as soon as threshold is exceeded. This kind of response pattern is often seen in situations where more than one intracellular effector molecule or complex bind to some target macromolecule to induce a response. For example, two or more Ca^{2+} ions must bind to calmodulin before it is activated, and in some steroid hormone-induced responses more than one hormone-receptor complex must bind simultaneously to specific regulatory sequences of the DNA to activate a particular gene. This type of response also can be seen when a ligand activates two enzymes, one that promotes the response and a second one that inhibits mechanisms that promote the opposite response. (5) In some cases positive feedback mechanisms exist downstream from the ligand-receptor interactions that can outlast receptor-ligand binding; these response systems display a memory (Miller & Kennedy, 1986).

VI. SIGNALING VIA ENZYME-LINKED CELL SURFACE RECEPTORS

Enzyme-linked receptors are single-pass transmembrane proteins, with their ligand-binding domain on the outer surface of the plasma membrane. Their cytosolic domains either have an intrinsic enzyme activity or they associate directly with an enzyme. There are five known classes of enzyme-linked receptors: (1) receptor guanylyl cyclases that catalyze cGMP in the cytosol; (2) receptor tyrosine kinases that phosphorylate specific tyrosine residues on a small set of intracellular signaling proteins; (3) tyrosine kinase-associated receptors that associate with proteins that have tyrosine kinase activity; (4) receptor tyrosine phosphatases that remove phosphate groups from tyrosine residues of specific intracellular signaling proteins; and (5) receptor serine/threonine kinases that phosphorylate specific serine or threonine residues on some intracellular proteins.

Receptor guanylyl cyclases catalyze GTP to form cGMP as an intracellular mediator. cGMP, in turn, binds to and activates cGMP-dependent protein kinase, which phosphorylates specific proteins on serine or threonine residues (Yuen & Garbers, 1992). Relatively few known receptors belong to this family of receptors. On the other hand, many receptors belong to the tyrosine kinase receptor family. Many of the receptors for growth and differentiation factors are in this family of receptors, including epidermal growth factor (EGF); platelet-derived growth factor (PDGF); fibroblast growth factor (FGF); insulin, insulin-like growth factor (IGF); nerve growth factor (NGF); and macrophage colony stimulating factor (M-CSF) (Carpenter, 1987; Schlessinger & Ullrich, 1992). After ligand binding to these types of receptors, the receptors themselves are phosphorylated to initiate the intracellular signaling cascade (reviewed in Carpenter, 1987; Fantl, Johnson, & Williams, 1993; Schlessinger & Ullrich, 1992; Ullrich & Schlessinger, 1990). In the case of EGF, ligand binding causes the receptor to assemble into dimers, which enables the two cytoplasmic domains to cross-phosphorylate each other on multiple tyrosine residues. This is referred to as autophosphorylation because it occurs within the receptor dimer. Ligand binding is believed to induce a conformational change in the extracellular domain of its receptors to induce receptor dimerization. This is thought to be the general mechanism for transducing ligand signals that use this type of receptor. However, in the case of PDGF receptors, the ligand is a dimer that cross-links two receptors. Tyrosine autophosphorylation of these receptors acts as a switch to trigger the transient assembly of an intracellular signaling complex, which serves to relay the signal into the cell interior. The activated receptor binds to a number of intracellular signaling proteins in the target cell. Each of these proteins binds to a different phosphorylated site on the activated receptor, recognizing surrounding features of the polypeptide chain in addition to the phosphotyrosine. Once bound, many of these proteins become phosphorylated themselves on tyrosines and are thereby activated.

Receptors for insulin and IGF-1 act in a slightly different way. These receptors are tetramers, and when activated there is an allosteric interaction of the two receptor halves. Ligand binding results in the phosphorylation of its catalytic domains, which then activates them to phosphorylate a separate protein, insulin receptor substrate-1 on multiple tyrosines. The phosphotyrosines on the insulin receptor substrate-1 molecules act as high-affinity binding sites for the docking and activation of other activated receptor tyrosine kinases.

Receptor tyrosine kinases, when activated, have a host of intracellular signaling proteins that bind to their phosphotyrosines, including a GTPase-activating protein (GAP), PLCγ, and the src-like nonreceptor protein tyrosine kinases (reviewed in Koch, Anderson, Moran, Ellis, & Pawson, 1991; Mayer & Baltimore, 1993; Pawson & Schlessinger, 1993). PLC-γ functions in the same way as PLC-β to activate the IP signaling pathway. The intracellular signaling proteins that bind to phosphotyrosine residues on activated receptor tyrosine kinases have varied structures and functions, but they usually share two highly conserved noncatalytic domains, called SH2 and SH3 for Src homology regions 2 and 3, because they were first found in the Src protein. The SH2 domains recognize phosphorylated tyrosines and enable proteins that contain them to bind to the activated receptor tyrosine kinases, as well as to other intracellular signaling proteins that have been transiently phosphorylated on tyrosines. The function of the SH3 domain is less clear, but is thought to bind to other proteins in the cells that lack the SH3 domain.

The Ras proteins belong to a large Ras superfamily of monomeric GTPases, which also contains two other subfamilies: (1) Rho and Rac proteins, involved in relaying signals form cell surface receptors to the actin cytoskeleton; and (2) the Rab family, involved in regulating the traffic of intracellular transport vesicles (reviewed in Bollag & McCormick, 1992; Hall, 1993; Lowy & Willumsen, 1993). The Ras proteins have a covalently bound prenyl group that helps to anchor the protein to the cytoplasmic face of the plasma membrane. Ras proteins aid in relaying signals from receptor tyrosine kinases to the nucleus to stimulate cell proliferation or differentiation. These proteins function as switches, cycling between two distinct conformational states, one that is active (when GTP is bound), and one that is inactive (when GDP is bound). Two classes of proteins regulate Ras activity: GAP, and guanine nucleotide releasing proteins (GNRPs). These proteins regulate the transition between the active and inactive states, the former increasing the rate of hydrolysis of bound GTP by Ras (promoting inactivation), the latter by promoting the exchange of bound GDP with GTP from the cytosol (promoting activation).

Activated receptor tyrosine kinases bind GAPs directly and bind GNRPs indirectly. The indirect binding of GNRPs is usually responsible for driving Ras into its active, GTP-bound state, rather than the inhibition of GAPs. Once activated, Ras relays the signal downstream by activating a serine/threonine phosphorylation cascade (reviewed in Nishida & Gotoh, 1993; Pelech, 1993; Ruderman, 1993). The effects of stimulating receptor tyrosine kinases at the cytoplasmic face of the plasma membrane are short-lived, the phosphorylations being quickly reversed by tyrosine phosphatases, and the Ras being inactivated by hydrolysis of its bound GTP to GDP. Stimulation of cell proliferation or differentiation occurs by converting these short duration signals into longer-lasting ones that can sustain the signal and relay it downstream to the nucleus. This relay system involves multiple, interacting cascades of serine/threonine phosphorylations, which are much longer-lived than tyrosine phosphorylations. Many serine/threonine kinases are involved in these cascades, but one family, which contains at least five members, plays a crucial role. This crucial component in these cascades is a novel type of protein kinase called mitogen-activated protein kinase (MAPK) or extracellular-signal regulated kinases (ERKs). These kinases are activated by a wide range of extracellular proliferation- and differentiation-inducing signals, some of which activate receptor tyrosine kinases, whereas others activate G protein-linked receptors. An unusual feature of MAPK is that they require phosphorylation of both a threonine and a tyrosine, separated by a single amino acid. MAPK-kinase phosphorylates MAPK. MAPK-kinase is itself activated by serine/threonine phosphorylation catalyzed by MAPK-kinase-kinase, which is thought to be activated by binding to activated Ras.

Once MAPK is activated, it relays signals downstream by phosphorylating various proteins, including other protein kinases and gene regulatory proteins. Transcription of a set of immediate early genes may be activated within minutes after cellular stimulation by a growth factor. One protein complex that is important for transcription activation is formed by the serum response factor (SRF) and Elk-1, which constitutively binds to a specific DNA sequence (the serum response element) found in the regulatory region of the fos gene and some other immediate early genes. When activated, MAPK move from the cytosol into the nucleus and phosphorylate Elk-1, thereby activating it to turn on the transcription of the fos gene. MAPK may also phosphorylate the Jun protein, which combines with the newly made Fos protein to form an active gene regulatory protein called AP-1. The AP-1 protein then turns on additional genes, although the exact role in stimulating cell proliferation is unknown. PKC also can phosphorylate Jun, and can activate MAPK-kinase-kinase, so that both Jun and MAPK-kinase-kinase are examples of integration points where several signaling pathways converge.

A large and heterogeneous class of receptors exists that is not ion channel- or G protein-linked, and that lacks an obvious catalytic domain. Most of the cytokine receptors whose ligands regulate proliferation and differentiation in the hemopoietic system, as well as receptors for some hormones (i.e., growth hormone and prolactin) and the antigen-specific receptors on T and B lymphocytes fall into this category of receptors (reviewed in Argetsinger et al., 1993; Miyajima, Hara, & Kitamura, 1992; Mustelin & Burn, 1993; Schreurs, Gorman, & Miyajima, 1993; Stahl & Yancopoulos, 1993). Many receptors in this category work through associated tyrosine kinases, which phosphorylate various target proteins when the receptor binds its ligand. The kinases involved in tyrosine kinase-associated receptors are largely members of the well-characterized Src family of nonreceptor protein tyrosine kinases, or of the Janus family of nonreceptor protein tyrosine kinases. Presumably these receptors function in much the same way as receptor tyrosine kinases, except that their kinase domain is encoded by a separate gene and is noncovalently associated with the receptor's polypeptide chain. Also like receptor tyrosine kinases, activation of these nonreceptor protein tyrosine kinases presumably are activated by ligand-induced dimerization.

The Src family of nonreceptor protein tyrosine kinases is composed of at least eight members: Src, Yes, Fgr, Fyn, Lck, Lyn, Hck, and Blk. They contain SH2 and SH3 domains and are all located on the cytoplasmic face of the plasma membrane through their interaction with transmembrane receptor proteins and, in part, through covalently attached lipid chains. Different family members associate with different receptors and phosphorylate overlapping, but distinct, sets of target proteins. For example, Lyn, Fyn, and Lck are each associated with different sets of receptors in lymphocytes. The Src-family tyrosine kinase is activated when an extracellular ligand binds to the appropriate receptor protein. The same Src-family kinase can interact both with receptors that do not have intrinsic tyrosine kinase activity and with receptors that do, so it is not surprising that receptor tyrosine kinases and Src-family-tyrosine kinase-associated receptors activate some of the same signaling pathways.

There is less information regarding the Janus family of nonreceptor protein tyrosine kinases, which include JAK1, JAK2, and Tyk2. They are involved in signaling of a number of tyrosine kinase-associated receptors, including those for growth hormone, prolactin, and various cytokines that act on hemopoietic cells. In many cases, ligand binding of tyrosine kinase-associated receptors causes the assembly of two or more different transmembrane receptor subunits. For example, the IL-2R is composed of three polypeptide chains (α, β, and γ), which presumably assemble after ligand binding to form a functional receptor complex.

Some receptors are protein tyrosine phosphatases that can rapidly dephosphorylate tyrosine residues from selective phosphotyrosines on particular types of proteins (reviewed in Koretzky, 1993; Walton & Dixon, 1993). These enzymes are structurally unrelated to the serine/threonine protein phosphatases. These are found in both soluble and membrane-bound forms, and come in greater varieties than the serine/threonine protein phosphatases. Their high specific activity ensures the tyrosine phosphorylations are very short-lived, and that the level of tyrosine phosphorylation in resting cells is very low. They do not simply reverse the effects of protein tyrosine kinases; instead, they are regulated to play specific roles in cell signaling and in the cell cycle. CD45 protein, a single-pass transmembrane glycoprotein, is an example of a regulated protein tyrosine phosphatase that is bound to the surface of white blood cells, and plays an essential part in the activation of both T and B lymphocytes by foreign antigens. When cross-linked by extracellular antibodies, its catalytic domain is activated to remove phosphate groups from tyrosine residues on specific target proteins, such as Lck, a tyrosine kinase, which then is activated to phosphorylate other proteins in the lymphocyte. Many of the genes that encode the proteins in the intracellular signaling cascades that are activated by receptor tyrosine kinases were first identified as oncogenes in cancer cells or tumor viruses, since their inappropriate activation causes a cell to proliferate excessively (Bishop, 1991; Gupta, Gallego, & Johnson, 1992).

Target cells can undergo adaptation or desensitization to a stimulus, such that when they are exposed to a stimulus for a prolonged period, their response to it decreases. This means that cells adjust their sensitivity to the stimulus. Adaptation enables cells to respond to changes in the concentration of a signaling ligand, rather than to the absolute concentration of the ligand, over a wide range of absolute concentrations. Adaptation is achieved through a negative feedback that operates with a delay. The delay is important, so that a sudden change in the stimulus is able to make itself felt strongly for a short period of time before the negative feedback has time to act. Adaptation to chemical signals occurs in a variety of ways. It may result from a gradual decrease in the number of receptors on the cell surface (occurs in hours), or it may result from a rapid inactivation of receptors (occurs in minutes). It may be due to changes in proteins involved in transducing the signal following receptor activation, which usually occurs with an immediate time course.

Slow adaptation depends on receptor down-regulation (Soderquist & Carpenter, 1986). After a protein hormone or growth factor binds to its receptors on the surface of a target cell, it is usually ingested by receptor-mediated endocytosis and delivered to endosomes. After discharging their ligand into the acidic environment of the endosome, the receptors are recycled back into the plasma membrane for reuse, and the ligand is degraded by the endosome. In some cases, a portion of the receptors fail to release their ligand and, thus, end up in the lysosomes, where they are degraded along with the ligand. Over time with high concentrations, the number of receptors on the surface decreases, and the cells become less sensitive to the ligand; this is called receptor down-regulation.

Rapid adaptation often involves ligand-induced phosphorylation of the receptor, in addition to the slower down-regulation of the number of receptor molecules on target cells (Hausdorff, Caron & Lefkowitz, 1990; Lefkowitz, 1993; Palczewski & Benovic, 1991). The best understood example of this is the β_2-AR, which activates adenylyl cyclase via the G_s. When cells are exposed to high concentration of NE, they can desensitize within minutes by two pathways that depend on β_2-AR receptor phosphorylation. In one, the rise in cAMP caused by NE binding activates PKA, which phosphorylates the β_2-AR on a serine residue, thereby interfering with the receptor's ability to activate G_s. In the other, the activated β_2-AR becomes a substrate to another, more specific protein kinase (called β-adrenergic kinase) that phosphorylates the carboxyl-terminal cytoplasmic tail of the activated receptor on multiple serine and threonine residues. This phosphorylated tail binds an inhibitory protein called β-arrestin, which blocks the receptor's ability to active G_s. The PKA-dependent mechanism that desensitizes β_2-AR operates whenever cAMP levels rise in the cell, so any type of receptor that activates adenylyl cyclase can desensitize the β_2-AR. This process, where one ligand desensitizes target cells to another, is called heterologous desensitization. The β-arrestin-dependent mechanism operates only when the β_2-AR itself is activated by ligand binding.

VII. LYMPHOCYTE ACTIVATION AND SIGNAL TRANSDUCTION PATHWAYS

Now that we have generally described the major types of receptors and the main features of their intracellular signaling pathways, we will turn our attention to a more detailed look at specific signal transduction pathways in lymphoid cells. In this section, a brief overview of lymphocyte activation will be presented, specifically focusing on T lymphocytes. We will describe the antigen receptor components and how these components interact with a known set of signal transduction pathways. Lastly, differential signaling through the TCR, achieved by qualitative differences in the effector pathways recruited by the TCR, will be reviewed. A number of excellent reviews of lymphocyte activation are available (Alberola-Ila, Takaki, Kerner, & Perlmutter, 1997; Altman, Coggeshall, & Mustelin, 1990).

Activation of T lymphocytes is initiated with binding of a ligand to the TCR which, in turn, generates an intracellular signal. Ultimately, this leads to a number of cellular responses. Lymphocyte activation can be regulated at various points, at the level of the receptor (i.e., availability of ligand, presence and affinity of receptors, etc.) and at points distal to the receptor complex (i.e., generation of second messengers, activation of specific genes, etc.). Ligand occupancy of antigen receptors need not necessarily provide identical responses in all instances. For example, ligation of antigen receptors may stimulate a proliferative response, induce a state of unresponsiveness to subsequent stimulation (anergy), or induce apoptosis. How does a single type of transmembrane receptor induce these very heterogeneous cellular responses? Existing evidence supports the view that the nature of ligand/receptor interaction directs the physical recruitment of signaling pathways differentially inside the lymphocyte, and hence defines the nature of the subsequent immune response.

The TCR is a transmembrane heterodimer composed of either α and β chains when associated with T helper (T_H) cells, or γ and δ chains, in association with cytotoxic T lymphocytes (CTLs). The TCR is of the tyrosine kinase-associated receptor class, because it interacts with intracellular protein tyrosine kinases, as well as a series of adaptor proteins that relay kinase-derived signals to appropriate effector pathways (Weiss, 1993) (see Figure 1). The specific intracellular signaling proteins are described below. Activation of T lymphocytes requires interactions of the multimeric TCR with a molecular complex carried on an antigen-presenting cell (APC), usually a macrophage (Clevers, Alarcon, Wileman, & Terhorst, 1988). This molecular

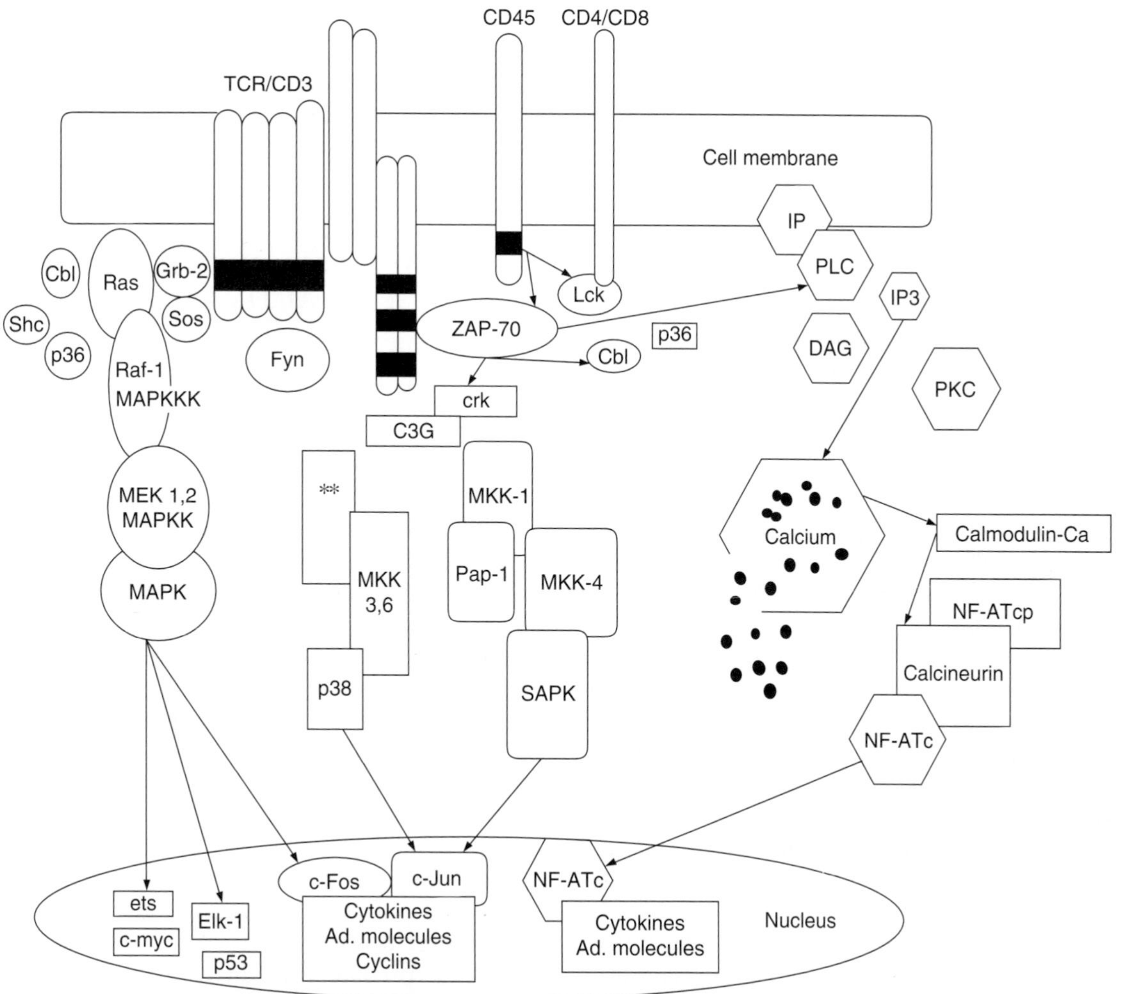

FIGURE 1 Schematic representation of the transmembrane signaling events activated by stimulation of the T cell receptor (TCR). The mitogen-activated protein kinase (MAPK) kinase-kinase enzyme of the p38 serine kinase cascade has not been identified to date. This is indicated by the ** in the figure. Abbreviations are defined in the text. (Figure was modified from Alberola-Ila et al., 1997).

complex contains processed antigen associated with a major histocompatibility (MHC) class I or class II molecule. This antigen-MHC complex allows for the dual recognition of "self" and antigen by the TCR. TCR will not recognize cells that contain antigens in association with foreign ("nonself") MHC molecules.

The products of the MHC are important for intercellular recognition and self/nonself discrimination. The MHC plays a central role in the development of both humoral and cell-mediated immune responses, since they present the antigenic peptides for recognition by the T cell repertoire. The MHC is a collection of proteins derived from genes found within a continuous stretch on chromosome 6 in humans, and chromosome 17 in mice. The MHC is referred to as the HLA complex and the H-2 complex in humans and mice, respectively. These MHC genes can be divided into three major groups. The third class of MHC genes generally encode secreted proteins associated with immune processes, including, but not limited to, soluble serum proteins, complement proteins, and some cytokines. Class I and Class II MHC are very similar in both structure and function. Class I MHC (MHC I) genes encode for glycoproteins expressed by almost all nucleated cells. MHC class I glycoproteins play a role in activating and presenting intracellular peptide antigens to mature cytotoxic T cells. Class II MHC (MHC II) genes encode glycoproteins expressed by APCs, where they present processed peptides derived from endocytosed antigens to T helper cell populations.

The cell surface glycoproteins, CD4 and CD8, are accessory molecules that restrict the interaction of T cell subsets to specific MHC molecules. CD4 protein is expressed by T_H cells and binds to MHC II. CD8 protein is expressed by CTLs subsets and binds to MHC I proteins. CTLs are CD4−, CD8+ cells that can interact with antigens presented by APC that express MHC I molecules. Binding of CTLs to the surface of target cells that express antigen-coupled MHC I molecules initiates a proteolytic cascade leading to target cell death. In contrast, T_H lymphocytes are CD4+, CD8- cells that interact with antigen coupled to MHC II antigen. Interaction of T_H cells with antigen-coupled MHC II molecules leads to secretion of lymphokines, such as IL-2 and interferon γ (IFNγ), which regulate the responses of other immune cells. Two specific subsets of T_H cells have been identified, T_{H1} and T_{H2} cells. These subtypes of T_H cells differ with respect to conditions for cell activation, lymphokine secretion, signal transduction (Gajewski, Schell & Fitch, 1990), and responses to NE (Sanders et al., 1997). T_{h1} cells produce IL-2, IL-8, TNFβ, and IFNγ. T_{h2} lymphocytes express IL-4, IL-5, IL-6, and IL-10. The different cytokine profiles of the two types of T cells are responsible for their different immune regulatory properties. In general, T_{h1} cells promote cell-mediated immunity, whereas T_{h2} cells promote humoral immunity by providing "help" for B cell antibody production.

For TCR activation and signal transduction, another group of integral membrane proteins, the CD3 complex, is required for interaction with the TCR. CD3 is a T cell-specific cell surface glycoprotein. The TCR and CD3 molecule form a complex that interacts with MHC I or II of the APC when it is bound to antigen. Thus, T cell-dependent immune responses require the simultaneous recognition of the foreign antigenic peptide by the T cell, and the recognition of MHC I or II antigens on the APC. Binding of the TCR-CD3 complex with the antigen-MHC complex that is presented by APC does not trigger a complete response in every circumstance; however, all responses are known to begin with activation of tyrosine kinases. Interaction of the TCR with its ligand induces activation of tyrosine kinases of the Src and Syk families. These protein signaling cascades are described below (Figure 1).

VIII. EARLY EVENTS IN T CELL ACTIVATION

A. Involvement of Src and Syk Nonreceptor Tyrosine Kinases

Activation of T lymphocytes with anti-CD3 antibodies, in vitro, initiates tyrosine kinase activity within a few seconds (Samelson, Patel, Weissman, Harford, & Klausner, 1986). This event leads to a cascade of biochemical changes that develop over many hours. T lymphocyte activation results in the expression of cytokine receptors (~2 h), secretion of cytokines (~6 h), initiation of DNA replication (~24 h), cell division (~48 h), and acquisition of an altered differentiative character (days) (Crabtree, 1989).

Three nonreceptor tyrosine kinases of the src and syk families have been implicated in the activation process: (1) $p56^{lck}$, which interacts physically and functionally with the CD4 and CD8 co-receptors (Shaw et al., 1990; Turner, Brodsky, Irving, Levin, Perlmutter & Littman, 1990); (2) Fyn kinase, which plays a pivotal role in directing the activation responses observed in mature thymocytes (Appleby et al., 1992); and (3) ZAP-70, a Syk-family member possessing tandemly repeated SH2 domains and lacking a known negative regulatory phosphorylation site (Appleby et al., 1992). Both Lck and Fyn are members of the Src family of tyrosine kinases, possessing N-terminal SH2 and SH3 domains involved in protein-protein interaction, and a C-terminal phosphorylation site that serves to regulate, in part, the activity of each (reviewed in Sawasdikosol, Ravichandran, Lee, Chang, & Burakoff, 1995). Highly selective Src family kinase inhibitors block TCR-induced IL-2 secretion and proliferation, supporting the view that phosphate transfer by Lck and Fyn stimulates subsequent events (Hanke et al., 1996).

Lck, Fyn, and ZAP-70 initiate TCR signaling by phosphorylating tyrosine residues of soluble cytoplasmic adaptor proteins, and tyrosine-containing motifs in the cytoplasmic tails of the TCR and CD3 protein chains, referred to as immunoreceptor tyrosine-based activation motifs (ITAMs) (reviewed in Alberola-Ila et al., 1997). Lck and Fyn appear to mediate the phosphorylation of tyrosine residues in the TCR ζ chain and CD3 subunits (γ, δ, and ε) (Gauen et al., 1994; van Oers, Killeen & Weiss, 1996; Watts et al., 1994; Weiss, 1993). The different ITAMS of the TCR/CD3 complex can interact with different cytosolic effectors (Osman, Lucas, & Cantrell, 1995; Romeo & Seed, 1991). Variations in the phosphorylation of individual ITAMs during T cell activation generate signaling diversity, and thus, diversity of T cell functions (Combadiere et al., 1996; Rozdzial, Malissen, & Finkel, 1995). In this way, activation of the TCR has the potential to deliver multiple independent signals. Phosphorylation of the ITAMs results in the recruitment and activation of ZAP-70 (van Oers & Weiss, 1995). Phosphorylation of ZAP-70 by Lck and/or Fyn augments its activity substantially (Chan et al., 1995; Iwashima, Irving, van Oers, & Chan, 1994; van Oers & Weiss, 1995).

B. Adaptor Proteins

Phosphorylation of the TCR complex by Lck and Fyn provides binding sites for a number of soluble intracellular polypeptides referred to as adaptor proteins. Adaptor proteins possess interaction domains and sites for tyrosine phosphorylation; however, they lack any enzymatic activity. These proteins are thought to function as primary mechanisms that regulate the recruitment of downstream signaling pathways after ligand-engagement of the TCR.

Grb2 is the best characterized adaptor protein. It contains a single SH2 domain flanked by two SH3 domains, that are constitutively bound by the GTP/GDP exchange factor, Sos. Following phosphorylation of ITAMS in the TCR complex, the SH2 domains of Grb-2 bind to the TCR, thus bringing Sos to the membrane where it activates Ras (Avruch, Zhang, & Kyriakis, 1994; Buday, Khwaja, Sipeki, Faragó, & Downward, 1996). Several other adaptor proteins (Sch, p36-38, and Cbl) also become tyrosine phosphorylated, and form a complex with Grb2 and/or the TCR complex after TCR/ligand interaction (Pelicci et al., 1992; Ravichandran et al., 1993). The p36-38 adaptor protein, appears as a 36-38 kD band in phosphotyrosine blots of activated T cell lysates (Buday, Egan, Rodriquez-Viciana, Cantrell & Downward, 1994; Motto et al., 1994; Sieh, Batzer, Schlessinger, & Weiss, 1994), and in addition to binding to Grb2 and the TCR complex, it also can associate with ZAP-70, Sos, PLCγ, and phosphatidylinositol-3 kinase (PI_3-K) (Sieh et al., 1994; Fukazawa et al., 1995). Evidence suggests that p36-38 plays a role in coupling the TCR to phosphoinositide metabolism (Motto, Musci, Ross, & Koretzky, 1996a). Tyrosine phosphorylation of p36-38 correlates well with inositol phosphate production, a measure of phospholipase activity (Motto, et al., 1996a).

SLP-76 is an additional adaptor protein that associates with Grb2 in T cells (Jackman et al., 1995). It has many potential tyrosine phosphorylation sites, an SH2 domain, and a proline-rich region that may interact with SH3-containing proteins. TCR ligation stimulates SLP-76 phosphorylation. Further, augmented expression of SLP-76 improves coupling of the TCR to translocation of the nuclear factor of activated T cells (NF-AT) transcription factor, a key regulatory event in IL-2 expression (Motto, Ross, Wu, Hendricks-Taylor, & Koretzky, 1996b).

Other adaptor proteins are phosphorylated with cross-linking of the TCR, including a 120 kDa protein identified as the product of the c-cbl protooncogene (Meisner, Conway, & Hartley, Czech, 1995). This adaptor protein associates with numerous signal molecules, including Grb-2, Fyn Lck, the Ras-GAP protein, PLC-γ, PI-3 kinase, and ZAP-70 (Donovan, Wange, Langdon, & Samelson, 1994; Fournel, Davidson, Weil, & Veillette, 1996). The significance of these interactions is unclear, but some evidence supports an active role for this molecule in TCR-mediated signal transduction (Blake, Heath, & Langdon, 1993). Numerous other adaptor proteins also may participate in TCR signaling, such as Crk (Buday et al., 1996; Gotoh et al., 1995; Reedquist et al., 1996; Ribon, Hubbell, Herrera, & Saltiel, 1996; Sawasdikosol et al., 1995), Vav (Fischer et al., 1999; Katzav, Sutherland, Packham, Yi, & Weiss, 1994; Tarakhovsky et al., 1995; Zhang, Alt, Davidson, Orkin, & Swat, 1995) and HS1 (Takemoto, Furuta, Li, Strong-Sparks, & Hashimoto, 1995; Taniuchi et al., 1995; Yamanashi et al., 1993).

Adaptor proteins bind to different domains of Grb2 (Motto et al., 1994). It has been proposed that these proteins compete for binding to Grb2, and that the proteins bound to one domain of Grb2 influence which proteins subsequently bind to other domains (Motto et al., 1994; Reif, Buday, Downward, & Cantrell, 1994). Intracellular signaling pathways may be differentially activated, depending on which proteins are bound to Grb2. The extraordinary potential for recruitment of diverse effector mechanisms by the TCR is, thus, possible through the recruitment of such a large group of adaptor proteins. Adaptor proteins are interposed between the signal-generating tyrosine kinases and more generic cellular control circuitry. Thus, subtle changes in the availability of adaptor proteins, their relative affinities for receptor polypeptides, and the time required for their binding to cognate ligands may greatly affect the nature of signaling through the TCR. Differences in signaling observed among subpopulations of lymphocytes at different times during their maturation are likely the result of tyrosine phosphorylation of the different ITAMs of the TCR/CD3 complex that can interact with different cytosolic effectors (Osman et al., 1995; Romeo & Seed, 1991). This suggests that variations in the phosphorylation of individual ITAMs during T cell activation will generate signaling diversity. Thus, the TCR signal transduction apparatus has the potential to deliver multiple independent signals.

C. Effector Signaling Cascades

The predominant effector systems involved in intracellular transmission of TCR signals resemble those defined in other systems and include calcium-dependent kinases and phosphatases and serine/threonine kinase cascades of the mitogen-activated protein kinase (MAPK) type. In this section, we briefly summarize what is known about their role in T lymphocyte activation.

1. *PLCγ and Calcium*

Following TCR ligation, PLC-γ is recruited to the plasma membrane and is activated by tyrosine phosphorylation. Activation of PLCγ stimulates the catabolism of membrane phospholipids and the release of the phosphoinositide second messengers, inositol 1, 4, 5, triphosphate (IP_3) and DAG (Noh, Shin, & Rhee, 1995). IP_3 stimulates the release of calcium from intracellular stores (Berridge, 1993) and is responsible for the early calcium increase observed following T cell activation. Most T cell responses require sustained increases in intracellular calcium. The sustained elevation in intracellular calcium is thought to be maintained by capacitative calcium entry (Fanger, Hoth, Crabtree, & Lewis, 1995; Putney, 1990; Serafini, Lewis, Clipstone & Bram, 1995).

Increases in intracellular calcium following T cell activation results in activation of calcineurin. Calcineurin is a calcium/calmodulin-dependent serine phosphatase. Calcineurin acts on transcription factors of the NF-AT family, which includes, NF-AT1, NF-ATc, NF-AT3, and NF-AT4. In response to calcium-dependent signals, NF-AT transcription factors translocate into the nucleus to interact with AP-1, and to bind cooperatively to the composite NF-AT/AP-1 site in the IL-2 gene. CaM-kinase II is another calcium-dependent enzyme that clearly plays a role in IL-2 induction (Hama, Paliogianni, Fessler, & Boumpas, 1995; Nghiem, Ollick, Gardner, & Schulman, 1994), however, little is understood about how these two competing calcium-regulated pathways interact. Activation of PLCγ following TCR ligand binding also results in generation of DAG. DAG directly activates PKC (Szamel & Resch, 1995). At present the importance of PKC activation in TCR signaling is unclear.

2. *GTP Binding Proteins*

Despite numerous studies that support a fundamental role for the Ras-GTP-binding protein in lymphocyte activation (Izquierdo, Pastro, Reif, & Cantrell, 1995), the mechanisms for Ras activation by TCR/CD3 complex following TCR ligation are poorly understood. Inhibition of the GAPs and activation of the guanine nucleotide exchange factor, Sos, participate in the regulation of Ras. Although Ras-GTP can directly stimulate a group of downstream effectors (reviewed in Marshall, 1995), studies in T lymphocytes have focused on the MAPK cascade (Kayne & Sternberg, 1995; Wassarman, Therrien, & Rubin, 1995).

Studies support a role for the Rho family of GTP-binding proteins, including Rho, Rac, and Cdc42, in growth regulation of fibroblasts (Olson, Ashworth, & Hall, 1995). Although less attention has been given to its role in T lymphocyte activation, studies suggest involvement of the Rho family GTP-binding proteins in CTL-mediated cytotoxic responses, apoptosis, and proliferation (Kolluri, Tolias, Carpenter, Rosen, & Kirchhausen, 1996; Lang et al., 1992; Molina, Sancho, Terhorst, Rosen, & Remold-O'Donnell, 1993; Moorman, Bobak, & Hahn, 1996; Qui, Chen, Kirn, McCormick, & Symons, 1995). Rho family proteins regulate stress-activated protein kinase (SAPK) and p38 kinase pathways (Vojtek & Cooper, 1995) which contribute to the control of T cell responsiveness. The role of this family of GTP-binding proteins in lymphocyte responses merits additional investigation.

3. *Serine/Threonine Kinase Cascades: General Features*

The MAPK cascade involves the successive phosphorylation of serine, threonine, or dual specificity kinases. The signaling cascade consists of three kinases: a MAPK; a MAPK-kinase, which phosphorylates the MAPK; and a MAPK-kinase, which phosphorylates the MAPK-kinase. Six MAPK signal transduction cascades with this basic format have been described in yeast (Graves, Campbell & Krebs, 1995; Waskiewicz & Cooper, 1995). Although at present only three MAPK signal transduction cascade pathways have been defined in detail in mammalian cells, the ERKS, the SAPKs, and p38 kinase, a similar or even larger group of related pathways, are likely to transmit signals in mammalian cells.

4. *Extracellular-Regulated Kinases (Erks)*

Numerous studies support a role for ERKS in the linkage of the TCR to the cell interior for signal transduction, which is required for cytokine gene transcription, T cell proliferation, and thymocyte differentiation (Alberola-Ila et al., 1995; Genot, Cleverley, Henning, & Cantrell, 1996; Izquierdo, Bowden, & Cantrell, 1994; Swan et al., 1995; Whitehurst & Geppert, 1996). The ERK pathway receives input from Ras-GTP. Ras-GTP binds directly to Raf-1, the MAPK-kinase-kinase in this pathway. Binding of Ras-GTP to Raf results in Raf becoming tyrosine phosphorylated and localized to the membrane. This stimulates its kinase activity. Once activated, Raf-1 phosphorylates and activates Mek-1 and Mek-2, the MAPK-kinases. Mek-1 and Mek-2 both act on the MAPKs, ERK-1 and ERK-2. Activated ERK-1 and ERK-2 then translocate to the nucleus and directly phosphorylate Fos and Jun transcriptional regulatory proteins and members of the ets family of transcription factors (Graves et al., 1995; Karin, 1995; Waskiewicz & Cooper, 1995).

5. *SAPKs*

The SAPKs are MAPKs that are activated by inhibitors of protein synthesis, inflammatory cytokines (e.g., TNF-α , and IL-1), and more generally by severe cellular stress (Davis, 1994; Kyriakis et al., 1994). The signaling cascade consists of MKK1 (the MAPK-kinase-kinase), MKK4/Sek-1 (the MAPK-kinase), and the SAPKs (the MAPK) (reviewed in Davis, 1994). In general, the SAPK signal transduction cascade is regulated by Rac 1 and Cdc24, small GTP-binding proteins, through activation of Pak-1, and in some cases through Ras activation (Minden et al., 1994). Phosphorylated SAPK activates the transcription factors c-Jun (Derijard et al., 1994) and ATF-2 (Gupta, Campbell, Derijard, & Davis, 1995), which then translocate to the nucleus. It has been suggested that this cascade could serve to mediate converging signals from accessory receptors that are required for satisfactory costimulation of T cells in vivo (Su et al., 1994). This is supported by recent evidence suggesting that activation of SAPKs and ERKS are blocked in T lymphocytes following TCR stimulation in the absence of costimulation (DeSilva, Feeser, Tancula, & Scherle, 1996). Additionally, experimental studies suggest a role for SAPK in signal transduction cascades involved with apoptosis (Verheij et al., 1996; Wilson et al., 1996). No studies have determined the consequences of a specific inhibition of the SAPK cascade in T lymphocytes.

6. *p38 Kinase*

Inflammatory cytokines and environmental stress also induce activity of the p38 kinase (Lee et al., 1994; Raingeaud et al., 1995). A serine kinase cascade regulates the activity of p38 kinase. This cascade involves MKK3, MKK6, and MKK4 (under some circumstances) as the MAPK-kinases (Raingeaud, Whitmarsh, Barrett, Derijard, & Davis, 1996). The MAPK-kinase-kinase enzyme of this serine kinase cascade has not been identified at present. Once activated, p38 kinase is capable of phosphorylating ATF-2 and MAPK-activated protein kinase 2. The activation of AFT-2 and MAPK-activated protein kinase 2 has been correlated with apoptosis (Xia, Dickens, Raingeaud, Davis, & Greenberg, 1995).

7. *PKC*

Numerous studies support that the in vivo regulation of Raf-1 activity may occur by more than one mechanism. Findings that a PKC inhibitor blocks Raf-1 activation, and that c-raf antisense oligodeoxyribonucleotide inhibits PKC-stimulated cell proliferation (Carroll & May, 1994; Riedel, Brennscheidt, Kiehntopf, Brach & Herrmann, 1993), support a role for PKC in regulating Raf-1 activity. Bryostatin 1, a pharmacologic activator of PKC, induces activation of Raf-1 in FDC-P1 cells. The PKC inhibitors, H7 and staurosporine, block both bryostatin- and IL-3-mediated Raf-1 phosphorylation and FDC-P1 cell proliferation (Reif et al., 1994). Purified PKC can phosphorylate Raf-1 serine residues and is sufficient to activate the enzymatic function of Raf-1 in vitro. PKCα was shown to directly phosphorylate and activate Raf-1 both in vitro and in vivo (Kolch et al., 1993). A similar PKC-mediated phosphorylation of Raf-1 occurs in murine hematopoietic cells (Chouaib, Welte, Mertelsmann, & Dupont, 1985). That ligation of the TCR/CD3 complex induces a PKC-dependent activation of Raf-1 (Siegel, Klausner, Rapp, & Samelson, 1990) further supports a role of PKC in T lymphocyte activation. However, activation of Raf-1 by PKC does not appear to be required for the induction of cell proliferation in all systems (Kolch et al., 1993) and p21ras is known to activate Raf-1 in an PKC-independent mechanism (Harwood & Cambier, 1993). In T lymphocytes, as well as other cell types, p21ras can trigger the ERK cascade and/or induce cell activation, in a PKC-independent mechanism (Avruch et al., 1994; Izquierdo, Downward, Graves, & Cantrell, 1992). The effects of PKC in T lymphocytes varies depending on the isoform and cell line being examined. For example, in EL4 thymoma cells, activated PKCα was a weak activator of AP-1, whereas PKCΘ was more potent (Baier-Bitterlich et al., 1996). In the Jurkat cell line, expression of activated PKCε helped to stimulate the NF-AT, AP-1, and NF-κB transcription factors. In contrast, PKCζ had no effect (Genot, Parker, & Cantrell, 1995). The use of specific PKC inhibitors should provide the necessary tools to evaluate the role of PKC more clearly during T cell activation. These results support a model in which activation of Raf-1 and/or the ERK cascade is regulated by a minimum of two independent pathways.

8. *Regulatory Enzymes — The Phosphatases*

Given the role of tyrosine phosphorylation in T cell activation, it has become increasingly clear that enzymes mediating dephosphorylation, i.e., phosphotyrosine phosphatase (PTPases) also participate in regulation of T cell activation. PTPases serve as both inhibitory and activating signals and have proven to be as diverse as the kinases (reviewed in Xia et al., 1995). The PTPases, CD45 and SHP1, are known to influence TCR signal transduction.

a. CD45

CD45 is a cell surface receptor expressed in extraordinarily high levels by hematopoietic cells. Alternative splicing of exons encoding the extracellular domain give rise to numerous isoforms of the CD45 receptor; however, the cytoplasmic domain of all CD45 molecules are identical and contain two PTPase domains. Some evidence exists for different functions of the CD45 isoforms (Chui, Ong, Johnson, Teh & Marth, 1994; Leitenberg, Novak, Farber, Smith, & Bottomly, 1996; McKenney, Onodera, Gorman, Mimura, & Rothstein, 1995; Novak et al., 1994), and the variable expression of these isoforms by different hematopoietic cell types supports this view. At present ligands specific for CD45 receptors have not been identified.

Activation of CD45, a transmembrane phosphatase, is required for T cell activation, since T cell lines deficient in CD45 do not respond to TCR-derived signals (Koretzky, Picus, Thomas, & Weiss, 1990; Pingel & Thomas, 1999). Studies suggest the PTPase domain of CD45 is required for normal TCR signaling (Byth et al., 1996; Desai, Sap, Silvennoinen, Schlessinger, & Weiss, 1994; Hovis et al., 1993), and that at least one target of PTPase activity is the C-terminal phosphorylation site of Lck (Y505) (McFarland et al., 1993; Ostergaard et al., 1989). Since phosphorylation of Lck at the Y505 position suppresses its activity, dephosphorylating the inhibitory residue may stimulate Lck function (Hurley, Hyman, & Sefton, 1993). Further, a physical association of CD45 and Lck has been reported (Gervais & Veillette, 1995; Ng, Watts, Aebersold, & Hohnson, 1996). Association of CD45 with TCR ζ chain also has been documented, and may serve to dephosphorylate the ITAM motifs (Furukawa, Itoh, Krueger, Streuli, & Saito, 1994). Although following antibody-mediated cross-linking of TCR, CD45 activity is not altered. Stover and Walsh (1994) reported a stimulatory effect of casein kinase II phosphorylation on the PTPase domain of CD45.

Ligand binding to the TCR/CD3 complex initiates a signal that activates CD45. Activated CD45 dephosphorylates the COOH-terminal tyrosine of inactive protein tyrosine kinases and converts the enzymes to an activated form. As mentioned previously, the three pivotal protein tyrosine kinases required for the initiation and transduction of a signal from the TCR/CD3 complex are Lck, Fyn, and ZAP-70 (Fields & Mariuzza, 1996; Fields et al., 1996; Heemels & Ploegh, 1995).

b. SHP

In contrast to CD45, the regulatory enzymes, SHP-1 (formerly designated SHPTP-1, SHP, HCP, and PTP1C) and SHP-2 (formerly designated SHPTP-2, SHPTP-3, syp, PTP2C, and PTP1D) suppress the flux of signals activated in TCR signaling pathways. SHP-1 is expressed solely in hematopoietic cells and associates with VAV, Grb-2, and Sos in these cells (Kon-Kozlowshi, Pani, Pawson, & Siminovitch, 1996).

Following T lymphocyte activation, SHP-1 binds and dephosphorylates ZAP-70 (Sells, Muthukumar, Sukhatme, Crist, & Rangnekar, 1995), supporting its proposed role as a suppressor of T cell activation. In motheaten mice, abnormalities in the SHP-1 gene result in the varied developmental and functional defects observed in white blood cells (Schultz et al., 1993), further supporting a role for SHP-1 in T cell development.

SHP-2 is widely distributed in mammalian cells, and associates with CTLA-4, a negative regulator of T cell activation in mouse T cells. It is thought that this phosphatase serves as a positive regulator of the MAPK cascade (Marengere et al., 1996). Further examination of the role of both SHP-1 and SHP-2 are clearly required to understand their importance in T cell signaling.

IX. B CELL ANTIGEN RECEPTOR AND MACROPHAGE CD14 RECEPTOR SIGNALING: AN ANALOGY

Although we have focused the present review on the TCR signaling, many similarities exist between the signaling pathways activated by TCR and pathways of the B cell antigen receptor (BCR) (Figure 2) and the macro-phage lipopolysaccharide (LPS) receptor, CD14 (Figure 3). For the BCR, different ligands can alter the signaling properties of the receptor, similar to the TCR. Membrane-bound immunoglobulins contain only three cytoplasmic disposed amino acids, indicating that these molecules, like their TCR counterparts, are not fully equipped to transmit signals alone. The signaling apparatus of the BCR appears to be contained in the cytoplasmic tails of Igα and Igβ. These are both homologous and functionally analogous to the ITAM-containing TCR components. Similarly, LPS at physiological concentrations binds to LPS-binding protein (LBP) present in the serum, and this complex then interacts with CD14 on macrophages or neutrophils (Ulevitch & Tobias, 1995). Although CD14 is a glycosylphosphatidylinositol-linked protein that lacks an intracellular domain, LPS-LBP binding to CD14 results in rapid phosphorylation of various proteins on tyrosyl residues (Ulevitch & Tobias, 1995). Ligation of the BCR and LPS binding to CD14 both activate Src and Syk family protein tyrosine kinases like those in T cells: the Btk, Fyn, Lyn, and ZAP-70 (Pleiman, D'Ambrosio, & Cambier, 1994) for BCR and Hck, Fgr, Lyn (Stefanova et al., 1993; Weinstein, June & DeFranco, 1993) and p38 (Lee & Young, 1996) for LPS/CD14 interaction. Phosphorylation of the ITAMs of Igα and Igβ and the CD14 LPS receptor directs subsequent downstream signaling events. These range from membrane phospholipid hydrolysis to activation of the Ras pathway. As for activation of T cells by stimulation of the TCR, activation of B cells (via BCR ligation) and macrophages (via LPS binding CD14) requires activation of the MAPK family cascades. BCR (reviewed in Hashimoto et al., 1998) and LPS/CD14 (Sweet & Hume, 1996; Ulevitch & Tobias, 1995) induce activation of all three known MAPK pathways. Since the signal transduction mechanisms leading from the BCR and the CD14 LPS receptor are analogous in all material respects to the TCR, neurotransmitters are likely to influence signal transduction pathways of each of these receptors at similar points in the MAPK pathways as indicated for the TCR.

X. MODULATION OF LYMPHOCYTE FUNCTION BY HORMONES THAT BIND NUCLEAR HORMONE RECEPTORS: GLUCOCORTICOIDS AS AN EXAMPLE

The mechanisms by which GC exert immunosuppressive and antiinflammatory properties have not been completely elucidated, but indicate that GC can affect T cell responses by interfering at multiple sites of the TCR activation cascade. GC can affect the growth, differentiation, and function of both lymphocytes and monocytes (Boumpas, Paliogianni, Anastassiou & Balow, 1991). GC affect T cell development and function through the induction of apoptotic death of immature thymocytes and the suppression of cytokine production by mature T cells (Barnes & Adcock, 1993; Cohen & Duke, 1984). GC suppress production of IL-2, a cytokine that plays a central role in the initiation of immune responses.

The mechanisms by which GC and other hormones bind nuclear hormone receptors are not entirely clear, but they do involve regulating gene expression. Nuclear hormone receptors regulate gene expression by two major modes of action: (1) by ligand-dependent DNA binding and transactivation, and (2) by cross-talk with other transcription factors. Both of these modes of action require binding of GC to a cytoplasmic glucocorticoid receptor (GR) within target cells. The GR has three main domains: (1) the N-terminal domain, which plays an important role in the transactivation activity of the GR; (2) the hormone-binding region, which resides in the C-terminal regions; and (3) the central basic domain,

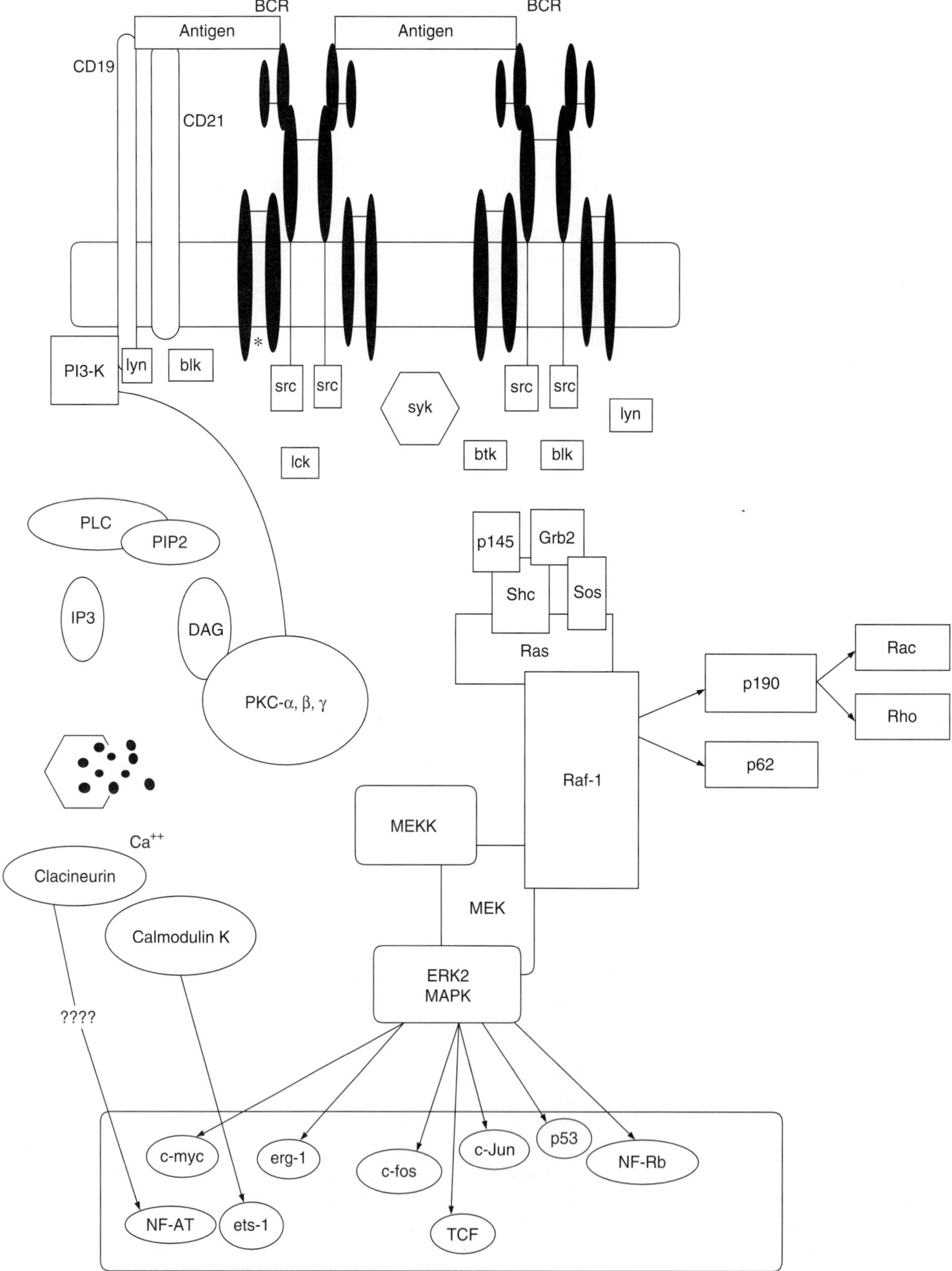

FIGURE 2 Mechanisms for B cell antigen receptor signaling, demonstrating that many similarities exist between this signaling pathway and that of the T cell receptor (TCR). Abbreviations are defined in the text.

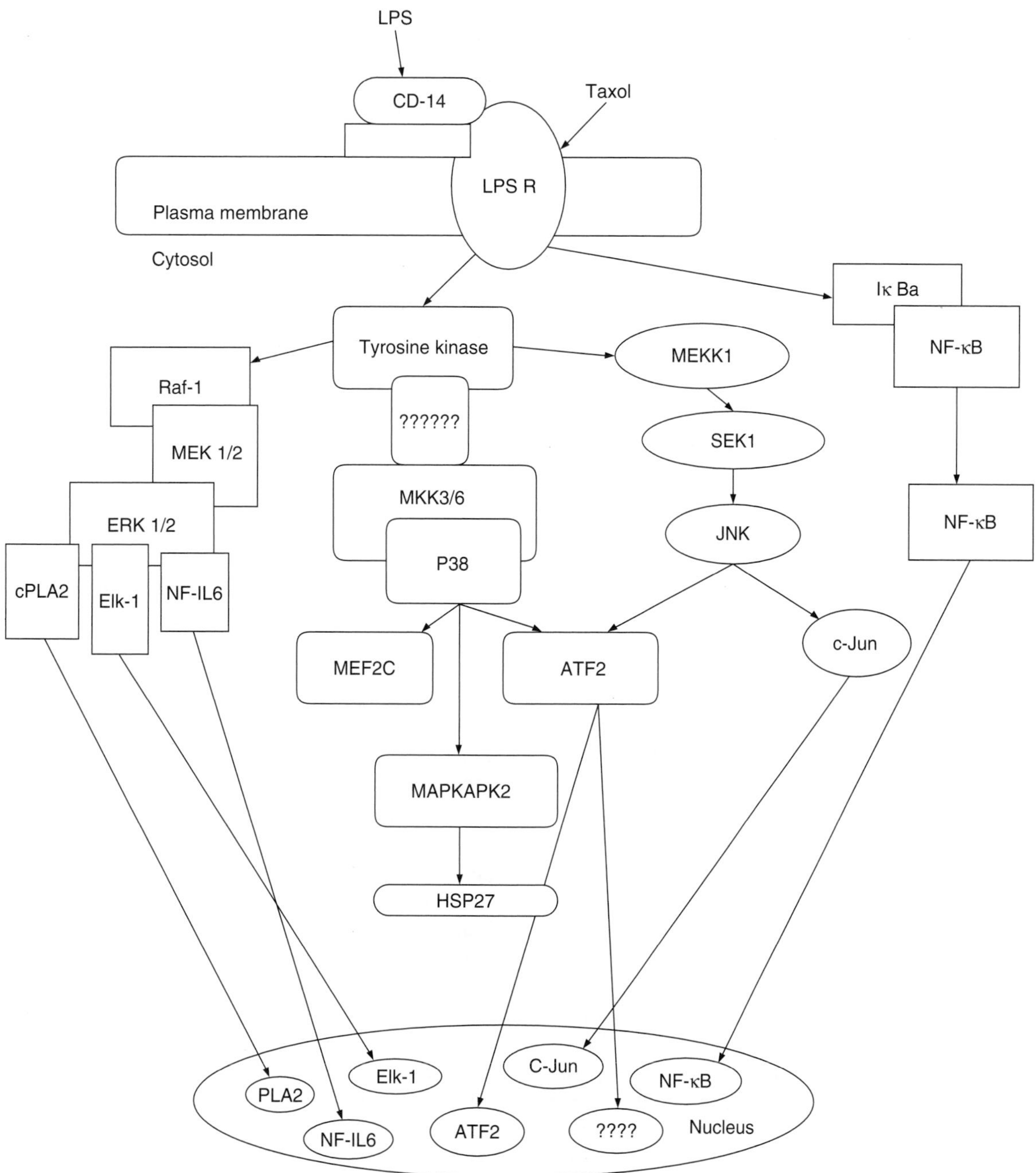

FIGURE 3 Model of the transmembrane signaling pathways elicited following activation of the macrophage lipopolysaccharide receptor (CD14). The signaling pathways employed by this receptor are similar to those stimulated following T cell receptor (TCR) activation. (This figure was modified from Tominaga, Saito, Matsuura, & Nakano, 1999). Abbreviations are defined in the text.

which possesses two zinc fingers and is responsible for the DNA-binding activity of the receptor (Truss & Beato, 1993). GC are small hydrophobic molecules that diffuse through the cell membrane and bind to GRs. Binding of GC to GRs allows rapid nuclear translocation of the GC-GR complex (Lapointe & Baxter, 1989). The classic model for steroid/thyroid hormone action proposes that binding of the ligand to the receptor induces an allosteric hinge that allows the receptor-hormone complex to bind to specific DNA sequences, termed GC response elements (GRE), upstream of the promoter region of GC-responsive genes (Truss & Beato, 1993). It is this binding that leads to positive or negative modulation of gene transcription (Lapointe & Baxter, 1989; Truss & Beato, 1993).

In addition to the classical mode of steroid receptor action, which involves binding as a dimer to regulatory sequences in target gene promoters and subsequent activation of transcription, a second mode of action is based predominantly on protein-protein interactions, referred to as transcriptional cross-talk. Transcriptional cross-talk refers to the observation that members of the steroid hormone receptor superfamily and the family of AP-1 transcription factors can interfere with each other's function. Thus activated, GRs directly interact with transcription factors such as AP-1 or NF-κB to reduce DNA binding by either protein (Jonat et al., 1990; Ray & Prefontaine, 1994; Schüle et al., 1990; Yang-Yen et al., 1990). This interference is usually inhibitory, but under some conditions can be synergistic. GC modulate the immune response by inhibiting gene transcription of cytokines, such as interleukin (IL)-1, IL-2, IL-6, and interferon-γ (Szefler, 1989; Vacca et al., 1992), and by inducing apoptosis in T lymphocytes (Schwartzman & Cidlowski, 1993). GC primarily inhibit cytokine production by transcriptional cross-talk. In contrast, GC regulate lymphocyte apoptosis by ligand-dependent DNA binding and transactivation.

A. Glucocorticoid-Induced Apoptosis

In cells of the immune system, GC particularly affect proliferation and the survival or apoptosis of T-cells (Ucker, 1987; Wyllie, 1980). Both the repression of survival or proliferation genes (Arya, Wong-Staal, & Gallo, 1984; Cupps & Fauci, 1982; Gillis, Crabtree, & Smith, 1979a, 1979b), and the induction of death genes have been suggested (Caron-Leslie & Cidlowski, 1991; Caron-Leslie, Schwartzman, Gaido, Compton, & Cidlowski, 1991; Dowd & Miesfeld, 1992; Gasson & Bourgeois, 1983; Shi, Kam, Powers, Aebersold, & Greenberg, 1992; Thulasi, Harbour, & Thompson, 1993). Studies using mutants of GR with altered recognition of the target DNA-element indicate that the sequence-specific recognition of GR target genes and presumably their transactivation are required to trigger apoptosis (Nazareth, Harbour, & Thompson, 1991). The N-terminal activation domain of the GR is required for steroid induction of lymphocyte apoptosis, supporting a role for transcription mediated by GR in lymphoid cell death (Dieken, Meese, & Miesfeld, 1990; Dieken & Miesfield, 1992). Examination of genes expressed specifically in GC-treated apoptotic immune cells have addressed the requirement for protein synthesis in the apoptosis process (Osborne & Schwartz, 1994). Eleven genes that are specifically induced by GCs have been isolated and characterized in WEHI- 7TG lymphomal cells (Harrigan, Baughman, Campbell & Bourgeois, 1989). Two other mRNAs associated with GC-induced programmed cell death, RP-2 and RP-8, also have been described (Owens, Hahn & Cohen, 1991). Induction of calmodulin (CaM) mRNA may serve as an example of such an induced gene that is required for GC-induced apoptosis (Dowd, MacDonald, Komm, Haussler, & Miesfeld, 1991).

Development of T cells occurs in the thymus and is directed by signals provided by the thymic microenvironment that can be divided into developmental signals and survival signals. Developmental signals induce differentiation of the cell from one stage to the next. One of the earliest developmental signals that thymocytes receive commits them to differentiate along the T lineage. Functional rearrangement of TCR β-chain genes induces differentiation to CD4+CD8+ dual-positive (DP) stage of T cell development. This is followed by rearrangement of the TCR α -chain. DP thymocytes that express TCR-α β are then subject to positive and negative selection signals that are provided by interaction of thymocytes with thymic stromal cells, cytokines, and hormones (reviewed in Kisielow & von Boehmer, 1995; Zuniga-Pflücker & Lenardo, 1996). Less than 5% of immature CD4/CD8 DP thymocytes are positively selected to survive and differentiate into single-positive CD4 and CD8 T cells, whereas the rest of the DP thymocytes undergo apoptosis (negative selection) without further differentiation. Both positive and negative selection events are processes that are regulated by the interaction of their TCR with peptide/MHC complexes and through some accessory molecules. Positive and negative selection differ quantitatively in the strength of the interaction between TCR and peptide/MHC molecules. Negative selection is thought to involve strong interactions of the TCR/CD3 complexes and self-MHC-encoded molecules (Alam et al., 1996). Apoptosis is induced in DP thymocytes by extensive crosslinking of TCR/CD3 complexes (Iwata, Hanaoka, & Sato, 1991; Smith, Williams, Kingston, Jenkinson, & Owen, 1989). Fas (CD95/Fas ligand) interactions are not required for the negative selection events in DP thymocytes (Singer & Abbas, 1994). GC also induce apoptosis of DP thymocytes (Claman, 1972; Cohen & Duke, 1984; Iwata et al., 1991), which is inhibited by proper stimulation of DP thymocytes through TCR/CD3 and costimulation through the coreceptor, CD4 or CD8, and the integrin-leukocyte-function associated antigen (LFA)-1 (Iwata et al., 1991; Zhao & Iwata, 1995). The antiapoptotic effects following TCR/CD3 ligation and accessory molecule stimulation are calcium- and PKCε-dependent (Iwata, Iseki & Kudo, 1993; Iwata,

Iseki, Sato, Tozawa, & Ohoka, 1994; Zhao, Tozawa, Iseki, Mukai, & Iwata, 1995) and induce differentiation and commitment of DP thymocytes to either $CD4^+$ or $CD8^+$ T cells (Iwata et al., 1994; Iwata, Kuwata, Mukai, Tozawa, & Yokoyama, 1996; Ohoka et al., 1996).

GC-induced apoptosis requires binding of GC to cytosolic GRs and protein synthesis. Inhibition of either mRNA or protein synthesis inhibits GC-induced apoptosis in thymocytes (Iwata et al., 1994). The binding of GC to GR stimulates translocation of the ligand-receptor complex from the cytosol to the nucleus. The ligand-receptor complex functions as a transcription regulatory factor and induces, enhances, or represses the expression of certain genes. Thus, the principal mechanism whereby they exert their powerful effects is through modulation of the transcription of specific sets of genes. GC-induced apoptosis in immature thymocytes is thought to involve GR-mediated activation of PKCε through de novo synthesis of macromolecules (Iwata et al., 1994). GC-induced apoptosis in DP thymocytes is inhibited by proper activation of PKC (Ca^{2+}-dependent cPKC) and a proper increase in $[Ca^{2+}]_i$ that requires calcineurin activation (Zhao et al., 1995). In contrast to mature T cells, GC-induced apoptosis in DP thymocytes is not dependent on p53, Nur77, or Fas/Fas ligand, apoptosis-related gene products.

Although the requirement has been established for functional GR in GC-induced apoptosis sensitivity, certain lymphoid cells resist apoptosis in vitro and in vivo despite having a GR content equivalent to or greater than GC-sensitive T cells and similar binding properties (Bourgeois, Newby, & Huet, 1978; Daaka, Luttrell & Lefkowitz, 1997; Homo, Duval, Hatzfeld, & Evrard, 1980; Kaspers et al., 1994; Soufi, Schneider, Beato, & Westphal, 1995; Thompson & Harmon, 1986). Clearly, other factors can control GC-induced apoptosis, such as secretion of protein factors that attenuate the lytic response (Sakuae, Bowtell, & Kasuga, 1992; Thompson, 1991). Immature CD4/CD8 double-negative cells (precursors of DP thymocytes) or mature T cells are much less sensitive to GC (Homo et al., 1980; Hugo, Boyd, Waanders, & Scollay, 1991). Although resistant, a significant number of mature splenic T cells do succumb to apoptotic death following treatment with dexamethasone, a synthetic GC, in the same concentration range that induces apoptosis in immature thymocytes (Ito, Satoh, Kaziro, & Itoh, 1995). However, the mechanism of GC-induced apoptosis in mature T cells differs from that of DP thymocytes. Apoptosis in mature T cells is modulated by T cell growth factors. IL-4 specifically rescues Th2 cells from GC-induced apoptosis. In contrast to Th2 cells where IL-2 and IL-1 rescues these cells, IL-2 is effective in inhibiting GC-induced apoptosis in Th1 cells. IL-4 or IL-2-dependent protection of Th cells against GC-induced apoptosis is PKC activation dependent (Zubiaga, Munoz, & Huber, 1992).

GC induce changes in expression of transcription factors and oncogenes, including cyclins, cyclin-dependent kinases, c-jun, and c-myc (that have been implicated in apoptosis) (Rhee, Bresnahan, Hirai, Hirai, & Thompson, 1995; Thompson, Thulasi, Saeed, & Johnson, 1995; Thulasi et al., 1993; Zhou & Thompson, 1996). Following GC treatment, down-regulation of c-myc is an early common response in arrested and/or killed cells (Eastman-Reks & Vedeckis, 1986; Helmberg, Auphan, Caelles, & Karin, 1995; Thompson et al., 1995; Thulasi et al., 1993). Additionally, others report that steroid hormones can modulate the activity of certain cAMP and G-protein-driven pathways (Gordeladze, Johansen, Paulssen, Paulssen, & Gautvic, 1994). For example, cAMP and GC synergistically induce cytolysis of T cells (Dowd & Miesfeld, 1992; Jondal, Xue, McConkey, & Okret, 1995; McConkey, Orrenius, Okret, & Jondal, 1993; Medh, Saeed, Johnson, & Thompson, 1998), and loss of PKA in WEHI-7 clones causes a significant decrease in GC sensitivity (Groul, Rajah, & Bourgeois, 1989). Conversely, GC-induced cellular responses can be modulated by other signal transduction pathways, including PKC (Schüle & Evans, 1991).

Activation- and GC-induced apoptotic signaling pathways in T cell hybridomas (Iseki, Mukai, & Iwata, 1991; Iwata et al., 1991; Zacharchuk, Mercep, Chakraborti, Simmons, & Ashwell, 1990) are mutually antagonistic. Activation-induced cell death in T cell hybridomas and in preactivated mature T cells requires Fas/Fas ligand interaction (Alderson et al., 1995; Brunner et al., 1995; Dhein, Walczak, Baumier, Debatin, & Krammer, 1995; Ju et al., 1995). GCs inhibit the expression of Fas ligand mRNA (Yang, Mercep, Ware, & Ashwell, 1995). As TCR/CD3-mediated stimulation activates calcineurin and PKC (Iseki et al., 1991; Zhao & Iwata, 1995), these pathways may antagonize each other in these cells. T cell activation results in a rapid activation of CaM kinase II and PKC activity. The increased activity of CaM kinase II, but not PKC, is blocked by treatment with dexamethasone (Paliogianni & Boumpas, 1995). Increased activity of CaM kinase II following T cell activation is the result of rapid phosphorylation of CaM kinase II, which is inhibited by dexamethasone treatment (Paliogianni, Hama, Balow, Valentine, & Boumpas, 1995). The inhibitory effect of dexamethasone on phosphorylation of CaM kinase II is reversed in the presence of a phosphatase inhibitor of a glucocorticoid antagonist. Collectively, these data suggest that GC inhibition following T cell activation requires both the GR and protein phosphatases. The regulation of mature T cell apoptosis is important for controlling the number of activated T cells, depleting self-reactive clones, and maintaining memory T cells. TCR- and steroid receptor-mediated stimulation influence regulation of apoptosis of mature T cells; however, further studies are necessary for fully elucidating the mechanisms by which these receptors modulate T cell death.

B. Glucocorticoid Modulation of IL-2 Production

Studies examining the mechanisms by which GC inhibit T cell proliferation and IL-2 production have focused on the interference of GC with the transcriptional activation of the IL-2 gene following activation of the TCR/CD3 complex. IL-2 production is mediated by at least two major activation pathways that are coupled to the TCR/CD3 complex via tyrosine phosphorylation events: those mediated by PLCγ1 and those mediated by the small G protein p21 ras (Pastor, Reif, & Cantrell, 1995; Secrist, Karnitz, & Abraham, 1991; Weiss, Koretzky, Schatzman, & Kadlecek, 1991). Tyrosine phosphorylation and the subsequent activation of PLCγ1 results in an increase in cytoplasmic levels of Ca^{2+}. This is a critical event for the activation of calcineurin, a calcium- and calmodulin-dependent serine/threonine phosphatase. Calcineurin mediates the dephosphorylation of NF-AT. NF-AT is a protein complex consisting of a cytosolic component, NF-ATp and AP-1 transcription factor (Flanagan, Corthesy, Bram, Crabtree, & 1991; Jain et al., 1993; Jain, McCaffrey, Valge-Archer, & Rao, 1992). NF-ATp is present in the cytoplasm of unstimulated T cell. NF-ATp is activated upon dephosphorylation by calcineurin following T-cell stimulation (Clipstone & Crabtree, 1992; Flanagan et al., 1991) and undergoes nuclear translocation where it combines with AP-1 to form the active IL-2 transcription complex NF-AT1 (McCaffrey, Perrino, Soderling, & Rao, 1993). The TCR/CD3 complex is coupled to the Ras pathway via tyrosine phosphorylated adaptor proteins, p36 and/or Shc, and results in the downstream activation of MAPK (Pastor et al., 1995; Weiss & Littman, 1994) as previously described. The activation of MAPK are critical for the induction of threshold levels of AP-1 required for formation of NF-AT1 (Weiss & Littman, 1994).

The effects of GC on cytokine production by lymphocytes have been addressed by analyzing the regulation of genes that code for the interleukins and interferons (reviewed in Parrillo & Fauci, 1979). Many of these genes are upregulated substantially by the AP-1, C/EBP, and especially, the NF-κB transcription factors (Arya et al., 1984; Caldenhoven et al., 1995; Jain et al., 1992; Mukaida et al., 1994; Northrop, Crabtree, & Mattila, 1992; Ray & Prefontaine, 1994; Serfling et al., 1989; Vacca et al., 1992; reviewed in Cato & Wade, 1996). GC, through interaction with GR, repress AP-1 and NF-κB transcription factors, and thus inhibit expression of interleukins. GC repress both NF-κB and AP-1 by inhibitory cross-talk through GR interaction. In the case of NF-κB, GC also activate IκB transcription, which further inhibits NF-κB. For example, studies examining the mechanisms by which GC inhibit T cell proliferation and IL-2 production have focused on the interference of GC with the transcriptional activation of the IL-2 gene. Although the IL-2 promoter lacks GRE, steroids on association with their intracellular receptor inhibit IL-2 gene transcription by interfering with the activity of AP-1 nuclear proteins that bind to the IL-2 promoter (Paliogianni, Raptis, Ahuja, Najjar, & Boumpas, 1993). GC also inhibit the activity of NF-κB by elevating transcription and protein synthesis of its cytoplasmic inhibitor, IκBα (Auphan, DiDonato, Rosette, Helmberg, & Karin, 1995; Scheinman, Cogswell, Lofquist, & Baldwin, 1995). Repression of AP-1 by the GR has been studied the most thoroughly. However, many other members of the nuclear hormone receptor superfamily, for example, progesterone and androgen receptors (Shemshedini, Knauthe, Sassone-Corsi, Pornon, & Gronemeyer, 1991), the estrogen receptor (Weisz & Rosales, 1990), and retinoic acid receptors (Lafyatis et al., 1990; Nicholson et al., 1990; Salbert et al., 1993; Schüle et al., 1990), act similarly. This suggests that mutual repression for AP-1 and nuclear hormone receptors is a general feature of this transcription factor family rather than a peculiarity of GR.

In addition to their known inhibitory effects on AP-1, GC also inhibit calcineurin-dependent pathways for T cell activation (Paliogianni & Boumpas, 1995). Calcineurin, a Ca^{2+}/calmodulin-dependent protein phosphatase, is an essential component of the T cell antigen receptor signal transduction pathway leading to IL-2 gene transcription. GC inhibit IL-2 promoter activation in Jurkat T cells cotransfected with plasmids containing the intact IL-2 promoter and a deletion mutant (delta CaM-AI) of calcineurin, known to have Ca^{2+}-independent constitutive phosphatase activity (Paliogianni & Boumpas, 1995). This GC effect is completely reversed by coincubation with a glucocorticoid antagonist, demonstrating that the effect was mediated through GR. Recently,

Baus and co-workers (Baus, Andris, Dobois, Urbain, & Leo, 1996) demonstrated that GC interfere with early steps of the TCR/CD3 signal transduction pathway. Treatment of murine T cell hybrids and activated peripheral T cells with dexamethasone inhibited TCR/CD3-mediated intracellular calcium mobilization, inositol phosphate production, and PLCγ1 tyrosine phosphorylation. Their data suggest that GC block anti-CD3-mediated calcium responses by interfering with a postreceptor signaling step prior to activation of PLCγ1. Thus, although GCs have been used for decades as clinical tools to suppress immune and inflammatory responses, the mechanisms by which they modulate immune functions still require further examination to be fully understood.

XI. G PROTEINS CAN MODULATE LYMPHOCYTE GROWTH AND DIFFERENTIATION

Although control of growth and differentiation traditionally has been associated with peptides acting through tyrosine kinase receptors to activate MAPK, it is now clear that many neurotransmitters and hormones coupled to G-proteins are important in these processes (Figure 4). MAPK pathways are activated by G protein-coupled receptors, as well as by growth factors with intrinsic tyrosine kinase activity. G protein-coupled receptors that signal by G_s (Faure, Voyno-Yasenetskaya, & Bourne, 1994; Wan & Huang, 1998), G_i (van Biesen et al., 1995), and G_q (Koch, Hawes, Allen, & Lefkowitz, 1994) have all been

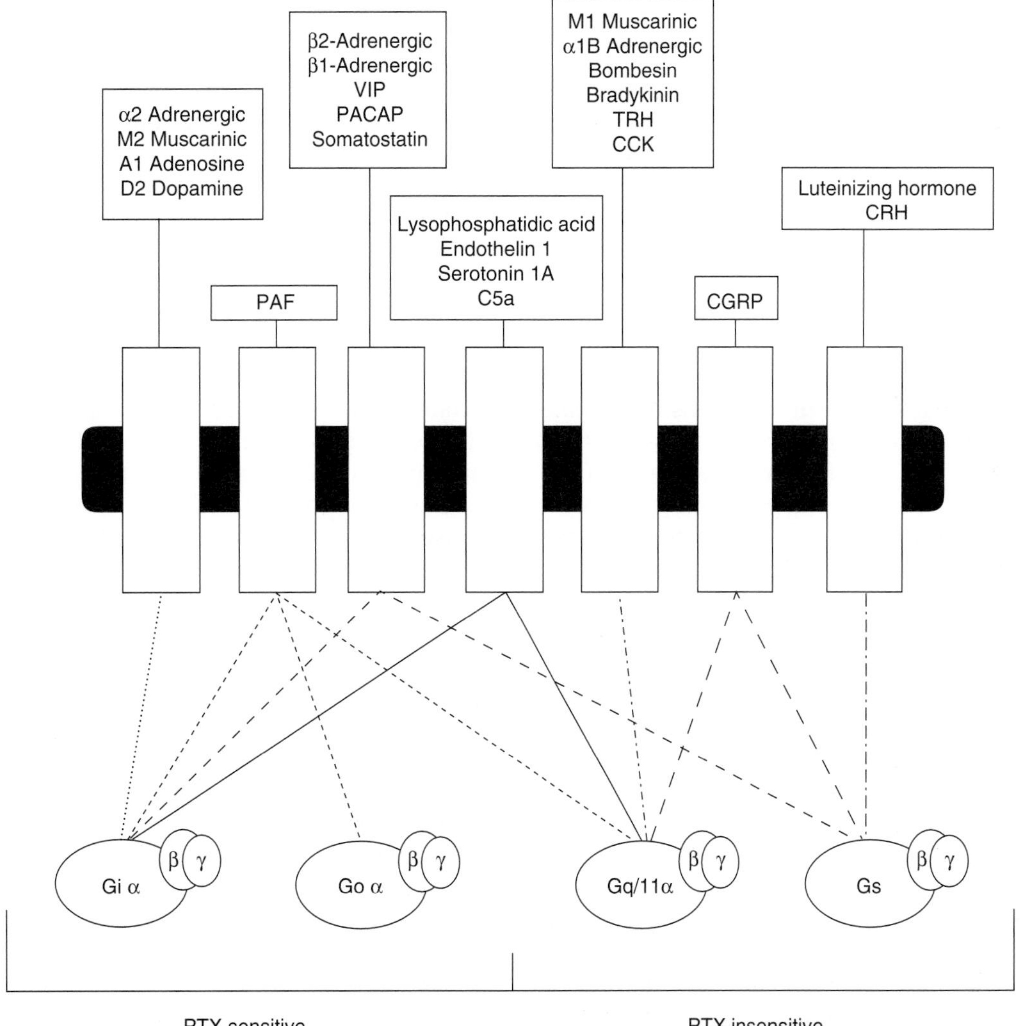

FIGURE 4 Schematic of the numerous neurotransmitters and hormones that are coupled to subsets of heterotrimeric G proteins. Neurotransmitters and hormones that interact with receptors coupled to G_i , G_q/11, and G_s family members of G proteins stimulate MAPK activity (see text for references and abbreviations). (This figure was modified from Luttrell et al., 1997).

shown to activate MAPK pathways, and thus have the ability to modulate TCR signaling. The signal pathways by which G protein-coupled receptors activate MAPK are complex and heterogeneous. MAPK activation by receptors coupled to various G proteins (G_s, G_q, and G_i) is mediated by second messengers, such as cAMP (Crespo, Cachero, Xu & Gutkind, 1995), Ca^{2+} (Dikic, Tokiwa, Lev, Courtneidge, & Schlessinger, 1996), and PKC (Della Rocca et al., 1997). MAPK activation also can occur, either directly or indirectly, through $G\alpha$ (Faure et al., 1994) or $G\beta\gamma$(Koch, et al., 1994; van Biesen et al., 1995), or directly through heterotrimeric G proteins (Feig & Cooper, 1988).

XII. MODULATION OF LYMPHOCYTE FUNCTION BY G_s PROTEINS USING THE β_2-AR AS AN EXAMPLE

A large number of neurotransmitters and modulators use cAMP as their second messenger. As an example of how these signaling molecules influence lymphocyte function, β_2-AR signaling, the most widely studied of this group, is described below. Despite the clear modulatory role of NA signaling in lymphocytes, there have been few studies aimed toward delineating how the intracellular signaling proteins activated by ligand binding with AR on the surface of lymphoid cells feed into the signaling protein cascades that operate in these cells to regulate cell function. Most of the research in this area has focused on the ability of ligand binding of β-adrenergic agents with β_2-AR to stimulate cAMP production and activation of PKA. In this section, we present a summary of what is known about catecholamine signaling in lymphoid cells, and where research still needs to be done to work out these mechanisms. We have already described how activation of β_2-AR stimulate cAMP production and activate PKA, so here we will focus our discussion on intracellular signaling by β_2-AR that is downstream to these events.

The stimulation of βAR and activation of lymphocytes via the antigen-MHC complex or mitogen leads to the initial induction of two entirely different signaling pathways (Figure 5). It is clear that a lymphocyte receives a number of signals from antigen-coupled MHC complex and cytokines that initiate a cascade of biochemical and molecular events leading to activation. It is in the context of these events that intracellular signals emanating from stimulation of adrenergic receptors must be interpreted and integrated. It is well-known that activation of the βAR on B cells (Bach, 1975; Bishopric et al., 1980; Niaudet et al., 1976), T cells (Bishopric et al., 1980; Geenen et al., 1986; Niaudet et al., 1976; Stachelin et al., 1985), and macrophages (Koff & Dunegan, 1986) results in a rapid increase in intracellular levels of cAMP. Stimulation of T cells through the TCR concurrent with activation of the βAR results in a synergistic rise in intracellular cAMP (Roszman & Carlson, 1991; Sakabe, Seiki, & Fujii, 1986). Increased intracellular cAMP levels in T cells has been demonstrated to inhibit antigen or mitogen driven proliferative responses (Boynton & Whitfield, 1983).

So, how does increased levels of cAMP and activation of PKA modulate signaling cascades elicited by stimulation of the TCR? These intracellular signaling proteins are capable of influencing other signaling proteins in the TCR signaling pathways. Before we go any further, we should point out that the data we are about to describe have been generated using nonphysiological means of stimulating intracellular cAMP concentrations. Agents that bypass adenylyl cyclase-linked receptors, such as forskolin or dibutyryl cAMP (dbcAMP), have been employed. Additionally, some of our understanding of cAMP-mediated effects has been gained from studies that use other neurotransmitters or growth factors to stimulate cAMP production. Although initially it was assumed that activated PKA interferes with the TCR-coupled PI turnover (Bismuth et al., 1988; Klausner et al., 1987; Lerner, Jacobson, & Miller, 1988), it soon became clear that PKA may affect multiple and independent steps along the activation pathways in T cells (Granja, Lin, Yunis, Relias & Dasgupta, 1991; Klausner et al., 1987; Tamir & Isakov, 1994; Wu et al., 1993b; Zaitsev et al., 1992). A common point of convergence for many, if not all neurotransmitters and growth factors that elevate intracellular cAMP and activate PKA, is the activation of the Ras proteins (Cook & McCormick, 1993b).

Ras signals activation of the cytosolic serine-threonine protein kinases, Raf-1, and MAPK (de Vries-Smits, Burgering, Leevers, Marshall & Bos, 1992; Robbins et al., 1992; Thomas, DeMarco, D'Arcangelo, Halegoua, & Brugge, 1992; Wood, Sarnecki, Roberts, & Blenis, 1992). Recent studies demonstrate that Raf-1 is an efficient in vitro substrate for PKA, and that treatment of cells with forskolin decreases Raf-1 binding affinity to p21ras (Wu et al., 1993a). Increased concentrations of cAMP are known to block activation of Raf-1, and Erk kinases in Rat1 fibroblasts (Cook & McCormick, 1993a; Wu et al., 1993a). These effects are accompanied by an increase in Raf-1 phosphorylation (Wu et al., 1993a). Further,

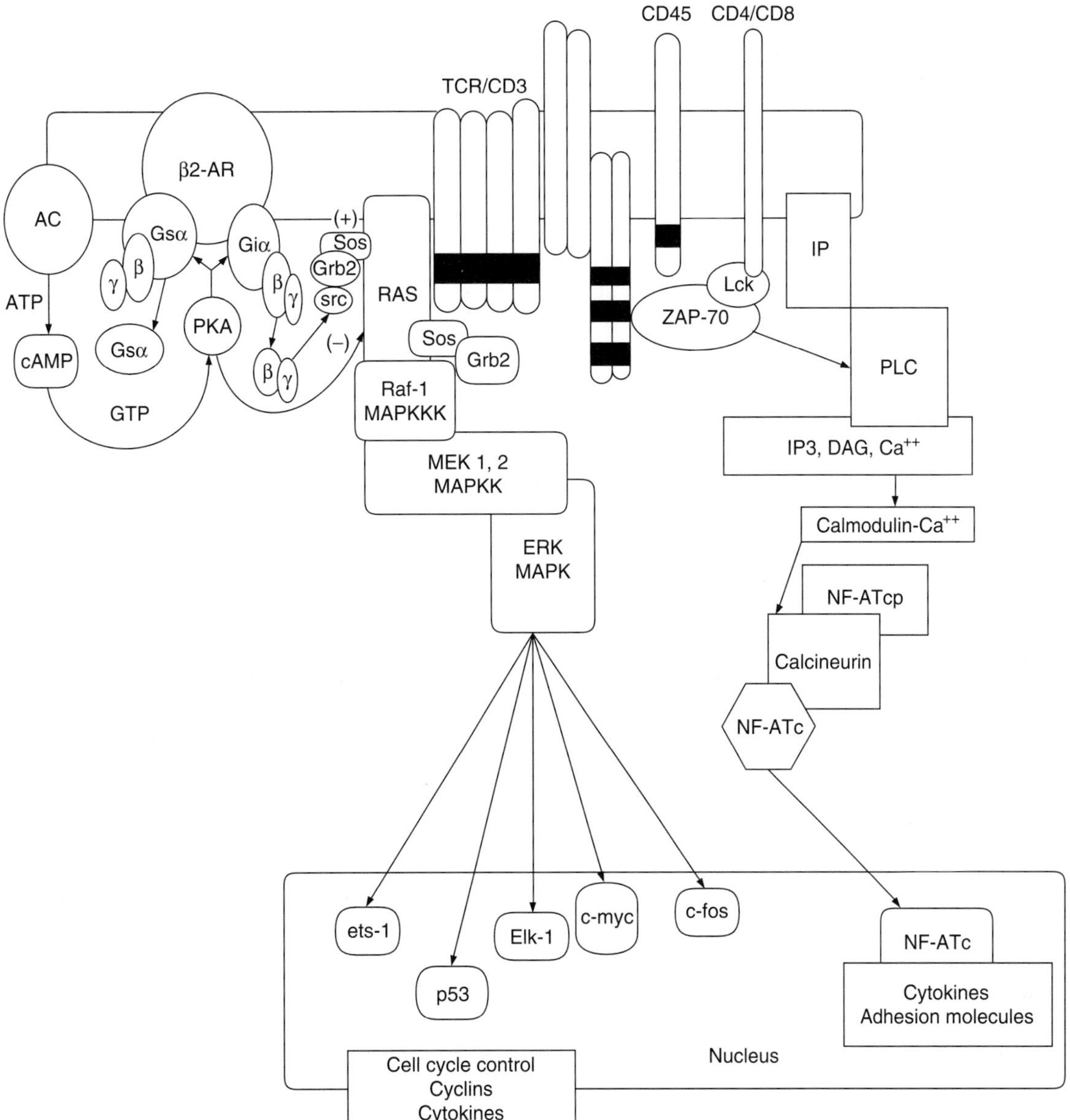

FIGURE 5 Schematic illustration of the transmembrane signaling events elicited by stimulation of β_2-AR and the T cell receptor (TCR). Activation of the β_2-adrenergic receptor (AR) and the TCR leads to the initial induction of two different signaling pathways. β_2-AR coupling to G_s proteins induces activation of protein kinase A (PKA). PKA interferes with Raf-1 binding to Ras, thus inhibiting downstream signaling of the TCR receptor. However, β_2-AR can switch their coupling from G_s proteins to G_i proteins, an effect that also is mediated by PKA. PKA phosphorylation of the β_2-AR leads to β_2-AR desensitization, reducing cAMP production in response to further stimulation, and causes the β_2-AR to be coupled to G_i proteins. The coupling of the β_2-AR with G_i proteins results in direct feedbeack inhibition of the G_s-mediated adenylyl cyclase signal that started the process. Coupling of the β_2-AR to G_i proteins then initiates a second wave of G_i-mediated signaling to activate mitogen-activated protein kinase (MAPK) pathways and promote functional responses iniated by TCR stimulation. Abbreviations are defined in the text.

the cAMP-dependent phosphorylation of Raf-1 in vitro and in vivo reduce the apparent affinity with which Raf-1 binds to Ras (Wu et al., 1993a). Subsequently, the specific sites of association between the Ras-GTP and Raf-1 proteins were identified (Marshall, 1995). The interaction between these contact points is essential for the membrane localization of Raf, and ultimately leads to kinase activation of Raf-1 by Ras. Schramm and co-workers (Schramm, Niehof, Radziwill, Rommel, & Moelling, 1994) reported that PKA phosphorylates the Ser43, and Ser259 of Raf-1 in vitro, as demonstrated by comparison of phosphopeptide maps of recombinant wild-type c-Raf-1 and corresponding mutants. In vivo, stimulation of the PKA pathway by treatment of A431 cells with forskolin results in an increase of phosphorylation in Ser43. The formation of Ras-GTP/Raf-1 complex is negatively regulated by PKA (Chuang et al., 1994; Hafner et al., 1994; Marshall, 1995; Schramm et al., 1994) (Figure 5). Phosphorylation of Raf by PKA on Ser43 resulted in significant inhibition of Ras binding demonstrating that the mechanism of cAMP down regulation results through structural changes occurring exclusively in this small Ras-binding domain (Chuang et al., 1994). Phosphorylation of c-Raf-1 on Ser43 is believed to cause an N-terminal cap structure to cover the Ras "docking site" (Marshall, 1995). Thus, PKA-phosphorylated Raf-1 exhibits a reduced affinity for GTP-loaded Ras.

In addition to weakening the interaction of Raf-1 binding to Ras, PKA inhibits Raf-1 function directly via phosphorylation of the Raf-1 kinase domain, down-regulating Raf-1 kinase activity, and thus, subsequent signaling of Erk (Hafner et al., 1994; Marshall, 1995; Mischak et al., 1996). This type of inhibition is dissociated from the ability of Raf-1 to associate with Ras because (1) the isolated Raf-1 kinase domain, which lacks the Ras binding domain, is susceptible to PKA inhibition; and (2) cAMP agonists inhibit Raf activity, which is Ras independent (Hafner et al., 1994). Data indicating recruitment of PKA to the TCR/CD3 complex (Skalhegg et al., 1994) of anti-CD3-activated T cells, where Raf-1 is found associated with the CD3γ and δ chain (Loh et al., 1994), may provide the appropriate conditions for the PKA-induced phosphorylation of Raf-1. Recently, $G_{s\alpha}$ was demonstrated to be required in βAR signaling to MAPK in a PKA-dependent pathway involving Raf-1 using $G_{s\alpha}$ and PKA-deficient S49 mouse lymphoma cells (Wan & Huang, 1998). These findings suggest that PKA may function to uncouple Ras from Raf-1 and inhibit Raf-1 activity.

Studies also suggest an affect of cAMP and PKA at additional sites in TCR signaling pathways. In NIH3T3 and rat-1 fibroblasts, an elevation of intracellular cAMP levels results in the inhibition of Erk2 activation induced by cAMP elevating agents (PDGF, EGF, and insulin) (Bergering, Pronk, Weeren, Chardin, & Bos, 1993). Analysis of various signaling intermediates reveals that cAMP interferes at a site downstream of p21ras, but upstream of Raf-1 kinase in these cell types. Inhibition by cAMP depends on both the cAMP concentration, and the absolute amount of p21ras molecules bound to GTP, suggesting a mechanism of competitive inhibition.

Bergering and co-workers (1993) observed that TPA-induced, p21ras-independent, activation of raf-1 kinase and Erk2 is inhibited by cAMP in fibroblast cell lines. They found that phosphorylation of the GTP/GDP exchange factor, mSos, as monitored by a mobility shift, is delayed with respect to p21ras and Erk2 activation and is inhibited by cAMP. Their results provide evidence for a model of p21ras-directed signaling toward Erk2 that feeds back on mSos by regulating its phosphorylation status. Further, they show that this pathway can be negatively modulated by PKA and positively modulated by PKC. Tamir and co-workers (Tamir, Granot, & Isakov, 1996) substantiated previous work showing that cAMP inhibits ERK activation in T cells, and demonstrated that both PKC-dependent and PKC-independent ERK activation can be inhibited by cAMP. Using a PKC-specific inhibitor, GF109203X, or PKC-depleted cells, they observed that a considerable portion of the anti-CD3-induced ERK activation is PKC dependent. Both the PKC-dependent and PKC-independent activation of ERK is blocked by forskolin or a cell-permeable cAMP analog, dbcAMP.

Activation of the TCR triggers protein tyrosine kinase activity of the src-family protein kinases ($p56_{lck}$ and $p59_{fyn}$) and the Syk-family member (ZAP-70). At least one study has explored potential effects of cAMP on the activity of these kinases, and observed that an increase in intracellular levels of cAMP following VIP treatment of resting thymocytes stimulates $p59_{fyn}$, but not $p56_{lck}$, kinase activity (Xin, Sun, & Ganea, 1997). The effect is dose dependent, and is reproduced by other cAMP-inducing agents, such as forskolin, PGE_2, and 8-bromo-cAMP, suggesting that cAMP alters the activity of this protein tyrosine kinase. This is consistent with reports that PKA activation inhibits the phosphorylation of the TCRγ and TCRε chains (Klausner et al., 1987; Patel, Samelson & Klausner, 1987).

XIII. cAMP AND COSTIMULATORY SIGNALS

Most studies examining signal transduction pathways required for activation of T cells use transformed T cell lines. However, transformed cell lines require only a single TCR/CD3-mediated signal for activation. Human CD4+ T cell clones require two distinct activating signals (TCR/CD4-mediated and a costimulatory signal) to trigger proliferation or cytokine production. Shanafelt and co-workers (Shanafelt et al., 1995) have established human T cell clones in which their activation is entirely dependent on costimulatory signals. These T cell clones have been used to distinguish between intracellular signals generated by TCR/CD3 complexes, and those generated by the costimulatory cell surface receptors, CD3 and CD28 (Lahesmaa et al., 1995). Lahesmaa and co-workers (1995) found that ligation of CD28, but not other costimulatory molecules, induced the tyrosine phosphorylation of two previously identified Grb2-binding proteins (pp76 and pp116). A third Grb2-binding protein (pp36) was extensively tryosine phosphorylated in response to combined CD3 and CD28 activation, but not in response to ligation of either receptor alone. Pretreatment of CD4+ T cell clones with cAMP affected tyrosine phosphorylation of proteins that associated with Grb2. Thus, in activated human T cell clones the composition of the Grb2 protein complex, a complex that is likely to be a critical intracellular control point, by determining which intracellular signal transduction pathways are activated, is modulated by costimulatory signals and cAMP.

Tamir and co-workers (1996) demonstrated that JNK (SAPK) activation also is inhibited by increases in intracellular cAMP. Activation of JNK (SAPK), another member of the MAPK family, requires CD3 and CD28 costimulation and is essential for the induction of T cell proliferation (Su et al., 1994). Consistent with these findings, Moule and Denton (1998) found that the βAR agonist, isoproterenol, increases the activity of the stress-activated kinase p38 MAPK over 10-fold in freshly isolated rat epididymal fat cells. Stimulation of the kinase was rapid, sustained for at least 60 min, and sensitive to the specific p38 MAPK inhibitor, SB203580. The cell permeable cAMP analog, chlorophenylthio-cyclic AMP, increased p38 MAPK activity to a similar extent as isoproterenol, suggesting that the effect of the βAR agonist is mediated via increased PKA activity . Isoproterenol had little or no effect on c-Jun N-terminal kinase activity, but isoproterenol and a number of other treatments which activated p38 MAPK, were found to stimulated PKA in fat cells. Despite these findings, activation of PKA and p38 MAPK were not found to be directly linked. Thus, evidence supports a negative effect for cAMP on T cell activation by interfering with multiple events along two MAPK signaling pathways, ERK pathways stimulated by TCR complexes, and SAPKs activated following CD3 and CD28 costimulation.

XIV. G_i PROTEINS ACTIVATE THE MAPK SIGNALING PATHWAY: α_{2A}-AR AS AN EXAMPLE

Pertussis toxin-sensitive G_i-coupled receptors (Figure 6) are known to activate MAPK in a Ras-dependent manner that is independent of phospholipase activation or inhibition of adenylyl cyclase (Alblas, van Corven, Hordijk, Milligan, & Moolenaar, 1993; Winitz et al., 1993). For example, stimulation of G_i-coupled α_{2A}-AR in CCL 39 cells with clonidine results in a pertussis-toxin-sensitive increase in DNA synthesis (Seuwen et al., 1990). This clonidine-induced increase in DNA synthesis is associated with activation of Ras, and is independent of phospholipase activation or inhibition of adenylyl cyclase (Alblas et al., 1993). Although agonist activation of α_{2A}-AR-coupled G_i protein signals is insensitive to PKC depletion, there is a marked attenuation of the agonist-induced MAPK activity by dominant negatives N17 Ras and ΔN Raf (Hawes, van Biesen, Koch, Luttrell, & Lefkowitz, 1995). Similarly, stimulation of G_i-coupled M_2-acetyl choline receptor (AChR) in Rat 1a fibroblasts with carbachol induces a pertussis toxin-sensitive activation of Ras, Raf, MEK, and MAPK (Winitz et al., 1993). Agonist activation of G protein-coupled receptors results in the dissociation of heterotrimeric G proteins into $G\alpha$ -GTP and $G\beta\gamma$ heterodimers. Recent studies have indicated a role for the $G\beta\gamma$ subunit in regulating activation of MAPK following activation of G_i-coupled receptors (Clapham & Neer, 1993). In contrast to G_q- and G_s-coupled receptors in COS-7 cells, where $G\alpha_q$ and $G\alpha_s$ activation is sufficient to activate MAPK, $G\alpha_i$ expression does not stimulate MAPK activity (Faure et al., 1994). However, expression of $G\beta\gamma$ subunits in these cells leads directly to MAPK activation (Faure et al., 1994; Hawes et al., 1995; Ito et al., 1995; Koch et al., 1994). Similarly, in Rat 1a fibroblasts, suppression of activated $G\alpha_{i2}$ mutants results in constitutive activation of the MAPK pathway, and causes neoplastic transformation (Gupta, Gallego, Johnson, & Heasley, 1992). These studies suggest that in these cells, MAPK activation by G_i-coupled receptors depends on the release of free $G\beta\gamma$ subunits. Consistent with a role for $G\beta\gamma$ in MAPK activation, the specific $G\beta\gamma$ subunit-binding peptide derived from the carboxyl-terminus of the βAR kinase 1 (βARK1ct) (Koch, Inglese, Stone, & Lefkowitz, 1993; Pitch et al., 1992) specifically antagonizes $G\beta\gamma$ Ras-dependent MAPK activation via pertussis-toxin sensitive G proteins, but not PKC-dependent and pertussis toxin-independent MAPK activation (Faure et al., 1994; van Biesen et al., 1995).

Growing evidence suggests that Ras-dependent MAPK activation by G_i protein-coupled receptors requires the tyrosine phosphorylation of "docking" proteins, which function as platforms for assembly of a Ras activation complex. Stimulation of α_{2A}-AR, or expression of $G\beta1\gamma2$ subunits, induces PKC-independent shc tyrosine phosphorylation and shc/Grb2

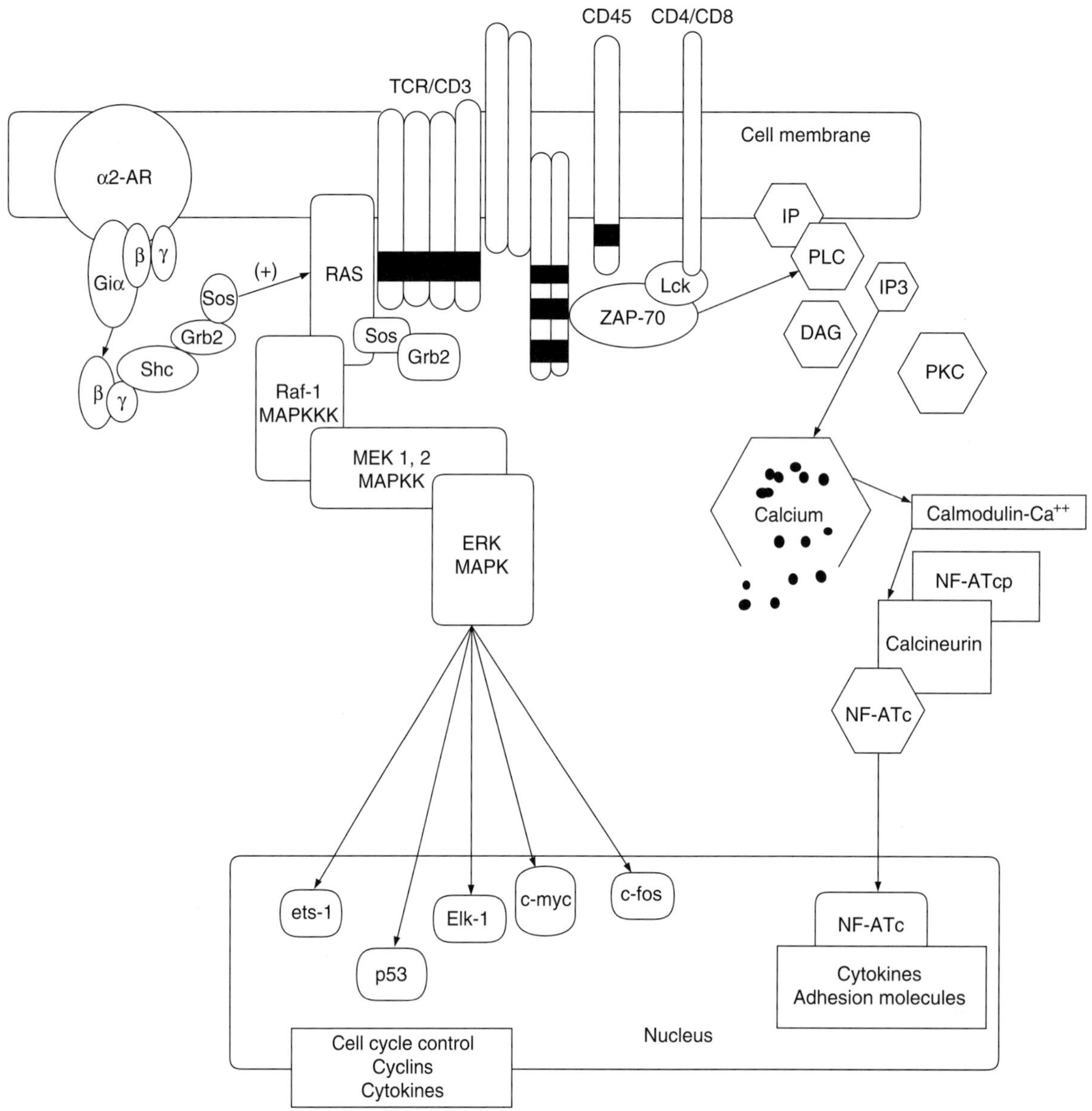

FIGURE 6 Model of the transmembrane signaling pathways elicited by activation of α_2-adrenergic receptors (AR) and the T cell receptor (TCR). Although these two receptors initiate different signaling pathways, α_2-AR stimuation can modulate functional reponses initated by TCR activation by impacting on downstream signaling at the level of Ras.

complex formation in COS-7 cells (Alblas et al., 1993; van Biesen et al., 1995). Tyrosine phosphorylation of shc is inhibited by treatment with pertussis toxin and coexpression of the $G\beta\gamma$ subunit-binding peptide, βARKct1. α_{2A}-AR-induced signals also are inhibited by genistein, an inhibitor of protein tyrosine kinases, at concentrations lower than those required to inhibit pertussis toxin-insensitive, Ras-dependent, MAPK activation by the EGF receptor tyrosine kinase (van Biesen et al., 1995). These studies suggest that phosphorylation of shc is mediated by the $G\beta\gamma$ subunits of pertussis toxin-sensitive G proteins. Thus, G_i-coupled receptors, such as the α_{2A}-AR, activate MAPK by a Ras-dependent mechanism that is sensitive to inhibitors of tyrosine protein kinases and converges on the MAPK pathways at the level of Raf 1 kinase.

Grb2-mediated recruitment of Sos1 is a required step in the signaling of G_i-coupled receptor activation of MAPK pathways. Coexpression of dominant negative mutants of Sos 1 (Δm-Sos1 and SOS-PRO) inhibit the G_i-coupled receptor- and $G\beta\gamma$-subunit-mediated MAPK activation (van Biesen et al., 1995; Sakuae et al., 1992). Functionally inactive Grb2/Sos mutant complexes, which disrupt the recruitment of wild-type Sos1 into shc/Grb2/Sos1 complexes, accumulate with expression of enzymatically inactive Sos1 (van Biesen et al., 1995). ΔmSos1 or SOS-PRO inhibits MAPK activation mediated by α_{2A}-AR or $G\beta1\gamma2$ subunits, with no effect on activation via constitutively activated mutant Ras (T24 Ras). Thus, Ras-dependent MAPK activation by G_i-coupled receptors, like the α_{2A}-AR, requires $G\beta\gamma$ subunit-mediated tyrosine phosphorylation of the shc adaptor protein and Grb2-mediated recruitment of Ras-guanine-nucleotide-exchange factor activity.

As indicated above, the TCR does not possess intrinsic tyrosine kinase activity and requires recruitment of src-family tyrosine kinases, Lck and Fyn, for tyrosine phosphorylation of the receptor (Cunningham & Lee, 1995). Similarly, recruitment of nonreceptor tyrosine kinases for phosphorylation of G_i-coupled receptors is required, and may be mediated by G_i proteins. Pertussis toxin-sensitive activation of Src, Fyn, and Yes by agonist-stimulated α_{2A}-AR, as well as α-thrombin receptor and M_2-AChR, have been documented (Elliott, Blum, Li, Metwali, & Weinstock, 1998).

XV. G_q PROTEINS ACTIVATE THE MAPK PATHWAY: THE G_q/11-COUPLED-α_1-AR AS AN EXAMPLE

Pertussis toxin-insensitive G_q/11-coupled receptors, such as α_{1B}-AR and M_1 muscarinic acetylcholine receptor (M_1-AChR), are known to activate PLC, which results in DAG and IP_3 generation (Figure 7). This is followed by IP_3-dependent increases in intracellular Ca^{2+} and activation of PKC by DAG. Activation of PKC results in MAPK activation (Hawes et al., 1995; Kolch et al., 1993). M_1-AChR-induced activation of MAPK is attenuated in PKC-depleted cells. Thus, G_q/11-coupled receptors mediate MAPK activation by PKC-dependent mechanisms. In addition, MAPK activation is inhibited by cells coexpressing M_1-AChR and a dominant negative mutant Raf protein (ΔN Raf) (Feig & Cooper, 1988; Luttrell et al., 1997). However, MAPK activation is not altered by cells coexpressing M_1-AChR and a dominant negative Ras protein (N17 Ras) in COS-7 (Luttrell et al., 1997). These studies indicate that G_q/11-coupled receptors stimulate MAPK activation in a Raf-1-dependent, but Ras-independent, manner.

Activated mutant $G\alpha$ subunits or $G\beta\gamma$ heterodimers have been used to determine if the effectors required for MAPK activation by G_q/11-coupled receptors are regulated by either $G\alpha$ or $G\beta\gamma$ subunits. Responses to G_q/11-linked receptors appear to involve both the $G\alpha$- and $G\beta\gamma$-subunits of G proteins; however, the $G\alpha1$-dependent activation of PKC is thought to play the predominant role (Crespo et al., 1995; Hawes et al., 1995).

XVI. G PROTEINS AND JNK/SAPK ACTIVATION

Similar mechanisms of $G\alpha$ and $G\beta\gamma$ activation of JNK/SAPK by G protein-coupled receptors have been reported (Coso, Chiariello, Kalinec, Kyriakis, Woodgett, & Gutkind, 1995; Daaka et al., 1997; Prasad, Dermott, Heasley, Johnson, & Dhanasekaran, 1995). JNK/SAPK is activated by stimulation of m_1 and m_2 muscarinic AChR coupled to G_i and G_q/11 proteins, respectively (Coso et al., 1996; Mitchell, Russell, & Johnson, 1995). The effect was not mimicked by expression of activated forms of $G\alpha_s$, $G\alpha_{12}$, or $G\alpha_{13}$ subunits (Coso et al., 1996); however, overexpression of $G\beta\gamma$ subunits did induce JNK/SAPK activation. Signaling from m_1 and m_2 muscarinic AChR to JNK/SAPK involving $G\beta\gamma$ subunits was Ras- and Rac-dependent (Coso et al., 1996). Involvement of $G\beta\gamma$ (Coso et al., 1996), as well as $G\alpha_q$/11, $G\alpha_{12}$, and $G\alpha_{13}$, was reported in JNK/SAPK activation (Collins, Minden, Karin, & Brown, 1996; Prasad et al., 1995; Voyno-Yasenetskaya, Faure, Ahn, & Bourne, 1996).

XVII. G PROTEINS AND p38 MAPK ACTIVATION

Little is known about the activation of p38 MAPK by G protein-coupled receptors. Recently, it was suggested that activation of p38 MAPK by G protein-coupled receptors involves $G\alpha_q$- as well as $G\beta\gamma$-subunits (Yamauchi, Nagao, Kaziro, & Itoh, 1997). Yamauchi and co-workers (1997) demonstrated that stimulation of G_q/11-coupled m_1 and G_i-coupled m_2 muscarinic AChR and G_s-coupled βAR activate p38 MAPK in human embryonic kidney 293 cells. Activation of p38 MAPK by m_2 AChR and βAR stimulation was completely inhibited by coexpression of $G\alpha_o$. In contrast, expression of $G\alpha_o$ following activation of the m_1 receptor only partially inhibited p38 MAPK activity. The overexpression of $G\beta\gamma$ or a constitutively activated mutant of $G\alpha_9$/11, but not $G\alpha_s$ or $G\alpha_i$, stimulated p38 MAPK. These results indicate that activation of p38 MAPK by G_i-coupled m_2 and βAR is mediated by $G\beta\gamma$. In contrast, activation of p38 MAPK by G_q/11-coupled m_1 receptor is mediated by both $G\beta\gamma$ and $G\alpha_q$/11. The

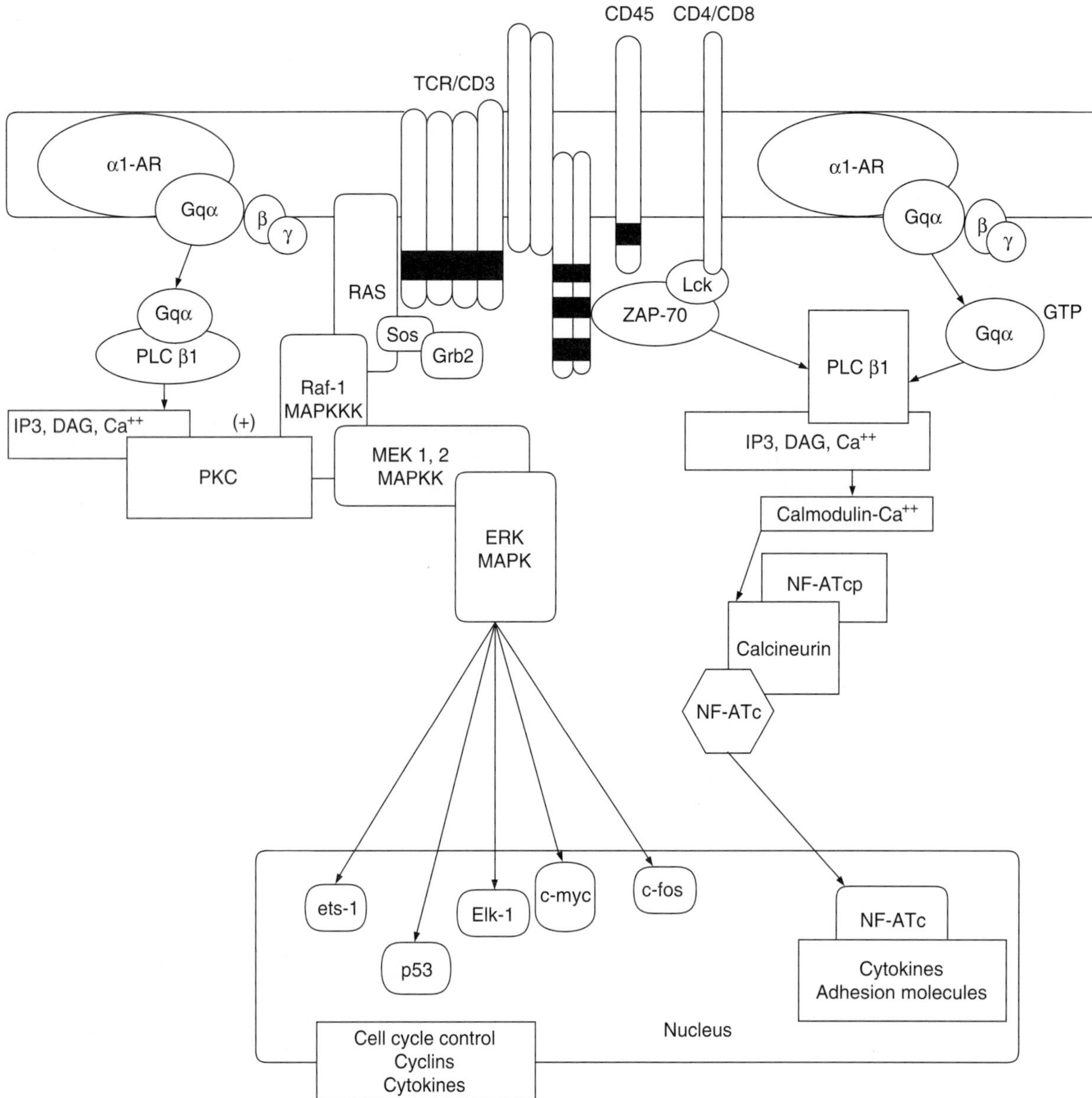

FIGURE 7 Diagramatic representation of the transmembrane signaling events activated by stimulation of α_1-adrenergic receptor (AR) and the T cell receptor (TCR). α_1-AR are coupled to the $G_q/11$ subfamily of G proteins. Agonist binding to the α_1-AR is known to activate phospholipase C (PLC), which results in diacylglycerol (DAG) and inositol triphosphate (IP_3) generation. IP_3 and DAG induce increases in intracellular Ca^{2+} and activation of protein kinase C (PKC), respectively. Activation of this signaling pathway can modulate TCR signaling by a PKC induced mitogen-activated protein kinase (MAPK) activation via PKC effect at the level of Raf-1. Further, activation of the α_1-AR also can impact on costimulatory signals by α_1-AR stimulation of nuclear factor of activated T cells (NF-AT) transcription factors.

physiological role of G protein-coupled receptor activation of p38 MAPK is unclear. The p38 MAPK pathway may be involved in the inhibition of cell growth and the promotion of cell death (Kyriakis & Avruch, 1996). Additional studies exploring the signal transduction cascade for G protein-induced activation of p38 MAPK may provide new insight into the functions of p38 MAPK.

XVIII. ADDITIONAL CONSIDERATIONS IN NEUROTRANSMITTER INFLUENCES ON IMMUNE FUNCTIONS

A. Receptor Desensitization

The density of βAR expressed by immunocytes, and thus the sensitivity to catecholamines, can be regulated by the presence (down-regulation) or absence (up-regulation) of ligand (Aarons & Molinoff, 1982; Aarons, Nies, Gerber & Molinoff, 1983; Miles et al., 1984). Local NE concentrations in the microenvironment are likely to vary depending on the exact spatial relationship between the target cell and the sites of NE release from NA nerve terminals. A lymphocyte or macrophage residing adjacent to a NA nerve terminal in a lymphoid organ is usually exposed to high concentrations of catecholamines. Immunocytes residing near these nerve terminals may have their βAR saturated and may be the most sensitive to changes in catecholamine levels during a decrease in sympathetic nerve activity. In contrast, immunocytes that reside away from NA nerve terminals are exposed to lower concentrations of NE and may have an up-regulation of βAR. These immunocytes would be expected to respond more to an increase in NE released during sympathetic nerve activation. Although no evidence exists for location-based in vivo regulation of βAR on immunocytes, several laboratories have demonstrated greater βAR densities on B cells compared with T cells (Fuchs, Albright & Albright, 1988a, 1988b; Genaro & Borda, 1989; Miles et al., 1984). This might be predicted based on the relative lack of innervation of B cell zones compared with T cell zones in the spleen.

Long-term activation of βAR has been studied using cells that express either β_2- or β_3 receptor subclasses by measuring adenylate cyclase activity, cAMP accumulation, and PKA activity in CWH cells and L cells (Nantel, Bouvier, Strosberg, & Marullo, 1995). Treatment of cells expressing β_2AR with 10 μM isoprenaline for 24 h resulted in a marked decrease in total receptor number and reduced the ability of the receptor to stimulate adenylyl cyclase. In contrast, one of the cell types expressing β_3AR and treated similarly was observed to have reduced β_3AR densities, the other cell type did not. Regardless of the cell type, Nantel and colleagues found that the β_3AR was more resistant than the β_2AR to long-term desensitization. Long-term desensitization may have functional effects on cell signaling depending on the βAR subtype and the cell type under consideration.

B. Activation State of the Target Cell

Expression of βAR and sensitivity to catecholamines depends on the activation state of the lymphocytes as well. The expression of βAR is regulated by intracellular signaling events initiated in lymphocytes (Cazaux, Sterin-Borda, Gorelik, & Cremashchi, 1995). The expression of βAR by murine lymphocytes stimulated with Con A was decreased at the peak of proliferation. Treatment of the cells with tyrosine kinases or protein kinase inhibitor blocked lymphocyte proliferation and reversed the decrease in βAR densities. Thus, mechanisms of βAR desensitization, by either exposure to elevated levels of catecholamines or by activation of lymphocytes, may affect the ability of the nervous system to modulate immune function.

C. Colocalization of Neurotransmitters and Circulating Hormones and Neurotransmitters

Colocalization of neuropeptides with catecholamines adds another level of complexity to the role of NA innervation in modulation of immune function. The efficacy of one neurotransmitter may be augmented or inhibited by the presence of another neurotransmitter. NA nerve terminals also may take up circulating catecholamines, both epinephrine and NE, via their high-affinity uptake carrier. This is likely to change the relative concentration of subsequently released catecholamines of which NE and epinephrine have different potencies with regard to β and αAR. Thus, behavioral responses that influence circulating catecholamines may alter responsiveness of immunocytes to catecholamines in this manner.

Similarly, hormones present in the local microenvironment also may alter the expression and sensitivity of catecholamines for their receptors expressed by immunocytes. GC may up-regulate or down-regulate AR subtypes. Recently, Rouppe van der Voort and co-workers (Rouppe van der Voort, Kavelaars, van de Pol, & Heijnen, 1999) have demonstrated that treatment of monocytes with the glucocorticoid dexamethasone induced the expression of functional α_{1b}- and α_{1d}-AR. They also report that the β_2AR agonist terbutaline induces expression of functional α_{1b}- and α_{1d}-AR in monocytes as well. Similarly, stimulation of β_3AR using the selective β_3AR agonist CL 316,243 has been demonstrated to selectively up-regulate α_{1a} receptor and mRNA expression in brown adipose tissue (Granneman, Zhai, & Lahners, 1997). This suggests that exposure of these cells to NA agonists is followed by a down-regulation of βAR and an increase in the expression of specific subclasses of αAR. Therefore, stress responses that result in an increase in the circulating levels of glucocorticoid and catecholamines are likely to alter the expression and sensitivity of neurotransmitters for their receptors on immune target cells.

D. Cytokine Secretion

Cytokines produced and secreted by immunocytes also may alter responsiveness of cells of the immune system to catecholamines. For example, dual stimulation of the TCR and βAR results in a synergistic increase in the elevation of intracellular cAMP (Carlson et al., 1989). Some evidence has been obtained that proinflammatory cytokines can induce expression of α_{1a}AR on human monocytes (C. Rouppe van der Voort et al., manuscript in preparation). Further, cytokines interact at the level of the central nervous system (hypothalamus) and in the periphery (the sympathetic nerve terminal) to provide a feedback mechanism for controlling sympathetic (and neuroendocrine) activity. Sympathetic activity may be altered by cytokines through changes in firing rates of the nerve terminals, increasing or decreasing neurotransmitter turnover, and changes in nerve fiber density by terminal degeneration or sprouting responses.

E. Efficacy of Adrenergic Receptor Subtype Subclasses Expressed

The sensitivity of immune cells to catecholamines also may depend on the relative density of the specific receptor subtype classes that are expressed on the immunocytes. Activation of closely related subclasses of αAR shows markedly different patterns of both functional responses and effectiveness in activating second messenger pathways. For example, in transfected PC12 cells expressing α_{1A}-, α_{1B}-, and α_{1D}-AR, NE increased inositol phosphate formation and intracellular Ca^{2+} levels and activated MAPK cascades in these cells in a manner dependent on receptor density (Zhong & Minneman, 1999). However, α_{1A}AR activated these second messenger pathways more effectively than α_{1B}AR. α_{1D}AR were the least effective. Although NE treatment activated Erks in cells expressing all three α_1AR, p38 MAPK was only activated in α_{1A}- and α_{1B}AR expressing cells and JNK was only activated in α_{1A}AR expressing cells. These differences in subclass expression of α_1AR corresponded to differences in the ability of NE to induce neurite outgrowth in PC12 cells. Only α_{1A}AR expressing cells differentiated in response to NE (Zhong & Minneman, 1999).

Similarly, epinephrine stimulation of α_{2D}-, α_{2B}-, and α_{2C}-AR subtypes expressed by stably transfected CHO cells induces a rapid activation of MAPK with subtype-specific differences in efficiencies (Flordellis et al., 1995). α_{2B}-AR induced MAPK activation with the greatest efficiency followed by α_{2D}AR and α_{2C}AR. Thus, closely related subtypes of AR show markedly different patterns of responses both functionally and by the intracellular signal pathways they induce.

F. Changes in Adrenergic Receptor Expression in Disease States

Disturbances in homeostasis in lymphoid tissues often results in changes in neurotransmitter turnover, or a more dramatic remodeling of nerves that distribute to them. The integrity of nerves in lymphoid organs changes over the life span of an individual (Ackerman, Bellinger, Felten, & Felten, 1991; Ackerman, Felten, Bellinger & Felten, 1987; Bellinger, Ackerman, Felten, & Felten, 1992; Bellinger, Ackerman, Felten, Lorton, & Felten, 1989; Bellinger, Felten, Collier, & Felten, 1987; Bellinger, Felten & Felten, 1988; Felten, Bellinger, Collier, Coleman, & Felten, 1987), with normal physiological events (Kendall et al., 1994), following immune activation (Molina et al., 1993; Novotny & Hsu, 1993; Yang, Wang, & Huang,1998), in response to disease states (Bellinger, Lorton, Felten, & Felten, 1992; Felten, Felten, Bellinger, & Olschowka, 1992; Hama et al., 1995; Izquierdo et al., 1995; Jackman et al., 1995; Levine, Dardick, Roizen, Helms, & Basbaum, 1986; Levine, Goetzl, & Basbaum, 1991; Lorton, Lubahn, Felten, & Bellinger, 1997; Mitchell, Kendall, Adam, & Schumacher, 1997; Schreurs, Versteeg, & Nijkamp, 1982; Szamel & Resch, 1995), and with injury, inflammatory, and reparative processes. Since the density of adrenergic receptors on target cells is determined in part by the concentration of neurotransmitter available for receptor interaction, receptor density on target cells is likely to change as well, and is likely to alter neural signaling to target cells of the immune system. For example, in an animal model for nasal allergy, the expression of muscarinic acetylcholine receptor is elevated in guinea pigs with hypersensitivity of the nasal mucosa (Namimatsu, Okazaki, Go, & Hata, 1992). Decreased density of βAR receptors occurs on peripheral blood mononuclear cells in patients with rheumatoid arthritis (Baerwald, Graefe, von Wichert, & Krause, 1992; Baerwald et al., 1997; Krause, Henrich, Beckh, von Wichert, & Baerwald, 1992) and asthma (Hataoka et al., 1993). In contrast, enhanced expression of β-AR densities on peripheral blood mononuclear cells has been observed in progressive multiple sclerosis patients in a number of independent studies (Arnason, Brown, Maselli, Karaszewski, & Reder, 1988; Karaszewski, Reder, Anlar, & Arnason, 1993; Karaszewski, Reder, Anlar, Kim, & Arnason, 1990; Karaszewski, Reder, Maselli, Brown, & Arnason, 1990; Zoukos, Leonard, Thomaides, Thompson, & Cuzner, 1992; Zoukos, Thomaides, Mathias, & Cuzner, 1994). It is likely that changes in receptor density on target immunocytes alter signaling between the nervous and immune systems, and that this phenomenon has an impact on disease outcome. These changes may reflect clonal expansion of specific cell populations, and changes in the trafficking of subpopulations of immunocytes to tissues, and thus change in the distribution of subpopulations of lymphocytes in the tissues or changes in the density of adrenergic receptors per lymphocyte.

Onset of disease also may induce expression of receptors not normally expressed by cells of the immune system. In patients suffering from the chronic inflammatory disease, juvenile rheumatoid arthritis, peripheral blood monocytes express functional α_1AR. Peripheral blood mononuclear cells of healthy donors do not express functional α_1AR. Stimulation of α_1AR on peripheral blood leukocytes of juvenile rheumatoid arthritis patients increases production of proinflammatory cytokines (Heijnen et al., 1996). Thus, expression of α_1AR receptors on leukocytes is likely to contribute to the disease process. Recently, Rouppe van der Voort and co-workers (1999) demonstrated that expression of α_1AR by human monocytes could be induced by treatment with dexamethasone or the β_2AR agonist terbutaline. This study suggests that glucocorticoid and stimulation of β_2AR can regulate the expression of α_1AR subtypes in human monocytes.

G. Alternate βAR Coupling to G_s and G_i Proteins

Depending on the cell type, an increase in intracellular cAMP levels may lead to cellular proliferation (Chambard, Paris, L'Allemain, & Pouysségur,1987; van Corven, Groenink, Jalik, Eichholtz, & Moolnenaar, 1989), differentiation (Cowley, Paterson, Kemp, & Marshal, 1994; Yarwood, Kilgour, & Anderson, 1996) or growth arrest (McKenzie & Pouysségur, 1996). This appears to result from activation of different signaling pathways in these cell types. Although most of the actions stimulated by activation of β_2AR are mediated through G_s proteins, increased cAMP and PKA pathways, βAR also can couple to G_i proteins (Abramson et al., 1988; Daaka et al., 1997; Xiao, Ji, & Lakatta, 1995). By coupling to different classes of G proteins, βAR can simultaneously activate several different signaling cascades depending on the cell type. For example, In fibroblasts, cAMP-dependent inhibition of Raf-1 antagonizes MAPK activation. However, in Cos-7 cells an increase in intracellular cAMP activates MAPK by a route not involving a receptor (Crespo et al., 1995; Faure et al., 1994) and in HEK293 cells induces an increase in cAMP, but also increases activation of MAPK by switching the G_s receptor coupling to an G_i-receptor coupling (Daaka et al., 1997).

Daaka and co-workers (1997) reported that β_2AR can switch coupling from G_s proteins to G_i proteins, an effect mediated by PKA. In HEK293 cells, agonist binding to β_2AR stimulates MAPK activity. This response is mediated by $\beta\gamma$ subunits of pertussis toxin-sensitive G proteins, suggesting a coupling of β_2AR to G_i proteins. Activation of the MAPK was blocked by an inhibitor of PKA, indicating that the receptor must be phosphorylated by PKA. Interaction of a βAR agonist with a mutant of the β_2AR lacking the sites normally phosphorylated by PKA, stimulates an increase in adenylyl cyclase activity leading to increased cAMP; however, MAPK is not activated. These results demonstrate that PKA-mediates uncoupling of the β_2AR from G_s proteins, leads to receptor desensitization, and then switches the coupling of this receptor from G_s to G_i to initiate a new set of signaling events.

Dual coupling of βAR to G_s and G_i pathways have been reported for other cells, including lymphoma cells (Abramson et al., 1988) and cardiac myocytes (Xiao et al., 1995). Additionally, β_3AR expressed in CHO/K1 cells specifically activates the MAPKs ERK1 and ERK2 coupling of the receptor to G_i proteins (Gerhardt, Gros, Strosberg, & Issad, 1999). Thus, PKA phosphorylation of the βAR plays an essential regulatory role in βAR signaling by decreasing receptor-coupling efficiency to G_s. PKA phosphorylation of the receptor leads to a heterologous receptor desensitization, reducing cAMP production in response to further stimulation. At the same time, the enhanced coupling efficiency to G_i proteins results in direct feedback inhibition of the G_s-mediated adenylyl cyclase signal that started the process. Coupling of the βAR to G_i proteins initiates a second wave of G_i-mediated signaling to activate MAPK. This event coincides with termination of the signal that started the initial response.

XIX. CONCLUSIONS

Neural-immune signaling is a dynamic and interactive process, the understanding of which requires integrative investigation of neurotransmitter, hormonal, and cytokine influences on multiple target cells. It is clear even at this early stage in studying neural-immune signaling, that (1) there is extensive cross-talk between the nervous and immune systems, (2) neurotransmitters and endocrine signals can profoundly alter immune function, (3) cytokines can profoundly influence nervous system function under normal conditions and in states of pathology, and (4) neural and immune mediators share common intracellular signaling pathways. Given the complexity of brain-immune signaling, elucidating mechanisms for this interaction will require both in vitro and in vivo approaches. These studies will require investigation at multiple hierarchical levels of immune function. We will need to evaluate neurotransmitter influences on (1) individual cell functions, (2) collective interactions of cells of the immune system, and (3) immune functions in the individual. Sharing of second messengers by neural and immunologic mediators and cross-talk between second messengers by T and B lymphocytes and macrophages will be important areas of future study that may lead to novel uses of pharmacological agents that target neural and endocrine systems to intervene in immmunologically mediated diseases. A better understanding of the interactions that occur between the central nervous system and immune system is essential for the development of effective strategies for the treatment of inflammation, infectious disease, autoimmune disease, and cancer.

References

Aarons, R. D., & Molinoff, P. B. (1982). Changes in the density of beta adrenergic receptors in rat lymphocytes, heart, and lung after chronic treatment with propranolol. *Journal of Pharmacology and Experimental Therapy, 221*, 439–443.

Aarons, R. D., Nies, A. S., Gerber, J. G., & Molinoff, P. B. (1983). Decreased beta adrenergic receptor density on human lymphocytes after chronic treatment with agonists. *Journal of Pharmacology and Experimental Therapy, 224*, 1–6.

Abramson, S. N., Martin, M. W., Hughes, A. R., Harden, T. K., Neve, K. A., Barrett, D. A., & Molinoff, P. B. (1988). Interaction of β-adrenergic receptors with the inhibitory guanine nucleotide-binding protein of adenylate cyclase in membranes prepared from *cyc*$^-$S49 lymphoma cells. *Biochemical Pharmacology, 37*, 4289–4297.

Ackerman, K. D., Bellinger, D. L., Felten, S. Y., & Felten, D. L. (1991). Ontogeny and senescence of noradrenergic innervation of the rodent thymus and spleen. In R. Ader, D. L. Felten, N. Cohen, (Eds.) *Psychoneuroimmunology* (2nd ed., pp. 72–125). New York: Academic Press.

Ackerman, K. D., Felten, S. Y., Bellinger, D. L., & Felten, D. L. (1987). Noradrenergic sympathetic innervation of the spleen: III. Development of innervation in the rat spleen. *Journal of Neuroscience Research, 18*, 49–54.

Alam, S. M., Travers, P. J., Wung, J. L., Nasholds, W., Redpath, S., Jameson, S. C., & Gascoigne, N. R. (1996). Cell-receptor affinity and thymocyte positive selection. *Nature, 381*, 616–620.

Alberola-Ila, J., Forbush, K. A., Seger, R., Krebs, E. G., Perlmutter, R. M., Avruch, J., & Woodgett, J. R. (1995). Selective requirement for MAPK activation in thymocyte differentiation. *Nature, 373*, 620–623.

Alberola-Ila, J., Takaki, S., Kerner, J. D., & Perlmutter, R. M. (1997). Differential signaling by lymphocyte antigen receptors. *Annual Review of Immunology, 15*, 125–154.

Alblas, J., van Corven, E. J., Hordijk, P. L., Milligan, G., & Moolenaar, W. H. (1993). Gi-mediated activation of the p21^{ras}-mitogen-activated protein kinase pathway by a_2-adrenergic receptors expressed in fibroblasts. *Journal of Biological Chemistry, 268*, 22235–22238.

Alderson, M. R., Tough, T. W., Davis-Smith, T., Braddy, S., Falk, B., Schooley, K. A., Goodwin, R. G., Smith, C. A., Ramsdell, F., & Lynch, D. H. (1995). Fas ligand mediates activation-induced cell death in human T lymphocytes. *Journal of Experimental Medicine, 181*, 71–77.

Altman, A., Coggeshall, K. M., & Mustelin, T. (1990). Molecular events mediating T cell activation. *Advances in Immunology, 48*, 227–360.

Appleby, M. W., Gross, J. A., Cooke, M. P., Levin, S. D., Qian, X., & Perlmutter, R. M. (1992). Defective T cell receptor signaling in mice lacking the thymic isoform of p59^{fyn}. *Cell, 70*, 751–763.

Argetsinger, L. S., Campbell, G. S., Yang, X., Witthuhn, B. A., Silvennoinen, O., Ihle, J. N., Carter-Su., C. (1993). Identification of JAK2 as a growth hormone receptor-associated tyrosine kinase. *Cell, 74*, 237–244.

Arnason, B. G. W., Brown, M., Maselli, R., Karaszewski, J., & Reder, A. (1988). Blood lymphocyte β-adrenergic receptors in multiple sclerosis. *Annals of the New York Academy of Sciences, 540*, 585–588.

Arya, S. K., Wong-Staal, F., & Gallo, R. C. (1984). Dexamethasone-mediated inhibition of human T cell growth factor in gamma-interferon messenger RNA. *Journal of Immunology, 133*, 273–276.

Asaoka, Y., Nakamura, S.-I., Yoshida, K., & Nishizuka, Y. (1992). Protein kinase C, calcium, and phospholipid degradation. *Trends in Biochemical Sciences, 17*, 414–387.

Auphan, N., DiDonato, J., Rosette, C., Helmberg, A., & Karin, M. (1995). Immunosuppression by glucocorticoids: Inhibition of NFκB activity through induction of IκB synthesis. *Science, 290*, 286–290.

Avruch, J., Zhang, X., & Kyriakis, J. M. (1994). Raf meets Ras: Completing the framework of a signal transduction pathway. *Trends in Biochemistry, 19*, 279–283.

Bach, M.- A. (1975). Differences in cyclic AMP changes after stimulation by prostaglandins and isoproterenol in lymphocyte subpopulations. *Journal of Clinical Investigation, 55*, 1074–1081.

Baerwald, C., Graefe, C., von Wichert, P., & Krause, A. (1992). Decreased density of beta-adrenergic receptors on peripheral blood mononuclear cells in patients with rheumatoid arthritis. *Journal of Rheumatology, 19*, 204–210.

Baerwald, C. G., Laufenberg, M., Specht, T., von Wichert, P., Burmester, G. R., & Krause, A. (1997). Impaired sympathetic influence on the immune response in patients with rheumatoid arthritis due to lymphocyte subset-specific modulation of beta 2-adrenergic receptors. *British Journal of Rheumatology, 36*, 1262–1269.

Baier-Bitterlich, G., Uberall, G., Bauer, R., Fresser, F., Wachter, H., Grunicke, H., Utermann, G., Altman, A., & Baier, G. (1996). Protein kinase C-θ isoenzyme selective stimulation of the transcription factor complex AP-1 in T lymphocytes. *Molecular and Cellular Biology, 16*, 1842–1850.

Bansal, V. S., & Majerus, P. W. (1990). Phosphatidylinositol-derived precursors and signals. *Annual Review of Cellular Biology, 6*, 41–67.

Barnes, P. J., & Adcock, I. (1993). Anti-inflammatory actions of steroids: Molecular mechanisms. *Trends in Pharmacological Science, 141*, 436–441.

Baus, E., Andris, F., Dobois, P. M., Urbain, J., & Leo, O. (1996). Dexamethasone inhibits the early steps of antigen receptor signaling in activated T lymphocytes. *Journal of Immunology, 156*, 4555.

Bellinger, D. L., Ackerman, K. D., Felten, S. Y., & Felten, D. L. (1992). A longitudinal study of age-related loss of noradrenergic nerves and lymphoid cells in the aged rat spleen. *Experimental Neurology, 116*, 295–311.

Bellinger, D. L., Ackerman, K. D., Felten, S. Y., Lorton, D., & Felten, D. L. (1989). Noradrenergic sympathetic innervation of thymus, spleen and lymph nodes: Aspects of development, aging and plasticity in neural-immune interactions. In G. Nistico, (Ed.) *Proceedings of a Symposium on Interactions Between the Neuroendocrine and Immune Systems* (pp. 35–66). Rome: Pythogora Press.

Bellinger, D. L., Felten, S. Y., Collier, T. J., & Felten, D. L. (1987). Noradrenergic sympathetic innervation of the spleen: IV. Morphometric analysis in adult and aged F344 rats. *Journal of Neuroscience Research, 18*, 55–63.

Bellinger, D. L., Felten, S. Y., & Felten, D. L. (1988). Maintenance of noradrenergic sympathetic innervation in the involuted thymus of the aged Fischer 344 rat. *Brain Behavior Immunity, 2*, 133–150.

Bellinger, D. L., Lorton, D., Felten, S. Y., & Felten, D. L. (1992). Innervation of lymphoid organs and implications in development, aging, and autoimmunity. *International Journal of Immunopharmacology, 14*, 329–344.

Bergering, B. M. T., Pronk, G. J., Weeren, P. C., Chardin, P., & Bos, J. L. (1993). cAMP antagonizes p21ras-directed activation of extracellular signal-regulated kinase 2 and phosphorylation of mSos nucleotide exchange factor. *EMBO Journal, 12*, 4211–4220.

Berridge, M. J. (1993). Inositol trisphosphate and calcium signalling. *Nature, 361*, 315–325.

Bidart, J. M., Motte, P.H., Assicot, M., Bohuon, C., & Bellett, D. (1983). Catechol-O-methyltransferase activity and aminergic binding sites distribution in human peripheral blood lymphocyte subpopulations. *Clinical Immunology Immunopathology, 26*, 1–9.

Birnbaumer, L. (1990). G proteins in signal transduction. *Annual Review of Pharmacology Toxicology, 30*, 675–705.

Birnbaumer, L. (1992). Receptor-to-effector signaling through G proteins: Roles for beta gamma dimers as well as alpha subunits. *Cell, 71*, 1069–1072.

Bishop, J. M. (1991). Molecular themes in oncogenes. *Cell, 64*, 235–248.

Bishopric, N. H., Cohen, H. J., & Lefkowitz, R. J. (1980). Beta adrenergic receptors in lymphocyte subpopulations. *Journal Allergy and Clinical Immunology, 65*, 29–33.

Bismuth, G., Theodorou, I., Gouy, H., Le Gouvello, S., Bernard, A., & Debre, P. (1988). Cyclic AMP-mediated alteration of the CD2 activation process in human T lymphocytes: Preferential inhibition of the phophoinositide cycle-related transduction pathway. *European Journal Immunology, 18*, 1351–1357.

Blake, T. J., Heath, K. G., & Langdon, W. Y. (1993). The truncation that generated the v-cbl oncogene reveals an ability for nuclear transport, DNA binding and acute transformation. *EMBO Journal, 12*, 2017–2026.

Bollag, G., & McCormick, F. (1992). Regulators and effectors of ras proteins. *Annual Review of Cellular Biology, 7*, 601–632.

Boumpas, D. T., Paliogianni, F., Anastassiou, E. D., & Balow, J. E. (1991). Glucocorticosteroid action on the immune system: Molecular and cellular aspects. *Clinical and Experimental Rheumatology, 9*, 413–423.

Bourgeois, S., Newby, R. F., & Huet, M. (1978). Glucocorticoid resistance in murine lymphoma and thymoma lines. *Cancer Research, 38*, 4279–4284.

Bourne, H.R., & Nichol, R. (1993). Molecular machines integrate coincident synaptic signals. *Cell, 72*, 65–75.

Bourne, H. R., Sanders, D. A., & McCormick, R. (1991). The GTPase superfamily: Conserved structure and molcular mechanism. *Nature, 349*, 117–127.

Boynton, A. L., & Whitfield, J. F. (1983). The role of cyclic AMP in cell proliferation: A critical assessment of the evidence. *Advances in Cyclic Nucleotide Research, 15*, 193–294.

Bredt, D. S., & Snyder, S. H. (1992). Nitric oxide, a novel neuronal messenger. *Neuron, 8*, 3–11.

Brindle, P. K., & Montminy, M. R. (1992). The CREB family of transcription activators. *Current Opinion in Genetic Development, 2*, 199–204.

Brown, A. M., & Birnbaumer, L. (1990). Ionic channels and their regulation by G protein subunits. *Annual Review of Physiology, 52*, 197–213.

Brunner, T., Mogil, R. J., LaFace, D., Yoo, N. J., Mahboubi, A., Echeverri, G., Martin, S. J., Force, W. R., Lynch, D. H., & War, C. F. (1995). Cell-autonomous Fas (CD95)/Fas-ligand interaction mediates activation-induced apoptosis in T cell hybridomas. *Nature, 373*, 441–444.

Buday, L., Egan, S. E., Rodriquez-Viciana, P., Cantrell, D. A., & Downward, J. (1994). A complex of Grb2 adaptor protein, Sos exchange factor, and a 36-kDa membrane-bound tyrosine phosphoprotein is implicated in ras activation in T cells. *Journal of Biological Chemistry, 269*, 9019–9023.

Buday, L., Khwaja, A., Sipeki, S., Faragó, A., & Downward, J. (1996). Interactions of Cbl with two adaptor proteins, Grb2 and Crk, upon T cell activation. *Journal of Biological Chemistry, 271*, 6159–6163.

Byth, K. F., Conroy, L. A., Howlett, S., Smith, A. J. H., May, J., Alexander, D. R., & Holmes, N. (1996). CD45-null transgenic mice reveal a positive regulatory role for CD45 in early thymocyte development, in the selection of CD4+CD8+ thymocytes, and in B cell maturation. *Journal of Experimental Medicine, 183*, 1707–1718.

Caldenhoven, E., Liken, J., Wissink, S., Van de Stolpe, A., Raaijmakers, J., Koenderman, L., Okret, S., Gustafsson, J. A., & Van der Saag, P. T. (1995). Negative cross-talk between RelA and the glucocorticoid receptor: A possible mechanism for the antiinflammatory action of glucocorticoids. *Molecular Endocrinology, 9*, 401–412.

Carafoli, E. (1987). Intracellular calcium homeostasis. *Annual Review of Biochemistry, 58*, 395–433.

Carlson, S. L., Brooks, W. H., & Roszman, T. L. (1989). Neurotransmitter-lymphocyte interactions: Dual receptor modulation of lymphocyte proliferation and cAMP production. *Journal of Neuroimmunology, 24*, 155.

Caron-Leslie, L. M., Schwartzman, R. A., Gaido, M. L., Compton, M. M., & Cidlowski, J. A. (1991). Identification and characterization of glucocorticoid-regulated nuclease(s) in lymphoid cells undergoing apoptosis. *Journal Steroid Biochemistry and Molecular Biology, 40*, 661–671.

Caron-Leslie, L. S., & Cidlowski, J. A. (1991). Similar actions of glucocorticoids and calcium on the regulation of apoptosis in S49 cells. *Molecular Endocrinology, 5*, 1169–1179.

Carpenter, G. (1987). Receptors for epidermal growth factor and other polypeptide mitogens. *Annual Review of Biochemistry, 56*, 881–914.

Carroll, M. P., & May, W. S. (1994). Protein kinase C-mediated serine phosphorylation directly activates Raf-1 in murine hematopoietic cells. *Journal Biological Science, 269*, 1249–1256.

Cato, A. C., & Wade, E. (1996). Molecular mechanisms of anti-inflammatory action of glucocorticoids. *Bioessays, 18*, 371–378.

Caveney, S. (1985). The role of gap junctions in development. *Annual Review of Physiology, 47*, 319–335.

Cazaux, C. A., Sterin-Borda, L., Gorelik, G., & Cremashchi, G. A. (1995). Down-regulation of beta-adrenergic receptors induced by mitogen activation of intracellular signaling events in lymphocytes. *FEBS Letters, 364*, 120–124.

Chambard, J. C., Paris, L., L'Allemain, G., & Pouysségur, J. (1987). Two growth factor signalling pathways in fibroblasts distinguished by pertussis toxin. *Nature, 326*, 800–803.

Chan, A. C., Dalton, M., Johnson, R., Kong, G. H., Wang, T., Thoma, R., & Kurosaki, T. (1995). Activation of ZAP-70 kinase activity by phosphorylation of tyrosine 493 is required for lymphocyte antigen receptor function. *EMBO Journal, 14*, 2499–2508.

Chouaib, S., Welte, K., Mertelsmann, R., & Dupont, B. (1985). Prostaglandin E2 acts at two distinct pathways of T lymphocyte activation: Inhibition of interleukin-2 production and down-regulation of transferrin receptor expression. *Journal of Immunology, 135*, 1172–1179.

Chuang, E., Barnard, D., Hettich, L., Zhang, X. F., Avruch, J., & Marshall, M. S. (1994). Critical binding and regulatory interactions between Ras and Raf occur through a small, stable N-terminal domain of Raf and specific Ras effector residues. *Molecular and Cellular Biology, 14*, 5318–5325.

Chui, D., Ong, C. J., Johnson, P., Teh, H., & Marth, J. D. (1994). Specific CD45 isoforms differentially regulate T cell receptor signaling. *EMBO Journal, 13*, 798–807.

Claman, H. N. (1972). Corticosteroids and lymphoid cells. *New England Journal of Medicine, 287*, 388–397.

Clapham, D. E., & Neer, E. J. (1993). New roles for G protein $\beta\gamma$-dimers in transmembrane signalling. *Nature, 365*, 159–161.

Clevers, H., Alarcon, B., Wileman, T., & Terhorst, C. (1988). The T cell receptor/CD3 complex: A dynamic protein ensemble. *Annual Review of Immunology, 6*, 629–662.

Clipstone, N.-A., & Crabtree, G.-R. (1992). Identification of calcineurin as a key signalling enzyme in T-lymphocyte activation. *Nature, 357*, 695–697.

Cohen, J. J., & Duke, R. C. (1984). Glucocorticoid activation of a calcium-dependent endonuclease in thymocyte nuclei leads to cell death. *Journal of Immunology, 132*, 38–42.

Cohen, P. (1988). Protein phosphorylation and hormone action. *Proceeding of the Royal Society of London, 234*, 115–144.

Cohen, P. (1989). Structure and regulation of protein phosphatase. *Annual Review of Biochemistry, 58*, 453–508.

Cohen, R. (1992). Signal integration at the level of protein kinases, protein phosphatases and their substrates. *Trends in Biochemical Science, 17*, 408–413.

Collins, L. R., Minden, A., Karin, M., & Brown, J. H. (1996). $G\alpha12$ stimulates c-Jun NH2-terminal kinase through the small G proteins Ras and Rac. *Journal of Biological Chemistry, 271*, 17349–17353.

Combadiere, B., Freedman, M., Chen, L., Shores, E. W., Love, P., & Lenardo, M. J. (1996). Qualitative and quantitative contributions of the T cell receptor ζ chain to mature T cell apoptosis. *Journal of Experimenatal Medicine, 183*, 2109–2117.

Cook, S. J., & McCormick, F. (1993a). Inhibition by cAMP of Ras-dependent activation of Raf. *Science, 262*, 1069–1072.

Cook, S. J., & McCormick, F. (1993b). Inhibition by cAMP of Ras-dependent activation of Raf. *Science, 262*, 1069–1072.

Coso, O. A., Chiariello, M., Kalinec, G., Kyriakis, J. M., Woodgett, J., & Gutkind, J. S. (1995). Transforming G protein-coupled receptors potently activate JNK (SAPK). Evidence for a divergence from the tyrosine kinase signaling pathway. *Journal of Biological Chemistry, 270*, 5620–5624.

Coso, O. A., Teramoto, H., Simonds, W. F., & Gutkind, J. S. (1996). Signaling from G protein-coupled receptors to c-Jun kinase involves beta gamma subunits of heterotrimeric G proteins acting on a Ras and Rac1-dependent pathway. *Journal of Biological Chemistry, 271*, 3963–3966.

Cowley, S., Paterson, H., Kemp, P., & Marshal, C. J. (1994). Activation of MAP kinase kinase is necessary and sufficient for PC12 differentiation and transformation of NIH 3T3 cells. *Cell, 77*, 841–852.

Crabtree, G. R. (1989). Contingent genetic regulatory events in T lymphocyte activation. *Science, 243*, 355–361.

Crespo, P., Xu, N., Daniotti, J. L., Troppmair, J., Rapp, U. R., & Gutkind, J. S. (1994). Signaling through transforming G protein-coupled receptors in NIH 3T3 cells involves c-Raf activation. Evidence for a protein kinase C-independent pathway. *Journal of Biological Chemistry, 269*, 21103–21109.

Crespo, P., Cachero, T. G., Xu, N., & Gutkind, J. S. (1995). Dual effect of β-adrenergic receptors on mitogen-activated protein kinase: Evidence for a $\beta\gamma$-dependent activation and $G\alpha s$-cAMP-mediated inhibition. *Journal of Biological Chemistry, 270*, 25259–25265.

Cunningham, S. M., & Lee, G. M. (1995). Neuropeptide Y in submucosal ganglia: Regional differences in the innervation of guinea-pig large intestine. *Journal of the Autonomic Nervous System, 55*, 135–145.

Cupps, T. R., & Fauci, A. S. (1982). Corticosteroid-mediated immunoregulation in man. *Immunological Review, 65*, 133–155.

Daaka, Y., Luttrell, L. M., & Lefkowitz, R. J. (1997). Switching of the coupling of the β_2-adrenergic receptor to different G proteins by protein kinase A. *Nature, 390*, 88–91.

Davis, R. J. (1994). MAPKs: new JNK expands the group. *Trends in Biochemical Sciences, 19*, 470–473.

de Vries-Smits, A. M., Burgering, B. M., Leevers, S. J., Marshall, C. J., & Bos, J. L. (1992). Involvement of p21ras in activation of extracellular signal-regulated kinase 2. *Nature, 357*, 602–604.

Della Rocca, G. J., van Biesen, T., Daaka, Y., Luttrell, D. K., Luttrell, L. M., & Lefkowitz, R. J. (1997). Ras-dependent mitogen-activated protein kinase activation by G protein-coupled receptors. Convergence of Gi-and Gq-mediated pathways on calcium/calmodulin, Pyk2, and Src kinase. *Journal of Biological Chemistry, 272*, 19125–19132.

Derijard, B., Hibi, M., Wu, I., Barrett, T., Su, B., Deng, T., Karin, M., & Davis, R. J. (1994). JNK1: A protein kinase stimulated by UV light and Ha-Ras that binds and phosphorylates the c-Jun activation domain. *Cell, 76*, 1025–1037.

Desai, D. M., Sap, J., Silvennoinen, O., Schlessinger, J., & Weiss, A. (1994). The catalytic activity of the CD45 membrane-proximal phosphatase domain is required for TCR signaling and regulation. *EMBO Journal, 13*, 4002–4010.

DeSilva, D. R., Feeser, W. S., Tancula, E. J., & Scherle, P. A. (1996). Anergic T cells are defective in both Jun NH2-terminal kinase and mitogen-activated protein kinase signaling pathways. *Journal of Experimental Medicine, 183*, 2017–2023.

Dhein, J., Walczak, H., Baumier, C., Debatin, K. M., & Krammer, P. H. (1995). Autocrine T cell suicide mediated by APO-1/(Fas/CD95). *Nature, 373*, 438–441.

Dieken, E. S., Meese, E. U., & Miesfeld, R. L. (1990). nt^i glucocorticoid receptor transcripts lack sequences encoding the amino-terminal transcriptional modulatory domain. *Molecular and Cellular Biology, 10*, 4574–4581.

Dieken, E. S., & Miesfield, R. L. (1992). Transcriptional transactivation functions localized to the glucocorticoid receptor N terminus are necessary for steroid induction of lymphocyte apoptosis. *Molecular and Cellular Biology, 12*, 589–597.

Dikic, I., Tokiwa, G., Lev, S., Courtneidge, S. A., & Schlessinger, J. (1996). A role for Pyk2 and Src in linking G-protein-coupled receptors with MAP kinase activation. *Nature, 383*, 547–550.

Donovan, J. A., Wange, R. L., Langdon, W. Y., & Samelson, L. E. (1994). The protein product of the c-cbl protooncogene is the 120-kDa tyrosine-phosphorylated protein in Jurkat cells activated via the T cell antigen receptor. *Journal of Biological Chemistry, 269,* 22921–22924.

Dowd, D. R., MacDonald, P. N., Komm, B. S., Haussler, M. R., & Miesfeld, R. (1991). Evidence for early induction of calmodulin gene expression in lymphocytes undergoing glucocorticoid-mediated apoptosis. *Journal of Biological Chemistry, 266,* 18423–18426.

Dowd, D. R., & Miesfeld, R. L. (1992). Evidence that glucocorticoid- and cyclic AMP-induced apoptotic pathways in lymphocytes share distal events. *Molecular and Cellular Biology, 12,* 3600–3608.

Eastman-Reks, S. B., & Vedeckis, W. V. (1986). Glucocorticoid inhibition of c-myc, c-myb, c-Ki-ras expression in a mouse lymphoma cell line. *Cancer Research, 46,* 2457–2462.

Elliott, D. E., Blum, A. M., Li, J., Metwali, A., & Weinstock, J. V. (1998). Preprosomatostatin messenger RNA is expressed by inflammatory cells and induced by inflammatory mediators and cytokines. *Journal of Immunology, 160,* 3997–4003.

Ernström, U., & Sandberg, G. (1973). Effects of adrenergic alpha- and beta-receptor stimulation on the release of lymphocytes and granulocytes from the spleen. *Scandinavian Journal of Haematology, 11,* 275–286.

Ernström, U., & Sandberg, G. (1974). Stimulation of lymphocyte release from the spleen by theophylline and isoproterenol. *Acta Physiologica Scandinavia, 90,* 202–209.

Ernström, U., & Söder, O. (1975). Influence of adrenaline on the dissemination of antibody-producing cells from the spleen. *Clinical and Experimental Immunology, 21,* 131–140.

Evans, R. M. (1988). The steroid and thyroid hormone receptor superfamily. *Science, 240,* 889–895.

Fanger, C. M., Hoth, M., Crabtree, G. R., & Lewis, R. S. (1995). Characterization of T cell mutants with defects in capacitative calcium entry: Genetic evidence for the physiological roles of CRAC channels. *Journal of Cell Biology, 131,* 655–667.

Fantl, W. J., Johnson, D. E., & Williams, L. T. (1993). Signalling by receptor tyrosine kinases. *Annual Review of Biochemistry, 62,* 453–481.

Faure, M., Voyno-Yasenetskaya, T. A., & Bourne H. R. (1994). cAMP and $\beta\gamma$ subunits of heterotrimeric G proteins stimulate the mitogen-activated protein kinase pathway in COS-7 cells. *Journal of Biological Chemistry, 269,* 7851–7854.

Feder, D., Im, M. J., Klein, H. W., Hekman, M., Holzhofer, A., Dees, C., Levitzki, A., Helmreich, E. J., & Pfeuffer, T. (1986). Reconstitution of beta1-adrenoceptor-dependent adenylate cyclase from purified components. *EMBO Journal, 5,* 1509–1514.

Feig, L. A., & Cooper, G. M. (1988). Inhibition of NIH3T3 cell proliferation by a mutant Ras protein with preferential affinity for GDP. *Molecular and Cellular Biology, 8,* 3235–3243.

Felten, D. L., Felten, S. Y., Bellinger, D. L., Carlson, S. L., Ackerman, K. D., Madden, K. S., Olschowka, J. A., & Livnat, S. (1987). Noradrenergic sympathetic neural interactions with the immune system: Structure and function. *Immunological Review, 100,* 225–260.

Felten, D. L., Felten, S. Y., Carlson, S. L., Olschowka, J. A., & Livnat, S. (1985). Noradrenergic and peptidergic innervation of lymphoid tissue. *Journal of Immunology, 135,* 755s–765s.

Felten, S. Y., Bellinger, D. L., Collier, T. J., Coleman, P. D., & Felten, D. L. (1987). Decreased sympathetic innervation of spleen in aged Fischer 344 rats. *Neurobiology of Aging, 8,* 159–165.

Felten, S. Y., Felten, D. L., Bellinger, D. L., & Olschowka, J. A. (1992). Noradrenergic and peptidergic innervation of lymphoid organs. In J. E. Blalock, (Ed.) *Chemical immunology: neuroimmunoendocrinology* (pp. 25–48). Basel: S. Karger.

Ferris, C. D., & Snyder, S. H. (1992). Inositol 1,4,5-trisphosphate-activated calcium channels. *Annual Review of Physiology, 54,* 469–488.

Fields, B. A., & Mariuzza, R. A. (1996). Structure and function of the T-cell receptor: insights from X-ray crystallography. *Immunology Today, 7,* 331–336.

Fields, B. A., Ober, B., Malchiodi, E. L., Lebedeva, M. I., Braden, B. C., Ysern, X., Kim, J. K., Shao, X., Ward, E. S., & Mariuzza, R. A. (1995). Crystal structure of Vα domain of a T cell antigen receptor. *Science, 270,* 1821–1824.

Fischer, K., Zmuidzinas, A., Gardner, S., Barbacid, M., Berstein, A., & Guidos, C. (1999). Defective T-cell receptor signalling and positive selection of Vav-deficient CD4+CD8+ thymocytes. *Nature, 347,* 474–477.

Flanagan, W.-M., Corthesy, B., Bram, R.-J., & Crabtree, G.-R. (1991). Nuclear association of T-cell transcription factor blocked by FK-506 and cyclosporine A. *Nature, 352,* 803–807.

Flordellis, C. S., Berguerand, M., Gouache, P., Barbu, V., Gavras, H., Handy, D. E., Bereziat, G., & Masliah, J. (1995). Alpha 2 adrenergic receptor subtypes expressed in Chinese hamster ovary cells activate differentially mitogen-activated protein kinase by a p21ras independent pathway. *Journal of Biological Chemistry, 270,* 3491–3494.

Fournel, M., Davidson, D., Weil, R., & Veillette, A. (1996). Association of tyrosine protein kinase Zap-70 with the protooncogene product p120$^{c\text{-}cbl}$ in T lymphocytes. *Journal of Experimental Medicine, 183,* 301–306.

Fuchs, B. A., Albright, J. W., & Albright, J. F. (1988a). β-adrenergic receptors on murine lymphocytes: Density varies with cell maturity and lymphocyte subtype and is decreased after antigen administration. *Cellular Immunology, 144,* 231–245.

Fuchs, B. A., Albright, J. W., & Albright, J. F. (1988b). β-Adrenergic receptors on murine lymphocytes: Density varies with cell maturity and lymphocyte subtype and is decreased after antigen administration. *Cellular Immunology, 114,* 231–245.

Fukazawa, T., Reedquist, K. A., Panchamoorthy, G., Soltoff, S., Trub, T., Drucker, B., Cantley, L., Shoelson, S. E., & Band, H. (1995). T cell activation-dependent association between the p85 subunit of the phosphatidylinositol 3-kinase and Grb2/phospholipase C-γ 1-binding phosphotyrosyl protein pp36/38. *Journal of Biological Chemistry, 270,* 20177–20182.

Furukawa, T., Itoh, M., Krueger, N. X., Streuli, M., & Saito, H. (1994). Specific interaction of the CD45 protein-tyrosine phosphatase with tyrosine-phosphorylated CD3 ζ chain. *Proceedings of the National Academy of Science USA, 91,* 10928–10932.

Gajewski, T. F., Schell, S. R., & Fitch, F. W. (1990). Evidence implicating utilization of different T cell receptor-associated signaling pathways by Th-1 and Th-2 clones. *Journal of Immunology, 144,* 4110–4220.

Gasson, J. C., & Bourgeois, S. (1983). A new determinant of glucocorticoid sensitivity in lymphoid cell lines. *Journal of Cell Biology, 96,* 409–415.

Gauen, L. K., Zhu, Y.; Letourneur, F., Hu, Q., Bolen, J. B., Matis, L. A., Klausner, R. D., & Shaw, A. S. (1994). Interactions of p59^{fyn} and ZAP-70 with T-cell receptor activation motifs: Defining the nature of a signalling motif. *Molecular and Cellular Biology, 14,* 3729–3741.

Geenen, V., Legros, J.-J., Franchimont, P., Baudrihaye, M., Defresne, M. P., & Boniver, J. (1986). The neuroendocrine thymus: Coexistence of oxytocin and neurophysin in the human thymus. *Science, 232,* 508–510.

Genaro, A. M., & Borda, E. (1989). Alloimmunization-induced changes in β-adrenoceptor expression and cAMP on B lymphocytes. *Immunopharmacology, 18*, 63–70.

Genot, E., Cleverley, S., Henning, S., & Cantrell, D. (1996). Multiple $p21^{ras}$ effector pathways regulate nuclear factor of activated T cells. *EMBO Journal, 15*, 3923–3933.

Genot, E. M., Parker, P. J., & Cantrell, D. A. (1995). Analysis of the role of protein kinase C-α, -ε, and -ζ in T cell activation. *Journal of Biological Chemistry, 270*, 9833–9839.

Gerhardt, C. C., Gros, J., Strosberg, A. D., & Issad, T. (1999). Stimulation of the extracellular signal-regulated kinase I/2 pathway by human β_3-adrenergic receptor: New pharmacological profile and mechanism of activation. *Molecular Pharmacology, 55*, 255–262.

Gervais, F. G., & Veillette, A. (1995). The unique amino-terminal domain of $p56^{lck}$ regulates interactions with tyrosine protein phosphatases in T lymphocytes. *Molecular and Cellular Biology, 15*, 2393–2401.

Gillis, S., Crabtree, G. R., & Smith, K. A. (1979a). Glucocorticoid-induced inhibition of T cell growth factor production. II. The effect on the in vitro generation of cytolytic T cells. *Journal of Immunology, 123*, 1632–1638.

Gillis, S., Crabtree, G. R., & Smith, K. A. (1979b). Glucocorticosteroid-induced inhibition of T cell growth factor production. I. The effect on mitogen-induced lymphocyte proliferation. *Journal of Immunology, 123*, 1624–1631.

Gordeladze, J. O., Johansen, P. W., Paulssen, R. H., Paulssen, E. J., & Gautvic, K. M. (1994). G-proteins: Implications for pathophysiology and disease. *European Journal of Immunology, 131*, 557–574.

Gotoh, T., Hattori, S., Nakamura, S., Kitayama, H., Noda, M., Takai, Y., Kaibuchi, I., Matsui, H., Hatase, O., & Takahashi, H. (1995). Identification of Rap1 as a target for the Crk SH3 domain-binding guanine nucleotide-releasing factor C3G. *Molecular and Cellular Biology, 15*, 6746–6753.

Granja, C., Lin, L.-L., Yunis, E. J., Relias, V., & Dasgupta, J. D. (1991). PLCg1, a possible mediator of T cell receptor function. *Journal of Biological Chemistry, 266*, 16277–16280.

Granneman, J. G., Zhai, Y., & Lahners, K. N. (1997). Selective up-regulation of alpha 1a-adrenergic receptor protein and mRNA in brown adipose tissue by neural and $beta_3$-adrenergic stimulation. *Molecular Pharmacology, 51*, 644–650.

Graves, J. D., Campbell, J. S., & Krebs, E. G. (1995). Protein serine/threonine kinases of the MAPK cascade. *Annals of the New York Academy of Science, 766*, 320–343.

Groul, D. J., Rajah, F.*M., & Bourgeois, S. (1989). Cyclic AMP-dependent protein kinase modulation of the glucocorticoid-induced cytolytic response in murine T-lymphoma cells. *Molecular Endocrinology, 3*, 2119–2127.

Gupta, S., Campbell, D., Derijard, B., & Davis, R. J. (1995). Transcription factor ATF2 regulation by the JNK signal transduction pathway. *Science, 267*, 389–393.

Gupta, S. K., Gallego, C., & Johnson, G. L. (1992). Mitogenic pathways regulated by G proteins oncogenes. *Molecular Biology and Cell, 3*, 123–128.

Gupta, S. K., Gallego, C., Johnson, G. L., & Heasley, L. E. (1992). MAP kinase is constitutively activated in Gip2 and src transformed Rat 1a fibroblasts. *Journal of Biological Chemistry, 267*, 7987–7990.

Hadden, J. W., Hadden, E. M., & Middleton, E., Jr. (1970). Lymphocyte blast transformation. I. Demonstration of adrenergic receptors in human peripheral lymphocytes. *Cellular Immunology, 1*, 583–595.

Hafner, S., Adler, H. S., Mischak, H., Janosch, P., Heidecker, G., Wolfman, A., Pippig, S., Lohse, M., Ueffing, M., & Kolch, W. (1994). Mechanism of inhibition of Raf-1 by protein kinase A. *Molecular and Cellular Biology, 14*, 6696–6703.

Hall, A. (1993). Ras-related proteins. *Current Opinions in Cellular Biology, 5*, 265–268.

Hama, N., Paliogianni, F., Fessler, B. J., & Boumpas, D. T. (1995). Calcium/calmodulin-dependent protein kinase II down-regulates both calcineurin and protein kinase C-mediated pathways for cytokine gene transcription in human T cells. *Journal of Experimental Medicine, 181*, 1217–1222.

Hanke, J. H., Gardner, J. P., Dow, R. L., Changelian, P. S., Brissette, W. H., Weringer, E. J., Pollok, B. A., & Connelly, P. A. (1996). Discovery of a novel, potent, and Src family-selective tyrosine kinase inhibitor. Study of Lck- and Fyn-T-dependent T cell activation. *Journal of Biological Chemistry, 271*, 695–701.

Hanson, P. I., & Schulman, H. (1992). Neuronal Ca^{2+}/calmodulin-dependent protein kinases. *Annual Review of Biochemistry, 61*, 559–601.

Harden, T. K. (1992). G-protein-regulated phospholipase C: identification of component proteins. *Advances in Second Messenger Phosphoprotein Research, 26*, 11–34.

Hardie, D. G. (1999). *Biochemical messengers: Hormones, neurotransmitters and growth factors.* London: Chapman and Hall.

Harrigan, M., Baughman, G., Campbell, N., & Bourgeois, S. (1989). Isolation and characterization of glucocorticoid- and cyclic AMP-induced genes in T lymphocytes. *Molecular and Cellular Biology, 9*, 3438–3446.

Harwood, A. E., & Cambier, J. H. (1993). B cell antigen receptor cross-linking triggers rapid protein kinase C independent activation of $p21^{ras}$. *Journal of Immunology, 151*, 4513–4522.

Hashimoto, Y., Katayama, H., Kiyokawa, E., Ota, S., Kurata, T., Gotoh, N., Otsuka, N., Shibata, M., & Matsuda, M. (1998). Phosphorylation of CrkII adaptor protein at tyrosine 221 by epidermal growth factor receptor. *Journal of Biological Chemistry, 273*, 17186–17191.

Hataoka, I., Okayama, M., Sugi, M., Inoue, H., Takishima, T., & Shirato, K. (1993). Decrease in beta-adrenergic receptors of lymphocytes in spontaneously occurring acute asthma. *Chest, 104*, 508–514.

Hausdorff, W. P., Caron, M. G., & Lefkowitz, R. J. (1990). Turning off the signal: Desensitization of β-adrenergic receptor function. *FASEB Journal, 4*, 2881–2889.

Hawes, B. E., van Biesen, T., Koch, W. J., Luttrell, L. M., & Lefkowitz, R. J. (1995). Distinct pathways of Gi-and Gq-mediated mitogen-activated protein kinase activation. *Journal of Biological Chemistry, 270*, 17148–17153.

Head, J. F. (1992). A better grip on calmodulin. *Currents in Biology, 2*, 609–611.

Heemels, M. T., & Ploegh, H. (1995). Generation translocation, and presentation of MHC class I-restricted peptides. *Annual Review of Biochemistry, 64*, 463–491.

Heijnen, C. J., Rouppe van der Voort, C., Walffraat, N., van der Net, J., Kuis, W., & Kavelaars, A. (1996). Functional α_1-adrenergic receptors on leukocytes of patients with polyarticular juvenile rheumatoid arthritis. *Journal of Neuroimmunology, 71*, 223–226.

Helmberg, A., Auphan, N., Caelles, C., & Karin, M. (1995). Glucocorticoid-induced apoptosis of human leukemic cells is caused by the repressive function of the glucorticoid receptor. *EMBO Journal, 14*, 452–460.

Hepler, J. R., & Gilman, A. G. (1992). G proteins. *Trends in Biochemical Sciences, 17*, 383–387.

Hille, B. (1992). G protein-coupled mechanisms and nervous signaling. *Neuron, 9*, 187–195.

Homo, F., Duval, D., Hatzfeld, J., & Evrard, C. (1980). Glucocorticoid sensitive and resistant cell populations in the mouse thymus. *Journal of Steroid Biochemistry, 13*, 135–143.

Hovis, R. R., Donovan, J. A., Musci, M. A., Motto, D. G., Goldman, F. D., Ross, S. E., & Koretzky, G. A. (1993). Rescue of signaling by a chimeric protein containing the cytoplasmic domain of CD45. *Science, 260*, 544–546.

Hugo, P., Boyd, R. L., Waanders, G. A., & Scollay, R. (1991). $CD4^{+}CD8^{+}CD3^{high}$ thymocytes appear transiently during ontogeny: Evidence from phenotype and functional studies. *European Journal of Immunology, 21*, 2655–2660.

Hurley, T. R., Hyman, R., & Sefton, B. M. (1993). Differential effects on expression of the CD45 tyrosine protein phosphatase on the tyrosine phosphorylation of the lck, fyn, and c-src tyrosine protein kinases. *Molecular and Cellular Biology, 13*, 1651–1656.

Iniguez-Lluhi, J., Kleuss, C., & Gilman, A. G. (1993). The importance of G-protein $\beta\gamma$ subunits. *Trends in Cell Biology, 3*, 230–235.

Iseki, R., Mukai, M., & Iwata, M. (1991). Regulation of T lymphocyte apoptosis: Signals for the antagonism between activation- and glucocorticoid-induced death. *Journal of Immunology, 147*, 4286–4292.

Ito, A., Satoh, T., Kaziro, Y., & Itoh, H. (1995). G protein $\beta\gamma$ subunit activates Ras, Raf, and MAP kinase in HEK 293 cells. *FEBS Letters, 368*, 183–187.

Iwashima, M., Irving, B. A., van Oers, N. S. C., & Chan, A. C. (1994). Sequential interactions of the TCR with two distinct cytoplasmic tyrosine kinases. *Science, 263*, 1136–1139.

Iwata, M., Hanaoka, S., & Sato, K. (1991). Rescue of thymocytes and T cell hybridomas from glucocorticoid-induced apoptosis by stimulation via the T cell receptor/CD3 complex: A possible in vitro model for positive selection of the T cell repertoire. *European Journal of Immunology, 21*, 643–648.

Iwata, M., Iseki, R., & Kudo, Y. (1993). Regulation of thymocyte apoptosis: Glucocorticoid-induced death and its inhibition by T cell receptor/CD3 complex-mediated stimulation. In M. L. Lavin, D. Watters, (Eds.) *Programmed cell Death: The cellular and molecular biology of apoptosis* (pp. 31–44). Chur, Switzerland: Harwood Academic Publishers.

Iwata, M., Iseki, R., Sato, K., Tozawa, Y., & Ohoka, Y. (1994). Involvement of protein kinase C-ε in glucocorticoid-induced apoptosis in thymocytes. *International Immunology, 6*, 431–438.

Iwata, M., Kuwata, T., Mukai, M., Tozawa, Y., & Yokoyama, M. (1996). Differential induction of helper and killer T cells from isolated $CD4^{+}CD8^{+}$ thymocytes in suspension culture. *European Journal of Immunology, 26*, 2081–2086.

Izquierdo, M., Bowden, S., & Cantrell, D. (1994). The role of Raf-1 in the regulation of extracellular signal-regulated kinase 2 by the T cell antigen receptor. *Journal of Experimental Medicine, 180*, 401–406.

Izquierdo, M., Downward, J., Graves, D., & Cantrell, D. A. (1992). Role of protein kinase C in T-cell antigen receptor regulation of $p21^{ras}$: Evidence that two $p21^{ras}$ regulatory pathways coexist in T cells. *Molecular and Cellular Biology, 12*, 3305–3312.

Izquierdo, M., Pastro, M., Reif, K., & Cantrell, D. (1995). The regulation and function of $p21^{ras}$ during T-cell activation and growth. *Immunology Today, 16*, 159–164.

Jackman, J. K., Motto, D. G., Sun, Q., Tanemoto, M., Turck, C. W., Peltz, G. A., Koretzky, G. A., & Findell, P. R. (1995). Molecular cloning of SLP-76, a 76-kDa tyrosine phosphoprotein associated with Grb2 in T cells. *Journal of Biological Chemistry, 270*, 7029–7032.

Jain, J., McCaffrey, P.-G., Miner, Z., Kerppola, T.-K., Lambert, J. -N., Verdine, G.-L., Curran, T., & Rao, A. (1993). The T-cell transcription factor NFATp is a substrate for calcineurin and interacts with c-Fos and c-Jun. *Nature, 365*, 352–355.

Jain, J., McCaffrey, P.-G., Valge-Archer, V.-E., & Rao, A. (1992). Nuclear Factor of activated T-cells contains Fos and Jun. *Nature, 356*, 801–804.

Jonat, C., Rahmsdorf, H. J., Park, K., Cato, A., Gebel, S., Pontaand, H., & Herrlich, P. (1990). Antitumor promotion and anti-inflammation: Down-modulation of AP-1 (fos/jun) activity by glucocorticoid hormone. *Cell, 62*, 1189–1204.

Jondal, M., Xue, Y., McConkey, D. J., & Okret, S. (1995). Thymocyte apoptosis by glucocorticoids and cAMP. In G. Kroemer, A. C. Martinez, (Eds.) *Current topics in microbiology and immunology: Apoptosis in immunology* (pp. 67–79). Berlin: Springer-Verlag.

Ju, S. T., Panka, D. J., Cui, H., Ettinger, R., el-Khatib, M., Sherr, D. H., Stanger, B. Z., & Marshak-Rothstein, A. (1995). Fas(CD95)/FasL interactions required for programmed cell death after T cell activation. *Nature, 373*, 444–448.

Kahn, C. R. (1976). Membrane receptors for hormones and neurotransmitters. *Journal of Cellular Biology, 70*, 261–286.

Karaszewski, J. W., Reder, A. T., Anlar, B., & Arnason, G. W. (1993). Increased high affinity beta-adrenergic receptor densities and cyclic AMP responses of CD8 cells in multiple sclerosis. *Journal of Neuroimmunology, 43*, 1–7.

Karaszewski, J. W., Reder, A. T., Anlar, B., Kim, W. C., & Arnason, G. W. (1990). Increased lymphocyte beta-adrenergic receptor density in progressive multiple sclerosis is specific for the CD8+, CD28-suppressor cell. *Annals of Neurology, 30*, 42–47.

Karaszewski, J. W., Reder, A. T., Maselli, R., Brown, M., & Arnason, B. G. (1990). Sympathetic skin responses are decreased and lymphocyte beta-adrenergic receptors are increased in progressive multiple sclerosis. *Annals of Neurology, 27*, 366–327.

Karin, M. (1995). The regulation of AP-1 activity by mitogen-activated protein kinases. *Journal of Biological Chemistry, 270*, 16483–16486.

Kaspers, G. J., Pieters, R., Klumper, E., DeWaal, R. C., & Veerman, A. J. (1994). Glucocorticoid resistance in childhood leukemia. *Leukocytes and Lymphomas, 13*, 187–201.

Katzav, S., Sutherland, M., Packham, G., Yi, T.-L., & Weiss, A. (1994). The protein-tyrosine kinase ZAP-70 can associate with the SH2 domain of proto-Vav. *Journal of Biological Chemistry, 269*, 32579–32585.

Kayne, P. S., & Sternberg, P. W. (1995). Ras pathways in *Caenorhabditis elegans*. *Current Opinion in Genetic Development, 5*, 38–43.

Kendall, M. D., Atkinson, B. A., Munoz, F. J., De La Riva, C., Clarke, A. G., & von Gaudecker, B. (1994). The noradrenergic innervation of the rat thymus during pregnancy and in the post-partum period. *Journal of Anatomy, 185*, 617–625.

Khan, M. M., Sansoni, P., Silverman, E. D., & Engleman, E. G. (1986). Beta-adrenergic receptors on human suppressor, helper, and cytolytic lymphocytes. *Biochemical Pharmacology, 35*, 1137–1142.

Kisielow, P., & von Boehmer, H. (1995). Development and selection of T cells: Facts and puzzles. *Advances in Immunology, 58*, 87–209.

Klausner, R. K., O'Shea, J. J., Luong, H., Ross, P., Bluestone, J. A., & Samelson, L. E. (1987). T cell receptor tyrosine phosphorylation, variable coupling for different ligands. *Journal of Biological Chemistry, 262*, 12654–12659.

Koch, C. A., Anderson, D., Moran, M. F., Ellis, C., & Pawson, T. (1991). SH2 and SH3 domains: Elements that control interactions of cytoplasmic signaling proteins. *Science, 252*, 668–674.

Koch, E. L. E. (1990). The endoplasmic reticulum and calcium storage. *Bioessays, 12*, 527–531.

Koch, W. J., Hawes, B. E., Allen, L. F., & Lefkowitz, R. J. (1994). Direct evidence that G_i-coupled receptor stimulation of mitogen-activated protein kinase is mediated by $G\beta\gamma$ activation of $p21^{ras}$. *Proceedings of the National Academy of Science USA, 91,* 12706–12710.

Koch, W. J., Inglese, J. I., Stone, W. C., & Lefkowitz, R. J. (1993). The binding site for the $\beta\gamma$ subunits of heterotrimeric G proteins of the β-adrenergic receptor kinase. *Journal of Biological Chemistry, 268,* 8256–8260.

Koff, W. C., & Dunegan, M. A. (1986). Neuroendocrine hormones suppress macrophage-mediated lysis of herpes simplex virus-infected cells. *Journal of Immunology, 136,* 705–709.

Kolch, W., Heidecker, G., Kochs, G., Hummel, R., Vahidi, H., Mischak, H., Finkenzeller, G., Marmé, D., & Rapp, U. R. (1993). Protein kinase $C\alpha$ activates RAF-1 by direct phosphorylation. *Nature, 364,* 249–252.

Kolluri, R., Tolias, K. R., Carpenter, C. L., Rosen, F. S., & Kirchhausen, T. (1996). Direct interaction of the Wiskott-Aldrich syndrome protein with the GTPase Cdc42. *Proceedings of the National Academy of Science USA, 93,* 5615–5618.

Kon-Kozlowshi, M., Pani, G., Pawson, T., & Siminovitch, K. A. (1996). The tyrosine phosphatase PTP1C associates with Vav, Grb2, and mSos1 in hematopoietic cells. *Journal of Biological Chemistry, 271,* 3856–3862.

Koretzky, G. A. (1993). Role of the CD45 tyrosine phosphatase in signal transduction in the immune system. *FASEB Journal, 7,* 420–426.

Koretzky, G. A., Picus, J., Thomas, M. L., & Weiss, A. (1990). Tyrosine phosphatase CD45 is essential for coupling T-cell antigen receptor to the phosphatidyl inositol pathway. *Nature, 346,* 66–68.

Krause, A., Henrich, A., Beckh, K. H., von Wichert, P., & Baerwald, C. (1992). Correlation between density of beta 2-adrenergic receptors on peripheral blood mononuclear cells and serum levels of soluble interleukin-2 receptors in patients with chronic inflammatory diseases. *European Journal of Clinical Investigation, 22*(Suppl 1), 47–51.

Krebs, E. G. (1989). Role of the cyclic AMP-dependent protein kinase in signal transduction. *Journal of the American Medical Association, 262,* 1815–1818.

Kyriakis, J. M., & Avruch, J. (1996). Sounding the alarm: Protein kinase cascades activated by stress and inflammation. *Journal of Biological Chemistry, 271,* 24313–24316.

Kyriakis, J. M., Banerjee, P., Nikolakaki, E., Dai, T., Rubi, E. A., Ahmad, M. F., Avruch, J., & Woodgett, J. R. (1994). The stress-activated protein kinases subfamily of c-Jun kinases. *Nature, 369,* 156–160.

Lafyatis, R., Kim, S. J., Angel, P., Roberts, A. B., Sporn, M. B., Karin, M., & Wilder, R. L. (1990). Interleukin-1 stimulates and all-trans-retinoic acid inhibits collagenase gene expression through its 5′ activator protein-1-binding site. *Molecular Endocrinology, 4,* 973–980.

Lahesmaa, R., Allusp, A., Soderberg, C., Jackman, J., Findell, P., & Peltz, G. (1995). Modulation of the Grb2-associated protein complex in human CD4+ T cells by receptor activation. *Journal of Immunology, 155,* 3815–3822.

Lai, C. Y. (1980). The chemistry and biology of cholera toxin. *CRC Critical Review of Biochemistry, 9,* 171–206.

Lamb, T. D., & Pugh, E. N., Jr. (1992). G-protein cascades: Gain and kinetics. *Trends in Neuroscience, 15,* 291–298.

Landmann, R., Bittiger, H., & Bühler, F. R. (1981). High affinity beta-2-adrenergic receptors in mononuclear leucocytes: Similar density in young and old subjects. *Life Sciences., 29,* 1761–1771.

Landmann, R., Burgisser, E., West, M., & Buhler, F. R. (1985). Beta adrenergic receptors are different in subpopulations of human circulating lymphocytes. *Journal of Receptor Research, 4,* 37–50.

Lang, P., Guizani, L., Vitte-Mony, I., Stancou, R., Dorseuil, O., Gacon, G., & Bertoglio, J. (1992). ADP-ribosylation of the ras-related, GTP-binding protein RhoA inhibits lymphocyte-mediated cytotoxicity. *Journal of Biological Chemistry, 267,* 11677–11680.

Lapointe, M. G., & Baxter, J. D. (1989). Molecular biology of glucocorticoid hormone action. In R. P. Schleimer, H. N. Claman, A. Oronsky, (Eds.) *Anti-inflammatory steroid action: Basic and clinical aspects* (pp. 3–23). New York: Academic Press.

Lee, J. C., Laydon, J. T., McDonnell, P. C., Gallagher, T. F., Kumar, S., Green, D., McNulty, D., Blumenthal, M. J., Heys, J. R., Landvatter, S. W., Strickler, J. E., McLaughlin, M. M., Siemens, I. R., Fisher, S. M., Livi, G. P., White, J. R., Adams, J. L., & Young, P. R. (1994). A protein kinase involved in the regulation of inflammatory cytokine biosynthesis. *Nature, 372,* 739–746.

Lee, J. C., & Young, P. R. (1996). Role of CSB/p38/Rk stress response kinase in LPS and cytokine signaling mechanisms. *Journal of Leukocyte Biology, 59,* 152–157.

Lefkowitz, R. J. (1993). G-protein-coupled receptor kinases. *Cell, 74,* 409–412.

Leitenberg, D., Novak, T. J., Farber, D., Smith, B. R., & Bottomly, K. (1996). The extracellular domain of CD45 controls association with the antigen-specific stimulation. *Journal of Experimental Medicine, 183,* 249–259.

Lerner, A., Jacobson, B., & Miller, R. (1988). Cyclic AMP concentrations modulate both calcium flux and hydrolysis of phophatidylinositol phosphates in mouse T lymphocytes. *Journal of Immunololgy, 140,* 936–940.

Levine, J. D., Dardick, S. J., Roizen, M. F., Helms, C., & Basbaum, A. L. (1986). Contribution of sensory afferents and sympathetic efferents to joint injury in experimental arthritis. *Journal of Neuroscience, 6,* 3423–3429.

Levine, J. D., Goetzl, E. J., & Basbaum, A. I. (1991). Contribution of the nervous system to the pathophysiology of rheumatoid arthritis and other polyarthritides. In *Rheumatic Disease Clinics of North America* (vol. 13, pp. 369–383). Philadelphia: W. B. Sounders.

Linder, M. E., & Gilman, A. G. (1992). G Proteins. *Scientific American, 267,* 36–43.

Livnat, S., Madden, K. S., Felten, D. L., & Felten, S. Y. (1987). Regulation of the immune system by sympathetic neural mechanisms. *Progress in Neuro-psychopharmacology & Biology Psychiatry, 11,* 145–152.

Loh, C., Romeo, C., Seed, B., Bruder, J. T., Rapp, U., & Rao, A. (1994). Association of Raf with the CD3 δ and γ chains of the T cell receptor-CD3 complex. *Journal of Biological Chemistry, 269,* 8817–8825.

Lorton, D., Lubahn, C., Felten, S. Y., & Bellinger, D. L. (1997). Norepinephrine content in primary and secondary lymphoid organs is altered in rats with adjuvant-induced arthritis. *Mechanisms of Ageing and Development, 94,* 145–63.

Loveland, B. E., Jarrott, B., & McKenzie, I. F. C. (1981). The detection of beta adrenoceptors on murine lymphocytes. *International Journal of Immunopharmacology, 3,* 45–55.

Lowenstein, C. J., & Snyder, S. H. (1992). Nitric oxide, a novel biological messenger. *Cell, 70,* 705–707.

Lowy, D. R., & Willumsen, B. M. (1993). Function and regulation of *Ras. Annual Review of Biochemistry, 62,* 851–891.

Luttrell, L. M., van Biesen, T., Hawes, B. E., Koch, W. J., Krueger, K. M., Touhara, K., & Lefkowitz, R. J. (1997). G-protein-coupled receptors and their regulation. Activation of the MAP kinase signaling pathway by G-protein-coupled receptors. In J. Corbin, S. Francis, (Eds.) *Signal transduction in health and disease. Advances in second messenger and phosphoprotein research* (pp. 263–277). Philadelpha: Lippincott-Raven.

Madden, K. S., Bellinger, D. L., Felten, S. Y., Synder, E., Maida, M. E., & Felten, D. L. (1997). Alterations in sympathetic innervation of thymus and spleen in aged mice. *Mechanisms of Ageing and Development, 94*, 165–175.

Madden, K. S., Felten, S. Y., Felten, D. L., Sundaresan, P. R., & Livnat, S. (1989). Sympathetic neural modulation of the immune system. I. Depression of T cell immunity in vivo and in vitro following chemical sympathectomy. *Brain, Behavior, and Immunity, 3*, 72–89.

Madden, K. S., Moynihan, J. A., Brenner, G. J., Felten, S. Y., Felten, D. L., & Livnat, S. (1994). Sympathetic nervous system modulation of the immune system. III. Alterations in T and B cell proliferation and differentiation in vitro following chemical sympathectomy. *Journal of Neuroimmunology, 49*, 77–87.

Madden, K. S., Sanders, V. M., & Felten, D. L. (1995). Catecholamine influences and sympathetic neural modulation of immune responsiveness. *Annual Review of Pharmacology and Toxicology, 35*, 417–448.

Marengere, L. E. M., Waterhouse, P., Duncan, G. S., Mittrücker, H., Feng, G., & Mak, T. W. (1996). Regulation of T cell receptor signaling by tyrosine phosphatase SYP association with CTLA-4. *Science, 272*, 1170–1173.

Marshall, M. S. (1995). Ras target proteins in eukaryotic cells. *FASEB Journal, 9*, 1311–1318.

Mayer, B. J., & Baltimore, D. (1993). signalling through SH2 and SH3 domains. *Trends in Cellular Biology, 3*, 8–13.

McCaffrey, P. G., Perrino, B. A., Soderling, T. R., & Rao, A. (1993). NF-ATp,a T lymphocyte DNA-binding protein that is a target for calcineurin and immunosuppressive drugs. *Journal of Biological Chemistry, 268*, 3747–3752.

McConkey, D. J., Orrenius, S., Okret, S., & Jondal, M. (1993). Cyclic AMP-induced apoptotic pathways in lymphocytes share distal events. *FASEB Journal, 7*, 580–585.

McFarland, E. D., Hurley, T. R., Pingel, J. T., Sefton, B. M., Shaw, A., & Thomas, M. L. (1993). Correlation between Src family member regulation by the protein-tyrosine-phosphatase CD45 and transmembrane signaling through the T cell receptor. *Proceeding of the National Academy of Science USA, 90*, 1402–1406.

McKenney, D. W., Onodera, H., Gorman, L., Mimura, T., & Rothstein, D. M. (1995). Distinct isoforms of the CD45 protein-tyrosine phosphatase differentially regulate interleukin 2 secretion and activation signal pathways involving Vav in T cells. *Journal of Biological Chemistry, 270*, 24949–24954.

McKenzie, F. R., & Pouysségur, J. (1996). cAMP-mediated growth inhibition in fibroblasts is not mediated via mitogen-activated protein (MAP) kinase (Erk) inhibition: cAMP-dependent protein kinase induces a temporal shift in growth factor-stimulated MAP kinases. *Science, 271*, 13476–13483.

Medh, R. D., Saeed, M. F., Johnson, B. H., & Thompson, E. B. (1998). Resistance of human leukemic CEM-C1 cells is overcome by synergism between glucocorticoid and protein kinase A pathways: correlation with c-Myc suppression. *Cancer Research, 58*, 3684–3693.

Meisner, H., Conway, B. R., Hartley, D., & Czech, M. P. (1995). Interactions of Cbl with Grb2 and phosophatidylinositol 3′-kinase in activated Jurkat cells. *Molecular and Cellular Biology, 15*, 3571–3578.

Michell, R. H. (1992). Inositol lipids in cellular signalling mechanisms. *Trends in Biochemical Sciences, 17*, 274–276.

Miles, K., Atweh, S., Otten, G., Arnason, B. G. W., & Chelmicka-Schorr, E. (1984). Beta-adrenergic receptors on splenic lymphocytes from axotomized mice. *International Journal of Immunopharmacology, 6*, 171–177.

Miller, SG., & Kennedy, M. B. (1986). Regulation of brain type II Ca^{2+}/calmodulin-dependent protein kinase by autophosphorylation: A Ca^{2+}-triggered molecular switch. *Cell, 44*, 861–870.

Minden, A., Lin, A., McMahon, M., Lange-Carter, C., Derijard, B., Davis, R. J., Johnson, G. L., & Karin, M. (1994). Differential activation of ERK and JNK mitogen-activated protein kinases by Raf-1 and MEKK. *Science, 266*, 1719–1723.

Mischak, H., Seitz, T., Janosch, P., Eulitz, M., Steen, H., Schellerer, M., Philipp, A., & Kolch, W. (1996). Negative regulation of Raf-1 by phosphorylation of serine 621. *Molecular and Cellular Biology, 16*, 5409–5418.

Mitchell, B., Kendall, M., Adam, E., & Schumacher, U. (1997). Innervation of the thymus in normal and bone marrow reconstituted severe combined immunodeficient (SCID) mice. *Journal of Neuroimmunology, 75*, 19–27.

Mitchell, F. M., Russell, M., & Johnson, G. L. (1995). Differential calcium dependence in the activation of c-Jun kinase and mitogen-activated protein kinase by muscarinic acetylcholine receptors in rat 1a cells. *Biochemical Journal, 309*, 381–384.

Miyajima, A., Hara, T., & Kitamura, T. (1992). Common subunits of cytokine receptors and the functional redundancy of cytokines. *Trends in Biochemical Sciences, 17*, 378–382.

Molina, I. J., Sancho, J., Terhorst, C., Rosen, F. S., & Remold-O'Donnell, E. (1993). T cells of patients with the Wiskott-Aldrich syndrome have a restricted defect in proliferative responses. *Journal of Immunology, 151*, 4383–4390.

Moncada, S., Palmer, R. M., & Higgs, E. A. (1991). Nitric oxide: Physiology, pathology and pharmacology. *Pharmacological Review, 43*, 109–142.

Moorman, J. P., Bobak, D. A., & Hahn, C. S. (1996). Inactivation of the small GTP binding protein Rho induces multinucleate cell formation and apoptosis in murine T lymphoma EL4. *Journal of Immunology, 156*, 4146–4153.

Motto, D. G., Musci, M. A., Ross, S. E., & Koretzky, G. A. (1996a). Tyrosine phosphorylation of Grb2-associated proteins correlates with phospholipase C-γ activation in T cells. *Molecular and Cellular Biology, 16*, 2823–2829.

Motto, D. G., Ross, E. S., Wu, J., Hendricks-Taylor, L. R., & Koretzky, G. A. (1996b). Implication of the GRB2-associated phosphoprotein SLP-76 in T cell receptor-mediated interleukin 2 production. *Journal of Experimental Medicine, 183*, 1937–1943.

Motto, D. G., Ross, S. E., Jackman, J. K., Sun, Q., Olson, A. L., Findell, P. R., & Koretzky, G. A. (1994). In vivo association of Grb2 with pp116, a substrate of the T cell antigen receptor-activated protein tyrosine kinase. *Journal of Biological Chemistry, 269*, 21608–21613.

Motulsky, H. J., Cunningham, E. M. S., Deblasi, A., & Insel, P. A. (1986). Desensitization and redistribution of β-adrenergic receptors on human mononuclear leukocytes. *American Journal of Physiology, 250*, E583–E590.

Moule, S. K., & Denton, R. M. (1998). The activation of p38 MAPK by the beta-adrenergic agonist isoproterenol in rat epididymal fat cells. *FEBS Letters, 439*, 287–290.

Mukaida, N., Morita, M., Ishikawa, Y., Rice, N., Okamoto, S., Kasahara, T., & Matsushima, K. (1994). Novel mechanism of glucocorticoid-mediated gene repression. Nuclear factor-kappa B is target for glucocorticoid-mediated interleukin 8 gene repression. *Journal of Biological Chemistry, 269*, 13289–13295.

Mulvihill, E. R., & Palmiter, R. D. (1997). Relationship of nuclear estrogen receptor levels to induction of ovalbumin and conalbumin mRNA in chick oviduct. *Journal of Biological Chemistry, 252*, 2060–2068.

Mustelin, T., & Burn, P. (1993). Regulation of *src* family tyrosine kinases in lymphocytes. *Trends in Biochemical Sciences, 18*, 215–220.

Namimatsu, A., Okazaki, R., Go, K., & Hata, T. (1992). Relationship between density of muscarinic receptors and nasal hypersecretion in a nasal allergic model. *Japanese Journal of Pharmacology, 59*, 427–434.

Nantel, F., Bouvier, M., Strosberg, A. D., & Marullo, S. (1995). Functional effects of long-term activation on human β_2- and β_3-adrenoceptor signalling. *British Journal of Pharmacology, 114*, 1045–1051.

Nazareth, L. V., Harbour, D. V., & Thompson, E. B. (1991). Mapping the human glucocorticoid receptor for leukemic cell death. *Journal of Biological Chemistry, 266*, 12976–12980.

Ng, D. H. W., Watts, J. D., Aebersold, R., & Hohnson, P. (1996). Demonstration of a direct interaction between p56*lck* and the cytoplasmic domain of CD45 in vitro. *Journal of Biological Chemistry, 271*, 1295–1300.

Nghiem, P., Ollick, T., Gardner, P., & Schulman, H. (1994). Interleukin-2 transcriptional block by multifunctional Ca2+/calmodulin kinase. *Nature, 371*, 374–350.

Niaudet, P., Beaurain, G., & Bach, M.-A. (1976). Differences in effect of isoproterenol stimulation on levels of cyclic AMP in human B and T lymphocytes. *European Journal of Immunology, 6*, 834–836.

Nicholson, R. C., Mader, S., Nagpal, S., Leid, M., Rochette-Egly, C., & Chambon, P. (1990). Negative regulation of the rat stromelysin gene promoter by retinoic acid is mediated by an AP1 binding site. *EMBO Journal, 9*, 4443–4454.

Nishida, E., & Gotoh, Y. (1993). The MAP kinase cascade is essential for diverse signal transduction pathways. *Trends in Biochemical Sciences, 18*, 128–130.

Nishizuka, Y. (1985). Signal transduction: Crosstalk. Trends in biochemical Science. *Trends in Biochemical Sciences, 17*, 367–443.

Nishizuka, Y. (1992). Intracellular signaling by hydrolysis of phopholipids and activation of protein kinase C. *Science, 258*, 607–614.

Noh, D. Y., Shin, S. H., & Rhee, S. G. (1995). Phosphoinositide-specific phospholipase C and mitogenic signaling. *Biochimica et Biophysica Acta, 1242*, 99–113.

Northrop, J. P., Crabtree, G. R., & Mattila, P. S. (1992). Negative regulation of interleukin 2 transcription by the glucocorticoid receptor. *Journal of Experimental Medicine, 175*, 1235–1245.

Novak, T. J., Farber, D., Leitenberg, D., Hong, S. C., Johnson, P., & Bottomly, K. (1994). Isoforms of the transmembrane tyrosine phosphatase CD45 differentially affect T cell recognition. *Immunity, 1*, 109–119.

Novotny, G. E., & Hsu, Y. (1993). The effect of immunostimulation on thymic innervation in the rat. *Journal fur Hirnforschung, 34*, 155–163.

O'Neil, K. T., & DeGrado, W. F. (1990). How calmodulin binds its targets: Sequence independent recognition of amphipathic α-helices. *Trends in Biochemical Sciences, 15*, 59–64.

Ohoka, Y., Kuwata, T., Tozawa, Y., Zhao, Y., Mukai, M., Motegi, Y., Suzuki, R., Yokoyama, M., & Iwata, M. (1996). In vitro differentiation and commitment of $CD4^+CD8^+$ thymocytes to the CD4 lineage without TCR engagement. *International Immunology, 8*, 297–306.

Olson, M. F., Ashworth, A., & Hall, A. (1995). An essential role for Rho, Rac, and Cdc42 GTPases in cell cycle progression through G1. *Science, 269*, 1270–1272.

Osborne, B. A., & Schwartz, L. M. (1994). Essential genes that regulate apoptosis. *Trends in Cellular Biology, 4*, 394–398.

Osman, N., Lucas, S., & Cantrell, D. (1995). The role of tyrosine phosphorylation in the interaction of cellular tyrosine kinases with the T cell receptor ζ chain tyrosine-based actvation motif. *European Journal of Immunology, 25*, 2863–2869.

Ostergaard, H. L., Shackelford, D. A., Hurley, T. R., Johnson, P., Hyman, R., Sefton, B. M., & Trowbridge, I. S. (1989). Expression of CD45 alters phosphorylation of the lck tyrosine protein kinase in murine lymphoma T cell lines. *Proceeding of the National Academy of Science USA, 86*, 8959–8963.

Owens, G. P., Hahn, W. E., & Cohen, J. J. (1991). Identification of mRNAs associated with programmed cell death in mature thymocytes. *Molecular and Cellular Biology, 11*, 4177–4188.

Palczewski, K., & Benovic, J. L. (1991). G-protein-coupled receptor kinases. *Trends in Biochemical Sciences, 16*, 387–391.

Paliogianni, F., & Boumpas, D. T. (1995). Glucocorticoids regulate calcineurin-dependent trans-activating pathways for interleukin-2 gene transcription in human T lymphocytes. *Transplantation, 59*, 1333–1339.

Paliogianni, F., Hama, N., Balow, J. E., Valentine, M. A., & Boumpas, D. T. (1995). Glucocorticoid-mediated regulation of protein phosphorylation in primary human T cells. Evidence for induction of phosphatase activity. *Journal of Immunology, 155*, 1809–1817.

Paliogianni, F., Raptis, A., Ahuja, S. S., Najjar, S. M., & Boumpas, D. T. (1993). Negative transcriptional regulation of human interleukin 2 (IL-2) gene by glucocorticoids through interference with nuclear transcription factors AP-1 and NF-AT. *Journal of Clinical Investigation, 91*, 1481–1489.

Parker, M. G. (1991). *Nuclear hormone receptors: Molecular mechanisms, cellular functions and clinical abnormalities*. London: Academic Press.

Parrillo, J. E., & Fauci, A. S. (1979). Mechanisms of glucorticoid action on immune processes. *Annual Review of Pharmacology and Toxicology, 19*, 179–201.

Pastor, M. I., Reif, K., & Cantrell, D. (1995). The regulation and function of p21ras during T-cell activation and growth. *Immunology Today, 16*, 159–164.

Patel, M. D., Samelson, L. E., & Klausner, R. D. (1987). T cell receptor tyrosine phosphorylation, variable coupling for different ligands. *Journal of Biological Chemistry, 262*, 12654.

Pawson, T., & Schlessinger, J. (1993). SH2 and SH3 domains. *Currents in Biology, 3*, 434–442.

Pelech, SL. (1993). Networking with protein kinases. *Currents in Biology, 3*, 513–515.

Pelicci, G., Lanfrancone, L., Grignani, F., McGlade, J., Cavallo, F., Forni, G., Nicoletti, I., Pawson, T., & Pelicci, P. G. (1992). A novel transforming protein (SHC) with an SH2 domain is implicated in mitogenic signal transduction. *Cell, 70*, 93–104.

Pingel, J. T., & Thomas, M. L. (1999). Evidence that the leukocyte-common antigen is required for antigen-induced T lymphocyte proliferaton. *Cell, 58*, 1055–1065.

Pitch, J. A., Inglese, J. I., Higgins, J. B. ., Arriza, J. L., Casey, P. J., Kim, C., Benovic, J. L., Kwatra, M. M., Caron, M. G., & Lefkowitz, R. J. (1992). Role of $\beta\gamma$ subunits of G proteins in targeting the b-adrenergic receptor kinase to membrane-bound receptors. *Science, 257*, 1264–1267.

Pleiman, C. M., D'Ambrosio, D., & Cambier, J. C. (1994). The B-cell antigen receptor complex: Structure and signal transduction. *Immunology Today, 15*, 393–399.

Pochet, R., & Delespesse, G. (1983). β-Adrenoreceptors display different efficiency on lymphocyte subpopulations. *Biochemical Pharmacology, 32*, 1651–1655.

Pochet, R., Delespesse, G., Gausset, P. W., & Collet, H. (1979). Distribution of beta-adrenergic receptors on human lymphocyte subpopulations. *Clinical and Experimental Immunology, 38*, 578–584.

Posada, J., & Cooper, J. A. (1992). Molecular signal integration. Interplay between serine, threonine, and tyrosine phosphorylation. *Molecular Biology and Cell, 3*, 583–592.

Prasad, M. V. V. S. V., Dermott, J. M., Heasley, L. E., Johnson, G. L., & Dhanasekaran, N. (1995). Activation of Jun kinase/stress-activated protein kinase by GTPase-deficient mutants of Gα12 and Gα13. *Journal of Biological Chemistry, 270*, 18655–18659.

Putney, J. W., Jr. (1990). Capacitative calcium entry revisited. *Cell Calcium, 11*, 611–624.

Qui, R., Chen, J., Kirn, D., McCormick, F., & Symons, M. (1995). An essential role for Rac in Ras transformation. *Nature, 374*, 457–459.

Raff, M. C. (1992). Social controls on cell survival and cell death. *Nature, 356*, 397–400.

Raingeaud, J., Gupta, S., Rogers, J. S., Dickens, M., Han, J., Ulevitch, R. J., & Davis, R. J. (1995). Pro-inflammatory cytokines and environmental stress cause p38 mitogen-activated protein kinase activation by dual phosphorylation on tyrosine and threonine. *Journal of Biological Chemistry, 270*, 7420–7226.

Raingeaud, J., Whitmarsh, A. J., Barrett, T., Derijard, B., & Davis, R. J. (1996). MKK3- and MKK6-regulated gene expression is mediated by the p38 mitogen-activated protein kinase signal transduction pathway. *Molecular and Cellular Biology, 16*, 1247–1255.

Ravichandran, K. S., Lee, K. K., Songyang, Z., Cantley, L. C., Burn, P., & Burakoff, S. J. (1993). Interaction of Shc with the ζ chain of the T cell receptor upon T cell activation. *Science, 262*, 902–925.

Ray, A., & Prefontaine, K. E. (1994). Physical association and functional antagonism between the p65 subunit of transcription factor NFκB and the glucocorticoid receptor. *Proceedings of the National Academy of Science USA, 91*, 752–760.

Reedquist, K. A., Fukazawa, T., Panchamoorthy, G., Langdon, W. Y., Shoelson, S. E., Druker, B. J., & Band, H. (1996). Stimulation through the T cell receptor induces Cbl association with Crk proteins and the guanine nucleotide exchange protein C3G. *Journal of Biological Chemistry, 271*, 8435–8442.

Reif, K., Buday, L., Downward, J., & Cantrell, D. A. (1994). SH3 domains of the adapter molecule Grb2 complex with two proteins in T cells: the guanine nucleotide exchange proteins Sos and a 75-kDa protein that is a substrate for T cell antigen receptor-activated tyrosine kinases. *Journal of Biological Chemistry, 269*, 14081–14087.

Rhee, K., Bresnahan, W., Hirai, A., Hirai, M., & Thompson, E. A. (1995). *c-myc* and cyclin D3 (*ConD3*) genes are independent targets for glucocorticoid inhibition of lymphoid cell proliferation. *Cancer Research, 55*, 4188–4195.

Ribon, V., Hubbell, S., Herrera, R., & Saltiel, A. R. (1996). The product of the *cbl* oncogene forms stable complexes in vivo with endogenous Crk in a tyrosine phophorylation-dependent manner. *Molecular and Cellular Biology, 16*, 45–52.

Riedel, D., Brennscheidt, U., Kiehntopf, M., Brach, M., & Herrmann, F. (1993). The mitogenic response of T cells to interleukin-2 requires Raf-1. *European Journal of Immunology, 23*, 3146–3150.

Robbins, D. J., Cheng, M., Zhen, E., Vanderbilt, C. A., Feig, L. A., & Cobb, M. H. (1992). Evidence for a Ras-dependent extracellular signal-regulated protein kinase (ERK) cascade. *Proceedings of the National Academy of Science USA, 89*, 6924–6928.

Romeo, C., & Seed, B. (1991). Cellular immunity to HIV activated by CD4 fused to T cell or Fc receptor polypeptides. *Cell, 64*, 1037–1046.

Roszman, T. L., & Carlson, S. L. (1991). Neurotransmitters and molecular signaling in the immune response. In R. Ader, D. L. Felten, N. Cohen, (Eds.) *Psychoneuroimmunology* (2nd ed., pp. 311). San Diego: Academic Press.

Rouppe van der Voort, C., Kavelaars, A., van de Pol, M., & Heijnen, C. J. (1999). Neuroendocrine mediators up-regulate alpha 1b- and alpha 1d-adrenergic receptor subtypes in human monocytes. *Journal of Neuroimmunology, 95*, 165–173.

Rozdzial, M. M., Malissen, B., & Finkel, T. H. (1995). Tyrosine-phosphorylated T cell receptor ζ chain associates with the actin cytoskeleton upon activation of mature T lymphocytes. *Immunity, 3*, 623–633.

Ruderman, J. V. (1993). MAP kinase and the activation of quiescent cells. *Current Opinions in Cellular Biology, 5*, 207–213.

Sakabe, K., Seiki, K., & Fujii, H. (1986). Histochemical localisation of progestin receptor in the rat thymus. *Thymus, 8*, 97–107.

Sakuae, M., Bowtell, D., & Kasuga, M. (1992). A dominant negative mutant of mSOS1 inhibits insulin-induced Ras activation and reveals Ras-dependent and -independent insulin signaling pathways. *Molecular and Cellular Biology, 15*, 379–388.

Salbert, G., Fanjul, A., Piedrafita, F. J., Lu, X. P., Kim, S. J., Tran, P., & Pfahl, M. (1993). Retinoic acid receptors and retinoid X receptor-alpha down-regulate the transforming growth factor-beta 1 promoter by antagonizing AP-1 activity. *Molecular Endocrinology, 7*, 1347–1356.

Samelson, L. E., Patel, M. D., Weissman, A. M., Harford, J. B., & Klausner, R. D. (1986). Antigen activation of murine T cells induces tyrosine phosphorylation of a polypeptide associated with the T cell antigen receptor. *Cell, 46*, 1083–1090.

Sanders, V. M., Baker, R. A., Ramer-Quinn, D. S., Kasprowicz, D. J., Fuchs, B. A., & Street, N. E. (1997). Differential expression of the β2-adrenergic receptor by Th1 and Th2 clones: Implications for cytokine production and B cell help. *Journal of Immunology, 158*, 4200–4210.

Sawasdikosol, S., Ravichandran, K. S., Lee, K. K., Chang, J. H., & Burakoff, S. J. (1995). Crk interacts with tyrosine-phosphorylated p116 upon T cell activation. *Journal of Biological Chemistry, 270*, 2893–2896.

Scheinman, R. I., Cogswell, P. C., Lofquist, A. K., & Baldwin, A. S., Jr. (1995). Role of transcriptional activation of I kappa B alpha in mediation of immunosuppression by glucocorticoids. *Science, 270*, 283–286.

Schimke, R. T. (1969). On the roles of synthesis and degradation in regulation of enzyme levels in mammalian tissues. *Current Topics in Cellular Regulation, 1*, 77–124.

Schlessinger, J., & Ullrich, A. (1992). Growth factor signaling by receptor tyrosine kinases. *Neuron, 9*, 383–391.

Schramm, K., Niehof, M., Radiziwill, G., Rommel, C., & Moelling, K. (1994). Phosphorylation of c-Raf-1 by protein kinase A interferes with activation. *Biochemical and Biophysical Research Communication, 201*, 740–747.

Schreurs, A. J. M., Versteeg, D. H. G., & Nijkamp, F. P. (1982). Involvement of catecholamines in Haemophilus influenzae induced decrease of β-adrenoceptor function. *Naunyn Schmiedebergs Archives of Pharmacology, 320*, 235–239.

Schreurs, J., Gorman, D. M., & Miyajima, A. (1993). Cytokine receptors: A new superfamily of receptors. *International Review of Cytology, 137B*, 121–155.

Schulman, H. (1993). The multifunctional Ca^{2+}/calmodulin-dependent protein kinases. *Current Opinions in Cellular Biology, 5*, 247–253.

Schultz, L. D., Schweitzer, P. A., Rajan, T. V., Yi, T., Ihle, J. N., Matthews, R. J., Thomas, M. L., & Beier, D. R. (1993). Mutations at the murine motheaten locus are within the hematopoietic cell protein-tyrosine phosphatase (*Hcph*) gene. *Cell, 73*, 1445–1454.

Schwartzman, R. A., & Cidlowski, J. A. (1993). Apoptosis: The biochemistry and molecular biology of programmed cell death. *Endocrinology Review, 14*, 133–151.

Schüle, R., & Evans, R. M. (1991). Cross-coupling of signal transduction pathways: Zinc finger meets leucine zipper. *Trends in Genetics., 7*, 377–381.

Schüle, R., Rangarajan, P., Kliewer, S., Ransone, L., Bolado, J., Yang, N., Verma, I., & Evan, R. (1990). Functional antagonism between oncoprotein c-Jun and the glucocorticoid receptor. *Cell, 62*, 1217–1226.

Secrist, J. P., Karnitz, L., & Abraham, R. T. (1991). T-cell antigen receptor ligation induces tyrosine phosphorylation of phospholipase C-gamma 1. *Journal of Biological Chemistry, 266*, 12135–12139.

Sekar, M. C., & Hokin, L. E. (1986). The role of phosphoinositides in signal transduction. *Journal of Membrane Biology, 89*, 193–210.

Sells, S. F., Muthukumar, S., Sukhatme, V. P., Crist, S. A., & Rangnekar, V. M. (1995). The zinc finger transcription factor EGR-1 impedes interleukin-1-inducible tumor growth arrest. *Molecular and Cellular Biology, 15*, 682–692.

Serafini, A. T., Lewis, R. S., Clipstone, N. A., & Bram, R. J. (1995). Isolation of mutant T lymphocytes with defects in capacitative calcium entry. *Immunity, 3*, 239–250.

Serfling, E., Barthelmas, R., Pfeuffer, I., Schenk, B., Zarius, S., Swoboda, R., Mercurio, F., & Karin, M. (1989). Ubiquitous and lymphocyte-specific factors are involved in the induction of the mouse interleukin 2 gene in T lymphocytes. *EMBO Journal, 8*, 465–473.

Seuwen, K., Magnaldo, I., Kobilka, B. K., Caron, M. G., Regan, J. W., Lefkowitz, & R. J., Pouyssegur, J. (1990). α_2-adrenergic agonists stimulate DNA synthesis in Chinese hamster lung fibroblasts transfected with a human α_2-adrenergic receptor gene. *Cell Regulation, 1*, 445–451.

Shanafelt, M. C., Soderberg, C., Allsup, A., Adelman, D., Peltz, G., & Lahesmaa, R. (1995). Costimulatory signals can selectively modulate cytokine production by subsets of CD4+ T cells. *Journal of Immunology, 154*, 1684–1690.

Shaw, A. S., Chalupny, J., Whitney, J. A., Hammond, C., Amrein, K. E., Kavathas, P., Sefton, B. M., & Rose, J. K. (1990). Short related sequences in the cytoplasmic domains of CD4 and CD8 mediated binding to the amino-terminal domain of the $p56^{lck}$ tyrosine kinase. *Molecular and Cellular Biology, 10*, 1853–1862.

Shemshedini, L., Knauthe, R., Sassone-Corsi, P., Pornon, A., & Gronemeyer, H. (1991). Cell-specific inhibitory and stimulatory effecs of Fos and Jun on transcription activation by nuclear receptors. *EMBO Journal, 10*, 3839–3849.

Shi, L., Kam, C. M., Powers, J. C., Aebersold, R., & Greenberg, A. H. (1992). Purification of three cytotoxic lymphocyte granule serine proteases that induce apoptosis through distinct substrate and target cell interactions. *Journal of Experimental Medicine, 176*, 1521–1529.

Siegel, J. N., Klausner, R. D., Rapp, U. R., & Samelson, L. E. (1990). T cell antigen receptor engagement stimulates *c-raf* phosphorylation and induces *c-raf*-associated kinase activity via a protein kinase C-dependent pathway. *Journal of Biological Chemistry, 265*, 18472–18480.

Sieh, M., Batzer, A., Schlessinger, J., & Weiss, A. (1994). GRB2 and phospholipase C-g-1 associate with a 36- to 38-kilodalton phosphotyrosine protein after T-cell -receptor stimulation. *Molecular and Cellular Biology, 14*, 4435–4442.

Singer, G. G., & Abbas, A. K. (1994). The Fas antigen is involved in peripheral but not thymic deletion of T lymphocytes in T cell receptor transgenic mice. *Immunity, 1*, 365–371.

Singh, U. (1979). Effect of catecholamines on lymphopoiesis in fetal mouse thymic explants. *Journal of Anatomy, 129*, 279–292.

Singh, U. (1984). Sympathetic innervation of fetal mouse thymus. *European Journal of Immunology, 14*, 757–759.

Skalhegg, B. S., Rasmussen, A. M., Tasken, K., Hansson, V., Jahnsen, T., & Lea, T. (1994). Cyclic AMP-sensitive signalling by the CD28 marker requires concomitant stimulation by the T-cell antigen receptor (TCR/CD3) complex. *Scandinavian Journal of Immunology, 40*, 201–208.

Smith, C. A., Williams, G. T., Kingston, R., Jenkinson, E. J., & Owen, J. J. (1989). Antibodies to CD3/T cell receptor complex induce death by apoptosis in immature T cells in thymic cultures. *Nature, 337*, 181–184.

Snyder, S. H. (1985). The molecular basis of communication between cells. *Scientific American, 253*, 132–140.

Soderquist, A. M., & Carpenter, G. (1986). Biosynthesis and metabolic degradation of receptors for epidermal growth factor. *Journal of Membrane Biology, 90*, 97–105.

Soufi, M., Schneider, A., Beato, M., & Westphal, H. M. (1995). The DNA steroid binding domains of the glucocorticoid receptor are not altered in mononuclear cells of treated CLL patients. *Experimental and Clinical Endocrinology and Diabetes, 103*, 175–183.

Stachelin, M., Müller, P., Portenier, M., & Harris, A. W. (1985). β-Adrenergic receptors and adenylate cyclase activity in murine lymphoid cell lines. *Journal of Cyclic Nucleotide and Protein Phosphorylation Research, 10*, 55–64.

Stahl, N., & Yancopoulos, G. D. (1993). The alphas, betas, and kinases of cytokine receptor complexes. *Cell, 74*, 587–590.

Stefanova, I., Corcoran, M. L., Horak, E. M., Wahl, L. M., Bolen, J. B., & Horak, I. D. (1993). Lipopolysaccharide induces activation of CD14-associated protein tyrosine kinase p53/56lyn. *Journal of Biological Chemistry, 268*, 20725–20728.

Sternweis, P. C., & Smrcha, A. V. (1992). Regulation of phospholipase C by G proteins. *Trends in Biochemical Sciences, 17*, 502–506.

Stevens, C. F. (1992). Just say NO. *Currents in Biology, 2*, 108–109.

Stover, D. R., & Walsh, K. A. (1994). Protein-tyrosine phosphatase activity of CD45 is activated by sequential phosphorylation by two kinases. *Molecular and Cellular Biology, 14*, 5523–5532.

Su, B., Jacinto, E., Hibi, M., Kallunki, T., Karin, M., & Ben-Neriah, Y. (1994). JNK is involved in signal integration during costimulation of T lymphocytes. *Cell, 77*, 727–736.

Swan, K. A., Alberola-Ila, J., Gross, J. A., Appleby, M. W., Forbush, D. A., Thomas, J. F., & Perlmutter, R. M. (1995). Involvement of $p21^{ras}$ distinguishes positive and negative selection in thymocyes. *EMBO Journal, 14*, 276–285.

Sweet, M. J., & Hume, D. A. (1996). Endotoxin signal transduction in macrophages. *Journal of Leukocyte Biology, 60*, 8–26.

Szamei, M., & Resch, K. (1995). T-cell antigen receptor-induced signal-transduction pathways. Activation and function of protein kinase C in T lymphocytes. *European Journal of Biochemistry, 228*, 1–15.

Szefler, S. J. (1989). General pharmacology of glucocorticoids. In R. P. Schleimer, H. N. Claman, A. Oronsky (Eds.), *Anti-inflammatory steroid action: Basic and clinical aspects* (pp. 353–370). New York: Academic Press.

Takemoto, Y., Furuta, M., Li, Z., Strong-Sparks, W. J., & Hashimoto, Y. (1995). LckBPI, a proline-rich protein expressed in haematopoietic lineage cells, directly associates with the SH3 domain of protein tyrosine kinse $p56^{lck}$. *EMBO Journal, 14*, 3403–3414.

Tamir, A., Granot, Y., & Isakov, N. (1996). Inhibition of T lymphocyte activation by cAMP is associated with down-regulation of two parallel mitogen-activated protein kinase pathways, the extracellular signal-related kinase and c-Jun N-terminal kinase. *Journal of Immunology, 157*, 1514–1522.

Tamir, A., & Isakov, N. (1994). Cyclic AMP inhibits phosphatidylinositol-coupled and -uncoupled mitogenic signals in T lymphocytes: Evidence that cAMP alters PKC-induced transcription regulation of members of the jun and fos family of genes. *Journal of Immunology, 152*, 3391–3399.

Taniuchi, I., Kitamura, D., Maekawa, Y., Fukuda, T., Kishi, H., & Watanabe, T. (1995). Antigen-receptor induced clonal expansion and deletion of lymphocytes are impaired in mice lacking HS1 protein, a substrate of the antigen-receptor-coupled tyrosine kinases. *EMBO Journal, 14*, 3664–3678.

Tarakhovsky, A., Turner, M., Schaal, S., Mee, P. J., Duddy, L. P., Rajewsky, K., & Tybulewicz, L. J. (1995). Defective antigen receptor-mediated proliferation of B and T cells in the absence of Vav. *Nature, 374*, 467–470.

Taylor, C. W., & Marshal, I. C. B. (1992). Calcium and inositol 1,4,5-triphosphate receptors: A complex relationship. *Trends in Biochemical Sciences, 17*, 403–407.

Taylor, S. S., Buechler, J. A., & Yonemoto, W. (1990). cAMP-dependent protein kinase: Framework for a diverse family of regulatory enzymes. *Annual Review of Biochemistry, 59*, 971–1005.

Thomas, S. M., DeMarco, M., D'Arcangelo, G., Halegoua, S., & Brugge, J. S. (1992). Ras is essential for nerve growth factor- and phorbol ester- induced tyrosine phosphorylation of MAP kinases. *Cell, 68*, 1031–1040.

Thompson, E. A. (1991). Glucocorticoid insensitivity of P1798 lymphoma cells is associated with production of a factor that attenuates the lytic response. *Cancer Research, 51*, 5551–5556.

Thompson, E. B., & Harmon, J. M. (1986). In G. P. Choursos, D. L. Louriaux, M. B. Lipsett, (Eds.), *Steroid hormone resistance* (pp. 111–127). New York: Plenum Publishing.

Thompson, E. B., Thulasi, R., Saeed, M. F., & Johnson, B. H. (1995). Glucocorticoid antagonist RU 486 reverses agonist-induced apoptosis and c-myc repression in human leukemic CEM-C7 cells. *Annals of the New York Academy of Science, 761*, 261–277.

Thulasi, R., Harbour, D. V., & Thompson, E. B. (1993). Suppression of c-myc is a critical step in glucocorticoid-induced human leukemic cell lysis. *Journal of Biological Chemistry, 268*, 18306–18312.

Tominaga, D., Saito, S., Matsuura, M., & Nakano, M. (1999). Lipopolysaccharide tolerance in murine peritoneal macrophages induces downregulation of the lipopolysaccharide signal transduction pathway through mitogen-activated protein kinase and nuclear factor-κB cascades, but not lipopolysaccharide-incorporation steps. *Biochimica et Biophysica Acta, 1450*, 130–144.

Truss, M., & Beato, M. (1993). Steroid hormone receptors: Interaction with deoxyribonucleic acid and transcription factors. *Endocrinology Review, 14*, 459–479.

Turner, J. M., Brodsky, M. H., Irving, B. A., Levin, S. D., Perlmutter, R. M., & Littman, D. R. (1990). Interaction of the unique N-terminal region of the tyrosine kinase $p56^{lck}$ with the cytoplasmic domains of CD4 and CD8 is mediated by cysteine motifs. *Cell, 60*, 755–765.

Ucker, D. S. (1987). Cytotoxic T lymphocytes and glucocorticoids activate an endogenous suicide process in target cells. *Nature, 327*, 62–64.

Ulevitch, R. J., & Tobias, P. S. (1995). Receptor-dependent mechanisms of cell stimulation by bacterial endotoxin. *Annual Review of Immunology, 13*, 437–457.

Ullrich, A., & Schlessinger, J. (1990). Signal transduction by receptors with tyrosine kinase activity. *Cell, 61*, 203–212.

Vacca, A., Felli, M. P., Farina, A. R., Martinotti, S., Maroder, M., Screpandi, I., Meco, D., Petrangeli, E., Frati, L., & Gulion, A. (1992). Glucocorticoid receptor-mediated suppression of the interleukin-2 gene expression through impairment of the cooperativity between NFAT and AP-1 enhancer elements. *Journal of Experiental Medicine, 175*, 637–646.

van Biesen, T., Hawes, B. E., Luttrell, D. K., Krueger, K. M., Touhara, K., Porfiri, E., Sakaue, M., Luttrell, L. M., & Lefkowitz, R. J. (1995). Receptor-tyrosine-kinase- and $G\beta\gamma$-mediated MAP kinase activation by a common signaling pathway. *Nature, 376*, 781–784.

van Corven, E. J., Groenink, A., Jalik, K., Eichholtz, T., & Moolnenaar, W. H. (1989). Lysophosphatidate-induced cell proliferation: Identification and dissection of signaling pathways mediated by G proteins. *Cell, 59*, 45–54.

van Oers, N. S. C., Killeen, N., & Weiss, A. (1996). Lck regulates the tyrosine phosphorylation of the T cell receptor subunits and ZAP-70 in murine thymocytes. *Journal of Experimental Medicine, 183*, 1053–1062.

van Oers, N. S. C., & Weiss, A. (1995). The Syk/Zap-70 protein tyrosine kinase connection to antigen receptor signalling processes. *Seminars in Immunology, 7*, 227–236.

Verheij, M., Bose, R., Lin, X. H., Yao, B., Jarvis, W. D., Grant, S., Birrer, M. F., Szabo, E., Zon, L. K., Kyriakis, J. M., Haimovitz-Friedman, A., Fuks, Z., & Kolesnick, R. N. (1996). Requirement for ceramide-initiated SAPK/JNK signalling in stress-induced apoptosis. *Nature, 380*, 75–79.

Vojtek, A. B., & Cooper, J. A. (1995). Rho family members: Activators of MAP kinase cascades. *Cell, 82*, 527–529.

Voyno-Yasenetskaya, T. A., Faure, M. P., Ahn, N. G., & Bourne, H. R. (1996). $G\alpha12$ and $G\alpha13$ regulate extracellular signal-regulated kinase and c-Jun kinase pathways by different mechanisms in COS-7 cells. *Journal of Biological Chemistry, 271*, 21081–21087.

Walton, K. M., & Dixon, J. E. (1993). Protein tyrosine phosphatases. *Annual Review of Biochemistry, 62*, 101–120.

Wan, Y., & Huang, X. Y. (1998). Analysis of the Gs/mitogen-activated protein kinase pathway in mutant S49 cells. *Journal of Biological Chemistry, 273*, 14533–14537.

Waskiewicz, A. J., & Cooper, J. A. (1995). Mitogen and stress response pathways: MAP kinase cascades and phosphatase regulation in mammals and yeast. *Current Opinions in Cellular Biology, 7*, 798–805.

Wassarman, D. A., Therrien, M., & Rubin, B. M. (1995). The Ras signaling pathway in *Drosophila*. *Current Opinion in Genetic Development, 5*, 44–50.

Watts, J. D., Affolter, M., Krebs, D. L., Wange, R. L., Samelson, L. E., & Aebersold, R. (1994). Identification by electrospray ionization mass spectrometry of the sites of tyrosine phosphorylation induced in activated Jurkat T cells on the protein tyrosine kinase ZAP-70 in murine thymocytes. *Journal of Biological Chemistry, 269*, 29520–29529.

Webber, R. H., DeFelice, R., Ferguson, R. J., & Powell, J. P. (1970). Bone marrow response to stimulation of the sympathetic trunks in rats. *Acta Anatatomica, 77*, 92–97.

Weinstein, S. L., June, C. H., & DeFranco, A. L. (1993). Lipopolysaccharide-induced protein tyrosine phosphorylation in human macrophages is mediated by CD14. *Journal of Immunology, 151*, 3829–3838.

Weiss, A. (1993). T cell antigen receptor signal transduction: A tale of tails and cytoplasmic protein-tyrosine kinases. *Cell, 73*, 209–212.

Weiss, A., Koretzky, G., Schatzman, R. C., & Kadlecek, T. (1991). Functional activation of T-cell antigen receptor induces tyrosine phosphorylation of phospholipase C-gamma 1. *Proceedings of the National Academy of Science USA, 88*, 5484–5488.

Weiss, A., & Littman, D. R. (1994). Signal transduction by lymphocyte antigen receptors. *Cell, 76*, 263–274.

Weisz, A., & Rosales, R. (1990). Identification of an estrogen response element upstream of the human c-fos gene that binds the estrogen receptor and the AP-1 transcription factor. *Nucleic Acids Research, 18*, 5097–5106.

Whitehurst, C. E., & Geppert, T. D. (1996). MEK1 and the extracellular signal-regulated kinases are required for the stimulation of IL-2 gene transcription in T cells. *Journal of Immunology, 156*, 1020–1029.

Williams, L. T., Snyderman, R., & Lefkowitz, R. J. (1976). Identification of β-adrenergic receptors in human lymphocytes by (–)[3H]-alprenolol binding. *Journal of Clinical Investigation, 57*, 149–155.

Wilson, D. J., Fortner, K. A., Lynch, D. H., Mattingly, R. R., Macara, I. G., Posada, J. A., & Budd, R. C. (1996). JNK, but not MAPK, activation is associated with Fas-mediated apoptosis in human T cells. *European Journal of Immunology, 26*, 989–994.

Winitz, S., Russell, M., Quian, N.-X., Gardner, A., Dwyer, L., & Johnson, G. L. (1993). Involvement of Ras and Raf in the Gi-coupled acetycholine muscarinic M2 receptor activation of mitogen-activated protein (MAP) kinase kinase and MAP kinase. *Journal of Biological Chemistry, 268*, 19191–19199.

Wood, K. W., Sarnecki, C., Roberts, T. M., & Blenis, J. (1992). Ras mediates nerve growth factor receptor modulation of three signal-transducing protein kinases: MAP kinase, Raf-1 and RSK. *Cell, 68*, 1041–1050.

Wu, J., Dent, P., Jelinek, T., Wolfman, A., Weber, M. J., & Sturgill, T. W. (1993a). Inhibition of the EGF-activated MAP kinase signaling pathway by adenosine 3′,5′-monophosphate. *Science, 262*, 1065–1069.

Wu, J., Dent, P., Jelinek, T., Wolfman, A., Weber, M. J., & Sturgill, T. W. (1993b). Inhibition of the EGF-actvated MAP kinase signaling pathway by adenosine 3′,5′-monophosphate. *Science, 262*, 1065–1069.

Wyllie, A. H. (1980). Glucocorticoid induced thymocytes apoptosis is associated with endogenous endonuclease activation. *Nature, 284*, 555–556.

Xia, Z, Dickens, M., Raingeaud, J., Davis, R. J., & Greenberg, M. E. (1995). Opposing effects of ERK and JNK-p38 MAP kinases on apoptosis. *Science, 270*, 1326–1331.

Xiao, R., Ji, X., & Lakatta, E. G. (1995). Functional coupling of the β_2-adrenoceptor to a pertussis toxin-sensitive G protein in cardiac myocytes. *Molecular Pharmacology, 47*, 322–329.

Xin, Z., Sun, L., & Ganea, D. (1997). Vasoactive intestinal peptide stimulates p59fyn kinase activity in murine thymocytes. *Peptides, 18*, 1151–1159.

Yamamoto, K. R. (1985). Steroid receptor regulated transcription of specific genes and gene networks. *Annual Review of Genetics, 19*, 209–252.

Yamanashi, Y., Okada, M., Semba, T., Yamori, T., Umemori, H., Tsunasawa, S., Toyoshima, K., Kitamura, D., Watanabe, T., & Yamamoto, T. (1993). Identification of HS1 protein as a major substrate of protein-tyrosine kinases(s) upon B-cell antigen receptor-mediated signaling. *Proceedings of the National Academy of Science USA, 90*, 3631–3635.

Yamauchi, J., Nagao, M., Kaziro, Y., & Itoh, H. (1997). Activation of p38 mitogen-activated protein kinase by signaling through G protein-coupled receptors. Involvement of $G\beta\gamma$ and $G\alpha q/11$ subunits. *Journal of Biological Chemistry., 272*, 27771–27777.

Yang, H., Wang, L., & Huang, C. S. (1998). Plasticity of GAP-43 innervation of the spleen during immune response in the mouse. Evidence for axonal sprouting and redistribution of the nerve fibers. *Neuroimmunomodulation, 5*, 53–60.

Yang, Y., Mercep, M., Ware, C. F., & Ashwell, J. D. (1995). Fas and activation-induced Fas ligand mediate apoptosis of T cell hybridomas: inhibition of Fas ligand expression by retinoic acid and glucocorticoids. *Journal of Experimental Medicine, 181*, 1673–1682.

Yang-Yen, H., Chambard, J. C., Sun, Y., Smeal, T., Schmidt, T. J., Drouin, J., & Karin, M. (1990). Transcriptional interference between c-jun and the glucocorticoid receptor: Mutual inhibition of DNA binding due to direct protein-protein interaction. *Cell, 62*, 1205–1215.

Yarwood, S. J., Kilgour, E., & Anderson, N. G. (1996). Cyclic AMP stimulates the phosphorylation and activation of p42 and p44 mitogen-activated protein kinases in 3T3-F442A preadipocytes. *Biochemical and Biophysical Researcj Communication, 224*, 734–739.

Yeh, P., Bellinger, D. L., Livnat, S., Ader, R., Felten, S. Y., & Felten, D. L. (1985). Noradrenergic innervation of mesenteric and popliteal lymph nodes in young and aging mice with autoimmune disorders. *Society for Neuroscience Abstract, 11*, 662.

Yuen, P. S. T., & Garbers, D. L. (1992). Guanylyl cyclase-linked receptors. *Annual Review of Neuroscience, 15*, 193–225.

Zacharchuk, C. M., Mercep, M., Chakraborti, PK., Simmons, S. S., Jr., & Ashwell, J. D. (1990). Programmed T lymphocyte death: Cell activation- and steroid-induced pathways are mutually antagonistic. *Journal of Immunology, 145*, 4037–4045.

Zaitsev, S. V., Khegia, L. A., Kim, B. B., Gavrilova, E. M., Yanovsky, O. G., & Zakharova, L. A. (1992). Involvement of opioid receptors in Met-enkephalin modulation of blast-transformation of mouse splenocytes. *Immunology Letters, 32*, 27–30.

Zhang, R., Alt, F. W., Davidson, L., Orkin, S. H., & Swat, W. (1995). Defective signalling through the T-and B-cell antigen receptors in lymphoid cells lacking the *vav* proto-oncogene. *Nature, 374*, 470–473.

Zhao, Y., & Iwata, M. (1995). Cross-linking of the TCR-CD3 complex with CD4, CD8 or LFA-1 induces an anti-apoptotic signal in thymocytes: the signal is cancelled by FK506. *International Immunology, 7*, 1387–1596.

Zhao, Y., Tozawa, Y., Iseki, R., Mukai, M., & Iwata, M. (1995). Calcineurin activation protects T cells from glucocorticoid-induced apoptosis. *Journal of Immunology, 154*, 6346–6354.

Zhong, H., & Minneman, K. P. (1999). Differential activation of mitogen-activated protein kinase pathways in PC12 cells by closely related α_1-adrenergic receptor subtypes. *Journal of Neurochemistry, 72*, 2388–2396.

Zhou, R., & Thompson, E. B. (1996). Role of c-jun induction in the glucocorticoid-evoked apoptotic pathway in human leukemic lymphoblasts. *Molecular Endocrinology, 10*, 306–316.

Zoukos, Y., Leonard, J. P, Thomaides, T., Thompson, A. J., & Cuzner, M. L. (1992). beta-Adrenergic receptor density and function of peripheral blood mononuclear cells are increased in multiple sclerosis: A regulatory role for cortisol and interleukin-1. *Annals of Neurology, 31*, 657–662.

Zoukos, Y., Thomaides, T., Mathias, C. J., & Cuzner, M. L. (1994). High beta-adrenoceptor density on peripheral blood mononuclear cells in progressive multiple sclerosis: A manifestation of autonomic dysfunction? *Acta Neurological Scandinavia, 90*, 382–387.

Zubiaga, A. M., Munoz, E., & Huber, B. T. (1992). IL-4 and IL-2 selectively rescue Th cell subsets from glucocorticoid-induced apoptosis. *Journal of Immunology, 149*, 107–112.

Zuniga-Pflücker, J. C., & Lenardo, M. J. (1996). Regulation of thymocyte development from immature progenitors. *Current Opinions in Immunology, 8*, 215–224.

CHAPTER

4

Neurotransmitter Receptors on Lymphocytes and Other Lymphoid Cells

VIRGINIA M. SANDERS, DEBORAH J. KASPROWICZ, ADAM P. KOHM, MICHELLE A. SWANSON

I. INTRODUCTION

Since a line of communication exists between the nervous system and immune system, as suggested by the findings from many experimental and clinical studies, then a mechanism must exist for the transfer of an extracellular neurotransmitter signal to the immune cell interior to affect either cell biochemistry or gene expression to bring about a change in immune cell function. The purpose of this chapter is to summarize the data that indicate the expression of adrenergic, cholinergic, serotonergic, and dopaminergic receptors on the cell surface of immune cells. The summary data will include both in vivo and in vitro findings collected at the functional level using pharmacological agonists and antagonists selective for specific neurotransmitter receptor subtypes. In addition, since functional data suggest merely the presence of a neurotransmitter receptor on a cell, this chapter also will include data that confirm directly the presence of the receptor at the cellular level by radioligand binding analysis, as well as at the molecular level using reverse transcription-polymerase chain reaction (RT-PCR) and Northern analysis. Finally, findings relevant to the receptor-specific signal transduction pathways associated with neurotransmitter receptors, as well as any receptor-specific changes in gene expression that may transpire following receptor stimulation, will be described.

II. ADRENERGIC RECEPTORS

A. Bone Marrow

A summary of the evidence for the presence of adrenergic receptors on cells in the bone marrow is presented in Table I. For the purposes of this review, details will not be included relating to either the concentration-dependent manner in which the neurotransmitter receptor effects were induced or the ability of an appropriate receptor antagonist to block the effects. Also, since many of the findings from studies using either human or animal cells were similar, we have not distinguished between species for most of the results. The authors refer the reader to the specific studies referenced herein for these types of detail.

TABLE I Summary of the Evidence for the Presence of Adrenergic Receptors on Bone Marrow Cells

Receptor	Response	Reference
Functional evidence		
α1AR agonist	In vitro - ↓ number of GM-CFU	(Maestroni et al., 1994a)
αAR antagonist	In vivo - Late protection against radiation-induced bone marrow cell death	(Byron & Fox 1969; Byron, 1972)
α1AR antagonist	In vivo - ↑ number of lymphocytes and platelets found in the peripheral blood	(Maestroni et al., 1992)
	In vivo - ↑ formation of GM-CFU	(Maestroni et al., 1992)
	In vivo - accelerated myelopoiesis	(Maestroni et al., 1992)
	In vivo - ↓ number of both thymocytes and splenic T cells and B cells	(Maestroni & Conti 1994b)
	In vitro (+NE) - ↓ number of GM-CFU	(Maestroni & Conti 1994b)
βAR agonist	In vivo - ↑ proliferation of bone marrow cells	(Lipski, 1980)
β2AR agonist	In vitro - ↓ CFU-E formation	(Beckman et al., 1980)
βAR antagonist	In vivo - early protection against radiation-induced bone marrow cell death	(Byron & Fox, 1969; Byron, 1972)
	In vivo (restraint stress) - ↑ number of specific bone marrow cell subpopulations	(Sudo et al., 1997)
β2AR antagonist	In vitro - ↓ bone marrow cell proliferation	(Dresch et al., 1981)
	In vitro - ↓ number of normal hematopoietic cells entering S phase	(Dresch et al., 1981)
	In vitro - Delayed the formation of GM-CFU	(Dresch et al., 1981)
NE-depletion in vivo via 6-OHDA	↑ Number of lymphocytes and platelets found in the peripheral blood	(Maestroni et al., 1992)
	↑ Formation of GM-CFU	(Maestroni et al., 1992)
	Accelerated myelopoiesis	(Maestroni et al., 1992)
NE-depletion in vivo via nerve cut	↑ Bone marrow progenitor cell mobilization	(Afan et al., 1997)
	↓ Bone marrow cellularity	(Afan et al., 1997)
Radioligand Binding		
α1AR	Kd = 0.98 nM; Bmax = 5 fM/mg protein (on lymphoid/stem cell fraction)	(Maestroni & Conti, 1994a)
	Kd = 55.9 nM; Bmax = 44 fM/mg protein (on unknown cell fraction)	(Maestroni & Conti, 1994a)
Signal Transduction		
βAR	↑ cAMP	(Lipski, 1976)
β2AR	↑ cAMP	(Beckman et al., 1980)

GM-CFU, granulocyte monocyte-colony forming unit; CFU-E, colony forming unit-erythrocyte; K_d, dissociation constant; B_{max}, binding maximum; CAMP, adenosine 3′,5′-monophosphate; NE, norepinephrine.

1. *Functional Evidence*

During the early 1970s, researchers proposed that the toxic effects of irradiation were due to the effects of an irradiation-induced release of norepinephrine and epinephrine that stimulated adrenergic receptors on bone marrow cells. The earliest studies to address the influence of the sympathetic nervous system (SNS) on bone marrow cell function showed that both alpha-adrenergic receptor (αAR) and beta-adrenergic receptor (βAR) antagonists provided protection to mice against radiation-induced bone marrow cell death, but that the timing of the antagonist treatment determined the efficiency of protection (Byron, 1972; Byron & Fox, 1969). For example, a βAR antagonist offered protection to irradiated mice if administered prior to irradiation, whereas an αAR antagonist was more effective if administered after irradiation. In another study, when irradiated mice were exposed to the β-agonist isoproterenol, an increase in bone marrow cell proliferation was measured 16 h later (Lipski, 1980). Thus, these studies suggested that if irradiation induced a release of norepinephrine and/or epinephrine, then the βAR on bone marrow cells would be stimulated to induce maximal proliferation and render the cells susceptible to the toxic effects of irradiation. Similarly, human bone marrow cells cultured in agar with either the βAR-nonselective antagonist propranolol or the β2AR-selective antagonist butoxamine decreased bone marrow cell proliferation, decreased the number of normal hematopoietic cells entering S phase, and delayed the formation of granulocyte-macrophage colonies (GM-CFU) (Dresch, Minc, Poirier, & Bouvet, 1981). In addition, the data suggested that both adrenergic receptor subtypes were expressed temporally, with the βAR being expressed predominantly during early stages of bone marrow activation and the αAR being expressed during later stages. Thus, the βAR appears to be expressed on cells in the bone marrow and stimulation of the receptor may enhance bone marrow cell proliferation and differentiation.

In addition to proliferation, stimulation of the βAR appears to affect bone marrow cell differentiation. For example, in vitro culture of bone marrow cells from Friend leukemia virus-infected mice with the β2AR-selective agonist albuterol suppresses the formation of erythroid colony forming units (CFU-E) (Beckman, Mirand, & Fisher, 1980) and this effect was blocked by the β2AR-selective antagonist butoxamine. Also, whereas restraint stress induced an increase in the number of specific bone marrow cell subpopulations, norepinephrine-depletion with 6-hydroxydopamine (6-OHDA) or exposure in vivo to the βAR-nonselective antagonist propranolol further enhanced the number of specific bone marrow cell subpopulations (Sudo, Yu, Sogawa, & Kubo, 1997), suggesting that the SNS exerted a suppressive effect on specific bone marrow cell subpopulations during acute stress through stimulation of the βAR. Thus, stimulation of the β2AR expressed on cells in the bone marrow may suppress bone marrow cell differentiation.

In a like manner to the effects induced in bone marrow cells from βAR stimulation, other reports suggested that the α1AR was expressed on bone marrow cells and that stimulation of this receptor modulated hematopoiesis [reviewed in (Maestroni, 1995)]. For example, the reconstitution of norepinephrine-depleted mice with syngeneic bone marrow cells increased the formation of granulocyte monocyte-colony forming unit (GM-CFU) and accelerated myelopoiesis. This effect from norepinephrine-depletion was mimicked in reconstituted norepinephrine-intact mice exposed to the α1AR-selective antagonist prazosin, but not to the βAR-nonselective antagonist propranolol (Maestroni, Conti, & Pedrinis, 1992). However, in bone marrow reconstituted norepinephrine-intact mice, prazosin decreased the differentiation of transferred precursor cells into thymocytes, splenic T cells, and splenic B cells (Maestroni & Conti, 1994b). In vitro, norepinephrine or the α1AR-selective agonist methoxamine decreased the number of GM-CFU that formed from bone marrow cells and this decrease was prevented by the α1AR-selective antagonist prazosin (Maestroni & Conti, 1994a, 1994b). Taken together, these findings suggest that the α1AR is expressed on cells in the bone marrow and that stimulation of this receptor may suppress myelopoiesis and enhance lymphopoiesis.

In addition to bone marrow cell proliferation and differentiation, a more recent study has examined the role of the SNS in the mobilization of cells from the bone marrow into the periphery. When the murine femoral nerve was mechanically severed, bone marrow progenitor cells were rapidly mobilized into the peripheral blood within 24 h and a decrease in bone marrow cellularity ensued (Afan, Broome, Nicholls, Whetton, & Miyan, 1997). These data suggest that the SNS influences the mobility of precursor cells from the bone marrow into the peripheral blood, but the data do not indicate the adrenergic receptor subtype responsible for mediating the norepinephrine-induced effect.

Thus, indirect functional evidence suggests that the β2AR is expressed on cells in the bone marrow and that stimulation of the receptor may enhance bone marrow cell proliferation, but suppress bone marrow cell differentiation. On the other hand, the functional data also suggest that the α1AR is expressed on bone marrow cells and that stimulation of this receptor may suppress myelopoiesis and enhance lymphopoiesis.

2. *Radioligand Binding*

To date, radioligand binding data supports the expression of the αAR on bone marrow cells. ^{3}H-labeled prazosin, an α1AR antagonist, was found to bind to both bone marrow cell membranes and intact bone marrow cells with a high and low affinity (Maestroni & Conti, 1994a). The high affinity binding site had a Kd of 0.98 nM and a Bmax of 5 fM/mg protein, whereas the low affinity binding site had a Kd of 55.9 nM and Bmax of 44 fM/mg protein. The high affinity α1AR binding site was found to be expressed on a lymphoid/stem cell fraction, but it remains unclear as to which cell subset expresses the lower affinity site. Thus, direct radioligand binding data suggest that the α1AR is expressed on lymphoid/stem cells in the bone marrow.

3. *Receptor-Specific Signal Transduction Pathways*

When mice were exposed to either norepinephrine, epinephrine, or isoproterenol, a biphasic increase in bone marrow cell adenosine 3′,5′-monophosphate (cAMP) content was measured at 1 min and at 15 min after drug exposure (Lipski, 1976). This increase in bone marrow cell cAMP content intracellularly was also measured in sublethally irradiated mice that were not exposed to any drugs. The βAR-antagonist propranolol prevented the increase in cAMP content in both cases, suggesting that the increase was mediated through stimulation of the βAR. In vitro studies showed similar results. In contrast, bone marrow cells from lethally irradiated mice did not show this biphasic change in cAMP content when exposed to the drugs. Thus, intracellular signaling data suggest that stimulation of the βAR on differentiated bone marrow cells elevates the level of cAMP, but does not affect the level of cAMP within stem cells. To date, we have not found data to indicate the presence of an α1AR-specific signal transduction pathway in bone marrow cells.

B. Thymus

A summary of the evidence for the presence of adrenergic receptors on cells in the thymus is presented in Table II.

1. *Functional Evidence*

In vivo exposure of mice to the βAR-nonselective agonist isoproterenol decreased thymic weight and thymocyte number (Durant, 1986). Likewise, catecholamines or the βAR-nonselective agonist isoproterenol decreased Con A- or LPS-induced proliferation of mouse thymus cells, whereas αAR agonists had no effect (Cook-Mills, Cohen, Perlman, & Chambers, 1995). Also, in vitro exposure of a purified population of rat thymic epithelial cells to the βAR-nonselective agonist isoproterenol decreased basal and serum-stimulated proliferation, without any change in the level of IL-1 production (Kurz et al., 1997). In addition, in vitro data suggested that βAR stimulation

TABLE II Summary of the Evidence for the Presence of Adrenergic Receptors on Cells in the Thymus

Receptor	Response	Reference
Functional evidence		
αAR agonist	In vitro - ↑ IL-6 by thymic epithelial cells	(von Patay et al., 1998)
βAR agonist	In vivo - ↓ thymic weight and cell number	(Durant, 1986)
	In vitro - ↓ proliferation	(Cook-Mills, Cohen, et al., 1995)
	In vitro - ↓ thymic epithelial cell proliferation	(Kurz et al., 1997)
NE-depletion in vivo via 6-OHDA	↓ Thymus weight and cellularity	(Kendall & al-Shawaf, 1991)
	↑ Apoptosis	
	↑ Proliferating cells in thymic cortex	
Radioligand binding		
βAR	Thymic epithelial cells	(Kurz et al., 1997)
β2AR	Thymic cell membranes	(Marchetti et al., 1994)
	Thymus cells	(Marchetti et al., 1992)
Northern		
β2AR	Thymus cells	(Morale et al., 1992; Marchetti et al., 1994)
RT-PCR		
β1AR	Thymic epithelial cells	(Kurz et al., 1997)
β2AR	Thymic epithelial cells	(Kurz et al., 1997)
Signal transduction		
αAR	In vitro - ↑ Mg++-dependent events	(Morgan et al., 1984)
βAR	In vivo - ↑ cAMP thymus cells	(Durant, 1986)
	In vitro - ↑ Ca++-dependent events	(Morgan et al., 1984)
β1AR	In vitro - ↑ cAMP thymic epithelial cells	(Kurz et al., 1997)
β2AR	In vitro - ↑ cAMP thymic epithelial cells	(Kurz et al., 1997)
	In vivo - ↑ cAMP thymus cells	(Morale et al., 1992)

cAMP, adenosine 3′,5′-monophosphate; Mg++, magnesium ion; Ca++, calcium ion; IL, interleukin.

by a mixed agonist induced thymocyte apoptosis, a cellular event that required both protein synthesis and the activation of proteases (Anderson, Anderson, Michell, Jenkinson, & Owen, 1996). In contrast, another study showed that culture of rat thymic epithelial cells alone, or with LPS, in the presence of an αAR agonist increased IL-6 production, but not IL-1 production, in a concentration-dependent manner and was blocked with an αAR antagonist (von Patay, Loppnow, Feindt, Kurz, & Mentlein, 1998). In comparison, another study reported that catecholamines exerted a positive effect on cell viability and function in the thymus since chemical sympathectomy of adult rats with 6-OHDA decreased thymus weight and cellularity, increased the level of apoptosis, and decreased the numbers of proliferating T cells in the periphery (Kendall & al-Shawaf, 1991). Thus, taken together, these data suggest that the βAR and αAR are expressed on cells within the thymus and that βAR stimulation of these cells may exert a suppressive effect, whereas αAR stimulation may exert a positive effect.

2. *Radioligand Binding*

Using the iodinated βAR-nonselective antagonist cyanopindolol and competitive displacement analysis with β1AR and β2AR antagonists and agonists, the β2AR was shown to be expressed by thymic cell membranes and the number of binding sites increased during the rat estrous cycle and pregnancy, but decreased after castration (Marchetti, Morale, Paradis, & Bouvier, 1994). Another study showed that cells in the rat thymus changed their level of β2AR cell surface expression during the course of an immune response (Morale, Gallo, Batticane, & Marchetti, 1992). Specifically, 3 days following exposure to the protein antigen bovine serum albumin, β2AR number was decreased on cells in the thymus without a change in affinity. However, at the peak of the immune response on days 7 and 15, receptor number was higher than that for unexposed control rats. In addition, using the radiolabeled βAR antagonist CGP 12177, binding sites were shown to be present on a defined population of rat thymic epithelial cells (Kurz et al., 1997). Thus, direct radioligand binding data suggest that the β2AR is expressed on cells in the thymus.

3. *Northern and RT-PCR*

Using Northern blot analysis, rat thymus cells were shown to express mRNA for the β2AR and that steady-state levels of receptor expression increased during the rat estrous cycle and pregnancy (Marchetti et al., 1994; Morale et al., 1992). However, there was a decrease in β2AR mRNA 3 days after immunization with bovine serum albumin, but an increase at the peak of the immune response on days 7 and 15 (Morale et al., 1992). Using RT-PCR, mRNA for both the β1AR and β2AR was detectable in rat thymic epithelial cells (Kurz et al., 1997). Thus, both Northern and RT-PCR data suggest that the β2AR is expressed on cells in the thymus and that both the β1AR and the β2AR may be expressed by thymic epithelial cells.

4. *Receptor-Specific Signal Transduction Pathways*

In vivo exposure of mice to the βAR-nonselective agonist isoproterenol induced a rapid increase in cAMP in cells within the thymus (Durant, 1986). However, another study reported that mice exposed to a β2AR-selective agonist had decreased cAMP content in thymic cells 3 days after immunization with bovine serum albumin, but increased cAMP at the peak of the immune response on days 7 and 15 (Morale et al., 1992). In vitro exposure of a defined population of rat thymic epithelial cells to catecholamines or the βAR-nonselective agonist isoproterenol increased intracellular cAMP levels in a concentration-dependent manner and appeared to be mediated by both the β1AR and β2AR, but not the β3AR (Kurz et al., 1997). Although there are no reports of a direct correlation between βAR stimulation, cAMP enhancement, and the induction of apoptosis, studies have shown that elevating intracellular cAMP in thymocytes leads to the induction of apoptosis (Anderson et al., 1996; McConkey, Orrenius, & Jondal, 1990; Suzuki, Tadakuma, & Kizaki, 1991).

In addition, when thymocytes were exposed to high concentrations of either epinephrine or the βAR agonist isoproterenol, magnesium-dependent events were initiated that led to cell division (Morgan, Wigham, & Perris, 1984). In contrast, when thymocytes were exposed to low concentrations of norepinephrine, calcium-dependent events were initiated that led to cell division. This finding suggested that a difference may exist between the signaling pathways induced by stimulation of the βAR or the αAR, assuming that norepinephrine stimulated the αAR in this study.

Thus, intracellular signaling data suggest that stimulation of the β2AR on cells within the thymus elevates the level of cAMP intracellularly, with the possibility that αAR stimulation by NE may induce a rise in Ca^{++} intracellularly.

C. T Lymphocytes

A summary of the evidence for the presence of adrenergic receptors on mature T lymphocytes is presented in Table III.

1. Functional Evidence

Studies have shown that stimulation of either the βAR or the β2AR inhibited either mitogen- or anti-CD3 antibody-induced T cell proliferation (Bartik, Bauman, Brooks, & Roszman, 1994; Bartik, Brooks, & Roszman, 1993; Bauman, Bartik, Brooks, & Roszman, 1994; Carlson, Brooks, & Roszman, 1989; Carlson, Trauth, Brooks, & Roszman, 1994; Hadden, Hadden, & Middleton, 1970; Johnson, Ashmore, & Gordon, 1981; Johnson & Gordon, 1981). Since T cell proliferation is promoted by the binding of IL-2 to the IL-2R expressed by the T cell, it was possible that the βAR-induced decrease in T cell proliferation was due to a decrease in either IL-2R expression or IL-2 production by the T cell. To address this possibility, studies with T cells showed that either βAR stimulation or a cAMP analog suppressed the expression of either one or both of the p55 and p75 chains of the IL-2 receptor (Feldman, Hunninghake, & McArdle, 1987; Krause & Deutsch, 1991) and decreased IL-2 production (Bartik et al., 1994; Bartik et al., 1993; Feldman et al., 1987; Krause & Deutsch, 1991; Mary, Peyron, Auberger, Aussel, & Fehlmann, 1989; Novak & Rothenberg, 1990; Ramer-Quinn, Baker, & Sanders, 1997; Selliah, Bartik, Carlson, Brooks, & Roszman, 1995; Wacholtz, Minakuchi, & Lipsky, 1991). More recent studies have attempted to determine the effect of βAR stimulation on CD4+ T cell subsets. In this regard, norepinephrine or the β2AR-selective agonist terbutaline decreased IL-2 production by both murine CD4+ naive T cells (Ramer-Quinn, Swanson, Lee, & Sanders, 2000) and clones of murine Th1 cells (Sanders et al., 1997; Ramer-Quinn et al., 1997). Thus, indirect functional evidence suggests that the β2AR is expressed on T lymphocytes and that stimulation of the receptor decreases IL-2 production.

In addition to IL-2 production, βAR stimulation also affected other cytokines produced by T cell subpopulations. CD4+ Th1 effector cells produce primarily the cytokines IL-2 and IFN-γ, whereas Th2 effector cells produce the cytokines IL-4, IL-5, IL-6, IL-10, and IL-13 (Mosmann, Cherwinski, Bond, Giedlin, & Coffman, 1986). Preexposure of Th1 clone cells with the β2AR-selective agonist terbutaline before their activation by antigen-presenting B cells decreased IFN-γ production (Sanders et al., 1997). Also, other pharmacological agents that increased the intracellular concentration of cAMP decreased IFN-γ production by Th1 clone cells (Betz & Fox, 1991; Gajewski, Schell, & Fitch, 1990). However, exposure of Th1 clone cells to the β2AR-selective agonist terbutaline either at the time of or after activation with immobilized anti-CD3 antibody induced no change in the amount of IFN-γ produced (Ramer-Quinn et al., 1997). Therefore, in contrast to IL-2 production, the timing of β2AR stimulation on Th1 cells appears to be important to the ability of that cell to produce IFN-γ.

Since CD4+ Th1 effector cells are derived from CD4+ naive T cells, it became important to determine if β2AR-stimulation of these naive cells would affect the development of Th1 effector cells or the ability of the resultant effector cells to produce IFN-γ. Under Th1-promoting culture conditions, naive T cells exposed to either norepinephrine or the β2AR-selective agonist terbutaline developed into Th1 effector cells that produced an increased level of IFN-γ on restimulation (Swanson, Lee, & Sanders, 2000). The ability of norepinephrine to modulate naive T cell differentiation was blocked by the addition of the βAR antagonist nadolol, but not by the αAR antagonist phentolamine, suggesting that norepinephrine stimulated the β2AR expressed on naive cells to influence Th1 cell development. In contrast, under Th2-promoting culture conditions, naive T cells exposed to either norepinephrine or the β2AR-selective agonist terbutaline developed into Th2 cells that produced equivalent amounts of IL-4 as compared with naive cells cultured without βAR stimulation (Swanson, Lee, & Sanders, 2000). Thus, indirect functional data suggest that the β2AR is expressed on CD4+ naive T cells and that stimulation of the receptor may enhance Th1 cell development, without affecting Th2 cell development.

The role of βAR stimulation on Th2 cell cytokine production remains unclear. A recent study showed that in either resting or activated Th2 cell clones, the β2AR-selective agonist terbutaline was unable to modulate the level of IL-4, IL-5, and IL-10 production (Ramer-Quinn et al., 1997; Sanders et al., 1997). Thus, a dichotomy appears to exist in the ability of β2AR stimulation to modulate the development of, and cytokine production by, Th1 cells, but not Th2 effector cells. Additional studies supported the finding that Th1 effector cell cytokines were susceptible to regulation by the elevation of cAMP levels, whereas Th2 effector cell cytokines were not (Betz & Fox, 1991; Gajewski et al., 1990; Katamura et al., 1995; Novak & Rothenberg, 1990; Paliogianni & Boumpas, 1996; Pochet & Delespesse, 1983; Yoshimura et al.,1998). However, other studies showed that cAMP elevation in Th2 cells was able to modulate the level of IL-4 production (Borger, Kauffman, Postma, & Vellenga,

TABLE III Summary of the Evidence for the Presence of Adrenergic Receptors on T Cells[a]

Receptor	Response	Reference
Functional evidence		
βAR agonist	↓ Proliferation induced by either mitogen- or anti-CD3 antibodies	(Hadden et al., 1970; Johnson & Gordon, 1981; Johnson et al., 1981; Bauman et al., 1994; Bartik et al., 1993, 1994; Carlson et al., 1994)
	↓ IL-2R α and β chain expression	(Feldman et al., 1987; Krause & Deutsch, 1991)
	↓ IL-2 production	(Wacholtz et al., 1991; Mary et al., 1989; Bartik et al., 1993, 1994; Ramer-Quinn et al., 1997; Novak & Rothenberg, 1990; Selliah et al., 1995)
	↓ CD8+ cytolytic activity	(Cook-Mills, Mokyr et al., 1995)
β2AR agonist	↓ Proliferation induced by either mitogen- or anti-CD3 antibodies	(Hadden et al., 1970; Johnson & Gordon, 1981; Johnson et al., 1981; Bauman et al., 1994; Bartik et al., 1993, 1994; Carlson et al., 1994
	↓ IL-2 production by CD4+ naive cells	(Ramer-Quinn et al., 2000)
	↓ IL-2 production by CD4+ Th1 clone cells	(Sanders et al., 1997; Ramer-Quinn et al., 1997)
	↓ IFN-γ production by CD4+ Th1 clone if receptor stimulated before cell activation	(Sanders et al., 1997)
	No change in IFN-γ production by CD4+ Th1 clone if receptor stimulated at time of or after cell activation	(Ramer-Quinn et al., 1997)
	↑ IFN-γ production by Th1 effector cells derived from β2AR-stimulated CD4+ naïve cells	(Swanson, Lee, & Sanders, 2000)
	IL-4, IL-5, and IL-10 production unchanged by Th2 clone cells	(Sanders et al., 1997; Ramer-Quinn et al., 1997)
	IL-4 production unchanged by Th2 effector cells derived from β2AR-stimulated CD4+ naive cells	(Swanson, Lee, & Sanders, 2000)
	↑CD8+ cytolytic activity	(Hatfield et al., 1986)
	↓CD8+ cytolytic activity	(Bender et al., 1993)
NE	↓CD8+ cytolytic activity	(Cook-Mills, Mokyr et al., 1995b; Strom et al., 1973)
	↓IL-2 production by CD Th1 clone cells	(Ramer-Quinn et al., 1997)
	No change in IFN-γ production by CD4+ Th1 clone if receptor stimulate at time of or after cell activation	(Ramer-Quinn et al., 1997)
	↑ IFN-γ production by Th1 effector cells derived from β2AR-stimulated CD4+ naive cells	(Swanson, Lee, & Sanders, 2000)
	IL-4, IL-5, and IL-10 production unchanged by Th2 clone cells	(Ramer-Quinn et al., 1997)
	IL-4 production unchanged by Th2 effector cells derived from β2AR-stimulated CD4+ naive cells	(Swanson, Lee, & Sanders, 2000)
NE-depletion in vivo via 6-OHDA	↓ Con A-induced proliferation of splenic and lymph node T cells in vitro	(Madden et al., 1994)
	↓ Con A-induced IL-2 and IFN-γ production by splenic T cells in vitro	(Madden et al., 1994)
	No change in Con A-induced IL-2 and IFN-γ production by lymph node T cells in vitro	(Madden et al., 1994)
	↓ CD8+ cells generated after DTH challenge	(Madden et al., 1989)
Radioligand binding		
βAR	CD4+ = 200 – 750 binding sites/cell CD8+ = 500 – 2500 binding sites/cell	(Williams et al., 1976; Pochet et al., 1979; Bishopric et al., 1980; Loveland et al., 1981; Krawietz et al., 1982; Pochet & Delespesse 1983; Bidart et al., 1983; Khan et al., 1986b; Westly & Kelley 1987; Fuchs, Albright et al., 1988; Van Tits et al., 1990; Radojcic et al., 1991)
β2AR	CD4+ = 200–750 binding sites/cell	(Conolly & Greenacre, 1977; Loveland et al., 1981; Meurs et al., 1982; Sanders et al., 1997; Ramer-Quinn et al., 1997; Bourne & Melmon, 1971; Pochet et al., 1979; Williams et al., 1976)

(Continues)

TABLE III (*Continued*)

Receptor	Response	Reference
	CD4+ Th1 clones = approx. 250 binding sites/cell; Kd = 100 pM	(Sanders et al., 1997; Ramer-Quinn et al., 1997)
	CD4+ Th2 clones = no detectable sites	(Sanders et al., 1997; Ramer-Quinn et al., 1997)
	↑ Binding sites after activation	(Sanders et al., 1985; Radojcic et al., 1991; Westly & Kelley, 1987)
	↑ Binding sites after activation of Th1 clones	(Ramer-Quinn et al., 1997)
	↓ Binding sites after activation	(Cazaux et al., 1995; Radojcic et al., 1991)
Immunofluorescence		
β2AR	CD4+ Th1 clones = low level expression	(Sanders et al., 1997)
	CD4+ Th2 clones = no detectable sites	(Sanders et al., 1997)
RT-PCR	CD4+ Th1 clones and newly-generated cells = β2AR	(Kohm, Swanson, & Sanders, 2000)
	CD4+ Th2 clones and newly-generated cells = no detectable expression	(Kohm, Swanson, & Sanders, 2000)
	CD4+ naive cells = β2AR	(Kohm, Swanson, & Sanders, 2000) (Swanson, Lee, & Sanders, 2000)
Signal transduction		
βAR, β2AR, or NE	↑ cAMP	(Brodde et al., 1984; Pochet et al., 1983; Khan et al., 1986a; Bauman et al., 1994; Makman, 1971; Williams et al., 1976; Conolly & Greenacre, 1977; Bishopric et al., 1980; Bourne & Melmon, 1971)
	↑ cAMP in Th1 clones	(Sanders et al., 1997)
	↑ Adenylate cyclase activity	(Baumen et al., 1984; Bartik et al., 1994)
Receptor-specific gene expression		
βAR or cAMP	↓ mRNA transcript for IL-2	(Chen & Rothenberg, 1994; Tamir & Isakov, 1994)
	↓ Stable protein binding factor interactions with portions of the DNA that are necessary for IL-2 transcription and expression	(Chen & Rothenberg, 1994)
	↓ Phosphatidyl inositol 4,5-bisphosphate hydrolysis	(Tamir & Isakov, 1994)
	↓ Transcription of the *jun* gene	(Tamir & Isakov, 1994)

[a]Data from CD8+ cells will be designated as such, otherwise data reflect CD4+ cells.

R, receptor; IL, interleukin; CD, cluster of designation; IFN, interferon; ConA, concanavalin A; Th, CD4+ T-helper cell; cAMP, adenosine 3′,5′-monophosphate; mRNA, messenger RNA; 6-OHDA, 6-hydroxy dopamine; NE, norepinephrine; DTH, delayed type hypersensitivity.

1996; Crocker, Townley, & Khan, 1996; Lacour et al., 1994; Wirth, Lacour, Jaunin, & Hauser, 1996). Thus, these functional data suggest that murine clones of Th1 cells, but not Th2 cells, express the β2AR, and that the ability of cAMP to modulate Th2 effector cell cytokine production may depend on the manner in which either the Th2 cells are activated or the level of cAMP is attained intracellularly.

In vivo studies indicated that norepinephrine stimulation of the βAR was important for Th1 effector cell-driven responses, such as delayed-type hypersensitivity. When mice were depleted of norepinephrine by chemical sympathectomy before sensitization with 2,4,6-trinitrochlorobenzene (TNCB), they showed decreased ear swelling on challenge with TNCB in comparison to controls (Madden, Felten, Felten, Sundaresan, & Livnat, 1989). An additional study found that splenic T cells from norepinephrine-depleted mice proliferated less and produced less IL-2 and IFN-γ in response to Con A in vitro, but that lymph node cells proliferated less, but produced more IL-2 and IFN-γ (Madden et al., 1994). In light of all the functional data suggesting that Th1 cells express a β2AR, these in vivo data suggest that norepinephrine stimulation of the β2AR may play a role in the generation of Th1 cell-driven cell-mediated immunity.

Studies also have identified expression of the βAR on CD8+ T cells. In the previously mentioned study in which mice were depleted of norepinephrine before sensitization with TNCB, the generation of hapten-specific cytotoxic T cells (CTL) was decreased on challenge with TNCB in comparison to controls (Madden et al., 1989). In vitro studies suggested that stimulation of the β2AR was important for optimal

CD8+ T cell lytic activity (Hatfield, Petersen, & Di Micco, 1986). In contrast, other in vitro studies showed that norepinephrine, epinephrine, the βAR-nonselective agonist isoproterenol (Cook-Mills, Mokyr, Cohen, Perlman, & Chambers, 1995; Strom et al., 1973), or the β2AR-selective agonist metaproterenol (Bender, Bell, Taylor, & Scarpace, 1993) decreased CTL activity. These data were supported by studies utilizing CTL clones that determined that an increase in cAMP inhibited the T cell receptor-dependent release of granules (Takayama, Trenn, & Sitkovsky, 1988). Thus, although the role of β2AR stimulation in modulating CD8+ CTL activities remains uncertain, the data do suggest that the receptor is expressed on CD8+ T cells.

Thus, taken together, these functional data suggest that both CD4+ and CD8+ T cells express the β2AR, but that the receptor may be differentially expressed by subsets of CD4+ cells. Also, stimulation of the β2AR on CD4+ T cells appears to inhibit cytokine production and proliferation, but this inhibitory effect may depend on the cell subset analyzed, the type of activation stimulus used, the time at which the β2AR is stimulated in relation to cell activation, and the intensity/duration of the second messenger signal.

2. *Radioligand Binding and Immunofluorescence*

The ability to enrich for subpopulations of T cells, as well as the ability to clone a specific T cell antigen specificity, has allowed for documentation of the presence of adrenergic receptors on T lymphocytes. Using radioligand binding analysis, the βAR was identified on both human and murine T cells (Bidart, Motte, Assicot, Bohuon, & Bellet, 1983; Bishopric, Cohen, & Lefkowitz, 1980; Fuchs, Albright, & Albright, 1988; Khan, Sansoni, Silverman, Engleman, & Melmon, 1986b; Krawietz et al., 1982; Loveland, Jarrott, & McKenzie, 1981; Pochet & Delespesse, 1983; Pochet, Delespesse, Gausset, & Collet, 1979; Radojcic, Baird, Darko, Smith, & Bulloch, 1991; Van Tits et al., 1990; Westly & Kelley, 1987; Williams, Snyderman, & Lefkowitz, 1976), with most characterized as being of the β2AR subtype (Bourne & Melmon, 1971; Conolly & Greenacre, 1977; Loveland et al., 1981; Meurs, Van Den Bogaard, Kauffman, & Bruynzeel, 1982; Pochet et al., 1979; Ramer-Quinn et al., 1997; Sanders et al., 1997; Williams et al., 1976). Thus far, no radioligand binding data have shown the presence of a high affinity β1AR or β3AR on T cells and, therefore, all previous studies may have reflected the presence of the β2AR. The absolute number of the βAR found per cell varied among the above-mentioned studies, but this variance might be explained by the use of either different T cell isolation techniques; different types of radiolabel, i.e., ^{3}H vs. ^{125}I; pharmacological ligands for which the receptor has differing affinities; or radioligand specific activity. However, on average, there were approximately 500–2500 βAR binding sites per CD8+ T cell, whereas there were approximately 200–750 binding sites per CD4+ T cell.

Resting clones of Th1 effector cells, but not clones of Th2 effector cells, have been shown to express a detectable level of the β2AR using both radioligand binding with iodopindolol and immunofluorescence staining with a polyclonal anti-β2AR antibody directed against the cytoplasmic region of the β2AR (Sanders et al., 1997). This study showed that the Th1 clone cells expressed approximately 250 binding sites/cell with a Kd = 100 pM. A subsequent study showed that following Th effector cell activation by stimulation of the CD3 complex associated with the TcR, the β2AR remained detectable on Th1 clones, but remained undetectable on Th2 clones, and that the β2AR number, but not affinity, may have increased as a function of time after initial activation (Ramer-Quinn et al., 1997). However, the specificity of this antibody is not dependable from batch to batch and care must be taken to perform appropriate positive and negative controls.

Other studies using activated cells showed that the level of β2AR expression on splenic or lymph node T cells either increased (Radojcic et al., 1991; Sanders & Munson, 1985; Westly & Kelley, 1987) or decreased (Cazaux, Sterin-Borda, Gorelik, & Cremaschi, 1995; Radojcic et al., 1991) 24 h after activation with either Con A or PMA/calcium ionophore. Also, after contact sensitization of mice, an increase was found in the level of expression of the βAR on draining lymph node cells (Madden et al., 1989). In contrast, immunization of mice with a Th cell-dependent antigen resulted in a significant decrease in the level of expression of the βAR on unfractionated splenocytes (Fuchs, Campbell, & Munson, 1988; Fuchs, Albright et al., 1988).

Thus, direct radioligand binding data suggest that the β2AR is expressed on CD4+ and CD8+ T cells, that the level of expression is greater on CD8+ cells, and that murine clones of Th1 and Th2 cells may express the receptor differentially.

3. *Northern and RT-PCR*

Confirmation of the presence of the β2AR on a panel of resting and activated Th1 clones, but not on Th2 clones, was confirmed by RT- PCR analysis using primers specific for the β2AR (Kohm, Swanson, &

Sanders, 2000). In addition, RT-PCR analysis showed that naive T cells also expressed the β2AR (Swanson, Lee, & Sanders, 2000). More importantly, recent RT-PCR data show that newly-generated Th1 and Th2 cells from naive cells also differentially express the β2AR (Kohm, Swanson, & Sanders, 2000).

4. *Receptor-Specific Signal Transduction Pathways*

Using CD4+ T cells, studies have shown that stimulation of the βAR with either norepinephrine, epinephrine, the βAR-nonselective agonist isoproterenol, or the β2AR-selective agonist terbutaline increased both the intracellular concentration of cAMP (Bartik et al., 1994; Bishopric et al., 1980; Bourne & Melmon, 1971; Brodde, Daul, & O'Hara, 1984; Conolly & Greenacre, 1977; Khan, Sansoni, Silverman, Engleman, & Melmon, 1986a; Makman, 1971; Pochet & Delespesse, 1983; Williams et al., 1976) and adenylate cyclase activity (Bartik et al., 1994; Bauman et al., 1994). Studies have also shown that an elevation in cAMP inhibited either mitogen- or anti-CD3 antibody-induced T cell proliferation (DeRubertis, Zenser, Adler, & Hudson, 1974; Diamantstein & Ulmer, 1975; Estes, Solomon, & Norton, 1971; Ledbetter et al., 1986; Smith, Steiner, Newberry, & Parker, 1971; Smith, Steiner, & Parker, 1971; Vischer, 1976; Weinstein, Segal, & Melmon, 1975) and, therefore, a βAR-induced increase in cAMP may explain the ability of βAR agonists to inhibit T cell proliferation as described above. In CD4+ T effector cells, the β2AR-selective agonist terbutaline induced an increase in the intracellular concentration of cAMP in clones of Th1 cells, but not in clones of Th2 cells (Sanders et al., 1997). Therefore, these data suggest that T cells express the β2AR and that this receptor is capable of increasing both the intracellular concentration of cAMP and the activity of PKA.

5. *Receptor-Specific Gene Expression*

Studies showed that the βAR-induced decrease in IL-2 production by T cells was occurring at the transcriptional level. Exposure of T cells to an agent that increased the intracellular concentration of cAMP resulted in lower levels of IL-2 mRNA transcript (Chen & Rothenberg, 1994; Tamir & Isakov, 1994). Recent findings have shown that elevations in intracellular cAMP concentration inhibit IL-2 production in Th cells by preventing the maintenance of stable protein binding factor interactions with portions of the DNA that are necessary for IL-2 transcription and expression (Chen & Rothenberg, 1994). Similarly, the elevation of cAMP in T cells activated with either anti-CD3 antibody or PMA/ionomycin decreased phosphatidyl inositol 4,5-bisphosphate hydrolysis, as well as IL-2 and IL-2 receptor expression (Tamir & Isakov, 1994). This study found that the elevation in cAMP interfered with the transcription of the *jun* gene and, therefore, altered the composition of *jun* in the AP-1 complex that binds to the IL-2 promoter site on the DNA, resulting in decreased IL-2 gene transcription.

Thus, taken together, the data suggest that stimulation of the β2AR on a T cell induces intracellular changes that allow for modulation of IL-2 gene expression.

D. B Lymphocyte

A summary of the evidence for the presence of adrenergic receptors on B lymphocytes is presented in Table IV.

1. *Functional Evidence*

Norepinephrine and β2AR stimulation inhibited B cell proliferation induced by LPS (Johnson, Ashmore et al., 1981; Kouassi, Li, Boukhris, Millet, & Revillard, 1988) or antiimmunoglobulin (Ig) antibodies (Holte et al., 1988; Kouassi, Li, & Revillard, 1990). In contrast, norepinephrine and β2AR stimulation has also been shown to enhance LPS-induced B cell proliferation (Kouassi et al., 1990). Similarly, in vitro studies using Th cell-dependent antigens and either norepinephrine, βAR-nonselective agonists, or β2AR-selective agonists to measure Th cell-dependent antibody production showed either an increase (Burchiel & Melmon, 1979a, 1979b; Kouassi et al., 1988; Roper, Conrad, Brown, Warner, & Phipps, 1990; Sanders & Munson, 1984a, 1984b; Sanders & Powell-Oliver, 1992; Shreurs, Versteeg, & Nijkamp, 1982; Stein & Phipps, 1991; Teh & Paetkau, 1976; Watson, Epstein, & Cohn, 1973) or decrease (Besedovsky, Del Rey, Sorkin, Da Prada, & Keller, 1979; Gilbert & Hoffman, 1985; Melmon et al., 1974; Patke, Orson, & Shearer, 1991; Watson et al., 1973). Thus, these data suggest that the β2AR is expressed on B lymphocytes and that β2AR stimulation of these cells may exert either immune enhancement or immune suppression.

However, data indicate that the signaling pathway induced in B cells by either LPS or crosslinking of surface Ig was qualitatively different from the signaling pathway induced in Th cells (Chartash, Imai, Gershengorn, Crow, & Friedman, 1988; Klaus & Parker, 1992). Moreover, another study showed that lower concentrations of cAMP inhibited B cell activation induced by anti-Ig than activation induced by contact with Th cells (Kawakami & Parker, 1993).

These results not only suggested that Ig-dependent cell activation induced different intracellular signaling pathways, but also suggested that these pathways were modulated differently by cAMP. Thus, any results obtained about the ability of individual Th cells and B cells to function following cell activation by mitogens or anti-Ig crosslinking antibodies may not be applicable to understanding the mechanism by which norepinephrine modulates Th cell-dependent B cell activation and antibody production. For these reasons, some researchers chose to study the mechanisms by which activation of the β2AR affect the functioning of both Th cells and B cells when they are stimulated by specific antigen and T cell-B cell interaction during a Th cell-dependent antibody response.

Following the identification of sympathetic nerve in the spleen, of the release of norepinephrine from these nerve terminals, and of the expression of the β2AR on lymphocytes in the spleen (reviewed in Madden, Sanders, & Felten, 1995), studies were designed to determine if Th cell-dependent antibody production was modulated by norepinephrine and β2AR stimulation. In vivo studies using adult rodents depleted of peripheral norepinephrine by 6-hydroxydopamine before antigen exposure showed either a decrease (Ackerman, Madden, Livnat, Felten, & Felten, 1991; Cross et al., 1986; Fuchs, Campbell et al., 1988; Hall et al., 1982; Kasahara, Tanaka, Ito, & Hamashima, 1977; Livnat, Felten, Carlson, Bellinger, & Felten, 1985; Madden et al., 1989) or increase (Besedovsky et al., 1979; Chelmicka-Schorr, Checinski, & Arnason, 1988; Miles, Quintans, Chelmicka-Schorr, & Arnason, 1981) in Th cell-dependent antibody production. Thus, the latter studies in vivo suggest that norepinephrine may be required to obtain an optimal level of antibody production and that either B cells and/or Th cells

TABLE IV Summary of the Evidence for the Presence of Adrenergic Receptors on B Lymphocytes

Receptor	Response	Reference
Functional evidence		
αAR agonist	In vitro - ↑ or ↓ TD antibody production	(Sanders & Munson, 1985; Heilig et al., 1993; Felsner et al., 1995; Besedovsky et al., 1979; Fuchs et al., 1991)
α1AR agonist	In vitro - ↑ TD IgM production	(Sanders & Munson, 1985)
α2AR agonist	In vitro - ↓ TD IgM production	(Sanders & Munson, 1985)
	In vitro - ↓ TD IgM production	(Besedovsky et al., 1979)
βAR agonist	In vitro - ↑ TD antibody production	(Shreurs et al., 1982; Burchiel & Melmon, 1979a, 1979b; Sanders & Munson, 1984a, 1984b; Kouassi et al., 1988; Sanders, & Powell-Oliver, 1992; Watson et al., 1973; Roper et al., 1990; Stein & Phipps, 1991; Teh & Paetkau, 1976)
	In vitro - ↓ TD antibody production	(Besedovsky et al., 1979; Melmon et al., 1974; Watson et al., 1973; Patke et al., 1991; Gilbert & Hoffman, 1985)
β2AR agonist	In vitro - ↓ LPS-induced proliferation	(Kouassi et al., 1990)
	In vitro - ↑ TD antibody production	(Shreurs et al., 1982; Burchiel & Melmon, 1979a, 1979b; Sanders & Munson, 1984a, 1984b; Kouassi et al., 1988; Sanders & Powell-Oliver, 1992; Watson et al., 1973; Roper et al., 1990; Stein & Phipps, 1991; Teh & Paetkau, 1976)
	In vitro - ↓ TD Antibody production	(Besedovsky et al., 1979; Melmon et al., 1974; Watson et al., 1973; Patke et al., 1991; Gilbert & Hoffman, 1985)
	In vitro - ↑ TD IgM production (Th2/B)	(Sanders & Powell-Oliver, 1992)
	In vitro - ↓ TD IgG2a if Th1 only is preexposed to agonist (Th1/B)	(Sanders et al., 1997)
	In vitro - ↑ TD IgG1, IgE if B cell only is preexposed to agonist (Th2/B)	(Kasprowicz et al., 2000)
	In vitro - ↑ B7-2 expression/signaling by B cell	(Kasprowicz et al., 2000)
	In vitro - ↑ IL-4 responsiveness of B cell	(Kasprowicz et al., 2000)
	In vitro - ↑ TD IgG2a, IgG1 if interacting Th1/B or Th2/B cells are exposed to agonist	(Swanson, Lee, & Sanders, 2000)

(Continues)

TABLE IV (*Continued*)

Receptor	Response	Reference
NE	In vitro - ↓ LPS-induced proliferation	(Kouassi et al., 1990)
	In vitro - ↑ TD antibody production	(Shreurs et al., 1982; Burchiel & Melmon, 1979a, 1979b; Sanders & Munson, 1984a, 1984b Kouassi et al., 1988; Sanders & Powell-Oliver, 1992; Watson et al., 1973; Roper et al., 1990; Stein & Phipps, 1991; Teh & Paetkau, 1976)
	In vitro - ↓ TD antibody production	(Besedovsky et al., 1979; Melmon et al., 1974; Watson et al., 1973; Patke et al., 1991; Gilbert & Hoffman 1985)
	In vitro - NE + αAR or βAR antagonists	(Sanders & Munson, 1984a, 1984b)
	In vitro - ↑ TD IgG1, IgE if B cell only is preexposed to agonist (Th2/B + NE + αAR or βAR antagonists)	(Kasprowicz et al., 2000)
	In vivo - ↓ in vitro proliferation of HEL-primed LN cells	(Heilig et al., 1993)
NE-depletion in vivo via 6-OHDA	↓ TD antibody production	(Kasahara et al., 1977; Hall et al., 1982; Livnat et al., 1985; Cross et al., 1986; Fuchs, Campbell et al., 1988; Ackerman et al., 1991; Madden et al., 1989)
	↑ TD antibody production	(Besedovsky et al., 1979; Miles et al., 1981; Chelmicka-Schorr et al., 1988)
	↑ IgG2a and IgG1 in Th1-slanted mouse	(Kruszewska et al., 1995)
	↑ IgG1 in Th2-slanted mouse	Kruszewska et al., 1995)
	↓ IgM and IgG1 primary and secondary response in Th2/B-reconstituted scid mouse	(Kohm & Sanders, 1999)
	↓ IgM and IgG2a primary and secondary response in Th1/B-reconstituted scid mouse	(Kohm & Sanders, 2000)
Radioligand binding		
αAR	Variable results	(Titinchi & Clark, 1984; McPherson & Summers, 1982; Goin et al., 1991)
βAR	Variable results	(Fuchs, Campbell, 1988; Miles et al., 1985; Krawietz et al., 1982; Pochet & Delespesse 1983; Bidart et al., 1983; Miles et al., 1984; Van Tits et al., 1990; Cremaschi et al., 1991)
β2AR	Variable results	(Fuchs, Campbell, 1988a; Krawietz et al., 1982; Pochet & Delespesse, 1983; Kohm & Sanders, 1998b)
Immunofluorescence		
β2AR		(Kohm & Sanders, 1999)
RT-PCR		
β2AR		(Kohm & Sanders, 1999)
Signal transduction		
βAR, β2AR, or NE	↑ cAMP	(Makman, 1971; Williams et al., 1976; Conolly & Greenacre, 1977; Bishopric et al., 1980; Bourne & Melmon, 1971; Pochet & Delepesse,1983; Kohm & Sanders, 1998b)
	↓ anti-Ig-induced phosphatidyl inositol hydrolysis and phosphorylation of the phospholipase C-γ1 subunit	(Blomhoff et al., 1987; Holte et al., 1988; Muthusamy et al., 1991)
	↑ PMA/ionomycin-induced B cell proliferation	(Cohen & Rothstein, 1989; Whisler et al., 1992; Li et al., 1989)
Receptor-specific gene expression		
cAMP	↑ CRE-dependent gene expression	(Xie et al., 1993)

TD, T-cell-dependent; I_g, immunoglobulin; LPS, lipopolysaccharide; IL, interleukin; Th, CD4+ T-helper cell; B, B cell; NE, norepinephrine; HEL, hen eggwhite lysozyme; cAMP, adenosine 3′,5′-monophosphate; PMA, phorbol myristate acetate; CRE, cAMP-responsive element.

that participate in the response may be affected directly by norepinephrine.

To determine the cellular mechanism by which norepinephrine enhances the cell-dependent antibody response in vitro, studies were designed to determine the adrenergic receptor subtype responsible for mediating the norepinephrine-induced enhancing effect. Murine spleen cells were cultured with a Th cell-dependent antigen in the presence of norepinephrine and either the αAR-nonselective antagonist phentolamine or the βAR-nonselective antagonist propranolol (Sanders & Munson, 1984a, 1984b). Cells cultured with either norepinephrine alone or norepinephrine in the presence of the αAR antagonist produced an enhanced number of IgM-secreting cells, whereas cells cultured with norepinephrine in the presence of the βAR antagonist produced a control level of antibody-secreting cells. These findings suggested that the norepinephrine-induced enhancement in IgM production was mediated through stimulation of the βAR. Using either AR-selective antagonists to either the β1AR or the β2AR selective agonist, results indicated that norepinephrine induced a concentration-dependent enhancement in the IgM response through stimulation of the β2AR. These studies also showed that the timing of β2AR stimulation in relation to IgM exposure was important for enhancing the magnitude of the IgM response. Addition of norepinephrine or the β2AR agonist terbutaline at either the time of antigen addition or shortly after the antigen addition enhanced IgM production, whereas the addition of agonist 24 h after antigen resulted in no change in the level of the antibody response in comparison to controls. Also, the norepinephrine-induced enhancement in IgM production was blocked by the addition of a β2AR antagonist during the first 6 h of agonist addition, suggesting that the effects of β2AR stimulation on the B cell were induced during the early stages of the IgM response. However, since this study used whole splenocyte cultures, the results suggested that either the B cell, the Th cell, the macrophage, or all three cell types were affected directly by β2AR stimulation.

Using limiting dilution analysis, cultures containing limiting numbers of murine naive trinitrophenyl (TNP)-specific B cells and nonlimiting numbers of keyhole limpet hemocyanin (KLH)-specific Th2 clone cells in the presence of the antigen TNP-KLH and the β2AR-selective agonist terbutaline showed a two-fold increase in the frequency of B cells that differentiated into IgM-secreting cells, but showed no change in burst size (Sanders & Powell-Oliver, 1992). Although these data suggested that more B cells became capable of differentiating into IgM-secreting cells following exposure to a β2AR agonist, it remained unclear as to whether the B cell, Th2 cell, or both were affected directly by β2AR stimulation. At the time of this study, it was assumed that both the B cell and Th2 cell clone expressed the β2AR. However, a later study showed that the Th2 cell clone, as opposed to the Th1 cell clone, did not express a detectable level of the β2AR in either the resting (Sanders et al., 1997) or activated (Ramer-Quinn et al., 1997) state. Therefore, these findings suggested that in a B cell-Th2 cell clone culture, the B cell may be affected directly by a β2AR-selective agonist, but this remains to be tested.

As part of the experimental design to test the above-mentioned hypothesis, it was found that the timing of β2AR stimulation in relation to Th cell or B cell activation in a Th cell-dependent antibody response appeared to be critical to the final outcome of antibody production. If Th cell exposure to the β2AR-selective agonist terbutaline occurred before activation by an unexposed antigen-presenting B cell, the Th1 or Th2 cell-dependent antibody response was either inhibited or unchanged, respectively (Sanders et al., 1997). However, if B cells were exposed to antigen and terbutaline before their interaction with Th2 cells, but during a time when the B cell was processing the antigen, they produced significantly more IgM, IgG1, and IgE in comparison with control cells (Kasprowicz et al., 2000). Furthermore, the enhancement in Th2 cell-dependent IgG1 and IgE production when β2AR stimulation of the B cell occurred before B cell interaction with a Th2 cell appeared to involve a β2AR-induced increase in B cell responsiveness to IL-4 and B7-2 expression/signaling (Kasprowicz et al., 2000). In contrast, exposure of B cells to antigen and terbutaline before their interaction with untreated Th1 cells did not change the level of either IgM or IgG2a production in comparison to controls. All of the above responses were prevented by the βAR antagonist nadolol. Thus, these data show that stimulation of the β2AR on B cells alone before interaction with either a Th1 or Th2 effector cell subset enhances the production of Th2 cell-dependent IgM, IgG1, and IgE, but does not affect the production of Th1 cell-dependent IgM and IgG2a.

In another study, antigen-specific Th clone cells were allowed to conjugate with antigen-specific B cells and the β2AR-selective agonist terbutaline was added to cultures at specific times after Th cell-B cell interaction. In either a Th1 or Th2 cell-dependent response, IgG2a and IgG1, respectively, were increased when terbutaline was added 12 h after T cell-B cell interaction, whereas no significant change from control was measured when terbutaline was added at other times (Swanson & Sanders, 2000). Again, in the Th2 cell-dependent cultures, it was concluded that the enhancing effect of terbutaline was mediated by the β2AR expressed by the B cell alone, but it remained unknown as to whether the β2AR expressed on either the B cell, Th1 clone cell, or both cells was responsible for mediating the enhancing effect induced by terbutaline.

A recent study in vivo showed that norepinephrine-depletion by chemical sympathectomy in a mouse strain slanted toward a Th1 profile (C57Bl/6) enhanced serum levels of both serum IgG2a and IgG1 after immunization with KLH, whereas in a mouse strain slanted toward a Th2 profile (Balb/c) the level of serum IgG1 was enhanced (Kruszewska, Felten, & Moynihan, 1995). This finding suggested that if norepinephrine was released in vivo, it played a down-modulatory role in Th1- and Th2-dependent antibody production. Although this finding is in contrast to other in vivo and in vitro findings, this study represented the first in vivo model system to address the effect of norepinephrine-depletion on Th1- and Th2 cell-dependent antibody production.

Another study reported a model system that used the severe combined immunodeficient (scid) mouse that was either norepinephrine-intact or norepinephrine-depleted with 6-hydroxydopamine before reconstitution with a murine clone of $\beta 2AR^{neg}$ KLH-specific Th2 clone cells and $\beta 2AR^{pos}$ splenic naive TNP-specific B cells (Kohm & Sanders, 1999). The ability of norepinephrine to maintain optimal Th2 cell-dependent IgM and IgG1 production in norepinephrine-intact reconstituted scid mice was suppressed by administration of the βAR-nonselective antagonist nadolol, but not by the administration of an αAR-selective antagonist phentolamine. Norepinephrine-depletion was found to suppress both IgM and IgG1 production during a primary response to antigen, but only IgG1 production was suppressed during a secondary response to antigen. In addition, the suppressive effect of norepinephrine-depletion on antibody production was partially reversed by the administration of the β2AR-selective agonists terbutaline or metaproterenol. As part of this study, it was found that splenic histology was comparable in norepinephrine-intact and norepinephrine-depleted mice prior to antigen exposure, but that follicle expansion and germinal center formation were suppressed in norepinephrine-depleted mice after antigen exposure in comparison to norepinephrine-intact control mice. Similar results were obtained with scid mice reconstituted with a murine clone of $\beta 2AR^{pos}$-KLH-specific Th1 cells and $\beta 2AR^{pos}$ splenic naive TNP-specific B cells (Kohm & Sanders, 2000). Taken together, these results suggested that norepinephrine stimulation of the β2AR expressed on B cells was necessary for the maintenance of an optimal primary and secondary Th2 cell-dependent antibody response in vivo.

In contrast to the plethora of studies that have examined the effect of norepinephrine and β2AR-selective agonists on B cell responses, few studies have shown an effect induced by norepinephrine that was mediated by stimulation of the αAR (Besedovsky et al., 1979; Felsner et al., 1995; Fuchs, McCall, & Munson, 1991; Heilig, Irwin, Grewal, & Sercarz, 1993; Sanders & Munson, 1985). In addition, norepinephrine suppressed the in vitro proliferation of hen eggwhite lysozyme (HEL)-primed lymph node (LN) cells through stimulation of the αAR by norepinephrine in vivo (Heilig et al., 1993). However, in this model system, amphetamine was used to stimulate the release of norepinephrine from sympathetic nerve terminals 9 days following antigen exposure. Thus, stimulation of the αAR during a later stage of the antibody response, as opposed to an early stage of the response, may provide a mechanism to limit the primary antibody response. In addition, in vitro studies by this same group suggested that addition of an αAR-nonselective agonist inhibited the ability of LN cells to proliferate. However, in both the in vitro and in vivo experiments described above, macrophages were present and were exposed to the chemical manipulations. Since macrophages have been reported to express the αAR, and since adrenergic receptor stimulation has been reported to suppress macrophage cell function (Brown et al., 1991), the results reported may not reflect a direct effect from norepinephrine stimulation of the αAR on T or B lymphocytes, but may reflect an indirect effect due to norepinephrine stimulation of the αAR expressed on the macrophage, perhaps to change a macrophage function that influenced the ability of T cells to proliferate or produce cytokines.

Thus, indirect functional evidence suggests that the β2AR is expressed on B lymphocytes and that stimulation of the receptor may either enhance or suppress B cell function. On the other hand, the functional data also suggest that the α1AR is expressed on bone marrow cells and that stimulation of this receptor may suppress myelopoiesis and enhance lymphopoiesis.

2. *Radioligand Binding and Immunofluorescence*

Using radioligand binding analysis, B cells were shown to express a higher level of the βAR than CD4+ Th cells (Bidart et al., 1983; Cremaschi, Fisher, & Boege, 1991; Fuchs, Albright et al., 1988; Krawietz et al., 1982; Miles, Atweh, Otten, Arnason, & Chelmicka-Schorr, 1984; Miles, Chelmicka-Schorr,

Atweh, Otten, & Arnason, 1985; Pochet & Delespesse, 1983; Van Tits et al., 1990). A few studies also showed that the AR expressed by the B cell was of the β2AR subtype (Fuchs, Albright et al., 1988; Krawietz et al., 1982; Pochet & Delespesse, 1983). Expression of the β2AR on murine naive TNP-specific B cells was confirmed recently using both radioligand binding with iodopindolol and immunofluorescence staining with a polyclonal anti-β2AR antibody directed against the cytoplasmic region of the β2AR (Kohm & Sanders, 1999).

Few radioligand binding studies have shown the presence of the αAR on B cells (Goin et al., 1991; McPherson & Summers, 1982; Titinchi & Clark, 1984). However, the results from these studies may be misleading since αAR-expressing platelets were not removed from lymphocyte samples and, therefore, may have complicated the interpretation of binding results. Thus, the most convincing radioligand binding data suggest that the β2AR is expressed on B lymphocytes.

3. *Northern and RT-PCR*

The presence of the β2AR on an enriched population of B cell was confirmed by RT-PCR analysis using primers specific for the β2AR (Kohm & Sanders, 1999). Thus, molecular data indicate that the β2AR is expressed by B lymphocytes.

4. *Receptor-Specific Signal Transduction Pathways*

Studies have shown that either βAR, β2AR, or norepinephrine stimulation on B cells enhanced the intracellular concentration of cAMP (Bishopric et al., 1980; Bourne & Melmon, 1971; Conolly & Greenacre, 1977; Kohm & Sanders, 1998a; Makman, 1971; Pochet & Delespesse, 1983; Williams et al., 1976). cAMP levels were also shown to increase intracellularly following exposure of naive TNP-specific B cells to the β2AR-selective agonist terbutaline (Kohm & Sanders, 1999). In one study, stimulation of the β2AR by terbutaline induced an increase in B7-2 expression that was inhibited in the presence of a PKA inhibitor, suggesting that the induction of B7-2 by stimulation of the β2AR on a B cell required cAMP-dependent activation of PKA (Kasprowicz & Sanders, 2000).

Likewise, stimulation of the β2AR and/or elevation of cAMP inhibited B cell proliferation induced by LPS (Diamantstein & Ulmer, 1975; Vischer, 1976) or antiimmunoglobulin antibodies (Blomhoff et al., 1987; Cohen & Rothstein, 1989; Muthusamy, Baluyut, & Subbarao, 1991; Whisler, Beiqing, Grants, & Newhouse, 1992) by mechanisms that involved an inhibition of early biochemical events, such as phosphatidyl inositol hydrolysis and phosphorylation of the phospholipase C-γ1 subunit (Blomhoff et al., 1987; Holte et al., 1988; Muthusamy et al., 1991). In contrast, other studies showed that activation of the β2AR and elevation of cAMP enhanced PMA/ionomycin-induced B cell proliferation (Cohen & Rothstein, 1989; Li, Kouassi, & Revillard, 1989; Whisler et al., 1992) but did not affect any earlier cell biochemistry (Li et al., 1989).

Thus, intracellular signaling data suggest that stimulation of the β2AR on B lymphocytes elevates the level of cAMP intracellularly.

5. *Receptor-Specific Gene Expression*

We were unable to find any specific studies that reported β2AR-specific gene expression in the B cell. However, one study showed that the transcription factor CREB was present in resting B cells and that CRE-dependent gene expression was synergistically regulated by B cell activation through both stimulation of the immunoglobulin receptor and an elevation in cAMP (Xie, Chiles, & Rothstein, 1993).

E. Macrophages

A summary of the evidence for the presence of adrenergic receptors on macrophages is presented in Table V.

1. *Functional Evidence*

Antigen encounter triggers a series of events in pulmonary macrophages, including the rapid consumption of oxygen and the generation of superoxide anions (O_2^-) and hydrogen peroxide. Although these events are used to combat foreign organisms, they were also shown to result in immunosuppression (Henricks, Verhoef, & Nijkamp, 1986). Studies using a β1AR- and a β2AR-selective agonist showed that the β1AR suppressed the production of H_2O_2 and other reactive oxygen species by macrophages (Henricks, van Esch, Van Oosterhout, & Nijkamp, 1988; Schopf & Lemmel, 1983). However, since the β1AR-induced suppression was not blocked by a βAR antagonist, it was likely that this suppressive effect was not induced by β1AR stimulation, but alternatively, that the agonist functioned as a scavenger of reactive oxygen species (Henricks et al., 1988). Despite this finding, other functional studies using human peritoneal macrophages exposed to catecholamines showed that the β2AR stimulation suppressed the generation of superoxide anions (O_2^-) and hydrogen peroxide (Fukushima et al., 1993), whereas a study of bovine pulmonary alveolar macrophages exposed to β1AR-

TABLE V Summary of the Evidence for the Presence of Adrenergic Receptors on Macrophages

Receptor	Response	Reference
Functional evidence		
αAR agonist	↑ phagocytosis ↑ LPS-induced TNF production	(Koff & Dunegan, 1985; Javierre et al., 1975) (Spengler et al., 1994; Balter & Schwartz, 1977)
α1AR agonist	↑ Production of complement cascade components	(Lappin & Whaley, 1982)
α2AR agonist	↑ TNF production ↓ Antimycobacterial activity	(Spengler et al., 1990) (Miles et al., 1996)
α2AR antagonist	In vitro - ↓ TNF production In vitro - ↑ antimycobacterial activity	(Ignatowski et al., 1996) (Miles et al., 1996)
βAR agonist	No effect on O_2^- generation ↑ Adhesiveness ↓ Phagocytosis ↓ LPS-induced TNF production	(Fuller et al., 1988) (Issaad et al., 1989) (Abrass et al., 1985; Serio et al., 1996) (Szabo et al., 1997)
β1AR agonist	↓ O_2^- and H_2O_2 generation ↓ H_2O_2 generation, but no effect on phagocytic ability	(Conlon et al., 1988) (Henricks et al., 1986)
β2AR agonist	↓ O_2^- and H_2O_2 generation No effect on H_2O_2 generation or phagocytosis No effect on O_2^- generation, but ↓ phagocytosis ↓ phagocytosis In vivo - ↓ phagocytosis	(Fukushima et al., 1993; Beusenberg et al., 1989) (Henricks et al., 1986) (Capelli et al., 1993) (Abrass et al., 1985) (Petty & Berg, 1988; Abrass et al., 1985)
NE	In vitro - ↓ LPS-induced TNF production	(Hjemdahl et al., 1990)
NE-depletion in vivo via 6-OHDA	↓ TNF production	(Chelmicka-Schorr et al., 1992a, 1992b)
Radioligand binding		
α2AR		(Spengler et al., 1990)
βAR	Binding sites = 1000; Kd = 50 pM	(Abrass et al., 1985; Rosati et al., 1986; Liggett, 1989; Hjemdahl et al., 1990)
β2AR	Binding sites = 23,000; Kd = 800 pM	(Henricks et al., 1988; van Esch et al., 1989)
Signal transduction		
α1AR agonist	↑ Activation of phospholipase C ↑ Activation of Ca2+ dependent K+ channel	(Hara et al., 1991) (Hara et al., 1991)
βAR, β2AR, or NE	↑ cAMP	(Weissman et al., 1971; Abrass et al., 1985; Higgins & David, 1976; Welscher & Cruchaud, 1976; Ikegami, 1977; Lavis et al., 1980; Rosati et al., 1986; Verghese & Snyderman 1983; Liggett, 1989; van Esch et al., 1989; Beusenberg et al., 1989)
	↑ Adenylate cyclase activity ↓ Activation of Ca2+ dependent K+ channels	(Beusenberg et al., 1990) (Rosati et al., 1986)
Receptor-specific gene expression		
βAR agonist	↓ LPS-induced TNF mRNA production	(Ignatowski et al., 1995)
αAR agonist	↑ LPS-induced TNF production	(Spengler et al., 1994)
α2AR agonist	↑ LPS-induced TNF mRNA production	(Spengler et al., 1990)

LPS, lipopolysaccharide; TNF, tumor necrosis factor; H_2O_2, hydrogen peroxide; O_2^-, oxygen free radical; Kd, dissociation constant; Ca ++, calcium ion; cAMP, adenosine 3′,5′-monophosphate; mRNA, messenger RNA.

and β2AR-selective agonists and antagonists showed that both β1AR and β2AR stimulation suppressed the ability of these cells to produce reactive oxygen species (Conlon et al., 1988). Likewise, exposure of alveolar macrophages to the βAR-nonselective agonist isoprenaline and the β1AR-selective agonist dobutamine decreased the PMA-induced production of hydrogen peroxide, whereas exposure to the β2AR-selective agonist salbutamol had no effect, and exposure to either agonist had no effect on phagocytic activity (Henricks, van Esch, & Nijkamp, 1986). In contrast, the βAR-nonselective agonist isoprenaline did not affect zymosan-induced activation or superoxide production by human alveolar macrophages (Fuller, O'Malley, Baker, & MacDermot, 1988) and the β2AR-selective agonists formoterol and salbutamol did not change the basal level of O_2^- production of human alveolar macrophages, but suppressed the phagocytic index (Capelli et al., 1993). Thus, indirect functional evidence suggests that both the β1AR and the β2AR are expressed on macrophages and that stimulation of the receptors may induce different effects on the production of H_2O_2 and other reactive oxygen species, depending on the macrophage type being stimulated.

Macrophages perform both microbicidal and tumoricidal activities through a variety of mechanisms besides the generation of reactive oxygen species, including phagocytosis and secretion of regulatory proteins, such as TNF (Balter & Schwartz, 1977). A βAR-nonselective agonist enhanced the adhesive properties of macrophages (Issaad, Ventura, & Thomopoulos, 1989), whereas the β2AR-selective agonist metaproterenol resulted in a suppression of phagocytic activity (Abrass, O'Connor, Scarpace, & Abrass, 1985). Likewise, stimulation of the βAR on macrophages inhibited the ability of cells to phagocytose (Abrass et al., 1985; Serio et al., 1996) and the ability of Ca2+ dependent K+ channels to function (Rosati, Hannaert, Dausse, Braquet, & Garay, 1986). Norepinephrine, epinephrine, and the βAR-nonselective agonist isoproterenol suppressed the LPS-induced increase in TNF production by rat spleen macrophages (Hjemdahl, Larsson, Johansson, Zetterlund, & Eklund, 1990). In contrast, although βAR stimulation suppressed TNF production in murine macrophages, an αAR-nonselective agonist and an α2AR-selective agonist enhanced LPS-induced TNF production by murine macrophages at both the message and protein level (Spengler, Chensue, Giacherio, Blenk, & Kunkel, 1994; Spengler, Allen, Remick, Strieter, & Kunkel, 1990). In vivo, a β2AR antagonist suppressed the phagocytic activity of mouse peritoneal macrophages to phagocytose (Abrass et al., 1985; Petty & Berg, 1988), whereas macrophages from chemically sympathectomized mice were suppressed in their ability to produce TNF (Chelmicka-Schorr, Kwasniewski, & Czlonkowska, 1992a,1992b). Furthermore, exposure of macrophages to low concentrations of norepinephrine resulted in enhanced macrophage phagocytosis and tumoricidal activity, suggesting the involvement of the αAR (Koff & Dunegan, 1985). Likewise, the αAR agonists metaraminol and phenylephrine, as well as norepinephrine, increased the phagocytic activity of peritoneal macrophages (Javierre, Pinto, Lima, & Sassine, 1975). Additional studies also suggested that stimulation of the α1AR on macrophages induced the production of components of the complement cascade (Lappin & Whaley, 1982). Thus, these data suggest that the β2AR and α2AR are expressed on macrophages and that β2AR stimulation of these cells may exert a suppressive effect on TNF and phagocytic activity, whereas α2AR stimulation may exert a positive effect.

As a result of extraneuronal uptake, macrophages have been shown to produce low levels of endogenous norepinephrine and epinephrine, 624 ± 120 and 284 ± 58 pg/10^8 cells, respectively, that decreased by approximately 50% following LPS-stimulation (Spengler et al., 1994). This finding may explain the report showing that the addition of either an αAR or a βAR antagonist alone to cultures of macrophages had the opposite effect on TNF production AR agonists (Balter & Schwartz, 1977). Also, another study showed that the antimycobacterial activity of mouse peritoneal macrophages against the growth of *Myobacterium avium* was inhibited by the α2AR agonist clonidine, but enhanced by the α2AR antagonist (Miles, Lafuse, & Zwilling, 1996). Interestingly, exposure of macrophages to both αAR and βAR antagonists further enhanced the antimycobacterial activity of macrophages (Miles et al., 1996). In addition, the α2AR antagonist yohimbine suppressed LPS-induced TNF production (Ignatowski, Gallant, & Spengler, 1996), suggesting, together with the previous result, that catecholamines may be taken up by macrophages and then released to serve an autoregulatory role during an immune response.

In general, however, the indirect functional data suggest that the β2AR and the α2AR are expressed on macrophages and that β2AR stimulation suppresses macrophage activity, whereas α2AR stimulation enhances macrophage activity.

2. *Radioligand Binding*

Functional evidence suggested the presence of adrenergic receptors on macrophages, but the first direct demonstration of the presence of adrenergic receptors on mouse peritoneal macrophages was made using insolubilized catecholamines (Nowell, Cruse, & Lewis, 1981). Radioligand binding analysis using the tritiated α2AR-selective antagonist yohimbine showed the presence of the α2AR on murine macrophages (Spengler et al., 1990). Radioligand binding studies on rat peritoneal macrophage using [^{125}I]-cyanopindolol showed the presence of the βAR at approximately 1,000 binding sites per cell with a Kd of 50 pM (Abrass et al., 1985). The radioligand binding curves followed the typical order of potency reported for the βAR with propranolol > isoproterenol > epinephrine > norepinephrine. However, this order of potency was not observed when using rat splenic macrophages or murine spleen lymphocytes (Hu, Goldmuntz, & Brosnan, 1991), suggesting that differences existed in AR subtype expression by macrophages, depending on their location and species of origin (Petty & Berg, 1988; Young, Ko, & Cohn, 1984). Rat (Abrass et al., 1985), mouse (Rosati et al., 1986), and human (Hjemdahl et al., 1990; Liggett, 1989) peritoneal macrophages have been shown to express the βAR using [^{125}I]-cyanopindolol. Guinea pig alveolar macrophages show expression of only the β2AR and at a very high number of 23,000 and a Kd of 800 pM (Henricks, van Esch, et al., 1988; van Esch, Henricks, Van Oosterhout, & Nijkamp, 1989). Thus, direct radioligand binding data suggest that the β2AR and the α2AR are expressed on macrophages.

3. *Receptor-Specific Signal Transduction Pathways*

Early studies performed in the 1970s first suggested the presence of the AR on guinea pig peritoneal macrophages by showing that catecholamines were able to increase both adenylate cyclase activity and the intracellular concentration of cAMP (Remold-O'Donnell, 1974). Other studies followed to show that intracellular cAMP levels were elevated in murine, rat, guinea pig, and human macrophages following exposure to catecholamines, βAR-nonselective agonists, and β2AR-selective agonists (Abrass et al., 1985; Higgins & David, 1976; Ikegami, 1977; Lavis, Strada, Ross, Hersh, & Thompson, 1980; Liggett 1989; Rosati et al., 1986; Verghese & Snyderman, 1983; Welscher & Cruchaud, 1976).

In addition, exposure of guinea pig alveolar macrophages to either the βAR-nonselective agonist isoproterenol or the β2AR-selective agonist salbutamol increased intracellular cAMP concentration in these cells from control levels of 7 pmol to 28 pmol and 14 pmol, respectively (van Esch et al., 1989). Both isoprenaline and salbutamol induced a concentration-dependent increase in cAMP levels in guinea pig and human alveolar macrophages, with cAMP levels two to threefold higher than controls at 10^{-6} M (Beusenberg, Adolfs, van Schaik-van Groningen, Hoogsteden, & Bonta, 1989). Likewise, both isoprenaline and salbutamol increased adenylyl cyclase activity in human alveolar macrophages in a concentration-dependent manner from 10^{-8}–10^{-4} M (Beusenberg, Van Amsterdam, van Schaik, Hoogsteden, & Bonta, 1990).

Also, stimulation of the βAR on macrophages inhibited activation of Ca2+ dependent K+ channels (Rosati et al., 1986). Stimulation of the α1AR on the macrophage activated the Ca2+ dependent K+ channel via the mobilization of intracellular Ca2+ stores, presumably via the activation of phospholipase C via a G-protein dependent mechanism (Hara, Ichinose, Sawada, & Maeno, 1991). The activation of Ca++-dependent K+ channels has been implicated in modulation of macrophage phagocytic activity and this may be the mechanism responsible for the αAR-induced enhancement in macrophage phagocytic activity (Young et al., 1984).

Thus, intracellular signaling data suggest that stimulation of the β2AR on macrophages elevates the level of cAMP, whereas stimulation of the αAR may affect intracellular Ca++ levels. To date, we have found no data to indicate the signal transduction pathway activated after stimulation of the α2AR on macrophages.

4. *Receptor-Specific Gene Expression*

The βAR-nonselective agonist isoproterenol suppressed LPS-induced TNF mRNA accumulation and production by macrophages (Ignatowski & Spengler, 1995), suggesting that βAR stimulation reduced TNF gene expression. An α2AR-selective agonist enhanced LPS-induced TNF production by murine macrophages at both the message and protein level (Spengler et al., 1990). Stimulation of the αAR increased LPS-induced TNF production and gene expression in murine macrophages, whereas βAR stimulation was suppressive (Spengler et al., 1994). However, the molecular mechanisms involved in the pathway from βAR and αAR stimulation to gene expression remain unknown.

F. Natural Killer Cells

A summary of the evidence for the presence of adrenergic receptors on natural killer (NK) cells is presented in Table VI.

1. *Functional Evidence*

Exposure of NK cells in vitro to either norepinephrine, epinephrine, or the βAR-nonselective agonist isoproterenol decreased NK cell lytic activity (Hellstrand, Hermodsson, & Strannegard, 1985; Maisel, Harris, Rearden, & Michel, 1990; Takamoto et al., 1991; Whalen & Bankhurst, 1990). One of these studies found that pretreatment of NK cells with

TABLE VI Summary of the Evidence for the Presence of Adrenergic Receptors on Natural Killer Cells

Receptor	Response	Reference
Functional evidence		
βAR agonist	In vitro - ↓ lytic activity	(Takamoto et al., 1991; Whalen & Bankhurst, 1990; Hellstrand et al., 1985; Maisel et al., 1990)
	In vitro - ↑ lytic activity if before target cell addition; ↓ if after target cell addition	(Hellstrand et al., 1985; Takamoto et al., 1991)
β2AR agonist	In vitro - ↓ lytic activity	(Maisel et al., 1990)
	In vitro - ↑ lytic activity	(Schedlowski et al., 1996; Murray et al., 1992)
	In vitro - ↓ adhesion to endothelial cells	(Benschop et al., 1997; Benschop et al., 1994)
	In vivo - ↓ lytic activity	(Shakhar & Ben-Eliyahu, 1998)
	In vivo - ↑ tumor metastasis	(Shakhar & Ben-Eliyahu, 1998)
	In vivo - ↓ lytic activity	(Irwin et al., 1988, 1990).
βAR antagonist	In vivo - ↓ stress or exercise-induced increase of NK cells in circulation	(Bachen et al., 1995)
NE-depletion in vivo via 6-OHDA	↑ Tumor metastasis, but no change in NK lytic activity	(Brenner et al., 1992)
Radioligand binding		
α1AR	Approximately 700 sites/cell	(Jetschmann et al., 1997)
α2AR	Approximately 400 sites/cell	(Jetschmann et al., 1997)
βAR	Approximately 200 sites/cell	(Van Tits et al., 1990)
β2AR	Approximately 1400 sites/cell	(Jetschmann et al., 1997)
Signal transduction		
βAR, β2AR, or NE	↑ cAMP	(Benschop et al., 1993)

NK, natural killer cell; cAMP, adenosine 3′,5′-monophosphate.

epinephrine, followed by removal of the adrenergic stimulus before the addition of target cells, increased cytolytic activity (Hellstrand et al., 1985). In contrast, adrenergic stimulation during the incubation of NK cells with target cells decreased NK-specific cytolytic activity (Hellstrand et al., 1985; Takamoto et al., 1991). In a later study, the β2AR was implicated as the adrenergic receptor responsible for mediating the suppressive effect of epinephrine since the β2AR-selective agonist terbutaline also decreased NK lytic activity (Maisel et al., 1990). However, β2AR stimulation of NK cells also has been reported to increase NK lytic activity, but the increase was transient and returned to control levels within 1 h (Murray et al., 1992; Schedlowski et al., 1996). Thus, indirect functional evidence suggests that the β2AR is expressed on NK cells and that stimulation of the receptor may either enhance or suppress NK cell lytic activity.

Additional in vitro studies determined that β2AR stimulation on NK cells suppressed their ability to adhere to cultured endothelial cells (Benschop, Nijkamp, Ballieux, & Heijnen, 1994; Benschop, Schedlowski, Wienecke, Jacobs, & Schmidt, 1997) These data may explain the ability of in vivo administered norepinephrine, epinephrine, or a βAR-specific agonist to increase the number of NK cells found in the circulation (Shakhar & Ben-Eliyahu, 1998; Schedlowski et al., 1996; Van Tits et al., 1990). Acute stress or exhaustive exercise that would increase circulating catecholamine levels also increased the number of NK cells in the circulation (Bachen et al., 1995; Benschop et al., 1994; Marsland et al., 1995; Murray et al., 1992) and this increase was blocked by preexposure to a β2AR-selective antagonist (Bachen et al., 1995), but not a β1AR-selective antagonist (Murray et al., 1992). Thus, these in vitro and in vivo data suggest that stimulation of a β2AR on NK cells decreases their ability to adhere to endothelial cells and, therefore, keeps these cells in the circulation and prevents their rapid localization to the site of infection.

In rats exposed to a βAR agonist, NK cell lytic activity was decreased ex-vivo and the ability of rats to inhibit the growth and metastasis of a NK-sensitive tumor was suppressed in vivo (Shakhar & Ben-Eliyahu, 1998). This finding was confirmed using NK-depleted mice that showed no difference in their susceptibility to tumor challenge in either the presence or absence of exposure to the β2AR-selective agonist metaproterenol (Shakhar & Ben-Eliyahu, 1998). Another study showed that mice depleted of norepinephrine and responding to tumor challenge had an increased number of metastases, but no change in NK cell lytic activity (Brenner, Felten, Felten, & Moynihan, 1992). Also, it was shown in vivo that CRH-induced activation of the sympathetic nervous system led to a β2AR-mediated decrease in NK cell lytic activity (Irwin, Hauger, Brown, & Britton, 1988; Irwin, Hauger, Jones, Provencio, & Britton, 1990). Thus, these data suggest that the β2AR-induced decrease in NK lytic activity in vivo results in an increase in tumor metastasis.

2. *Radioligand Binding*

Using radioligand binding, an early study determined that NK cells expressed the βAR (Van Tits et al., 1990), whereas a more recent study confirmed that CD16+ NK cells expressed the α1AR, α2AR, and β2AR (Jetschmann et al., 1997). The latter study also determined that administration of epinephrine decreased the level of β2AR receptor expression on NK cells.

3. *Receptor-Specific Signal Transduction Pathways*

The β2AR-induced decrease in the ability of NK cells to adhere to cultured endothelial cells was shown to be cAMP dependent (Benschop, Oostveen, Heijnen, & Ballieux, 1993).

Taken together, these studies show that NK cells express predominantly the β2AR and that stimulation of this receptor induces an accumulation of cAMP that suppresses NK cell activity.

III. CHOLINERGIC RECEPTORS

In this section, we have attempted to summarize more recent studies addressing the presence of cholinergic receptors on immune cells. We refer the reader to the following review that discusses the earlier work in this area of research (Qiu, Peng, & Wang, 1996). A summary of the more recent evidence for the presence of cholinergic receptors on immune cells is presented in Table VII.

A. Acetylcholine Synthesis by Immune Cells

Before summarizing the functional data that suggest the presence of cholinergic receptors on immune cells, it is important to emphasize that immune cells possess the enzyme choline acetyltransferase that is involved in acetylcholine synthesis and that acetylcholine appears to be synthesized and released by certain immune cells, particularly T cells. If these data are accurate, then previous data using cholinergic receptor antagonists must be reexamined and reinterpreted. Using RT-PCR, choline acetyltransferase mRNA was found to be expressed in PHA-activated human mononuclear lymphocytes (Fujii et al., 1998), PHA-activated human leukemic T cell lines (Kawashima, Fujii, Watanabe, & Misawa, 1998), and PHA-activated leukemic T cell lines and leukemic lymphoblastoid Th line Jurkat (Fujii et al., 1996). Choline acetyltransferase protein was also expressed in these cells (Fujii et al., 1996; Rinner et al., 1995) and acetylcholine was released (Kawashima, Fujii, Watanabe, & Misawa, 1998; Fujii et al., 1996). Thus, T lymphocytes appear to synthesize and release acetylcholine, which may play an autoregulatory role during an immune response.

B. Functional Evidence

In vitro exposure of rat thymocytes to the cholinergic receptor nonselective agonist carbachol induced apoptosis (Yamada, Murayama, & Nomura, 1997), whereas carbachol reduced the level of thymocyte apoptosis induced by culturing them with thymic epithelial cell lines (Rinner et al., 1995). When thymocytes were collected from rats exposed in vivo to the acetylcholine degradation inhibitor physostigmine, there was no change in thymocyte apoptosis; whereas, thymocytes collected from rats exposed to physostigmine in combination with the muscarinic receptor antagonist atropine showed an increased level of apoptosis and a decreased number of CD3+ cells (Rinner et al., 1995). In the same study, spleen cells collected from rats exposed in vivo to the acetylcholine degradation inhibitor physostigmine and activated in vitro with Con A showed no change in their ability to proliferate when compared with control rat cells; whereas, spleen cells from rats exposed to physostigmine in combination with the muscarinic receptor antagonist atropine showed a decreased ability to proliferate (Rinner et al., 1995). Pretreatment of human peripheral blood CD3+ T cells with the muscarinic-1 subtype (M1)-selective agonist oxotremorine increased PHA-induced IL-2 mRNA, IL-2 protein, IL-2R α- and β-chain mRNA, but not IL-2R α- and β-chain protein (Fujino, Kitamura, Yada, Uehara, & Nomura, 1997), but did not increase the level of expression of any other surface molecule (Fujino et al., 1997). Taken together, these studies suggest that thymocytes and mature CD3+ peripheral blood T cells express the muscarinic receptor and

TABLE VII Summary of the Evidence for the Presence of Cholinergic Receptors on Immune Cells

Receptor	Response	Reference
Functional evidence		
M agonist	In vitro - ↑ thymocyte apoptosis	(Yamada et al., 1997)
	In vitro - ↓ thymocyte apoptosis	(Rinner et al., 1995)
M1 agonist	In vitro - increased PHA-induced IL-2 mRNA and IL-2 protein in huPBL	(Fujino et al., 1997)
	In vitro - ↑ IL-2R α- and β-chain mRNA, but no change in IL-2R α- and β-chain protein in huPBL	(Fujino et al., 1997)
	In vitro - no change in other molecules on huPBL	(Fujino et al., 1997)
	↑ Secretion rate of IgG	(Brink et al., 1994)
Physostigmine - Ach degradation inhibitor	In vivo - no change in thymocyte apoptosis	(Rinner et al., 1995)
	In vivo - no change in thymocyte proliferation	(Rinner et al., 1995)
	↓ Serum IL-6	(Rinner et al., 1995)
Physostigmine + M antagonist	In vivo - ↑ thymocyte apoptosis	(Rinner et al., 1995)
	In vivo - ↓ number thymocyte CD3+ cells	(Rinner et al., 1995)
	In vivo - ↓ thymocyte proliferation	(Rinner et al., 1995)
Radioligand binding		
Muscarinic	↑ Number on rat thymocytes by electrolytic lesion in anterior hypothalamus	(Guschin et al., 1994)
	Murine number on CD8+ > CD4+	(Genaro et al., 1993)
	Murine B, none detectable	(Genaro et al., 1993)
	Human peripheral blood lymphocytes; 57–127 sites/cell; Kd = 45–133 pM	(Meurs et al., 1993)
M1 and M3	Rat thymocytes = 3000 with a Kd of 80 nM	(Yamada et al., 1997)
	↑ Number on rat thymocytes by hydrocortisone	(Yamada et al., 1997)
M2, M3, and M4	Bursa of Fabricius in pigeons; 38 fmol/mg protein; Kd = 0.31 nM	(Ricci et al., 1996)
	Human peripheral blood lymphocytes; 2.33 fmol/2 × 10^6 cells; Kd = 0.6 nM	(Bronzetti et al., 1996)
M3	Jurkat = 45,000 sites/cell; Kd = 14.1 nM	(Kaneda et al., 1993)
Northern and RT-PCR		
M3	Human Jurkat cell line	(Kaneda et al., 1993)
	Rat PBML	(Costa, Castoldi et al., 1994; Costa, Traver, 1994)
M3 and M5	Human leukemic line Peer	(Hellstrom-Lindahl & Nordberg, 1996)
M3, M4, and M5	Human PBML	(Costa et al., 1995)
	Human T	(Hellstrom-Lindahl & Nordberg, 1996)
	Human B	(Hellstrom-Lindahl & Nordberg, 1996)
M4	Rat T and B	(Costa, Castoldi, 1994; Costa Traver, 1994a)
M4 and M5	Human leukemic line HL-60	(Hellstrom-Lindahl & Nordberg 1996)
Signal transduction		
Muscarinic agonist	↑ IP3, [Ca++]I from intracellular stores	(Laskowska-Bozek et al., 1995, 1996)
	CD8+ - ↑ cGMP and IP3	(Genaro et al., 1993)
	CD4+ - no change cGMP and IP3	(Genaro et al., 1993)
	↑ [Ca++] from voltage-dependent Ca++ channel	(Brink et al., 1994)
M1 agonist	↑ Activation of phospholipase C, protein kinase C, c-Raf-1	(Siegel et al., 1993)
M3 agonist	↑ Phospholipase C and IP3	(Kaneda et al., 1993)

PHA, phytohemaglutinin; mRNA, messenger RNA; IL, interleukin; huPBL, human peripheral blood lymphocytes; CD, cluster of designation; Ig, immunoglobulin; Kd, dissociation constant; PBML, peripheral blood mononuclear leukocytes; T, T cell; B, B cell; IP, inositol phosphate; Ca++, calcium ion; cGMP, guanosine 3′,5′-monophosphate.

that stimulation of the receptor maintains cell viability and the proliferative capacity of these cells in vivo.

The ability of B cells to respond to cholinergic receptor stimulation was shown in a study in which the cholinergic nonselective agonist carbachol increased the secretion rate of IgG by exposed avian lacrimal gland plasma cells (Brink et al., 1994). On the other hand, no change in the murine primary humoral response was seen in mouse lymphocytes exposed to cholinergic agonists (Pruett, Han, Munson, & Fuchs, 1992). In a study in which rats were exposed in vivo to LPS and the acetylcholine degradation inhibitor physostigmine showed a suppression in the serum level of IL-6 that was blocked by the presence of the muscarinic receptor antagonist atropine (Rinner et al., 1995). Thus, a limited amount of functional data suggest that B cells and macrophages may express the muscarinic receptor, but the functional relevance of the stimulation of this receptor on these cells remains unclear.

C. Radioligand Binding

Using a radiolabeled muscarinic antagonist, rat thymocytes were shown to express approximately 3,000 muscarinic binding sites that were of both the M1 and M3 subtype, with a Kd of 80 nM (Yamada et al., 1997). In the same study, pretreatment of rats with hydrocortisone increased the number of muscarinic sites by 82% (Yamada et al., 1997). In another study with rats, an electrolytic lesion in the area of the anterior hypothalamus increased the number of thymocyte muscarinic binding sites within 7 days of lesioning, but did not change the number of sites on spleen or peripheral blood lymphocytes; exposure of the lesioned rats to either Th cell-dependent or -independent antigens increased the number of binding sites on spleen lymphocytes, but not on peripheral blood lymphocytes (Gushchin et al., 1994). Murine CD8+ and CD4+ cells were shown to also express muscarinic binding sites with the CD8+ expressing more binding sites than the CD4+ cell, but with both cells having a similar Kd (Genaro, Cremaschi, & Borda, 1993). In contrast, B cells did not express a detectable number of binding sites (Genaro et al., 1993) despite the functional data cited above suggesting that binding sites might exist on B cells.

Human peripheral blood lymphocytes showed muscarinic receptors of the M2, M3, and M4 subtype with a density of 2.33 fmol per 2×10^6 cells and a Kd of 0.6 nM (Bronzetti et al., 1996). In contrast, human Jurkat cells showed muscarinic receptors of the M3 subtype with a maximum of 45,000 sites per cell and a Kd of 14.1 nM (Kaneda, Kitamura, & Nomura, 1993). Using ^{3}H-N-methyl-scopolamine, human peripheral blood lymphocytes showed at least 57–127 muscarinic binding sites per cell with a Kd of 45-133 pM, whereas peripheral mononuclear cells expressed no detectable binding sites (Meurs, Timmermans, de Monchy, Zaagsma, & Kauffman, 1993). Cells within the bursa of Fabricius in pigeons showed muscarinic receptors of the M2, M3, and M4 subtypes with a binding density of 38 fmol/mg protein and a Kd of 0.31 nM (Ricci et al., 1996). In this study, autoradiography was also used to show localization of binding sites within the medulla, follicular septa, corticomedullary border, and cortical layer (Ricci et al., 1996). Thus, direct radioligand binding data suggest that the M1, M2, M3, and M4 subtypes are expressed on immune cells, but that the particular cell type and species of origin may determine the subtype distribution.

D. Northern and RT-PCR

Using RT-PCR, human peripheral blood mononuclear cells were shown to express mRNA for the M3, M4, and M5 muscarinic subtypes and this was the first report of the M5 subtype being expressed outside of the CNS (Costa, Auger, Traver, & Costa, 1995). In another study, purified T lymphocytes were shown to express mRNA for the M3, M4, and M5 muscarinic subtypes, whereas purified B cells and macrophages expressed no message (Hellstrom-Lindahl & Nordberg, 1996). Using RT-PCR, the leukemic cell line Peer expressed mRNA for the M3 and M5 subtypes, whereas the leukemic cell line HL-60 expressed the M4 and M5 subtypes (Hellstrom-Lindahl & Nordberg, 1996), but the human Jurkat cell line expressed only the M3 subtype as determined by Northern blot analysis (Kaneda et al., 1993). Using both RT-PCR and Northern blot analysis, rat peripheral blood macrophages expressed only the M3 subtype, whereas T and B cells expressed only the M4 subtype (Costa, Castoldi, Traver, & Costa, 1994; Costa, Traver, Auger, & Costa, 1994). Therefore, molecular data suggest that the M3, M4, and M5 subtypes are expressed at the message level in immune cells, but again, the particular cell type and species of origin may determine the subtype distribution. The data also suggest that the M5 subtype may be expressed at the message level, but not at the protein level on the cell surface, as suggested by the radioligand binding data summarized above.

E. Receptor-Specific Signal Transduction Pathways

Single cell analysis of human peripheral blood mononuclear cells, the T leukemic Jurkat cell line, and the B leukemic Raji cell line loaded with Indo-1 showed that the muscarinic nonselective agonist carbachol or the nicotinic receptor agonist nicotine increased the free cytoplasmic concentration of Ca++ as a result of an increase in the concentration of IP3 to induce Ca++ release from intracellular stores (Laskowska-Bozek, Bany, Stokarska, & Ryzewski, 1995; Laskowska-Bozek et al., 1996). Using the Jurkat cell line, M3 agonists transiently elevated the free cytosolic Ca++ concentration from intracellular stores and this effect involved a bacteria toxin-insensitive GTP-binding protein, phospholipase C activation, and IP3 formation (Kaneda et al., 1993). It was also found in this study that activation of protein kinase C negatively modulated the expression of the M3 receptor protein.

Murine CD8+ cells exposed to the muscarinic nonselective agonist carbachol showed an increase in both cGMP and IP3, whereas CD4+ cells showed no change in either cGMP or IP3 (Genaro et al., 1993). On the other hand, human T cells exposed to an M1-selective agonist activated a G-protein that subsequently activated phospholipase C, protein kinase C, and c-Raf-1 via a tyrosine kinase-independent mechanism (Siegel, June, Yamada, Rapp, & Samelson, 1993). An additional study indicated that a third mechanism may be involved in a muscarinic receptor-induced response since avian lacrimal gland plasma cells exposed to the cholinergic nonselective agonist carbachol increased the secretion rate of IgG through a mechanism that required Ca ++ influx mediated by a voltage-dependent Ca ++ channel (Brink et al., 1994). Thus, intracellular signaling data suggest that stimulation of the muscarinic receptor on T cells elevates the level of Ca ++ intracellularly by either the release of Ca ++ from intracellular stores or the activation of a voltage-dependent Ca ++ channel.

IV. SEROTONERGIC RECEPTORS

In this section, we have attempted to summarize the most recent studies addressing the presence of serotonergic receptors on immune cells. We refer the reader to the following review that discusses the earlier work in this area of research (Qiu et al., 1996). A summary of the evidence for the presence of serotonergic receptors on immune cells is presented in Table VIII.

A. Serotonin (5-HT) Uptake by Immune Cells

Human peripheral blood mononuclear cells and murine spleen cells have been reported to make and release 5-HT (Aune, Golden, & McGrath, 1994) and express a 5-HT-specific transporter (Faraj, Olkowski, & Jackson, 1994, 1997) that was identical to one shown in neuronal tissue using RT-PCR (Faraj et al., 1997). The functional significance of these findings are unclear, but recovering alcoholics in long-term abstinence had a significantly increased level of ^{3}H-5-HT uptake (Faraj et al., 1997), and when the 5-HT uptake inhibitor fluoxetine was given to monkeys in infancy, they showed an increased number of CD4+ and CD8+ cells in the CSF 2 years later in adolescence, whereas the CD4+ and CD8+ cell profile in the blood was unaffected (Coe, Hou, & Clarke, 1996). If these data are accurate, then previous data using 5-HT receptor antagonists must be reexamined and reinterpreted.

B. Functional Evidence

The Con A-induced response of teleost fish lymphocytes was suppressed following addition of the 5-HT3 agonist 2-methyl-5-HT was added to the cell cultures due to a block in cell cycle progression from G0/G1 to S (Meyniel, Khan, Ferriere, & Deschaux, 1997). Likewise, rainbow trout peripheral blood lymphocytes exposed to 5-HT were suppressed in their proliferative response to LPS and PHA and this effect was reversed by the 5-HT1A-selective antagonist spiperone (Ferriere, Khan, Troutaud, & Deschaux, 1996). In contrast, another study showed that 5-HT1A receptor stimulation was responsible for the enhancement of LPS-induced proliferation in rat and murine B cells which was blocked by the 5-HT1A-selective antagonist WAY 100135 (Iken, Chheng, Fargin, Goulet, & Kouassi, 1995). In addition, the monocyte-induced inhibition of IFN-γ production by NK cells was abrogated by exposure of purified human monocytes and NK cells to a 5-HT1A-selective agonist (Hellstrand et al., 1993; Hellstrand & Hermodsson, 1993). Other data suggested that immune cells store exogenous 5-HT and that 5-HT antagonists blocked T cell proliferation, decreased Th1 cytokine production, decreased the DTH response to oxazalone, and had no effect on the antibody response to oxazalone (Aune et al., 1994). Thus, taken together, these functional data suggest that predominantly the 5-HT1A receptor is expressed on T cells, B cells, and macrophages and that stimulation of this receptor either enhances or suppresses immune cell function.

C. Radioligand Binding

Teleost fish lymphocytes were shown to express 5-HT3 receptors when the 5-HT3 agonist 2-methyl-5-HT

TABLE VIII Summary of the Evidence for the Presence of Serotonergic Receptors on Immune Cells

Receptor	Response	Reference
Functional evidence		
5-HT	↓ Proliferation	(Ferriere et al., 1996)
	↑ Proliferation	(Iken et al., 1995)
5-HT1A antagonist	Reversed 5-HT-induced ↓ in proliferation	(Ferriere et al., 1996)
	Reversed 5-HT-induced ↑ in proliferation	(Iken et al., 1995)
	↓ Monocyte-induced inhibition of IFN-γ production by NK cells	(Hellstrand et al., 1993; Hellstrand & Hermodsson, 1993)
	↓ T cell proliferation	(Aune et al., 1994)
	Th1 cytokine production	(Aune et al., 1994)
	↓ DTH response to oxazalone	(Aune et al., 1994)
	No effect on the antibody response to oxazalone	(Aune et al., 1994)
5-HT3 agonist	↓ Proliferation	(Meyniel et al., 1997)
	Block cell progression from G0/G1 to S	(Meyniel et al., 1997)
Radioligand binding		
5-HT1A	Activated lymphocytes only	(Ferriere et al., 1996)
	B cells	(Iken et al., 1995)
	Human leukemic cells; Bmax of 2.8 fmol/106 cells; Kd of 20 nM	(Khan et al., 1995)
	Human PBMC, no detectable receptors	(Marazziti et al., 1995)
5-HT3	Teleost fish lymphocytes	(Meyniel et al., 1997)
In situ hybridization		
5-HT1A	Human PBMC, detectable	(Marazziti et al., 1995)
Signal transduction		
5-HT	↓ [Ca ++]i by opening outward Ca ++ channels	(Khan et al., 1995)
5-HT1A	↓ Adenylate cyclase activity	(Aune et al., 1994)
5-HT3	↑ Inward movement of Na+	(Meyniel et al., 1997)
	↑ [Ca ++]i from extracellular stores through L-type, but not N-type Ca ++ channels	(Ferriere et al., 1997)

5-HT, 5-hydroxy trytamine; NK, natural killer cell; DTH, delayed type hypersensitivity; Kd, dissociation constant; B_{max}, binding maximum; PBMC, peripheral blood mononuclear cell; Ca ++, calcium ion; IFN, interferon.

displaced the binding of ^{3}H-serotonin (Meyniel et al., 1997). On the other hand, rainbow trout lymphocytes were shown to express 5-HT1A receptors that were not detectable on resting cells, but only on LPS- or PHA-activated cells (Ferriere et al., 1996). Mouse and rat B cells were shown to express 5-HT1A receptors (Iken et al., 1995), whereas studies using human leukemia cells expressed a 5-HT1A receptor with a Bmax of 2.8 fmol/10^6 cells and a Kd of 20 nM (Khan, Ferriere, & Deschaux, 1995). In contrast, human peripheral blood mononuclear cells showed no detectable level of 5-HT1A receptors even though they expressed 5-HT1A receptor mRNA as determined by in situ hybridization (Marazziti, et al., 1995). Thus, direct radioligand binding data suggest that predominantly the 5-HT1A receptor is expressed on lymphocytes.

D. Receptor-Specific Signal Transduction Pathways

The 5-HT3 agonist 2-methyl-5-HT increased the inward movement of Na+ in teleost fish lymphocytes that was blocked by an antagonist (Meyniel et al., 1997), whereas rainbow trout lymphocytes increased [Ca++]i via stimulation of 5-HT3 receptors, but not 5-HT-1A or 5-HT-2, and the Ca++ was mobilized from extracellular stores through L-type, but not N-type Ca++ channels (Ferriere, Khan, Meyniel, & Deschaux, 1997). 5-HT caused human leukemia cells to decrease [Ca++]i and this effect was blocked by verapramil, indicating that 5-HT opened Ca++ channels (Khan, Ferriere, & Deschaux, 1995). And finally, stimulation of 5-HT1A receptors decreased the activation of adenylate cyclase (Aune et al., 1994).

Thus, stimulation of 5-HT1A receptors on lymphocytes appears to induce signal transduction pathways that involve either the activation of L-type Ca++ channels to increase the intracellular Ca++ concentration or the suppression of adenylate cyclase activity.

V. DOPAMINERGIC RECEPTORS

A summary of the evidence for the presence of adrenergic receptors on immune cells is presented in Table IX.

A. Functional Evidence

Currently, the level and subtypes of the dopamine receptor (DR) expressed on lymphocytes remains unclear. Early functional studies investigating DR stimulation and the modulation of lymphocyte function suggested a variety of roles for dopamine or dopamine agonist stimulation in modulating immune cell functions, including lymphocyte proliferation (Boukhris, Kouassi, & Revillard, 1988; Ferguson, Schmidtke, & Simmons, 1975; Kouassi et al., 1987; Nahas, Desoize, & Leger, 1979; Scorza-Smeraldi et al., 1983; Waterfield, Hammarstrom, & Smith, 1976), cytokine production (Boukhris et al., 1988), and lymphocyte subset numbers (Kouassi et al., 1987). In addition, more recent studies showed that administration of 1-methyl-4-phenyl-1,2,3,6-tetrahydropyridine (MPTP), a drug that lowers endogenous dopamine levels in the periphery, suppressed in vitro LPS- and Con A-induced splenocyte proliferation; administration of D1R- and D2R-selective agonists enhanced proliferation (Tsao, Lin, & Cheng, 1997). Thus, these studies suggest that lymphocytes express the DR and that an agonist appears to enhance proliferation of immune cells, whereas an antagonist appears to suppress proliferation.

Unfortunately, more recent studies provide other explanations for the results described above. For example, some studies dispute the expression of the DR by splenocytes, since administration of either a DR agonist or antagonist consistently produced a pronounced inhibitory effect on the in vivo alloantigen-induced immune response and in vitro splenocyte IL-2 production (Maloteaux, Waterkein, & Laduron, 1982; Panajotova, 1997). Thus, since the addition of either a DR agonist or antagonist produced the same suppression in IL-2 production, the authors suggested that the immunosuppressive action of these agents was independent of DR binding. These findings were further supported by a study showing that although dopamine inhibited anti-μ-induced proliferation of murine B cells in vitro, both the mixed D2R and D3R antagonist haloperidol and D2R-selective antagonist spiperone enhanced anti-μ-induced B cell proliferation (Liu & Wolfe, 1996). However, since this study was unable to mimic the effects of haloperidol and spiperone with selective antagonists of any of the DR subtypes, it was concluded by the author that these drugs may exert an effect independent of DR stimulation. Therefore, although earlier studies support a functional role for the DR expressed on lymphocytes, other studies suggest that pharmacologic agents may be acting independently of a specific DR to modulate immune cell function.

Functional data also suggested a role for DR stimulation in modulating macrophage and NK cell function. For example, in vivo stimulation of the DR enhanced macrophage phagocytosis (Ali, Qureshi, & McCorkle, 1994; Sternberg, Wedner, Leung, & Parker, 1987) and IFN-γ-induced Ia expression (Sternberg, Trial, & Parker, 1986). Unfortunately, to our knowledge, no recent studies have added to these findings. In a manner similar to macrophages, DR stimulation enhanced NK cell function. In vivo administration of the mixed DR antagonist haloperidol for 5 days suppressed NK cell activity without altering NK cell number, and this effect was not blocked by supplementation of animals with prolactin, suggesting that the effects of haloperidol on NK cell activity were prolactin-independent (Nozaki, Hozumi, Nishimura, & Habu, 1996). However, similar to the conflicting results obtained about DR function in lymphocytes, another study showed that the effects of various dopaminergic receptor antagonists on NK cell cytotoxicity and effector-target cell conjugation were inconsistent and most likely mediated by mechanisms unrelated to the dopaminergic pathway (Won, Chuang, Huang, Liu, & Lin, 1995). Thus, although data support a functional role for DR expression in modulating lymphocyte, macrophage, and NK cell activity, other studies suggest that the pharmacological agents used in previous studies may have mediated their effects on cellular function independently of DR binding.

B. Radioligand Binding

Similar to the functional studies discussed above, conflicting reports of radioligand binding data exist concerning the expression of the DR on immune cell populations. Early studies observed [^{3}H]-spiroperidol binding sites in mammalian lymphocytes (Le Fur, Phan, & Uzan, 1980) and murine B cells (Uzan, Phan, & Le Fur, 1981). In addition, rat thymocytes bound [^{3}H]-dopamine with high affinity receptors with a

TABLE IX Summary of the Evidence for the Presence of Dopaminergic Receptors on Immune Cells

Receptor	Response	Reference
Functional evidence		
DR agonist	Lymphocyte proliferation	(Boukhris et al., 1988; Ferguson et al., 1975; Waterfield et al., 1976; Nahas et al., 1979; Scorza-Smeraldi et al., 1983; Kouassi et al., 1987a)
	Cytokine production	(Boukhris et al., 1988)
	Lymphocyte subset numbers	(Kouassi et al., 1987)
	In vivo - ↓ in vivo alloantigen response	(Panajotova, 1997; Maloteaux et al., 1982)
	↓ IL-2 production	(Panajotova, 1997; Maloteaux et al., 1982)
	↓ Anti-μ-induced proliferation	(Liu & Wolfe, 1996)
	↑ Macrophage phagocytosis	(Sternberg et al., 1987; Ali et al., 1994)
	↑ IFN-γ-induced macrophage Ia expression	(Sternberg et al., 1986)
D1R- and D2R agonists	↑ Splenocyte proliferation	(Tsao et al., 1997)
DR antagonist	↓ In vivo alloantigen response	(Panajotova, 1997; Maloteaux et al., 1982)
	↓ IL-2 production	(Panajotova, 1997; Maloteaux et al., 1982)
Mixed DR antagonist	↑ Anti-μ-induced proliferation	(Liu & Wolfe, 1996)
	In vivo - ↓ NK cell activity	(Nozaki et al., 1996)
MPTP to lower endogenous dopamine levels	↓ splenocyte proliferation	(Tsao et al., 1997)
Radioligand binding		
DR		(Le Fur et al., 1980; Uzan et al., 1981)
D2R and D3R	Kd = 0.9 nM	(Chi et al., 1992)
D3R or D4R	Kd = 1.6×10^{-8} M	(Ovadia et al., 1987)
D3R and D5R	Age-dependent ↑ in D3R, but not D5R	(Barili et al., 1996)
		(Ricci, Mariotta et al., 1997)
D4R		(Ricci, Bronzetti et al., 1997)
Northern and RT-PCR		
D1R		(Dearry et al., 1990; Zhou et al., 1990)
D2R		(Bunzow et al., 1988)
D3R		(Sokoloff et al., 1990; Giros et al., 1990; Vile & Strange, 1996)
D4R		(Van Tol et al., 1991; Bondy et al., 1996)
D5R		(Sunahara et al., 1991)
D1R, D3R, and D5R		(Caronti et al., 1998)
D3R and D5R	↓ D3R in Parkinson's disease	(Nagai et al., 1996)
Signal transduction		
Dopamine agonist	↑ Intracellular levels of cAMP	(Kouassi & Revillard, 1987; Stepien et al., 1981; Santambrogio et al., 1993)

IL, interleukin; IFN, interferon; NK, natural killer cell; Kd, dissociation constant; cAMP, adenosine 3′,5′-monophosphate; DR, dopamine receptor.

Kd = 1.6×10^{-8} M (Ovadia, Lubetzki-Korn, & Abramsky, 1987) which was displaced by low concentrations of either dopamine or the mixed DR selective-agonist apomorphine, but not by either the D2R-selective antagonist sulpiride, the D2R-selective agonist bromocriptine, or the mixed antagonist haloperidol, suggesting the presence of the D3R subtype. However, a more recent study has been reported that haloperidol binds the D3R subtype, thus the previous results may have shown the presence of the D4R and D5R subtype. Other studies using (-)-[^{3}H]sulpiride suggested the presence of the D2R and the D4R on lymphocytes with a Kd of 0.9 nM, rather than the D3R subtype (Chi, Gong, Daigneault, & Kostrzewa, 1992).

More recent studies supported the findings of earlier studies since they confirmed the existence of D4R on human peripheral blood lymphocytes through the use of [^{3}H]-clozapine (Ricci, Bronzetti, Felici, Tayebati, & Amenta, 1997). Other studies not only confirmed the existence of D3R and D5R receptors on human peripheral blood lymphocytes, but also reported an age-dependent decrease in the level of the D3R, but not the D5R, expression on lymphocytes (Barili et al., 1996). Finally, another recent study demonstrated the presence of the D3R and D5R in sections of rat thymus and on peripheral rat lymphocytes (Ricci, Mariotta, Greco, & Bisetti, 1997). Thus, radioligand binding data support the expression of a variety of DR subtypes on lymphocytes.

However, other radioligand binding data dispute the expression of specific DR subtypes on lymphocytes. In disagreement with functional studies, one study did not detect the D1R on mouse spleen or thymus cells using [^{3}H]-labeled-2-amino-6,7-dihydroxy-1,2,3,4-tetrahydronaphtalene (ADTN), a selective D1R agonist (Shaskan, Ballow, Lederman, Margoles, & Melchreit, 1984). In addition, a more recent study by Vile and Strange did not detect D2R-like receptors on human blood lymphocytes through the use of [^{3}H]-nemonapride (Vile & Strange, 1996). Thus, while the majority of radioligand binding studies support the expression of the DR protein on lymphocytes, a few studies have been unable to detect specific subtypes of this receptor on the surface of lymphocytes.

C. Northern and RT-PCR

Currently, five different subtypes of the DR have been described at the molecular level: D1R (Dearry et al., 1990; Zhou et al., 1990), D2R (Bunzow et al., 1988), D3R (Sokoloff, Giros, Martres, Bouthenet, & Schwartz, 1990; Giros, Martres, Sokoloff, & Schwartz, 1990), D4R (Van Tol et al., 1991), and the D5R (Sunahara et al., 1991). Recent data have confirmed the expression of D3R and D5R mRNA in human peripheral blood lymphocytes and have shown a decrease in D3R mRNA in Parksinson's disease that correlated with the severity of the disease (Nagai et al., 1996). Another study confirmed the expression of D4R mRNA in peripheral human lymphocytes using RT-PCR (Bondy, de Jonge, Pander, Primbs, & Ackenheil, 1996). However, others have detected D3R mRNA in lymphocytes, but could not D2R mRNA expression (Vile & Strange, 1996). Finally, one study showed the expression of mRNA for the D1R, D3R, and D5R in rat lymphocytes, but was unable to detect D2R or D4R mRNA in rat lymphocytes (Caronti, Calderaro, Passarelli, Palladini, & Pontieri, 1998). Thus, as with functional and radioligand binding studies, the majority of studies confirm the expression of the DR on lymphocytes at the message level, but do not agree on the subtypes of the DR expressed.

D. Receptor-Specific Signal Transduction Pathways

Dopamine agonists have been reported to increase the intracellular concentration of cAMP in lymphocytes (Kouassi & Revillard, 1987; Santambrogio, Lipartiti, Bruni, & Dal Toso, 1993; Stepien, Kunert-Radek, Karasek, & Pawlikowski, 1981).

VI. SUMMARY

The purpose of this chapter is to summarize the data that indicate the presence of adrenergic, cholinergic, serotonergic, and dopaminergic receptors on the cell surface of immune cells. Although the data summarized herein may not be all encompassing, they do provide both indirect and direct evidence for the presence of these neurotransmitter receptors on the cells surface of immune cells. The challenge to the neuroimmunologist in future research endeavors is to enter the immune cell interior to identify the molecular changes induced in gene expression by neurotransmitter receptor stimulation and to understand how these changes in gene expression influence immune cell function within the context of a whole organism.

For example, in the bone marrow, we need to understand if the αAR and βAR are differentially expressed on subsets of bone marrow and thymus cells and if the stimulation of these receptors affects the production of new-migrant cells that occupy lymphoid organs in the periphery. For both T and B lymphocytes, a better understanding is needed about the expression of neurotransmitter receptors by naive, effector, and memory cells, as well as the mechanisms by which stimulation of these receptors on each cell subset may affect the outcome of both cell-mediated and humoral immune responses. For macrophages and NK cells, we need to understand the mechanisms by which receptor stimulation affects the ability of these cells to protect the organism from microbial attack and tumor development and progression.

It remains unclear in many clinical examples of proposed nervous system-immune system interactions as to the cellular immune mechanisms that contribute to clinical outcome. For example, the Th cell and B cell play an important role in the development of antitumor humoral immunity. HER-2/neu is a growth factor receptor that is overexpressed on cells in breast, ovarian, and uterine cancers. Serum antibodies directed against HER-2/neu are found in a high frequency of patients with early stage cancer and these antibodies are known to limit tumor growth and metastasis by preventing activation of the growth factor receptor. The B cell is responsible for binding low levels of tumor antigen and, for eventually, producing antibody against it. However, most of the detectable anti-HER-2/neu antibodies made by the B cell are of the IgG isotype, indicating that B cell activation, proliferation, and differentiation to antibody production depends on help provided to the B cell by the Th cell through both contact- and cytokine-mediated signals. Therefore, it is essential that we gain a better understanding of the mechanism by which an endogenous neurotransmitter that is within the microenvironment of both Th cells and B cells, such as norepinephrine, either augments or suppresses the generation of the Th cell-dependent antibody response that helps to maintain homeostasis.

Also, as mammals age, the tendency to develop infections and autoimmune-type disorders increases, whereas the effectiveness of the humoral immune response decreases. Antibodies of low affinity are proportionally greater in the aged individual and the efficacy of vaccination is poor. Therefore, it will be important to determine the mechanisms by which stimulation of a neurotransmitter receptor on aged immune cells may influence the production of new immune cells from bone marrow precursors, the migration of new immune cells to the periphery, and the functional responsiveness of the new immune cells produced.

An understanding of the effects from neurotransmitter receptor stimulation on bone marrow cells will provide better insight into the development of therapeutic approaches for more effective and efficient recovery following bone marrow replacement therapy and chemotherapy. Studies that assess the importance of β2AR stimulation in Th1 cell-mediated in vivo disease models, such as experimental allergic encephalitis and autoimmune diabetes, will provide better insight into the mechanisms by which adrenergic receptor stimulation influences the development and progression of multiple sclerosis and Type I diabetes. An understanding of the mechanism by which neurotransmitter receptor stimulation influences the level and isotype of antibody produced against an antigen will suggest approaches that can be used to either enhance the efficacy of vaccination protocols or block specific pathways identified as key modulators in the production of specific antibody isotypes, such as IgE in allergy and asthma patients.

Acknowledgments

The authors are indebted to the editors for providing us with the opportunity of updating our database and then organizing our thoughts about the data. The experiments that were underway while we were writing this review were supported by a grant from the National Institute of Health (AI37326) and the American Cancer Society (RPG-96-067-03-CIM).

References

Abrass, C. K., O'Connor, S. W., Scarpace, P. J., & Abrass, I. B. (1985). Characterization of the beta-adrenergic receptor of the rat peritoneal macrophage. *Journal of Immunology, 135*, 1338–1341.

Ackerman, K. D., Madden, K. S., Livnat, S., Felten, S. Y., & Felten, D. L. (1991). Neonatal sympathetic denervation alters the development of in vitro spleen cell proliferation and differentiation. *Brain Behavior Immunity, 5*, 235–261.

Afan, A. M., Broome, C. S., Nicholls, S. E., Whetton, A. D., & Miyan, J. A. (1997). Bone marrow innervation regulates cellular retention in the murine haemopoietic system. *British Journal Haematology, 98*, 569–577.

Ali, R. A., Qureshi, M. A., & McCorkle, F. M. (1994). Profile of chicken macrophage functions after exposure to catecholamines in vitro. *Immunopharmacology and Immunotoxicology, 16*, 611–625.

Anderson, K. L., Anderson, G., Michell, R. H., Jenkinson, E. J., & Owen, J. J. (1996). Intracellular signaling pathways involved in the induction of apoptosis in immature thymic T lymphocytes. *Journal of Immunology, 156*, 4083–4091.

Aune, T. M., Golden, H. W., & McGrath, K. M. (1994). Inhibitors of serotonin synthesis and antagonists of serotonin 1A receptors inhibit T lymphocyte function in vitro and cell-mediated immunity in vivo. *Journal of Immunology, 153*, 489–498.

Bachen, E. A., Manuck, S. B., Cohen, S., Muldoon, M. F., Raible, R., Herbert, T. B., & Rabin, B. S. (1995). Adrenergic blockade ameliorates cellular immune responses to mental stress in humans. *Psychosomatic Medicine, 57*, 366–372.

Balter, N. J. & Schwartz, S. L. (1977). Accumulation of norepinephrine by macrophages and relationships to known uptake processes. *Journal of Pharmacology and Experimental Therapeutics, 201*, 636–630.

Barili, P., Bronzetti, E., Felici, L., Ferrante, F., Ricci, A., Zaccheo, D., & Amenta, F. (1996). Age-dependent changes in the expression of dopamine receptor subtypes in human peripheral blood lymphocytes. *Journal of Neuroimmunology, 71*, 45–50.

Bartik, M. M., Bauman, G. P., Brooks, W. H., & Roszman, T. L. (1994). Costimulatory signals modulate the antiproliferative effects of agents that elevate cAMP in T cells. *Cellular Immunology, 158*, 116–130.

Bartik, M. M., Brooks, W. H., & Roszman, T. L. (1993). Modulation of T cell proliferation by stimulation of the beta-adrenergic receptor: Lack of correlation between inhibition of T cell proliferation and cAMP accumulation. *Cellular Immunology, 148*, 408–421.

Bauman, G. P., Bartik, M. M., Brooks, W. H., & Roszman, T. L. (1994). Induction of cAMP-dependent protein kinase (PKA) activity in T cells after stimulation of the prostaglandin E2 or the beta-adrenergic Receptors: Relationship between PKA activity and inhibition of anti-CD3 monoclonal antibody-induced T cell proliferation. *Cellular Immunology, 158*, 182–194.

Beckman, B., Mirand, E., & Fisher, J. W. (1980). Effects of beta adrenergic agents and prostaglandin E1 on erthyroid colony (CFU-E) growth and cyclic AMP formation in Friend erythroleukemic cells. *Journal of Cellular Physiology, 105*, 355–361.

Bender, B. S., Bell, W. E., Taylor, S., & Scarpace, P. J. (1993). Decreased sensitivity to cAMP in the in vitro generation of memory splenic cytotoxic T-lymphocytes from aged mice: Role of phosphodiesterase. *Journal of Pharmacology and Experimental Therapeutics, 264,* 1381–1386.

Benschop, R. J., Oostveen, F. G., Heijnen, C. J., & Ballieux, R. E. (1993). Beta 2-adrenergic stimulation causes detachment of natural killer cells from cultured endothelium. *European Journal of Immunology, 23,* 3242–3247.

Benschop, R. J., Nieuwenhuis, E. E., Tromp, E. A., Godaert, G. L., Ballieux, R. E., & van Doornen, L. J. (1994). Effects of beta-adrenergic blockade on immunologic and cardiovascular changes induced by mental stress. *Circulation, 89,* 762–769.

Benschop, R. J., Nijkamp, F. P., Ballieux, R. E., & Heijnen, C. J. (1994). The effects of beta-adrenoceptor stimulation on adhesion of human natural killer cells to cultured endothelium. *British Journal of Pharmacology, 113,* 1311–1316.

Benschop, R. J., Schedlowski, M., Wienecke, H., Jacobs, R., & Schmidt, R. E. (1997). Adrenergic control of natural killer cell circulation and adhesion. *Brain, Behavior, and Immunity, 11,* 321–332.

Besedovsky, H. O., Del Rey, A., Sorkin, E., Da Prada, M., & Keller, H. H. (1979). Immunoregulation mediated by the sympathetic nervous system. *Cellular Immunology, 48,* 346–355.

Betz, M. & Fox, B. S. (1991). Prostaglandin E2 inhibits production of Th1 lymphokines but not of Th2 lymphokines. *Journal of Immunology, 146,* 108–113.

Beusenberg, F. D., Adolfs, M. J., van Schaik-van Groningen, J. M., Hoogsteden, H. C., & Bonta, I. L. (1989). Regulation of cyclic AMP levels in alveolar macrophages of guinea pigs and man by prostanoids and beta-adrenergic agents. *Agents Actions, 26,* 105–107.

Beusenberg, F. D., Van Amsterdam, J. G., van Schaik, J. M., Hoogsteden, H. C., & Bonta, I. L. (1990). Adenyl cyclase activity in human alveolar macrophages. *Agents Actions, 31* (Suppl), 123–126.

Bidart, J. M., Motte, Ph., Assicot, M., Bohuon, C., & Bellet, D. (1983). Catechol-O-methyltransferase activity and aminergic binding sites distribution in human peripheral blood lymphocyte subpopulations. *Clinical Immunology and Immunopathology, 26,* 1–9.

Bishopric, N. H., Cohen, H. J., & Lefkowitz, R. J. (1980). Beta-adrenergic receptors in lymphocyte subpopulations. *Journal of Allergy and Clinical Immunology, 65,* 29–33.

Blomhoff, H. K., Smeland, E. B., Beiske, K., Blomhoff, R., Ruud, E., Bjoro, T., Pfeifer-Ohlsson, S., Watt, R., Funderud, S., Godal, T., & Ohlsson, R. (1987). Cyclic AMP-mediated suppression of normal and neoplastic B cell proliferation is associated with regulation of *myc* and Ha-*ras* protooncogenes. *Journal of Cellular Physiology, 131,* 426–433.

Bondy, B., de Jonge, S., Pander, S., Primbs, J., & Ackenheil, M. (1996). Identification of dopamine D4 receptor mRNA in circulating human lymphocytes using nested polymerase chain reaction. *Journal of Neuroimmunology, 71,* 139–144.

Borger, P., Kauffman, H. F., Postma, D. S., & Vellenga, E. (1996). Interleukin-4 gene expression in activated human T lymphocytes is regulated by the cyclic adenosine monophosphate-dependent signaling pathway. *Blood, 87,* 691–698.

Boukhris, W., Kouassi, E., & Revillard, J. P. (1988). Differential effect of mixed D1/D2 and selective D2 dopaminergic antagonists on mouse T and B lymphocyte proliferation and interleukin production in vitro. *Immunopharmacology and Immunotoxicology, 10,* 501–512.

Bourne, H. R. & Melmon, K. L. (1971). Adenyl cyclase in human leukocytes: Evidence for activation by separate beta adrenergic and prostaglandin receptors. *Journal of Pharmacology and Experimental Therapeutics, 178,* 1–7.

Brenner, G. J., Felten, S. Y., Felten, D. L., & Moynihan, J. A. (1992). Sympathetic nervous system modulation of tumor metastases and host defense mechanisms. *Journal of Neuroimmunology, 37,* 191–201.

Brink, P. R., Walcott, B., Roemer, E., Grine, E., Pastor, M., Christ, G. J., & Cameron, R. H. (1994). Cholinergic modulation of immunoglobulin secretion from avian plasma cells: The role of calcium. *Journal of Neuroimmunology, 51,* 113–121.

Brodde, O. E., Daul, A., & O'Hara, N. (1984). Beta-adrenoceptor changes in human lymphocytes, induced by dynamic exercise. *Naunyn-Schmiedeberg's Archives of Pharmacology, 325,* 190–192.

Bronzetti, E., Adani, O., Amenta, F., Felici, L., Mannino, F., & Ricci, A. (1996). Muscarinic cholinergic receptor subtypes in human peripheral blood lymphocytes. *Neuroscience Letters, 208,* 211–215.

Brown, R., Li, Z., Vriend, C., Nirula, R., Janz, L., Falk, J., Nance, D. M., Dyck, D. G., & Greenburg, A. H. (1991). Suppression splenic macrophage interleukin-1 secretion following intracerebroventricular injection of interleukin-1 beta: Evidence for pituitary-adrenal and sympathetic control. *Cellular Immunology, 132,* 84–93.

Bunzow, J. R., Van Tol, H. H., Grandy, D. K., Albert, P., Salon, J., Christie, M., Machida, C. A., Neve, K. A., & Civelli, O. (1988). Cloning and expression of a rat D2 dopamine receptor cDNA [see comments]. *Nature, 336,* 783–787.

Burchiel, S. W. & Melmon, K. L. (1979a). Augmentation of the in vitro humoral immune responseby pharmacologic agents. I: An explanation of the differential enhancement of humoral immunity via agents that elevate cAMP. *Immunopharmacology, 1,* 137–150.

Burchiel, S. W. & Melmon, K. L. (1979b). Augmentation of the in vitro humoral immune response by pharmacologic agents. II: The comparison of the effects of antiproliferative agents with dibutyryl cAMP. *Immunopharmacology, 1,* 151–163.

Byron, J. W. (1972). Evidence for a beta-adrenergic receptor initiating DNA synthesis in haemopoietic stem cells. *Experimental Cell Research, 71,* 228–232.

Byron, J. W. & Fox, M. (1969). Adrenergic receptor blocking agents modifying the radioprotective action of T.A.B. *British Journal of Radiology, 42,* 400.

Capelli, A., Lusuardi, M., Carli, S., Zaccaria, S., Trombetta, N., & Donner, C. F. (1993). In vitro effect of beta 2-agonists on bacterial killing and superoxide anion (O2-) release from alveolar macrophages of patients with chronic bronchitis. *Chest, 104,* 481–486.

Carlson, S. L., Brooks, W. H., & Roszman, T. L. (1989). Neurotransmitter-lymphocyte interactions: Dual receptor modulation of lymphocyte proliferation and cAMP production. *Journal of Neuroimmunology, 24,* 155–162.

Carlson, S. L., Trauth, K., Brooks, W. H., & Roszman, T. L. (1994). Enhancement of beta-adrenergic-induced cAMP accumulation in activated T-cells. *Journal of Cellular Physiology, 161,* 39–48.

Caronti, B., Calderaro, C., Passarelli, F., Palladini, G., & Pontieri, F. E. (1998). Dopamine receptor mRNAs in the rat lymphocytes. *Life Sciences, 62,* 1919–1925.

Cazaux, C. A., Sterin-Borda, L., Gorelik, G., & Cremaschi, G. A. (1995). Down-regulation of beta-adrenergic receptors induced by mitogen activation of intracellular signaling events in lymphocytes. *FEBS Letters, 364,* 120–124.

Chartash, E. K., Imai, A., Gershengorn, M. C., Crow, M. K., & Friedman, S. M. (1988). Direct human T helper cell-mediated B cell activation is not mediated by inositol lipid hydrolysis. *Journal of Immunology, 140*, 1974–1981.

Chelmicka-Schorr, E., Checinski, M., & Arnason, B. G. W. (1988). Chemical sympathectomy augments the severity of experimental allergic encephalomyelitis. *Journal of Neuroimmunology, 17*, 347–350.

Chelmicka-Schorr, E., Kwasniewski, M. N., & Czlonkowska, A. (1992a). Sympathetic nervous system modulates macrophage function. *International Journal of Immunopharmacology, 14*, 841–846.

Chelmicka-Schorr, E., Kwasniewski, M. N., & Czlonkowska, A. (1992b). Sympathetic nervous system and macrophage function. *Annals of the New York Academy of Sciences, 650*, 40–45.

Chen, D. & Rothenberg, E. V. (1994). Interleukin 2 transcription factors as molecular targets of cAMP inhibition: Delayed inhibition kinetics and combinatorial transcription roles. *Journal of Experimental Medicine, 179*, 931–942.

Chi, D. S., Gong, L., Daigneault, E. A., & Kostrzewa, R. M. (1992). Effects of MPTP and vitamin E treatments on immune function in mice. *International Journal of Immunopharmacology, 14*, 739–746.

Coe, C. L., Hou, F. Y., & Clarke, A. S. (1996). Fluoxetine treatment alters leukocyte trafficking in the intrathecal compartment of the young primate. *Biological Psychiatry, 40*, 361–367.

Cohen, D. P. & Rothstein, T. L. (1989). Adenosine 3′, 5′-cyclic monphosphate modulates the mitogenic responses of murine B lymphocytes. *Cellular Immunology, 121*, 113–124.

Conlon, P. D., Ogunbiyi, P. O., Black, W. D., & Eyre, P. (1988). Beta-adrenergic receptor function and oxygen radical production in bovine pulmonary alveolar macrophages. *Canadian Journal of Physiology and Pharmacology, 66*, 1538–1541.

Conolly, M. E. & Greenacre, J. K. (1977). The beta-adrenoceptor of the human lymphocyte and human lung parenchyma. *British Journal of Pharmacology, 59*, 17–23.

Cook-Mills, J. M., Cohen, R. L., Perlman, R. L., & Chambers, D. A. (1995). Inhibition of lymphocyte activation by catecholamines: Evidence for a non-classical mechanism of catecholamine action. *Immunology, 85*, 544–549.

Cook-Mills, J. M., Mokyr, M. B., Cohen, R. L., Perlman, R. L., & Chambers, D. A. (1995). Neurotransmitter suppression of the in vitro generation of a cytotoxic T lymphocyte response against the syngeneic MOPC-315 plasmacytoma. *Cancer Immunology Immunotherapy, 40*, 79–87.

Costa, P., Auger, C. B., Traver, D. J., & Costa, L. G. (1995). Identification of m3, m4 and m5 subtypes of muscarinic receptor mRNA in human blood mononuclear cells. *Journal of Neuroimmunology, 60*, 45–51.

Costa, P., Castoldi, A. F., Traver, D. J., & Costa, L. G. (1994). Lack of m2 muscarinic acetylcholine receptor mRNA in rat lymphocytes. *Journal of Neuroimmunology*, 49, 115–124.

Costa, P., Traver, D. J., Auger, C. B., & Costa, L. G. (1994). Expression of cholinergic muscarinic receptor subtypes mRNA in rat blood mononuclear cells. *Immunopharmacology, 28*, 113–123.

Cremaschi, G. A., Fisher, P., & Boege, F. (1991). Beta-adrenoceptor distribution in murine lymphoid cell lines. *Immunopharmacology, 22*, 195–206.

Crocker, I. C., Townley, R. G., & Khan, M. M. (1996). Phosphodiesterase inhibitors suppress proliferation of peripheral blood mononuclear cells and interleukin-4 and -5 secretion by human T-helper type 2 cells. *Immunopharmacology, 31*, 223–235.

Cross, R. J., Jackson, J. C., Brooks, W. H., Sparks, D. L., Markesbery, W. R., & Roszman, T. L. (1986). Neuroimmunomodulation: Impairment of humoral immune responsiveness by 6-hydroxydopamine treatment. *Immunology, 57*, 145–152.

Dearry, A., Gingrich, J. A., Falardeau, P., Fremeau, R. T., Jr., Bates, M. D., & Caron, M. G. (1990). Molecular cloning and expression of the gene for a human D1 dopamine receptor. *Nature, 347*, 72–76.

DeRubertis, F. R., Zenser, T. V., Adler, W. H., & Hudson, T. (1974). Role of cyclic adenosine 3′,5′-monophosphate in lymphocyte mitogenesis. *Journal of Immunology, 113*, 151–161.

Diamantstein, T. & Ulmer, A. (1975). The antagonistic action of cyclic GMP and cyclic AMP on proliferation of B and T lymphocytes. *Immunology, 28*, 113–119.

Dresch, C., Minc, J., Poirier, O., & Bouvet, D. (1981). Effect of beta adrenergic agonists on beta blocking agents on hemopoiesis in human bone marrow. *Biomedicine, 34*, 93–98.

Durant, S. (1986). In vivo effects of catecholamines and glucocorticoids on mouse thymic cAMP content and thymolysis. *Cellular Immunology, 102*, 136–143.

Estes, G., Solomon, S. S., & Norton, W. L. (1971). Inhibition of lymphocyte stimulation by cyclic and non-cyclic nucleotides. *Journal of Immunology, 107*, 1489–1492.

Faraj, B. A., Olkowski, Z. L., & Jackson, R. T. (1994). Expression of a high-affinity serotonin transporter in human lymphocytes. International. *Journal of Immunopharmacology, 16*, 561–567.

Faraj, B. A., Olkowski, Z. L., & Jackson, R. T. (1997). Prevalence of high serotonin uptake in lymphocytes of abstinent alcoholics. *Biochemical Pharmacology, 53*, 53–57.

Feldman, R. D., Hunninghake, G. W., & McArdle, W. (1987). Beta-adrenergic receptor-mediated suppression of interleukin 2 receptors in human lymphocytes. *Journal of Immunology, 139*, 3355–3359.

Felsner, P., Hofer, D., Rinner, I., Porta, S., Korsatko, W., & Schauenstein, K. (1995). Adrenergic suppression of peripheral blood T cell reactivity in the rat is due to activation of peripheral alpha 2-receptors. *Journal of Neuroimmunology, 57*, 27–34.

Ferguson, R. M., Schmidtke, J. R., & Simmons, R. L. (1975). Concurrent inhibition by chlorpromazine of concanavalin A-induced lymphocyte aggregation and mitogenesis. *Nature, 256*, 744–745.

Ferriere, F., Khan, N. A., Meyniel, J. P., & Deschaux, P. (1997). 5-Hydroxytryptamine-induced calcium-channel gating in rainbow trout (*Oncorhynchus mykiss*) peripheral blood lymphocytes. *Biochemical Journal, 323*, 251–258.

Ferriere, F., Khan, N. A., Troutaud, D., & Deschaux, P. (1996). Serotonin modulation of lymphocyte proliferation via 5-HT1A receptors in rainbow trout (*Oncorhynchus mykiss*). *Developmental and Comparative Immunology, 20*, 273–283.

Fuchs, B. A., Albright, J. W., & Albright, J. F. (1988). Beta-adrenergic receptor on murine lymphocytes: Density varies with cell maturity and lymphocyte subtype and is decreased after antigen administration. *Cellular Immunology, 114*, 231–245.

Fuchs, B. A., Campbell, K. S., & Munson, A. E. (1988). Norepinephrine and serotonin content of the murine spleen: Its relationship to lymphocyte beta-adrenergic receptor density and the humoral immune response in vivo and in vitro. *Cellular Immunology, 117*, 339–351.

Fuchs, B. A., McCall, C. O., & Munson, A. E. (1991). Enhancement of the murine primary antibody response by phenylephrine in vitro. *Drug and Chemical Toxicology, 14*, 67–82.

Fujii, T., Tsuchiya, T., Yamada, S., Fujimoto, K., Suzuki, T., Kasahara, T., & Kawashima, K. (1996). Localization and synthesis of acetylcholine in human leukemic T cell lines. *Journal of Neuroscience Research, 44*, 66–72.

Fujii, T., Yamada, S., Watanabe, Y., Misawa, H., Tajima, S., Fujimoto, K., Kasahara, T., & Kawashima, K. (1998). Induction of choline acetyltransferase mRNA in human mononuclear leukocytes stimulated by phytohemagglutinin, a T-cell activator. *Journal of Neuroimmunology, 82*, 101–107.

Fujino, H., Kitamura, Y., Yada, T., Uehara, T., & Nomura, Y. (1997). Stimulatory roles of muscarinic acetylcholine receptors on T cell antigen receptor/CD3 complex-mediated interleukin-2 production in human peripheral blood lymphocytes. *Molecular Pharmacology, 51*, 1007–1014.

Fukushima, T., Sekizawa, K., Jin, Y., Yamaya, M., Sasaki, H., & Takishima, T. (1993). Effects of beta-adrenergic receptor activation on alveolar macrophage cytoplasmic motility. *American Journal of Physiology, 265*, L67–L72.

Fuller, R. W., O'Malley, G., Baker, A. J., & MacDermot, J. (1988). Human alveolar macrophage activation: inhibition by forskolin but not beta-adrenoceptor stimulation or phosphodiesterase inhibition. *Pulmunary Pharmacology and Therapeutics, 1*, 101–106.

Gajewski, T. F., Schell, S. R., & Fitch, F. W. (1990). Evidence implicating utilization of different T cell receptor-associated signaling pathways by Th-1 and Th-2 clones. *Journal of Immunology, 144*, 4110–4120.

Genaro, A. M., Cremaschi, G. A., & Borda, E. S. (1993). Muscarinic cholinergic receptors on murine lymphocyte subpopulations. Selective interactions with second messenger response system upon pharmacological stimulation. *Immunopharmacology, 26*, 21–29.

Gilbert, K. M. & Hoffman, M. K. (1985). cAMP is an essential signal in the induction of antibody production by B cells but inhibits helper function of T cells. *Journal of Immunology, 135*, 2084–289.

Giros, B., Martres, M. P., Sokoloff, P., & Schwartz, J. C. (1990). Gene cloning of human dopaminergic D3 receptor and identification of its chromosome. *Comptes Rendus de L Academie Des Sciences, Series III, 311*, 501–508.

Goin, J. C., Sterin-Borda, L., Borda, E. S., Finiasz, M., Fernandez, J., & de Bracco, M. M. (1991). Active alpha 2 and beta adrenoceptors in lymphocytes from patients with chronic lymphocytic leukemia. *International Journal of Cancer, 49*, 178–181.

Gushchin, G. V., Jakovleva, E. E., Kataeva, G. V., Korneva, E. A., Gajewski, M., Grabczewska, E., Laskowska-Bozek, H., Maslinski, W., & Ryzewski, J. (1994). Muscarinic cholinergic receptors of rat lymphocytes: Effect of antigen stimulation and local brain lesion. *Neuroimmunomodulation, 1*, 259–264.

Hadden, J. W., Hadden, E. M., & Middleton, E. (1970). Lymphocyte blast transformation. I. Demonstration of adrenergic receptors in human peripheral lymphocytes. *Cellular Immunology, 1*, 583–595.

Hall, N. R., McClure, J. E., Hu, S., Tare, S., Seals, C. M., & Goldstein, A. L. (1982). Effects of 6-hydroxydopamine upon primary and secondary thymus dependent immune responses. *Immunopharmacology, 5*, 39–48.

Hara, N., Ichinose, M., Sawada, M., & Maeno, T. (1991). The activation of Ca(2+)-dependent K+ conductance by adrenaline in mouse peritoneal macrophages. *Pflugers Archives: European Journal of Physiology, 419*, 371–379.

Hatfield, S. M., Petersen, B. H., & Di Micco, J. A. (1986). Beta adrenoceptor modulation of the generation of murine cytotoxic T lymphocytes in vitro. *Journal of Pharmacology and Experimental Therapeutics, 239*, 460–466.

Heilig, M., Irwin, M., Grewal, I., & Sercarz, E. (1993). Sympathetic regulation of T-helper cell function. *Brain, Behavior, and Immunity, 7*, 154–163.

Hellstrand, K., Czerkinsky, C., Ricksten, A., Jansson, B., Asea, A., Kylefjord, H., & Hermodsson, S. (1993). Role of serotonin in the regulation of interferon-gamma production by human natural killer cells. *Journal of Interferon Research, 13*, 33–38.

Hellstrand, K. & Hermodsson, S. (1993). Serotonergic 5-HT1A receptors regulate a cell contact-mediated interaction between natural killer cells and monocytes. *Scandanavian Journal of Immunology, 37*, 7–18.

Hellstrand, K., Hermodsson, S., & Strannegard, O. (1985). Evidence for a beta-adrenoceptor-mediated regulation of human natural killer cells. *Journal of Immunology, 134*, 4095–4099.

Hellstrom-Lindahl, E. & Nordberg, A. (1996). Muscarinic receptor subtypes in subpopulations of human blood mononuclear cells as analyzed by RT-PCR technique. *Journal of Neuroimmunology, 68*, 139–144.

Henricks, P. A., van Esch, B., & Nijkamp, F. P. (1986). Beta-agonists can depress oxidative metabolism of alveolar macrophages. *Agents and Actions, 19*, 353–354.

Henricks, P. A., van Esch, B., Van Oosterhout, A. J., & Nijkamp, F. P. (1988). Specific and non-specific effects of beta-adrenoceptor agonists on guinea pig alveolar macrophage function. *European Journal of Pharmacology, 152*, 321–330.

Henricks, P. A. J., Verhoef, J., & Nijkamp, F. P. (1986). Modulation of phagocytic cell function. *Veterinary Research Communications, 10*, 165–188.

Higgins, T. J. & David, J. R. (1976). Effect of isoproterenol and aminophylline on cyclic AMP levels of guinea pig macrophages. *Cellular Immunology, 27*, 1–10.

Hjemdahl, P., Larsson, K., Johansson, M. C., Zetterlund, A., & Eklund, A. (1990). Beta-adrenoceptors in human alveolar macrophages isolated by elutriation. *British Journal of Clinical Pharmacology, 30*, 673–682.

Holte, H., Torjesen, P., Blomhoff, H. K., Ruud, E., Funderud, S., & Smeland, E. B. (1988). Cyclic AMP has the ability to influence multiple events during B cell stimulation. *European Journal of Immunology, 18*, 1359–1366.

Hu, X., Goldmuntz, E. A., & Brosnan, C. F. (1991). The effect of norepinephrine on endotoxin-mediated macrophage activation. *Journal of Neuroimmunology, 31*, 35–42.

Ignatowski, T. A., Gallant, S., & Spengler, R. N. (1996). Temporal regulation by adrenergic receptor stimulation of macrophage-derived tumor necrosis factor (TNF) production post-LPS challenge. *Journal of Neuroimmunology, 65*, 107–117.

Ignatowski, T. A. & Spengler, R. N. (1995). Regulation of macrophage-derived tumor necrosis factor production by modification of adrenergic receptor sensitivity. *Journal of Neuroimmunology, 61*, 61–70.

Ikegami, K. (1977). Modulation of adenosine 3',5'-monophosphate contents of rat peritoneal macrophages mediated by beta2-adrenergic receptors. *Biochemical Pharmacology, 26*, 1813–1816.

Iken, K., Chheng, S., Fargin, A., Goulet, A. C., & Kouassi, E. (1995). Serotonin upregulates mitogen-stimulated B lymphocyte proliferation through 5-HT1A receptors. *Cellular Immunology, 163*, 1–9.

Irwin, M., Hauger, R. L., Brown, M., & Britton, K. T. (1988). CRF activates autonomic nervous system and reduces natural killer cytotoxicity. *American Journal of Physiology, 255*, R744–R747.

Irwin, M., Hauger, R. L., Jones, L., Provencio, M., & Britton, K. T. (1990). Sympathetic nervous system mediates central corticotropin-releasing factor induced suppression of natural killer cytotoxicity. *Journal of Pharmacology and Experimental Therapeutics, 255*, 101–107.

Issaad, C., Ventura, M. A., & Thomopoulos, P. (1989). Biphasic regulation of macrophage attachment by activators of cyclic adenosine monophosphate-dependent kinase and protein kinase C. *Journal of Cellular Physiology, 140*, 317–322.

Javierre, M. Q., Pinto, L. V., Lima, A. O., & Sassine, W. A. (1975). Immunologic phagocytosis by macrophages: Effect by stimulation of alpha adrenergic receptors. *Revista Brasileira Pesquisas Medicas E Biologicas, 8*, 271–274.

Jetschmann, J. U., Benschop, R. J., Jacobs, R., Kemper, A., Oberbeck, R., Schmidt, R. E., & Schedlowski, M. (1997). Expression and in-vivo modulation of alpha- and beta-adrenoceptors on human natural killer (CD16+) cells. *Journal of Neuroimmunology, 74*, 159–164.

Johnson, D. L., Ashmore, R. C., & Gordon, M. A. (1981). Effects of beta-adrenergic agents on the murine lymphocyte response to mitogen stimulation. *Journal of Immunopharmacology, 3*, 205–219.

Johnson, D. L. & Gordon, M. A. (1981). Effect of chronic beta-adrenergic therapy on the human lymphocyte response to concanavalin A. *Research Communications in Chemical Pathology and Pharmacology, 32*, 377–380.

Kaneda, T., Kitamura, Y., & Nomura, Y. (1993). Presence of M3 subtype muscarinic acetylcholine receptors and receptor-mediated increases in the cytoplasmic concentration of Ca2+ in Jurkat, a human leukemic helper T lymphocyte line. *Molecular Pharmacology, 43*, 356–364.

Kasahara, K., Tanaka, S., Ito, T., & Hamashima, Y. (1977). Suppression of the primary immune response by chemical sympathectomy. *Research Communications in Chemical Pathology and Pharmacology, 16*, 687–694.

Kasprowicz, D. J., Kohm, A. P., Berton, M. T., Chruscinski, A. J., Sharpe, A., & Sanders, V. M. (2000). Stimulation of the B cell receptor, CD86 (B7-2), and the beta2-adrenergic receptor intrinsically modulates the level of IgG1 and IgE produced per B cell. *Journal of Immunology, 165*, 680–690.

Katamura, K., Shintaku, N., Yamauchi, Y., Fukui, T., Ohshima, Y., Mayumi, M., & Furusho, K. (1995). Prostaglandin E2 at priming of naive CD4+ T cells inhibits acquisition of ability to produce IFN-gamma and IL-2, but not IL-4 and IL-5. *Journal of Immunology, 155*, 4604–4612.

Kawakami, K. & Parker, D. C. (1993). Antigen and helper T lymphocytes activate B lymphocytes by distinct signaling pathways. *European Journal of Immunology, 23*, 77–84.

Kawashima, K., Fujii, T., Watanabe, Y., & Misawa, H. (1998). Acetylcholine synthesis and muscarinic receptor subtype mRNA expression in T-lymphocytes. *Life Sciences, 62*, 1701–1705.

Kendall, M. D. & al-Shawaf, A. A. (1991). Innervation of the rat thymus gland. *Brain, Behavior, and Immunity, 5*, 9–28.

Khan, N. A., Ferriere, F., & Deschaux, P. (1995). Serotonin-induced calcium signaling via 5-HT1A receptors in human leukemia (K 562) cells. *Cellular Immunology, 165*, 148–152.

Khan, M. M., Sansoni, P., Silverman, E. D., Engleman, E. G., & Melmon, K. L. (1986a). Beta-adrenergic receptors on human suppressor, helper, and cytolytic lymphocytes. *Biochemical Pharmacology, 35*, 1137–1142.

Khan, M. M., Sansoni, P., Silverman, E. D., Engleman, E. G., & Melmon, K. L. (1986b). Beta-adrenergic receptors on human suppressor, helper, and cytolytic lymphocytes. *Biological Psychiatry, 35*, 1137–1142.

Klaus, S. J. & Parker, D. C. (1992). Inducible cell contact signals regulate early activation gene expression during B-T lymphocyte collaboration. *Journal of Immunology, 149*, 1867–1875.

Koff, W. C. & Dunegan, M. A. (1985). Modulation of macrophage-mediated tumoricidal activity by neuropeptides and neurohormones. *Journal of Immunology, 135*, 350.

Kohm, A. P. & Sanders, V. M. (2000). Suppression of antigen-specific Th2 cell-dependent IgM and IgG1 production following norepinephrine depletion in vivo., *162*, 5299–5308.

Kohm, A.P. & Sanders, V. M. (2000). Suppression of Th1 cell-dependent IgM and IgG2a production following norepinephrine depletion in vivo. Manuscript in preparation.

Kohm, A. P., Swanson, M. A., & Sanders, V. M. (2000). The role of histone acetylation and DNA methylation in modulating the differential expression of the beta2-adrenergic receptor in $CD4^+$, Th1 and Th2 cells. Manuscript submitted for publication.

Kouassi, E., Boukhris, W., Descotes, J., Zukervar, P., Li, Y. S., & Revillard, J. P. (1987). Selective T cell defects induced by dopamine administration in mice. *Immunopharmacology and Immunotoxicology, 9*, 477–488.

Kouassi, E., Li, Y. S., Boukhris, W., Millet, I., & Revillard, J.-P. (1988). Opposite effects of the catecholamines dopamine and norepinephrine on murine polyclonal B-cell activation. *Immunopharmacology, 16*, 125–137.

Kouassi, E., Li, Y. S., & Revillard, J.-P. (1990). Catecholamine regulation of mouse B cell activation. Functional dichotomy between LPS and anti-immunoglobulin antibody responses. *Annals New York Academy of Science, 594*, 391–392.

Kouassi, E. & Revillard, J. P. (1987). Contribution of beta-adrenoceptors to the dopamine-induced elevation of cyclic 3′,5′-adenosine monophosphate levels in mouse lymphocytes. *European Journal of Pharmacology, 144*, 97–100.

Krause, D. S. & Deutsch, C. (1991). Cyclic AMP directly inhibits IL-2 receptor expression in human T cells: Expression of both p55 and p75 subunits is affected. *Journal of Immunology, 146*, 2285–2294.

Krawietz, W., Werdan, K., Schober, M., Erdmann, E., Rindfleisch, G. E., & Hannig, K. (1982). Different numbers of beta-receptors in human lymphocyte subpopulations. *Biochemical Pharmacology, 31*, 133–136.

Kruszewska, B., Felten, S. Y., & Moynihan, J. A. (1995). Alterations in cytokine and antibody production following chemical sympathectomy in two strains of mice. *Journal of Immunology, 155*, 4613–4620.

Kurz, B., Feindt, J., von Gaudecker, B., Kranz, A., Loppnow, H., & Mentlein, R. (1997). Beta adrenoceptor-mediated effects in rat cultured thymic epithelial cells. *British Journal of Pharmacology, 120*, 1401–1408.

Lacour, M., Arrighi, J. F., Muller, K. M., Carlberg, C., Saurat, J. H., & Hauser, C. (1994). cAMP up-regulates IL-4 and IL-5 production from activated CD4+ T cells while decreasing IL-2 release and NF-AT induction. *International Immunology, 6*, 1333–1343.

Lappin, D. & Whaley, K. (1982). Adrenergic receptors on monocytes modulate complement component synthesis. *Clinical and Experimental Immunology, 47*, 606–612.

Laskowska-Bozek, H., Bany, U., Burakowski, T., Janiak, R., Lewartowski, B., & Ryzewski, J. (1996). Effect of cholinergic stimulation on free intracellular Ca2+ concentration in human lymphocytes. *Neuroimmunomodulation, 3*, 247–253.

Laskowska-Bozek, H., Bany, U., Stokarska, G., & Ryzewski, J. (1995). Level of inositol-1,4,5-trisphosphate after cholinergic stimulation of human lymphocytes. *Neuroimmunomodulation, 2*, 25–30.

Lavis, V. R., Strada, S. J., Ross, C. P., Hersh, E. M., & Thompson, W. J. (1980). Comparison of the responses of freshly isolated and cultured human monocytes and P388D1 cells to agents affecting cyclic AMP metabolism. *Journal of Laboratory and Clinical Medicine, 96*, 551–550.

Le Fur, G., Phan, T., & Uzan, A. (1980). Identification of stereospecific [3H]spiroperidol binding sites in mammalian lymphocytes. *Life Sciences, 26*, 1139–1148.

Ledbetter, J. A., Parsons, M., Martin, P. J., Hansen, J. A., Rabinovitch, P. S., & June, C. H. (1986). Antibody binding to CD5 (Tp67) and Tp44 T cell surface molecules: Effects on cyclic nucleotides, cytoplasmic free calcium, and cAMP-mediated suppression. *Journal of Immunology, 137*, 3299–3305.

Li, Y. S., Kouassi, E., & Revillard, J.-P. (1989). Cyclic AMP can enhance mouse B cell activation by regulating progression into late G_1/S phase. *European Journal of Immunology, 19*, 1721–1725.

Liggett, S. B. (1989). Identification and characterization of a homogeneous population of beta 2-adrenergic receptors on human alveolar macrophages. *American Review of Respiratory Disease, 139*, 552–555.

Lipski, S. (1976). Effects of beta-adrenergic stimulation on bone-marrow function in normal and sublethally irradiated mice. I. The effect of isoproterenol on cAMP content in bone-marrow in vivo and in vitro. *International Journal of Radiation Biology and Related Studies in Physical and Chemical Medicine, 29*, 359–366.

Lipski, S. (1980). Effect of beta-adrenergic stimulation by isoproterenol on proliferation and differentiation of mouse bone marrow cells in vivo. *Polish Journal of Pharmacology and Pharmacy, 32*, 281–287.

Liu, Y. & Wolfe, S. A., Jr. (1996). Haloperidol and spiperone potentiate murine splenic B cell proliferation. *Immunopharmacology, 34*, 147–159.

Livnat, S., Felten, S. Y., Carlson, S. L., Bellinger, D. L., & Felten, D. L. (1985). Involvement of peripheral and central catecholamine systems in neural-immune interactions. *Journal of Neuroimmunology, 10*, 5–30.

Loveland, B. E., Jarrott, B., & McKenzie, I. F. C. (1981). The detection of beta-adrenoceptors on murine lymphocytes. *International Journal of Immunopharmacology, 3*, 45–55.

Madden, K. S., Felten, S. Y., Felten, D. L., Sundaresan, P. R., & Livnat, S. (1989). Sympathetic neural modulation of the immune system. I. Depression of T cell immunity in vivo and in vitro following chemical sympathectomy. *Brain, Behavior and Immunity, 3*, 72–89.

Madden, K. S., Moynihan, J. A., Brenner, G. J., Felten, S. Y., Felten, D. L., & Livnat, S. (1994). Sympathetic nervous system modulation of the immune system. III. Alterations in T and B cell proliferation and differentiation in vitro following chemical sympathectomy. *Journal of Neuroimmunology, 49*, 77–87.

Madden, K. S., Sanders, V. M., & Felten, D. L. (1995). Catecholamine influences and sympathetic neural modulation of immune responsiveness. *Annual Review of Pharmacology and Toxicology, 35*, 417–448.

Maestroni, G. J. M. (1995). Adrenergic regulation of haematopoiesis. *Pharmacological Research, 32*, 249–253.

Maestroni, G. J. M. & Conti, A. (1994a). Modulation of hematopoiesis via alpha-1-adrenergic receptors on bone marrow cells. *Experimental Hematology, 22*, 313–320.

Maestroni, G. J. M. & Conti, A. (1994b). Noradrenergic modulation of lymphohematopoiesis. *International Journal of Immunopharmacology, 16*, 117–122.

Maestroni, G. J. M., Conti, A., & Pedrinis, E. (1992). Effect of adrenergic agents on hematopoiesis after syngeneic bone marrow transplantation in mice. *Blood, 80*, 1178-1182.

Maisel, A. S., Harris, T., Rearden, C. A., & Michel, M. C. (1990). Beta-adrenergic receptors in lymphocyte subsets after exercise. Alterations in normal individuals and patients with congestive heart failure. *Circulation, 82*, 2003–2010.

Makman, M. H. (1971). Properties of adenylate cyclase of lymphoid cells. *Proceedings of the National Academy of Sciences, 68*, 885–889.

Maloteaux, J. M., Waterkein, C., & Laduron, P. M. (1982). Absence of dopamine and muscarinic receptors on human lymphocytes. *Archives of Pharmacodynamics and Therapeutics, 258*, 174–176.

Marazziti, D., Palego, L., Dal Canto, B., Rotondo, A., Pasqualetti, M., Gino, G., Lucacchini, A., Ladinsky, H., Nardi, I., & Cassano, G. B. (1995). Presence of serotonin1A (5-HT1A) receptor mRNA without binding of [3H]-8-OH-DPAT in peripheral blood mononuclear cells. *Life Sciences, 57*, 2197–2203.

Marchetti, B., Morale, M. C., Paradis, P., & Bouvier, M. (1994). Characterization, expression, and hormonal control of a thymic beta-2-adrenergic receptor. *American Journal of Physiology, 267*, E718–E731.

Marsland, A. L., Manuck, S. B., Wood, P., Rabin, B. S., Muldoon, M. F., & Cohen, S. (1995). Beta 2-adrenergic receptor density and cardiovascular response to mental stress. *Physiological Behavior, 57*, 1163–1167.

Mary, D., Peyron, J.-F., Auberger, P., Aussel, C., & Fehlmann, M. (1989). Modulation of T cell activation by differential regulation of the phosphorylation of two cytosolic proteins. *Journal of Biological Chemistry, 264*, 14498-14502.

McConkey, D. J., Orrenius, S., & Jondal, M. (1990). Agents that elevate cAMP stimulate DNA fragmentation in thymocytes. *Journal of Immunology, 145*, 1227–1230.

McPherson, G. A. & Summers, R. J. (1982). Characteristics and localization of 3H-clonidine binding in membranes prepared from guinea pig spleen. *Clinical and Experimental Pharmacology & Physiology, 9*, 77–87.

Melmon, K. L., Bourne, H. R., Weinstein, Y., Shearer, G. M., Kram, J., & Bauminger, S. (1974). Hemolytic plaque formation by leukocytes in vitro: Control by vasoactive amines. *Journal of Clinical Investigation, 53*, 13–21.

Meurs, H., Van Den Bogaard, W., Kauffman, H. F., & Bruynzeel, P. L. B. (1982). Characterization of (−)-[^{3}H]Dihydroalprenolol binding to intact and broken cell preparations of human peripheral blood lymphocytes. *European Journal of Pharmacology, 85*, 185–194.

Meurs, H., Timmermans, A., de Monchy, J. G., Zaagsma, J., & Kauffman, H. F. (1993). Lack of coupling of muscarinic receptors to phosphoinositide metabolism and adenylyl cyclase in human lymphocytes and polymorphonuclear leukocytes: Studies in healthy subjects and allergic asthmatic patients. *International Archives of Allergy and Immunology, 100*, 19–27.

Meyniel, J. P., Khan, N. A., Ferriere, F., & Deschaux, P. (1997). Identification of lymphocyte 5-HT3 receptor subtype and its implication in fish T-cell proliferation. *Immunology Letters, 55*, 151–160.

Miles, B. A., Lafuse, W. P., & Zwilling, B. S. (1996). Binding of alpha-adrenergic receptors stimulates the anti-mycobacterial activity of murine peritoneal macrophages. *Journal of Neuroimmunology, 71*, 19–24.

Miles, K., Atweh, S., Otten, G., Arnason, B. G. W., & Chelmicka-Schorr, E. (1984). Beta-adrenergic receptors on splenic lymphocytes from axotomized mice. *International Journal of Immunopharmacology, 6*(3), 171–177.

Miles, K., Chelmicka-Schorr, E., Atweh, S., Otten, G., & Arnason, B. G. W. (1985). Sympathetic ablation alters lymphocyte membrane properties. *Journal of Immunology, 135*, 797s–801s.

Miles, K., Quintans, J., Chelmicka-Schorr, E., & Arnason, B. G. W. (1981). The sympathetic nervous system modulates antibody response to thymus-independent antigens. *Journal of Neuroimmunology, 1*, 101–105.

Morale, M. C., Gallo, F., Batticane, N., & Marchetti, B. (1992). The immune response evokes up- and down-modulation of beta-2-adrenergic messenger RNA concentration in the male rat thymus. *Molecular Endocrinology, 6*, 1513–1524.

Morgan, J. I., Wigham, C. G., & Perris, A. D. (1984). The promotion of mitosis in cultured thymic lymphocytes by acetylcholine and catecholamines. *Journal of Pharmacy and Pharmacology, 36*, 511–515.

Mosmann, T. R., Cherwinski, H., Bond, M. W., Giedlin, M. A., & Coffman, R. L. (1986). Two types of murine helper T cell clones. I. Definition according to profiles of lymphokine activities and secreted proteins. *Journal of Immunology, 136*, 2348.

Murray, D. R., Irwin, M., Rearden, C. A., Ziegler, M., Motulsky, H., & Maisel, A. S. (1992). Sympathetic and immune interactions during dynamic exercise. Mediation via a beta 2-adrenergic-dependent mechanism. *Circulation, 86*, 203–213.

Muthusamy, N., Baluyut, A. R., & Subbarao, B. (1991). Differential regulation of surface Ig- and Lyb2-mediated B cell activation by cyclic AMP. I. Evidence for alternative regulation of signaling through two different receptors linked to phosphatidylinositol hydrolysis in murine B cells. *Journal of Immunology, 147*, 2483–2492.

Nagai, Y., Ueno, S., Saeki, Y., Soga, F., Hirano, M., & Yanagihara, T. (1996). Decrease of the D3 dopamine receptor mRNA expression in lymphocytes from patients with Parkinson's disease. *Neurology, 46*, 791–795.

Nahas, G. G., Desoize, B., & Leger, C. (1979). Effects of psychotropic drugs on DNA synthesis in cultured lymphocytes. *Proceedings of the Society for Experimental Biology and Medicine, 160*, 344–348.

Novak, T. J. & Rothenberg, E. V. (1990). cAMP inhibits induction of interleukin 2 but not of interleukin 4 in T cells. *Proceedings of the National Academy of Sciences, 87*, 9353–9357.

Nowell, G. H., Cruse, J. M., & Lewis, R.E. (1981). Detection of beta-adrenergic receptors on mouse peritoneal macrophages by binding to insolubilized hormone preparation. *Federation Proceedings, 40*, 81a–810.

Nozaki, H., Hozumi, K., Nishimura, T., & Habu, S. (1996). Regulation of NK activity by the administration of bromocriptine in haloperidol-treated mice. *Brain, Behavior, and Immunity, 10*, 17–26.

Ovadia, H., Lubetzki-Korn, I., & Abramsky, O. (1987). Dopamine receptors on isolated membranes of rat thymocytes. *Annals of the New York Academy of Sciences, 496*, 211–216.

Paliogianni, F. & Boumpas, D. T. (1996). Prostaglandin E2 inhibits the nuclear transcription of the human interleukin 2, but not the Il-4, gene in human T cells by targeting transcription factors AP-1 and NF-AT. *Cellular Immunology, 171*, 95–101.

Panajotova, V. (1997). The effect of dopaminergic agents on cell-mediated immune response in mice. *Physiological Research, 46*, 113–118.

Patke, C. L., Orson, F. M., & Shearer, W. T. (1991). Cyclic AMP-mediated modulation of immunoglobulin production in B cells by prostaglandin E1. *Cellular Immunology, 137*, 36–45.

Petty, H. R. & Berg, K. A. (1988). Combinative ligand-receptor interactions: Epinephrine depresses RAW264 macrophage antibody-dependent phagocytosis in the absence and presence of met-enkephalin. *Journal of Cellular Physiology, 134*, 281–286.

Pochet, R. & Delespesse, G. (1983). Beta-adrenoceptors display different efficiency on lymphocyte subpopulations. *Biochemical Pharmacology, 32*, 1651–1655.

Pochet, R., Delespesse, G., Gausset, P. W., & Collet, H. (1979). Distribution of beta-adrenergic receptors on human lymphocyte subpopulations. *Clinical Experimental Immunology*, 38, 578–584.

Pruett, S. B., Han, Y., Munson, A. E., & Fuchs, B. A. (1992). Assessment of cholinergic influences on a primary humoral immune response. *Immunology, 77*, 428–435.

Qiu, Y., Peng, Y., & Wang, J. (1996). Immunoregulatory role of neurotransmitters. *Advances in Neuroimmunology, 6*, 223–231.

Radojcic, T., Baird, S., Darko, D., Smith, D., & Bulloch, K. (1991). Changes in beta-adrenergic receptor distribution on immunocytes during differentiation: An analysis of T cells and macrophages. *Journal Neuroscience Research, 30*, 328–335.

Ramer-Quinn, D. S., Baker, R. A., & Sanders, V. M. (1997). Activated Th1 and Th2 cells differentially express the beta-2-adrenergic receptor: A mechanism for selective modulation of Th1 cell cytokine production. *Journal of Immunology, 159*, 4857–4867.

Ramer-Quinn, D. S., Swanson, M. A., Lee, W. T., & Sanders, V. M. (2000). Cytokine production by naive and primary effector $CD4^+$ T cells exposed to norepinephrine. Manuscript submitted for publication.

Remold-O'Donnell, E. (1974). Stimulation and desensitization of macrophage adenylate cyclase by prostaglandins and catecholamines. *Journal of Biological Chemistry, 249*, 311–321.

Ricci, A., Bronzetti, E., Felici, L., Ciriaco, E., Vega, J. A., & Germana, G. (1996). Muscarinic cholinergic receptor subtypes in the pigeon bursa of Fabricius: A radioligand binding and autoradiographic study. *Journal of Neuroimmunology, 66*, 23–28.

Ricci, A., Bronzetti, E., Felici, L., Tayebati, S. K., & Amenta, F. (1997). Dopamine D4 receptor in human peripheral blood lymphocytes: a radioligand binding assay study. *Neuroscience Letters, 229*, 130–134.

Ricci, A., Mariotta, S., Greco, S., & Bisetti, A. (1997). Expression of dopamine receptors in immune organs and circulating immune cells. *Clinical Experimental Hypertension, 19*, 59–71.

Rinner, I., Felsner, P., Falus, A., Skreiner, E., Kukulansky, T., Globerson, A., Hirokawa, K., & Schauenstein, K. (1995). Cholinergic signals to and from the immune system. *Immunology Letters, 44*, 217–220.

Roper, R. L., Conrad, D. H., Brown, D. M., Warner, G. L., & Phipps, R. P. (1990). Prostaglandin E2 promotes IL-4-induced IgE and IgG1 synthesis. *Journal of Immunology, 145*, 2644–2651.

Rosati, C., Hannaert, P., Dausse, J. P., Braquet, P., & Garay, R. (1986). Stimulation of beta-adrenoceptors inhibits calcium-dependent potassium- channels in mouse macrophages. *Journal of Cellular Physiology, 129*, 310–314.

Sanders, V. M. & Munson, A. E. (1984a). Kinetics of the enhancing effect produced by norepinephrine and terbutaline on the murine primary antibody response in vitro. *Journal of Pharmacology and Experimental Therapeutics, 231*, 527–531.

Sanders, V. M. & Munson, A. E. (1984b). Beta-adrenoceptor mediation of the enhancing effect of norepinephrine on the murine primary antibody response in vitro. *Journal of Pharmacology and Experimental Therapeutics, 230*, 183–192.

Sanders, V. M. & Munson, A. E. (1985). Role of alpha adrenoceptor activation in modulating the murine primary antibody response in vitro. *Journal of Pharmacology and Experimental Therapeutics, 232*, 395–400.

Sanders, V. M. & Powell-Oliver, F. E. (1992). Beta-2-adrenoceptor stimulation increases the number of antigen-specific precursor B lymphocytes that differentiate into IgM-secreting cells without affecting burst size. *Journal of Immunology, 148*, 1822–1828.

Sanders, V. M., Baker, R. A., Ramer-Quinn, D. S., Kasprowicz, D. J., Fuchs, B. A., & Street, N. E. (1997). Differential expression of the beta-2-adrenergic receptor by Th1 and Th2 clones: Implications for cytokine production and B cell help. *Journal of Immunology, 158*, 4200–4210.

Santambrogio, L., Lipartiti, M., Bruni, A., & Dal Toso, R. (1993). Dopamine receptors on human T- and B-lymphocytes. *Journal of Neuroimmunology, 45*, 113–119.

Schedlowski, M., Hosch, W., Oberbeck, R., Benschop, R. J., Jacobs, R., Raab, H. R., & Schmidt, R. E. (1996). Catecholamines modulate human NK cell circulation and function via spleen-independent beta 2-adrenergic mechanisms. *Journal of Immunology, 156*, 93–99.

Schopf, R. E. & Lemmel, E. M. (1983). Control of the production of oxygen intermediates of human polymorphonuclear leukocytes and monocytes by beta adrenergic receptors. *Journal of Immunopharmacology, 5*, 208–216.

Scorza-Smeraldi, R., Sabbadini Villa, M. G., Fabio, G., Bonara, P., Vanoli, M., Resele, L., & Zanussi, C. (1983). HLA antigens and the reactivity of lymphocytes to some drugs and PHA. *International Journal of Immunopharmacology, 5*, 145–149.

Selliah, N., Bartik, M. M., Carlson, S. L., Brooks, W. H., & Roszman, T. L. (1995). cAMP accumulation in T-cells inhibits anti-CD3 monoclonal antibody-induced actin polymerization. *Journal of Neuroimmunology, 56*, 107–112.

Serio, M., Potenza, M. A., Montagnani, M., Mansi, G., Mitolo-Chieppa, D., & Jirillo, E. (1996). Beta-adrenoceptor responsiveness of splenic macrophages in normotensive and hypertensive rats. *Immunopharmacology and Immunotoxicology, 18*, 247–265.

Shakhar, G. & Ben-Eliyahu, S. (1998). In vivo beta-adrenergic stimulation suppresses natural killer activity and compromises resistance to tumor metastasis in rats. *Journal of Immunology*, 160, 3251–3258.

Shaskan, E. G., Ballow, M., Lederman, M., Margoles, S. L., & Melchreit, R. (1984). Spiroperidol binding sites on mouse lymphoid cells. Effects of ascorbic acid and psychotropic drugs. *Journal of Neuroimmunology, 6*, 59–66.

Shreurs, A. J. M., Versteeg, D. H. G., & Nijkamp, F. P. (1982). Involvement of catecholamines in Haemophilus influenzae induced decrease of beta-adrenoceptor function. *Naunyn-Schmiedeberg's Archives of Pharmacology, 320*, 235–239.

Siegel, J. N., June, C. H., Yamada, H., Rapp, U. R., & Samelson, L. E. (1993). Rapid activation of C-Raf-1 after stimulation of the T-cell receptor or the muscarinic receptor type 1 in resting T cells. *Journal of Immunology, 151*, 4116–4127.

Smith, J. W., Steiner, A. L., Newberry, M., & Parker, C. W. (1971). Cyclic adenosine 3′,5′-monophosphate in human lymphocytes. Alterations after phytohemagglutinin stimulation. *Journal of Clinical Investigation, 50*, 432–441.

Smith, J. W., Steiner, A. L., & Parker, C. W. (1971). Human lymphocyte metabolism. Effects of cyclic and noncyclic nucleotides on stimulation by phytohemagglutinin. *Journal of Clinical Investigation, 50*, 442–448.

Sokoloff, P., Giros, B., Martres, M. P., Bouthenet, M. L., & Schwartz, J. C. (1990). Molecular cloning and characterization of a novel dopamine receptor (D3) as a target for neuroleptics. *Nature, 347*, 146–151.

Spengler, R. N., Allen, R. M., Remick, D. G., Strieter, R. M., & Kunkel, S. L. (1990). Stimulation of alpha-adrenergic receptor augments the production of macrophage-derived tumor necrosis factor. *Journal of Immunology, 145*, 1430–1434.

Spengler, R. N., Chensue, S. W., Giacherio, D. A., Blenk, N., & Kunkel, S. L. (1994). Endogenous norepinephrine regulates tumor necrosis factor-alpha production from macrophages in vitro. *Journal of Immunology, 152*, 3024–3031.

Stein, S. H. & Phipps, R. P. (1991). Antigen-specific IgG2a production in response to prostaglandin E_2, immune complexes, and IFN-gamma. *Journal of Immunology, 147*, 2500–2506.

Stepien, H., Kunert-Radek, J., Karasek, E., & Pawlikowski, M. (1981). Dopamine increases cyclic AMP concentration in the rat spleen lymphocytes in vitro. *Biochememical and Biophysical Research Commununications, 101*, 1057–1063.

Sternberg, E. M., Trial, J., & Parker, C. W. (1986). Effect of serotonin on murine macrophages: Suppression of Ia expression by serotonin and its reversal by 5-HT2 serotonergic receptor antagonists. *Journal of Immunology, 137*, 276–282.

Sternberg, E. M., Wedner, H. J., Leung, M. K., & Parker, C. W. (1987). Effect of serotonin (5-HT) and other monoamines on murine macrophages: modulation of interferon-gamma induced phagocytosis. *Journal of Immunology, 138*, 4360–4365.

Strom, T. B., Carpenter, C. B., Garovoy, M. R., Austen, K. F., Merrill, J. P., & Kaliner, M. (1973). The modulating influence of cyclic nucleotides upon lymphocyte-mediated cytotoxicity. *Journal of Experimental Medicine, 138*, 381–393.

Sudo, N., Yu, X. N., Sogawa, H., & Kubo, C. (1997). Restraint stress causes tissue-specific changes in the immune cell distribution. *Neuroimmunomodulation, 4*, 113–119.

Sunahara, R. K., Guan, H. C., O'Dowd, B. F., Seeman, P., Laurier, L. G., Ng, G., George, S. R., Torchia, J., Van Tol, H. H., & Niznik, H. B. (1991). Cloning of the gene for a human dopamine D5 receptor with higher affinity for dopamine than D1. *Nature, 350*, 614–619.

Suzuki, K., Tadakuma, T., & Kizaki, H. (1991). Modulation of thymocyte apoptosis by isoproterenol and prostaglandin E2. *Cellular Immunology, 134*, 235–240.

Swanson, M. A., Lee, W. T., & Sanders, V. M. (2000). Neuromodulation of IL-12-dependent naive CD4+ T cell differentiation. Manuscript submitted for publication.

Swanson, M. A. & Sanders, V. M. (2000). IgG2a and IgG1 production by Th1/B and Th2/B cell cultures exposed to a beta-2-adrenergic receptor agonist after cell-cell interaction. Manuscript in preparation.

Szabo, C., Hasko, G., Zingarelli, B., Nemeth, Z. H., Salzman, A. L., Kvetan, V., Pastores, S. M., & Vizi, E. S. (1997). Isoproterenol regulates TNF, IL-10, IL-6, and nitric oxide production and protects against the development of vascular hyporeactivity in endotoxemia. *Immunology, 90*, 95–100.

Takamoto, T., Hori, Y., Koga, Y., Toshima, H., Hara, A., & Yokoyama, M. M. (1991). Norepinephrine inhibits human natural killer cell activity in vitro. *International Journal of Neuroscience, 58*, 127–131.

Takayama, H., Trenn, G., & Sitkovsky, M. V. (1988). Locus of inhibitory action of cAMP-dependent protein kinase in the antigen receptor-triggered cytotoxic T lymphocyte activation pathway. *Journal of Biological Chemistry, 263*, 2330-2336.

Tamir, A. & Isakov, N. (1994). Cyclic AMP inhibits phosphatidylinositol-coupled and -uncoupled mitogenic signals in T lymphocytes. Evidence that cAMP alters PKC-induced transcription regulation of members of the jun and fos family of genes. *Journal of Immunology, 152*, 3391–3399.

Teh, H. S. & Paetkau, V. (1976). Regulation of immune responses. II. The cellular basis of cyclic AMP effects on humoral immunity. *Cellular Immunology, 24*, 220–229.

Titinchi, S. & Clark, B. (1984). Alpha-2 -adrenoceptors in human lymphocytes: Direct Characterization by [3H]Yohimbine binding. *Biochememical and Biophysical Research Commununications, 121*(1), 1–7.

Tsao, C. W., Lin, Y. S., & Cheng, J. T. (1997). Effect of dopamine on immune cell proliferation in mice. *Life Sciences, 61*, PL 361–PL 371.

Uzan, A., Phan, T., & Le Fur, G. (1981). Selective labelling of murine B lymphocytes by [3H]spiroperidol. *Journal of Pharmacy and Pharmacology, 33*, 102–103.

van Esch, B., Henricks, P. A., Van Oosterhout, A. J., & Nijkamp, F. P. (1989). Guinea pig alveolar macrophages possess beta-adrenergic receptors. *Agents Actions, 26*, 123–124.

Van Tits, L. J. H., Michel, M. C., Grosse-Wilde, H., Happel, M., Eigler, F.-W., Soliman, A., & Brodde, O.-E. (1990). Catecholamines increase lymphocyte beta-2-adrenergic receptors via a beta-2-adrenergic, spleen-dependent process. *American Journal of Physiology, 258*, E191–E202.

Van Tol, H. H., Bunzow, J. R., Guan, H. C., Sunahara, R. K., Seeman, P., Niznik, H. B., & Civelli, O. (1991). Cloning of the gene for a human dopamine D4 receptor with high affinity for the antipsychotic clozapine. *Nature, 350*, 610–614.

Verghese, M. W. & Snyderman, R. (1983). Hormonal activation of adenylate cyclase in macrophage membranes is regulated by guanine nucleotides. *Journal of Immunology, 130*, 869–873.

Vile, J. M. & Strange, P. G. (1996). D2-like dopamine receptors are not detectable on human peripheral blood lymphocytes. *Biological Psychiatry, 40*, 881–885.

Vischer, T. L. (1976). The differential effect of cAMP on lymphocyte stimulation by T- or B-cell mitogens. *Immunology, 30*, 735–739.

von Patay, B., Loppnow, H., Feindt, J., Kurz, B., & Mentlein, R. (1998). Catecholamine and lipopolysaccharide synergistically induce the release of interleukin-6 from thymic epithelial cells. *Journal of Neuroimmunology, 86*, 182–189.

Wacholtz, M. C., Minakuchi, R., & Lipsky, P. E. (1991). Characterization of the 3′,5′-cyclic adenosine monophosphate-mediated regulation of IL2 production by T cells and Jurkat cells. *Cellular Immunology, 135*, 285–298.

Waterfield, J. D., Hammarstrom, L., & Smith, E. (1976). The effect of membrane stabilizing agents on induction of the immune response. I. Effect of lymphocyte activation in mixed lymphocyte reactions. *Journal of Experimental Medicine, 144*, 562–567.

Watson, J., Epstein, R., & Cohn, M. (1973). Cyclic nucleotides as intracellular mediators of the expression of antigen-sensitive cells. *Nature, 246*, 405–409.

Weinstein, Y., Segal, S., & Melmon, K. L. (1975). Specific mitogenic activity of 8-Br-guanosine 3′,5′-monophosphate (Br-cyclic GMP) on B lymphocytes. *Journal of Immunology, 115*, 112–117.

Weissmann, G., Dukor, P., & Zurier, R. B., (1971). Effect of cyclic AMP on release of lysosomal enzymes from phagocytes. *Nature New Biology, 231*, 131–135.

Welscher, H. D. & Cruchaud, A. (1976). The influence of various particles and 3′, 5′ cyclic adenosine monophosphate on release of lysosomal enzymes by mouse macrophages. *Journal of the Reticuloendothelial Society, 20*, 405–420.

Westly, H. J. & Kelley, K. W. (1987). Down-regulation of glucocorticoid and beta-adrenergic receptors on lectin-stimulated splenocytes. *Proceedings of the Society for Experimental Biology and Medicine, 185*, 211–218.

Whalen, M. M. & Bankhurst, A. D. (1990). Effects of beta-adrenergic receptor activation, cholera toxin and forskolin on human natural killer cell function. *Biochemical Journal, 272*, 327–331.

Whisler, R. L., Beiqing, L., Grants, I. S., & Newhouse, Y. G. (1992). Cyclic AMP modulation of human B cell proliferative responses: role of cAMP-dependent protein kinases in enhancing B cell responses to phorbol diesters and ionomycin. *Cellular Immunology, 142*, 398–415.

Williams, L. T., Snyderman, R., & Lefkowitz, R. J. (1976). Identification of beta adrenergic receptors in human lymphocytes by (−)^{3}H-alprenolol binding. *Journal of Clinical Investigation, 57*, 149–155.

Wirth, S., Lacour, M., Jaunin, F., & Hauser, C. (1996). Cyclic adenosine monophosphate (cAMP) differentially regulates IL-4 in thymocyte subsets. *Thymus, 24*, 101–109.

Won, S. J., Chuang, Y. C., Huang, W. T., Liu, H. S., & Lin, M. T. (1995). Suppression of natural killer cell activity in mouse spleen lymphocytes by several dopamine receptor antagonists. *Experientia, 51*, 343–348.

Xie, H., Chiles, T. C., & Rothstein, T. L. (1993). Induction of CREB activity via the surface Ig receptor of B cells. *Journal of Immunology, 151*, 880–889.

Yamada, T., Murayama, T., & Nomura, Y. (1997). Muscarinic acetylcholine receptors on rat thymocytes: their possible involvement in DNA fragmentation. *Japanese Journal of Pharmacology, 73*, 311–316.

Yoshimura, T., Nagao, T., Nakao, T., Watanabe, S., Usami, E., Kobayashi, J., Yamazaki, F., Tanaka, H., Inagaki, N., & Nagai, H. (1998). Modulation of Th1- and Th2-like cytokine production from mitogen- stimulated human peripheral blood mononuclear cells by phosphodiesterase inhibitors. *General Pharmacology, 30*, 175–180.

Young, J. D.-E., Ko, S. S., & Cohn, Z. A. (1984). The increase in intracellular free calcium associated with IgGgamma2b/gamma1 Fc receptor-ligand interactions: role in phagocytosis. *Proceedings of the National Academy of Sciences, 81*, 5430–5434.

Zhou, Q. Y., Grandy, D. K., Thambi, L., Kushner, J. A., Van Tol, H. H., Cone, R., Pribnow, D., Salon, J., Bunzow, J. R., & Civelli, O. (1990). Cloning and expression of human and rat D1 dopamine receptors. *Nature, 347*, 76–80.

C H A P T E R

5

Catecholamines, Sympathetic Nerves, and Immunity

KELLEY S. MADDEN

I. INTRODUCTION

Exogenous and endogenous stimuli, including physical stressors, behavioral conditioning, lipopolysaccharide (LPS), and opioids can modulate immune and inflammatory processes through sympathetic nervous system (SNS) activation, release of catecholamines, and interactions with adrenergic receptors (AR) (Cunnick, Lysle, Kucinski, & Rabin, 1990; Elenkov, Haskó, Kovács, & Vizi, 1995; Exton et al., 1998; Fecho, Maslonek, Dykstra, & Lysle, 1996; Sheridan et al., 1998). The range of stimuli that can alter immune function through SNS activation suggests that this pathway is important for appropriate removal of infectious agents and malignancies, while minimizing reactivity to self-antigens. This chapter reviews recent advances in catecholamine regulation of immune reactivity in vivo, and discusses the relevance of sympathetic neural-immune interactions to disease processes.

II. SYMPATHETIC NERVOUS SYSTEM: NEUROTRANSMITTERS AND RECEPTORS

A. Sources of NE and EPI

Cells of the immune system may encounter norepinephrine (NE) and epinephrine (EPI) from several sites in vivo. NE is released from sympathetic noradrenergic (NA) nerve fibers present in primary and secondary lymphoid organs (Stevens-Felten & Bellinger, 1997). The adrenal medulla can release primarily EPI, but also NE, into the blood stream (Qi, Zhou, Wurster, & Jones, 1991). More recently, it has been postulated that lymphocytes and macrophages may contain catecholamines, either by uptake or by synthesis (Bergquist, Tarkowski, Ekman, & Ewing, 1994; Chou, Dong, Noble, Knight, & Spengler, 1998; Spengler, Chensue, Giacherio, Blenk, & Kunkel, 1994) that can be released and regulate lymphocyte function in an autocrine fashion.

B. Co-localized transmitters

Neuropeptide Y (NPY) is present in NA nerve terminals in a variety of tissues, including the spleen

(Lundberg, Anggard, Pernow, & Hokfelt, 1985; Romano, Felten, Felten, & Olschowka, 1991). Adenosine triphosphate (ATP) is released from adrenal chromaffin cells and sympathetic nerve terminals, and is stored in large core vesicles with NE (Lundberg, 1996). Receptors that recognize NPY and ATP (the purinergic receptors) are present on cells of the immune system (De La Fuente, Bernaez, Del Rio, & Hernanz, 1993; Petitto, Huang, & McCarthy, 1994). Release of colocalized transmitters with NE depends on the intensity of the stimulus (Lundberg, 1996; Lundberg, Rudehill, Sollevi, Theodorsson-Norhein, & Hamberger, 1986), but the impact of the release of these colocalized neurotransmitters on immune reactivity has yet to be examined systematically.

C. Presynaptic Regulation of NE Release

In lymphoid organs, the release of NE, NPY, and ATP is inhibited by stimulation of presynaptic α_2-AR (Lundberg, 1996). By radioligand binding, α_2-AR were detected in splenic nerve of the dog, and were reduced following splenic nerve ligation (Schoups, Annaert, & De Potter, 1990). In rat spleen and thymus, stimulation-evoked release of NE from nerve terminals was potentiated by the highly selective α_2-AR antagonist CH 38083 (Elenkov & Vizi, 1991; Haskó, Elenkov, & Vizi, 1995; Vizi, Orsó, Osipenko, Haskó, & Elenkov, 1995). In the spleen, α_2-AR-mediated inhibition of NE release was stimulation frequency-dependent; α_2-blockade was not effective at high frequency (Elenkov & Vizi, 1991). In thymus preparations, release of NE was inhibited by adenosine and prostaglandin E_2, and increased by 1,1-di-methyl-4-phenylpiperazinium (DMPP), an N-nicotinic receptor agonist that stimulates postganglionic NA nerve fibers (Haskó et al., 1995). Therefore, NE release in lymphoid organs is regulated by a variety of agents, indicating that the microenvironment can determine the local concentration of released NE.

D. Adrenergic Receptors

By radioligand binding studies, mature lymphocytes express high-affinity β-AR, mainly of the β_2-subclass (reviewed in Landmann, 1992). The density of β-AR in B cells is greater than T cells; CD8+ T cells express more than CD4+ T cells; NK cells express more than CD4+ or CD8+ T cells. Recent evidence suggests that heterogeneity of βAR may be present within T helper (Th) cell populations (Sanders et al., 1997, see Sanders et al., this volume). Most reports indicate that receptor density, but not affinity, differs between lymphocyte populations, although human T cells may contain more agonist-induced high affinity β-AR compared with B cells (Griese et al., 1988).

In rat spleen and lymph nodes, α_2-AR have been demonstrated autoradiographically, but were absent in compartments containing lymphocytes (Fernández-López & Pazos, 1994), suggesting that the majority of rodent lymphocytes do not express α-AR. By radioligand binding techniques, adjuvant-elicited macrophages have been demonstrated to express β-AR and α_2-AR (Abrass, O'Connor, Scarpace, & Abrass, 1985; Spengler, Allen, Remick, Strieter, & Kunkel, 1990). AR expression by resting macrophages and dendritic cells has not been widely reported, because of the difficulties in obtaining purified populations in sufficient quantities. Recently, methods for obtaining large numbers of dendritic cells have been developed, making these important antigen presenting cells more amenable to study (Banchereau & Steinman, 1998). For example, dendritic cells were purified from mouse spleen 10 days after treatment with granulocyte-macrophage colony stimulating factor (GM-CSF), a method that generates a large quantity of mature dendritic cells with potent antigen presenting capabilities (Banchereau & Steinman, 1998). Radioligand binding with the non-selective β-AR antagonist [^{125}I]-cyanopindolol demonstrated that these dendritic cells express saturable and specific β-AR (Figure 1). Scatchard analysis revealed that β-AR density was about 850 sites per cell, with an affinity similar to that of lymphocytes. This finding, combined with in vitro evidence that dendritic cell interleukin (IL)-12 production is reduced by β-agonist stimulation (Panina-Bordignon et al., 1997), indicates that catecholamines can regulate dendritic cell function.

III. ROLE OF THE SYMPATHETIC NERVOUS SYSTEM IN VIVO

In vivo, investigators have used ablation of sympathetic NA innervation, infusion with AR agonists/antagonist, and sympathetic activation to examine the role of the SNS in modulating immune function. As will be seen, different experimental approaches are necessary because none is without interpretational difficulties or alternative explanations. These experiments demonstrate that the SNS regulates all aspects of immune function in vivo, including proliferation, cytokine production, antibody production, and lymphocyte migration.

A. Ablation of NA Nerve Fibers

Removal of peripheral sympathetic NA nerve fibers by treatment with 6-hydroxydopamine (6-

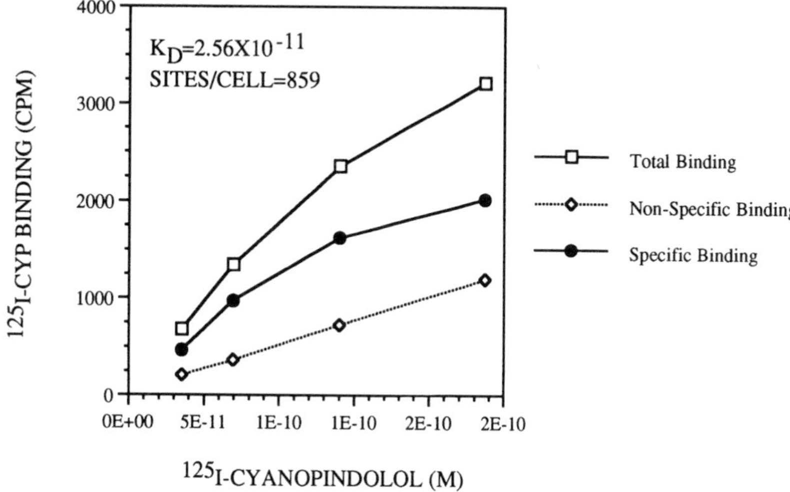

FIGURE 1 β-Adrenergic receptor (β-AR) expression by activated dendritic cells. Dendritic cells were purified from mouse spleen 10 days after treatment with granulocyte-macrophage colony stimulating factor (GM-CSF). Radioligand binding of the nonselective β-AR antagonist ^{125}I-cyanopindolol in the presence (nonspecific binding) or absence (total binding) of the β-AR antagonist 10^{-6} M CGP 12177. Specific binding was calculated by subtracting nonspecific cpm from total cpm. Affinity (K_D) and sites per cell were determined by Scatchard analysis.

OHDA) has been used to assess immune function in the absence of the SNS. The advantage of 6-OHDA is that it is highly selective for NA nerve fibers, and it does not cross the blood-brain barrier when administered to adults (Kostrzewa & Jacobwitz, 1974). A single intraperitoneal injection rapidly (<6 h) destroys most NA nerve fibers in 6-OHDA-sensitive tissues; NE is depleted by 75–85% in spleen and lymph nodes for at least 2 weeks (De Champlain, 1971; Madden, Felten, Felten, Hardy, & Livnat, 1994). It is taken up by the high affinity catecholamine uptake I system, and is blocked by uptake I blockers, such as the tricyclic antidepressant desipramine (De Champlain, 1971). On uptake, 6-OHDA rapidly destroys the integrity of the nerve terminal by a mechanism that is not well understood, resulting in the release of NE and other intracellular components from the nerve terminal. In adults, NA cell bodies are not destroyed, and reinnervation of the spleen begins as early as 5 days after 6-OHDA treatment (Lorton, Hewitt, Bellinger, Felten, & Felten, 1990). A gradual return of NA innervation occurs over the next several weeks, with complete recovery of the spleen observed 60 days after 6-OHDA treatment.

Because of the mechanism of action of 6-OHDA, several alternative interpretations must be assessed experimentally to conclude that the absence of NA nerve fibers was responsible for 6-OHDA-induced alterations in immune function. In vitro, very high levels of 6-OHDA can be toxic to lymphocytes, but the concentrations required are not likely to be attained in vivo. For example, 6-OHDA in vitro ($> 5 \times 10^{-5}$ M) inhibited T cell proliferation, cytokine production, and B cell differentiation (Josefsson, Månsson, Blennow, & Tarkowski, 1994), but as will be seen, 6-OHDA-induced changes in immune function in vivo are not unidirectional. To address the possibility of 6-OHDA toxicity in vivo, pretreatment with the tricyclic catecholamine uptake blocker desipramine has been used to prevent 6-OHDA uptake (and thus NE depletion), but allow direct interactions of 6-OHDA and its by-products with cells of the immune system. Desipramine pretreatment blocked 6-OHDA-induced alterations in T and B cell responses (Kruszewska, Felten, & Moynihan, 1995; Madden, Felten et al., 1994; Madden, Felten, Felten, Sundaresan, & Livnat, 1989; Madden, Moynihan et al., 1994). However, a 6-OHDA-induced decrease in macrophage phagocytosis was not blocked by desipramine pretreatment, evidence that phagocytic macrophages may be directly affected by 6-OHDA (Lyte, Ernst, Driemeyer, & Baissa, 1991). Scavenging and removal of the metabolic by-products of 6-OHDA may be mediated by these macrophages.

The degeneration of NA neurons that occurs immediately following 6-OHDA treatment may also influence immune reactivity. When these nerve fibers are destroyed, the cell contents, including NE and colocalized neurotransmitters, are rapidly released into the surrounding environment. The possibility exists that the transient release of NE may contribute to 6-OHDA-induced effects on immune function. For example, Josefsson et al. (1994) suggested that NE release may be responsible for the antiinflammatory effects of 6-OHDA administered just prior to an inflammatory agent. To address this issue, we have treated animals with the β-blocker propranolol prior to 6-OHDA to prevent interaction of NE with β-AR. This pretreatment had no effect on the sympathectomy-induced changes in delayed type hypersensitivity (Madden et al., 1989) and cellular proliferation in vivo (Madden, Felten et al., 1994). A chronic denervation approach has also been used to address this issue, in which denervated mice were immunized several weeks after 6-OHDA injection and the initial exposure to NE (Kruszewska et al., 1995). The effects of sympathectomy were the same in the chronically denervated state as in the acutely denervated state. Both of these approaches suggest that the release of intracellular contents following 6-OHDA treatment cannot induce significant changes in immune function, but it may not be possible to experimentally eliminate the potential for NE and colocalized neurotransmitter-induced alterations in immune reactivity following 6-OHDA treatment.

One advantage of 6-OHDA, besides its selectivity for NA nerve fibers, is its inability to cross the blood-brain barrier when administered to adults (Kostrzewa & Jacobwitz, 1974). Thus, destruction of central catecholaminergic pathways will not contribute to 6-OHDA-induced effects in the periphery. However, this does not imply that the central nervous system (CNS) is unaware that destruction of NA nerve fibers has occurred in the periphery. Recently, 6-OHDA treatment was shown to induce c-fos, an early-intermediate gene indicative of neuronal activation, in specific brain regions of C57BL/6 mice (Callahan, Moynihan, & Piekut, 1998). No c-fos was present in the circumventricular organs, confirming that 6-OHDA cannot cross the blood-brain barrier, and indicating that 6-OHDA did not induce c-fos directly. These results suggest that the CNS does detect the dramatic loss of sympathetics in the periphery, and that 6-OHDA-induced alterations in immune reactivity may be related to changes in signaling from the CNS, perhaps in the form of elevated glucocorticoid levels. Several investigators have attempted to determine if elevated glucocorticoids contribute to 6-OHDA-induced changes in immune reactivity (Kruszewska, Felten, Stevens, & Moynihan, 1998; Leo, Callahan, & Bonneau, 1998). It is also possible that the compensatory up-regulation of EPI from the adrenals after sympathectomy is induced by the 6-OHDA-induced activation of specific brain regions (Mueller, Thoenen, & Axelrod, 1969).

Recent findings using chemical sympathectomy have contributed to a greater understanding of SNS modulation of immune function. In many of these studies, experiments were conducted to address the potential confounding factors inherent in the use of 6-OHDA, and thus convincingly demonstrate that loss of NA innervation and NE depletion were responsible for altered immune reactivity following 6-OHDA treatment.

1. *Th Dominance and Effects of Sympathectomy*

The effects of sympathectomy in mice have been demonstrated to be dependent on the predominant Th cytokine pattern produced following antigenic stimulation. In adult C57BL/6 mice (a Th1 predominant strain) sympathectomized prior to intraperitoneal immunization, the primary antibody response to keyhole limpet hemocyanin (KLH) was elevated (Kruszewska et al., 1995). IgM and IgG anti-KLH antibody titers were increased following sympathectomy, including the isotypes IgG1 (Th2-associated) and IgG2a (Th1-associated). In BALB/c mice (a Th2 predominant strain), anti-KLH IgM and IgG responses were not altered by sympathectomy. Of the IgG subtypes, IgG1 was slightly increased, but only at a single time point postimmunization. Spleen cell KLH-induced proliferation in vitro was increased by sympathectomy in both strains, as were the KLH-induced cytokines, IL-2 and IL-4, although BALB/c mice produced much more IL-4 than C57BL/6, as expected in a Th2 predominant strain. KLH-induced interferon (IFN)-γ production was increased by sympathectomy only in the Th1 strain, C57BL/6 (Kruszewska et al., 1998).

Several experiments were conducted to determine that sympathectomy and NE depletion were responsible for the 6-OHDA-induced effects. First, desipramine pretreatment completely blocked the 6-OHDA-induced enhancement of KLH-induced proliferation and cytokine production, indicating that loss of sympathetics, and not direct effects of 6-OHDA, account for the 6-OHDA-induced effects (Kruszewska et al., 1995). Second, to determine if the initial release of NE immediately following destruction of sympathetic nerve terminals induced changes in immune function, mice were treated with 6-OHDA once a week, 16 days before antigen challenge, to ensure that all released NE had dissipated at the time of immunization. Elevated KLH-induced responses were observed in the chronically denervated mice, similar to the acutely denervated mice. Because reinnervation was prevented by weekly administration of 6-OHDA, this experiment also eliminated the possibility that regrowth of splenic NA innervation contribute to the 6-OHDA-induced effects

(Kruszewska et al., 1995). Finally, plasma corticosterone levels were elevated for 1–2 days in both strains of mice following the initial 6-OHDA treatment (Kruszewska et al., 1998). In chronically denervated BALB/c mice, glucocorticoid levels had returned to baseline at the time of immunization, and the enhancing effects of sympathectomy were still observed. Furthermore, in both strains of mice, implantation of the glucocorticoid receptor blocker RU 486 did not alter the denervation-induced changes in immune reactivity (Kruszewska et al., 1998). These results indicate that increased glucocorticoid levels did not mediate the sympathectomy-induced enhancement in immune reactivity to KLH. Taken together, these results demonstrated that sympathetic NA ablation was responsible for the 6-OHDA-induced increase in KLH-induced immune reactivity. Th dominance determined the impact of NA ablation on specific components of the response, including the effector (antibody) stage.

2. *Differences in Sympathectomy Related to Lymphoid Organs and Activational Signaling*

The enhancing effects of chemical sympathectomy in KLH-immunized mice suggest that intact NA innervation inhibits the immune response to KLH (Kruszewska et al., 1995, 1998). Similarly, Esquifino and Cardinali (1994) demonstrated increased antibody production in surgically denervated submaxillary lymph nodes relative to sham-denervated lymph nodes. However, delayed type hypersensitivity, a cell-mediated response, was inhibited by chemical sympathectomy in mice, including reduced cytotoxic T lymphocyte generation and IL-2 production by draining lymph node cells in vitro (Madden et al., 1989). Desipramine pretreatment blocked the 6-OHDA-induced effects, and propranolol pretreatment had no effect, leading to the conclusion that the SNS can promote cell-mediated immune responses. Contradictory effects of sympathectomy on immune reactivity have been discussed previously (Madden & Livnat, 1991), some of which may be explained by differences in the Th cytokine response. Other explanations for these differences may reside in the lymphoid organ draining the site of antigen challenge, as well as the nature of lymphocyte activation.

We have demonstrated differences in the response to sympathectomy in spleen versus inguinal lymph nodes of nonimmunized mice. For example, in sympathectomized animals, mitogen-induced B cell proliferation was dramatically increased in the lymph nodes, but decreased in the spleen (Madden, Moynihan et al., 1994). Spleen cell concanavalin A (Con A)-induced T cell proliferation in vitro was reduced in association with decreased IL-2 and IFN-γ production. In the lymph nodes, IL-2 production was not altered by sympathectomy, and IFN-γ production was dramatically increased. These differences may be related to sympathectomy-induced changes in lymphocyte migration patterns. The inguinal lymph nodes, but not the spleen, appeared to be susceptible to sympathectomy-induced changes in lymphocyte migration (Madden, Felten et al., 1994). Finally, Callahan and Moynihan (personal communication) have shown that sympathectomy in mice reduced spleen cell Con A-induced T cell proliferation, but increased antigen-specific proliferation by the same spleen cells, suggesting that the immunological stimulus may also determine the outcome of sympathectomy.

Together, these data suggest that the SNS regulates effector immune responses through alterations in such functions as lymphocyte proliferation, cytokine production, and migratory behavior, the net effect depending on genetic factors, such as Th dominance, as well as the lymphoid organ involved in the immune response, and even the nature of the activational signal received by lymphocytes. Investigators using different experimental approaches have drawn similar conclusions regarding the complex nature of interactions between the SNS and the immune system.

B. Administration of AR Agonists and Antagonists

To mimic a high level of sympathetic activation and β-AR signaling, Murray and colleagues implanted miniosmotic pumps containing two doses of the β-AR nonselective agonist, isoproterenol (ISO) into rats (Murray et al., 1993). Both doses of ISO induced cardiac hypertrophy from 1 to 4 days after receiving the implant, but spleen weight and splenocyte number were only transiently reduced day 2 after implant. The most dramatic change in percentage of leukocyte subsets was a reduction in the percentage of natural killer (NK) cells in the spleen, and a corresponding increase in NK cells in the blood, suggesting that the increase in circulating NK cells was in part due to NK cells entering the blood from the spleen. ISO-induced changes in the percentage of lymphocytes were not present in peripheral blood and were very small in the spleen. Functionally, spleen cell Con A-induced proliferation was reduced only at the highest ISO dose on day 2 after ISO implant. In immunized animals, ISO did not alter the antibody response in the spleen. The relatively small magnitude and transiency of the ISO-induced effects on lymphocyte function is most likely related to the rapid down-regulation of lymphocyte β-AR and subsequent receptor desensitization (Murray et al., 1993).

Felsner et al. demonstrated an α-AR-mediated reduction in peripheral blood T cell proliferation in vitro (Felsner et al. 1992). Using implantable pellets, a 20 h infusion of NE, but not EPI, reduced T lymphocyte proliferation by peripheral blood, but not spleen cells. In the presence of propranolol, both NE and EPI markedly inhibited peripheral blood Con-A-induced T cell proliferation; again, spleen cell proliferation was not altered by this treatment. The inhibitory effect observed with the combination of catecholamine and β-blockade was blocked by simultaneous administration of the α-AR antagonist, phentolamine. Coadministration of the α_2-agonist clonidine with propranolol or nadolol, a nonselective β-antagonist that does not cross the blood-brain barrier, also inhibited Con A-induced proliferation (Felsner et al., 1995). β-blockade was required for this effect; phentolamine administered alone or concurrently with EPI or NE did not alter peripheral blood T cell proliferation. In β-blocked animals, nighttime release of melatonin from the pineal gland is reduced; in animals receiving NE and propranolol, melatonin administration abolished the inhibition of Con A-induced proliferation (Liebmann, Hofer, Felsner, Wölfler, & Schauenstein, 1996). These results demonstrate site-specific changes in immune reactivity following AR stimulation (blood, but not spleen). In this case, the interaction of the SNS and the pineal gland appeared to evoke changes in T cell function.

These results and those reported by Murray et al., (1993) demonstrate that in young animals, catecholamine alterations in lymphocyte function are not easily induced experimentally. This tight regulation of catecholamine-lymphocyte signaling suggests that a disruption of the homeostatic tendency may contribute to immune dysfunction.

C. Lymphocyte Migration

1. *Lymphocyte Circulation*

Circulating lymphocytes are responsible for recognition of foreign entities, and on detection, induction of a rapid mobilization of the appropriate leukocytes (Westermann & Pabst, 1990). The SNS may be an important regulator of lymphocyte trafficking. Following physical exercise or exposure to mental or physical stressors, a rapid and transient leukocytosis occurs, consisting of increased NK cells, lymphocytes, and monocytes in the blood. These effects are blocked by β-AR blockers and can be mimicked by injection of EPI or ISO (Mills, Karnik, & Dillon, 1997; Schedlowski et al., 1996; reviewed by Benschop, Rodriquez-Feuerhahn, & Schedlowski, 1996). The mechanism behind this catecholamine-induced leukocytosis has been investigated, but is still not well understood. In vitro, β_2-AR agonists reduced adhesion of T cells and NK cells to endothelial cells (Benschop, Schedlowski, Wienecke, Jacobs, & Schmidt, 1997; Carlson, Beiting, Kiani, Abell, & McGillis, 1996), suggesting that cells in the marginal pool (attached to the endothelium of blood vessels) would be less likely to attach firmly to the endothelium in the presence of catecholamines. In vivo and in vitro, NE or EPI did not alter expression of a variety of cell adhesion molecules (Benschop et al., 1997; Carlson et al., 1996; Schedlowski et al., 1996), although affinity was not examined. Exercise to exhaustion increased plasma levels of intracellular adhesion molecule-1 (ICAM-1) by a β–AR-dependent mechanism (Rehman et al., 1997).

2. *Lymphocyte Entry and Exit from Lymphoid Organs*

Lymphocytes must enter draining lymphoid organs to encounter antigen; evidence suggests that the SNS and catecholamines alter entrance into lymphoid organs. Migration of adoptively transferred lymphocytes to Peyer's patch, mesenteric and inguinal lymph nodes was altered in chemically sympathectomized animals (González-Ariki & Husband, 1998; Madden, Felten et al., 1994). Incubation of lymphocytes with ISO in vitro increased homing of these cells to spleen and lymph nodes (Carlson, Fox, & Abell, 1997). Emigration from the spleen is also regulated by catecholamines. Early studies demonstrated that direct infusion of catecholamines into the spleen resulted in increased leukocyte output by either β- or α-AR-mediated mechanisms in the absence of changes in blood flow (Ernström & Sandberg, 1973). Using an in vivo perfusion method in rats, Besedovsky's group has recently demonstrated that sympathetic innervation of the spleen can regulate leukocyte output by altering flow resistance and by inducing cell output through a flow resistance-independent, β-AR mediated pathway (Rogausch, del Rey, Oertel, & Besedovsky, 1999). Together, these results suggest that the SNS and NE can regulate cell entry, retention and release from lymphoid organs. Understanding the mechanism underlying catecholamine-induced changed in lymphocyte trafficking may help provide the means by which cells can be mobilized or immobilized during local immune and inflammatory responses.

D. Thymus

The thymus is the primary site for differentiation of immature T cells into mature T cells that recognize and respond appropriately to foreign antigen. In the thymus of young animals, networks of NA nerve fibers are localized in the subcapsular, cortical, and corticomedullary regions associated with blood vessels and intralobular septa (Ackerman, Bellinger, Felten, & Felten, 1991; Kurz et al., 1997; Kendall & Al-Shawaf, 1991; Vizi et al., 1995), see Bellinger and Felten, this volume. Striking alterations in thymic NA innervation have been reported with age and pregnancy (Bellinger, Felten, & Felten, 1988; Kendall et al., 1994; Madden et al., 1997), but the functional significance is unknown.

When examined by radioligand binding assays, unfractionated thymocytes express very low levels of high affinity β-AR compared to mature T cells (Figures 2A, 2B). Mature corticosterone-resistant thymocytes express β-AR at levels equivalent to peripheral T cells (Fuchs, Albright, & Albright, 1988;

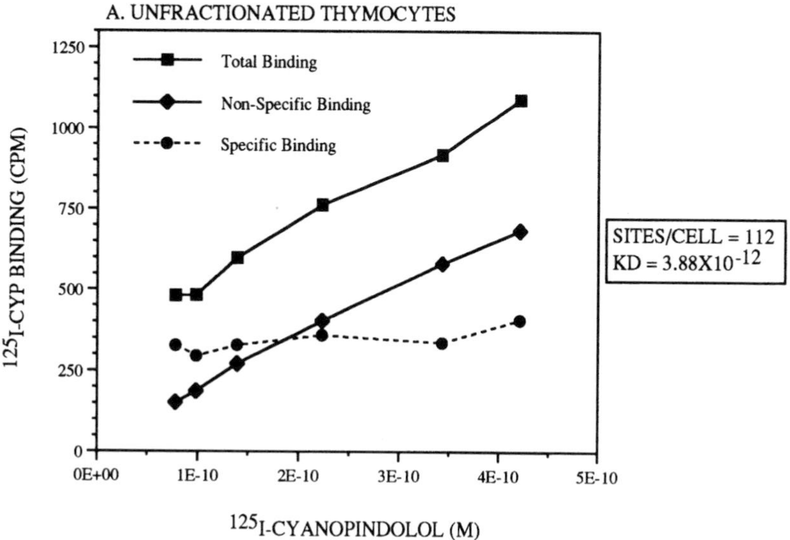

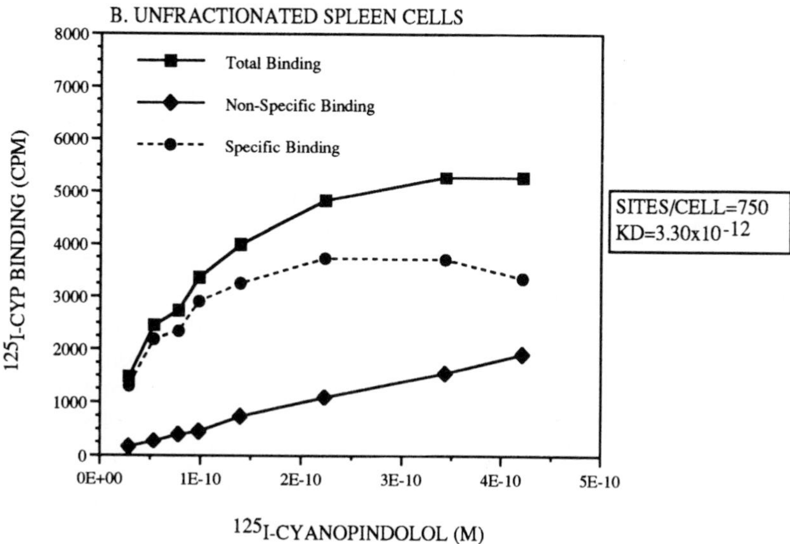

FIGURE 2 β- Adrenergic receptor (β-AR) expression by unfractionated thymocytes and splenocytes. ^{125}I-cyanopindolol binding to unfractionated (A) thymocytes and (B) spleen cells in the presence (nonspecific binding) or absence (total binding) of the β-AR antagonist 10^{-6} M CGP 12177. Specific binding was calculated by subtracting nonspecific cpm from total cpm. Affinity (K_D) and sites per cell were determined by Scatchard analysis.

Radojcic, Baird, Darko, Smith, & Bulloch, 1991), suggesting that immature T cells express very low levels of β-AR, and that β-AR expression is upregulated later in the differentiation process. Consistent with this notion of maturation-dependent regulation of β-AR expression in thymocytes is the localization of β_2-AR primarily to the medullary region of the rat thymus by autoradiography (Marchetti, Morale, Paradis, & Bouvier, 1994). When β-agonist-induced intracellular cAMP production was examined in vitro, the efficiency of receptor-coupling to adenylate cyclase was reported to be greater in unfractionated thymocytes when compared with spleen or lymph nodes (Bach, 1975). Similarly, we have found that unfractionated thymocytes generate an ISO-induced cAMP response that is equivalent to that of spleen cells, and yet spleen cells express far more β-AR (Table I, Figure 2). This suggests that the thymocytes that do express β-AR are exquisitely sensitive to β-AR agonist signaling. Furthermore, thymic epithelial cells, essential to the process of positive and negative selection in the thymus, may also express β-AR. Rat cultured thymic epithelial cells possess functional β-AR, as assessed by mRNA, radioligand binding, and cAMP induction (Kurz et al., 1997).

Very little is known about the functional role of NA innervation in the thymus. Older studies have alluded to enhanced thymocyte differentiation following β-AR stimulation and inhibition of thymocyte proliferation in the presence of intact NA innervation (Singh, 1985; Singh & Owen, 1976). More recently, chemical sympathectomy was reported to increase the number of proliferating cells, as detected by bromodeoxyuridine uptake, in the thymic cortex (Kendall & Al-Shawaf, 1991). Treatment of mice with 6-OHDA also increased apoptosis in the thymus, decreased thymus cellularity, and reduced spontaneous thymocyte proliferation in vitro (Delrue-Perollet, Li, Vitiello, & Neveu, 1995; Tsao, Cheng, Shen, & Lin, 1996). The 6-OHDA-induced increased apoptosis was prevented by desipramine pretreatment, demonstrating that ablation of NA nerve fibers induced this response (Tsao et al., 1996). However, 6-OHDA (10^{-5} M) also induced apoptosis in vitro, and co-incubation of 6-OHDA with desipramine in vitro prevented this effect (Tsao et al., 1996). This finding suggests that thymocytes may possess catecholamine uptake mechanisms, but further investigation is required. Chemical sympathectomy-induced changes in the thymus must be interpreted cautiously, because the thymus is not depleted of NE as completely as other tissues, such as the spleen (Kostrzewa & Jacobwitz, 1974). The possibility that the effects of 6-OHDA in the thymus may be induced by elevated corticosterone levels has not been addressed adequately. For example, Delrue-Perollet et al. (1995) demonstrated that corticosterone levels were not altered in sympathectomized animals at the time of sacrifice, 3 days after the first injection of 6-OHDA, but earlier time points were not examined. These results suggest that NA innervation in the thymus may influence thymocyte development, but studies using a variety of pharmacological approaches are necessary.

TABLE I Intracellular cAMP in Unfractionated Thymocytes and Spleen Cells

Drug	Spleen	Thymocytes
0	0.50[a]	0.56
ISO (10^{-4})	3.11	2.80
Stimulation Index[b]	6.2	5.0

Note: ISO = isoproterenol
[a] pMol/10^6 cells/10 min
[b] Stimulation index = cAMP (ISO)/cAMP (0 Drug)

E. Bone Marrow

The bone marrow is responsible for differentiation and maturation of erythrocytes, neutrophils, megakaryocytes, and B lymphocytes. NA and peptidergic innervation of sinuses and tissue parenchyma has been demonstrated (Afan, Broome, Nicholls, Whetton, & Miyan, 1997; Müller & Weihe, 1991; Tabarowski, Gibson-Berry, & Felten, 1996; Weihe, Müller, Fink, & Zentel, 1989), but the function of this innervation has not been extensively investigated, and is somewhat controversial. For example, neither neonatal 6-OHDA treatment (to permanently remove NA nerve fibers) nor unilateral surgical denervation of the sciatic nerve in mice had any effect on the percentage of granulocytes or GM-CFU obtained from bone marrow, leading Benestad and colleagues to postulate that NA innervation does not significantly influence differentiation of hematopoietic cells (Benestad, Strøm-Gundersen, Iversen, Haug, & Njå, 1998). Furthermore, only one report has characterized AR expression on bone marrow cells (Maestroni & Conti, 1994). Nonetheless, several investigators have reported that pharmacological manipulation of the SNS can alter bone marrow cellularity and cell mobilization.

Chemical sympathectomy in adult mice reduced bone marrow cellularity and increased the number of nucleated cells in the peripheral blood, suggesting that cells were driven out of the bone marrow following 6-OHDA treatment (Afan et al., 1997).

Progenitor cells did not appear to emigrate in response to NE depletion; in sympathectomized animals the number of GM-CFU increased, suggesting that they were either retained and/or were induced to proliferate. Increased cellular proliferation in the bone marrow has been observed following chemical sympathectomy in mice, suggesting that an intact SNS may inhibit spontaneous cell proliferation in the bone marrow (Madden et al., 1994).

Maestroni and co-workers reported that the $\alpha1/\alpha2b$-AR antagonist, prazosin, enhanced myelopoiesis and inhibited lymphopoiesis in normal mice and following syngeneic bone marrow transfer (Maestroni & Conti, 1994; Maestroni, Conti, & Pedrinis, 1992). In vitro, NE and the α_1-AR agonist methoxamine inhibited the growth of GM-CFU colonies (Maestroni & Conti, 1994). This corresponded well with the finding that unfractionated bone marrow cells possess high and low affinity ^{3}H-prazosin binding sites; the rank order of potency for inhibition of binding classified the high affinity site as α_1-AR (Maestroni & Conti, 1994). In addition, unlike in the spleen (Kelley, Grota, Felten, Madden, & Felten, 1996), NE and its metabolites in the bone marrow were greater at night compared with the day (Maestroni et al., 1998), suggesting that sympathetic NA innervation may direct those bone marrow functions that exhibit diurnal variation. Finally, quantifiable levels of NE were measured in tissue culture medium obtained following short-term culture of bone marrow cells and human pre-B lymphoblastoid lines, suggesting that NE in the bone marrow may be derived from neuronal and from non-neuronal cells (Maestroni et al., 1998). Closer examination of the function of sympathetic NA innervation of the bone marrow may lead to novel therapies to stimulate hematopoiesis following bone marrow transplant and chemotherapy (Maestroni, Togni, & Covacci, 1997).

IV. SYMPATHETIC ACTIVATION AND IMMUNOMODULATION

Sympathetic activation generally, but not always, inhibits T cell function and NK cell activity, especially in the spleen. Administration of the ganglionic stimulant DMPP inhibited T cell function and NK cell activity in the spleen, but did not alter T cell function in mesenteric lymph nodes (Fecho, Maslonek, Dykstra, & Lysle, 1993). Acute morphine and central administration of IFN-α, IL-1β, and corticotropin releasing factor (CRF) similarly reduced mitogen-induced T cell proliferation and NK cell activity in the spleen; these effects were blocked by peripheral β-AR blockade or ganglionic blockade (Fecho, Dykstra, & Lysle, 1993; Fecho et al., 1996; Irwin, Hauger, Brown, & Britton, 1988; Katafuchi, Take, & Hori, 1993; Sundar, Cierpial, Kilts, Ritchie, & Weiss, 1990; Take, Mori, Katafuchi, & Hori, 1993). In contrast, IL-2 administered concurrently with sheep red blood cells (SRBC) enhanced the IgM anti-SRBC response in rats and mice. Splenic nerve dissection and β-AR blockade prevented the IL-2-induced increase, suggesting that IL-2 acted through activation of splenic NA innervation (Zalcman et al., 1994).

Recently, significant progress has been made in the area of LPS-induced sympathetic activation and catecholamine regulation of proinflammatory and antiinflammatory cytokine mediators of endotoxic shock. The information obtained from experimental models of endotoxic shock, a potentially lethal condition, may contribute to understanding sympathetic regulation of cytokine production following more typical, nonlethal encounters with antigen and in pathogenic disease states involving these cytokines.

V. SYMPATHETIC ACTIVATION AND ENDOTOXIC SHOCK

Endotoxic shock is induced in laboratory animals by administration of LPS. Within 30 min of intraperitoneal LPS administration, plasma EPI and NE are elevated and splenic nerve activity and NE turnover are increased (MacNeil, Jansen, Greenberg, & Nance, 1996; Qi et al., 1991; Zhou, Wurster, & Jones, 1992). Many peripheral and central responses to endotoxin are mediated through the CNS by signaling of afferent vagal neurons (Goehler et al., 1999), but the precise pathway by which LPS induces sympathetic activation is still under investigation (MacNeil, Jansen, Janz, Greenberg, & Nance, 1997). Surprisingly, chlorisondamine treatment prior to LPS administration did not alter plasma tumor necrosis factor (TNF)-α concentration (Elenkov et al., 1995), but treatment with AR agonists and antagonists before LPS can alter serum levels of cytokine agents of inflammation, and can influence mortality (Fessler, Otterbein, Chung, & Choi, 1996; reviewed in Haskó & Szabó, 1998).

A. Antiinflammatory Effects of β-AR Stimulation

TNF-α is the primary proinflammatory cytokine induced in endotoxic shock. In laboratory animals and in human subjects a reduction in plasma TNF-α levels is associated with reduced mortality (Tracey et al., 1987). Elenkov et al. (1995) suggested that sympathetic activation inhibits TNF-α production through β-AR stimulation, based on the following evidence from LPS-treated mice: (1) propranolol pretreatment increased plasma TNF-α, (2) ISO pretreatment inhibited plasma TNF-α, and (3) α_2-AR blockade with the highly selective α_2-antagonist CH 38083 reduced plasma TNF-α. Pretreatment with chlorisondamine blocked the CH 38083-induced effect, suggesting that sympathetic activity was required. Furthermore, the nonselective β-blocker propranolol and the β_1-selective antagonist atenolol, but not the β_2-selective antagonist ICI 118,551, prevented the CH 38083-induced reduction in TNF-α, suggesting that the inhibitory effect of the α_2-antagonist was mediated by β_1-AR (Elenkov et al., 1995). Together, these data suggest a dual role for SNS activation following LPS administration: (1) reduction of TNF-α through β-AR, and (2) inhibition of NE release through presynaptic α_2-AR. Pharmacological disinhibition of α_2-AR, or agonist-induced β-AR stimulation, shifts the balance of AR stimulation toward β-AR mediated down-regulation of TNF-α production.

Other investigators have demonstrated similar inhibitory effects of β-stimulation on the inflammatory response induced by LPS in mice and humans. EPI and ISO administration in vivo reduced plasma levels of TNF-α, nitric oxide, IL-12, and IFN-γ, but enhanced IL-6 and IL-10 (Haskó, Szabó, Németh, Salzman, & Vizi, 1998; Monastra & Secchi, 1993; Szabó et al., 1997; van der Poll, Coyle, Barbosa, Braxton, & Lowry, 1996; van der Poll, Jansen, Endert, Sauerwein, & van Deventer, 1994). These in vivo results are consistent with in vitro evidence demonstrating that macrophages can participate directly in the β-AR-mediated inhibition of TNF-α (Chou et al., 1996; Haskó, Szabó et al., 1998; Ignatowski & Spengler, 1995; Severn, Rapson, Hunter, & Liew, 1992; Spengler et al., 1994).

IL-10 can down-regulate an inflammatory response by reducing TNF-α production; e.g., increasing plasma levels of IL-10 decreased mortality in endotoxemic mice by inhibition of TNF-α (Gérard et al., 1993). To determine if the β-agonist-induced decrease in plasma TNF-α was mediated by increased IL-10, LPS was administered to IL-10-deficient (IL-10−/−) mice (Haskó, Szabó et al., 1998). In both wildtype (IL-10+/+) and IL-10−/− mice, β-AR stimulation inhibited plasma TNF-α, IL-12, and IFN-γ, indicating that IL-10 is not required for the antiinflammatory effects of β-AR stimulation. IL-10 was also not required for a β-AR-induced enhancement of IL-8 production in vitro (Kavelaars, van de Pol, Zijlstra, & Heijnen, 1997). Nonetheless, regulation of IL-10 by β-AR stimulation may indeed influence the inflammatory response. In vivo β-blockade with oxprenolol reduced LPS-induced plasma IL-10 in mice, and ISO and EPI increased LPS-induced IL-10 mRNA and protein by macrophages in vitro (Suberville, Bellocq, Fouqueray, Philippe, Lantz, Perez, & Baud, 1996; van der Poll et al., 1996). ISO- and EPI-induced inhibition of TNF-α production in vitro was partially blocked by neutralizing anti-IL-10 antibodies (Suberville et al., 1996; van der Poll et al., 1996). NE also modestly increased LPS-induced IL-10 production in vitro, mainly through β-AR (van der Poll et al., 1996).

IL-10 is significant not only as a potent antiinflammatory cytokine; it also serves as an indicator of the Th2 (humoral) response. In vivo, β-AR-stimulation increased plasma IL-10, and decreased plasma concentrations of the Th1 cytokines IL-12 and IFN-γ (Haskó, Szabó et al., 1998), indicative of a shift to a predominantly Th2 response following LPS treatment. In vitro, IL-12 production by activated monocytes and dendritic cells was reduced by a β-agonist at much lower concentrations than was required to inhibit TNF-α production (Panina-Bordignon et al., 1997). Furthermore, in vitro differentiation of neonatal naive T cells shifted from a predominantly Th1 pattern of cytokine production to a predominantly Th2 pattern in the presence of the β-agonist salbutamol (Panina-Bordignon et al., 1997). Together, these results suggest that Th1-mediated responses are inhibited by β-AR stimulation, and conversely, that Th2-mediated responses are promoted by β_2-agonists. If this hypothesis is true, then clinical diseases that exhibit a Th subset predominance may benefit therapeutically by manipulating catecholamine regulation of cytokine production.

B. Are Macrophage α_2-AR Proinflammatory in Vivo?

In contrast to the inhibitory effects of β-agonist stimulation on TNF-α production, α_2-AR stimulation of macrophages in vitro can increase LPS-induced TNF-α production (Spengler et al., 1990, 1994). In vivo, evidence for pro-inflammatory effects of macrophage α_2-AR stimulation is sparse. The α_2-AR agonists UK 14304 and dexmedetomidine administered before LPS reduced plasma TNF-α (Elenkov et al., 1995). Ganglionic blockade with chlorisondamine did not prevent the UK 14304-induced inhibition of TNF-α, suggesting that sympathetic activation and presynaptic neuronal α_2-AR do not mediate this response. Fessler et al. (1996) reported that mortality was increased in rats treated with the α_2-agonists xylazine and UK 14304 prior to LPS, but plasma TNF-

α levels were not measured in these animals. In contrast, pretreatment with the α_2-antagonist rauwolscine protected all rats from an LD100 dose of LPS (Fessler et al., 1996). In these animals, α_2-blockade not only reduced plasma TNF-α levels, but also increased arterial pressure, reduced liver enzymes and bilirubin, and prevented bowel hemorrhage, suggesting that many tissues are targets for α_2-AR stimulation.

These results demonstrate that following exposure to endotoxin, and possibly other inducers of inflammation (Le Tulzo et al., 1997), sympathetic activation inhibits proinflammatory cytokine production by β-AR stimulation. At the same time, the increase in sympathetic outflow is dampened by catecholamine stimulation of α_2-AR. Further work is required to determine if macrophage α_2-AR play a significant role in cytokine production in vivo. It should be emphasized that catecholamine signaling also will be influenced by the presence of other regulators of the inflammatory response, such as glucocorticoids and prostaglandins. For example, in an in vitro study, preexposure of macrophages to ISO reduced the ability of both ISO and prostaglandin E_2 to inhibit TNF-α production, suggesting that under certain conditions catecholamine signaling capacity will be reduced (Ignatowski & Spengler, 1995). Basic studies clarifying the role for AR and the temporal relationship between endotoxin administration and catecholamine-induced alterations in cytokine production in vivo may lead to clinical studies that maximize the benefits and minimize unwanted side effects of stimulation of AR receptors.

The regulation of pro- and antiinflammatory cytokines by catecholamines indicate that pharmacological manipulation of the interface between the nervous system and immune system may be therapeutically beneficial in autoimmune diseases that have a significant inflammatory component, including multiple sclerosis (MS) and rheumatoid arthritis. Evidence of a role for the SNS in animal models of autoimmune disease and in clinical disease will be discussed below.

VI. SYMPATHETIC REGULATION OF AUTOIMMUNE DISEASES

Experimental animal models have been developed to mimic a variety of autoimmune diseases present in the human population. In these animal models, alterations in sympathetic innervation, NE levels, and lymphocyte AR expression have been demonstrated. Removal of sympathetic NA innervation or stimulation of AR can alter the clinical severity of autoimmune disease, evidence that modulation of the SNS influences autoimmune disease pathology.

A. Animal Models

1. *Changes in Sympathetics during the Course of Disease*

In MRL-*lpr*/*lpr* mice, a genetic model for systemic lupus erythematosus, reduced splenic NA innervation and decreased splenic NE levels were observed just prior to onset of disease symptoms (Breneman, Moynihan, Grota, Felten, & Felten, 1993). A similar reduction in splenic NE concentration was reported in experimental allergic encephalomyelitis (EAE), an MS-like disease induced in rats by injection of myelin basic protein in complete Freund's adjuvant (Mackenzie, Leonard, & Cuzner, 1989). The reduction in splenic NE concentration appeared early after EAE induction, and was accompanied by an increase in the density of splenic β-AR at the time of maximal antigen-induced lymphocyte proliferation. In a chronic-relapsing form of EAE (CREAE) in rats, splenocyte β-AR density correlated positively with the severity of CREAE, and splenic β-AR density increased with each relapse, suggesting that NE levels were reduced in the spleen, similar to EAE (Wiegmann, Muthyala, Kim, Arnason, & Chelmicka-Schorr, 1995). Together, these results suggest that a reduction in NE concentration may promote the disease process by removal of an inhibitory signal for lymphocyte proliferation.

2. *Catecholamine Manipulation Alters Disease Severity*

In adjuvant-induced arthritis in rats, systemic removal of sympathetic input, either by β-AR blockade or by chemical sympathectomy with 6-OHDA or guanethidine, reduced arthritic symptoms, suggesting that the SNS promotes arthritis development (Levine, Coderre, Helms, & Basbaum, 1988). In contrast, localized denervation of draining lymph nodes, with sparing of the nerves innervating the joint, was shown to exacerbate disease (Lorton, Bellinger, Duclos, Felten, & Felten, 1996). These results suggest that the SNS has different functions at the site of induction of the disease (the draining lymph nodes) compared with the inflammatory site (the joint). The SNS may inhibit the generation of antigen-specific T cells in draining lymph nodes, but promote inflammation in the joints. Administration of a high dose of EPI reduced severity of experimental arthritis by an α_2-AR mediated mechanism, but a low dose of EPI exacerbated joint injury (Coderre, Basbaum, Helms, &

Levine, 1991). These results indicate that care must be used in manipulating the SNS therapeutically in complex diseases.

In contrast to the inhibitory effects of systemic sympathectomy on arthritis, chemical sympathectomy with 6-OHDA enhanced the severity of symptoms in experimental autoimmune myasthenia gravis (Agius, Checinski, & Arnason, 1987) and in EAE (Chelmicka-Schorr, Checinski, & Arnason, 1988). Administration of ISO or the β_2-selective agonist terbutaline reduced the severity of symptoms in EAE and CREAE (Chelmicka-Schorr, Kwasniewski, Thomas, & Arnason, 1989; Wiegmann et al., 1995). In CREAE, treatment with terbutaline also reduced the number of relapses (Wiegmann et al., 1995). Terbutaline administered after disease induction also reduced the clinical severity in experimental autoimmune myasthenia gravis (Chelmicka-Schorr, Wollmann, Kwasniewski, Kim, & Dupont, 1993) and in experimental allergic neuritis, an induced inflammation of peripheral nerves similar to Guillain-Barré disease (Kim et al., 1994).

3. *SNS Can Alter Lymphocyte Function in EAE*

Alteration of autoimmune disease pathology by the SNS may be mediated by lymphoid or nonlymphoid mechanisms (for example of the latter, see Goldmuntz, Brosnan, & Norton, 1986). To determine if sympathectomy altered the ability of antigen-specific T cells to induce disease, adoptive transfer of myelin basic protein-sensitized T cells was employed (Chelmicka-Schorr, Kwasniewski, & Wollmann, 1992). When donor T cells were obtained from sympathectomized animals and transferred into intact animals, EAE was more severe in recipients of T cells from sympathectomized animals, demonstrating a functional alteration in T cells. EAE was also more severe when the recipients of antigen-specific T cells had been sympathectomized, suggesting that the environment in a sympathectomized animals is more conducive to induction of EAE. Together, these results suggest that sympathectomy affects the disease process at several levels, including the antigen-specific T cell. TNF-α, IL-12, and IL-10 are thought to be key mediators of adjuvant-induced arthritis and EAE (Chou et al., 1998; Leonard, Waldburger, & Goldman, 1995; Rott, Fleischer, & Cash, 1994). Given the potent regulatory effects of the SNS on LPS-induced production of these cytokines (see Section V), it is reasonable to suggest that catecholamines may act via T cells and/or macrophages to influence autoimmune processes through altered cytokine production. An investigation of in vivo catecholamine regulation of cytokines contributing to these autoimmune disease models should prove fruitful.

B. Clinical Evidence

Collectively, the evidence from a variety of animal models indicates that the SNS may influence induction and progression of autoimmune disease. Similarly, evidence suggests that the SNS can influence autoimmune processes in humans.

1. *Juvenile Chronic Arthritis and Rheumatoid Arthritis*

a. *Altered Sympathetic Activity*

In children with active juvenile chronic arthritis (JCA), increased resting heart rate and high levels of urinary 3-methoxy-4-hydroxy-phenylglycol (MHPG, an NE metabolite) were observed, evidence that increased sympathetic activity is associated with this disease (Kuis et al., 1996). Adults with rheumatoid arthritis also develop autonomic dysfunction, depending on the severity of the disease (Leden, Eriksson, Lilja, Sturfelt, & Sundkvist, 1983; Perry, Heller, Kamiya, & Levine, 1989). Furthermore, regional removal of sympathetic input by guanethidine treatment improved arthritic symptoms, possibly by removing a pro-inflammatory component in the joint itself (Levine, Fye, Heller, Basbaum, & Whiting-O'Keefe, 1986). These results imply that autonomic dysfunction in patients with active arthritis may contribute to the underlying inflammatory process.

b. *Changes in Lymphocyte AR Expression and/or Sensitivity*

In patients with active JCA, the increase in sympathetic outflow is associated with hyporesponsiveness to an orthostatic stress test; this reduced responsiveness to SNS activation is also present at the level of the lymphocyte (Kuis et al., 1996; Kavelaars, de Jong-de Vos van Steenwijk, Kuis, & Heijnen, 1998). Intracellular cAMP production in response to stimulation with the β-agonist isoprenaline was reduced in lymphocytes from JCA patients compared with healthy controls and patients with nonactive JCA. Furthermore, peripheral blood mononuclear cells from patients with polyarticular JCA (the more severe form of the disease), but not oligoarticular patients, produced IL-6 in vitro in the presence of the α_1-AR agonist, phenylephrine; no other stimulant was required (Heijnen et al., 1996). This effect was blocked by the α_1-AR-selective antagonist doxazosin, suggesting that α_1-AR are expressed with disease progression; α_1-AR are not normally present in peripheral blood monocytes from healthy human subjects. In adults with rheumatoid arthritis, Baerwald et al. reported that β-AR density was decreased on peripheral blood mononuclear cells, with a corresponding decrease in affinity (Baerwald, Graefe, von Wichert, & Krause, 1992). This decrease did not correlate with plasma catecholamines, but it did correlate positively with disease activity. By contrast, Zoukos et al. reported increased β-AR expression in lymphocytes from rheumatoid arthritis patients, similar to changes in MS patients (Zoukos, Leonard, Thomaides, Thompson, & Cuzner, 1992). Determining β-AR signaling capacity of lymphocytes from rheumatoid arthritis patients may help resolve these differences. A clinical investigation of the in vivo effects of α-antagonists and/or β-AR agonist stimulation may be fruitful, for example, to determine if TNF-α production can be reduced in rheumatoid arthritis (Saxne, Palladino, Heinegård, Talal, & Wollheim, 1988).

2. *Multiple Sclerosis*

a. Altered Sympathetic Activity and Lymphocyte AR Expression

Reduced sympathetic tonus has been demonstrated in MS patients with active disease (Karaszewski, Reder, Maselli, Brown, & Arnason, 1990). Increased β-AR expression on CD8+ T cells have been reported in MS patients undergoing relapse and in patients with chronic progressive multiple sclerosis, and is associated with elevated intracellular cAMP in response to β-AR stimulation (Karaszewski, Reder, Anlar, & Arnason, 1993; Zoukos et al., 1992). Zoukos et al. have proposed that increased lymphocyte β-AR density may be induced by, and thus be an indicator of, inflammation. First, the increased lymphocyte β-AR correlated with increased high affinity IL-2 receptors on T cells and also correlated with worsening of disease, as assessed by clinical observations and MRI activity. Second, increased lymphocyte β-AR were present in patients with rheumatoid arthritis, presumably reflective of an underlying inflammation. Third, IL-1 and cortisol, which may be present during inflammation, increased β-AR in normal cells in vitro (Zoukos et al., 1992, 1994). It should be noted that the finding of increased β-AR on peripheral blood lymphocytes of rheumatoid arthritis patients is not universally reported (Baerwald et al., 1992).

The functional significance of the increased lymphocyte β-AR sensitivity in MS disease progression is unknown. β-agonist stimulation of normal lymphocytes in vitro reduced IL-2 receptor expression and suppressed mitogen-induced proliferation, suggesting that increased β-AR expression may be an attempt to mute the proliferative response of T cells by increasing sensitivity to endogenous catecholamines (Zoukos et al., 1994). If IL-12 and IL-10 play central roles in MS (Balashov, Smith, Khoury, Hafler, & Weiner, 1997; van Boxel-Dezaire et al., 1999), then administration of β-agonists may reduce the Th1 component of the disease and slow disease progression in MS patients.

The evidence from clinical studies of human autoimmune disease points to a role for the SNS in regulating disease progression, but further research is necessary to determine if changes in sympathetic tone or AR expression contribute to induction of the disease process, or if these alterations occur in response to the inflammation underlying these diseases. The association of stressful life events with MS relapse suggests that catecholamines may play a role in initiating the disease process (Kroencke & Denney, 1999). Alternatively, if the increased lymphocyte β-AR represents a mechanism to attenuate the disease process, β-AR stimulation may provide a means of restoring homeostatic balance. Effective therapies may be devised to slow disease progression and minimize pathology in MS, rheumatoid arthritis, and other diseases associated with dysregulation of the immune system and inflammation.

VII. SYMPATHETIC REGULATION OF TUMOR GROWTH AND METASTASES

Very few reports exist demonstrating that the SNS can modulate tumor growth. Mammary tumor cells grew more slowly in the ear in which sympathetic input had been ablated by unilateral surgical removal of the superior cervical ganglia (Romeo et al., 1991). Tumor size in the denervated animals was approximately 50% that of the contralateral sham controls with no change in tumor metastases. In denervated submaxillary lymph nodes, a 60% increase in ornithine decarboxylase activity, an indicator of increased lymphocyte metabolism, was observed. These results suggest an immunological mechanism may mediate the reduced tumor growth, but other nonimmunological mechanisms are also possible. ThyagaRajan et al. demonstrated that treatment with deprenyl, a monoamine oxidase B inhibitor, reduced spontaneous mammary and pituitary tumor growth in old rats (ThyagaRajan, Meites, & Quadri, 1995). Deprenyl can partially restore of splenic NA innervation and improve immune function in old animals, but the antitumor mechanism of deprenyl treatment has yet to be determined (ThyagaRajan, Felten, & Felten, 1998; ThyagaRajan, Madden et al., 1998).

Increased tumor metastasis was mediated by β-AR-induced inhibition of NK cell activity in rats (Shakhar & Ben-Eliyahu, 1998). Metaproterenol (MET), a β-AR nonselective agonist, was administered subcutaneously 1 h prior to intravenous injection of the NK cell-sensitive adenocarcinoma MADB106. Lung tumor retention, measured 24 h posttumor cell injection, and lung metastases, measured 3 weeks after tumor cell injection, were both increased in MET-treated rats; peripheral β-blockade with nadolol prevented these effects. One hour after MET administration, peripheral blood NK cell activity was decreased, an effect that was blocked by propranolol and nadolol. In vivo NK cell depletion by treatment of rats with anti-NKR-P1 antibody, prevented the MET-induced increase in lung tumor retention, suggesting that MET acted via NK cell β-AR. These results indicate that sympathetic activation can attenuate elimination of tumor cell metastases by inhibiting NK cell activity.

In contrast, increased metastasis of an alveolar adenocarcinoma, Line 1, to the lung was observed in chemically sympathectomized mice, an effect that was independent of changes in NK cell activity (Brenner, Felten, Felten, & Moynihan, 1992). The increased metastasis occurred when 6-OHDA was administered prior to, but not following, Line 1 injection. No sympathectomy-induced change in NK cell activity was detected in vivo in the lung, spleen, and liver, or by a standard spleen cell in vitro assay. Furthermore, in vivo priming with irradiated Line 1 cells abrogated Line 1 metastases, but ablation of NA innervation prior to priming did not alter this T cell-mediated reduction in Line 1 metastases. These results suggest that intact NA innervation can decrease tumor metastases through a nonimmunological mechanism. The influence of the SNS on tumor metastases is complex and depends on factors such as the type of tumor and species. To begin to determine the relative importance of these factors, it might be interesting to test whether mice with elevated splenic NK cell activity following chemical sympathectomy (Delrue-Perollet et al., 1995) exhibit enhanced or reduced tumor metastases following sympathectomy.

VIII. NEW METHODOLOGIES AND FUTURE DIRECTIONS

Several laboratories have been developing ex-vivo model systems that maintain the three-dimensional structure of lymphoid organs, but allow control of the extracellular environment and easy access to secreted or released substances. In the superfusion technique described by Straub and colleagues, electrically stimulated and K^+-stimulated NE release from spleen sections were dependent on calcium and were inhibited by tetrodotoxin, similar to in vivo NE release (Straub, Lang, Falk, Scholmerich, & Singer, 1995). A three-dimensional bone marrow system has been developed by Wu and his group in which collagen microbeads are used to support bone marrow hematopoiesis (Felten, Gibson-Berry, & Wu, 1996). ISO (10^{-7} to 10^{-5} M) increased hematopoietic cell output two- to threefold, equivalent to erythropoietin in the same system. Maintenance of the three-dimensional structure in combination with a controlled microenvironment may be particularly useful in examining the functional significance of neural–immune interactions in the bone marrow and thymus.

Transgenic mice or rats may be designed to disable the tendency toward homeostasis in the normal animal. For example, engineering a transgenic mouse that is unable to down-regulate lymphocyte β_2-AR in response to agonist may provide a means of assessing lymphocyte β_2-AR functions under a variety of conditions (stress/nonstress/disease). If tissue-specific transgene expression is achieved, with temporal control of gene expression, many interpretational difficulties may be minimized (Yu, Redfern, & Fishmore, 1996). Altered expression of the genes regulating NA nerve fiber activity and target cell responsiveness may be valuable in dissecting the mechanism(s) underlying SNS modulation of immune reactivity.

In vivo, the interactions between the SNS and cells of the immune system always occur in the context of other potent immunomodulators, such as glucocorticoids. Many experimental manipulations that alter immune function have an adrenal-dependent and nonadrenal-dependent component (Bonneau, Sheridan, Feng, & Glaser, 1993; Dobbs, Vasquez, Glaser, & Sheridan, 1993; Fecho et al., 1996), indicating that several pathways interact to generate an immune response of the proper magnitude and duration (Sheridan et al., 1998). Future research should focus on how glucocorticoids and colocalized neurotransmitters interact with the SNS to regulate immune reactivity under normal and disease conditions.

In the previous edition of *Psychoneuroimmunology*, a model of catecholamine modulation of antigen-induced immune reactivity was proposed, incorporating in vivo and in vitro evidence (Madden & Livnat,

1991). This model hypothesized that NE plays a key role in orchestrating the response to antigen, permitting proliferation when required, but subsequently inhibiting the proliferative and effector phase of the response to prevent unwanted self-reactivity. We have yet to prove or disprove this hypothesis adequately in vivo. Furthermore, we now have a more complex view of the immune system, and we must incorporate recent advances in lymphocyte/accessory cell signaling and cytokine diversity into this model. We have yet to precisely integrate the SNS into immune reactivity in vivo, especially in the bone marrow and thymus.

IX. CONCLUSIONS

We now have evidence in vivo that the immunomodulatory effects of sympathetic NA innervation depend on Th predominance, and that inflammatory processes, as exemplified by endotoxemia, can be very sensitive to modulation by catecholamines. We have seen that sympathetic activation can significantly reduce T cell and NK cell activity, at least in the spleen, and may influence tumor metastases. Experimental manipulation of the SNS often leads to transient effects of small magnitude, suggesting that compensatory mechanisms rapidly restore homeostasis. In vivo experimental approaches that incapacitate these compensatory mechanisms may be valuable in determining how the SNS contributes to immune dysfunction. Inflammatory and disease models are invaluable to our understanding of the relevance of SNS-immune system interactions in vivo. The potential therapeutic benefit of modulating catecholamine signaling in human disease states affirms the importance of achieving a greater understanding of SNS modulation of immune function.

Acknowledgments

The author thanks Dr. Barbara Kruszewska for critical reading of this manuscript, and Dr. David Felten for his support and encouragement.

References

Abrass, C. K., O'Connor, S. W., Scarpace, P. J., & Abrass, I. B. (1985). Characterization of the beta-adrenergic receptor of the rat peritoneal macrophage. *Journal of Immunology, 135,* 1338–1341.

Ackerman, K. D., Bellinger, D. L., Felten, S. Y. & Felten, D. L. (1991). Ontogeny and senescence of noradrenergic innervation of the rodent thymus and spleen. In R. Ader, D. L. Felten & N. Cohen (Eds.), *Psychoneuroimmunology* (2nd ed., pp. 71–125). San Diego: Academic Press.

Afan, A. M., Broome, C. S., Nicholls, S. E., Whetton, A. D., & Miyan, J. A. (1997). Bone marrow innervation regulates cellular retention in the murine haemopoietic system. *British Journal of Haematology, 98,* 569–577.

Agius, M. A., Checinski, M. E., & Arnason, B. G. W. (1987). Sympathectomy enhances the severity of experimental autoimmune myasthenia gravis. *Journal of Neuroimmunology, 16,* 11–12.

Bach, M.-A. (1975). Differences in cyclic AMP changes after stimulation by prostaglandins and isoproterenol in lymphocyte subpopulations. *Journal of Clinical Investigations, 55,* 1074–1081.

Baerwald, C., Graefe, C., von Wichert, P., & Krause, A. (1992). Decreased density of βadrenergic receptors on peripheral blood mononuclear cells in patients with rheumatoid arthritis. *Journal of Rheumatology, 19,* 204–210.

Balashov, K. E., Smith, D. R., Khoury, S. J., Hafler, D. A., & Weiner, H. L. (1997). Increased interleukin 12 production in progressive multiple sclerosis: induction by activated CD4+ T cells via CD40 ligand. *Proceedings of the National Academy of Sciences of the United States of America, 94,* 599–603.

Banchereau, J. & Steinman, R. M. (1998). Dendritic cells and the control of immunity. *Nature, 392,* 245–252.

Bellinger, D. L., Ackerman, K. D., Felten, S. Y., & Felten, D. L. (1992). A longitudinal study of age-related loss of noradrenergic nerves and lymphoid cells in the rat spleen. *Experimental Neurology, 116,* 295–311.

Bellinger, D. L., Felten, S. Y., & Felten, D. L. (1988). Maintenance of noradrenergic sympathetic innervation in the involuted thymus of the aged Fischer 344 rat. *Brain, Behavior, and Immunity, 2,* 133–150.

Benestad, H. B., Strøm-Gundersen, I., Iversen, P. O., Haug, E., & Njå, A. (1998). No neuronal regulation of murine bone marrow function. *Blood, 91,* 1280–1287.

Benschop, R. J., Rodriquez-Feuerhahn, M., & Schedlowski, M. (1996). Catecholamine-induced leukocytosis. Early Observations, current research, and future directions. *Brain, Behavior, and Immunity, 10,* 77–91.

Benschop, R. J., Schedlowski, M., Wienecke, H., Jacobs, R., & Schmidt, R. E. (1997). Adrenergic control of natural killer cell circulation and adhesion. *Brain, Behavior, and Immunity, 11,* 321–332.

Bergquist, J., Tarkowski, A., Ekman, R., & Ewing, A. (1994). Discovery of endogenous catecholamine in lymphocytes and evidence for catecholamine regulation of lymphocyte function via an autocrine loop. *Proceedings of the National Academy of Sciences of the United States of America, 91,* 12912–12916.

Bonneau, R. H., Sheridan, J. F., Feng, N., & Glaser, R. (1993). Stress-induced modulation of the primary cellular immune response to herpes simplex virus infection is mediated by both adrenal-dependent and independent mechanisms. *Journal of Neuroimmunology, 42,* 167–176.

Breneman, S. M., Moynihan, J. A., Grota, L. J., Felten, D. L., & Felten, S. Y. (1993). Splenic norepinephrine is decreased in MRL-lpr/lpr mice. *Brain, Behavior, and Immunity, 7,* 135–143.

Brenner, G. J., Felten, S. Y., Felten, D. L., & Moynihan, J. A. (1992). Sympathetic nervous system modulation of tumor metastases and host defense mechanisms. *Journal of Neuroimmunology, 37,* 191–202.

Callahan, T. A., Moynihan, J. A., & Piekut, D. T. (1998). Central nervous system activation following peripheral chemical sympathectomy: Implications for neural-immune interactions. *Brain, Behavior, and Immunity, 12,* 230–241.

Carlson, S. L., Beiting, D. J., Kiani, C. A., Abell, K. M., & McGillis, J. P. (1996). Catecholamines decrease lymphocyte adhesion to cytokine-activated endothelial cells. *Brain, Behavior, and Immunity, 10,* 55–67.

Carlson, S. L., Fox, S., & Abell, K. M. (1997). Catecholamine modulation of lymphocyte homing to lymphoid tissues. *Brain, Behavior, and Immunity, 11*, 307–320.

Chelmicka-Schorr, E., Checinski, M., & Arnason, B. G. W. (1988). Chemical sympathectomy augments the severity of experimental allergic encephalomyelitis. *Journal of Neuroimmunology, 17*, 347–350.

Chelmicka-Schorr, E., Kwasniewski, M. N., Thomas, B. E., & Arnason, B. G. W. (1989). The β-adrenergic agonist isoproterenol suppresses experimental allergic encephalomyelitis in Lewis rats. *Journal of Neuroimmunology, 25*, 203–207.

Chelmicka-Schorr, E., Kwasniewski, M. N., & Wollmann, R. L. (1992). Sympathectomy augments adoptively transferred experimental allergic encephalomyelitis. *Journal of Neuroim-munology, 37*, 99–103.

Chelmicka-Schorr, E., Wollmann, R. L., Kwasniewski, M. N., Kim, D. H., & Dupont, B. L. (1993). The β-adrenergic agonist terbutaline suppresses acute passive transfer experimental autoimmune myasthenia gravis (EAMG). *International Journal of Immunopharmacology, 15*, 19–24.

Chou, R. C., Dong, X. L., Noble, B. K., Knight, P. R., & Spengler, R. N. (1998). Adrenergic regulation of macrophage-derived tumor necrosis factor-α generation during a chronic polyarthritis pain model. *Journal of Neuroimmunology, 82*, 140–148.

Chou, R. C., Stinson, M. W., Noble, B. K., & Spengler, R. N. (1996). β-adrenergic receptor regulation of macrophage-derived tumor necrosis factor-α production from rats with experimental arthritis. *Journal of Neuroimmunology, 67*, 7–16.

Coderre, T. J., Basbaum, A. I., Helms, C., & Levine, J. D. (1991). High-dose epinephrine acts at α-adrenoceptors to suppress experimental arthritis. *Brain Research, 544*, 325–328.

Cunnick, J. E., Lysle, D. T., Kucinski, B. J., & Rabin, B. S. (1990). Evidence that shock-induced immune suppression is mediated by adrenal hormones and peripheral β-adrenergic receptors. *Pharmacology Biochemistry & Behavior, 36*, 645–651.

De Champlain, J. (1971). Degeneration and regrowth of adrenergic nerve fibers in the rat peripheral tissues after 6-hydroxydopamine. *Canadian Journal of Physiology and Pharmacology, 49*, 345–355.

De La Fuente, M., Bernaez, I., Del Rio, M., & Hernanz, A. (1993). Stimulation of peritoneal macrophage function by neuropeptide Y and peptide YY. Involvement of protein kinase C. *Immunology, 80*, 259–265.

Delrue-Perollet, C., Li, K.-S., Vitiello, S., & Neveu, P. J. (1995). Peripheral catecholamines are involved in the neuroendocrine and immune effects of LPS. *Brain, Behavior, and Immunity, 9*, 149–162.

Dobbs, C. M., Vasquez, M., Glaser, R., & Sheridan, J. F. (1993). Mechanisms of stress-induced modulation of viral pathogenesis and immunity. *Journal of Neuroimmunology, 48*, 151–160.

Elenkov, I. J., Haskó, G., Kovács, K. J., & Vizi, E. S. (1995). Modulation of lipopolysaccharide-induced tumor necrosis factor-α production by selective α- and β-adrenergic drugs in mice. *Journal of Neuroimmunology, 61*, 123–131.

Elenkov, I. J. & Vizi, E. S. (1991). Presynaptic modulation of release of noradrenaline from the sympathetic nerve terminals in the rat spleen. *Neuropharmacology, 30*, 1319–1324.

Ernström, U. & Sandberg, G. (1973). Effects of alpha- and beta-receptor stimulation on the release of lymphocytes and granulocytes from the spleen. *Scandinavian Journal of Haematology, 11*, 275–286.

Esquifino, A. I. & Cardinali, D. P. (1994). Local regulation of the immune response by the autonomic nervous system. *Neuroimmunomodulation, 1*, 265–273.

Exton, M. S., von Hörsten, S., Schult, M., Vöge, J., Strubel, T., Donath, S., Steinmüller, C., Seeliger, H., Nagel, E., Westermann, J., & Schedlowski, M. (1998). Behaviorally conditioned immunosuppression using cyclosporine A: Central nervous system reduces IL-2 production via splenic innervation. *Journal of Neuroimmunology, 88*, 182–191.

Fecho, K., Dykstra, L. A., & Lysle, D. T. (1993). Evidence for beta adrenergic receptor involvement in the immunomodulatory effects of morphine. *Journal of Pharmacology and Experimental Therapeutics, 265*, 1079–1087.

Fecho, K., Maslonek, K. A., Dykstra, L. A., & Lysle, D. T. (1993). Alterations of immune status induced by the sympathetic nervous system: Immunomodulatory effects of DMPP alone and in combination with morphine. *Brain, Behavior, and Immunity, 7*, 253–270.

Fecho, K., Maslonek, K. A., Dykstra, L. A., & Lysle, D. T. (1996). Evidence for sympathetic and adrenal involvement in the immunomodulatory effects of acute morphine treatment in rats. *Journal of Pharmacology and Experimental Therapeutics, 277*, 633–645.

Felsner, P., Hofer, D., Rinner, I., Mangge, H., Gruber, M., Korsatko, W., & Schauenstein, K. (1992). Continuous in vivo treatment with catecholamines suppresses in vitro reactivity of rat peripheral blood T-lymphocytes via α-mediated mechanisms. *Journal of Neuroimmunology, 37*, 47–57.

Felsner, P., Hofer, D., Rinner, I., Porta, S., Korsatko, W., & Schauenstein, K. (1995). Adrenergic suppression of peripheral blood T cell reactivity in the rat is due to activation of peripheral α-receptors. *Journal of Neuroimmunology, 57*, 27–34.

Felten, D. L., Gibson-Berry, K. L. & Wu, J. H. D. (1996). Innervation of bone marrow by tyrosine hydroxylase-immunoreactive nerve fibers and hemopoiesis modulating activity of a β-adrenergic agonist in mouse. In N. G. Abraham (Ed.), *Molecular biology of hematopoiesis 5* (pp. 627–636). New York: Plenum Press.

Fernández-López, A. & Pazos, A. (1994). Identification of α-adrenoceptors in rat lymph node and spleen: An autoradiographic study. *European Journal of Pharmacology, 252*, 333–336.

Fessler, H. E., Otterbein, L., Chung, H. S., & Choi, A. M. K. (1996). Alpha-2 adrenoceptor blockade protects rats against lipopolysaccharide. *American Journal of Respiratory and Critical Care Medicine, 154*, 1689–1693.

Fuchs, B. A., Albright, J. W., & Albright, J. F. (1988). β-adrenergic receptors on murine lymphocytes: Density varies with cell maturity and lymphocyte subtype and is decreased after antigen administration. *Cellular Immunology, 114*, 231–245.

Goehler, L. E., Gaykema, R. P. A., Nguyen, K. T., Lee, J. E., Tilders, F. J. H., Maier, S. F., & Watkins, L. R. (1999). Interleukin-1β in immune cells of the abdominal vagus nerve: A link between the immune and nervous systems? *Journal of Neuroscience, 19*, 2799–2806.

Goldmuntz, E. A., Brosnan, C. F., & Norton, W. T. (1986). Prazosin treatment suppresses increased vascular permeability in both acute and passively transferred experimental autoimmune encephalomyelitits in the Lewis rat. *Journal of Immunology, 137*, 3444–3450.

González-Ariki, S. & Husband, A. J. (1998). The role of sympathetic innervation of the gut in regulating mucosal immune responses. *Brain, Behavior, and Immunity, 12*, 53–63.

Griese, M., Körholz, U., Körholz, D., Seeger, K., Wahn, V., & Reinhardt, D. (1988). Density and agonist-promoted high and low affinity states of the β-adrenoceptor on human B- and T-cells. *European Journal of Clinical Investigations, 18*, 213–217.

Gérard, C., Bruyns, C., Marchant, A., Abramowicz, D., Vandenabeele, P., Delvaux, A., Friers, W., Goldman, M., & Velu, T. (1993). Interleukin 10 reduces the release of tumor necrosis factor and prevents lethality in experimental endotoxemia. *Journal of Experimental Medicine, 177*, 547–550.

Haskó, G., Elenkov, I. J., & Vizi, E. S. (1995). Presynaptic receptors involved in the modulation of release of noradrenaline from the sympathetic nerve terminals of the rat thymus. *Immunology Letters, 47*, 133–137.

Haskó, G., Németh, Z. H., Szabó, C., Zsilla, G., Salzman, A. L., & Vizi, E. S. (1998). Isoproterenol inhibits IL-10, TNF-α, and nitric oxide production in RAW 264.7 macrophages. *Brain Research Bulletin, 45*, 183–187.

Haskó, G. & Szabó, C. (1998). Regulation of cytokine and chemokine production by transmitters and co-transmitters of the autonomic nervous system. *Biochemical Pharmacology, 56*, 1079–1087.

Haskó, G., Szabó, C., Németh, Z. H., Salzman, A. L., & Vizi, E. S. (1998). Stimulation of β-adrenoceptors inhibits endotoxin-induced IL-12 production in normal and IL-10 deficient mice. *Journal of Neuroimmunology, 88*, 57–61.

Heijnen, C. J., van der Voort, C. R., Wulffraat, N., van der Net, J., Kuis, W., & Kavelaars, A. (1996). Functional α_1-adrenergic receptors on leukocytes of patients with polyarticular juvenile rheumatoid arthritis. *Journal of Neuroimmunology, 71*, 223–226.

Ignatowski, T. A. & Spengler, R. N. (1995). Regulation of macrophage-derived tumor necrosis factor production by modification of adrenergic receptor sensitivity. *Journal of Neuroimmunology, 61*, 61–70.

Irwin, M., Hauger, R. L., Brown, M., & Britton, K. T. (1988). CRF activates autonomic nervous system and reduces natural killer cytotoxicity. *American Journal of Physiology, 255*, R744–R747.

Josefsson, E., Månsson, J.-E., Blennow, K., & Tarkowski, A. (1994). Immunomodulating and anti-inflammatory properties of the sympatholytic compound 6-hydroxydopamine. *Journal of Neuroimmunology, 55*, 161–169.

Karaszewski, J. W., Reder, A. T., Anlar, B., & Arnason, B. G. W. (1993). Increased high affinity beta-adrenergic receptor densities and cyclic AMP responses of CD8 cells in multiple sclerosis. *Journal of Neuroimmunology, 43*, 1–8.

Karaszewski, J. W., Reder, A. T., Maselli, R., Brown, M., & Arnason, B. G. W. (1990). Sympathetic skin responses are decreased and lymphocyte beta-adrenergic receptors are increased in progressive multiple sclerosis. *Annals of Neurology, 27*, 366–372.

Katafuchi, T., Take, S., & Hori, T. (1993). Roles of sympathetic nervous system in the suppression of cytotoxicity of splenic natural killer cells in the rat. *Journal of Physiology, 465*, 343–357.

Kavelaars, A., de Jong-de Vos van Steenwijk, T., Kuis, W., & Heijnen, C. J. (1998). The reactivity of the cardiovascular system and immunomodulation by catecholamines in juvenile chronic arthritis. *Annals of the New York Academy of Sciences, 840*, 698–704.

Kavelaars, A., van de Pol, M., Zijlstra, J., & Heijnen, C. J. (1997). β-Adrenergic activation enhances interleukin-8 production by human monocytes. *Journal of Neuroimmunology, 77*, 211–216.

Kelley, S. P., Grota, L. J., Felten, S. Y., Madden, K. S., & Felten, D. L. (1996). Norepinephrine in mouse spleen shows minor strain differences and no diurnal variation. *Pharmacology Biochemistry & Behavior, 53*, 141–146.

Kendall, M. D. & Al-Shawaf, A. A. (1991). Innervation of the rat thymus gland. *Brain, Behavior, and Immunity, 5*, 9–28.

Kendall, M. D., Atkinson, B. A., Munoz, F. J., De La Riva, C., Clarke, A. G., & von Gaudecker, B. (1994). The noradrenergic innervation of the rat thymus during pregnancy and in the post partum period. *Journal of Anatomy, 185*, 617–625.

Kim, D. H., Muthyala, S., Soliven, B., Wiegmann, K., Wollmann, R., & Chelmicka-Schorr, E. (1994). The β-adrenergic agonist terbutaline suppresses experimental allergic neuritis in Lewis rats. *Journal of Neuroimmunology, 51*, 177–183.

Kostrzewa, R. M. & Jacobwitz, D. M. (1974). Pharmacological actions of 6-hydroxydopamine. *Pharmacological Reviews, 26*, 199–288.

Kroencke, D. C. & Denney, D. R. (1999). Stress and coping in multiple sclerosis: Exacerbation, remission and chronic subgroups. *Multiple Sclerosis, 5*, 89–93.

Kruszewska, B., Felten, D. L., Stevens, S. Y., & Moynihan, J. A. (1998). Sympathectomy-induced immune changes are not abrogated by the glucocorticoid receptor blocker RU-486. *Brain, Behavior, and Immunity, 12*, 181–200.

Kruszewska, B., Felten, S. Y., & Moynihan, J. A. (1995). Alterations in cytokine and antibody production following chemical sympathectomy in two strains of mice. *Journal of Immunology, 155*, 4613–4620.

Kuis, W., de Jong-de Vos van Steenwuk, C. C. E., Sinnema, G., Kavelaars, A., Prakken, B., Helders, P. J. M., & Heijnen, C. J. (1996). The autonomic nervous system and the immune system in juvenile rheumatoid arthritis. *Brain, Behavior, and Immunity, 10*, 387–398.

Kurz, B., Feindt, J., von Gaudecker, B., Kranz, A., Loppnow, H., & Mentlein, R. (1997). β-adrenoceptor-mediated effects in rat cultured thymic epithelial cells. *British Journal of Pharmacology, 120*, 1401–1408.

Landmann, R. (1992). Beta-adrenergic receptors in human leukocyte subpopulations. *European Journal of Clinical Investigations, 22*, 30–36.

Le Tulzo, Y., Shenkar, R., Kaneko, D., Moine, P., Fantuzzi, G., Dinarello, C. A., & Abraham, E. (1997). Hemorrhage increases cytokine expression in lung mononuclear cells in mice Involvement of catecholamine in nuclear factor-KB regulation and cytokine expression. *Journal of Clinical Investigations, 99*, 1516–1524.

Leden, I., Eriksson, A., Lilja, B., Sturfelt, G., & Sundkvist, G. (1983). Autonomic nerve function in rheumatoid arthritis of varying severity. *Scandinavian Journal of Rheumatology, 12*, 166–170.

Leo, N. A., Callahan, T. A., & Bonneau, R. H. (1998). Peripheral sympathetic denervation alters both the primary and memory cellular immune responses to herpes simplex virus infection. *Neuroimmunomodulation, 5*, 22–35.

Leonard, J. P., Waldburger, K. E., & Goldman, S. J. (1995). Prevention of experimental autoimmune encephalomyelitis by antibodies against interleukin 12. *Journal of Experimental Medicine, 181*, 381–386.

Levine, J. D., Coderre, T. J., Helms, C., & Basbaum, A. I. (1988). β-2 adrenergic mechanisms in experimental arthritis. *Proceedings of the National Academy of Sciences of the United States of America, 85*, 4553–4556.

Levine, J. D., Fye, K., Heller, P., Basbaum, A. I., & Whiting-O'Keefe, Q. (1986). Clinical response to regional intravenous guanethidine in patients with rheumatoid arthritis. *Journal of Rheumatology, 13*, 1040–1043.

Liebmann, P. M., Hofer, D., Felsner, P., Wölfler, A., & Schauenstein, K. (1996). Beta-blockade enhances adrenergic immunosuppression in rats via inhibition of melatonin release. *Journal of Neuroimmunology, 67*, 137–142.

Lorton, D., Bellinger, D. L., Duclos, M., Felten, S. Y., & Felten, D. L. (1996). Application of 6-hydroxydopamine into the fatpads surrounding the draining lymph nodes exacerbates adjuvant-induced arthritis. *Journal of Neuroimmunology, 64*, 103–113.

Lorton, D., Hewitt, D., Bellinger, D. L., Felten, S. Y., & Felten, D. L. (1990). Noradrenergic reinnervation of the rat spleen following chemical sympathectomy with 6-hydroxydopamine: Pattern and time course of reinnervation. *Brain, Behavior, and Immunity, 4,* 198–222.

Lundberg, J. M. (1996). Pharmacology of cotransmission in the autonomic nervous system: Integrative aspects on amines, neuropeptides, adenosine triphosphate, amino acids, and nitric oxide. *Pharmacological Reviews, 48,* 113–178.

Lundberg, J. M., Anggard, A., Pernow, J., & Hokfelt, T. (1985). Neuropeptide Y-, substance P- and VIP-immunoreactive nerves in cat spleen in relation to autonomic vascular and volume control. *Cell and Tissue Research, 239,* 9–18.

Lundberg, J. M., Rudehill, A., Sollevi, A., Theodorsson-Norhein, E., & Hamberger, B. (1986). Frequency- and reserpine-dependent chemical coding of sympathetic transmission: Differential release of noradrenaline and neuropeptide Y from pig spleen. *Neuroscience Letters, 63,* 96–100.

Lyte, M., Ernst, S., Driemeyer, J., & Baissa, B. (1991). Strain-specific enhancement of splenic T cell mitogenesis and macrophage phagocytosis following peripheral axotomy. *Journal of Neuroimmunology, 31,* 1–8.

Mackenzie, F. J., Leonard, J. P., & Cuzner, M. L. (1989). Changes in lymphocyte β-adrenergic receptor density and noradrenaline content of the spleen are early indicators of immune reactivity in acute experimental allergic encephalomyelitis in the Lewis rat. *Journal of Neuroimmunology, 23,* 93–100.

MacNeil, B. J., Jansen, A. H., Greenberg, A. H., & Nance, D. M. (1996). Activation and selectivity of splenic sympathetic nerve electrical activity response to bacterial endotoxin. *American Journal of Physiology, 270,* R264–R270.

MacNeil, B. J., Jansen, A. H., Janz, L. J., Greenberg, A. H., & Nance, D. M. (1997). Peripheral endotoxin increases splenic sympathetic nerve activity via central prostaglandin synthesis. *American Journal of Physiology, 273,* R609–R614.

Madden, K. S., Bellinger, D. L., Felten, S. Y., Snyder, E., Maida, M. E., & Felten, D. L. (1997). Alterations in sympathetic innervation of thymus and spleen in aged mice. *Mechanisms of Ageing and Development, 94,* 165–175.

Madden, K. S., Felten, S. Y., Felten, D. L., & Bellinger, D. L. (1995). Sympathetic nervous system-immune system interactions in young and old Fischer 344 rats. *Annals of the New York Academy of Sciences, 771,* 523–534.

Madden, K. S., Felten, S. Y., Felten, D. L., Hardy, C. A., & Livnat, S. (1994). Sympathetic nervous system modulation of the immune system II. Induction of lymphocyte proliferation and migration in vivo by chemical sympathectomy. *Journal of Neuroimmunology, 49,* 67–75.

Madden, K. S., Felten, S. Y., Felten, D. L., Sundaresan, P. R., & Livnat, S. (1989). Sympathetic neural modulation of the immune system. I. Depression of T cell immunity in vivo and in vitro following chemical sympathectomy. *Brain, Behavior, and Immunity, 3,* 72–89.

Madden, K. S. & Livnat, S. (1991). Catecholamine action and immunologic reactivity. In R. Ader, D.L. Felten & N. Cohen (Eds.), *Psychoneuroimmunology* (2nd ed., pp. 283–310). San Diego: Academic Press.

Madden, K. S., Moynihan, J. A., Brenner, G. J., Felten, S. Y., Felten, D. L., & Livnat, S. (1994). Sympathetic nervous system modulation of the immune system III. Alterations in T and B cell proliferation and differentiation in vitro following chemical sympathectomy. *Journal of Neuroimmunology, 49,* 77–87.

Maestroni, G. J. M. & Conti, A. (1994). Modulation of hematopoiesis via α_1-adrenergic receptors on bone marrow cells. *Experimental Hematology, 22,* 313–320.

Maestroni, G. J. M., Conti, A., & Pedrinis, E. (1992). Effect of adrenergic agents on hematopoiesis after syngeneic bone marrow transplantation in mice. *Blood, 80,* 1178–1182.

Maestroni, G. J. M., Cosentino, M., Marino, F., Togni, M., Conti, A., Lecchini, S., & Frigo, G. (1998). Neural and endogenous catecholamines in the bone marrow. Circadian association of norepinephrine with hematopoiesis? *Experimental Hematology, 26,* 1172–1177.

Maestroni, G. J. M., Togni, M., & Covacci, V. (1997). Norepinephrine protects mice from acute lethal doses of carboplatin. *Experimental Hematology, 25,* 491–494.

Marchetti, B., Morale, M. C., Paradis, P., & Bouvier, M. (1994). Characterization, expression, and hormonal control of a thymic β-adrenergic receptor. *American Journal of Physiology, 267,* E718–E731.

Mills, P. J., Karnik, R. S., & Dillon, E. (1997). L-selectin expression affects T-cell circulation following isoproterenol infusion in humans. *Brain, Behavior, and Immunity, 11,* 333–342.

Monastra, G. & Secchi, E. F. (1993). β-Adrenergic receptors mediate in vivo the adrenaline inhibition of lipopolysaccharide-induced tumor necrosis factor release. *Immunology Letters, 38,* 127–130.

Mueller, R. A., Thoenen, H., & Axelrod, J. (1969). Adrenal tyrosine hydroxylase—Compensatory increase in activity after chemical sympathectomy. *Science, 163,* 468–469.

Murray, D. R., Polizzi, S. M., Harris, T., Wilson, N., Michel, M. C., & Maisel, A. S. (1993). Prolonged isoproterenol treatment alters immunoregulatory cell traffic and function in the rat. *Brain, Behavior, and Immunity, 7,* 47–62.

Müller, S. & Weihe, E. (1991). Interrelation of peptidergic innervation with mast cells and ED1-positive cells in rat thymus. *Brain, Behavior, and Immunity, 5,* 55–72.

Panina-Bordignon, P., Mazzeo, D., Di Lucia, P., D'Ambrosio, D., Lang, R., Fabbri, L., Self, C., & Sinigaglia, F. (1997). β-agonists prevent Th1 development by selective inhibition of IL-12. *Journal of Clinical Investigations, 100,* 1513–1519.

Perry, F., Heller, P. H., Kamiya, J., & Levine, J. D. (1989). Altered autonomic function in patients with arthritis or with chronic myofascial pain. *Pain, 39,* 77–84.

Petitto, J. M., Huang, Z., & McCarthy, D. B. (1994). Molecular cloning of NPY-Y1 receptor cDNA from rat splenic lymphocytes: Evidence of low levels of mRNA expression and [^{125}INPY binding sites. *Journal of Neuroimmunology, 54,* 81–86.

Qi, M., Zhou, Z., Wurster, R. D., & Jones, S. B. (1991). Mechanisms involved in the rapid dissipation of plasma epinephrine response to bacterial endotoxin in conscious rats. *American Journal of Physiology, 261,* R1431–R1437.

Radojcic, T., Baird, S., Darko, D., Smith, D., & Bulloch, K. (1991). Changes in β-adrenergic receptor distribution on immunocytes during differentiation: An analysis of T cells and macrophages. *Journal of Neuroscience Research, 30,* 328–335.

Rehman, J., Mills, P. J., Carter, S. M., Chou, J., Thomas, J., & Maisel, A. S. (1997). Dynamic exercise leads to an increase in circulating ICAM-1: Further evidence for adrenergic modulation of cell adhesion. *Brain, Behavior, and Immunity, 11,* 343–351.

Rogausch, H., del Rey, A., Oertel, J., & Besedovsky, H. O. (1999). Norepinephrine stimulates lymphoid cell mobilization from the perfused rat spleen via β-adrenergic receptors. *American Journal of Physiology, 276,* R724–R730.

Romano, T. A., Felten, S. Y., Felten, D. L., & Olschowka, J. A. (1991). Neuropeptide-Y innervation of the rat spleen: Another potential immunomodulatory neuropeptide. *Brain, Behavior, and Immunity, 5,* 116–131.

Romeo, H. E., Colombo, L. L., Esquifino, A. I., Rosenstein, R. E., Chuluyan, H. E., & Cardinali, D. P. (1991). Slower growth of tumours in sympathetically denervated murine skin. *Journal of the Autonomic Nervous System, 32*, 159–164.

Rott, O., Fleischer, B., & Cash, E. (1994). Interleukin-10 prevents experimental allergic encephalomyelitis. *European Journal of Immunology, 24*, 1434–1440.

Sanders, V. M., Baker, R. A., Ramer-Quinn, D. S., Kasprowicz, D. J., Fuchs, B. A., & Street, N. E. (1997). Differential expression of the β_2-adrenergic receptor by Th1 and Th2 clones. *Journal of Immunology, 158*, 4200–4210.

Saxne, T., Palladino, M. A., Jr., Heinegård, D., Talal, N., & Wollheim, F. A. (1988). Detection of tumor necrosis factor α but not tumor necrosis factor β in rheumatoid arthritis synovial fluid and serum. *Arthritis and Rheumatology, 31*, 1041–1045.

Schedlowski, M., Hosch, W., Oberbeck, R., Benschop, R. J., Jacobs, R., Raab, H.-R., & Schmidt, R. E. (1996). Catecholamines modulate human NK cell circulation and function via spleen-independent β-adrenergic mechanisms. *Journal of Immunology, 156*, 93–99.

Schoups, A. A., Annaert, W. G., & De Potter, W. P. (1990). Presence and subcellular localization of α-adrenoceptors in dog splenic nerve. *Brain Research, 517*, 308–314.

Severn, A., Rapson, N. T., Hunter, C. A., & Liew, F. Y. (1992). Regulation of tumor necrosis factor production by adrenaline and β-adrenergic agonists. *Journal of Immunology, 148*, 3441–3445.

Shakhar, G. & Ben-Eliyahu, S. (1998). In vivo β-adrenergic stimulation suppresses natural killer activity and compromises resistance to tumor metastasis in rats. *Journal of Immunology, 160*, 3251–3258.

Sheridan, J. F., Dobbs, C., Jung, J., Chu, X., Konstantinos, A., Padgett, D., & Glaser, R. (1998). Stress-induced neuroendocrine modulation of viral pathogenesis and immunity. *Annals of the New York Academy of Sciences, 840*, 803–808.

Singh, U. (1985). Lymphopoiesis in the nude fetal mouse thymus following sympathectomy. *Cellular Immunology, 93*, 222–228.

Singh, U. & Owen, J. J. T. (1976). Studies on the maturation of thymus stem cells - The effects of catecholamines, histamine, and peptide hormones on the expression of T alloantigens. *European Journal of Immunology, 6*, 59–62.

Spengler, R. N., Allen, R. M., Remick, D. G., Strieter, R. M., & Kunkel, S. L. (1990). Stimulation of alpha-adrenergic receptor augments the production of macrophage-derived tumor necrosis factor. *Journal of Immunology, 145*, 1430–1434.

Spengler, R. N., Chensue, S. W., Giacherio, D. A., Blenk, N., & Kunkel, S. L. (1994). Endogenous norepinephrine regulates tumor necrosis factor-α production from macrophages in vitro. *Journal of Immunology, 152*, 3024–3031.

Stevens-Felten, S. Y. & Bellinger, D. L. (1997). Noradrenergic and peptidergic innervation of lymphoid organs. *Chemical Immunology, 69*, 99–131.

Straub, R. H., Lang, B., Falk, W., Scholmerich, J., & Singer, E. A. (1995). In vitro superfusion method for the investigation of nerve-immune cell interaction in murine spleen. *Journal of Neuroimmunology, 61*, 53–60.

Suberville, S., Bellocq, A., Fouqueray, B., Philippe, C., Lantz, O., Perez, J., & Baud, L. (1996). Regulation of interleukin-10 production by β-adrenergic agonists. *European Journal of Immunology, 26*, 2601–2605.

Sundar, S. K., Cierpial, M. A., Kilts, C., Ritchie, J. C., & Weiss, J. M. (1990). Brain IL-1-induced immunosuppression occurs through activation of both pituitary-adrenal axis and sympathetic nervous system by corticotropin-releasing factor. *Journal of Neuroscience, 10*, 3701–3706.

Szabó, C., Haskó, G., Zingarelli, B., Németh, Z. H., Salzman, A. L., & Kvetan, V. (1997). Isoproterenol regulates tumour necrosis factor, interleukin-10, interleukin-6 and nitric oxide production and protects against the development of vascular hyporeactivity in endotoxaemia. *Immunology, 90*, 95–100.

Tabarowski, Z., Gibson-Berry, K., & Felten, S. Y. (1996). Noradrenergic and peptidergic innervation of the mouse femur bone marrow. *Acta Histochemica, 98*, 453–457.

Take, S., Mori, T., Katafuchi, T., & Hori, T. (1993). Central interferon-α inhibits natural killer cytotoxicity through sympathetic innervation. *American Journal of Physiology, 265*, R453–R459.

ThyagaRajan, S., Felten, S. Y., & Felten, D. L. (1998). Restoration of sympathetic noradrenergic nerve fibers in the spleen by low doses of L-deprenyl treatment in young sympathectomized and old Fischer 344 rats. *Journal of Neuroimmunology, 81*, 144–157.

ThyagaRajan, S., Madden, K. S., Kalvass, J. C., Dimitrova, S. S., Felten, S. Y., & Felten, D. L. (1998). L-deprenyl-induced increase in IL-2 and NK cell activity accompanies restoration of noradrenergic nerve fibers in the spleens of old F344 rats. *Journal of Neuroimmunology, 92*, 9–21.

ThyagaRajan, S., Meites, J., & Quadri, S. K. (1995). Deprenyl reinitiates estrous cycles, reduces serum prolactin, and decreases the incidence of mammary and pituitary tumors in old acyclic rats. *Endocrinology, 136*, 1103–1110.

Tracey, K., Fong, Y., Hesse, D. G., Manogue, K. R., Lee, A. T., Kuo, G. C., Lowry, S. F., & Cerami, A. (1987). Anti-cachectin/TNF monoclonal antibodies prevent septic shock during lethal bacteraemia. *Nature, 330*, 662–664.

Tsao, C.-W., Cheng, J.-T., Shen, C.-L., & Lin, Y.-S. (1996). 6-hydroxydopamine induces thymocyte apoptosis in mice. *Journal of Neuroimmunology, 65*, 91–95.

van Boxel-Dezaire, A. H., Hoff, S. C., van Oosten, B. W., Verweij, C. L., Drager, A. M., Ader, H. J., van Houwelingen, J. C., Barkhof, F., Polman, C. H., & Nagelkerken, L. (1999). Decreased interleukin-10 and increased interleukin-12p40 mRNA are associated with disease activity and characterize different disease stages in multiple sclerosis. *Annals of Neurology, 45*, 695–703.

van der Poll, T., Coyle, S. M., Barbosa, K., Braxton, C. C., & Lowry, S. F. (1996). Epinephrine inhibits tumor necrosis factor-α and potentiates interleukin 10 production during human endotoxemia. *Journal of Clinical Investigations, 97*, 713–719.

van der Poll, T., Jansen, J., Endert, E., Sauerwein, H. P., & van Deventer, S. J. H. (1994). Noradrenaline inhibits lipopolysaccharide-induced tumor necrosis factor and interleukin 6 production in human whole blood. *Infection and Immunity, 62*, 2046–2050.

Vizi, E. S., Orsó, E., Osipenko, O. N., Haskó, G., & Elenkov, I. J. (1995). Neurochemical, electrophysiological and immunocytochemical evidence for a noradrenergic link between the sympathetic nervous system and thymocytes. *Neuroscience, 68*, 1263–1276.

Weihe, E., Müller, S., Fink, T., & Zentel, H. J. (1989). Tachykinins, calcitonin gene-related peptide and neuropeptide Y in nerves of the mammalian thymus: Interactions with mast cells in autonomic and sensory neuroimmunomodulation. *Neuroscience Letters, 100*, 77–82.

Westermann, J. & Pabst, R. (1990). Lymphocyte subsets in the blood: A diagnostic window on the lymphoid system? *Immunology Today, 11*, 406–410.

Wiegmann, K., Muthyala, S., Kim, D. H., Arnason, B. G. W., & Chelmicka-Schorr, E. (1995). β-adrenergic agonists suppress chronic/relapsing experimental allergic encephalomyelitis (CREAE) in Lewis rats. *Journal of Neuroimmunology, 56*, 201–206.

Yu, Z., Redfern, C. S., & Fishmore, G. I. (1996). Conditioned transgene expression in the heart. *Circulation Research, 79*, 691–697.

Zalcman, S., Green-Johnson, J. M., Murray, L., Wan, W., Nance, D. M., & Greenberg, A. H. (1994). Interleukin-2-induced enhancement of an antigen-specific IgM plaque-forming cell response is mediated by the sympathetic nervous system. *Journal of Pharmacology and Experimental Therapeutics, 271*, 977–982.

Zhou, Z. Z., Wurster, R. D., & Jones, S. B. (1992). Arterial baroreflexes are not essential in mediating sympathoadrenal activation in conscious endotoxic rats. *Journal of the Autonomic Nervous System, 39*, 1–12.

Zoukos, Y., Kidd, D., Woodroofe, M. N., Kendall, B. E., Thompson, A. J., & Cuzner, M. L. (1994). Increased expression of high affinity IL-2 receptors and β-adrenoceptors on peripheral blood mononuclear cells is associated with clinical and MRI activity in multiple sclerosis. *Brain, 117*, 307–315.

Zoukos, Y., Leonard, J. P., Thomaides, T., Thompson, A. J., & Cuzner, M. L. (1992). β-adrenergic receptor density and function of peripheral blood mononuclear cells are increased in multiple sclerosis: A regulatory role for cortisol and interleukin-1. *Annals of Neurology, 31*, 657–662.

CHAPTER

6

Regulation of Immune and Inflammatory Reactions in Local Microenvironments by Sensory Neuropeptides

JOSEPH P. McGILLIS, STEFAN FERNANDEZ, MELISSA A. KNOPF

I. INTRODUCTION

One of the best adapted systems for dynamic efferent communication between the nervous system and the immune system is the sensory nervous system. In considering the vast array of hypothetical mediators of immune system–nervous system communication and models that have been proposed over the last 20 years, there are a number of issues that are difficult to reconcile with our current knowledge of how both the innate and specific immune systems function. It is clear that the central nervous system (CNS) and immune system depend on bi-directional communication, and many of the afferent aspects are fairly well documented (i.e., fever induction by cytokines, influence on protective and adaptive behaviors, etc.). In contrast, the vast literature on efferent mechanisms can be confusing and is frequently contradictory. One of the specific difficulties with understanding the role of many mediators is that although we can show that they have effects in in vitro assay systems, there is no evidence that these mediators are present in the specific anatomical compartments where they could influence immune and inflammatory processes.[1] This is complicated by the continued misconception that immune and inflammatory responses occur in the bloodstream. Inflammatory responses occur in localized areas in response to injury or infection. Specific immune responses are initiated by antigen processing in the affected tissue and antigen presentation in the regional lymph node. This is done largely by tissue dendritic cells or macrophages that drain to regional lymph nodes via the lymphatic system. Lymphocyte activation and expansion then occur inside the regional lymph nodes. Subsequently, activated cells are released into the bloodstream where they home to their target sites. In the case of an activated cytotoxic T cell, this might be a virally infected mucosal surface. In contrast, terminally differentiated immunoglobulin

[1]*Inflammatory response* is used synonymously with *innate immunity* in this chapter, as opposed to *specific immunity*. It should be recognized that there are inflammatory responses that do not have specific immune components, and that immune responses generally involve both inflammatory or innate immunity and specific lymphocyte mediate immune responses.

producing B lymphocytes (plasma cells) migrate to the bone marrow. Thus, for the most part, the bloodstream is merely a superhighway that allows a mobilized immune system to travel where it is needed. One might suggest that septicemia (bacterial infection in the bloodstream) is an exception. However, closer consideration of the response reveals that antigen presenting cells in septicemia end up in lymph nodes and the recognition and expansion phases are similar to a localized response. In this case the bloodstream is the localized microenvironment, or infected tissue, targeted by activated and expanded effector cells. For these reasons it is sometimes difficult to reconcile how neuroendocrine and endocrine hormones might play a dynamic role in the normal regulation of immune and inflammatory responses. This is not to say that there are not well established examples of detrimental neuroendocrine and endocrine effects on immune and inflammatory functions. The question is whether they are actually involved in dynamic control of protective responses, or whether their significance is in their potential pathologic effects on innate and specific immunity. We will argue that there is a much stronger rationale for efferent communication by neuropeptides released at local sites of immune and inflammatory processes. Ultimately, many of the detrimental effects of stress, anxiety, and so forth, correlated by alterations in function of systems such as the hypothalamic-pituitary-adrenal endocrine system, may result in part from their effects on the functions of local innervation.

The sensory neuropeptides described in this chapter, calcitonin gene-related peptide (CGRP) and substance P (SP), are well suited for an efferent role in CNS–immune system communication. The underlying hypothesis is that these sensory neuropeptides function to place immune and inflammatory responses in the proper temporal and spatial contexts. This hypothesis is founded in part on the concept of neurogenic inflammation. *Neurogenic inflammation* is a term first used to describe the contribution of sensory nerves to local dermatologic inflammatory processes. The first observations on this response were in the late 1800s, and the process has been well reviewed by Foreman (reviewed in Foreman, 1987). There are several factors that support the role of sensory neuropeptides in the neurogenic aspects of inflammation. First, they are released from nociceptive nerve endings in a highly localized manner. The classic stimuli for their release includes trauma or any condition that causes pain or even mild discomfort. Recent studies have shown that they can also be released in response to proinflammatory cytokines produced by inflammatory cells at local sites (Herbert & Holzer, 1994a, 1994b). Once released, their longer half-lives give them a distinct advantage over the smaller, less stable, amine neurotransmitters. This is important in that biogenic amines have very short half-lives and that to influence the activities of cells in a prolonged inflammatory or immune response, they would need to be present at elevated levels for a longer temporal window. Finally, in conceptualizing the effects of amine neurotransmitters (i.e., epinephrine, acetyl choline, etc.), it is necessary to reconcile their effects on other target tissues such as smooth and skeletal muscle with potential effects on immune and inflammatory cells. Where many neurotransmitters have key dynamic roles in regulating muscle tension, etc., most neuropeptides do not seem to play dynamic roles in these processes. In fact many reviews suggest that SP, which can cause smooth muscle relaxation and vasodilation, plays an integrating role in immune and inflammatory responses (McGillis & Fernandez, 1999; McGillis & Figueiredo, 1996; McGillis, Mitsuhashi, & Payan, 1991; Payan, 1992). Under normal conditions, it is not thought to play a dynamic role in smooth muscle tonicity (reviewed in Pernow, 1983). However, under conditions driven by neurogenic inflammation, it can cause smooth muscle relaxation that is coordinated with other proinflammatory effects including edema, chemoattraction, and regulation of inflammatory cell functions at a local site (rev. in Brain, 1997; Maggi, 1997; McGillis & Fernandez, 1999; Payan, 1992). The remainder of this review will consider some facets of the role of these peptides in immune and inflammatory responses and will consider more recent information on some of their functions.

II. THE SENSORY NEUROPEPTIDES SP AND CGRP

Neuropeptides are synthesized in the cell body and transported to the nerve ending where they are released when the neuron is depolarized. Once released, they can bind to specific receptors, diffuse out of the tissue into the lymph or blood, or be cleaved into fragments by cell surface or soluble proteases. Sensory neuropeptides that regulate local inflammatory and immune functions are present in unmyelinated C-type and small myelinated A-δ-type nerve fibers. They have a wide variety of functions ranging from effects on local vasculature to effects on leukocytes (Brain, 1997; Maggi, 1997; McGillis & Fernandez, 1999; Payan, 1992). They are synthesized in cells of the dorsal root ganglia and there is frequently more than one neuropeptide produced and released by a single neuron. With respect to neurogenic inflammation, the principal mediators CGRP and SP are commonly colocalized in sensory neurons (Lee et al., 1985). Neuropeptides are produced as prohormone precursors that undergo proteolytic processing within secretory granules to yield the smaller active forms. To date, there are at least 40 mammalian neuropeptides that have been identified and grouped in structural or functional classes. This review will focus on only 2 neuropeptides in particular, CGRP and SP, which are the primary mediators of sensory nervous system influences on immune and inflammatory reactions.

A. SP

SP, the original prototype member of the tachykinin family, is an 11 amino acid neuropeptide that was discovered in 1931 (Von Euler & Gaddum, 1931). SP is widely distributed throughout the CNS and is also present in peripheral sensory neurons. Sites where it can influence immune and inflammatory responses include nerve endings around blood vessels, lymphoid tissue, bone marrow, and the skin (Hukkanen et al., 1992; Kar, Rees, & Quirion, 1994; Larsson, Ekblom, Henriksson, Lundebert, & Theodorsson, 1991; Marksteiner et al., 1994). SP is usually colocalized with CGRP in nerve endings, although it can also be found alone. SP has also been observed in endocrine cells of the gut, parenchymal cells of the carotid body, the adrenal gland, the anterior pituitary, and eosinophils (Maggi, 1997).

The tachykinin family, which also includes neurokinin A (NKA)[2] and neuromedin K (NMK), has a conserved C-terminal domain that consists of the sequence -Phe-X-Gly-Leu-Met-NH_2 where X is a branched aromatic or aliphatic amino acid (McGillis, Mitsuhashi et al., 1991). Two genes encode mammalian tachykinins, preprotachykinin A (PPT-A) and PPT-B (reviewed in Nussdorfer & Malendowicz, 1990). SP and NKA are derived from differential splicing of PPT-A mRNA. Alternative splicing of PPT-A results in the production of three distinct mRNAs: PPTA-α, PPTA-β, and PPTA-γ. PPTA-α is found predominantly in the CNS, whereas PPTA-β, PPTA-γ, and PPTB are found in both the CNS and peripheral nervous system (PNS). Precursor prohormones translated from PPTA-α mRNA contain one single copy of SP, whereas those translated from PPTA-β and PPTA-γ mRNA have a copy of both SP and NKA. PPT-A also encodes NPK and NPγ, whereas PPT-B only encodes NKB. NPK is derived from PPTA-β and NPγ is encoded by PPTA-γ. Precursors that can give rise to both SP and NKA are expressed in the CNS. In contrast, precursors expressed in the periphery only give rise to a single peptide.

[2]There is some debate on the nomenclature for the tachykinin peptides. NKA was originally called substance K, and NMK is sometimes referred to as NKB.

Many functions have been attributed to SP, and it is likely that more will be discovered. It has potent excitatory effects, which are generally long lasting. Its antidromic release from sensory neurons can affect vascular and inflammatory tissues. Vascular effects include vasodilation, increase in venular permeability, plasma leakage leading to edema, and smooth muscle contraction (Brain, 1997). In the CNS, SP affects a variety of systems including neuroendocrine secretion, pain, memory processing, spinal and ganglionic reflexes, and pituitary hormone secretion (Maggi, Patacchini, Rovero, & Giachetti, 1993). SP promotes vascular smooth muscle relaxation by promoting release of nitric oxide (Maggi et al., 1993). In other tissues such as the urinary system, pulmonary system, and uterus, it can stimulate muscle contraction (Regoli, Boudon, & Fauchere, 1994). These contractile events can induce effects such as constriction of bronchial tubes, contraction of the bladder, uterus, etc. This constriction has been shown to be dependent on the induction of IP3 and increased intracellular Ca^{2+} (Regoli et al., 1994). SP induces secretion of saliva and activates various exocrine glands such as the pancreas and intestinal secretory glands (Regoli et al., 1994). SP is also responsible for the release of some chemical agents from various cell types including histamine release from mast cells (Pernow, 1983). It also causes release of interleukin(IL)-1 in the brain and IL-6 from a human astrocytoma cell line (Martin, Charles, Sanderson, & Merrill, 1992; Merrill et al., 1992). These effects may indicate that SP plays a role in inflammatory responses of the brain.

B. CGRP

CGRP is a 37-amino-acid neuropeptide that is located in nociceptive nerve endings throughout the body (reviewed in Tache, Holzer, & Rosenfeld, 1992). It was first identified in 1982 as a result of molecular cloning of the calcitonin gene (Amara, Jones, Rosenfeld, Ong, & Evans, 1982). There are two isoforms of CGRP, α and β, that differ by one amino acid in rats and by three in humans. CGRP-α results from differential splicing of the calcitonin/CGRP gene. This gene contains six exons in rats and humans. Exons 1–3 code for the 5′ untranslated region, exon 4 codes for calcitonin, and exons 5–6 encode CGRP. The calcitonin mRNA consists of exons 1–4 and the CGRP mRNA includes exons 1–3, 5, and 6. The CGRP containing precursor is produced in neural tissues and the calcitonin precursor is produced in endocrine tissues. CGRP-β is produced from a second gene that encodes only CGRP (Amara et al., 1985). The CGRP-β gene appears to have arisen by gene duplication and is lacking a functional fourth exon (calcitonin encoding). There are no clear functional differences between the two CGRP's, although there may be some differences in the function of their cleavage products (Davies, Medeiros, Keen, Truner, & Haynes, 1992; Manley & Haynes, 1989).

CGRP is a member of the amylin family, which also includes amylin and adrenomedullin (ADM) (reviewed in Tache et al., 1992). There is approximately 20% homology between CGRP and ADM and 40% homology between CGRP and amylin. Amylin-like peptides have six to seven amino acids in a common N-terminal disulfide ring that is required for biological activity, an amidated C-terminal, and some conserved amino acids in the middle of the peptide. CGRP has a disulfide linkage between Cys2 and Cys7, an amphipathic alpha-helix between residues 8 and 18, a β-turn formed by residues 19–20, and a C-terminal amide. These basic similarities probably account for a certain degree of cross-reactivity between CGRP and ADM.

CGRP is found throughout the CNS and PNS. In the periphery it is present in the nerve endings of sensory nerve fibers, where it is usually coexpressed with SP. It is present in nerve endings in all body surfaces, around all blood vessels, in lymphoid tissue, and in bone and dental pulp (Bjurholm, 1991; Bjurholm, Kreicbergs, Brodin, & Schultzberb, 1988; Bjurholm, Kreicbergs, Dahlberg, & Schultzberg, 1990; Kimberly & Byers, 1988; Kruger, Silverman, Mantyh, Sternini, & Brecha, 1991; Lee et al., 1985; Popper, Mantyh, Vigna, Maggio, & Mantyh, 1988; Popper & Micevych, 1989; Rodrigo et al., 1985; Weihe, Muller, Fink, & Zentel, 1989). About 80% of neurons contain both CGRP and SP, but CGRP can be found without SP in some motor and enteric neurons (Rodrigo et al., 1985).

CGRP has numerous functions; perhaps most notably, it is one of the most potent vasodilators known (Brain, Williams, Tippins, Morris, & MacIntyre, 1985). It is released by voltage-dependent calcium uptake in response to noxious stimuli and generally acts in restricted local microenvironments. It has been shown that the addition of the proinflammatory cytokine IL-1 can cause release of CGRP and SP from nerve endings (Herbert & Holzer, 1994a, 1994b). In the cardiovascular system, CGRP functions to increase vasodilation and therefore decrease arteriolar blood pressure and increase muscle contractility (reviewed in Preibisz, 1993). In the renal system, it can stimulate renin secretion and can influence renal blood flow and glomerular filtration (Gnaedinger et al., 1989; Kurtz, Muff, & Fischer, 1989). It enhances the effects of tachykinins, such as SP, on edema via its vasodilitory effects (Brain, 1997; Brain & Williams, 1985). CGRP more recently has been shown to have effects on the immune system (reviewed in McGillis & Fernandez, 1999; McGillis & Figueiredo, 1996). Some of these include altering responses to T cell mitogens, inhibiting IL-2 production by T cells, inhibiting differentiation of the pre-B cell line 70Z/3, inhibiting production of H_2O_2 by interferon (IFN)-γ in macrophages, and blocking antigen presentation by macrophages (Asahina, Moro et al., 1995; Boudard & Bastide, 1991; Fox et al., 1997; McGillis, Humphreys, Rangnekar, & Ciallella, 1993b; Nong, Titus, Ribeiro, & Remold, 1989; Owan & Ibaraki, 1994; Torii et al., 1997; Umeda, Takamiya, Yoshizaki, & Arisawa, 1988).

C. SP Receptors

The tachykinin receptors are seven transmembrane domain, G-protein linked receptors (reviewed in Maggi et al., 1993; Regoli et al., 1994). They activate phospholipase C (PLC), which then catalyzes the cleavage of phosphotidylinositol into IP_3 and diacylglycerol (DAG). IP_3 is responsible for the mobilization of Ca^{2+} whereas DAG activates PKC. Genes for three tachykinin receptors that have about 65% homology have been identified: neurokinin-1 (*NK1*), *NK2*, and *NK3* (Hershey & Krause, 1990; Masu et al., 1987; Shigemoto, Yokota, Tsuchida, & Nakanishi, 1990; Yokata et al., 1990). These three receptors are capable of binding all members of the tachykinin family; however, they do so with distinct affinities. *NK1* preferentially binds SP, *NK2* binds NKA with the highest affinity, and *NK3* binds NKB. *NK1* and *NK2* have two different isoforms that are differentially expressed in specific tissues. When SP binds to *NK1* there is a clathrin-dependent endocytosis of the receptor ligand complex (Garland, Grady, Payan, Vigna, & Bunnett, 1994; Grady et al., 1995). The SP:*NK1* complex is internalized by acidic endosomes where SP is degraded and *NK1* is recycled and returned to the cell surface. This process occurs within minutes of ligand binding, such that the cellular response to SP is limited and there is rapid desensitization. Selectivity of SP for NK1 is largely conferred by the region spanning from transmembrane domain 2 to the second extracellular loop and partly by the extracellular N-terminal portion of the receptor (Yokota, Akazawa, Ohkubo, & Nakanishi, 1992). The extracellular domain of the receptor recognizes the C-terminal sequence of SP, consistent with the necessity of the ligand to retain this portion to be biologically active. Amino acid mutational analysis of transmembrane region 2 found that three conserved amino acids, asn85, asn89, and tyr92, and one non-conserved residue, asn96, are important for high affinity binding of SP (Huang, Yu, Strader, & Fong, 1994). Additionally, the proline residue at position 4 of SP may be necessary for its selective binding to *NK1* (Yokata et al., 1990).

Only one copy of the *NK1* gene has been found in all species from which it has been cloned, but multiple forms of the protein are generated through differential splicing (Quartara & Maggi, 1997). The shorter version binds SP with lower affinity than the full length (Quartara & Maggi, 1997). The relevance of having two isoforms of *NK1* has yet to be determined. Stimulation of the *NK1* receptor can generate distinct second messengers that will in turn lead to various effector functions. Some second messengers activated by SP include PLC that will lead to Ca^{2+} mobilization and arachidonic acid metabolism by phospholipase A2 (Mitsuhashi et al., 1992; Mochizuki-Oda, Nakajima, & S, 1994; Nakajima, Tsuchida, Negishi, Ito, & Nakanishi, 1992). There is a difference in effector mechanisms activated depending on the ligand that binds *NK1* in that it has been shown that NKA will activate different second messengers than will SP (Nakajima et al., 1992; Sagan, Chassaing, Pradier, & Lavielle, 1996).

The NK1 receptor is located throughout the central and peripheral nervous systems. In the peripheral nervous system, it functions in vasodilation, increasing vascular permeability, stimulation of salivary and airway secretions, and contraction of smooth muscles (Lembeck & Holzer, 1979; Lembeck & Starke, 1968; Von Euler & Gaddum, 1931). The receptor is also present outside of the nervous system and has been found in places such as the immune system (Payan, Brewster, & Goetzl, 1984; Payan, Brewster, Nissirian-Bastian, & Goetzl, 1984; Payan, McGillis, & Organist, 1986; Stanisz, Schiccitano, Dazin, Bienenstock, & Payan, 1987). There is differential expression of SP receptors on T cell subsets. In human peripheral blood lymphocytes (PBL) the receptor is found on about 10–20% of CD4+ and CD8+ T cells (Payan, Brewster, Nissiran-Bastian et al., 1984).

D. CGRP Receptors

The CGRP receptor is also a seven transmembrane domain G-protein linked receptor. One CGRP receptor, calcitonin receptor-like receptor (CRLR), was cloned in 1993 and initially identified as an orphan receptor related to the calcitonin receptor (Chang, Pearse, O'Connell, & Rosenfeld, 1993; Njuki et al., 1993). Subsequently, the human homologue to CRLR was identified and then found to be the receptor for CGRP (Aiyar et al., 1996). The molecular weights for the receptor differ somewhat in various species. In the human neuroblastoma cell line, SK-N-MC, the MW is 56,000 d, but is reduced to 44,000 d after deglycosylation (Muff, Born, & Fischer, 1995). On rat lymphocytes the weight is 74,500 d, whereas on the murine pre-B cell line 70Z/3, the weight is 103,000 d (McGillis et al., 1993b; McGillis, Humphreys, & Reid, 1991). These inconsistencies could be attributed to species differences, differences in posttranslational processing or expression of different CGRP receptor genes. Two CGRP receptor subtypes have been suggested, CGRP1 and CGRP2, based on differences in affinity for the binding of specific peptide fragments (Quirion, Van Rossum, Dumont, St-Piere, & Fournier, 1992). This was discovered using the C-terminal fragment antagonist $CGRP_{8-37}$ (Dennis et al., 1990). $CGRP_{8-37}$ was found to be an effective antagonist in guinea pig atria, but less effective in rat vas deferens. The linear CGRP agonist [Cys(acetomethoxy)^{2,7}] CGRP is a more potent agonist on rat vas deferens than on guinea pig atria (Quirion et al., 1992). The placement of the CGRP receptor into two different categories has been controversial because binding studies using $CGRP_{8-37}$ as an antagonist have not demonstrated a clear consistent difference in affinities in all studies. The differences in affinities observed may also be complicated by species differences. Further characterization of CGRP receptor genes and receptor isoforms will be necessary to resolve the issue of functional CGRP receptor classification.

Presently, three CGRP receptor candidates have been cloned, and more clones may yet be identified (Aiyar et al., 1996; Chang et al., 1993; Kapas & Clark, 1995; Libert et al., 1989; Luebke, Dahl, Roos, & Dickerson, 1996; Njuki et al., 1993). These clones include CRLR, RDC-1, and CGRP-RCP. CRLR and RDC-1 are both G-protein linked receptors initially reported as orphan receptors (Chang et al., 1993; Libert et al., 1989; Njuki et al., 1993). CGRP-RCP is a GPI anchored external membrane protein (Luebke et al., 1996). Other than the initial report of its cloning, there is no further information on its localization, function, etc. It has been thought that ADM and CGRP can bind the same receptor because there is a certain degree of cross-reactivity in binding assays. ADM can compete with CGRP with about sevenfold lower affinity, and can therefore act as an agonist. A possible explanation for this has recently been reported by McLatchie et al. (1998) They reported that the type of functional receptor expressed on a $CRLR^+$ cell, whether it is CGRP or ADM depends on the expression of a coprotein. These proteins are called receptor activity modulating proteins (RAMP). If the receptor is expressed with RAMP1 it acts as a CGRP receptor; however, if it is expressed with RAMP2 it acts as an ADM receptor (McLatchie et al., 1998).

CGRP receptors are widely located throughout the body, including the nervous system, cardiovascular system, and endocrine system (Dennis, Fournier, St. Pierre, & Quirion, 1989; Haegerstrand, Dalsgaard, Jonzon, Larsson, & Nilsson, 1990; Hirata et al., 1988; Seifert, Chesnut, De Souza, Rivier, & Vale, 1985; Seifert, Sawchenko et al., 1985; Sexton et al., 1986; Sexton, McKenzie, & Mendelsohn, 1988; Sigrist et al., 1986; Tschopp et al., 1985). In the CNS, both high and low affinity receptors have been identified, whereas in the cardiovascular system only one affinity class has been found. The CGRP receptor is also found in the immune system. This was first discovered using whole spleen preparations (Nakamuta et al., 1986; Sigrist et al., 1986), but has since been positively identified on rat T and B cells, monocytes, and macrophages, in mouse bone marrow, and various lymphoid cell lines (Abello, Kaiserlian, Cuber, Revillard, & Chayvialle, 1991; Bulloch et al., 1991; McGillis, Humphreys, Rangnekar, & Ciallella, 1993a; McGillis, Humphreys et al., 1991; Mullins, Ciallella, Rangnekar, & McGillis, 1993; Owan & Ibaraki, 1994; Ullman, Northrop, Vereiji, & Crabtree, 1990; Vignery, Wang, & Ganz, 1991). At present, however, it is not known what particular populations of T and B cells express the CGRP receptors. We have found that in the mouse bone marrow, there are more CGRP receptors than on mature B cells (3,000/cell vs. 700/cell). In addition, the murine pre-B cell 70Z/3 has approximately 20,000 receptors/cell (McGillis et al., 1993a). This data implies a role for CGRP on development of B cells. We have attempted to further characterize the specific populations of B cells to determine whether they have functional receptors. Traditionally, ligand binding assays are performed to determine if a particular cell type expresses the receptor. This has been problematic because a large number of cells are required for these assays and purifying a sufficient number is very expensive and difficult. Thus, we purified cells from multiple fractions and tested for the receptor using RT-PCR. This has shown that the CRLR version of the receptor is present from the very earliest B cell progenitors through mature (IgM^+, IgD^+) B cells (unpublished observation).

III. INFLAMMATORY AND IMMUNOREGULATORY EFFECTS OF SP AND CGRP

A. Sensory Innervation in Immune Organs

It is recognized in the field of neural–immune interactions that physical connections between the immune and nervous systems are critical. Sensory nerve fibers containing the sensory neuropeptides CGRP and SP are present in primary and secondary lymphoid organs including the thymus, bone marrow, and lymph nodes (Bjurholm, 1991; Bjurholm et al., 1988; Kimberly & Byers, 1988; Pereira da Silva & Carmo-Fonseca, 1990; Popper et al., 1988; Weihe et al., 1989). The presence of SP in the thymus is corroborated in functional studies by Geppetti and co-workers showing that the thymus could be depleted of SP by treatment with capsaicin, a sensory neuron-specific neurotoxin (Geppetti et al., 1987). CGRP has been identified in the thymus of all mammalian species studied so far, always in discrete sites (Bulloch et al., 1991; Weihe et al., 1989). The bone marrow, site of B-cell lymphopoiesis in the adult mammal, also contains $CGRP^+$ and SP^+ sensory fibers (Bjurholm et al., 1988; Bjurholm et al., 1990; Goto, Yamaza, Kido, & Tanaka, 1998; Hukkanen et al., 1992). Using immunohistochemical analysis of lymph nodes, Popper and co-workers could show CGRP and SP immunoreactivity in the medullary cord, in the blood vessels and in the deep cortex (Popper et al., 1988). In addition, CGRP and SP are present around all blood vessels and in all internal and external surfaces, where they can influence local inflammatory and immune responses.

B. Effect of Substance P on Immune Functions

The effect of SP on the immune system has been studied for almost 20 years and has been reviewed recently (Brain, 1997; Maggi, 1997; McGillis, & Fernandez, 1999; McGillis, Mitsuhashi et al., 1991; Payan, 1992). Therefore, this chapter will only highlight some of the effects of SP, especially more recent work. Experimental data gathered so far characterizes SP as a neuropeptide capable of up-regulating and enhancing different aspects of both innate and specific immune responses. SP can regulate cytokine production by immune cells, immunoglobulin production by B-lymphocytes and the migration of cells into sites of infection (Lotz, Vaughn, & Carson, 1988; Matis, Lavker, & Murphy, 1990; Nakagawa, Sano,

& Iwamoto, 1995; Quinlan et al., 1998, 1999; Rameshwar, Ganea, & Gascon, 1994; Rameshwar & Gascon, 1995, 1996; Serra, Calzetti, Ceska, & Cassatella, 1994; Smith, Barker, Morris, MacDonald, & Lee, 1993; Stanisz, Befus, & Bienenstock, 1986; Takahashi, 1996). This last function involves regulatory effects that influence the ability of activated T-cells and other leukoctyes to leave blood venules and penetrate infected sites. Extravasation depends on the expression of adhesion molecules on the surface of these cells and on the cells lining the walls of blood vessels. SP up-regulates adhesion molecules that facilitate activated T-cell extravassation. Ansel and co-workers found that SP up-regulates VCAM-1 and ICAM-1 adhesion molecule expression (required for activated T-cell migration) in human endothelial cells in a concentration and time-dependent manner (Quinlan et al., 1998, 1999). These effects were neutralized with the use of SP receptor (NKR1) antagonists, underscoring their specificity. These observations have been corroborated by other researchers (Lambert et al., 1998; Nakagawa et al., 1995). Nakagawa and co-workers show that SP significantly increases neutrophil transendothelial migration through ICAM-1-dependent mechanisms (Nakagawa et al., 1995). Members of the selectin family of adhesion molecules are also regulated by SP. SP has been shown to up-regulate P- and E-selectin expression and translocation to cytoplasmic membranes in endothelial cells (Matis et al., 1990; Smith et al., 1993). Eosinophil migration is also upregulated in the presence of SP (El-Shazly, Masuyama, Eura, & Ishikawa, 1996).

SP also regulates humoral responses by acting directly on T and B-lymphocytes. SP receptors are found in specific subsets of T-lymphocytes as well as in B-lymphocytes (Payan, Brewster, & Goetzl, 1984; Payan, Brewster, Nissirian-Bastian et al., 1984; Stanisz et al., 1987). SP enhances proliferation of T-lymphocytes in response to mitogens and production of IgA by B-lymphocytes isolated from the mesenteric lymph nodes, spleen, and Peyer's patches (Payan, Brewster, & Goetzl, 1983; Stanisz et al., 1986). More recent studies also suggest that SP has a role in hematopoiesis. The presence of SP-containing nerve endings in the bone marrow suggests that SP plays a regulatory role in blood cell development (Goto et al., 1998; Hukkanen et al., 1992). Colony forming assays showed that SP increases the number of colonies of myeloid lineage (macrophage and granulocyte) (Rameshwar et al., 1993). In contrast, NKA inhibits myeloid colony formation (Rameshwar & Gascon, 1996). The effect of SP is at least partially due to its induction of IL-3 and granulocyte-macrophage colony-stimulating factor (GM-CSF), whereas the counter-effects of NKA appear to be due to its induction of MIP-1α and TGF-β (Rameshwar, Ganeo, & Gascon, 1994; Rameshwar & Gascon, 1995).

C. Effect of CGRP on Lymphocytes

CGRP has been reported to affect T-cells in different ways. The effects of CGRP on T-lymphocytes were first described in 1988 by Umeda et al. CGRP was shown to inhibit mitogen-induced proliferation of cells from mouse spleen and lymph nodes in a dose-dependent manner. The optimal CGRP concentrations were about 10^{-9} M, which are similar to the reported dissociation constants for the CGRP receptor. This inhibitory effect correlates with a strong induction of cAMP by CGRP. The inhibitory effect of CGRP on proliferation has been confirmed and extended by several investigators. Boudard and Bastide show that spleen T-cell inhibition by CGRP is probably due to down-regulation of the proliferative cytokine IL-2, a fact that was later confirmed by Wang et al. (Boudard & Bastide, 1991; Wang, Millet, Bottomly, & Vignery, 1992) CGRP has also been shown to inhibit concanavalin A (Con A) induced proliferation of thymocytes (Bulloch et al., 1991). This inhibition was suggested to be the consequence of an enhancement in the rate of apoptosis in the presence of CGRP (Bulloch, McEwen, Nordberg, Diwa, & Baird, 1998). This CGRP-induced apoptosis is more evident among $CD8^+/CD4^+$ cells. It is interesting to notice that this group of cells normally undergoes selection in the thymus, suggesting that CGRP plays a role in development and selection of T-cells. Although the concentration levels of CGRP used in these experiments are within the physiological levels, it is not clear why the use of $CGRP_{8-37}$ does not block the CGRP effect in these studies. In most other studies with CGRP in lymphocytes, $CGRP_{8-37}$ blocks the effects of CGRP, suggesting that some effects of CGRP may be mediated through different receptors that are not sensitive to $CGRP_{8-37}$.

The effects of CGRP on specific subsets of T-lymphocytes have shown that its effect varies depending on the cell phenotype. Using T-cell clones it was possible to show that although CGRP had no apparent effect on Th_2 clones, it does induce a transient, if strong accumulation of cAMP in Th_1 clones (Levite, 1998). However, it should be noted that these results were based on analysis of three cell lines. Elevation of cAMP has been reported to activate mechanisms that down-regulate expression of IL-2 (Chen & Rothenberg, 1994). This effect was specific, since the use of the CGRP antagonist $CGRP_{8-37}$

prevented it. In contrast, Levite has reported that CGRP, as well as other neuropeptides like substance P and somatostatin may have more profound effects in Th_1 and Th_2 cell clones, inducing a wide array of changes in their cytokine secretion profile (Levite, 1998). Although the cytokines produced contradict the previous reports, more controls need to be included to corroborate these results and to test for the specificity of these effects. Interestingly, a recent study with transgenic NOD mice expressing CGRP in the pancreas found a delay in the onset of insulin dependent diabetes mellitus (IDDM) (Khachatryan et al., 1997). IDDM is an autoimmune disease mediated by Th_1 cells. It is possible that a CGRP inhibition of Th1 cells could account for the delayed onset of IDDM in this model.

CGRP also affects B-lymphocyte function and development. We found that the pre-B-cell line 70Z/3 expresses a high number of high affinity CGRP receptors on the surface (McGillis et al., 1993a). In the study of the expression of the immunoglobulin gene, 70Z/3 cells have been used extensively. Although they have rearranged μ (heavy chain) and κ (light chain) immunoglobulin genes, they only express cytoplasmic μ protein. Treatment of 70Z/3 with LPS or IL-1 induces a differentiation process that leads to the expression of surface immunoglobulin (sIg) (McGillis et al., 1993b). We have shown that CGRP in nanomolar concentration inhibits the differentiation process induced by LPS. This inhibition is abrogated with the use of $CGRP_{8\text{-}37}$. Inhibition of LPS-induced differentiation can be mimicked by use of the protein kinase A (PKA) activator dibutyryl cAMP, pointing to cAMP and PKA as intermediates of CGRP-induced inhibition (McGillis et al., 1993b). We have also shown that CGRP prevents the LPS-induced translocation on NF-$\kappa\beta$ transcription factor into the nucleus of the cell (unpublished observation).

The process of differentiation and surface expression of Ig in 70Z/3 cells resembles that of developing B-lymphocytes in the bone marrow (Paige, Kincade, & Ralph, 1978). Immature B cells undergo a rapid change in the expression of surface markers as they mature from the most primitive population (with unrearranged Ig genes) to naive but immunocompetent B cells expressing sIg. This process is regulated by several cytokines produced and secreted by the stromal cell matrix that regulates lymphopoiesis in the bone marrow. The most important cytokine in this group is IL-7. IL-7 is required to induce proliferation and differentiation in those cells that have successfully completed rearrangement of their heavy chain Ig genes reviewed in (Candejas, Muegge, & Durum, 1997). We have conducted experiments to gauge the effect of CGRP in IL-7 induced proliferation of bone marrow-derived pre-B cells (manuscript submitted). We found that CGRP strongly inhibits the ability of pre-pro-B cells to expand in response to IL-7. CGRP acts directly on IL-7 responding pre-pro-B cells and also acts indirectly by inducing the secretion of a second inhibitory factor from stromal cells. It is not clear whether CGRP and the second inhibitory factor act at the same stages in B cell development. A goal of this research is to elucidate the ultimate function of CGRP in the bone marrow. A critical aspect in the regulation of B cell lymphopoiesis is the process of eliminating cells with the potential of reacting to self-peptides, a source of autoimmunity. During an immune response the immune system secretes cytokines that can accelerate B-cell development to levels that may override the selective machinery that eliminates self-reactive clones. CGRP can thus be thought of as a protective regulatory element designed to prevent developing B-lymphocytes from expanding to levels that threaten the body integrity.

D. Effect of CGRP on Macrophages

Macrophages have several key roles in both innate and specific immune responses including phagocytosis of pathogens, generation of reactive radicals that kill microbes, antigen presentation to T cells, and production of cytokines. The expression of functional CGRP receptors on macrophages suggested that CGRP might regulate macrophage functions (Owan & Ibaraki, 1994; Vignery et al., 1991). Nong et al. reported that human peripheral blood monocytes preincubated with nanomolar concentrations of CGRP failed to produce H_2O_2 in response to IFN-γ (1989). A similar result was reported by Taylor et al., who found that the aqueous humor from the eye in rabbits contains CGRP (Taylor, Yee, & Streilein, 1998). In this system exogenously added CGRP also inhibited nitric oxide synthase (NOS2) activity in a macrophage cell line, thus inhibiting the production of nitric oxide (NO). A caveat in this report is that the concentration of CGRP found in the aqueous humor (and therefore used in the experiments) was higher than the physiological levels. These results have been somewhat contradicted by Tang and co-workers, who reported that CGRP increases NO production in mouse peritoneal macrophages, which is required to increase IL-6 synthesis in the same cells (Tang, Feng, & Wang, 1997; Tang, Han, & Wang, 1999). This effect is cAMP and PKA-dependent and is specific, as $CGRP_{8\text{-}37}$ can suppress this induction. Furthermore, when NOS2-specific inhibitors were used, IL-6 synthesis was stopped, suggesting that CGRP may be using

NO as a mediator in macrophages. These data show a strong correlation between CGRP and NO induction.

Although phagocytosis (a prerequisite for antigen presentation) in peritoneal macrophages has been reported to be enhanced by CGRP (Ichinose & Sawada, 1996), CGRP has been shown to act as an inhibitor of antigen presentation in these cells (Nong et al., 1989; Torii et al., 1997). This observation also has been made regarding Langerhans cells (LC) (Asahina, Hosoi, Grabbe, & Granstein, 1995). Langerhans cells, although related to macrophages, retained the ability to engulf pathogens and antigens in the skin and to serve as APCs in secondary lymphoid organs. In these experiments, treatment of LCs resulted in an accumulation of cytoplasmic cAMP, although this increase alone could not account for the inhibition in antigen presentation in these cells (Asahina, Hosoi et al., 1995).

Further investigation into the inhibition of antigen presentation in macrophages and LCs revealed that CGRP affects cytokine secretion in LCs (Fox et al., 1997; Torii et al., 1997). CGRP enhances LPS and GM-CSF induced production of IL-10, whereas it inhibits IL-1β and the p40 subunit of IL-12. In peritoneal macrophages, secretion of LPS-induced IL-10 is also increased, though IL-1β is down-regulated (Torii et al., 1997). In the same report, it was shown that CGRP could also down-regulate expression of B7-2, a surface protein required for antigen presentation to T-cells. The down-regulation of B7-2 appears to be due to the increased levels of IL-10 since using neutralizing antibodies against IL-10 abrogates the inhibition in B7-2 expression. The same group reports similar findings in human peripheral blood mononuclear cells (PBMC) (Fox et al., 1997). Anti-IL-10 antibodies restores the level of IL-12 p40, of IFN-γ and proliferation in CGRP-treated PBMC.

E. Effects of CGRP on Neutrophils and Eosinophils

Neutrophils and eosinophils are members of the innate immune system. They infiltrate infected tissues where they engulf antibody-coated pathogens and parasites, respectively. The ability of eosinophils and neutrophils to target sites of infection depends of two factors: the production and recognition of chemotactic factors, and expression of adhesion molecules. Neuropeptides can influence the production of adhesion molecules in the endothelial cells lining the blood vessels and can also regulate the rate at which chemotactic factors are produced. Injection of CGRP enhances IL-1 induced edema formation and neutrophil infiltration at the site of injection (Buckley, Brain, Collins, & Williams, 1991). Eosinophil chemotaxis to platelet-activating factor and to leukotriene B4 is also enhanced in the presence of CGRP (Numao & Agrawal, 1992). Further studies into this phenomenon revealed that amino acids 32–35 of CGRPα are identical to the eosinophil chemotactic factor of anaphylaxis (Manley & Haynes, 1989). Products of the digestion of CGRP with trypsin exhibited chemotactic activity. The neutral endopeptidase 24.11 cleaves several peptides (including CGRP) and is present on the surface of many cell types. CGRP is cleaved by neutral endopeptidase 24.11, releasing fragments 32–35 (Davies et al., 1992), increasing chemotatic activity. CGRP seems to act as a chemotactic factor after cleavage by peptidases present on the surrounding cells at the site of infection. Interestingly, the structure of the chemotactic factor can only be derived from CGRP α. It is not clear whether similar chemotactic fragments can be derived from CGRP β . Thus, this may be the first example of different functions of the α and β isoforms of CGRP.

CGRP induces secretion of secondary granules from neutrophils (Richter, Andersson, Edvinsson, & Gullberg, 1992). Data suggests that CGRP acts through chemotactic factor (FMLP) receptors since the CGRP concentrations used in these experiments were substantially above physiological levels. In addition, adhesion of neutrophils to endothelial cells is induced by CGRP in vitro (Zimmerman, Anderson, & Granger, 1992). It is not clear whether CGRP is acting through adhesion molecules on the endothelial cells or directly through the neutrophils.

IV. CONCLUSION AND FUTURE PERSPECTIVES

Inflammatory and immunoregulatory activities for the sensory neuropeptides SP and CGRP are well supported by experimental data. There is ample evidence to suggest that they have multiple roles on different cells in different environments and under different conditions. These range from regulating microvascular components of inflammation to influencing lymphocyte functions in local sites to roles in hematopoiesis in the bone marrow. Although this may seem like an artificially broad range of activities, they all have the common feature of local regulation by sensory nerve products in specific microenvironments. In this context, one might argue that the immune system has adapted to recognize nervous system signals common to virtually any local microenvironment undergoing immune and/or inflammatory processes. Thus, the specific response of a T cell vs. a B cell to SP or CGRP is a reflection of what that cell is programmed to do in its target environment. This view supports the initial hypothesis that these mediators play an integrating role in local responses. They do this by allowing many different highly differentiated cells to recognize common signals in a local context that can specifically influence their discreet functions. Although there has been considerable interest in these two peptides in the last 10 to 20 years, we are just beginning to understand how they mediate the efferent arm of nervous system–immune system communication. Research over the next decade will need to focus on more specific roles for these peptides at the cellular and molecular levels. Ultimately, this knowledge may provide a better understanding for how protective immune and inflammatory processes are integrated within the body. Such knowledge would facilitate our comprehension of disease processes and of how they can be affected by behavioral phenomena.

References

Abello, J., Kaiserlian, D., Cuber, J. C., Revillard, J. P., & Chayvialle, J. A. (1991). Characterization of calcitnonin gene-related peptide receptors and adenylate cyclase response in the murine macrophage cell line P388 D1. *Neuropeptides, 19*, 43–49.

Aiyar, N., Rand, K., Elshourgagy, N. A., Zeng, A., Adamou, J. E., Bergsma, D. J., & Li, Y. (1996). A cDNA encoding the calcitonin gene-related peptide type 1 receptor. *Journal of Biological Chemistry, 271*, 11325–11329.

Amara, S. G., Arriza, J. L., Leff, S. E., Swanson, L. W., Evans, R. M., & Rosenfeld, M. G. (1985). Expression in brain of a messenger RNA encoding a novel neuropeptide homologous to calcitonin gene-related peptide. *Science, 229*, 1094–1097.

Amara, S. G., Jones, V., Rosenfeld, M. G., Ong, E. S., & Evans, R. M. (1982). Alternative RNA processing in calcitonin gene expression generates mRNAs encoding different polypeptide products. *Nature, 298*, 240–244.

Asahina, A., Hosoi, J., Grabbe, S., & Granstein, R. D. (1995). Modulation of Langerhans cell function by epidermal nerves. *Journal of Allergy and Clinical Immunology, 96*, 1178–1182.

Asahina, A., Moro, O., Hosoi, J., Lerner, E. A., Xu, S., Takashima, A., & Granstein, R. D. (1995). Specific induction of cAMP in Langerhans cells by calcitonin gene-related peptide: Relevance to functional effects. *Proceedings of the National Academy of Sciences USA, 92*, 8323–8327.

Bjurholm, A. (1991). Neuroendocrine peptides in bone. *International Orthopedics, 15*, 325–329.

Bjurholm, A., Kreicbergs, A., Brodin, E., & Schultzberb, M. (1988). Substance P- and CGRP-immunoreactive nerves in bone. *Peptides, 9*, 166–171.

Bjurholm, A., Kreicbergs, A., Dahlberg, L., & Schultzberg, M. (1990). The occurrence of neuropeptides at different stages of DPM-induced heterotopic bone formation. *Bone and Mineral, 10*, 95–98.

Boudard, F., & Bastide, M. (1991). Inhibition of mouse T-cell proliferation by CGRP and VIP: Effects of these neuropeptides on IL-2 production and cAMP systhesis. *Journal of Neuroscience Research, 29*, 29–41.

Brain, S. D. (1997). Sensory neuropeptides: Their role in inflammation and wound healing. *Immunopharmacology, 37*, 133–52.

Brain, S. D., & Williams, T. J. (1985). Inflammatory oedema induced by synergism between calcitonin gene-releated peptide (CGRP) and mediators of increased vascular permeability. *British Journal of Pharmacology, 86*, 855–860.

Brain, S. D., Williams, T. J., Tippins, J. R., Morris, H. R., & MacIntyre, I. (1985). Calcitonin gene-related peptide is a potent vasodilator. *Nature, 313*, 54–56.

Buckley, T. L., Brain, S. D., Collins, P. D., & Williams, T. J. (1991). Inflammatory edema induced by interactions between IL-1 and the neuropeptide calcitonin gene-related peptide. *Journal of Immunology, 146*, 3424–3430.

Bulloch, K., McEwen, B. S., Nordberg, J., Diwa, A., & Baird, S. (1998). Selective regulation of T-cell development and function by calcitonin gene-related peptide in thymus and spleen. *Annals of the New York Acadamy Sciences USA, 840*, 551–562.

Bulloch, K., Radojcic, T., Yu, R., Hausman, J., Lenhard, L., & Baird, S. (1991). The distribution and function of calcitonin gene-related peptide in the mouse thymus and spleen. *Progress in Neuroendocrinimmunology, 4*, 186–194.

Candejas, S., Muegge, K., & Durum, S. K. (1997). IL-7 Receptor and VDJ Recombination: Trophic versus mechanistic actions. *Immunity, 6*, 501–508.

Chang, C. P., Pearse, R. V., O'Connell, S., & Rosenfeld, M. G. (1993). Identification of a seven transmembrane helix receptor for corticotropin-releasing factor and sauvagine in mammalian brain. *Neuron, 11*, 11187–1195.

Chen, D., & Rothenberg, E. V. (1994). Interleukin 2 transcription factors as molecular targets of cAMP inhibition: Delayed inhibition kinetics and combinatorial transcription roles. *Journal of Experimental Medicine, 179*, 931–942.

Davies, D., Medeiros, M. S., Keen, J., Truner, A. J., & Haynes, L. W. (1992). Endopeptidase-24.11 cleaves a chemotactic factor from alpha-calcitonin gene-related peptide. *Biochemical Pharmacology, 43*, 1753–1756.

Dennis, T., Fournier, A., Cadieux, A., Pomerleau, F., Jolicoeur, F. B., St. Pierre, S., & Quirion, R. (1990). hCGRP8-37, a calcitonin gene-related peptide antagonist revealing calcitonin gene-related peptide receptor heterogeneity in brain and periphery. *Journal of Pharmacology and Experimental Therapeutics, 254*, 123–128.

Dennis, T., Fournier, A., St. Pierre, S., & Quirion, R. (1989). Structure-activity profile of calcitonin gene-related peptide in peripheral and brain tissues. Evidence for receptor multiplicity. *Journal of Pharmacology and Experimental Therapeutics, 251*, 718–725.

El-Shazly, A. E., Masuyama, K., Eura, M., & Ishikawa, T. (1996). Immunoregulatory effect of substance P in human eosinophil migratory function. *Immunological Investigations, 25*, 191–201.

Foreman, J. C. (1987). Peptides and neurogenic inflammation. *British Medical Bulletin, 43*, 386–400.

Fox, F. E., Kubin, M., Cassin, M., Niu, Z., Hosoi, J., Torii, H., Granstein, R. D., Trinchieri, G., & Rook, A. H. (1997). Calcitonin gene-related peptide inhibits proliferation and antigen presentation by human peripheral blood mononuclear cells: Effects on B7, interleukin 10, and interleukin 12. *Journal of Investigative Dermatology, 108*, 43–48.

Garland, A. M., Grady, E. F., Payan, D. G., Vigna, S. R., & Bunnett, N. W. (1994). Agonist-induced internalization of the substance P (NK1) receptor expressed in epithelial cells. *Biochemical Journal, 303*, 177–186.

Geppetti, P., Maggi, C. A., Zecchi-Orlandini, S., Santicioli, P., Meli, A., Frilli, S., Spillantini, M. G., & Amenta, F. (1987). Substance P-like immunoreactivity in capsaicin-sensitive structures of the rat thymus. *Regulatory Peptides, 18*, 321–329.

Gnaedinger, M. P., Uehlinger, D. E., Weidmann, P., Sha, S. G., Muff, R., Born, W., Rascher, W., & Fischer, J. A. (1989). Distinct hemodynamic and renal effects of calcitonin gene-related peptide and calcitonin in men. *American Journal Physiology, 257,* 870–875.

Goto, T., Yamaza, T., Kido, M. A., & Tanaka, T. (1998). Light- and electron-microscopic study of the distribution of axons containing substance P and the localization of neurokinin-1 receptor in bone. *Cell and Tissue Research, 293,* 87–93.

Grady, E. F., Garland, A. M., Gamp, P. D., Lovett, M., Payan, D. G., & Bunnett, N. W. (1995). Delineation of the endocytic pathway of substance P and its seven-transmembrane domain NK1 receptor. *Molecular and Cellular Biology, 6,* 509–524.

Haegerstrand, A., Dalsgaard, C.-J., Jonzon, B., Larsson, O., & Nilsson, J. (1990). Calcitonin gene-related peptide stimulates proliferation of human endothelial cells. *Proceedings of the National Acadamy of Sciences, USA, 87,* 3299–3303.

Herbert, M. K., & Holzer, P. (1994a). Interleukin-1 beta enhances capsaicin-induced neurogenic vasodilatation in the rat skin. *British Journal of Pharmacology, 111,* 681–686.

Herbert, M. K., & Holzer, P. (1994b). Nitric oxide mediates the amplification by interleukin-1a of neurogenic vasodilatation in the rat skin. *European Journal of Pharmacology, 260,* 89–93.

Hershey, A. D., & Krause, J. E. (1990). Molecular characterization of a functional cDNA encoding the rat substance P receptor. *Science, 247,* 958–962.

Hirata, Y., Takagi, Y., Takata, S., Fukuda, Y., Yoshimi, H., & Fujita, T. (1988). Calcitonin gene-related peptide receptor in cultured vascular smooth muscle and endothelial cells. *Biochemical and Biophysical Research Communications, 151,* 1113–1121.

Huang, R. R., Yu, H., Strader, C. D., & Fong, T. M. (1994). *Biochemistry, 15,* 3007–3013.

Hukkanen, M., Konttinin, Y., Rees, R. G., Gibson, S. J., Santavirta, S., & Polak, J. M. (1992). Innervation of bone from healthy and arthritic rats by substance P and calcitonin gene related peptide containing sensory fibers. *Journal of Rheumatology, 19,* 1252–1259.

Ichinose, M., & Sawada, M. (1996). Enhancement of phagocytosis by calcitonin gene-related peptide (CGRP) in cultured mouse peritoneal macrophages. *Peptides, 17,* 1405–1414.

Kapas, S., & Clark, A. J. L. (1995). Identification of an orphan receptor gene as a type 1 calcitonin gene-related peptide receptor. *Biochemical and Biophysical Resesearch Communications, 217,* 832–838.

Kar, S., Rees, R. G., & Quirion, R. (1994). Altered calcitonin gene-related peptide, substance P and enkephalin immunoreactivities and receptor binding sites in the dorsal spinal cord of the polyarthritic rat. *European Journal of Neuroscience, 6,* 345–354.

Khachatryan, A., Guerder, S., Palluault, F., Cote, G., Solimena, M., Valentijn, K., Millet, I., Flavell, R. A., & Vignery, A. (1997). Targeted expression of the neuropeptide calcitonin gene-related peptide to beta cells prevents diabetes in NOD mice. *Journal of Immunology, 158,* 1409–1416.

Kimberly, C. L., & Byers, M. R. (1988). Inflammation of rat molar pulp and periodontium causes increased calcitonin gene-related peptide and axonal sprouting. *Anatomical Record, 222,* 289–300.

Kruger, L., Silverman, J. D., Mantyh, P. W., Sternini, C., & Brecha, N. C. (1991). Peripheral patterns of calcitonin-gene-related peptide general somatic sensory innervation: Cutaneous and deep terminations. *Journal of Comparative Neurology, 280,* 291–302.

Kurtz, A., Muff, R., & Fischer, J. A. (1989). *Kidney International, 36,* 222–227.

Lambert, N., Lescoulie, P. L., Yassine-Diab, B., Enault, G., Mazieres, B., & De Preval, C. (1998). Substance P enhances cytokine-induced vascular cell adhesion molecule-1 (VCAM-1) expression on cultured rheumatoid fibroblast-like fibroblasts. *Clinical and Experimental Immunology, 113,* 269–275.

Larsson, J., Ekblom, A., Henriksson, K., Lundebert, T., & Theodorsson, E. (1991). Concentration of substance P, neurokinin A, calcitonin gene-related peptide, neuropeptide Y and vasoactive intestinal polypeptide in synovial fluid from knee joints in patients suffering from rheumatoid arthritis. *Scandinavian Journal of Rheumatology, 20,* 326–335.

Lee, Y., Takami, K., Kawai, Y., Girgis, S., Hillyard, C. J., MacIntyre, I., Emson, P. C., & Tohyama, M. (1985). Distribution of calcitonin gene-releated peptide in the rat peripheral nervous sytem with reference to its coexistence with substance P. *Neuroscience, 15,* 1227–1237.

Lembeck, F., & Holzer, P. (1979). Substance P as neurogenic mediator of antidromic vasodilation and neurogenic plasma extravasation. *Naunyn-Schmiedeberg's Archives of Pharmacology, 310,* 175–183.

Lembeck, F., & Starke, K. (1968). Substanz P und Speichelsekretion. *Naunyn-Schmiedeberg's Archives of Pharmacology, 259,* 375–385.

Levite, M. (1998). Neuropeptides, by direct interaction with T cells, induce secretion and break the commitment to a distinct T helper phenotype. *Proceedings of the National Academy of Sciences USA, 95,* 12544–12549.

Libert, F., Parmentier, M., Lefort, A., Dinsart, C., Van Sande, J., Maenhaut, C., Simons, M. J., Dumont, J. E., & Vassart, G. (1989). Selective amplification and cloning of four new members of the G protein-coupled receptor family. *Science, 244,* 569–572.

Lotz, M., Vaughn, J. H., & Carson, D. A. (1988). Effects of neuropeptides on production of inflammatory cytokines by human monocytes. *Science, 241,* 1218–1221.

Luebke, A. E., Dahl, G. P., Roos, B. A., & Dickerson, I. M. (1996). Identification of a protein that confers calcitonin gene-related peptide responsiveness to oocytes by using a cystic fibrosis transmembrane conductance regulator assay. *Proceedings of the National Academy of Sciences USA, 93,* 3455–3460.

Maggi, C. A. (1997). The effects of tachykinins on inflammatory and immune cells. *Regulatory Peptides, 70,* 75–90.

Maggi, C. A., Patacchini, R., Rovero, P., & Giachetti, A. (1993). Tachykinin receptors and tachykinin receptor antagonists. *Journal of Autonomic Pharmacology, 13,* 13–23.

Manley, H. C., & Haynes, L. W. (1989). Eosinophil chemotactic response to rat CGRP-1 is increased after exposure to trypsin or guinea-pig lung particulate fraction. *Neuropeptides, 13,* 29–34.

Marksteiner, J., Mahata, S. K., Pycha, R., Mahata, M., Saria, A., Fischer-Colbrie, R., & Winkler, H. (1994). Distribution of secretoneurin immunoreactivity in the spinal cord and lower brainstem in comparison with that of substance P and calcitonin gene-related peptide. *Journal of Comparative Neurology, 340,* 243–254.

Martin, F. C., Charles, A. C., Sanderson, M. J., & Merrill, J. E. (1992). Substance P stimulates IL-1 production by astrocytes via intracellular calcium. *Brain Research, 599,* 13–18.

Masu, Y., Nakayama, K., Tamaki, H., Harada, Y., Kuno, M., & Nakanishi, S. (1987). cDNA cloning of bovine substance-K receptor through oocyte expression system. *Nature, 329,* 836–838.

Matis, W. L., Lavker, R. M., & Murphy, G. M. (1990). Substance P induces the expression of an endothelial-leukocyte adhesion molecule by microvascular endothelium. *Journal of Investigative Dermatology, 94,* 492–495.

McGillis, J. P., & Fernandez, S. (1999). Sensory Neuropeptides, Neurogenic Inflammation and Inflammatory Cells. In S. D. Brain & P.K. Moore (Eds.), *Progress in inflammation research: Pain and neurogenic inflammation.* (pp. 115–135). Basel: Birkhauser.

McGillis, J. P., & Figueiredo, H. F. (1996). Sensory neuropeptides: The role of calcitonin gene-related peptide (CGRP) in modulating inflammation and immunity. In J. A. Marsh & M. D. Kendall (Eds.), *The physiology of immunity* (pp. 127–143). Boca Raton, FL: CRC Press.

McGillis, J. P., Humphreys, S., Rangnekar, V., & Ciallella, J. (1993a). Modulation of B lymphocyte differentiation by calcitonin gene related peptide (CGRP) I: Characterization of high affinity CGRP receptors on murine 70Z cells. *Cellular Immunology, 150,* 391–404.

McGillis, J. P., Humphreys, S., Rangnekar, V., & Ciallella, J. (1993b). Modulation of B lymphocyte differentiation by calcitonin gene related peptide (CGRP) II: Inhibition of LPS induced kappa light chain expression by CGRP. *Cellular Immunology, 150,* 405–416.

McGillis, J. P., Humphreys, S., & Reid, S. (1991). Characterization of functional calcitonin gene-related peptide receptors on rat lymphocytes. *Journal of Immunology, 147,* 3482–3489.

McGillis, J. P., Mitsuhashi, M., & Payan, D. G. (1991). Immunologic properties of substance P. In R. Ader, D. L. Felten, & N. Cohen (Eds.), *Psychoneuroimmunology* (2nd ed., pp. 209–224). San Diego: Academic Press.

McLatchie, L. M., Fraser, N. J., Main, M. J., Wise, A., Brown, J., Thompson, N., Solari, R., Lee, M. G., & Foord, S. M. (1998). RAMPs regulate the transport and ligand specificity of the calcitonin-receptor like receptor. *Nature, 393,* 333–339.

Merrill, J. E., Koyanagi, Y., Zack, J., Thomas, L., Martin, F., & Chen, I. S. (1992). Induction of interleukin-1 and tumor necrosis factor alpha in brain cultures by human immunodeficiency virus type 1. *Journal of Virology, 66,* 2217–2225.

Mitsuhashi, M., Ohashi, Y., Shichijo, S., Christian, C., Sudduth-Klinger, J., Harrowe, G., & Payan, D. G. (1992). Multiple intracellular signaling pathways of the neuropeptide substance P receptor. *Journal of Neuroscience Research, 32,* 437–443.

Mochizuki-Oda, N., Nakajima, Y., & S, N. S. I. (1994). Characterization of the substance P receptor-mediated calcium influx in cDNA transfected Chinese hamster ovary cells. A possible role of inositol 1,4,5-trisphosphate in calcium influx. *Journal of Biological Chemistry, 269,* 9651–9658.

Muff, R., Born, W., & Fischer, J. A. (1995). Calcitonin, calcitonin gene related peptide, adrenomedullin and amylin: Homologous peptides, separate receptors and overlapping biological actions. *European Journal of Endocrinlogy, 133,* 17–20.

Mullins, M. S., Ciallella, J., Rangnekar, V., & McGillis, J. P. (1993). Characterization of a calcitonin gene-related peptide (CGRP) receptor on mouse bone marrow cells. *Regulatory Peptides, 49,* 65–72.

Nakagawa, N., Sano, H., & Iwamoto, I. (1995). Substance P induces the expression of intercellular adhesion molecule-1 on vascular endothelial cells and enhances neutrophil transendothelial migration. *Peptides, 16,* 721–725.

Nakajima, Y., Tsuchida, K., Negishi, M., Ito, S., & Nakanishi, S. (1992). Direct linkage of three tachykinin receptors to stimulation of both phosphatidylinositol hydrolysis and cyclic AMP cascades in transfected Chinese hamster ovary cells. *Journal of Biological Chemistry, 267,* 2437–2442.

Nakamuta, H., Fukuda, Y., Koida, M., Fufii, N., Otaka, A., Funakoshi, S., Mitsuyasu, N., & Orlowski, R. C. (1986). Binding sites of calcitonin gene-related peptide (CGRP): Abundant occurrence in visceral organs. *Japan J. Pharmacol., 42,* 175–180.

Njuki, F., Nicholl, C. G., Howard, A., Mak, J. C., Barnes, P. J., Girgis, S. I., & Legon, S. (1993). A new calcitonin-receptor-like sequence in rat pulmonary blood vessels. *Clinical Science Colchester, 85,* 385–388.

Nong, Y. H., Titus, R. G., Ribeiro, J. M. C., & Remold, H. G. (1989). Peptides encoded by the calcitonin gene inhibit macrophage function. *Journal of Immunology, 143,* 45–49.

Numao, T., & Agrawal, D. K. (1992). Neuropeptides modulate human eosinophil chemotaxis. *Journal of Immunology, 149,* 3309–3315.

Nussdorfer, G. G., & Malendowicz, L. K. (1990). Role of tachykinins in the regulation of the hypothalamo-pituitary-adrenal axis. *Peptides, 19,* 949–968.

Owan, I., & Ibaraki, K. (1994). The role of calcitonin gene-related peptide (CGRP) in macrophages: The presence of functional receptors and effects on proliferation and differentiation into osteoclast-like cells. *Bone and Mineral, 24,* 151–164.

Paige, C. J., Kincade, P. W., & Ralph, P. (1978). Murine B cell leukemia line with inducible surface immunoglobulin expression. *Journal of Immunology, 121,* 641–647.

Payan, D. G. (1992). The role of neuropeptides in inflammation. In J. I. Gallin, I. M. Goldstein, & R. Snydermann (Eds.), *Inflammation: Basic principles and clinical correlates* (2nd ed., pp. 177–192). New York: Raven Press.

Payan, D. G., Brewster, D. R., & Goetzl, E. J. (1983). Specific stimulation of human T lymphocytes by substance P. *Journal of Immunology, 131,* 1613–1615.

Payan, D. G., Brewster, D. R., & Goetzl, E. J. (1984). Stereospecific receptors for substance P on cultured human IM-9 lymphoblasts. *Journal of Immunology, 133,* 3260–3265.

Payan, D. G., Brewster, D. R., Nissirian-Bastian, A., & Goetzl, E. J. (1984). Subtance P recognition by a subset of human T lymphocytes. *Journal of Clinical Investigation, 74,* 1532–1539.

Payan, D. G., McGillis, J. P., & Organist, M. L. (1986). Binding characteristics and affinity labeling of protein constituents of the human IM-9 lymphoblast receptor for substance P. *Journal of Biological Chemistry, 261,* 14321–14329.

Pereira da Silva, J. A., & Carmo-Fonseca, M. (1990). Peptide containing nerves in human synovium: Immunohistochemical evidence for decreased innervation in rheumatoid arthritis. *Journal of Rheumatology, 17,* 1592–1599.

Pernow, B. (1983). Substance P. *Pharmacological Reviews, 5,* 85–141.

Popper, P., Mantyh, C. R., Vigna, S. R., Maggio, J. E., & Mantyh, P. W. (1988). The localization of sensory nerve fibers and receptor binding sites for sensory neuropeptides in canine mesenteric lymph nodes. *Peptides, 9,* 257–267.

Popper, P., & Micevych, P. E. (1989). Localization of calcitonin gene-related peptide and its receptors in a striated muscle. *Brain Research, 496,* 180–186.

Preibisz, J. J. (1993). Calcitonin gene-related peptide and regulation of human cardiovascular homeostasis. *American Journal of Hypertension.*

Quartara, L., & Maggi, C. A. (1997). The tachykinin NK1 receptor. Part I: Ligands and mechanisms of cellular activation. *Neuropeptides, 31,* 537–563.

Quinlan, K. L., Song, I. S., Bunnett, N. W., Letran, E., Steinhoff, M., Harten, B., Olerud, J. E., Armstrong, C. A., Wright Caughman, S., & Ansel, J. C. (1998). Neuropeptide regulation of human dermal microvascular endothelial cell ICAM-1 expression and function. *American Journal Physiology, 275,* C1580–C1590.

Quinlan, K. L., Song, I. S., Naik, S. M., Letran, E. L., Olerud, J. E., Bunnett, N. W., Armstrong, C. A., Caughman, S. W., & Ansel, J. C. (1999). VCAM-1 expression on human dermal microvascular endothelial cells is directly and specifically up-regulated by substance P. *Journal of Immunology, 162,* 1656–1661.

Quirion, R., Van Rossum, D., Dumont, Y., St-Piere, S., & Fournier, A. (1992). Characterization of CGRP1 and CGRP2 receptor subtypes. *Annals of the New York Acadamy Sciences, 657,* 88–105.

Rameshwar, P., Ganea, D., & Gascon, P. (1993). In vitro stimulatory effect of substance P on hematopoiesis. *Blood, 81,* 391–398.

Rameshwar, P., Ganea, D., & Gascon, P. (1994). Induction of IL-3 and granulocyte-macrophage colony-stimulating factor by substance P in bone marrow cells is partially mediated through the release of IL-1 and IL-6. *Journal of Immunology, 152*, 4044–4054.

Rameshwar, P., & Gascon, P. (1995). Substance P (SP) mediates production of stem cell factor and interleukin-1 in bone marrow stroma: Potential atuoregulatory role for these cytokines in SP receptor expression and induction. *Blood, 86*, 482–490.

Rameshwar, P., & Gascon, P. (1996). Induction of negative hematopoietic regulators by neurokinin-A in bone marrow stroma. *Blood, 88*, 98–106.

Regoli, D., Boudon, A., & Fauchere, J. L. (1994). Receptors and antagonists for substance P and related peptides. *Pharmacology Reviews, 46*, 551–599.

Richter, J., Andersson, R., Edvinsson, L., & Gullberg, U. (1992). Calcitonin gene-related peptide (CGRP) activates human neutrophils—inhibition by chemotactic paptide antagonist BOC-MLP. *Immunology, 77*, 416–421.

Rodrigo, J., Polak, J. M., Fernandez, L., Ghatei, M. A., Mulderry, P., & Bloom, S. R. (1985). Calcitonin gene-related peptide immunoreactive sensory and motor nerves of the rat, cat, and monkey esophagus. *Gastroenterology, 88*, 444–451.

Sagan, S., Chassaing, G., Pradier, L., & Lavielle, S. (1996). Tachykinin peptides affect differently the second messenger pathways after binding to CHO-expressed human NK-1 receptors. *Journal of Pharmacology and Experimental Therapeutics, 276*, 1039–1048.

Seifert, H., Chesnut, J., De Souza, E., Rivier, J., & Vale, W. (1985). Binding sites for calcitonin gene-related peptide in distinct areas of rat brain. *Brain Research, 346*, 195–198.

Seifert, H., Sawchenko, P., Chesnut, J., Rivier, J., Vale, W., & Pandol, S. J. (1985). Receptor for calcitonin gene-related peptide: Binding to exocrine pancreas mediates biological actions. *American Journal of Physiology, 249*, G147–G151.

Serra, M. C., Calzetti, F., Ceska, M., & Cassatella, M. A. (1994). Effect of substance P on superoxide anion and IL-8 production by human PMNL. *Immunology, 82*, 63–69.

Sexton, P. M., McKenzie, J. S., Mason, R. T., Moseley, J. M., Martin, T. J., & Mendelsohn, F. A. O. (1986). Localization of binding sites for calcitonin gene-related peptide in rat brain by in vitro autoradiography. *Neuroscience, 19*, 1235–1245.

Sexton, P. M., McKenzie, J. S., & Mendelsohn, F. A. O. (1988). Evidence for a new subclass of calcitonin/calcitonin gene-related peptide binding site in rat brain. *Neurochemistry International, 12*, 323–335.

Shigemoto, R., Yokota, Y., Tsuchida, K., & Nakanishi, S. (1990). Cloning and expression of a rat neuromedin K receptor cDNA. *Journal of Biological Chemistry, 265*, 623–628.

Sigrist, S., Franco-Cereceda, A., Muff, R., Henke, H., Lundberg, J. M., & Fischer, J. A. (1986). Specific receptor and cardiovascular effects of calcitonin gene-related petide. *Endocrinology, 119*, 381–389.

Smith, C. H., Barker, J. N., Morris, R. W., MacDonald, D. M., & Lee, T. H. (1993). Neuropeptides induce rapid expression of endothelial cell adhesion molecules and elicit granulocytic infiltration in human skin. *Journal of Immunology, 151*, 3274–3282.

Stanisz, A. M., Befus, D., & Bienenstock, J. (1986). Differental effects of vasoactive intestinal peptide, subtance P, and somatostatin on immunoglobulin synthesis and proliferation by lymphocytes from Peyer's patches, mesenteric lymph nodes, and spleen. *Journal of Immunology, 136*, 152–156.

Stanisz, A. M., Schiccitano, R., Dazin, P., Bienenstock, J., & Payan, D. G. (1987). Distribution of subtance P receptors on murine spleen and Peyer's patch T and B cells. *Journal of Immunology, 139*, 749–754.

Tache,Y., Holzer, P., & Rosenfeld, M. G. (Eds.) (1992). *Calcitonin gene-related peptide, the first decade of a novel pleiotropic neuropeptide.* (1992) New York: New York Academy of Sciences.

Takahashi, M., Ikeda, U., Masuyama, J., Funayama , H., Kano, S., & Shimada, K. (1996). Substance P selectively activates TNF-alpha gene expression in murine mast cells. *Cytokine, 8*, 817–821.

Tang, Y., Feng, Y., & Wang, X. (1997). Calcitonin gene-related peptide potentiates LPS-induced IL-6 release from mouse peritoneal macrophages. *Journal of Neuroimmunology, 84*, 207–212.

Tang, Y., Han, C., & Wang, X. (1999). Role of nitric oxide and prostaglandins in the potentiating effects of calcitonin gene-related peptide on lipopolysaccharide-induced interleukin-6 release from mouse peritoneal macrophages. *Immunology, 96*, 171–175.

Taylor, A. W., Yee, D. G., & Streilein, J. W. (1998). Suppression of nitric oxide generated by inflammatory macrophages by calcitonin gene-related peptide in aqueous humor. *Investigative Ophthalmology, 39*, 1372–1378.

Torii, H., Hosoi, J., Beissert, S., Xu, S., Fox, F. E., Asahina, A., Takashima, A., Rook, A. H., & Granstein, R. D. (1997). Regulation of cytokine expression in macrophages and the Langerhans cell-like line XS52 by calcitonin gene-related peptide. *Journal of Leukocyte Biology, 61*, 216–223.

Tschopp, F. A., Henke, H., Petermann, J. B., Tobler, P. H., Janzer, R., Hokfelt, T., Lundberg, J. M., Cuello, C., & Fisher, J. A. (1985). Calcitonin gene-related peptide and its binding sites in the human central nervous system and pituitary. *Proceedings of the National Acadamy of Sciences USA, 82*, 248–252.

Ullman, K., Northrop, J. P., Vereiji, C. L., & Crabtree, G. R. (1990). Transmission of signals from the T-lymphocyte antigen receptor to the genes responsible for cell proliferation and immune function: The missing link. *Annual Review of Immunology, 8*, 421–452.

Umeda, Y., Takamiya, M., Yoshizaki, H., & Arisawa, M. (1988). Inhibition of mitogen-stimulated T lymphocyte proliferation by calcitonin gene-related petide. *Biochemical and Biophysical Research Communications, 154*, 227–235.

Vignery, A., Wang, F., & Ganz, M. B. (1991). Macrophages express functional receptors for calcitonin-gene-related peptide. *J. Cell. Physiol., 149*, 301–306.

Von Euler, V. S., & Gaddum, J. H. (1931). An unidentified depressor substance in certain tissue extracts. *Journal of Physiology, 72*, 577–593.

Wang, F., Millet, I., Bottomly, K., & Vignery, A. (1992). Calcitonin gene-related peptide inhibits interleukin 2 production by murine T lymphocytes. *Journal of Biological Chemistry, 267*, 21052–21057.

Weihe, E., Muller, S., Fink, T., & Zentel, H. J. (1989). Tachykinins, calcitonin gene-related peptide and neuropeptide Y in nerves of the mammalian thymus: Interactions with mast cells in autonomic and sensory neuroimmunomodulation. *Neuroscience Letters, 100*, 77–82.

Yokata, Y., Sasai, Y., Tanaka, K., Fujiwara, T., Tsuchida, K., Shigemoto, R., Kakizuka, A., Ohkubo, H., & Nakanishi, S. (1990). Molecular characterization of a functional cDNA for rat substance P receptor. *Journal of Biological Chemistry, 264*, 17649–17652.

Yokota, Y., Akazawa, C., Ohkubo, H., & Nakanishi, S. (1992). Delineation of structural domains involved in the subtype specificity of tachykinin receptors through chimeric formation of substance P/substance K receptors. *EMBO Journal, 11*, 3585–3591.

Zimmerman, B. J., Anderson, D. C., & Granger, D. N. (1992). Neuropeptides promote neutrophil adherence to endothelial cell monolayers. *American Journal of Physiology, 263*, G678–G682.

CHAPTER

7

Neural Influences on Cell Adhesion Molecules and Lymphocyte Trafficking

SONIA L. CARLSON

I. INTRODUCTION

Leukocyte migration between lymphoid tissues and inflammatory sites is essential for the process of immune surveillance and for ensuring the cell-cell interactions that are necessary for generating an effective immune response. Over the past decade, much has been learned of the mechanisms that are used by the immune system to specifically direct cells to the appropriate sites. It is now known that the process of lymphocyte homing to lymphoid tissue or inflammatory sites is a dynamic process where the production of proinflammatory substances and the expression of adhesion molecules play a major role in regulating what cells enter the site, as well as the time course over which they enter. It is also now recognized that in addition to the classic immune mediators that regulate leukocyte homing and migration, products of the nervous system also are able to be powerful modulators. Thus, this chapter will explore the role of the peripheral nervous system in directly modulating leukocyte migration and homing. In particular, it will focus on the neurotransmitters released by the sympathetic and sensory nerves that have been shown to affect the influx or retention of lymphoid cells in lymphoid tissues and sites of inflammation.

A. Leukocyte Migration to Lymphoid Tissues

Leukocytes from the blood enter lymph nodes and other secondary lymphoid tissues at postcapillary venules where the endothelial cells are specialized into high endothelial cells (high endothelial venules, HEVs). These endothelial cells have a more cuboidal morphology than typical endothelial cells, and also express adhesion molecules that help to direct lymphocyte extravasation at this site. HEVs are particularly located in the medullary region of lymph nodes. In studies monitoring the in vivo migration of fluorescently-labeled lymphocytes, we have noted that the labeled cells rapidly adhere to the HEV and appear lined up within HEVs (Carlson, Fox, & Abell, 1997). Subsequently, the cells migrate into appropriate compartments in the cortex. Lymphocyte migration, particularly of memory cells, shows tissue specificity that is dependent on the adhesion molecules, or homing receptors, expressed by the lymphocytes

(Jutila, 1994). Migration into the spleen appears to be under a slightly different mechanism since this tissue does not have the typical HEVs found in other lymphoid tissues and is not dependent on L-selectin interactions (Mackay, 1995; Mackay & Imhof, 1993; Pabst & Binns, 1989). Lymphocytes first enter the spleen at the marginal zone and flow into the red pulp (Carlson et al., 1997). Subsequently, these cells cross the marginal zone to enter appropriate T and B-cell compartments within the white pulp. Lyons and colleagues (Lyons & Parish, 1995) have shown that marginal zone macrophages are involved in regulating the migration of lymphocytes from the red pulp into the white pulp. The migration of lymphocytes and macrophages to specific compartments within the lymphoid tissues is critical for ensuring efficient antigen presentation and stimulation of lymphocytes such that an appropriate immune response is generated.

B. Leukocyte Interactions with Endothelial Cells and Migration to Inflammatory Sites

The patterns and mechanisms for leukocyte adhesion to endothelial cells and subsequent migration in tissues have been characterized extensively in the last decade and have been the subject of numerous detailed reviews (Dunon, Piali, & Imhof, 1996; Imhof & Dunon, 1997; Jutila, 1994). The initial step leading to leukocyte extravasation from the blood is the interaction of selectin adhesion molecules expressed by leukocytes and endothelial cells (Figure 1). Selectins promote the initial low-affinity adhesion of leukocytes to the endothelial cell surface, which results in the leukocytes rolling along the endothelial cell layer because of the sheer force of the flowing blood. Subsequently, signaling associated with adhesion molecule interactions and with stimulation from chemoattractants present at the site causes activation of the integrin adhesion molecules on leukocytes that stops the rolling and promotes firm adhesion to immunoglobulin superfamily adhesion molecules on endothelial cells. Firm adhesion is achieved with the interaction of the integrin/adhesion molecule pairs including LFA-1/ICAM-1, LFA-1/ICAM-2, VLA-4/VCAM-1, and Mac-1/ICAM-1. These interactions lead to the subsequent process of diapedesis in which the leukocytes migrate between endothelial cells to enter the tissue. The entire process of rolling-adhesion-diapedesis occurs within a few minutes. Adhesion molecules are chronically expressed by HEV of the secondary lymphoid tissues, but are induced on endothelial cells at inflammatory sites, thus targeting leukocyte migration to particular sites. At inflammatory sites, adhesion molecule expression is rapidly induced by proinflammatory cytokines such as interleukin-1, tumor necrosis factor alpha, and gamma interferon. Some selectins, such as P-selectin, can be expressed within minutes from intracellular pools. The enhanced expression of other adhesion molecules such as ICAM-1 and VLA-4 can occur within a few hours. Thus, site directed migration of the various leukocyte subsets can occur rapidly in response to an immune stimulus.

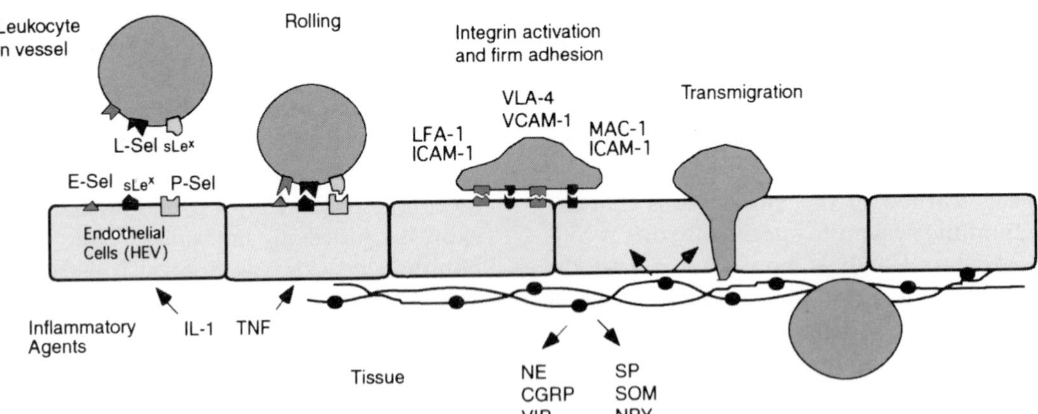

FIGURE 1 Leukocyte adhesion to endothelial cells and migration into tissues. Leukocyte adhesion and migration is a multistep process that initially involves (a) leukocyte rolling, (b) stimulation of integrins and firm adhesion, and (c) diapedesis into the tissues. Catecholamines such as norepinephrine (NE) and neuropeptides (calcitonin gene-related peptide [CGRP], substance P [SP], somatostatin [SOM], neuropeptide Y [NPY], vasoactive intestianl peptide [VIP] present in nerve terminals surrounding blood vessels or contained in the tissue parenchyma can modulate this process.

C. Potential for Interactions between the Nervous and Immune Systems

As discussed in other chapters in this volume, there are numerous sites in the body where nerve fibers and the transmitters they release can interact with and influence the behavior of leukocytes. Lymphoid tissues are richly innervated with sympathetic fibers, particularly surrounding blood vessels and in specific tissue compartments (see Felten and Bellinger, this volume). Nerve fibers in lymphoid tissues also contain numerous neuropeptides including substance P, vasoactive intestinal peptide, neuropeptide Y (NPY), and calcitonin gene-related peptide (CGRP). Thus, catecholamines and neuropeptides are in a position to readily influence leukocyte migration into, and efflux from, lymphoid tissues. In addition to localized innervation, the sympathetic nervous system releases catecholamines systemically that can influence leukocytes in a more generalized way. The nervous system also can modulate leukocyte accumulation at inflammatory sites. This could be through the innervation that exists surrounding blood vessels, or through the sensory innervation found in areas such as skin, joints, or tissue parenchyma. As will be discussed, this innervation can modulate the accumulation of leukocytes during an inflammatory response.

II. CATECHOLAMINE MODULATION OF LEUKOCYTE MIGRATION AND ADHESION

A. Catecholamine Effects on Peripheral Blood Leukocytes

Numerous studies have examined the influence of catecholamines on the number of circulating leukocytes present in the blood. Early studies showed that increased systemic catecholamines resulted in increased numbers of leukocytes in peripheral blood, which has been recently been reviewed by Benschop and colleagues (Benschop, Rodriguez-Feuerhahn, & Schedlowski, 1996). These studies have shown that catecholamines stimulate a rapid increase in peripheral blood lymphocytes that is maximal within 30 min (Erickson & Hedfors, 1977; Gader & Cash, 1975; Steel, French, & Aitchison, 1971). Lymphocyte changes return to normal rapidly after catecholamine administration is discontinued. Neutrophils are also increased, but with a time course that is more sustained, with levels remaining elevated at least 4 h (Steel et al., 1971). A difference was found in the potency between epinephrine and norepinephrine; epinephrine stimulates a greater response than norepinephrine (Gader & Cash, 1975).

In the past decade, studies have further characterized the response of leukocyte subsets as identified by antibody staining for specific cell surface markers. Catecholamine administration results in increased numbers of peripheral blood natural killer (NK) cells and neutrophils (Burns, Keogan, Donaldson, Brown, & Park, 1997; Kappel, Poulsen, Galbo, & Pedersen, 1998; Schedlowski et al., 1993), with variable effects found on CD3, CD4, and CD8-positive T cells (Burns et al., 1997; Schedlowski et al., 1993). The increase in NK cell number is also associated with an increase in NK activity (Kappel et al., 1998; Schedlowski et al., 1993). The effects of epinephrine on NK number and cytotoxicity are more sustained than the effects produced by norepinephrine (Schedlowski et al., 1993). Prolonged administration of catecholamines can result in different effects on lymphocyte populations in the blood. Patients with congestive heart failure, which is associated with a chronic elevation of catecholamines, or volunteers administered a β-adrenergic agonist for 7 days, have decreased numbers of suppressor/cytotoxic T-cells (Ts/c) and NK cells (Maisel et al., 1990). Conversely, withdrawal of sympathetic tone by 7-day administration of a β-adrenergic antagonist results in an increase in T-cells, but no change in other leukocytes, including NK cells (Maisel et al., 1991). Collectively, these studies show that alterations in catecholamine levels, whether acute or chronic, can modulate the number and subset composition of leukocytes present in the peripheral blood.

Physiologically, systemic catecholamine levels can be dramatically altered by events such as stress or dynamic exercise. Vigorous exercise causes a rapid increase in peripheral blood leukocytes, particularly NK cells and $CD8^+$ cells (Baum, Geitner, & Liesen, 1996; Landmann, Portenier, Staehelin, Wesp, & Box, 1988; Maisel et al., 1990; Murray et al., 1992; Strasner et al., 1997). Smaller and more variable effects have been found on the numbers of $CD4^+$ T-cells and B cells (Baum et al., 1996; Hedfors, Holm, Ivansen, & Wahren, 1983; Landmann et al., 1988; Murray et al., 1992). Exercise also can cause elevated numbers of granulocytes and monocytes (Shinkai, Watanabe, Asai, & Shek, 1996). In general, the cell numbers return to normal within 30–60 min after exercise is stopped. Studies using antagonists show that the effect is at least partly dependent on β-adrenergic receptors (Murray et al., 1992). Supporting this, the expression of β-adrenergic receptors is highest on the leukocyte subsets that respond with altered numbers in the blood (Landmann et al., 1988).

A variety of stressors also have been shown to result in rapid and transient increases in NK and Ts/c cells in the blood (Benschop, Brosschot et al., 1994; Brosschot, Nijkamp, Ballieux, & Heijnen, 1992; Hammami, Bouchama, Shail, Aboul-Enein, & Al-Sedairy, 1998; Landmann et al., 1984; Mills et al., 1995; Schedlowski et al., 1993). The effects on $CD4^+$ T-helper (Th) cells and on B cells was again more variable, perhaps related to the intensity or duration of the stressor (Hammami et al., 1998; Landmann et al., 1984; Mills et al., 1995; Schedlowski et al., 1993). Although the cell numbers generally return to normal levels in a short time, cell numbers can actually decrease below basal levels (Schedlowski et al., 1993). Decreases in peripheral T and NK cells are also found with chronic daily life stress (Brosschot et al., 1992). Diurnal variations in catecholamine levels also are associated with changes in the number and proportion of peripheral blood lymphocyte subsets (Infante et al., 1996; Suzuki et al., 1997). Those subsets with the greatest number of β-adrenergic receptors increased with the daily increase in catecholamines, including granulocytes, macrophages, NK cells, $CD8^+$ cells and γ/δ T-cells.

B. Catecholamine Modulation of Leukocyte Trafficking, Adhesion to Endothelial Cells, and Adhesion Molecule Expression

Studies using animals have allowed assessment of the effect of catecholamine changes on tissue as well as blood leukocyte composition. As in human studies, acute stress or β-adrenergic agonist administration results in increased peripheral blood leukocyte and NK cell numbers (Dhabhar & McEwen, 1997; Dhabhar, Miller, McEwen, & Spencer, 1995; Shakhar & Ben-Eliyahu, 1998). With stress, the leukocyte changes are at least in part related to the plasma corticosterone levels (Dhabhar et al., 1995), and the effects on lymphocyte mobilization into the blood become attenuated if the stress is chronic (Dhabhar & McEwen, 1997). Acute catecholamine administration results in an increase in lymphocyte egress from peripheral lymph nodes (Moore, 1984) and spleen (Ernstrom & Sandberg, 1973). Continuous systemic catecholamine administration also stimulates a cell loss in spleen, particularly of NK cells, which appear to move into the general circulation (Murray et al., 1993). Inescapable shock stress was found to particularly alter the T-cell composition of mesenteric lymph nodes, with an increase in the percentage of $CD4^+$ and a decrease in $CD8^+$ cells in these lymph nodes (Fleshner et al., 1992). This in turn was associated with a decrease in antibody production specifically from these tissues.

In vivo studies of lymphocyte homing to lymphoid tissues suggest that catecholamines act to inhibit lymphocyte homing and accumulation in spleen and lymph nodes. We have found that prestimulation of T-cells with catecholamines, which desensitizes the β-adrenergic receptor, results in enhanced migration of these cells to spleen and lymph node during the first 2 h after intravenous infusion of the cells into a host animal (Carlson et al., 1997). Consistent with this hypothesis, Madden and colleagues (Madden, Felten, Felten, Hardy, & Livnat, 1994) have found that lymphocytes show enhanced homing to peripheral lymph nodes after injection into catecholamine-depleted mice compared to intact mice. Conversely, lymphocytes from sympathectomized mice, which are likely to have upregulation of β-adrenergic receptors, do not home as well to lymph nodes of normal mice as controls. Collectively, studies done in vivo suggest that catecholamines tend to decrease retention of lymphocytes in lymphoid tissues. It is likely that effects are most prominently found on specific subsets of cells, which needs to be studied in greater depth in further research.

The increase in peripheral blood leukocytes after catecholamines, stress, or exercise could be from cells released from tissues or from marginated pools of cells bound to endothelial cells. As indicated above, studies in animals have shown that catecholamines can influence the release of leukocytes from the spleen or lymph nodes (Moore, 1984; Murray et al., 1993). In human studies, splenectomized patients had similar changes in blood leukocyte subsets in response to catecholamines or exercise as controls, so the spleen does not appear to be the source of the additional cells (Baum et al., 1996; Schedlowski et al., 1996; Steel et al., 1971). Several studies have examined the hypothesis that catecholamines modulate the adhesion of lymphocytes to endothelial cells. Benschop and colleagues have shown that catecholamines, particularly epinephrine, can inhibit NK cell adhesion to unstimulated endothelial cells and can induce detachment even if the cells have adhered (Benschop, Nijkamp et al., 1994; Benschop, Oostveen, Heijnen, & Ballieux, 1993; Benschop, Schedlowski, Wienecke, Jacobs, & Schmidt, 1997). We have shown that catecholamines also decrease T-cell adhesion to IL-1-activated endothelial cells (Carlson, Beiting, Kiani, Abell, & McGillis, 1996). In all of these studies, the catecholamines must be present during the adhesion assay, as pretreatment of the lymphocytes or endothelial cells is not effective.

To further define the mechanism of catecholamine action, several studies have examined whether catecholamines can modulate adhesion molecules. Catecholamines have not been found to alter the expression of LFA-1, VLA-4, ICAM-1, or VCAM-1 on lymphocytes or endothelial cells (Carlson et al., 1996; Mills, Karnik & Dillon, 1997). In like manner, catecholamine infusion does not alter serum levels of soluble sVCAM-1, sICAM-1, or sE-Selectin (Benschop et al., 1997). Exhaustive exercise, however, is associated with increased sICAM-1, an effect that can be blocked with β-adrenergic antagonists (Rehman et al., 1997). Soluble E-selectin was not altered in this study. Further examination of lymphocyte subsets divided by level of adhesion molecule expression may be helpful in sorting out the catecholamine effects, as Mills and colleagues (1997) found different effects of catecholamines on specific lymphocyte subsets in peripheral blood when the level of L-selectin was taken into account. In general, the above studies on adhesion and adhesion molecule expression suggest that the effect of catecholamines may relate more to modulation of the strength or affinity of adhesion molecule interactions, rather than modulation of the amount of adhesion molecule expression. The data also emphasize that catecholamine effects on leukocytes are not global, but depend on the level of β-adrenergic receptor expression and the specific subsets of leukocytes being examined.

III. NEUROPEPTIDE MODULATION OF LEUKOCYTE ADHESION AND MIGRATION

Numerous neuropeptide neurotransmitters that are associated with lymphoid innervation or with sensory nerves have been shown to modulate leukocyte migration and homing. As opposed to the well-established systemic effects of catecholamines, neuropeptides have predominantly been studied through in vitro adhesion or migration assays, or through migration assays related to specific tissues.

A. CGRP

CGRP is associated with C-type sensory fibers in skin and is also a proinflammatory mediator. In vitro, CGRP can stimulate mononuclear cell migration and chemotaxis (Foster, Mandak, Kromer, & Rot, 1992; Schratzberger et al., 1997). In chemotaxis assays, it is effective for CD4 and CD8-positive T cells, but not B cells (Foster et al., 1992). It also enhances T-cell adhesion to fibronectin, which is a major glycoprotein component of extracellular matrix (Levite, Cahalon, Hershkoviz, Steinman, & Lider, 1998). CGRP has also been shown to potentiate the IL-1 induced extravasation of neutrophils (Ahluwalia & Perretti, 1994) and to enhance the recruitment of Th, Ts/c, and macrophages to the inflamed skin during allergic contact dermatitis (Goebeler, Henseleit, Roth, & Sorg, 1994). The latter effect of CGRP did not involve enhanced expression of ICAM-1 or VCAM-1 by the endothelial cells.

B. NPY

NPY can be found to be colocalized with norepinephrine in sympathetic nerve fibers. As with CGRP, it can increase T-cell adhesion to fibronectin (Levite et al., 1998). NPY appears to be able to act at the level of the endothelial cell to modulate migration because preincubation of endothelial cultures with NPY increases neutrophil adhesion to endothelial cells (Sung, Arleth, & Feuerstein, 1991). The effect is found within 30 min and continues for at least 48 h. This effect was not mediated by a change in endothelial cell ICAM-1 expression, nor did it require new protein synthesis.

C. Secretoneurin

Secretoneurin (SN) is associated with sensory afferent C-fibers. In contrast to most of the other neuropeptides, its effects appear to be predominantly on monocytes and eosinophils. SN can stimulate eosinophil chemotaxis with a potency similar to interleukin-8 (Dunzendorfer, Schratzberger, Reinisch, Kahler & Wiedermann, 1998). Several studies have shown that SN can stimulate chemotactic migration of monocytes (Reinisch et al., 1993; Schratzberger et al., 1997; Schratzberger, Woll, Reinisch, Kahler, & Wiedermann, 1996). In contrast, it does not show chemotactic effects on peripheral blood leukocytes (Schratzberger et al., 1997).

E. Somatostatin

A few studies have examined effects of somatostatin (SOM) on leukocyte chemotaxis and adhesion. SOM can induce chemotaxis of neutrophils and monocytes, but high concentrations are required (Partsch, & Matucci-Cerinic, 1992; Wiedermann, Reinisch, & Braunsteiner, 1993). As seen with some of the other neuropeptides, SOM can decrease the migration of leukocytes toward other chemotactic agents (Pawlikowski, Stepien, Kunert-Radek, Zelazowski, & Schally, 1987; Pawlikowski, Zelazowski, Stepien, &

Schally, 1987; Wiedermann, Reinisch et al., 1993). This effect may be through stimulation of the formation or activity of leukocyte migration inhibiting factor (LMIF). Levite and colleagues (Levite, 1998) showed that SOM, along with CGRP and vasoactive intestinal peptide (VIP), can increase T-cell adhesion to fibronectin, an effect that is blocked by substance P. T-cell adhesion to fibronectin is mediated by the beta-1 integrin.

F. Substance P

Substance P (SP) has been studied more extensively than other neuropeptides in relation to leukocyte trafficking. In numerous studies SP has been shown to alter migration of leukocytes, particularly neutrophils. Neutrophil migration and chemotaxis are stimulated by SP, particularly at high doses (Carolan & Casale, 1993; Jarpe et al., 1998; Nakagawa, Sano, & Iwamoto, 1995; Partsch & Matucci-Cerinic, 1992; Shipp, Stefano, Switzer, Griffin, & Reinherz, 1991; Thomsen, 1991). These effects may in part be due to effects of SP to increase ICAM-1 expression on endothelial cells (Nakagawa et al., 1995) and CD11b/CD18 on neutrophils (Shipp et al., 1991), thus enhancing adhesion and migration. SP also induces shedding of LAM-1 (Shipp et al., 1991). Interactions between SP and the proinflammatory substances IL-1, tumor necrosis factor alpha, and leukotrienes may also be involved in the mechanism of enhanced migration of neutrophils (Perretti, Ahluwalia, Flower, & Manzini, 1993; Saban, Saban, Bjorling, & Haak-Frendscho, 1997). In contrast to these effects, low levels of SP can decrease the chemotactic response of neutrophils to f-MLP or IL-8 (Wiedermann, Kahler, Reinisch, & Wiedermann, 1993). Like effects on neutrophils, SP also has been shown to stimulate chemotaxis of monocytes (Ottaway, 1984; Ruff, Schiffmann, Terranova, & Pert, 1985) and eosinophils (Wiedermann, Kahler et al., 1993).

Several studies have examined the effects of SP on lymphocytes. Heerwagen and colleagues (Heerwagen, Pabst, & Westermann, 1995) found no evidence for SP effects on trafficking of thoracic duct lymphocytes; however, other studies related to specific tissues have found modulatory effects. Stimulation of the sciatic nerve, which stimulates SP release into the footpad, results in increased numbers of T-cells in that tissue (Herzberg, Murtaugh, Mullet & Beitz, 1995). Infusion of SP into afferent lymph results in an initial decrease in $CD4^+$ T-cell release from a peripheral lymph node, with a subsequent large increase after 18 h (Moore, 1984). SP can cause chemotaxis of T and B cells (Schratzberger et al., 1997), and promotes the migration of leukocytes through microvessel walls when applied locally in the tissue (Ohlen, Thureson-Klein, Lindbom, Persson, & Hedqvist, 1989). In contrast, SP can block the effect of the neuropeptides CGRP, NPY and SOM to promote T-cell adhesion to fibronectin (Levite et al., 1998). Overall, the effects of SP on leukocyte adhesion and migration are mediated through the NK-1 receptor (Levite et al., 1998; Perretti et al., 1993; Schratzberger et al., 1997). In general, it appears that SP alone can have stimulatory effects on chemotaxis and migration, but can act to decrease the activity of other mediators that promote chemotaxis or adhesion.

G. VIP

VIP has been shown to modulate the migration and adhesion of lymphocytes and monocytes, but has little effect on neutrophils (Carolan & Casale, 1993; Johnston et al., 1994). Infusion of VIP into the afferent lymph reduces lymphocyte efflux from the lymph node, particularly of $CD4^+$ T-cells (Moore, 1984; Moore, Spruck, & Said, 1988). Studies on in vivo migration suggest that VIP normally enhances T-cell migration to mesenteric lymphoid tissues. Ottaway (1984; 1985) found that prestimulation of T-cells with VIP, which decreases the cellular expression of VIP receptors, reduced the subsequent migration of these cells to Peyer's patches and mesenteric lymph nodes. This was due to a specific reduction in the clearance of these cells from the blood into the mesenteric lymphoid tissues since migration to other lymphoid tissues was not altered. This has been further studied by using intravital fluorescence microscopy to monitor the migration of fluorescently labeled T-cells to Peyer's patches after VIP stimulation of the cells or infusion of VIP (Miura et al., 1997). Although the initial interaction with postcapillary venule endothelial cells was not altered, the subsequent migration of cells into the tissue parenchyma and lymphatics was decreased. In vitro studies have shown that VIP stimulates chemotaxis of CD4 and $CD8^+$ T-cells, monocytes, and B-cells (Johnston et al., 1994; Schratzberger et al., 1997; Xia, Gaufo, Wang, Sreedharan & Goetzl, 1996). This effect of VIP may be mediated by both VIP receptors type I and II, although the ratio of VIPR1 and VIPR2 may be important (Schratzberger et al., 1997; Xia et al., 1996).

IV. CONCLUSION

This chapter has focused on evidence for catecholamines and neuropeptide modulation of leukocyte trafficking and adhesion to endothelial cells. The immune system depends on the interaction of many different cell types to generate an appropriate immune response, thus the migration of these cells to appropriate locations is critical to immune function. Evidence from the literature shows that the nervous system can modulate this trafficking, which in numerous studies has been associated with alterations in immune responses. A more thorough understanding of the effects of the nervous system on leukocyte migration to tissues and inflammatory sites may help to unravel some of the functional data that at times can appear contradictory if the specific cellular subtypes present are not taken into account.

In the past few years knowledge of the mechanisms and signaling involved in leukocyte migration and adhesion has vastly increased. Much more work needs to be done in the area of neuroimmunology to examine potential effects on specific adhesion molecules and their signaling pathways and affinity for adhesion to counter receptors. This review dealt predominantly with direct effects of catecholamines and neuropeptides on lymphocyte adhesion and migration. It is becoming clear, however, that interactions exist between some neurotransmitters and inflammatory cytokines in which they can modulate each other's production. For example, if a neuropeptide stimulates the production and release of a proinflammatory cytokine that can increase adhesion molecule expression or affinity, this in turn will affect leukocyte trafficking to the site. Thus, future studies will need to look in greater depth at the neurotransmitters, cytokines, adhesion molecules, and signaling pathways involved in sorting out the complex neural–immune interactions that take place in lymphoid tissues and at inflammatory sites.

References

Ahluwalia, A., & Perretti, M. (1994). Calcitonin gene-related peptides modulate the acute inflammatory response induced by interleukin-1 in the mouse. *European Journal of Pharmacology, 264*, 407–415.

Baum, M., Geitner, T., & Liesen, H. (1996). The role of the spleen in the leucocytosis of exercise: Consequences for physiology and pathophysiology. *International Journal of Sports Medicine, 17*, 604–607.

Benschop, R. J., Brosschot, J. F., Godaert, G. L., De Smet, M. B., Geenen, R., Olff, M., Heijnen, C. J., & Ballieux, R. E. (1994). Chronic stress affects immunologic but not cardiovascular responsiveness to acute psychological stress in humans. *American Journal of Physiology, 266*(1 Pt 2), R75–R80.

Benschop, R. J., Nijkamp, F. P., Ballieux, R. E., & Heijnen, C. J. (1994). The effects of beta-adrenoceptor stimulation on adhesion of human natural killer cells to cultured endothelium. *British Journal of Pharmacology, 113*, 1311–1316.

Benschop, R. J., Oostveen, F. G., Heijnen, C. J., & Ballieux, R. E. (1993). Beta 2-adrenergic stimulation causes detachment of natural killer cells from cultured endothelium. *European Journal of Immunology, 23*, 3242–3247.

Benschop, R. J., Rodriguez-Feuerhahn, M., & Schedlowski, M. (1996). Catecholamine-induced leukocytosis: Early observations, current research, and future directions. *Brain, Behavior, and Immunity, 10*, 77–91.

Benschop, R. J., Schedlowski, M., Wienecke, H., Jacobs, R., & Schmidt, R. E. (1997). Adrenergic control of natural killer cell circulation and adhesion. *Brain, Behavior, and Immunity, 11*, 321–332.

Brosschot, J. F., Benschop, R. J., Godaert, G. L., de Smet, M. B., Oliff, M., Heijnen, C. J., & Ballieux, R. E. (1992). Effects of experimental psychological stress on distribution and function of peripheral blood cells. *Psychosomatic Medicine, 54*, 394-406.

Burns, A. M., Keogan, M., Donaldson, M., Brown, D. L., & Park, G. R. (1997). Effects of inotropes on human leucocyte numbers, neutrophil function and lymphocyte subtypes. *British Journal of Anaesthesia, 78*, 530–535.

Carlson, S. L., Beiting, D. J., Kiani, C. A., Abell, K. M., & McGillis, J. P. (1996). Catecholamines decrease lymphocyte adhesion to cytokine-activated endothelial cells. *Brain, Behavior, and Immunity, 10*, 55–67.

Carlson, S. L., Fox, S., & Abell, K. M. (1997). Catecholamine modulation of lymphocyte homing to lymphoid tissues. *Brain, Behavior, and Immunity, 11*, 307–320.

Carolan, E. J., & Casale, T. B. (1993). Effects of neuropeptides on neutrophil migration through noncellular and endothelial barriers. *Journal of Allergy and Clinical Immunology, 92*, 589–598.

Dhabhar, F. S., & McEwen, B. S. (1997). Acute stress enhances while chronic stress suppresses cell-mediated immunity in vivo: A potential role for leukocyte trafficking. *Brain, Behavior, and Immunity, 11*, 286–306.

Dhabhar, F. S., Miller, A. H., McEwen, B. S., & Spencer, R. L. (1995). Effects of stress on immune cell distribution. Dynamics and hormonal mechanisms. *Journal of Immunology, 154*, 5511–5527.

Dunon, D., Piali, L., & Imhof, B. A. (1996). To stick or not to stick: The new leukocyte homing paradigm. *Current Opinion in Cell Biology, 8*, 714–723.

Dunzendorfer, S., Schratzberger, P., Reinisch, N., Kahler, C. M., & Wiedermann, C. J. (1998). Secretoneurin, a novel neuropeptide, is a potent chemoattractant for human eosinophils. *Blood, 91*, 1527–1532.

Erickson, B., & Hedfors, E. (1977). The effect of adrenaline, insulin and hydrocortisone on human peripheral blood lymphocytes studied by cell surface markers. *Scandinavian Journal of Haematology, 18*, 121–128.

Ernstrom, U., & Sandberg, G. (1973). Effects of alpha- and beta-receptor stimulation on the release of lymphocytes and granulocytes from the spleen. *Scandinavian Journal of Haematology, 11*, 275–286.

Fleshner, M., Watkins, L. R., Lockwood, L. L., Bellgrau, D., Laudenslager, M. L., & Maier, S. F. (1992). Specific changes in lymphocyte subpopulations: A potential mechanism for stress-induced immunomodulation. *Journal of Neuroimmunology, 41*, 131–142.

Foster, C. A., Mandak, B., Kromer, E., & Rot, A. (1992). Calcitonin gene-related peptide is chemotactic for human T lymphocytes. *Annals of the New York Academy of Sciences, 657*, 397–404.

Gader, A. M. A., & Cash, J. D. (1975). The effect of adrenaline, noradrenaline, isoprenaline and salbutamol on the resting levels of white blood cells in man. *Scandinavian Journal of Haematology, 14*, 5–10.

Goebeler, M., Henseleit, U., Roth, J., & Sorg, C. (1994). Substance P and calcitonin gene-related peptide modulate leukocyte infiltration to mouse skin during allergic contact dermatitis. *Archives of Dermatology Research, 286*, 341–346.

Hammami, M. M., Bouchama, A., Shail, E., Aboul-Enein, H. Y., & Al-Sedairy, S. (1998). Lymphocyte subsets and adhesion molecules expression in heatstroke and heat stress. *Journal of Applied Physiology, 84*, 1615–1621.

Hedfors, E., Holm, G., Ivansen, M., & Wahren, J. (1983). Physiological variation of blood lymphocyte reactivity: T-cell subsets, immunoglobulin production, and mixed-lymphocyte reactivity. *Clinical Immunology and Immunopathology, 27*, 9–14.

Heerwagen, C., Pabst, R., & Westermann, J. (1995). The neuropeptide substance P does not influence the migration of B, T, CD8+ and CD4+ ("naive" and "memory") lymphocytes from blood to lymph in the normal rat. *Scandinavian Journal of Immunology, 42*, 480–486.

Herzberg, U., Murtaugh, M. P., Mullet, M. A., & Beitz, A. J. (1995). Electrical stimulation of the sciatic nerve alters neuropeptide content and lymphocyte migration in the subcutaneous tissue of the rat hind paw. *Neuroreport, 6*, 1773–1777.

Imhof, B. A., & Dunon, D. (1997). Basic mechanism of leukocyte migration. *Hormone and Metabolic Research, 29*, 614–621.

Infante, J. R., Peran, F., Martinez, M., Poyatos, R., Roldan, A., Ruiz, C., & Garrido, F. (1996). Lymphocyte subpopulations and catecholamines; daytime variations and relationships. *Revista Espaniol de Fisiologia, 52*, 143–148.

Jarpe, M. B., Knall, C., Mitchell, F. M., Buhl, A. M., Duzic, E., & Johnson, G. L. (1998). [D-Arg1,D-Phe5,D-Trp7,9,Leu11]Substance P acts as a biased agonist toward neuropeptide and chemokine receptors. *Journal of Biologic Chemistry, 273*, 3097–3104.

Johnston, J. A., Taub, D. D., Lloyd, A. R., Conlon, K., Oppenheim, J. J., & Kevlin, D. J. (1994). Human T lymphocyte chemotaxis and adhesion induced by vasoactive intestinal peptide. *Journal of Immunology, 153*, 1762–1768.

Jutila, M. A. (1994). Function and regulation of leukocyte homing receptors. *Journal of Leukocyte Biology, 55*, 133–140.

Kappel, M., Poulsen, T. D., Galbo, H., & Pedersen, B. K. (1998). Influence of minor increases in plasma catecholamines on natural killer cell activity. *Hormone Research, 49*, 22–26.

Landmann, R., Portenier, M., Staehelin, M., Wesp, M., & Box, R. (1988). Changes in β-adrenoceptors and leucocyte subpopulations after physical exercise in normal subjects. *Archives of Pharmacology, 337*, 261–266.

Landmann, R. M. A., Müller, F. B., Perini, C., Wesp, M., Erne, P., & Bühler, F. R. (1984). Changes of immunoregulatory cells induced by psychological and physical stress: Relationship to plasma catecholamines. *Clinical and Experimental Immunology, 58*, 127–135.

Levite, M., Cahalon, L., Hershkoviz, R., Steinman, L., & Lider, O. (1998). Neuropeptides, via specific receptors, regulate T cell adhesion to fibronectin. *Journal of Immunology, 160*, 993–1000.

Lyons, A. B., & Parish, C. R. (1995). Are murine marginal-zone macrophages the splenic white pulp analog of high endothelial venules. *European Journal of Immunology, 25*, 3165–3172.

Mackay, C. (1995). Lymphocyte migration. A new spin on lymphocyte homing. *Current Biology, 5*, 733–736.

Mackay, C. R., & Imhof, B. A. (1993). Cell adhesion in the immune system. *Immunology Today, 14*, 99–102.

Madden, K. S., Felten, S. Y., Felten, D. L., Hardy, C. A., & Livnat, S. (1994). Sympathetic nervous system modulation of the immune system. II. Induction of lymphocyte proliferation and migration in vivo by chemical sympathectomy. *Journal of Neuroimmunology, 94*, 67–75.

Maisel, A. S., Knowlton, K. U., Fowler, P., Rearden, A., Ziegler, M. G., Motulsky, H. J., Insel, P. A., & Michel, M. C. (1990). Adrenergic control of circulating lymphocyte subpopulations. Effects of congestive heart failure, dynamic exercise, and terbutaline treatment. *Journal of Clinical Investigation, 85*, 462–467.

Maisel, A. S., Murray, D., Lotz, M., Rearden, A., Irwin, M., & Michel, M. C. (1991). Propranolol treatment affects parameters of human immunity. *Immunopharmacology, 22*, 157–164.

Mills, P. J., Berry, C. C., Dimsdale, J. E., Ziegler, M. G., Nelesen, R. A., & Kennedy, B. P. (1995). Lymphocyte subset redistribution in response to acute experimental stress: Effects of gender, ethnicity, hypertension, and the sympathetic nervous system. *Brain, Behavior, and Immunity, 9*, 61–69.

Mills, P. J., Karnik, R. S., & Dillon, E. (1997). L-selectin expression affects T-cell circulation following isoproterenol infusion in humans. *Brain, Behavior, and Immunity, 11*(4), 333–342.

Miura, S., Serizawa, H., Tsuzuki, Y., Kurose, I., Suematsu, M., Higuchi, H., Shigematsu, T., Hokari, R., Hirokawa, M., Kimura, H., & Ishii, H. (1997). Vasoactive intestinal peptide modulates T lymphocyte migration in Peyer's patches of rat small intestine. *American Journal of Physiology, 272*(1 Pt 1), G92–G99.

Moore, T. C. (1984). Modification of lymphocyte traffic by vasoactive neurotransmitter substances. *Immunology, 52*, 511–518.

Moore, T. C., Spruck, C. H., & Said, S. I. (1988). Depression of lymphocyte traffic in sheep by vasoactive intestinal peptide (VIP). *Immunology, 64*, 475–478.

Murray, D. R., Irwin, M., Rearden, A., Ziegler, M., Motulsky, H., & Maisel, A. S. (1992). Sympathetic and immune interactions during dynamic exercise. Mediation via a β2-adrenergic-dependent mechanism. *Circulation, 86*, 203–213.

Murray, D. R., Polizzi, S. M., Harris, T., Wilson, N., Michel, M. C., & Maisel, A. S. (1993). Prolonged isoproterenol treatment alters immunoregulatory cell traffic and function in the rat. *Brain, Behavior, and Immunity, 7*, 47–62.

Nakagawa, N., Sano, H., & Iwamoto, I. (1995). Substance P induces the expression of intercellular adhesion molecule-1 on vascular endothelial cells and enhances neutrophil transendothelial migration. *Peptides, 16*, 721–725.

Ohlen, A., Thureson-Klein, A., Lindbom, L., Persson, M. G., & Hedqvist, P. (1989). Substance P activates leukocytes and platelets in rabbit microvessels. *Blood Vessels, 26*(2), 84–94.

Ottaway, C. A. (1984). In vitro alteration of receptors for vasoactive intestinal peptide changes the in vivo localization of mouse T cells. *Journal of Experimental Medicine, 160*, 1054–1069.

Ottaway, C. A. (1985). Evidence for local neuromodulation of T cell migration in vivo. *Advances in Experimental Medicine and Biology, 186*, 637–645.

Pabst, R., & Binns, R. M. (1989). Heterogeneity of lymphocyte homing physiology: Several mechanisms operate in the control of migration to lymphoid and non-lymphoid organs in vivo. *Immunology Review, 108*, 83–109.

Partsch, G., & Matucci-Cerinic, M. (1992). Effect of substance P and somatostatin on migration of polymorphonuclear (PMN) cells in vitro. *Inflammation, 16*, 539–547.

Pawlikowski, M., Stepien, H., Kunert-Radek, J., Zelazowski, P., & Schally, A. V. (1987). Immunomodulatory action of somatostatin. *Annals of the New York Academy of Sciences, 496*, 233–239.

Pawlikowski, M., Zelazowski, P., Stepien, H., & Schally, A. V. (1987b). Somatostatin and its analog enhance the formation of human leukocyte migration inhibiting factor: Further evidence for immunomodulatory action of somatostatin. *Peptides, 8*, 951–952.

Perretti, M., Ahluwalia, A., Flower, R. J., & Manzini, S. (1993). Endogenous tachykinins play a role in IL-1-induced neutrophil accumulation: Involvement of NK-1 receptors. *Immunology, 80,* 73–77.

Rehman, J., Mills, P. J., Carter, S. M., Chou, J., Thomas, J., & Maisel, A. S. (1997). Dynamic exercise leads to an increase in circulating ICAM-1: Further evidence for adrenergic modulation of cell adhesion. *Brain, Behavior, and Immunity, 11,* 343–351.

Reinisch, N., Kirchmair, R., Kahler, C. M., Hogue-Angeletti, R., Fischer-Colbrie, R., Winkler, H., & Wiedermann, C. J. (1993). Attraction of human monocytes by the neuropeptide secretoneurin. *FEBS Letters, 334,* 41–44.

Ruff, M., Schiffmann, E., Terranova, V., & Pert, C. B. (1985). Neuropeptides are chemoattractants for human tumor cells and monocytes: A possible mechanism for metastasis. *Clinical Immunology and Immunopathology, 37,* 387–396.

Saban, M. R., Saban, R., Bjorling, D., & Haak-Frendscho, M. (1997). Involvement of leukotrienes, TNF-alpha, and the LFA-1/ICAM-1 interaction in substance P-induced granulocyte infiltration. *Journal of Leukocyte Biology, 61,* 445–451.

Schedlowski, M., Falk, A., Rohne, A., Wagner, T. O. F., Jacobs, R., Tewes, U., & Schmidt, R. E. (1993). Catecholamines induce alterations of distribution and activity of human natural killer (NK) cells. *Journal of Clinical Immunology, 13,* 344–351.

Schedlowski, M., Hesch, W., Oberbeck, R., Benschop, R. J., Jacobs, R., Raab, H. R., & Schmidt, R. E. (1996). Catecholamines modulate human NK cell circulation and function via spleen-independent beta 2-adrenergic mechanisms. *Journal of Immunology, 156,* 93–99.

Schratzberger, P., Reinisch, N., Prodinger, W. M., Kahler, C. M., Sitte, B. A., Bellmann, R., Fischer-Colbrie, R., Winkler, H., & Wiedermann, C. J. (1997). Differential chemotactic activities of sensory neuropeptides for human peripheral blood mononuclear cells. *Journal of Immunology, 158,* 3895–3901.

Schratzberger, P., Woll, E., Reinisch, N., Kahler, C. M., & Wiedermann, C. J. (1996). Secretoneurin-induced in vitro chemotaxis of human monocytes is inhibited by pertussis toxin and an inhibitor of protein kinase C. *Neuroscience Letters, 214,* 208–210.

Shakhar, G., & Ben-Eliyahu, S. (1998). In vivo beta-adrenergic stimulation suppresses natural killer activity and compromises resistance to tumor metastasis in rats. *Journal of Immunology, 160,* 3251–3258.

Shinkai, S., Watanabe, S., Asai, H., & Shek, P. N. (1996). Cortisol response to exercise and post-exercise suppression of blood lymphocyte subset counts. *International Journal of Sports Medicine, 17,* 597–603.

Shipp, M. A., Stefano, G. B., Switzer, S. N., Griffin, J. D., & Reinherz, E. L. (1991). CD10 (CALLA)/neutral endopeptidase 24.11 modulates inflammatory peptide-induced changes in neutrophil morphology, migration, and adhesion proteins and is itself regulated by neutrophil activation. *Blood, 78,* 1834–1841.

Steel, C. M., French, E. B., & Aitchison, W. R. C. (1971). Studies on adrenaline-induced leucocytosis in normal man. I. The role of the spleen and of the thoracic duct. *British Journal of Haematology, 21,* 413–421.

Strasner, A., Davis, J. M., Kohut, M. L., Pate, R. R., Ghaffar, A., & Mayer, E. (1997). Effects of exercise intensity on natural killer cell activity in women. *International Journal of Sports Medicine, 18*(1), 56–61.

Sung, C. P., Arleth, A. J., & Feuerstein, G. Z. (1991). Neuropeptide Y upregulates the adhesiveness of human endothelial cells for leukocytes. *Circulation Research, 68*(1), 314–318.

Suzuki, S., Toyabe, S., Moroda, T., Tada, T., Tsukahara, A., Iiai, T., Minagawa, M., Maruyama, S., Hatakeyama, K., Endoh, K., & Abo, T. (1997). Circadian rhythm of leucocytes and lymphocytes subsets and its possible correlation with the function of the autonomic nervous system. *Clinical and Experimental Immunology, 110,* 500–508.

Thomsen, M. K. (1991). Substance P: A neurogenic mediator of acute cellular inflammation in the dog? *Journal of Veterinary Pharmacology and Therapeutics, 14,* 250–256.

Wiedermann, C. J., Reinisch, N., & Braunsteiner, H. (1993). Stimulation of monocyte chemotaxis by human growth hormone and its deactivation by somatostatin. *Blood, 82,* 954–960.

Wiedermann, F. J., Kahler, C. M., Reinisch, N., & Wiedermann, C. J. (1993). Induction of normal human eosinophil migration in vitro by substance P. *Acta Haematolgica, 89,* 213–215.

Xia, M., Gaufo, G. O., Wang, Q., Sreedharan, S. P., & Goetzl, E. J. (1996). Transduction of specific inhibition of HuT 78 human T cell chemotaxis by type I vasoactive intestinal peptide receptors. *Journal of Immunology, 157,* 1132–1138.

CHAPTER

8

Age-Related Alterations in Neural–Immune Interactions and Neural Strategies in Immunosenescence

DENISE L. BELLINGER, KELLEY S. MADDEN, DIANNE LORTON, SRINIVASAN THYAGARAJAN, DAVID L. FELTEN

I. INTRODUCTION

The innervation of lymphoid organs is not static in its response to a changing lymphoid microenvironment (see chapter 2, Innervation of Lymphoid Tissues, in this volume), although nerves usually maintain their compartmentation in specific regions of lymphoid tissue. As an organism ages, there are changes in the structure and cellularity of lymphoid organs, changes in receptor expression and intracellular function of immunocytes, changes in neural structure and function, and overall changes in the capacity of the immune system to mount a response to many specific types of challenges, such as viral infections and tumors.

It is difficult to determine whether neural changes induce immunologic changes, whether an altered immunologic microenvironment induces nerve changes, or whether both process occur simultaneously, the most likely possibility. Work from our laboratories and from other laboratories suggests that the interplay between nerves and the target lymphoid environment is extensive, continuous, and gradually shifts as the organism ages. It is possible that strategies directed toward neural–immune communication and signaling may be useful as tools to forestall immune senescence, and to enhance host defenses as the organism ages. These issues are discussed in depth in this chapter.

II. BURSA OF FABRICIUS

Age-dependent changes in the innervation of the pigeon bursa of Fabricius have been studied using fluorescence histochemistry for localizing catecholamines, and with acetylcholinesterase (AChE) staining (Ciriaco, Ricci, Bronzetti, Mammola, Germana, & Vega, 1995). The density of noradrenergic (NA) and $AChE^{+}$ nerves associated with the vasculature increases from the time of hatching through 30 days of age, when the adult pattern of innervation is achieved. NA nerves form perivascular plexuses in the perimuscular connective tissue, muscle, and mucosa, often in close proximity to autofluorescent cells. Fine linear fibers travel between the lymphoid nodules, but do not enter the nodules. NA fibers are not present in the epithelium. The distribution pattern and the density of NA and AChE$^+$ nerves remains unchanged through postnatal day 75; the density of nerves then progressively increases between 90 and 120 days of age.

Peptidergic innervation of the bursa of Fabricius from young adult birds has been reported, and includes nerve staining for tachykinins such as substance P (SP) and substance K, vasoactive intestinal polypeptide (VIP), galanin, and calcitonin gene-related peptide (CGRP). These peptide-containing nerves are distributed throughout the different bursal compartments, except for the medulla of the bursal follicles, where the early stages of lymphocyte maturation occur (Zentel & Weihe, 1991). The plasticity of these peptidergic nerves in the bursa of Fabricius with age has not been investigated.

III. BONE MARROW

A. Maturation

In young adult rodents, NA and neuropeptide Y (NPY)$^+$ nerves course in small nerve bundles that extend into the bone through the nutrient foramena, along with the vasculature. The majority of NA/NPY$^+$ nerves (Figure 1) form dense plexuses along the vasculature (S. Felten & Felten, 1991; D. Felten, Felten, Carlson, Olschowka, & Livnat, 1985; Tabarowski, Gibson-Berry, & Felten, 1996). From these vascular plexuses, NA/NPY$^+$ nerve fibers course into the surrounding parenchyma among hemopoietic cells in the marrow. AChE$^+$ nerves have been reported in the bone marrow, but have not been confirmed as cholinergic nerves (DePace & Webber, 1975).

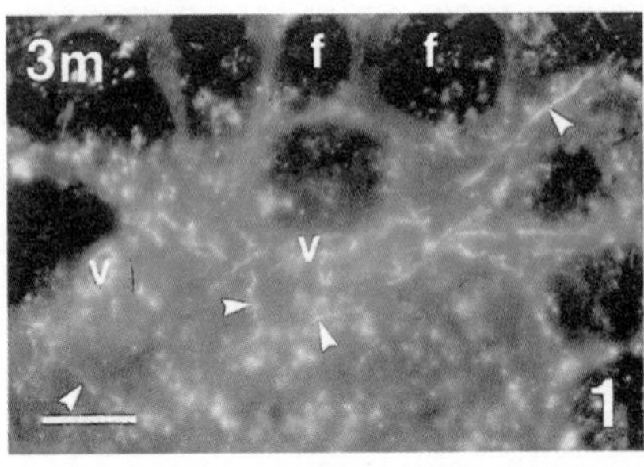

FIGURE 1 Noradrenergic (NA) nerve fibers are present along the vasculature (v) and in the parenchyma (arrowheads) of bone marrow from the 3-month-old (3m) rat femur. Glyoxylic acid-induced histofluorescence (HF) for catecholamines (CAs). X43. Calibration bar = 100 μm.

B. Ontogeny

A few studies examining the ontogeny of nerves into bone marrow have been undertaken in rodents (Calvo & Forteza-Vila, 1969; Calvo & Haas, 1969) and rabbits (Miller & McCuskey, 1973). In the Wistar rat (Calvo & Haas, 1969) and the New Zealand rabbit (Miller & McCuskey, 1973), NA nerves in the bone marrow appear late in fetal life, just prior to the onset of hemopoietic activity (Miller & McCuskey, 1973), suggesting a role of sympathetic innervation of bone marrow in the subsequent development of hematopoiesis. This possible role is strengthened by three-dimensional bone marrow cultures showing catecholamine modulation of hematopoiesis and synergism of growth factors (D. Felten, Gibson-Berry, & Wu, 1996).

C. Senescence

Normal aging results in changes in the morphology of bone marrow. The fat content in the bone marrow increases with advancing age. The proportion of myeloid cells increase, and the proportion of lymphoid cells decrease, notable at the onset of thymic involution (at the time of puberty) (Dominguez-Gerpe & Rey-Mendez, 1998b). A loss in lymphoid cells with advancing age is a consistent finding in both primary and secondary lymphoid organs. Despite the changes in bone marrow histology that occur with normal aging, NA innervation of the bone marrow from 21-month-old Fischer 344 (F344) rats remains intact (Figures 1 and 2). Maintenance of NA sympathetic nerves in primary lymphoid organs appears to be a consistent feature of aging. It is not known whether changes in norepinephrine (NE) metabolism occur in NA nerves in bone marrow of aging animals, or whether altered nerve function or neurotransmitter receptor expression on bone marrow cells contributes to the age-related cellular changes that occur in the bone marrow.

Data from several studies in young adult animals are consistent with a contributory role of NA sympathetic nerves in determining the cellular make-up of the bone marrow. NE and dopamine concentrations in mouse bone marrow display diurnal rhythmicity, peaking at night (Maestroni, Cosentino, Marino, Togni, Conti, Lecchini, & Frigo, 1998), which positively correlates with the G2/M and S phases of the cell cycle (Maestroni et al., 1998; Cosentino, Marino, Bombelli, Ferrari, Maestroni, Conti, Rasini, Lecchini, &

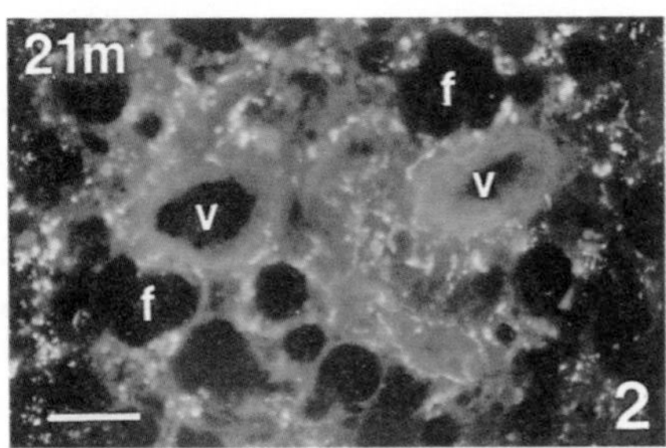

FIGURE 2 With normal aging there is decreased cellularity in the bone marrow and an increase in fat cells (f). Despite these morphological changes the density and distribution of NA sympathetic nerves in the bone marrow from the rat femur at 21 months of age (21m) is similar to that seen at 3 months of age (see Figure 1). NA nerve fibers course along the blood vessels (v) and in the bone marrow parenchyma (arrowheads). Glyoxylic acid-induced HF for CAs. X43. Calibration bar = 100 μm.

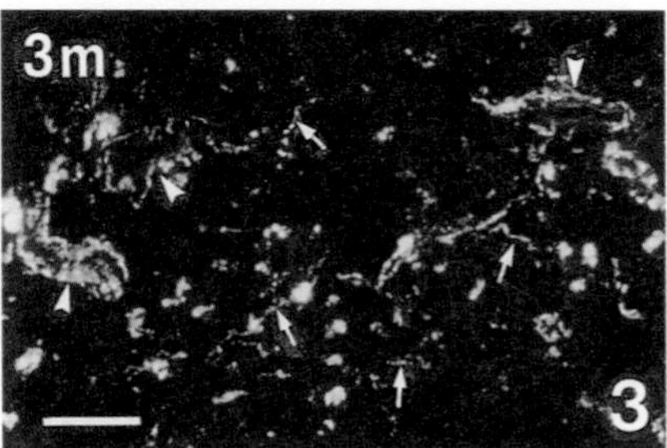

FIGURE 3 In the thymus of a 3-month-old rat (3m), dense vascular plexuses (arrowheads) of NA fibers course in the thymic cortex near the corticomedullary junction. NA nerve fibers also course as free fluorescent profiles (arrows) among cortical thymocytes, stromal cells, and yellow cortical autofluorescent cells. Glyoxylic acid-induced HF for X43. Calibration bar = 100 μm.

Frigo, 1998), suggesting a possible neural association. Further, chemical sympathectomy with 6-hydroxydopamine (6-OHDA), or administration of the α_1-adrenergic antagonist, prazosin, enhances myelopoiesis and inhibits lymphopoiesis (Maestroni & Conti, 1994; Maestroni, Conti, & Pedrinis, 1992). The effects induced by blocking sympathetic neurotransmission, however, are directionally opposite from what would be predicted from the robust density of NA nerves present in old animals, unless age-related defects in NE signal transduction in myeloid and hematopoietic cells are also proposed.

IV. THYMUS

A. Maturation

A variety of neurotransmitter-specific nerves have been demonstrated in the young adult thymus from a variety of species (reviewed in chapter 2, Volume 1, of this book). In young adult rodents, NA fibers enter the thymus with large blood vessels as moderately dense plexuses, and travel in the capsule and interlobular septa, or continue with the vasculature into the cortex (Bellinger, Felten, & Felten, 1988; Bulloch & Pomerantz, 1984; D. Felten et al., 1985; Nance, Hopkins, & Bieger, 1987; Williams & Felten, 1981; Williams, Peterson, Shea, Schmedtje, Bauer, & Felten, 1981). With fluorescence histochemistry for catecholamines, individual NA nerve fibers are seen extending into cortical regions of the rat thymus, where they reside adjacent to thymocytes and cortical yellow autofluorescent cells (CAF cells) (Figure 3). In the septa, NA nerves course in close proximity to mast cells. The most prominent location of NA sympathetic fibers is in the interlobular septa and in the cortex, with a high density near the corticomedullary junction. At the corticomedullary junction, NA nerves associate with the medullary sinuses, which are continuous with the system of vessels in the septa; some nerve fibers extend from these plexuses into the surrounding parenchyma. Neurochemical studies indicate that catecholamine innervation of the thymus is virtually all NA.

Immunohistochemical studies have demonstrated thymic nerves that utilize a variety of neuropeptides, including NPY, tachykinins (SP, neurokinin A and neurokinin B, collectively), SP, CGRP, and VIP (Bellinger, Lorton, Romano, Olschowka, Felten, & Felten, 1990; D. Felten & Felten, 1989; S. Felten & Felten, 1991; D. Felten et al., 1985; Geppetti, Frilli, Renzi, Santicioli, Maggi, Theodorsson, & Fanciulacci, 1988; Geppetti, Maggi, Zecchi-Orlandini, Santicioli, Meli, Frilli, Spillantini, & Amenta, 1987; Lorton, Bellinger, Felten, & Felten, 1990a; Romano, Felten, Olschowka, & Felten, 1994; Sergeeva, 1974; Weihe, Müller, Fink, & Zentel, 1989). The distribution of NPY^+ nerves in the rat thymus overlaps with the pattern of nerves expressing tyrosine hydroxylase (TH, the rate-limiting enzyme in the synthesis of NE); similarly, SP^+ and $CGRP^+$ have overlapping distributions. $SP^+/CGRP^+$ nerves occur in the capsule and septal system, and less frequently in the cortical regions. In the rodent thymus, VIP^+ fibers are present in the capsule, interlobular septa, in the cortex, and along blood vessels at the corticomedullary junction and in the medulla (Bellinger, Lorton, Horn, Felten, & Felten, 1997; Müller & Weihe, 1991).

B. Ontogeny

The development of NA sympathetic innervation of the thymus occurs mainly postnatally (Ackerman,

1989; Ackerman, Bellinger, S. Felten, & D. Felten, 1991; Kranz, Kendall, & von Gaudecker, 1997). Fluorescence histochemical studies reveal NA sympathetic nerves in the rodent thymus by day 17 to 18 of gestation (full term is 20 to 21 days) (Bulloch, Cullen, Schwartz, & Longo, 1987; Singh, 1984). At this time point, only a few NA fibers can be found in the cortex and along arterioles at the corticomedullary junction. In thymus from 1-day-old F344 rat pups, the density of NA nerves is sparse, and the intensity of the fluorescence is dull compared with the innervation of the adult thymus (Ackerman, 1989; Ackerman, Bellinger, S. Felten, & D. Felten, 1991). Most of the NA nerve fibers in 1-day-old pups course in nerve bundles traveling in the capsule and interlobular septa, which extends to the boundary of the corticomedullary junction. Only a few nerve profiles can be found in the cortex adjacent to the capsule, whereas at the corticomedullary junction, relatively dense plexuses of fine fibers associate with medium-sized arteries. Some NA nerve fibers extend from these vascular plexuses a short distance into the surrounding parenchyma.

The thymus rapidly increases in size through day 7, and becomes divided into lobules by the septal system (Ackerman, 1989; Ackerman, Bellinger et al., 1991). At this stage of development, NA nerves form a much denser plexus in the interlobular septa than is seen in newborn rats. Also there is an increase in the density of NA nerves traveling along arteries in the septa and along their branches that extend deep into the cortex by postnatal day 7. Fluorescent nerve fibers arborize in the cortical parenchyma among thymocytes. It is common to find NA fibers in close proximity to CAF cells that are scattered throughout the cortex. In the adult thymus, CAF cells form a zone near the corticomedullary boundary, an area that receives the greatest density of NA nerves. The phenotype and function of CAF cells has not been elucidated. By day 7, the large venous sinuses in the medulla also are innervated.

Between 7 and 14 days, there is an increase in both the density and intensity of NA nerves associated with the vasculature (Ackerman, 1989; Ackerman, Bellinger et al., 1991). Septal arteries and penetrating arteries of the thymus are surrounded by a dense, tangled plexus of varicose fibers, similar to that seen in the adult. Individual NA nerve fibers exit these plexuses deep in the cortex, forming close associations with thymocytes and CAF cells. Similarly, the adult pattern of NA innervation of the venous sinuses and septal systems are realized by day 14. Consistent with the adult distribution and density of fibers at day 14, thymic NE content reaches adult concentrations.

NA nerves associated with the septa, cortical arterioles, sinuses, and capsule continue to keep pace with the rapid growth of the thymus from 14 to 56 days of age (Ackerman, 1989; Ackerman, Bellinger et al., 1991). The predominant feature at this time point is in the organization of the corticomedullary junction. CAF cells now form a concentrated zone of cells in this region of the thymus, accompanied by a dense plexus of NA nerves, either associated with blood vessels in the corticomedullary junction or as free nerve fibers. In contrast, NA nerve fibers in the medulla predominate along the arteries and sinuses with few parenchymal fibers.

Receptor bindings studies indicate that unfractionated thymocytes express very low levels of β-adrenoceptors, and that β-adrenoceptor expression appears to increase with thymocyte maturation (Fuchs, Albright, & Albright, 1988; Radojcic, Baird, Darko, Smith, & Bulloch, 1991). Enriched populations of thymocytes (cortisone-resistant or peanut nonagglutinating thymocytes) express equivalent numbers of β-adrenoceptors as mature T lymphocytes in the periphery (Fuchs et al., 1988). In vitro autoradiographic studies by Marchetti and co-workers (Marchetti, Morale, & Pelletier, 1990) have revealed β-adrenoceptors present predominantly in the medulla of the rat thymus, a site that receives fewer fibers compared with the cortex. Stromal elements of the thymus, which include epithelial cells, macrophages, and dendritic cells, may express α- or β-adrenoceptors, and are possible targets of NA innervation.

These studies suggest that NE is available to interact with thymocytes early in ontogeny. During early development of the thymus, NA innervation may modulate several important functions, such as promoting the entry of thymic stem cells into the thymus, and/or regulating proliferation and differentiation of thymocytes. Singh and colleagues have provided evidence that catecholamines can influence proliferation and differentiation of thymocytes in culture (Singh, 1979a, 1979b, 1984, 1985; Singh & Owen, 1976). NE also may influence thymocyte entry into the organ, either directly through an interaction with adrenoceptors on thymocytes, or indirectly by influencing thymic stromal cells, thymocyte chemotaxis and/or migration, and regulating blood flow through the thymus.

Wiedmeier et al. (Wiedmeier, Burnham, Singh, & Daynes, 1987) examined the role of NA sympathetic nerves in T lymphocyte ontogeny from thymic epithelial grafts into the anterior chamber of the eye. They found that deoxyguanosine-treated thymic epithelial grafts implanted into the anterior chamber of the eye are receptive to host lymphoid progenitor cells. Further, thymic epithelial grafts are capable of supporting T lymphocyte maturational processes, and are able to export mature T cells to the secondary lymphoid organs of a previously deficient host. In addition, intact NA sympathetic innervation of the anterior chamber reduced the number of lymphoid cells recovered from thymic epithelial grafts compared with grafts from a sympathetically denervated anterior chamber. This finding further supports a role for sympathetic nerves in proliferation and differentiation of thymocytes. At later stages in development, NA innervation may modulate maturation and emigration of thymocytes for the seeding of secondary lymphoid organs.

C. Senescence

In humans and experimental animals, the thymus reaches its maximum size at sexual maturation, and then begins to atrophy shortly after puberty. Histologically, involution of the thymus is represented by a progressive shrinking of the thymic cortex that results from a loss of thymocytes, the appearance of Hassal's corpuscles, and an infiltration of fat. This normal degenerative process continues into old age (Bellinger et al., 1988; Boyd, 1932). Thymic involution occurs in parallel with a decline in thymic hormone secretion, which appears to be regulated by the hypothalamus (Hall, O'Grady, & Farah, 1991). Neuropeptide innervation of the aged thymus has not been extensively investigated; only a short report describing CGRP-containing nerves in thymuses from old mice is available (Bulloch, Hausman, Radojcic, & Short, 1991).

Age-related changes in NA sympathetic innervation of the murine and rat thymus have been investigated by our laboratories (Bellinger et al., 1988; Madden et al., 1997). The distribution and density of NA innervation of the thymus of 3-month-old rats (Figure 3) (Bellinger et al., 1988) is consistent with earlier studies in young adult rodents, as described above (Bulloch & Pomerantz, 1984; D. Felten et al., 1985; S. Felten, Felten, Bellinger, Carlson, Ackerman, Madden, Olschowka, & Livnat, 1988; Nance et al., 1987; Sergeeva, 1974; Williams & Felten, 1981; Williams et al., 1981). By 8 months of age, thymic involution is apparent, notable by a decline in thymic weight of approximately 35%. Fluorescence histochemistry for catecholamines demonstrates intact NA innervation of the thymus from 8-month-old animals (Figure 4). The most remarkable feature at this age is an increase in the density of NA sympathetic nerves in the thymic cortex and paracortex. NA fibers in these regions commonly appear as linear and punctate profiles in these regions, in addition to their association with the vasculature. NA fibers in the thymic parenchyma of the inner cortex form close associations with CAF cells at the corticomedullary junction with increasing frequency compared with that seen at 3 months of age.

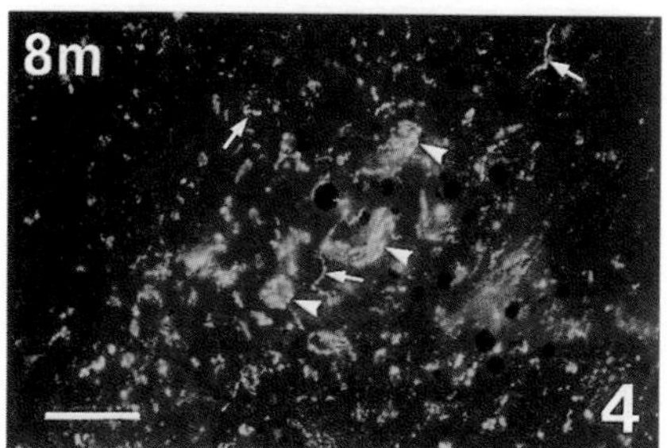

FIGURE 4 At 8 months of age (8m), the rat thymus as an abundance of periarteriolar NA plexuses (arrowheads) and individual fibers (arrows) in the cortex. At this age, NA innervation appears to be more robust compared with the density of innervation of the thymus from 3-month-old rats (see Figure 3). Glyoxylic acid-induced HF for CAs. X85. Calibration bar = 100 μm.

Between 8 and 27 months of age the density of NA nerve fibers in all compartments of the thymus progressively increases as the thymus continues to involute (Figures 4–6) (Bellinger et al., 1988). NA innervation is especially dense in the cortex and at the corticomedullary junction of the aged thymus. In this region, the NA nerves form plexuses that are denser than those noted anywhere else in the body, with the possible exception of the vas deferens. Dense tangles of NA nerve fibers engulf the vasculature and course as free fibers through the parenchyma of the cortex and paracortex (Figure 6). Free fibers often form long longitudinal arrays oriented parallel to the long axis of the thymic surface. Corresponding to the increase in NA nerve fiber density, there are more CAF cells in the thymus, not just at the corticomedullary junction, but also throughout the cortex (Figures 4–6). The density of NA nerves in the medulla is not as markedly altered with advancing age, making the boundary between the cortex and medulla much more distinct than in

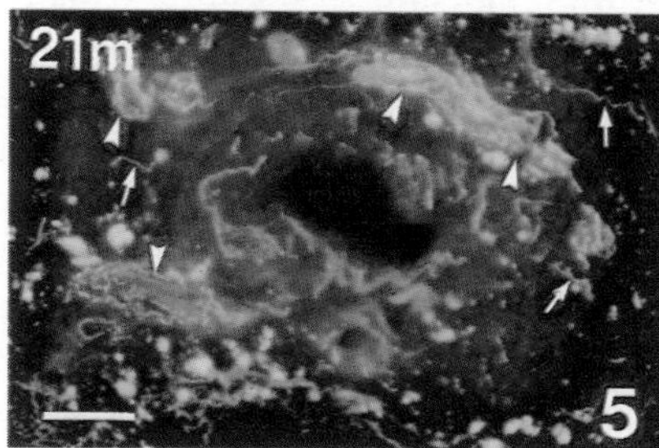

FIGURE 5 In 21-month-old (21m) rats, NA nerve fibers form dense vascular plexuses (arrowheads). Abundant NA nerve fibers (arrows) course as individual fibers among thymocytes, CAF cells, and stromal cells in the thymic cortex. Glyoxylic acid-induced HF for CAs. X85. Calibration bar = 100 μm.

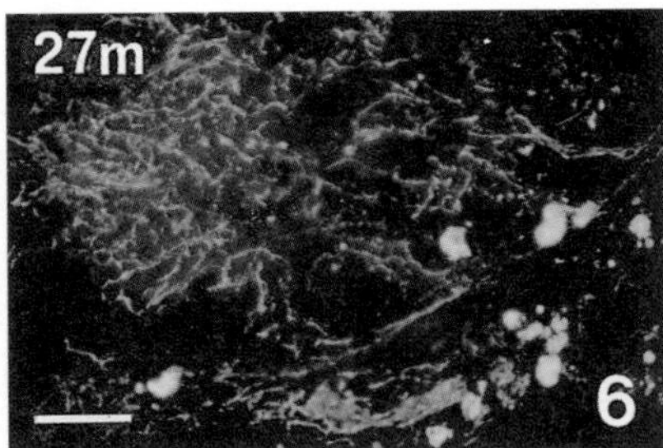

FIGURE 6 By 27 months of age (27m), A dense tangle of NA fibers associated with the vasculature, and parallel arrays of linear parenchymal fibers are present in the involuted thymus. NA nerves frequently reside in close proximity to CAF cells. Glyoxylic acid-induced HF for CAs. X85. Calibration bar = 100 μm.

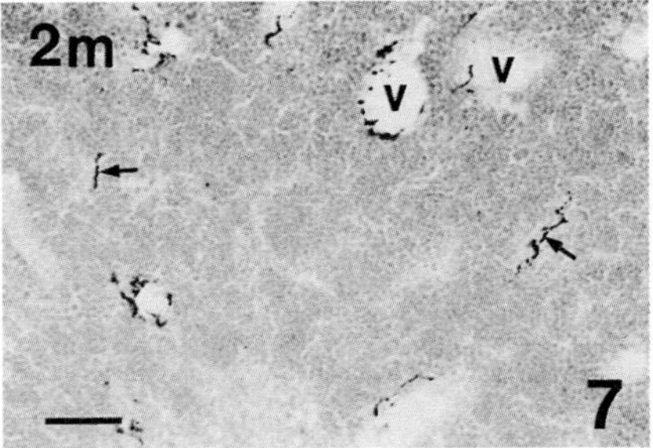

FIGURE 7 TH^+ nerve fibers travel along blood vessel (v) and as individual linear fibers in the parenchyma of the thymic cortex (arrows) in a 2-month-old (2m) BALB/c mouse. Single-label immunocytochemistry (ICC) for TH counterstained with thionin. X43. Calibration bar = 200 μm.

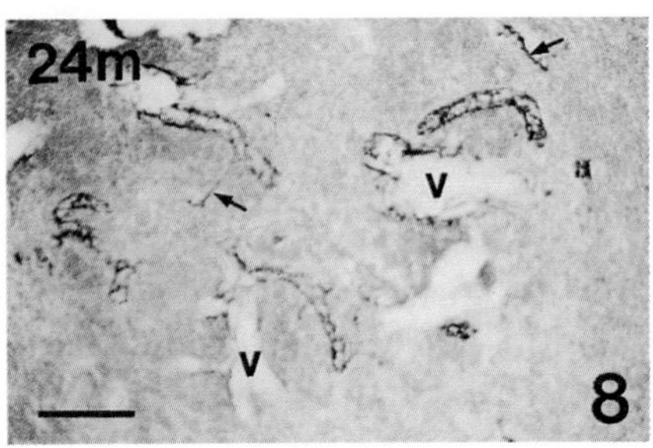

FIGURE 8 By 24 months of age (21m), TH^+ nerve fibers have a similar distribution in the involuted thymus, but the density of nerves in these compartments in significantly increased. Dense vascular plexuses of TH^+ nerve fibers are present in the cortex. TH^+ nerve fibers (arrows) exit these plexuses and course in the surrounding parenchyma. v, blood vessels. Single-label ICC for TH counterstained with thionin. X43. Calibration bar = 200 μm.

younger animals. It is noteworthy that in some cortical regions, where only minimal cortex remains and a few CAF cells are present, NA innervation also is lost. It is tempting to hypothesize from this observation that a critical threshold of thymic cells must be present to maintain NA nerves in the cortex, and when thymic cell density drops below that threshold, the nerves degenerate.

Neurochemical data also indicate that NA innervation increases in density with age because the full complement of nerve fibers is maintained in the increasingly diminishing thymic cortex as it involutes (Bellinger et al., 1988). NE content per whole thymus is relatively stable throughout the life span, whereas thymic NE concentration per milligram wet weight shows a progressive increase from 3 to 17 months of age with a small decline to a second plateau from 21 to 27 months of age. Based on hematoxylin and eosin staining, an increase in wet weight occurs over this time period, in which we attribute the decline in NE concentration between 21 and 27 months to infiltration of fat into thymus that is not as well innervated as the remaining thymic tissue.

Recently, we have extended this work to examine alterations in NA sympathetic innervation of the thymus from 2-, 12-, and 24-month-old male BALB/c mice using fluorescence histochemistry for catecholamines and immunocytochemistry for TH (Figures 7 and 8) (Madden et al., 1997). Findings from this study are in agreement with those in the rat. With advancing age and thymic involution, NA nerves increase in density (Figures 7 and 8). By 24 months of age, dense plexuses occur among septa and blood vessels, and numerous linear, varicose nerves course in the cortical parenchyma (Figure 8). Thymic NE concentrations (pmol per mg wet weight) increase by approximately fourfold in 12-month-old animals and 15-fold in 24-month-old animals. Total NE content in the whole thymus from 24-month-old mice is not different from that measured in 2-month-old mice, again suggesting that NA innervation is maintained as the thymus involutes.

Collectively, these studies reveal the remarkable ability of NA nerves to accommodate to the loss of cellularity in the cortex and conform to the changing geometry of the aged thymus. Even though there does not appear to be an increase in the total innervation of the aged thymus, the thymus becomes hyperinnervated with age by progressively shrinking in volume. The increased thymic NE concentration that occurs with advancing age suggests an increase in NE availability in the thymic cortex for interaction with remaining thymocytes and other target cells of the immune system.

Since mature thymocyte subpopulations appear to possess adrenergic receptors (Fuchs et al., 1988; Marchetti et al., 1990), they may be capable of responding to NE that is released by these nerve fibers; however, we have found no peer-reviewed reports indicating whether the presence and transduction capacity of these receptors on thymocytes are functional in the aged thymus. Preliminary studies

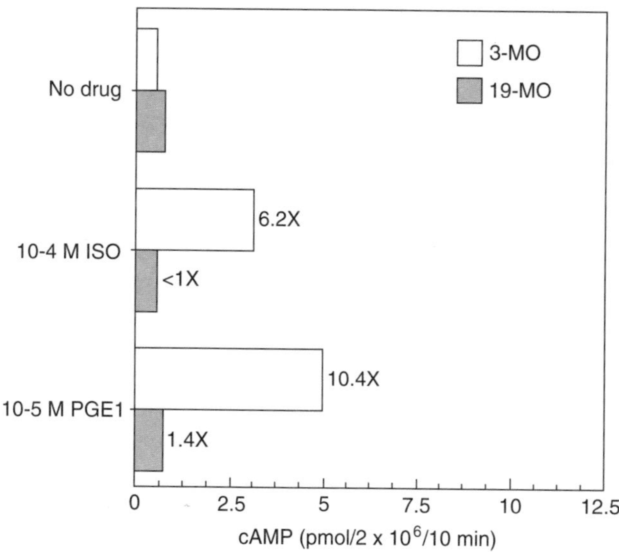

FIGURE 9 cAMP generation in thymocytes (expressed as pmol/10^6 cells) from 3- (3-MO) and 19-month-old (19-MO) BALB/c mice after β-adrenoceptor stimulation with no drug (control), 10^{-4} M isoproterenol (ISO), or 10^{-5} M prostaglandin E_1 (PGE_1) (which also uses cAMP as its second messenger). In thymocytes from young mice, addition of 10^{-4} M ISO or 10^{-5} M PGE_1 to the culture media resulted in a 6.2- or 10.4-fold increase in cAMP generation, respectively, over that seen in wells with no drug added. In old mice, ISO- and PGE_1-stimulated cAMP generation in thymocytes was reduced 1X or 1.4X, respectively, over that seen in wells in which no drug was added.

from our laboratory using unfractionated thymocytes from young and old BALB/c mice indicate an age-related reduction in cAMP production after stimulation with isoproterenol, a nonselective β-adrenoceptor agonist (Figure 9). This finding suggests a decreased ability of thymocytes to respond to NA sympathetic stimulation with advancing age.

In BALB/c and C57Bl/6 mice stressed by immobilization for 1 h/day for up to 14 consecutive days, stress-induced thymic involution was more pronounced in older animals (Dominguez-Gerpe & Rey-Mendez, 1998a). These data suggest that increased sympathetic outflow and/or activation of the hypothalamo-pituitary-adrenal axis may be contributory to thymic involution. It is well known that glucocorticoids can induce apoptosis of thymocytes. Several recent studies have reported that NE can regulate lymphocyte proliferation by inducing apoptosis in lymphocytes (Josefsson, Bergquist, Ekman, & Tarkowski, 1996). In the report by Josefsson et al. (1996), exposure of lymphocytes to catecholamines at concentrations as low as 10 nM were found to decrease proliferation and differentiation. This catecholamine-dependent inhibition of T and B lymphocyte activity is mediated via an induction of a Bcl-2/Bax and Fas/FasL involved in apoptosis, suggesting a novel mechanism for regulation of lymphocyte activity (Berquist, Josefsson, Tarkowski, Ekman, & Ewing, 1997). If similar regulatory mechanisms for proliferation exist in thymocytes, then perhaps sympathetic hyperinnervation and increased NE availability may promote apoptosis of thymocytes contributing to the decrease in cellularity of the thymus with aging.

In a preliminary study (K. Madden, unpublished data), we have found that chronic β- or α-adrenoceptor blockade has no effect on thymocyte differentiation in 2- or 12-month-old BALB/c mice, but significantly alters thymocyte CD4/CD8 coexpression in 24-month-old animals, suggesting a role for NE in thymocyte maturation. Further, these findings suggest that the sympathetic innervation may have more profound regulatory influences on thymic function in old animals than in young animals. Age-related changes in adrenoceptor expression on thymocytes, or the ability of NE to signal old thymocytes, needs to be investigated more thoroughly.

D. Age-Related Changes in Other Neurotransmitter-Specific Nerves

Age-associated changes in other neurotransmitter-specific nerves have not been examined extensively in the thymus. There is one report examining CGRP innervation of the murine thymus during development and in old animals (Bulloch et al., 1991). CGRP-ir nerves are present in close proximity to blood vessels in the corticomedullary junction of the thymus as early as embryonic day 17 in the mouse. With increasing maturity the density of $CGRP^+$ nerves increases in density, and nerve fibers exit these vascular plexuses into the surrounding cortical and medullary regions among cells of the thymus. In 18-month-old mice, this pattern of innervation appears to be maintained (Bulloch et al., 1991).

V. LYMPH NODES

A. Maturation

Fluorescence histochemical studies of lymph nodes in rats (D. Felten et al., 1985; D. Felten, Felten, Bellinger, Carlson, Ackerman, Madden, Olschowka, & Livnat, 1987; Giron, Crutcher, & Davis, 1980) and several strains of mice (Bellinger, Ackerman, Felten, Lorton, & Felten, 1989; D. Felten, Livnat, Felten, Carlson, Bellinger, & Yeh, 1984; Livnat, Felten, Carlson, Bellinger, & Felten, 1985) demonstrate dense plexuses of NA nerves along blood vessels at the hilus, the presumed point of entry of NA nerve fibers. In

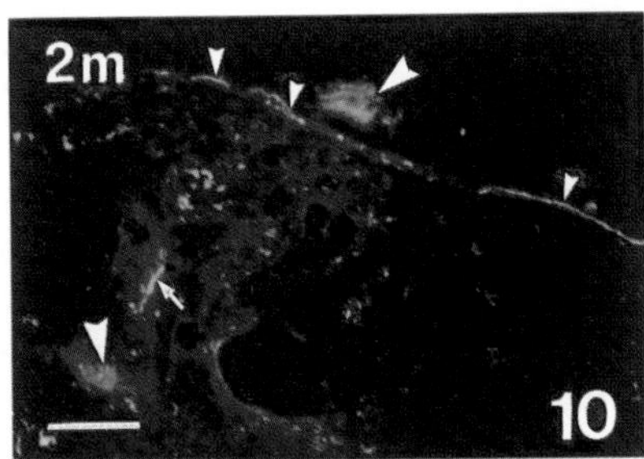

FIGURE 10 In mesenteric lymph nodes from a 2-month-old (2m) C57Bl/6 mouse, NA nerve fibers are seen coursing in the capsule (small arrowheads), along blood vessels (large arrowheads), and as single fluorescent profiles (arrow) in the cortex. Glyoxylic acid-induced HF for CAs. X85. Calibration bar = 100 μm.

lymph nodes, NA nerves distribute either into a subcapsular plexus (Figure 10) or continue in vascular plexuses through the medullary cords. These fibers course adjacent to both vascular and lymphatic channels in the medulla and continue with small vessels into the paracortical regions, which are rich in T lymphocytes. Individual varicose fibers branch from these vascular plexuses and travel in the paracortical parenchyma. NA nerves from the subcapsular plexus continue along small vessels into the cortex, and single varicose profiles course in the cortical parenchyma. Parenchymal fibers are present in cortical and paracortical regions, among T lymphocytes, but are absent from nodular regions and germinal centers where B lymphocytes predominate.

The compartmentation of NA nerves in lymph nodes shows many similarities with NA innervation of the spleen, suggesting a common functional role in both organs. For example, the marginal zone of the spleen receives abundant NA innervation and serves as a site of lymphocyte entry, antigen capture, and antigen presentation. Similarly, in lymph nodes the corticomedullary junction, subcapsular sinus, and the paracortex and medullary cords are sites also innervated by NA nerves, sites that subserve similar lymphocyte entry, antigen capture and antigen presentation, respectively. A role for NA at sites of antigen capture, antigen-presentation, and lymphocyte activation is suggested from studies demonstrating a decline in primary and secondary plaque-forming cell (PFC) responses in spleen and lymph nodes following sympathetic denervation (Livnat et al., 1985). Egress of activated lymphocytes into the circulation (functions that occur in the outer marginal zone of the spleen and in the medullary sinuses of the lymph nodes) occur after infusion of catecholamines (D. Felten et al., 1987; Ernström & Sandberg, 1974; Ernström & Söder, 1975), indicating an additional functional role for NE at this site.

A few preliminary observations of AChE$^+$ staining in nerve profiles that supply lymph nodes (Bellinger, Felten, Coleman, Yeh, & Felten, 1985) exist, but it is not clear that these nerves are cholinergic. Peptidergic nerves also are present in lymph nodes from mature animals. NPY innervation is similar in the pattern of distribution and nerve density to that described for NA innervation of lymph nodes. NPY$^+$ nerves course along blood vessels in the hilus, in the medulla, and interfollicular regions of lymph nodes. Some NPY$^+$ fibers are present as linear profiles in the parenchyma in paracortical and cortical regions, where they end among fields of lymphocytes. SP+/CGRP+ nerves are present in the hilus, beneath the capsule, at the corticomedullary junction, in medullary regions, and in internodal regions of the lymph nodes. SP$^+$ and CGRP$^+$ nerve fibers travel along the vasculature, from which they branch into the parenchyma among lymphocytes and accessory cells. VIP$^+$ nerves course along the vasculature in internodal regions of the cortex, and along medullary cords (Figure 22) (Fink & Weihe, 1988; Popper, Mantyh, Vigna, Magioos, & Mantyh, 1988). VIP and peptide histidine isoleucine (PHI) staining overlap in their distribution and may be colocalized. In the rat, VIP$^+$ nerves are found in mesenteric lymph nodes but not in popliteal lymph nodes (Bellinger et al., 1997).

B. Ontogeny

No studies have examined the ontogeny of innervation in lymph nodes from animals with a normal genetic makeup. Development of NA nerves into lymph nodes of nerve growth factor (NGF) transgenic mice (NGF overexpression in the skin, but not in lymphoid tissue) has been investigated by Carlson et al. (Carlson, Johnson, Parrish, & Cass, 1998). They report hyperinnervation of peripheral lymph nodes at an early postnatal age compared with age-matched control mice; development of NA nerves into mesenteric lymph nodes was not different from control animals.

C. Senescence

We have examined cervical, mesenteric, and popliteal lymph nodes from several strains of aged mice, including C3H, C57Bl/6, BALB/c, New Zealand White (NZW), New Zealand Black (NZB), and NZB × NZW F1 (NZBW), and in aged F344 rats with fluorescence histochemistry for catecholamines (Bellinger, Ackerman et al., 1989). In cervical and popliteal lymph nodes from rats and mice, NA innervation in all compartments of lymph nodes is diminished with age (Bellinger, Ackerman et al., 1989). The time course of diminished NA innervation varies, depending on the strain, and correlates with the expected life span of the animals. In mesenteric lymph nodes from C57Bl/6 mice, the density of NA nerve fibers increases in the cortex and paracortex, present among an increasing density of yellow autofluorescent cells (Figures 11 and 12). However, in mesenteric lymph nodes from old BALB/c mice (Figure 13), NA nerve fiber density is strikingly lower in old mice compared with that seen in 2-month-old animals (similar to NA innervation seen in Figure 10). These findings indicate that there may be differences in aging patterns of NA sympathetic innervation depending on the location of the lymph node in the body, and in the species examined.

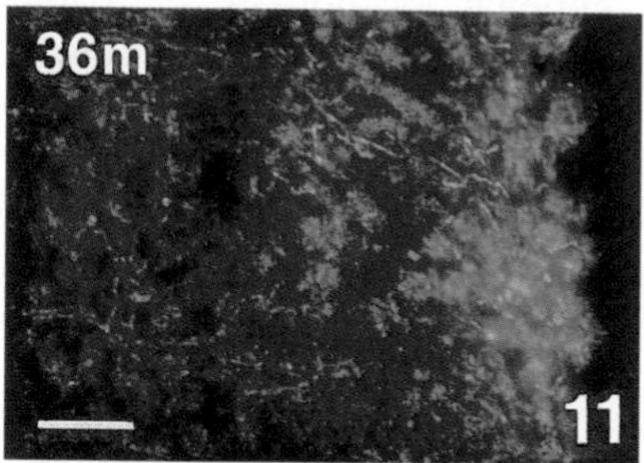

FIGURE 11 A dense array of NA nerve fibers are present in the outer cortex of a mesenteric lymph node from a 36-month-old (36m) C57Bl/6 mouse. These NA nerve fibers are scattered among clusters of yellow autofluorescent cells. Glyoxylic acid-induced HF for CAs. X85. Calibration bar = 100 μm.

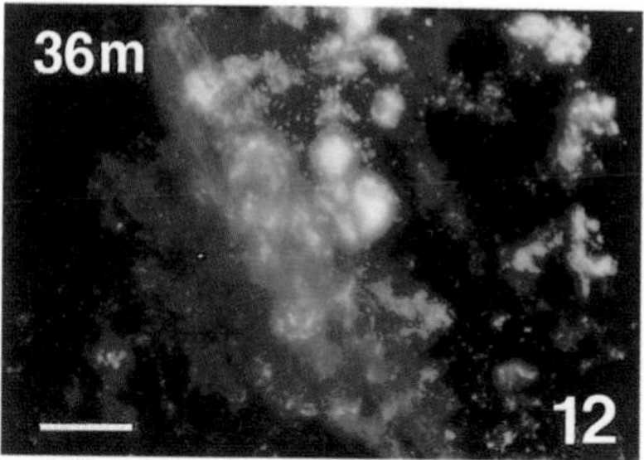

FIGURE 12 Higher magnification of the cortex in mesenteric lymph nodes from an old C57Bl/6 mice (36m) reveals NA nerve fibers in a vascular plexus that are closely apposed to yellow autofluorescent cells. Glyoxylic acid-induced HF for CAs. X170. Calibration bar = 50 μm.

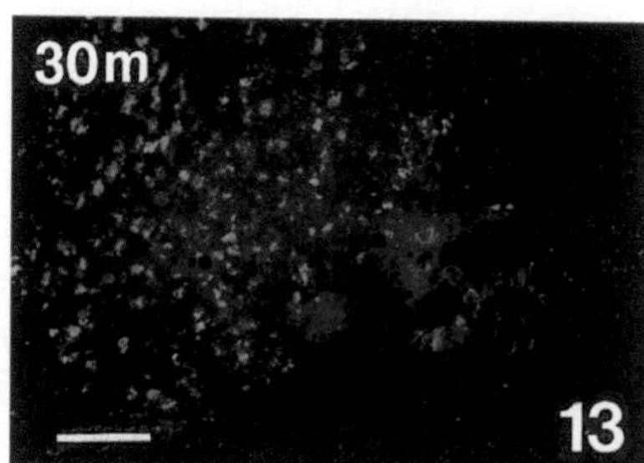

FIGURE 13 In the cortex of a mesenteric lymph node from a 30-month-old (36m) BALB/c mouse there is an increase in the density of yellow autofluorescent cells, and a loss of NA nerve fibers. X85. Glyoxylic acid-induced HF for CAs. Calibration bar = 100 μm.

Szewczuk and Wade (1983) reported no age-associated immune dysfunction in mucosal-associated lymph nodes. Mesenteric and mediastinal lymph nodes PFC responses of old mice after immune challenge do not decline in magnitude, and are highly heterogeneous with regard to antibody affinity. In addition, there are no appreciable antiidiotype-blocked, hapten-augmentable PFCs. In contrast, the number of splenic, and draining peripheral lymph node immunoglobulin (Ig)M, IgG, and IgA antitrinitrophenol (TNP) PFC responses to TNP-BGG decreases in old animals with a preferential loss of high affinity PFC. This decline in immune activity coincides with increased antiidiotype-blocked, hapten-augmentable PFC. The differential effect of aging on in vivo immune responses of mucosal and systemic lymphoid tissues implies a site preference for age-related changes in immune function, and a division of the immune system into regulatory compartments during the normal immune response to antigens in old mice. The findings in this study are consistent with our hypothesis that the age-related loss in NA innervation of peripheral lymph nodes and the spleen is causally related to diminished immune responses in these sites with advancing age.

Maintenance of NA innervation in mucosal-associated lymphoid tissue may be restricted to mesenteric lymph nodes. In the enteric nervous system of the murine gut, there is an age-related decline in PGP 9.5^+ neurons in the myenteric and submucosal plexuses in the antrum, duodenum, and colon from 12- and 24-month-old mice compared with 3-month-old animals (El-Salhy, Sandstrom, & Holmlund, 1999; El-Salhy & Sandstrom, 1999). At 12 and 24 months of age, the concentrations of gastrin, somatostatin, VIP, SP, NPY, galanin, and neurotensin decrease in the antrum compared with levels seen in 3-month-old mice. In the duodenum of old mice, somatostatin, VIP, gastrin, motilin, VIP, NPY, and galanin decrease as well. In the colon of 12-month-old mice, the concentrations of peptide YY, somatostatin, VIP, NPY, galanin, and neurotensin decrease, and at 24 months of age, VIP decreases, whereas SP increases.

Similarly, an examination of the distribution of nerves and mast cells in the lacrimal glands of 3-, 5-, 14- and 24-month-old rats with light microscopic histochemical and immunohistochemical techniques reveals an age-related loss in innervation (Sung, Arleth, & Feuerstein, 1991). In 14-month-old, and to a greater extent, 24-month-old rats, signs were noted of chronic inflammation and patchy destruction of acinar, ductal, and vascular tissue. The lacrimal glands from animals of all ages contained nerves staining for AChE, VIP, NPY, CGRP, TH, SP, and phosphoprotein B-50. A loss in the number and intensity of staining of TH^+ and NPY^+ nerves was seen by 24 months of age, associated with damage to the gland. Mast cells staining with histamine and $5\text{-}HT^+$, and alcian blue/safranin or toluidine blue, mostly associated with neurovascular tissue. An increase in the number of SP, CGRP, VIP, and NPY nerves apposed to mast cells was found in lacrimal glands from 24-month-old rats compared with animals at 3–5 months of age. The role of these changes in peptide innervation of the gut and other mucosal-associated lymphoid tissues in influencing immune function at these sites needs to be investigated further.

VI. SPLEEN

A. Maturation

Innervation of the mature spleen has been studied more extensively than any other lymphoid organ. In rodents (Ackerman, Felten, Bellinger, & Felten, 1987; Ackerman, Felten, Bellinger, Livnat, & Felten, 1987; Ackerman, Felten, Dijkstra, Livnat, & Felten, 1989; Bellinger, Ackerman, Felten, & Felten, 1992a; Bellinger, Felten, Collier, & Felten, 1987; Bellinger, Felten, Lorton, & Felten, 1989b; Besedovsky, del Rey, Sorkin, Burri, Honegger, Schlumpf, & Lichtensteiger, 1987; S. Felten, Felten et al., 1988; S. Felten, Bellinger, Collier, Coleman, & Felten, 1987; Fillenz & Pollard, 1976; Williams & D. Felten, 1981; Williams et al., 1981) NA nerves enter the spleen as a dense vascular plexus associated with the splenic artery. The site at which the splenic artery penetrates the capsule of the spleen is referred to the hilus or hilar region; NA nerves enter at the hilus and continue to course along branches from this artery to form subcapsular and trabecular plexuses. NA nerves continue to travel with the vasculature, which eventually give rise to central arterioles, surrounded by the lymphoid compartment of the spleen, the white pulp (Figure 14).

In the white pulp, NE-containing nerves exit the central arteriole into the surrounding parenchyma, the periarteriolar lymphatic sheath (PALS), which is composed primarily of T lymphocytes (Figure 14). Double-label immunocytochemistry reveal close association between TH^+ nerves and T lymphocytes in the PALS (Figure 14). TH^+ nerve fibers also are present along blood vessels, in nerve bundles, or as individual fibers in the marginal zone (Figure 16). S. Felten and Olschowka (1987) confirmed this association with immunocytochemistry for TH at the electron microscopic level. They reported direct contacts between lymphocytes and TH-immunoreactive nerves along the distal face of the central artery of the white pulp and in deeper zones of the PALS, in addition to the more conventional location of sympathetic nerves adjacent to smooth muscle of the central arteriole. TH^+ nerves also reside among B cell and macrophages in the marginal zone, the outer region of the white pulp (Figure 16). In the follicles of the white pulp, predominantly a region of B lymphocytes, only occasional NA nerve fibers are present (Figure 18).

Neuropeptide innervation also has been described in the spleen. NPY^+ is colocalized with NE in sympathetic nerves that innervate the rat spleen as indicated by a loss of NPY^+ fibers in chemically sympathectomized animals (Romano, Felten, Felten, & Olschowka, 1991; Romano et al., 1994). Nerve fibers staining for SP, CGRP, met-enkephalin, VIP, cholecystokinin, neurotensin, and interleukin (IL)-1 have been demonstrated in the spleen (Bellinger et al., 1997; D. Felten et al., 1985; Fried, Terenius, Brodin, Efendic, Dockray, Fahrenkrug, Goldstein, & Hökfelt, 1986; Lorton, Bellinger, Felten, & Felten, 1989, 1991; Lundberg, Änggård, Pernow, & Hökfelt, 1985; Schultzberg, Svenson, Unden, & Bartfai, 1987). These neuropeptide-containing nerves differ in their distribution in the spleen from sympathetic fibers.

SP and CGRP have overlapping distributions in the spleen, but $CGRP^+$ nerves occur more frequently than SP^+ nerves, indicating a subset of $CGRP^+$ nerves that do not contain SP. $SP^+/CGRP^+$ nerves are present predominantly in red pulp compartments of the spleen, including the capsular/trabecular compartments, and also are found as free fibers in the red pulp parenchyma of the red pulp. However, refinement of our immunocytochemical staining procedure has revealed additional $SP/CGRP^+$ nerves along the central arterioles, and as free fibers in the surrounding PALS and marginal zone (reviewed in chapter 2, volume 1, of this book). These nerves reside adjacent to $OX19^+$ T lymphocytes, $ED3^+$ macrophages, and IgM^+ B cells. $SP^+/CGRP^+$ nerves are absent in the follicles of the white pulp. VIP^+ nerve fibers course along large arteries and central arterioles, and in the white pulp, venous/trabecular system, and red pulp of the rat spleen (Bellinger et al., 1997). VIP innervation is more robust in Long-Evans hooded rats than in F344 rats (Bellinger et al., 1997).

B. Ontogeny

NA sympathetic innervation of the developing rodent spleen has been investigated, but no studies are available that have examined neuropeptidergic nerves during the ontogeny of the spleen. The first detectable NA sympathetic nerve in the developing rat spleen occur by 17 to 19 days of gestation, and further development largely occurs postnatally (Ackerman, 1989; Ackerman, Bellinger et al., 1991; Ackerman, Felten, Bellinger, & Felten et al., 1987; Ackerman, Felten, Bellinger, Livnat et al., 1987; Ackerman et al., 1989; Bellinger, Ackerman et al., 1989; D. Felten, Felten, Carlson, Bellinger, Ackerman, Romano, & Livnat, 1988; D. Felten, Felten, Madden, Ackerman, & Bellinger, 1989; S. Felten, Olschowka, Ackerman, & Felten, 1988). On postnatal days 1 to 3, NA nerves enter the hilar region in bundles that travel with the splenic artery and its branches. Some NA fibers are present in the white pulp of the spleen. TH^+ nerve bundles in the white pulp course among IgM^+ B lymphocytes at the outer border of the PALS. These TH^+ profiles encircle the zone containing T- and B-lymphocytes, and occasionally branch from this plexus into the developing PALS. The most striking feature at this time point is a total lack of TH^+ nerves associated with the central arteriole.

Ultrastructural study of spleens from newborn rats reveals direct contacts between TH^+ nerve terminals and lymphocytes (Ackerman, 1989; Ackerman, Bellinger et al., 1991; Ackerman, Felten, Bellinger, & Felten, 1987; Ackerman, Felten, Bellinger, Livnat et al., 1987; Ackerman et al., 1989; Bellinger, Ackerman et al., 1989; D. Felten et al., 1988; D. Felten, Felten et al., 1989; S. Felten, Olschowka et al., 1988) that are similar to those observed in young adult rats (S. Felten & Olschowka, 1987; S. Felten, Felten et al., 1988; S. Felten, Olschowka et al., 1988), as well as direct appositions between TH^+ terminals and an unidentified reticular-like cell (Ackerman, 1989; Ackerman, Bellinger et al., 1991; Ackerman, Felten, Bellinger, & Felten, 1987; Ackerman, Felten, Bellinger, Livnat et al., 1987; Ackerman et al., 1989; Bellinger, Ackerman et al., 1989; D. Felten et al., 1988; D. Felten, Felten et al., 1989; S. Felten, Olschowka et al., 1988) not present in the inner PALS of the adult rat spleen. Despite the sparcity of TH^+ nerves at this time point, NE concentration in the spleen is approximately 25% of levels in the adult spleen. Still, NE turnover in the spleens from 1-day-old rats is low, but progressively increases from 0 to 7 days of age.

By day 7 the four compartments of the PALS are distinguishable as the central and peripheral PALS, the marginal sinus, and the marginal zone (Ackerman, Felten, Bellinger, & Felten, 1987; Ackerman, Felten, Bellinger, Livnat et al., 1987; Ackerman, 1989; Ackerman, Bellinger et al., 1991; Ackerman et al., 1989; Bellinger, Ackerman et al., 1989; D. Felten et al., 1988; D. Felten, Felten et al., 1989; S. Felten, Olschowka et al., 1988). T lymphocytes occur throughout the PALS, intermixed with B lymphocytes in the outer PALS. B lymphocytes also reside in the marginal zone of the 7-day-old spleen, separated from the PALS by the marginal sinus. Surrounding the central arteriole is a dense plexus of TH^+ nerves, with numerous TH^+ fibers appearing to exit this plexus to travel in the PALS among T and B cells; however, the early presence of TH^+ nerve fibers in the PALS, but not along the central artery raises the possibility that these two compartments may be innervated by separate NA cell bodies in the ganglia. Unlike the adult rat spleen, where B cell compartments such as the follicle are not well innervated by sympathetic nerves, TH^+ nerve fibers arborize extensively among B cells in the outer PALS and inner marginal zone of the neonatal spleen. At birth, $ED3^+$ macrophages are scattered throughout the spleen, but become confined to the marginal zone by 7 to 10 days of age. Likewise, these cells also occur in proximity with TH^+ nerve fibers in the marginal zone. One prominent characteristic of this time point is that the density of nerves and the intensity of TH staining is more robust than at any other age examined.

The PALS reorganizes between 7 and 14 days, forming more adult-like boundaries between T and B lymphocytes (Ackerman, 1989; Ackerman, Bellinger et al., 1991; Ackerman, Felten, Bellinger, & Felten, 1987; Ackerman, Felten, Bellinger, Livnat et al., 1987; Ackerman et al., 1989; Bellinger, Ackerman et al., 1989; D. Felten et al., 1988; D. Felten, Felten et al., 1989; S. Felten, Olschowka et al., 1988). T and B cells become oriented to the inner and outer PALS, respectively, and B lymphocytes aggregate to form follicles. B cells also are present in the marginal zone adjacent to the marginal sinus. Coinciding with this cellular reorganization of the white pulp, NA nerves redistribute to the inner PALS, forming dense, tangled nerve plexuses among T lymphocytes. TH^+ nerves also reside in the parafollicular and marginal zones among B cells and macrophages, and in the marginal sinus. By postnatal day 14, the pattern of innervation resembles that seen in the young adult spleen, and between 10 and 14 days splenic NE concentration dramatically increases, approaching young adult levels.

Between 14 and 28 days of age, there is a shift in the relative sizes of the splenic white pulp compartments, such that the inner PALS becomes thin and elongated, and the follicles and marginal zones expand (Ackerman, 1989; Ackerman, Bellinger et al., 1991; Ackerman, Felten, Bellinger, & Felten, 1987; Ackerman, Felten, Bellinger, Livnat et al., 1987; Ackerman et al., 1989; Bellinger, Ackerman et al., 1989; D. Felten et al., 1988; D. Felten, Felten et al., 1989; S. Felten, Olschowka et al., 1988). NA nerve fibers adjust to the remodeled compartmentation, distributing to the inner one-third of the PALS, similar to distribution of sympathetic nerves in the adult spleen. NA nerves also remain in the marginal and parafollicular zones among a more abundant rim of $ED3^+$ macrophages. The outer marginal zone receives TH^+ nerves that extend from nerve plexuses of the venous sinuses and trabeculae. Some of the nerves in the parafollicular region enter into the follicle, as is seen in young adult rats.

The most striking change in sympathetic innervation between 21 and 28 days is a marked increase in the density of TH^+ nerves along the venous sinuses and trabeculae (Ackerman, 1989; Ackerman, Bellinger et al., 1991; Ackerman, Felten, Bellinger, & Felten, 1987; Ackerman, Felten, Bellinger, Livnat et al., 1987; Ackerman et al., 1989; Bellinger, Ackerman et al., 1989; D. Felten et al., 1988; D. Felten, Felten et al., 1989; S. Felten, Olschowka et al., 1988). Relatively few fibers extend into the surrounding red pulp from these plexuses. The mature pattern of NA innervation of the rat spleen is observed by 28 days after birth. From 28 days to adulthood, all compartments of the spleen increase in volume, which is accompanied by a parallel growth of NA innervation. Between 14 and 56 days of age, NE levels show a second increase, followed by a more gradual increase to adult levels. Adult proportions in the spleen are attained by 56 days of age.

Radioligand binding studies in spleen tissue from developing F344 rats reveal two plateaus in β-adrenoceptor receptor density on splenocytes over the first 90 days of life (Figure 19A) (Ackerman, 1989; Ackerman, Bellinger et al., 1991; Ackerman, Felten, Bellinger, & Felten, 1987; Ackerman, Felten, Bellinger, Livnat et al., 1987; Ackerman et al., 1989; Bellinger, Ackerman et al., 1989; D. Felten et al., 1988; D. Felten, Felten et al., 1989; S. Felten, Olschowka et al., 1988). Splenocytes from 1- to 10-day-old rats express a B_{max} of 400 to 500 sites per cell, whereas splenocytes from 14- to 90-day-old animals express adult levels of 800 to 1000 sites per cell (Figure 19A). This shift in receptor density may reflect a change in spleen cell populations or the development of immunocompetent cells, with splenocytes maturing toward a more activated state in which they possess more receptors. The existence of NA nerve in developing compartments of the spleen from birth through adulthood indicates that NE is available for signaling target cells of the immune system toward immunocompetence, perhaps at critical periods during their development. β-Adrenoceptor expression on immunocytes early in development supports this hypothesis.

Collectively, these findings suggest a role for NE in the formation and maturation of splenic lymphoid compartments through selective migration of specific populations of cells into the spleen, by modulating proliferation and maturation of lymphocytes, and by the activation of specific cell functions at critical time points during splenic development. Conversely, lymphoid and nonlymphoid cells that reside near nerve fibers in the marginal sinus may influence the growth and maturation of NA nerves. Several lines of research support this contention. A variety of cytokines and neurotrophic factors that are synthesized and released by cells of the immune system can promote the growth and differentiation of neurons (Araujo & Cotman, 1993; Awatsuji, Furukawa, Nakajima, Furukawa, & Hayashi, 1993; Brenneman, Schultzberg, Bartfai, & Gozes, 1992; Carnahan, Patel, & Miller, 1994; Haugen & Letourneau, 1990; Kannan, Bienenstock, Ohta, Stanisz, & Stead, 1996; Kushima, Hama, & Hatanaka, 1992; Mehler, Rozental, Dougherty, Spray, & Kessler, 1993; Murphy, Reid, Brown, & Bartlett, 1993; Torii, Yan, Hosoi, & Granstein, 1997; van Coelln, Unsicker, & Krieglstein, 1995).

In transgenic mice that overexpress NGF in the skin but not in immune tissues, development of NA nerves into the spleen has been examined (Carlson et al., 1998). NGF content in spleen from 1- to 2-day-old transgenic mice is higher than controls, at a time when little NA innervation is present, and then splenic NGF content gradually declines with increasing maturity. Splenic innervation in NGF transgenic mice gradually diverged from controls during the first 2 postnatal weeks, with the greatest change occurring between postnatal days 13 and 16, when the splenic organization matures to the adult pattern. These findings suggest that the spleen can uptake and store NGF produced and secreted from the skin, which in turn leads to an altered pattern of NA nerve development into spleens from NGF transgenic mice.

C. Senescence in F344 Rats

1. *Sympathetic Nerve Density and NE Content*

With advancing age, NA innervation of spleens from F344 rats declines progressively, manifested as a decline in the density of fluorescent NA nerves and TH^+ nerves by approximately 75%, and by a decline in splenic NE content by approximately 50%, by 27 months of age (Bellinger et al., 1987; S. Felten et al., 1987). It appears that the discrepancy in nerve density and splenic NE concentration results from an increase in NE synthesis in age-resistant nerves in the spleen, and an increase in the ability of remaining NA nerve terminals to reuptake NE. These age-resistant nerves reside near the hilus; the more extensive nerve depletion is apparent distal from the hilus. Turnover studies indicate that NE synthesis is enhanced in age-resistant NA nerves. Additionally, an increase in circulating NE with age has been reported (Esler, Skews, Leonard, Jackman, Bobik, & Korner, 1981; Krall, Connelly, Weisbart, & Tuck, 1981; Lake, Zeigler, Coleman, & Kopin, 1977; Ziegler, Lake, & Kopin, 1976), which may contribute to maintaining the NE content of the spleen at a level a bit higher than loss of nerve fibers would predict.

Longitudinal studies using fluorescence histochemistry, double-label immunocytochemistry (Figures 14–18), and neurochemistry for measuring NE have been performed by our laboratory (Bellinger, Ackerman et al., 1992). Data from these studies indicate that NA innervation is maintained through 12 months of age (Figure 14 and 16), and then gradually begins to decline through 27 months of age (Figures 15, 17, and 18). At 12 months of age, TH$^+$ nerve fibers are densely packed in the PALS. Double-label immunocytochemistry further reveals a gradual decline in the density of T lymphocytes in the PALS (Figure 15), and ED3$^+$ macrophages in the marginal zone (Figure 17) that parallel the decline in NA innervation. In 12-month-old rats, the PALS and marginal zone are reduced as a result of this cell loss. At this time point, however, NA innervation of these compartments is still robust. NA nerves retract into the smaller lymphoid compartments to maintain their anatomical distribution within these shrinking lymphoid compartments, giving the appearance of hyperinnervation. By 17 months of age,

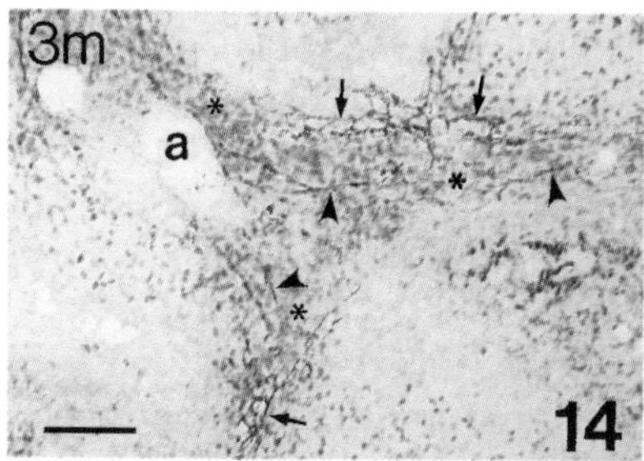

FIGURE 14 In this spleen section from a 3-month-old (3m) F344 rat, a dense plexus of TH$^+$ nerve fibers (black) (arrows) course along the central arteriole (a), and linear black profiles (arrowheads) can be seen in the adjacent periarteriolar lymphatic sheath (*), stained here with OX19 (brown), a marker for T lymphocytes. Double-label ICC for TH and OX19. mz, marginal zone. X85. Calibration bar = 100 μm.

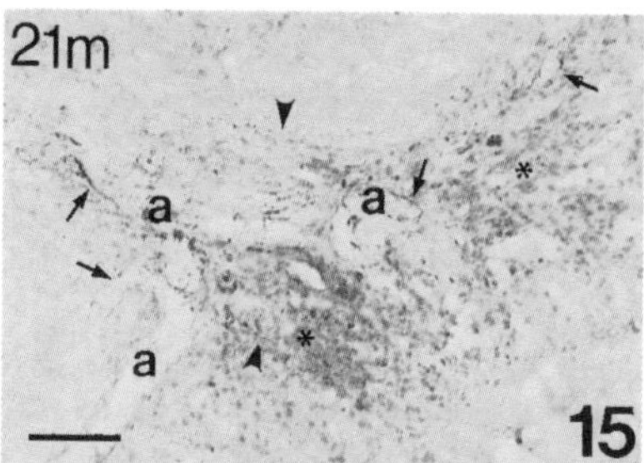

FIGURE 15 In spleens from rats at 21 months of age (21m), the density of TH$^+$ nerves (black) (arrows) in vascular plexuses around the central arterioles (a) declines, and the intensity of the immunoreaction product in age-resistant nerves is reduced. An occasional TH$^+$ nerve fiber (arrowheads) can still be found in the surrounding periarteriolar lymphatic sheath (*). Corresponding to the loss of NA sympathetic innervation, the density of OX19$^+$ T cells (brown) in the periarteriolar lymphatic sheath is diminished by 21 months of age. mz, marginal zone. Double-label ICC for TH and OX19. X85. Calibration bar = 100 μm.

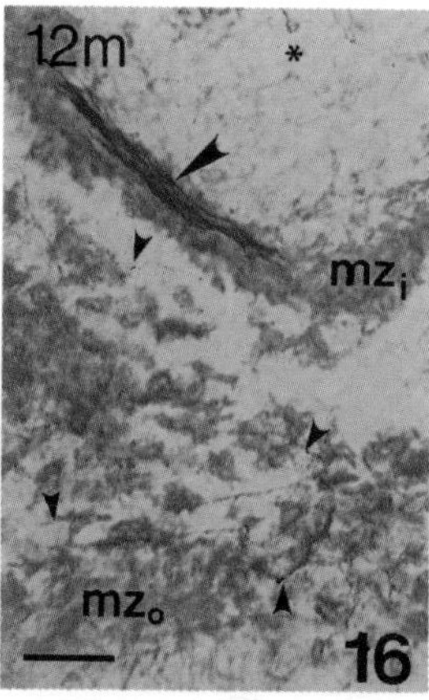

FIGURE 16 In the inner (mz_i) and outer (mz_o) marginal zone in spleens from 3-month-old (3m) rats, ED3$^+$ macrophages (brown) are present as inner dense cluster around the periarteriolar lymphatic sheath, and an outer more diffuse network of cells, respectively. Bundles of TH$^+$ nerves (black) (large arrowheads) are often found in the inner marginal zone. TH$^+$ nerve fibers, either associated with blood vessels or as single profiles, also travel in the inner and outer marginal zone (small arrowheads). Double-label ICC for TH and ED3, a marker for marginal macrophages. X170. Calibration bar = 50 μm.

a further loss of T lymphocytes and ED3$^+$ macrophages is apparent; at this time point there also is a decline in density of TH$^+$ nerves associated with these compartments. This parallel decline in the density of specific populations of cells of the immune system and in NA innervation continues through 27 months of age.

The pattern of NA nerve loss and the decline in T lymphocytes and ED3$^+$ macrophages in these two splenic compartments occur in a precise manner, with nerve fibers first lost in lymphoid compartments that

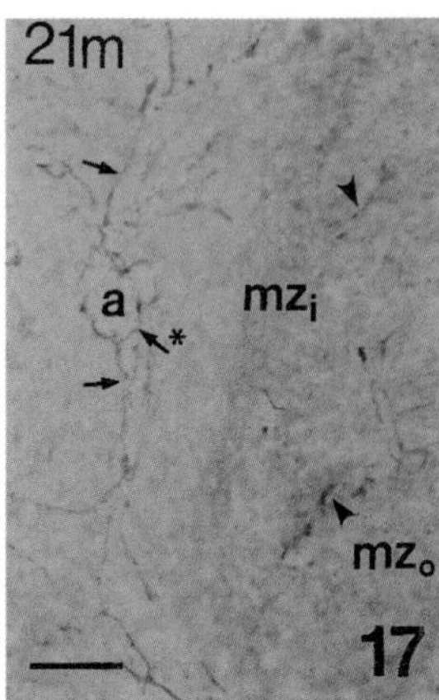

FIGURE 17 By 21 months of age (21m), there is a marked decline in the density of ED3$^+$ macrophages (brown) in the inner (mz$_i$) and outer (mz$_o$) marginal zone. This loss of macrophages corresponds with a loss of TH$^+$ nerve fibers (black) long the central arterioles (a), periarteriolar lymphatic sheath (*), and in the inner and outer marginal zone (mz$_i$ and mz$_o$, respectively) (arrowheads). Double-label ICC for TH and ED3. X85. Calibration bar = 100 μm.

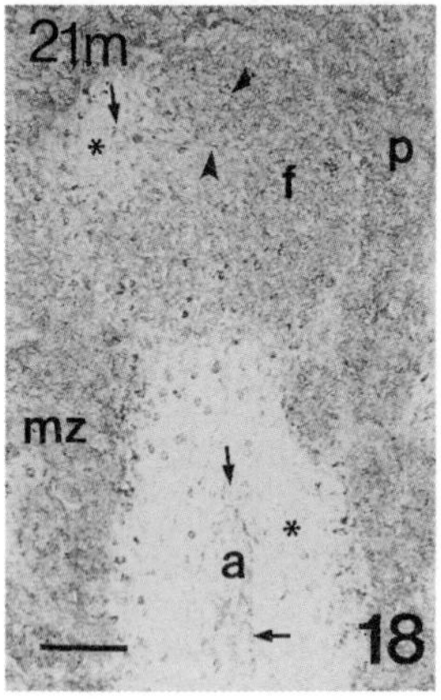

FIGURE 18 There are no remarkable age-related differences in the density or the staining intensity of IgM$^+$ B lymphocytes (brown) in the follicle (f), the parafollicular zone (p), or the marginal zone (mz) in spleens from 21-month-old (21m) rats. However, the loss of TH$^+$ nerve fibers (black) (is apparent in compartments of the spleen where IgM$^+$ lymphocytes reside (arrowheads), along the central arteriole (a) (fibers indicated by arrows), and in the adjacent (unstained) periarteriolar lymphatic sheath (*) where T lymphocytes predominate. X85. Calibration bar = 100 μm.

reside most distal from the hilar region, the site of entry of the NA sympathetic nerves (Bellinger, Ackerman et al., 1992). NA innervation continues to decline in this distal-to-proximal fashion with respect to the hilus until the only appreciable remaining NA nerves in the 27-month-old spleen are distributed near the hilus. The density of T lymphocytes in the PALS and ED3$^+$ macrophages in the marginal zone display a similar pattern of loss that closely overlaps the loss of NA innervation. Cell loss in these compartments occurs first at sites distal to the hilus, with progressive loss nearer to the hilus with advancing age.

Whether the loss in NA innervation is causally related to the reduced cellularity of T lymphocytes and macrophages in the spleen is not known. Preliminary studies by S.Y. Stevens (unpublished data; personal communications) examining the ability of sympathetic nerves to innervate spleen fragments from young and old rats transplanted into the anterior chamber of the eye suggest that macrophages may be important for ingrowth and maintenance of sympathetic nerves. Additionally, macrophages synthesize NGF and other neurotrophic factors, consistent with a neuroprotective role for these cells in the spleen. Further, support for this hypothesis comes from preliminary studies from Lorton and colleagues (unpublished data; personal communications) showing dramatically reduced immunoreactivity for NGF in the PALS and marginal zone of spleens from Lewis rats with experimental arthritis, in which NA sympathetic nerve fiber density declines as the disease progresses (see chapter 2, volume 1, of this book). In severe combined immunodeficient (SCID) mice, which are deficient in T and B lymphocytes, NA sympathetic innervation of the spleen (S.Y. Stevens, unpublished data; personal communications) and thymus (Mitchell, Kendall, Adam, & Schumacher, 1997) are still robust. These findings suggest that T lymphocytes may not be critical in providing neurotrophic support necessary to maintain NA nerves in the spleen in these mice. Furthermore, NA innervation of the young adult murine spleen following lymphocyte depletion using hydrocortisone or cyclophosphamide in young adults does not decline acutely (Carlson, Felten, Livnat, & Felten, 1987). Collectively, these findings suggesting that NA denervation may not be compensatory to the loss of T lymphocytes in the white pulp of the spleen with age, although we cannot dismiss the possibility that it could, in conjunction with other aging changes, be contributory. T and B lymphocytes express mRNA for NGF (Santambrogio, Benedetti, Chao, Muzaffar, Kulig, Gabellini, & Hochwald, 1994), making it possible, at least under some conditions, to provide trophic support to NA nerve fibers in lymphoid tissues.

The density and distribution of B lymphocytes in the follicles and the marginal zone, on the other hand, do not change remarkably with advancing age (Figure 18) (Bellinger, Ackerman et al., 1992). The boundary between B cells in the follicle and the marginal zone, and between the marginal zone and the PALS, becomes less distinct with age. TH$^+$ nerve density in the marginal zone diminishes with age. Only an occasional TH$^+$ nerve profile occurs in the follicle, so age-related changes in nerve density in this compartment are more difficult to discern; however, TH^+ nerve can still be found in the follicles near the hilus of spleens from old rats (Figure 18).

A loss of staining of sympathetic innervation of the spleen could result from (1) deficits in the synthetic machinery for these neurotransmitters reducing the stainability of these nerves with our histochemical methods or (2) an absence of nerves. In support of the second hypothesis, administration of α-methylnorepinephrine (100 mg/kg body weight, i.p.) a compound that is taken up by high-affinity carriers into NA terminals, persists because it cannot be catabolized, and fluoresces with histofluorescent staining methods, reveals no change in the density of fluorescent profiles in spleens from α-methylnorepinephrine-treated 27-month-old animals compared with vehicle-treated, age-matched rats (Ackerman, Bellinger et al., 1991). These results cannot be attributed to a defect in the high-affinity uptake system in the aged spleen, since we have found that NE uptake per nerve terminal in the old spleen is enhanced compared with that seen in young adults (Bellinger, unpublished data). Kinetic analysis of these data indicate an increase in the density of high-affinity uptake binding site for NE in age-resistant NA nerve terminals in spleens from old rats, probably as a compensatory mechanism resulting from reduced NE concentration and/or reduced nerve density.

2. *β-Adrenoceptor Density on Splenocytes with Aging*

The density of β-adrenoceptors on splenocytes increases in aging F344 rats (Figure 19A), consistent with up-regulation of β-adrenoceptors in response to declining NE levels from an age-related loss of innervation (Ackerman, Bellinger et al., 1991). Alternatively, increased β-adrenoceptor expression on old splenocytes may reflect age-related changes in specific subsets of cells in the spleen. No difference in receptor affinity was detected in old rats (Figure 19B). Measurement of β-adrenoceptor density alone, however, is not a sufficient indicator of the ability of these cells to respond to NA stimulation. Several studies have shown impaired lymphocyte responsiveness to NE, resulting from a defect in the coupling of β-adrenoceptors with adenylate cyclase or in the catalytic capacity of adenylate cyclase (Feldman, Limbird, Nadeau, Robertson, & Wood, 1984; O'Hara, Daul, Fesel, Siekmann, & Brodde, 1985). These studies have been performed using peripheral blood lymphocytes from mice. Similar findings of defective intracellular signaling by β-adrenoceptors have been reported for old rat myocardium and lung (Kusiak & Pitha, 1983; Kostrouch, Raska, Felt, Nedvídková, & Holecková, 1987; O'Connor, Scarpace, & Abrass, 1983; Scarpace & Abrass, 1983).

Studies from our laboratory do not entirely support a defect in NE signaling in splenocytes from F344 rats. First, if NE signaling is defective, we would predict that mechanisms important for regulating β-adrenoceptor density on splenocytes from old rats also would be defective. Our finding of enhanced β-adrenoceptor expression in the face of diminished NA innervation (Ackerman, Bellinger et al., 1991) suggests that β-adrenoceptor surface expression is intact in F344 rats. A progressive decline in β-adrenoceptors expression on splenocytes from 3- and 17-month-old rats occurs between 1 and 3 days after chemical sympathectomy with 6-OHDA treatment (Bellinger, Felten, & Felten, 1992). This initial decline in β-adrenoceptor expression on splenocytes is likely to result from bolus release of NE after nerve destruction. In 3-month-old rats, the decline in β-adrenoceptor density is followed by a progressive rise in density above control values, apparent 5 days after treatment, and continues through day 21 posttreatment. By 56 days after sympathectomy, β-adrenoceptor expression on splenocytes from 3-month-old rats returns to normal density, corresponding with reinnervation of the spleen and a return to normal splenic NE concentrations.

β-adrenoceptor expression on splenocytes from 17-month-old animals increases between 3 to 5 days postsympathectomy, at a time when the spleen is denervated and NE concentrations are extremely low (Bellinger, Felten et al., 1992). However, β-adrenoceptor density rapidly declines to levels below controls by day 10 and remain low through day 21, before a gradual increase in β-adrenoceptor density occurs that parallels the reinnervation of the spleen and rising splenic NE concentrations. NE concentrations in spleens from old denervated rats return to the same concentrations as that seen in young denervated rats, but β-adrenoceptor density elevates past normal levels and remains at this higher concentration. These findings suggest that old splenocytes respond appropriately to diminished NE concentrations in the spleen, but β-adrenoceptor expression becomes dysregulated at higher splenic NE concentrations. Consistent with this interpretation, De Blasi, Lipartiti, Algeri, Sacchetti, Costantini, Fratelli, & Cotecchia, 1986 have shown that after a stressful event (restraint stress), used as a mechanism to increase NE availability, β-adrenoceptor down-regulation is impaired in aged rats. Again, these changes also could be explained by shifts in the percentage of lymphocytes subsets that differentially express β-adrenoceptors in the old spleen.

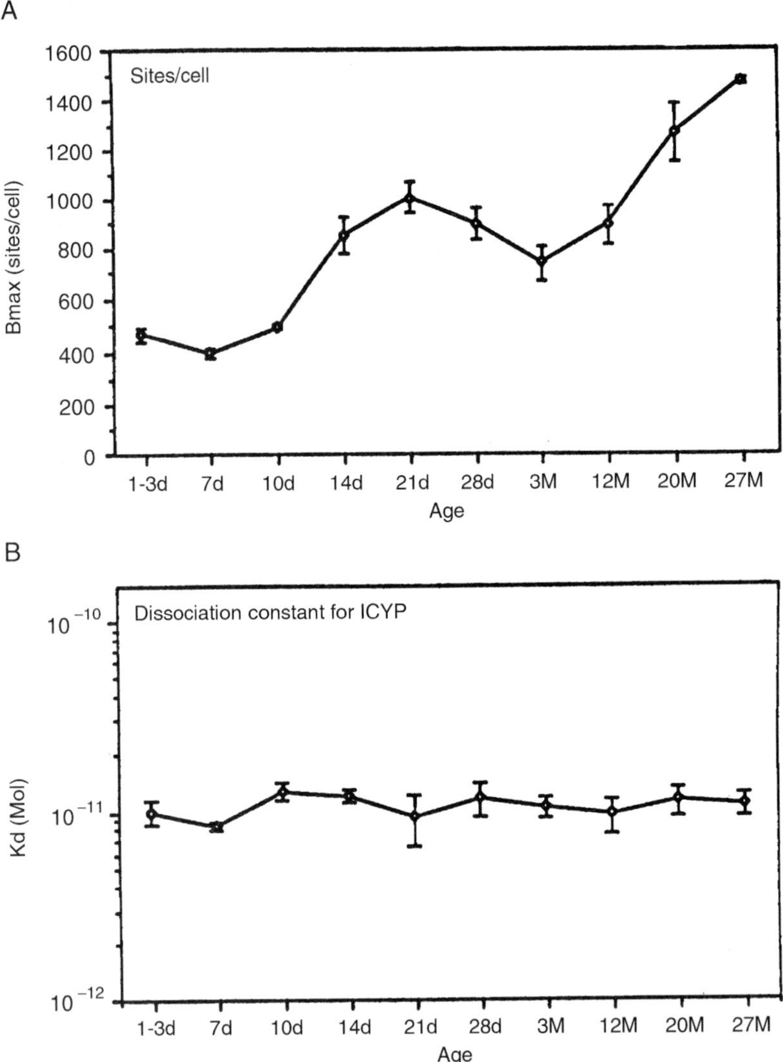

FIGURE 19 Radioligand binding analysis of β-adrenoceptor expression on intact splenocytes. Spleen cells were incubated for 60 min at 37°C with different concentrations of $[^{125}I]$CYP ranging from 0.1 to 2 pM. Nonspecific binding was determined using parallel assays incubated in the presence of 1 μm CGP-12177, a hydrophilic β-adrenoceptor antagonist. The data were analyzed using Scatchard analysis and represent the mean ± SEM of at least three pools of animals. A. β-Adrenoceptor density is expressed as sites per cell. The apparent increase in receptor density from 12 to 27 months of age was detected only in healthy aged animals. Sick animals (not included in this study) showed either no changes or a reduced density of β-adrenoceptors compared with young adult controls, but had consistently lower density than healthy aged animals. B. Dissociation constant (K_D) expressed in moles per liter (moles), plotted on log scale, for $[^{125}I]$CYP binding to intact splenocytes. (Taken from Ackerman et al., 1991).

Age-related changes in the ability of the central nervous system to modulate sympathetic outflow also may be impaired. Irwin and colleagues (Irwin, Hauger, & Brown, 1992) found that central administration of CRH produced a greater elevation in NE and NPY plasma concentrations, which persisted longer in aged rats compared with responses in young animals. The CRH-induced increase in sympathetic outflow in old rats correlates with an increased suppression of natural killer (NK) cell activity, suggesting a role of the sympathetic nervous system, and the descending central neural circuits that regulate sympathetic outflow, in abnormal regulation of NK cytotoxicity in vivo.

3. *Aging and Sympathetic Influence on Immune Function*

Functional studies using sympathectomized young and old rats, both immunized and naive, indicate that

TABLE I. Summary of Effects of Sympathectomy on Rat Spleen Cell Responsiveness

Days after 6-OHDA[b] treatment	Young (3 months old)	Old (17 months old)
Con A-Induced T Cell Proliferation[a]		
1	NC	⇑
3	NC/⇓	NC/⇓[d]
5	NC	⇓⇓
10	NC	NC/⇓
15	NC	NC
21	⇓⇓	NC
30	NC	NC
56	NC	NC
IL-2 Production[c]		
1	NC	⇑
3	NC	NC/⇑
5	NC	NC
10	NC	NC
15	NC	NC
21	NC	NC
30	NC	NC
56	NC	NC
IFN-γ Production[e]		
1	NC	NC
3	NC	NC
5	NC	NC
10	NC	NC
15	NC	NC
21	⇓⇓	NC
30	NC	NC
56	NC	NC

Note: Summary of data published in Madden, Felten, Felten, & Bellinger (2000) *Journal of Neuroimmunology, 103*, 131–145.
[a]Assessed by incorporaion of tritiated-thymidine into cultured splenocytes for the last 18 h of culture.
[b]6-OHDA treatment was 80 mg/kg, i.p. on day -4, and 40 mg/kg, i.p., on days -2 and 0; this produces maximal depletion from 1 to 5 days after the last 6-OHDA injection to a level <20% of vehicle controls.
[c]Measured with a bioassay (ability of supernatants to support the growth of the cell line, CTLL-2).
[d]Also seen in vehicle-treatment controls in this experimental repetition.
[e]Measured with a bioassay (ability of supernatants to protect the fibroblast line, L929, from infection with vesicular stomatitis virus).
Abbreviations: Con-A, concanavalin A; 6-OHDA, 6-hydroxydopamine; IL-2, interleukin-2; IFN-γ, interferon-γ; NC, no change.

old splenocytes are still responsive to NA stimulation (Madden, Felten, Felten, & Bellinger, 1995, 2000). In 3-month-old rats, no alterations in spleen cell concanavalin A (Con A)-induced T cell proliferation, IL-2 production, or interferon-γ (IFN-γ) production occur up to 15 days after sympathectomy, when splenic NE concentrations are maximally depleted (see Table I). By 21 days after sympathectomy, when NE levels partially recover to approximately 40% of vehicle controls, Con A-induced proliferation and IFN-γ production, but not IL-2 production, is reduced (see Table I). This delayed effect of sympathectomy was transient; at days 30 and 56 postsympathectomy, no alterations in Con A-induced proliferation or IL-2 production were observed. These delayed effects on T cell proliferation may result from ingrowth of NA nerves back into the spleen.

In 17-month-old rats, the extent of NE depletion after 6-OHDA treatment relative to vehicle controls are similar to that seen in young rats. Con A-induced T cell proliferation was enhanced 1 day after sympathectomy compared with controls (see Table I), and correlated with an increase in the percentage of $CD5^+$ T cells. T cell proliferation in old sympathectomized animals was not altered 3 days after denervation in the first experiment, but was reduced in the second experiment. At day 1 and 3, splenic T cell responsiveness by vehicle controls was altered compared with untreated controls, suggesting that the variability may be related to differences in the stress response to handling during drug administration. Spleen cell Con A-stimulated proliferation was reduced 5 days after sympathectomy in 17-month-old animals in the absence of significant changes in $CD5^+$ T cells, IL-2 production or IFN-γ production (see Table I). Desipramine pretreatment, preventing 6-OHDA uptake and subsequent sympathectomy, completely blocked the 6-OHDA-induced reduction in T cell proliferation, demonstrating that the decrease in proliferative response requires the destruction of NA nerve fibers. From 5 to 56 days after denervation, no sympathectomy-induced changes in Con A-induced T cell functions were found in old animals.

These results suggest that young rats can rapidly evoke compensatory mechanisms to maintain T lymphocyte activity following NE depletion. In old rats, sympathectomy-induced changes in T cell function are more readily apparent, indicating that compensatory mechanisms are limited. The transient reduction in T cell proliferation at day 5, a time point when NA innervation has not recovered, suggests that splenic NA innervation in old animals, though diminished, still exerts a positive regulatory influence on T cell function.

Sympathectomy followed by immunization with keyhole-limpet hemocyanen (KLH) (150 μg/rat, i.p.) increases serum IgM anti-KLH response in both young and old F344 rats (Figure 20). This effect is much greater in old rats (Figure 20B) than it is in young rats (Figure 20A). Sympathectomy also enhanced serum IgG anti-KLH response in old rats (Figure 21B), but not young animals (Figure 21A). The ability of splenocytes from KLH-immune animals to respond to KLH in vitro was assessed to examine whether proliferative

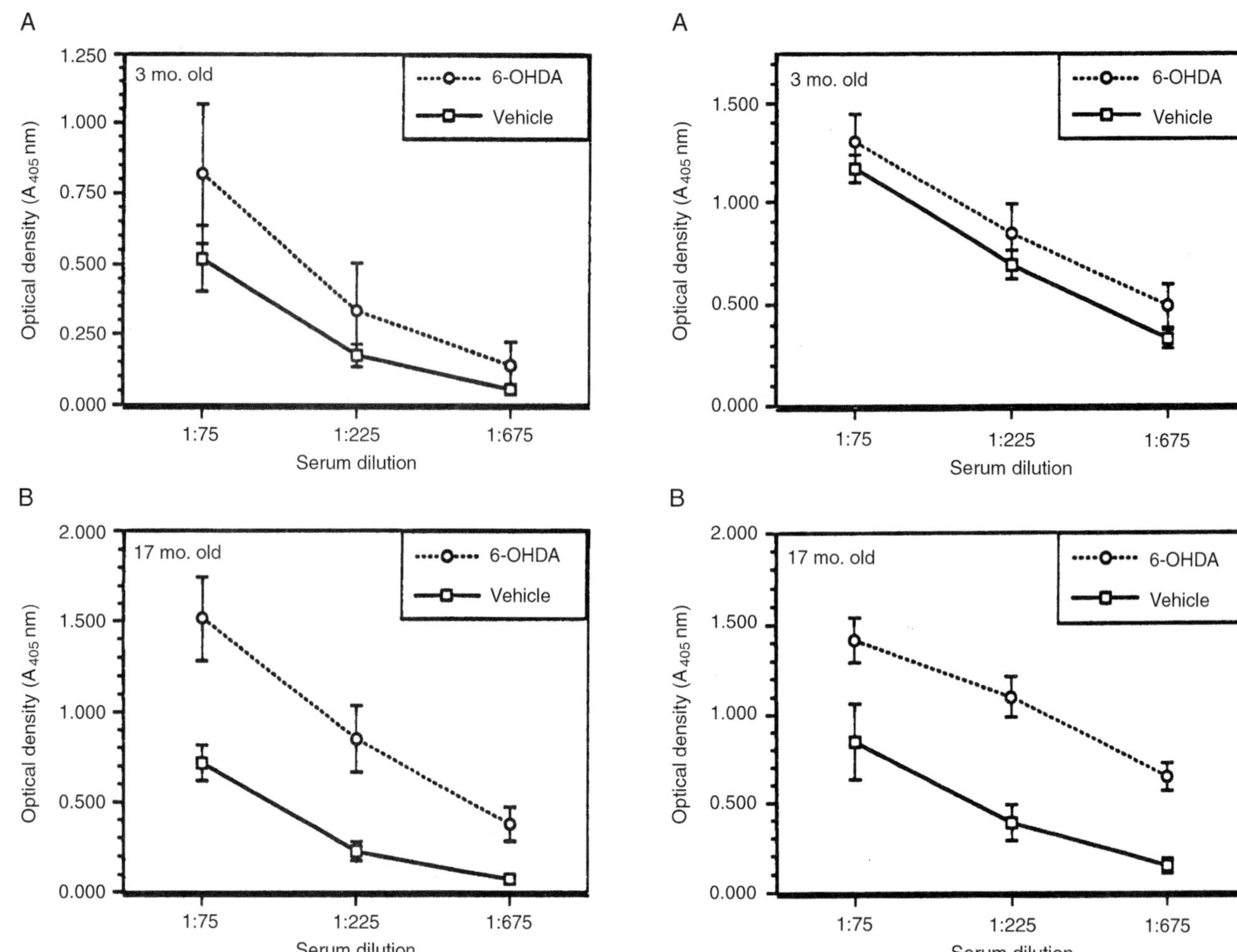

FIGURE 20 Serum IgM anti-KLH antibody response in 3-month-old (A) and 17-month-old (B) F344 rats is elevated in both young and old sympathectomized animals (open circle-dashed line) compared with vehicle-treated controls (open squares-solid line), that is more striking in old animals. Control or 6-OHDA-treated animals ($n = 6$–7 per treatment per age) were immunized with 150 μg KLH and bled 14 days later. Analysis of variance (ANOVA) was conducted with age and treatment as dependent variables. Serum dilution was treated as a repeated measure. There was a main effect of age and treatment ($p < -0.05$). (Taken from Madden et al., 1995.)

FIGURE 21 Serum IgG anti-KLH antibody response in 3-month-old (A) and 17-month-old (B) F344 rats is augmented in old sympathectomized animals compared with vehicle-treated old rats. Control or 6-OHDA-treated animals ($n = 6$–7 per treatment per age) were immunized with 150 μg KLH and bled 14 days later. ANOVA was conducted with age and treatment as dependent variables. If a significant main effect or interaction was identified ($p < 0.05$), post hoc analysis by Neuman-Keuls or simple effects, respectively, was used for comparison between groups. Serum dilution was treated as a repeated measure. There was a main effect of treatment and a treatment × age interaction. (Taken from Madden et al., 1995.)

responses to KLH were altered with sympathectomy. Sympathectomy enhances KLH-induced proliferation by spleen cells from young and old rats (greater effect in old) (Figure 22A and 22B), suggesting that antigen-specific T and B cell proliferation are altered by sympathectomy. Sympathectomy elevates Con A-induced T cell proliferation (Figure 23A) and lipopolysaccharide (LPS)/dextran sulfate (DxS)-stimulated B cell proliferation (Figure 23B) in 17-month-old, but not in 3-month-old immunized rats. Enhanced proliferation is not the result of enhanced IL-2 production (Figure 24), suggesting that other cytokines that regulate T cell proliferation may be responsible for this sympathectomy-induced enhancement. These changes also do not result from alterations in the proportions of T and B cells in the spleen, since the percentages of T and B cells do not change after sympathectomy in either age group (Figure 25). Collectively, these findings suggest that NA sympathetic innervation in aged rats, though diminished compared with young rats, is capable of modulating immune reactivity. Elevated antibody production and

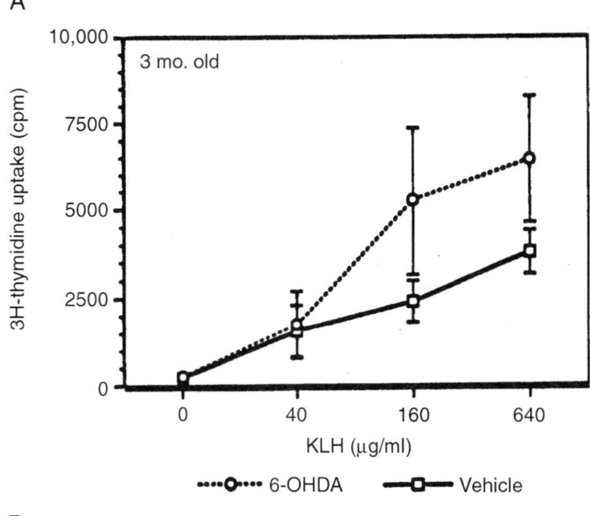

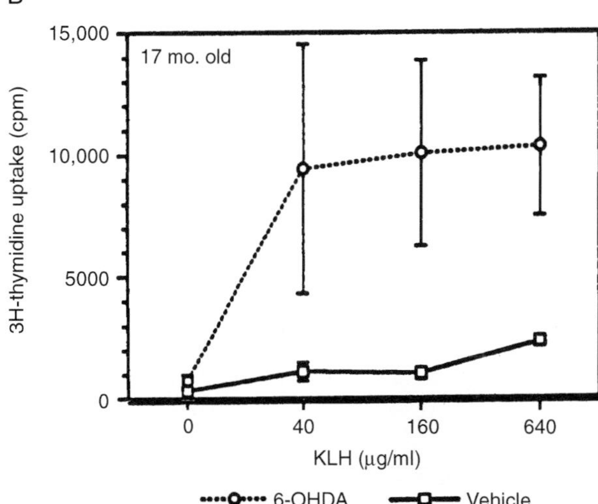

FIGURE 22 Sympathectomy increased KLH-induced proliferation in spleen cells from 3-month-old (A) and 17-month-old (B) F344 rats, an effect that was greater in old animals. Spleen cells were cultured with varying concentrations of KLH for 5 days. ANOVA was conducted with age and treatment as dependent variables. If a significant main effect or interaction was identified ($p < 0.05$), post hoc analysis by Neuman-Keuls or simple effects, respectively, was used for comparison between groups. KLH concentration was treated as a repeated measure. There was a significant main effect of treatment. (Taken from Madden et al., 1995.)

lymphocyte proliferation following sympathectomy suggests that in immunized rats, sympathetic innervation may provide an inhibitory signal to humoral responses.

When effects of sympathectomy are observed in young rats, the effects are qualitatively similar to that seen in old rats, although less dramatic, suggesting that immunomodulatory effects of the SNS are similar in young and old rats. It is likely that compensatory mechanisms after NA nerve loss are more robust in young spleens compared with old spleens. The

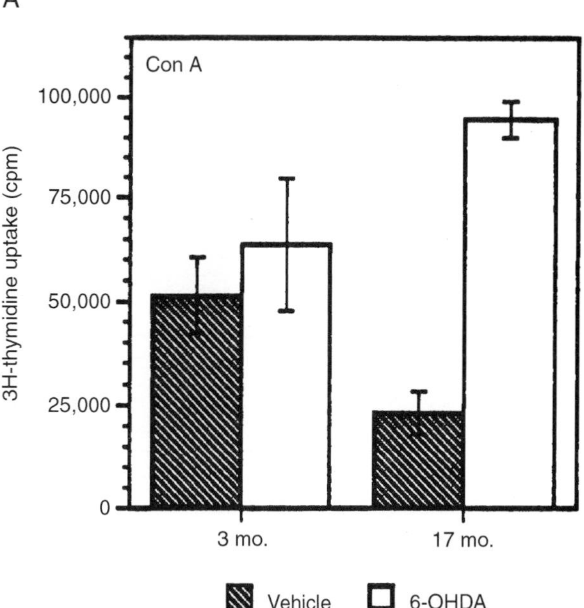

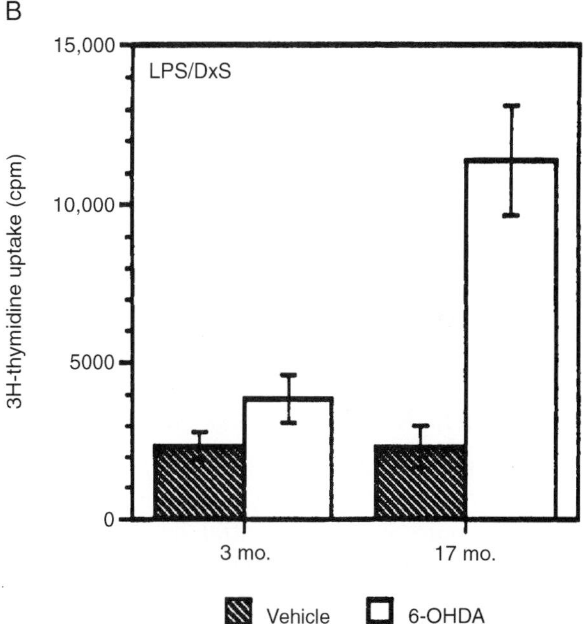

FIGURE 23 Mitogen-induced proliferation was examined in spleen cells cultured with 1.25 μg/mL Con A (A) or 5 μg/mL LPS + 5 μg/mL D × S (B) for 3 days. 6-OHDA treatment increases mitogen-induced T and B cell proliferation in only the 17-month-old animals. ANOVA was conducted with age and treatment as dependent variables. If a significant main effect or interaction was identified ($p < 0.05$), post hoc analysis by Neuman-Keuls or simple effects, respectively, was used for comparison between groups. Mitogen concentration was treated as a repeated measure. There was an age × treatment interaction for both mitogen responses. (Taken from Madden et al., 1995.)

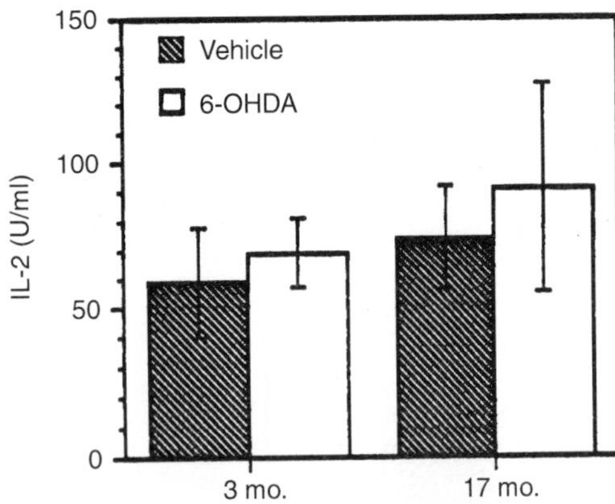

FIGURE 24 Con A-stimulated IL-2 production in spleen cells cultured with 1.25 μ/mL Con A was performed, and the supernatants harvested 24 h later to test for IL-2 activity using the IL-2-dependent cell line, CTLL. IL-2 production was not altered by sympathectomy regardless of age. ANOVA was conducted with age and treatment as dependent variables, but no significant main effect or interaction was identified ($p > 0.05$). (Taken from Madden et al., 1995.)

constant ratio of T or B cells suggest that sympathectomy-induced changes occur by mechanisms that directly alter the ability of lymphocytes to proliferate and/or produce antibody. In immunized rats, splenic T cell proliferation is decreased following sympathectomy, an effect that is directionally opposite to that seen in nonimmune rats and in immunized mice. These findings suggest that immunomodulatory effects of SNS may depend on a variety of factors, including activational state of the immune system, lymphoid microenvironment, and species.

D. Senescence in Mice

1. *Sympathetic Nerve Density and NE Content*

In spleens from 2-month-old BALB/c (Figure 26) and C57Bl/6J (Figure 30) mice, NA innervation enters the white pulp with the central arteriole and its branches (Madden et al., 1997). NA nerves extends into the surrounding PALS and marginal zone. At 12 months of age, histologically (Figures 27 and 31) and neurochemically (Figure 34) there is no change in splenic NA innervation. By 24 months of age, NE increase significantly (Figure 34), independent of changes in spleen weight. With advancing age, histochemical analysis reveals an increase in the density of NE-containing nerves in the parenchyma of the white pulp (Figures 28, 29, 32, and 33), especially near the hilus. More distal from the hilus NA innervation of the white pulp is variable, with some white pulp regions containing a density of nerve similar to that seen at 2 months of age, and other white pulp regions showing a depletion of NA nerves.

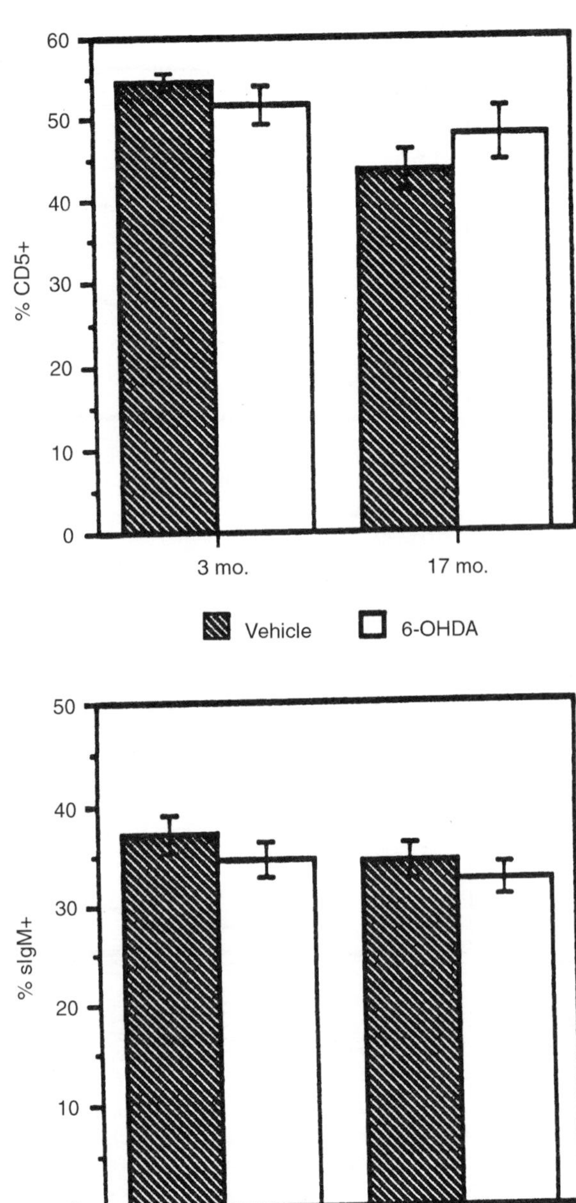

FIGURE 25 Percentage of $CD5^+$ T cells and $sIgM^+$ B cells. Sympathectomy did not alter the number of splenic T or B cells. ANOVA was conducted with age and treatment as dependent variables, but no significant main effect or interaction was identified ($p > 0.05$). (Taken from Madden et al., 1995.)

These findings indicate that overall NA innervation of the spleen is enhanced with advancing age. These observations are directionally opposite to the marked diminution in splenic NA innervation in old F344 rats.

We have extended our investigation up to 33 months of age in C57Bl/6 mice, and still find robust NA sympathetic innervation of the murine spleen

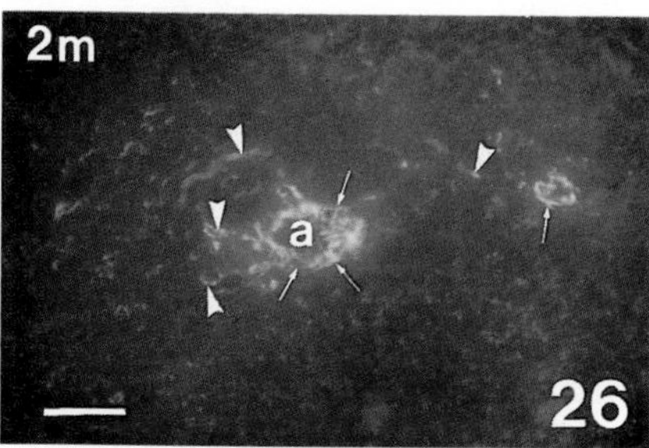

FIGURE 26 An abundance of NA sympathetic nerves travels along the central arteriole (a) (arrows), and as single, linear, varicose profiles (arrowheads) in the surrounding periarteriolar lymphatic sheath in the spleen of a 2-month-old (2m) BALB/c mouse. Glyoxylic acid-induced HF for CAs. X85. Calibration bar = 100 μm.

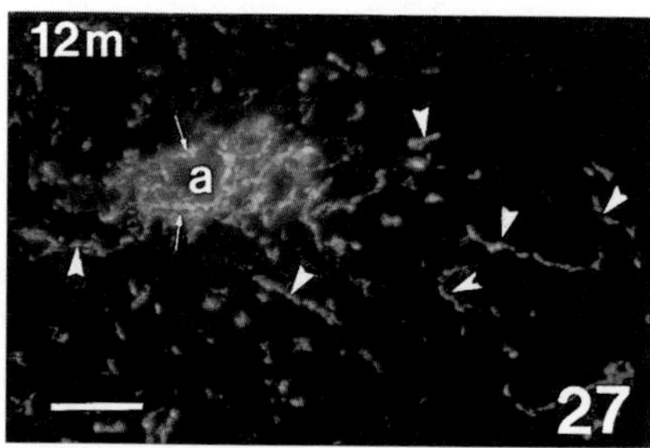

FIGURE 27 A dense plexus of NA sympathetic nerve fibers are intimate with the central arteriole (a) (arrows) in the white pulp of the spleen from a 12-month-old (12m) BALB/c mice. Long, linear, varicose, fluorescent profiles (arrowheads) radiate from this vascular plexus into the adjacent periarteriolar sheath in which T lymphocytes predominate. Glyoxylic acid-induced HF for CAs. X85. Calibration bar = 100 μm.

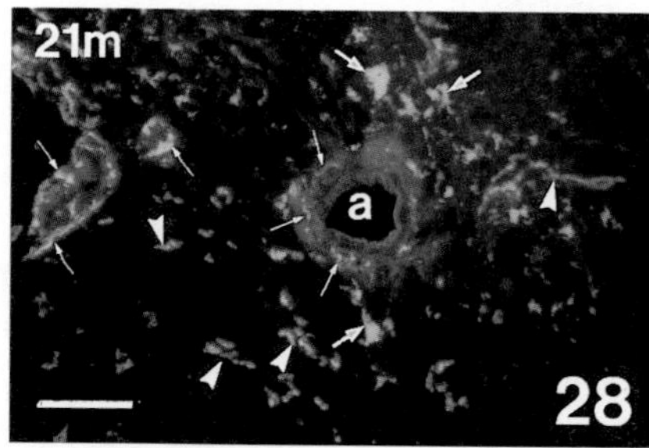

FIGURE 28 At 21 months of age (21m), NA sympathetic nerve fibers (small arrows) are still robust along the central arterioles (a) in the white pulp of the spleen from BALB/c mice; however, there is great variability in the density of nerve fibers in this compartment depending on there location relative to the hilus of the spleen. This photomicrograph demonstrates the density of NA innervation associated with the central arteriole that is distal to the hilus. At this age, abundant NA nerve fibers (arrowheads) and yellow autofluorescent cells (large arrows) are prominent in the periarteriolar lymphatic sheath. Glyoxylic acid-induced HF for CAs. X170. Calibration bar = 50 μm.

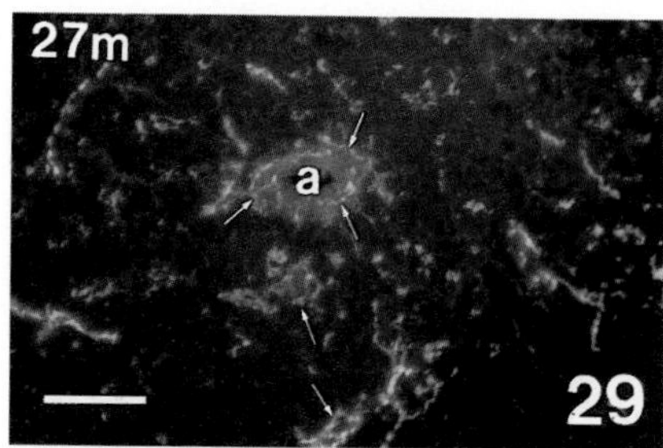

FIGURE 29 In 27-month-old BALB/c mice, the density of NA nerve plexuses (arrows) along the central arterioles (a) is remarkably robust, and the periarteriolar lymphatic sheath is well-innervated by NA nerve fibers (arrowheads). Glyoxylic acid-induced HF for CAs. X85. Calibration bar = 100 μm.

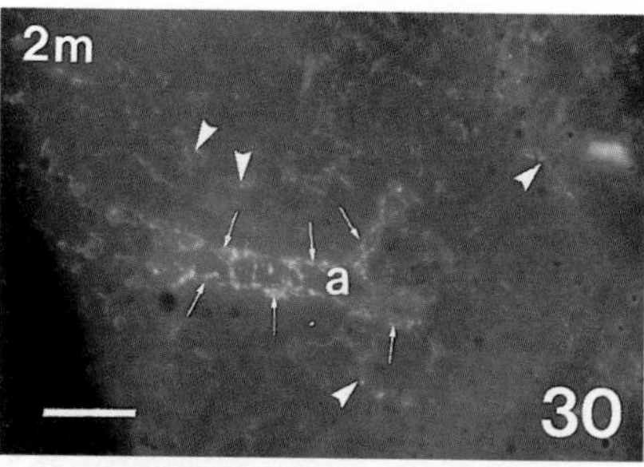

FIGURE 30 NA sympathetic nerve plexuses (arrows) course along a central arteriole cut in longitudinal section in a spleen from a 2-month-old (2m) C57Bl/6 mouse. Numerous NA nerve fibers also are seen in the surrounding periarteriolar lymphatic sheath. Glyoxylic acid-induced HF for CAs. X85. Calibration bar = 100 μm.

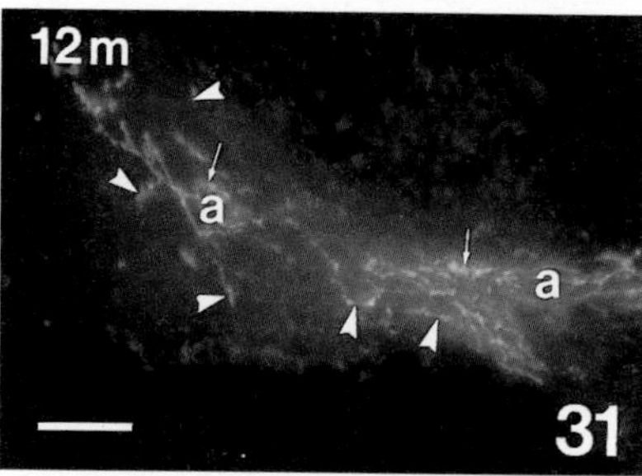

FIGURE 31 NA sympathetic innervation of the white pulp from a 12-month-old (12m) C57Bl/6 mouse is remarkably similar to that seen in mice at 2 months of age. An abundance of NA nerve fibers travel along the central arteriole (a) (arrows), and in the adjacent periarteriolar lymphatic sheath (arrowheads). Glyoxylic acid-induced HF for CAs. X85. Calibration bar = 100 μm.

(Figure 33). The variable density of NA nerves in white pulp regions distal to the hilus suggest that there may be, at least to some limited extent, some loss of NA nerves in these sites with possible reorganization of these lymphoid areas. The enhanced splenic NE concentration in spleens from old mice, despite the possible loss of some NA nerves, raises the additional possibility that NE metabolism is altered in spleens from these aging mouse strains.

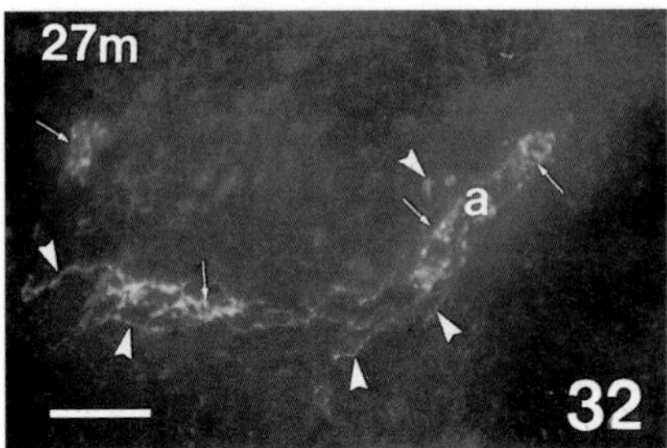

FIGURE 32 At 27 months of age (27m), the white pulp of spleens from C57Bl/6 mice receive a dense population of NA sympathetic nerves that course with the central arteriole (a) (arrows), and extend from this plexus into the periarteriolar lymphatic sheath among fields of T lymphocytes (arrowheads). Glyoxylic acid-induced HF for CAs. X85. Calibration bar = 100 μm.

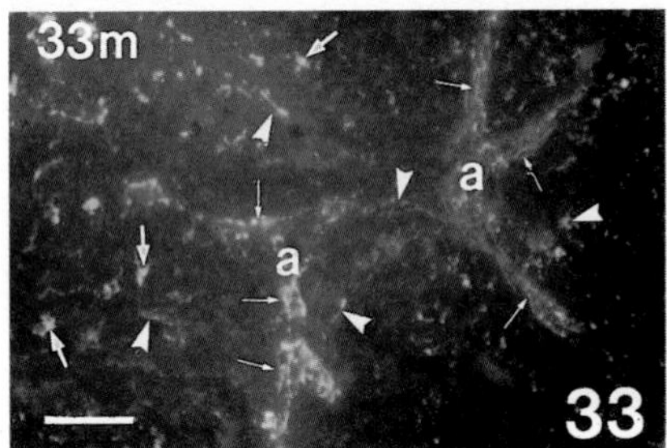

FIGURE 33 Even at the age of 33 months (33m), NA sympathetic innervation remains robust, with a dense nerve plexus (small arrows) along the central arteriole (a), and individual nerve fibers (arrowheads) coursing in the white pulp. The density of yellow autofluorescent cells (large arrows) also is increased by 33 months of age. Glyoxylic acid-induced HF for CAs. X85. Calibration bar = 100 μm.

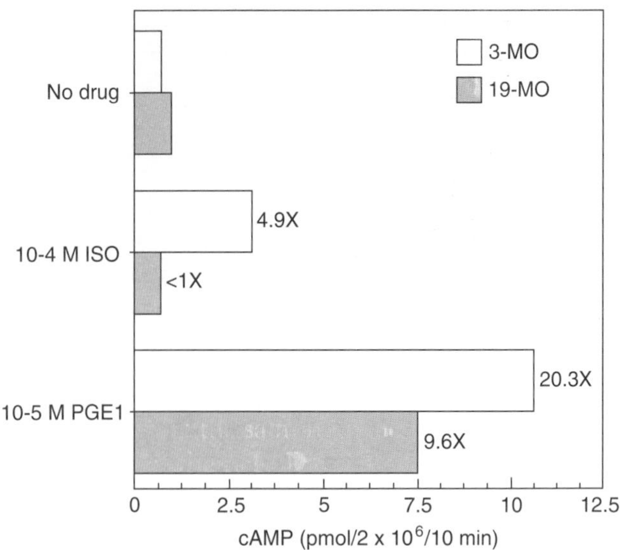

FIGURE 34 cAMP generation in splenocytes (expressed as pmol/10^6 cells) from 3- (3-MO) and 19-month-old (19-MO) BALB/c mice was measured in control wells (no drug), and after β-adrenoceptor stimulation with 10^{-4} M isoproterenol or 10^{-5} M prostaglandin E_1 (PGE_1) (which also uses cAMP as its second messenger). Addition of 10^{-4} M ISO to the medium caused a 4.9-fold increase in cAMP concentration in splenocytes from 3-month-old mice above no drug concentrations, but only a slight (1-fold) increase in splenocytes from old mice. cAMP generation also is blunted in spleen cells from 19-month-old mice stimulated with PGE_1 compared with young adult control values.

We also have studied the influence of age on NA sympathetic innervation of spleens from several autoimmune strains of mice. With the normal aging process, the density and intensity of fluorescence in NA nerves diminishes in spleens from NZB, NZW, and NZBW mice; however, the time course of decline varies with each strain (Bellinger, Ackerman et al., 1989). In spleens from NZW mice, NA innervation is maintained through 10 weeks of age. By 17 to 18 months of age, NA innervation is markedly reduced in all compartments of the spleen. The remaining NA nerves distribute in the same compartments as seen in young adult NZW mice, but a gradient exist, such that a higher density of nerves is present close to the hilar region and the density progressively declines with distance from the hilus. The size of the white pulp is diminished in the aged spleen, and often is difficult to delineate clearly from the red pulp. Progressive loss of NA nerves in the spleen continues through 24 months of age. In NZB mice loss of NA innervation of the spleen is accelerated compared with NZW mice. It is evident by 4 months of age and continues to decline through 10 months of age, at which time only an occasional faintly fluorescing profile remains in the white pulp; in sites distal from the hilus no NA fibers could be detected. NA innervation of spleens from NZBW mice shows a course of age-associated loss in the density of nerve fibers that is more slowly progressing than in the other two strains. A slight loss of NA nerves is apparent in spleens from 17 to 18-month-old NZBW mice, but clearly not to the extent that occurs by this age in spleens from NZB mice. By 35 months of age the hilar-to-distal gradient loss of NA fibers is prominent in NZBW spleens.

The MRL-lpr/lpr (lpr) mouse is a murine model for systemic lupus erythematosus (Andrew et al., 1978). Both the lpr and the congenic MRL-+/+ (+/+) mice develop autoimmune disease; the presence of the lpr gene profoundly accelerates disease progression. In lpr mice, splenomegaly, an indicator of disease, is apparent by 12 weeks of age. Splenomegaly does not occur in +/+ mice. Histofluorescence for localizing catecholamines reveals an age-associated reduction in the density of NA nerves and reduced fluorescence intensity in age-resistant nerves in spleens from lpr mice compared with +/+ mice in which the density and fluorescent intensity appears to remain constant (Breneman, Moynihan, Grota, Felten, & Felten, 1993).

By 24 weeks of age, virtually no detectable fluorescence is found in spleens from lpr mice. At this time point, there is generally 50% mortality in populations of lpr mice resulting from renal failure and vasculitis (Theofilopoulos & Dixon, 1985). The NE concentration in spleens (pmol NE/g wet weight) from lpr mice is significantly lower than the NE concentration in age-matched +/+ mice at every time point. The magnitude of these differences increases with advancing age, because the NE concentration in spleens of lpr and +/+ mice decreases and increases over time, respectively. Because the spleen weight increases dramatically in lpr mice as the disease progresses, total splenic NE may be more representative of differences between the two strains. Total splenic NE is significantly less in spleens from lpr mice compared with age-matched, +/+ mice. In addition, there is no change in the whole spleen NE content, whereas there is a progressive increase in NE in whole spleen from +/+ mice.

Collectively, these studies indicate an age-related denervation of the spleen in all autoimmune strains of mice thus far examined. Furthermore, the time course of this decline in innervation correlates with the general life span of each strain, and with the time of onset of the autoimmune disease. Besedovsky and colleagues (del Rey, Besedovsky, Sorkin, Da Prada, & Arrenbrecht, 1981) have reported that the basal NE concentration in the spleen is inversely related to immunological activity. After immunologic challenge, NE concentrations decrease, which has been attributed to an increase in NE turnover (Besedovsky, del Rey, Sorkin, Da Prada, & Keller, 1979). Additionally, the magnitude of change in splenic NE concentration is proportional to the magnitude of the immune response (del Rey, Besedovsky, Sorkin, Da Prada, & Bondiolotti, 1982). If this is indeed the case, then one explanation for the decline in NA innervation is the enhanced immunological activity in autoimmune animals that increases sympathetic activity. Such chronic activation of sympathetic outflow to the spleen may promote damage to nerve terminals from an increase in neurotoxic oxidative metabolites that occurs with the higher activity level (Felten, Felten, Steece-Collier, Date, & Clemens, 1992). Other factors that may be important in determining the fate of NA sympathetic nerves in the aging mouse spleen include changes in the splenic microenvironment, production of autoantibodies that target sympathetic neurons, and differences in genetic programming.

Lastly, loss of NA sympathetic nerves with disease progression may be an inherent protective mechanism to slow disease progression. Conversely, it is possible that reduction in NA innervation of the spleen contributes to the onset and progression of autoimmune disease. The role of catecholamines in the course and severity of autoimmune disease has been examined by several laboratories. Colburn et al. (1990) reported that administration of isoproterenol promotes increased anti-DNA antibody titers in MRL-lpr/lpr mice, a measure often used an index of disease severity. On the other hand, in the Lewis rat model of induced autoimmune demyelination, experimental allergic encephalitis (EAE), Chelmicka-Schorr et al. (Chelmicka-Schorr, Kwasniewski, Thomas, & Arnason, 1989) found that propranolol, a β-adrenergic antagonist, increases the severity of disease and susceptibility of Lewis rats to EAE, whereas administration of isoproterenol, a β-adrenergic agonist, decreases susceptibility and disease severity. In the Lewis rat model for rheumatoid arthritis, systemic chemical sympathectomy, or β-antagonist administration, attenuates joint pain and inflammation (Levine, Coderre, Helms, & Basbaum, 1988; Levine, Dardick, Basbaum, & Scipio, 1985). However, we have found that local sympathectomy of lymphoid tissue that drains relevant antigen important in the initiation of disease exacerbates the severity and onset of arthritis (Lorton, Bellinger, Duclos, Felten, & Felten, 1996). As is the case with the autoimmune mice, NA innervation of the spleen is diminished as the disease progresses in Lewis rats given complete Freund's adjuvant to induce experimental arthritis (Lorton, Lubahn, Felten, & Bellinger, 1997). In summary, it appears that NE may play different roles in induced and genetic autoimmune models, or in the progression and severity of autoimmune disease in different strains of rodents.

2. *β-Adrenoceptor Function on Murine Splenocytes with Aging*

Unfractionated splenocytes from young adult BALB/c mice incubated with 10^{-4} M isoproterenol, a β-adrenoceptor agonist, are capable of generating cAMP. This response is significantly reduced in splenocytes from old mice (Figure 34), suggesting that old splenocytes are less responsive to NA signaling. There also is a slight age-related reduction in cAMP production in unfractionated splenocytes stimulated with prostaglandin E_1 (10^{-5} M) (Figure 34), suggesting that signaling through other receptors that couple with adenylate cyclase may be impaired with aging. Reduced cAMP production could result from uncoupling of β-adrenoceptors from G_s protein or from decreased or impaired adenylate cyclase activity. In support of this hypothesis, the agonist affinity and the high affinity state of agonist-β-adrenoceptor-G_s protein complex are decreased in several tissues, including heart (Scarpace & Abrass, 1986), lung (Scarpace, 1986), peripheral blood lymphocytes (Montamant & Davies, 1989), parotid gland (Miyamato, Kowatch, & Roth, 1993), and vascular smooth muscle (Briggs & Lefkowitz, 1980) with normal aging. In the aging heart, there is evidence that β-adrenoceptors uncouple from G_s proteins, making them less able to form the active ternary complex, resulting in impaired signal transduction (Briggs & Lefkowitz, 1980; Miyamoto, Kawana, Kimura, & Ohskika, 1994). One mechanism that has been suggested to account for this phenomenon is decreased membrane fluidity with age, interfering with the β-adrenoceptor-G_s protein interaction (Benedetti, Ferretti, Curatola, Jezequel, & Orlandi, 1988; Briggs & Lefkowitz, 1980; Caldirini, Bonetti, Battistella, Crews, & Toffano, 1983; Jagadeesh, Tian, Gupta, & Deth, 1990; Orly & Schramm, 1975; Petkova, Momchilova, & Koumanov, 1986; Rasenick, Stein, & Bitensky, 1981; Rimon, Hanski, Braun, & Levitzki, 1978). Bypassing the receptor complex by directly activating adenylyl cyclase with forskolin often restores age-related changes in cAMP-mediated functions (Tsujimoto, Lee, & Hoffman, 1986; Vacca et al., 1992). Chronically high concentrations of NE, as seen in the old C57Bl/6 and BALB/c mouse spleen (Madden et al., 1997), as well as in the rodent thymus, may be contributory to impaired β-adrenoceptor signal transduction in splenocytes (Collins, 1993; Hausdorff, Caron, & Lefkowitz, 1990).

3. *Aging and Sympathetic Influence on Immune Function in Mice*

Functional studies with splenocytes from chemical sympathectomized young and old BALB/c and C56Bl/6 mice in our laboratories are preliminary, but have revealed striking differences in how old mice respond to chemical sympathectomy with 6-OHDA (Figures 35–42). Sympathectomy reduces KLH anti-

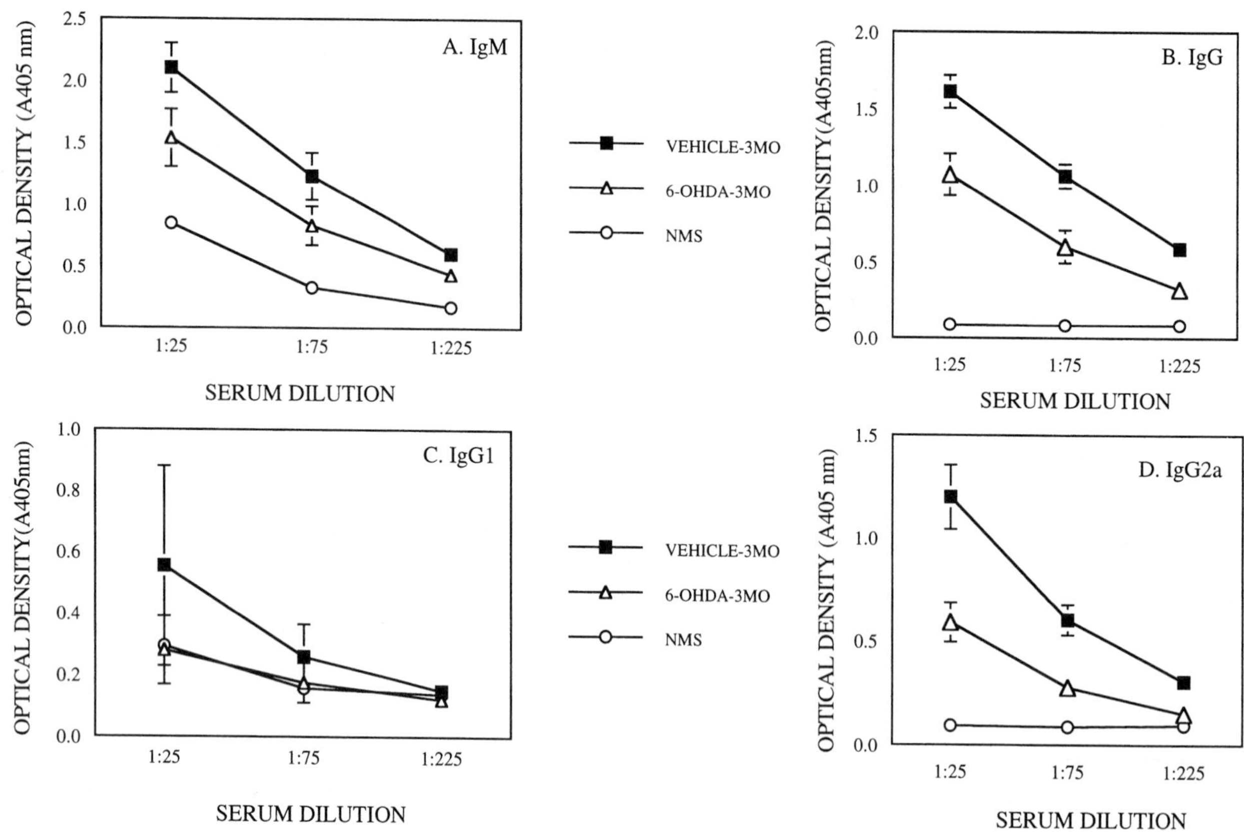

FIGURE 35 Serum anti-KLH antibody response in 3-month-old BALB/c mice: (A) IgM; (B) IgG; (C) IgG_1; and (D) IgG_{2a}. 6-OHDA treatment reduces anti-KLH antibody response (IgM, IgG, IgG_1, and IgG_{2a}) in young mice. Mice were sympathectomized on day 0. Two days later, animals were immunized with 100 μg KLH, i.p. Six days after immunization, animals were bled, and serum anti-KLH titers were determined by enzyme-linked immunoabsorbent assay (ELISA). An $n = 6$-7 per treatment per age was used for this experiment. Vehicle treatment, solid squares; 6-OHDA treatment, open triangles; normal mouse serum (NMS), open circles.

body response (IgM, IgG, IgG_1, and IgG_{2a}) in young BALB/c mice 6 days after immunization with KLH (Figure 35). KLH-induced proliferation in splenocytes from young sympathectomized BALB/c mice is enhanced 6 days after challenge (Figure 39A). These sympathectomy-induced effects are not likely to be due to changes in T cell migration, since there are no changes in the percentages of $CD4^+$ or $CD8^+$ T cells in spleens from sympathectomized mice (Figure 41A). The percentages of naive and memory $CD4^+$ and $CD8^+$ T cells also are not altered by chemical sympathectomy, although changes in the density of naive and memory T cells do occur with age (Figure 42A and 42C). Sympathectomy-induced changes in antibody response, however, may result from increases in IL-2 (Figure 40A), IL-4 (Figure 40E), and IFN-γ (Figure 40 C) production. Our data showing the effects of chemical sympathectomy on primary antibody response in young BALB/c mice are consistent with previous reports by Kruszewska and colleagues (Kruszewska, Felten, & Moynihan, 1995; Kruszewska, Felten, Stevens, & Moynihan, 1998). Sympathectomy-induced effects that are seen in young BALB/c mice do not occur in old sympathectomized, immunized mice; there are no significant effects of sympathectomy on KLH-induced immune parameters, (Figures 36, 39A), even though there are changes in cytokine production (increased IL-2 at 24 and 48 hours and increased IFN-γ 72 hours after incubation with Con A).

In contrast, no effects of chemical sympathectomy on KLH antibody response (Figure 37 and 38) or KLH-induced proliferation (Figure 39) were observed in either young (Figure 37 and 39), as previously reported by Kruszewska et al. (Kruszewska et al., 1995; 1998), or old (Figure 38 and 39) C57Bl/6 mice. However, there was an increase in IL-4 production in young, sympathectomized animals (Figure 43), an effect not seen in old, denervated mice (Figure 40F). There were no effects of sympathectomy on the

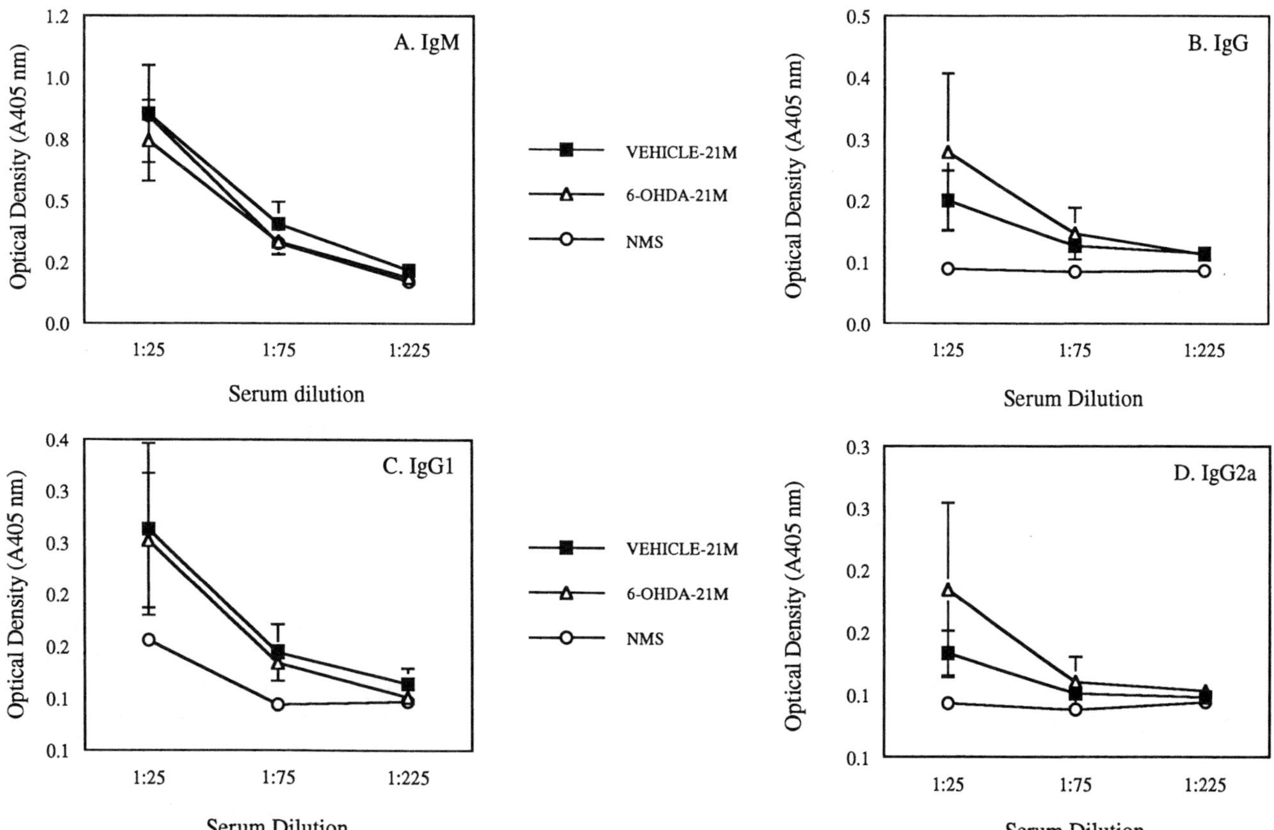

FIGURE 36 Serum anti-KLH antibody response in 21-month-old BALB/c mice: (A) IgM; (B) IgG; (C) IgG_1; and (D) IgG_{2a}. Sympathectomy does not alter anti-KLH antibody response in old mice. Mice were sympathectomized on day 0. Two days later, animals were immunized with 100 μg KLH, i.p. Six days after immunization, animals were bled, and serum anti-KLH titers were determined by ELISA. An $n = 6$-7 per treatment per age was used for this experiment. Vehicle treatment, solid squares; 6-OHDA treatment, open triangles; normal mouse serum (NMS), open circles.

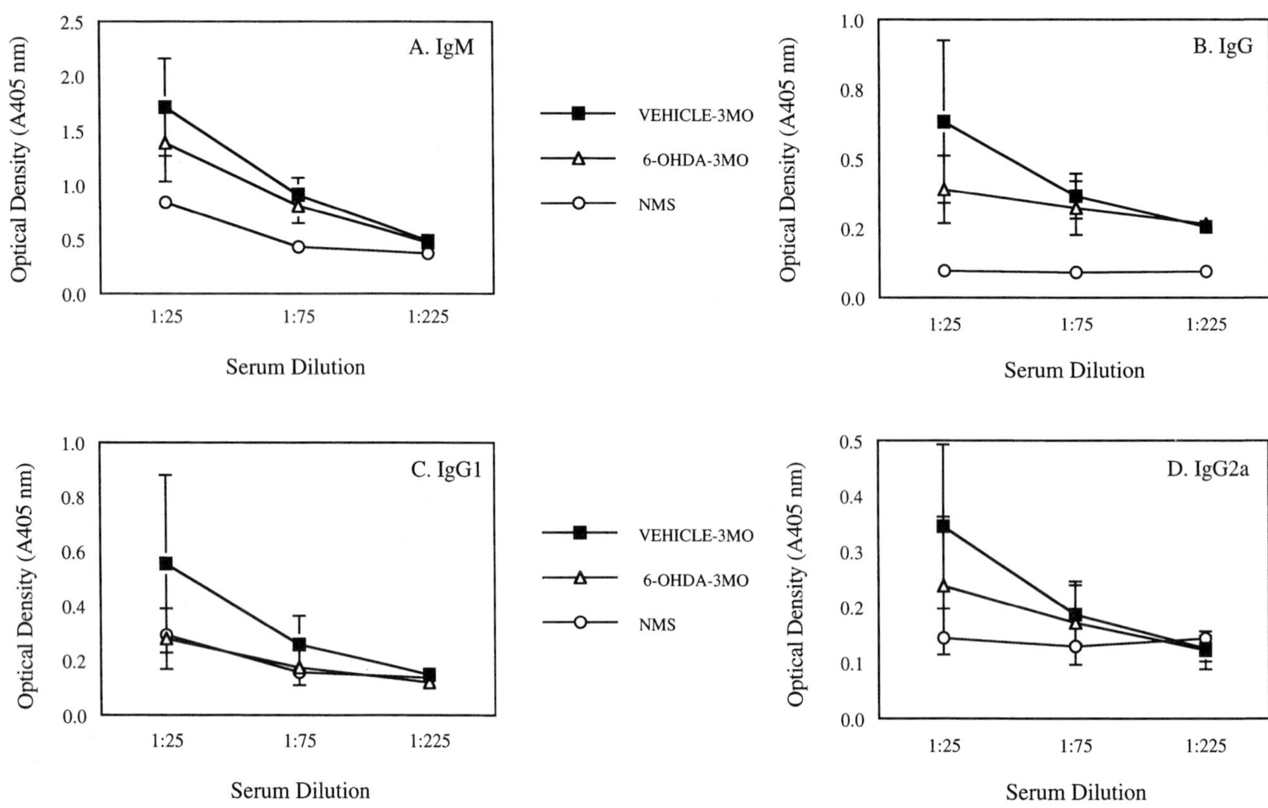

FIGURE 37 Serum anti-KLH antibody response in 3-month-old C57Bl/6 mice: (A) IgM; (B) IgG; (C) IgG_1; and (D) IgG_{2a}. 6-OHDA treatment has no effect on anti-KLH antibody response (IgM, IgG, IgG_1, and IgG_{2a}) in young mice. Mice were sympathectomized on day 0. Two days later, animals were immunized with 100 μg KLH, i.p. Six days after immunization, animals were bled, and serum anti-KLH titers were determined by ELISA. An $n = 6$–7 per treatment per age was used for this experiment. Vehicle treatment, solid squares; 6-OHDA treatment, open triangles; normal mouse serum (NMS), open circles.

percentages of $CD4^+$ or $CD8^+$ T lymphocytes, or in the percentages of $CD4^+$ or $CD8^+$ naive and memory T cells from young or old C57Bl/6 mice (Figure 42B and 42D). At the time these immune measures were made, chemical sympathectomy depleted splenic NE concentrations by approximately 63% in BALB/c mice and 79% in C57Bl/6 mice, regardless of age. Serum anti-KLH antibody titers are significantly lower in old compared with young BALB/c and C57Bl/6 mice; 6-OHDA treatment had no effect on this measure. Collectively, our functional data are consistent with our cAMP data, showing a severely blunted response in cAMP generation in splenocytes from old BALB/c mice.

E. Senescence in Other Strains of Rats

Because we did not find a dramatic age-related decline in NA sympathetic innervation in the spleen from strains of mice that do not develop autoimmune disease, we have examined several other strains of aging rats to determine whether the aging changes we have reported in F344 rats are selective for this strain or whether such changes occur across rat strains. In Brown-Norway (Figures 43 and 44) and Brown-Norway X F344 (F_1) (Figure 45) rats, age-related changes in NA sympathetic innervation of the spleen is similar to the alterations described in aging spleens from C57Bl/6 and BALB/c mice. Neurochemistry for NE has revealed an increase in splenic NE content in 21-month-old rats from both strains of approximately 15 to 20%. NA nerves in white pulps course along the central arteriole, into the PALS, and marginal zones, with an apparent hyperinnervation of white pulps in the hilar regions, and variable density of nerves in white pulps distal to the hilus. Conversely, the profile of age-related changes in NA sympathetic innervation of spleens from Lewis rats (Figure 46) is similar to that described in spleens from F344 rats (Figure 47). The loss of NA nerves in spleens from Lewis rats is apparent by 17 months of age, with splenic NE content reduced to approximately 50 to 60% in 24-month-old spleens compared with that seen in spleens from 3-month-old animals. These findings suggest that

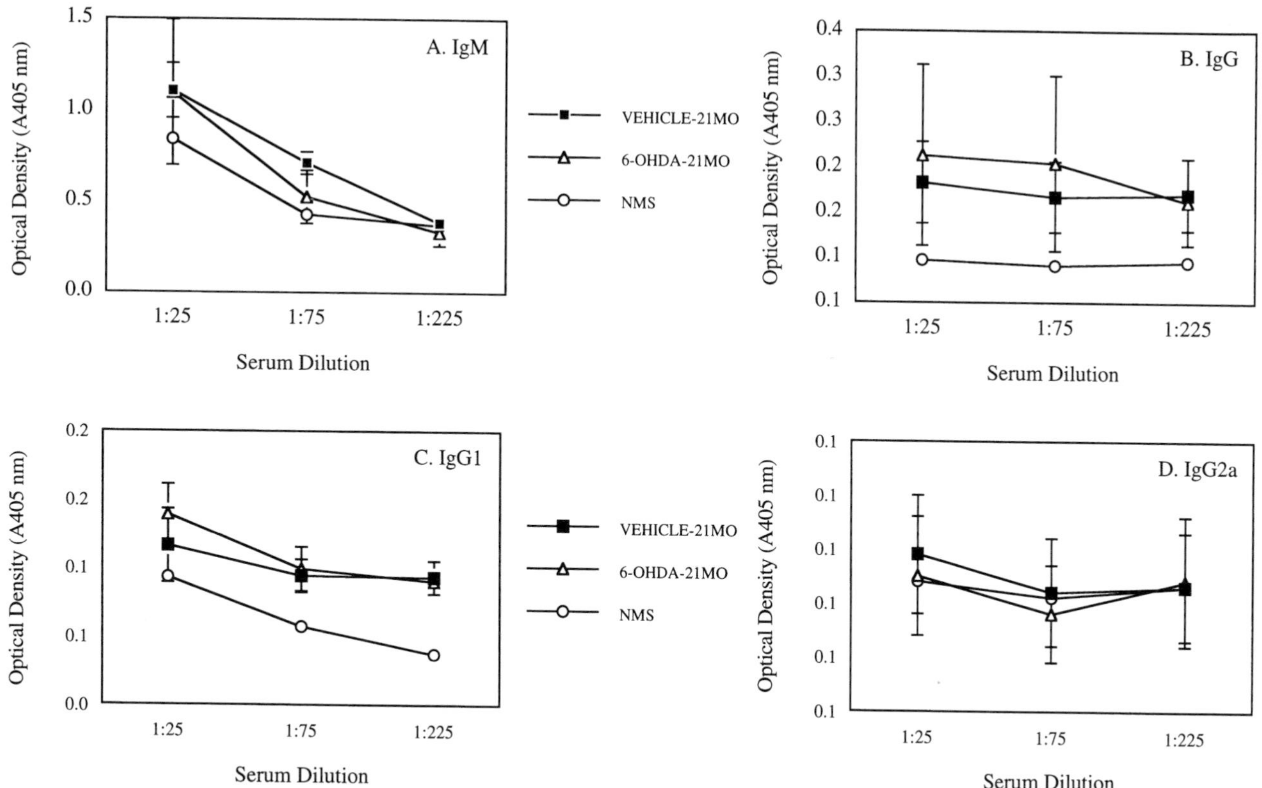

FIGURE 38 Serum anti-KLH antibody response in 21-month-old C57Bl/6 mice: (A) IgM; (B) IgG; (C) IgG_1; and (D) IgG_{2a}. 6-OHDA treatment has no effect on anti-KLH antibody response (IgM, IgG, IgG_1, and IgG_{2a}) in old mice. Mice were sympathectomized on day 0. Two days later, animals were immunized with 100 μg KLH, i.p. Six days after immunization, animals were bled, and serum anti-KLH titers were determined by ELISA. An $n = 6–7$ per treatment per age was used for this experiment. Vehicle treatment, solid squares; 6-OHDA treatment, open triangles; normal mouse serum (NMS), open circles.

age-related changes in sympathetic innervation of the spleen is species- and strain-dependent.

We have described several scenarios for age-related changes in NA innervation of the secondary lymphoid tissues. In scenario one, there is substantial loss of sympathetic nerves and NE content. In spite of these dramatic changes, splenocytes remain responsive to sympathetic stimulation, and appear to be more sensitive to NE signals. This progression is seen in the spleen of aging F344 rats. In scenario two, NA nerves remodel, with hyperinnervation of hilar lymphoid tissue and variable innervation of distal lymphoid tissue, associated with an increase in NE content. Splenocytes from spleens with this pattern of innervation generate substantially less cAMP in the presence of NA agonists, and splenocytes are functionally unresponsive to manipulation of sympathetic nerves in scenario two. It is not known how aging influences sympathetic innervation of the human spleen, or the consequences of altered innervation on immune function. However, it is conceivable that both scenarios of NA nerve remodeling with advancing age and the age-related decline in immune function could occur in humans concurrently. This awaits further investigation.

In autoimmune-prone mice and rats, we generally find a decline in sympathetic innervation, and from functional studies using chemical sympathectomy it appears that the immune system is still capable of responding to sympathetic signals. However, this pattern of sympathetic aging is not unique to autoimmune-prone animals, since sympathetic innervation of spleens from F344 rats also show declining NA innervation with age; this strain is relatively resistant to induced autoimmune reactivity. Differences in age-related changes in NA innervation are likely to reflect microenvironmental differences that occur in spleens from different strains and species, factors important in determining the fate of NA nerve fibers in the spleen. Perhaps a factor as straight-forward as heightened capacity for anti-oxidant protection of NE-derived oxidative derivatives would be sufficient to prevent the age-related loss of NA nerve fibers by auto-oxidative destruction.

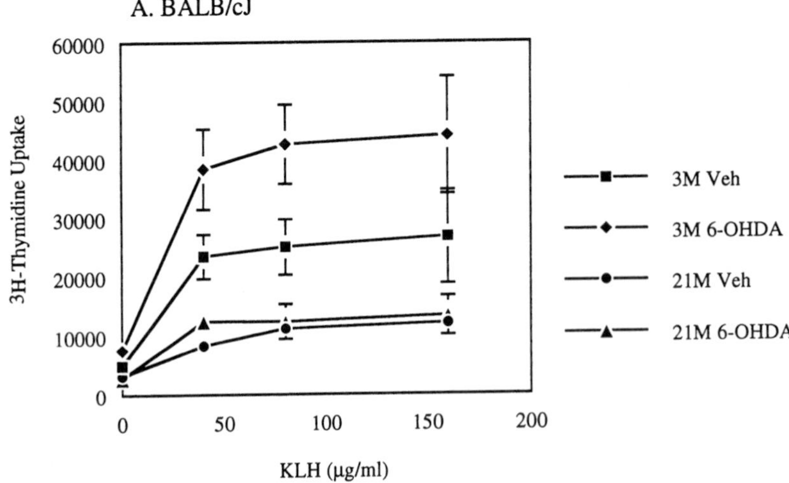

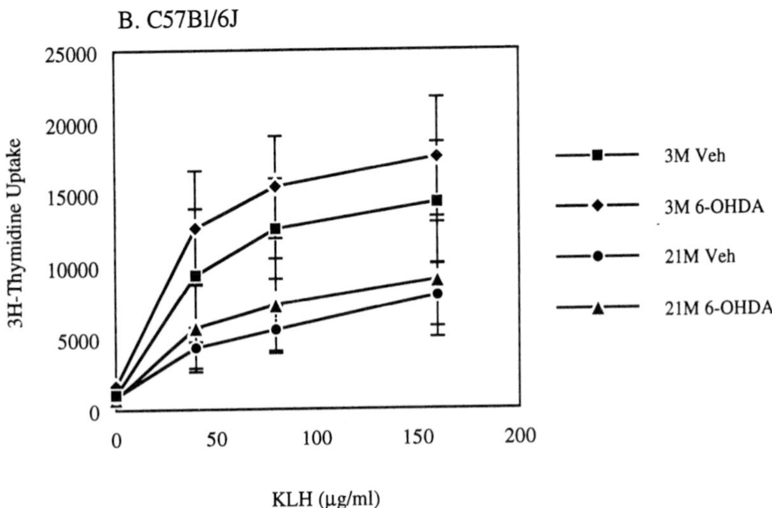

FIGURE 39 KLH-induced proliferation in 3- and 24-month-old BALB/c (A) and C57Bl/6 (B) mice. Proliferation was reduced in old BALB/c and C57Bl/6 mice. Sympathectomy enhanced KLH-induced proliferation in young BALB/c mice, an effect that was not seen in old BALB/c or C57Bl/6 mice. Mice were sympathectomized on day 0. Two days later, animals were immunized with 100 μg KLH, i.p. Six days after immunization, animals were bled, and serum anti-KLH titers were determined by ELISA. An $n = 6$–7 per treatment per age was used for this experiment. 3M, 3 months of age; 21M, 21 months of age; Veh, vehicle treatment; 6-OHDA, 6-OHDA treatment.

F. Age-Related Changes in Peptidergic-Specific Nerves

Age-associated changes in peptidergic nerves in the spleen have not been examined extensively. We have examined the effect of age on NPY^+ (Figures 48–57) and SP^+ (Figures 58–65) innervation of the spleen in F344 rats (Bellinger, Lorton, Felten, & Felten, 1989). Similar aging changes occur for NPY^+ innervation of the F344 rat spleen (D. Felten, Bellinger, & Felten, 1989), in regard to density and distribution of nerves that is seen for NA sympathetic nerves. There is an age-related decline in the density of nerve fibers (and staining intensity) that is apparent by 17 months of age and continue with advancing age (Figures 48–51). The decline in NPY nerve density also parallels the loss of T cells in the PALS (Figures 52 and 53), and the loss of $ED3^+$ macrophages in the marginal zones (Figures 54 and 55). IgM^+ B cell density appears to be unaffected by aging, but there are fewer NPY+ nerve fibers are B cell compartments of the aged F344 rat spleen (Figures 56 and 57). Neurochemical measurement of NPY is not

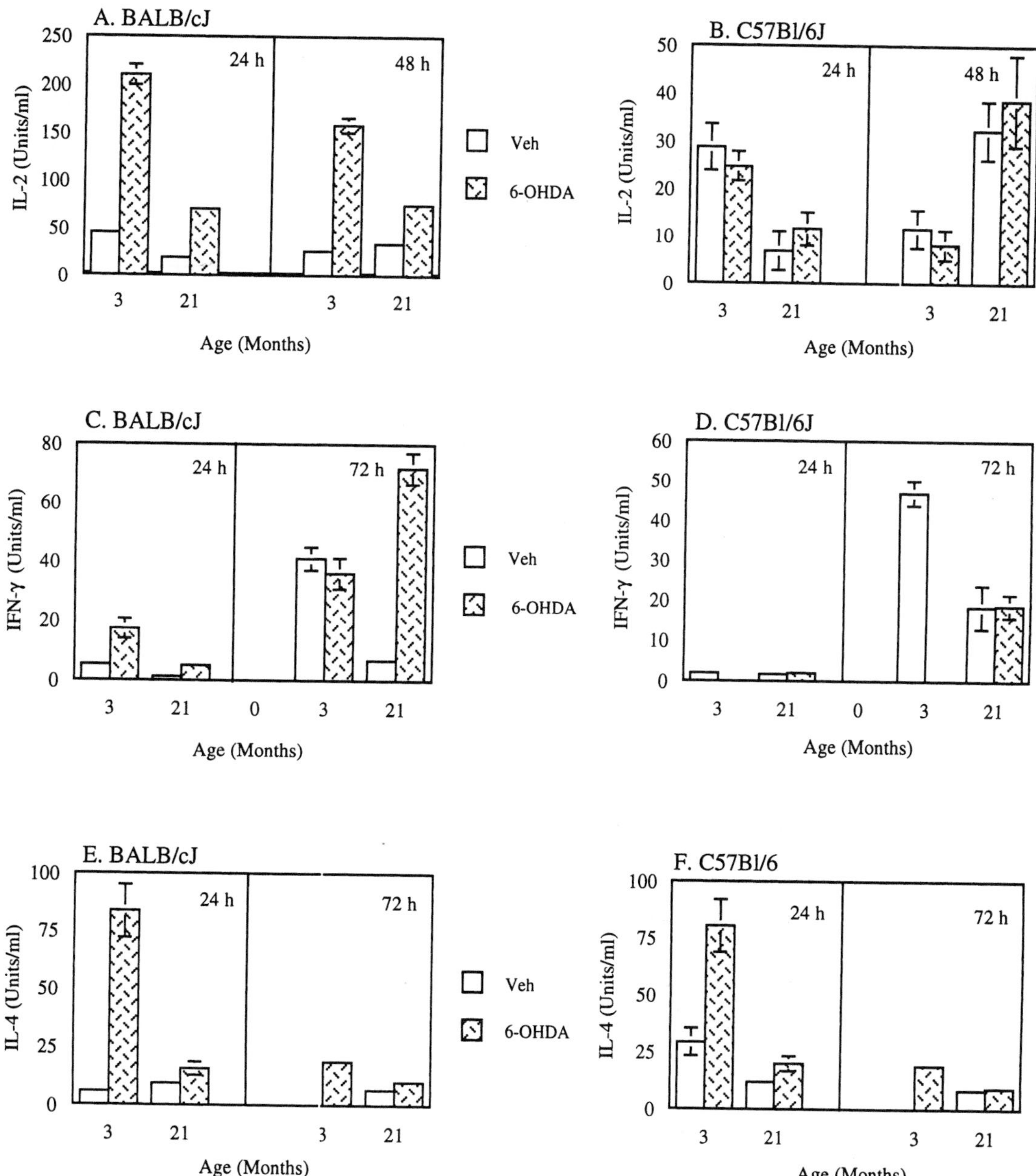

FIGURE 40 Cytokine production in 2- and 21-month-old BALB/c and C57Bl/6 mice: (A, B) IL-2; (C, D) IFN-γ; and (E, F) IL-4. Cytokine levels were measured 24 or 48 h after incubation with 1.25 μg/mL Con A. Mice were sympathectomized on day 0. Two days later, animals were immunized with 100 μg KLH, i.p. Six days after immunization, animals were bled, and serum anti-KLH titers were determined by ELISA. An $n = 6$–7 per treatment per age was used for this experiment. Veh, vehicle treatment; 6-OHDA, 6-OHDA treatment.

useful in these studies, because a large amount of NPY in the spleen occurs in platelets, megakaryocytes, and other cell types (Ericsson et al., 1987), obscuring any changes in NPY in neural compartments.

The paucity of SP$^+$ nerves in the rat makes it somewhat difficult to assess changes in the density of these nerves with aging. However, our impression from examining SP$^+$ stained sections in spleens from rats at 3, 8, 12, 17, 21, and 27 months of age is that the density of SP$^+$ nerves to aging spleen is relatively unaltered by advancing age (Figures 58–65). One of the most striking features in SP$^+$ innervation of the spleen in old animals is an apparent increase in the frequency of SP$^+$ nerves that course in the inner and outer white pulp as single fibers (Figures 64 and 65), and along smaller vasculature in the inner white pulp

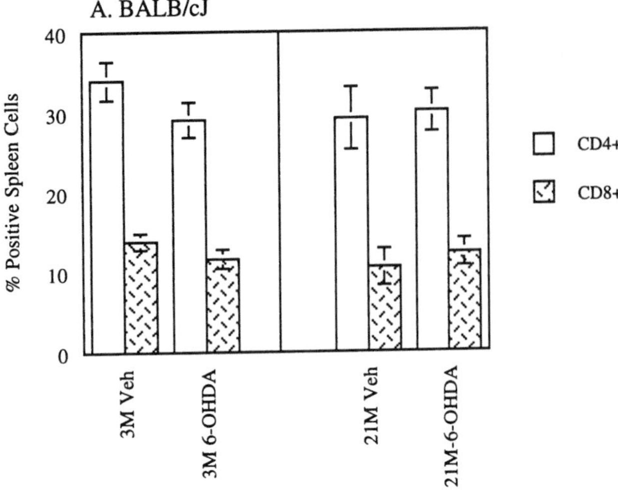

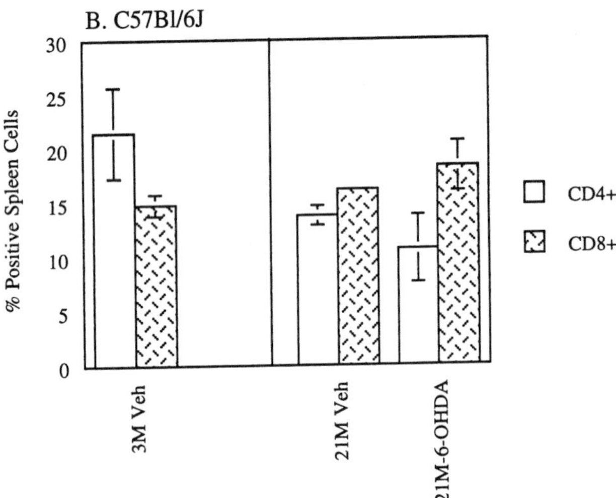

FIGURE 41 Percentage of $CD4^+$ and $CD8^+$ T cells in 3- (3M) and 21-month-old (21M) BALB/c (A) and C57Bl/6 (B) mice. Sympathectomy did not alter the number of splenic $CD4^+$ or $CD8^+$ T cells from young or old animals.

(Figure 65). One explanation for this finding could be an increase in SP synthesis in SP^+ nerves present in spleens from old animals makes these nerve fibers detectable with current immunocytochemical methods.

VII. PLASTICITY OF SPLENIC NA INNERVATION

A. Maturation

Acute administration of 6-OHDA also produces profound depletion of NE concentration in lymphoid tissues from adult rodents, but does not deplete catecholamines from the central nervous system (Laverty, Sharman & Vogt, 1965; Malmfors & Sachs, 1968). The degree of depletion after 6-OHDA treatment is variable, depending on age, strain of animal, drug regimen, and tissue. In some tissue such as vas deferens, sympathetic ganglia, and thymus, NA nerve terminals appear to be more resistant to this neurotoxin than those in the spleen (Kostrzewa & Jacobwitz, 1974; Malmfors & Sachs, 1968; Williams et al., 1981). Acute chemical sympathectomy in young adult rats, 1 day after treatment, produces approximately a 70 to 95% reduction in thymic and splenic NE concentration, respectively, compared with vehicle controls (Ackerman, 1989; Bellinger, Felten et al., 1989b; Lorton, Hewitt, Bellinger, S. Felten & D. Felten, 1990). In spleens from young adult denervated rats, loss of NE content persists through day 10 posttreatment, followed by a gradual increase in splenic NE concentrations that returns to normal values 56 days later (Lorton, Hewitt et al., 1990).

The time course and pattern of reinnervation of NA sympathetic nerves into the spleen after acute 6-OHDA treatment in young adult F344 rats was examined using glyoxylic acid histofluorescence for localization of catecholamines (Lorton, Hewitt et al., 1990). A few 6-OHDA-resistant NA nerves were present in spleens 1 to 3 days after denervation. By day 5, reinnervation by an ingrowth of NA nerves proceeded initially along the splenic artery as it enters the hilar region of the spleen. Ten days after denervation, abundant nerves regrowing into the hilus of the spleen were apparent, and between 21 and 56 days posttreatment the ingrowth of NA fibers extended into regions of the spleen distal from the hilus. NA nerves reinnervating the spleen distributed to the same splenic compartments as seen in saline-injected and nontreated controls; however, the density of nerves in these compartments displayed a high-to-low gradient from the hilus to regions distally.

At 56 days posttreatment, splenic compartments distal to the hilus contained fewer NA profiles than nondenervated controls, suggesting that the anatomical process of reinnervation does not restore the full complement of nerves back to the spleen, even though NE content returns to normal ranges in pieces of spleen at the hilus as well as distal to it. These findings suggest that functional restoration of splenic sympathetic innervation may involve metabolic and receptor up-regulation in returning NA nerves as a compensatory mechanism for the lack of complete fiber regrowth into denervated spleens. Additionally, adrenal compensation has been reported with long-term chemical sympathectomy, resulting in increased TH activity, greater catecholamine turnover from

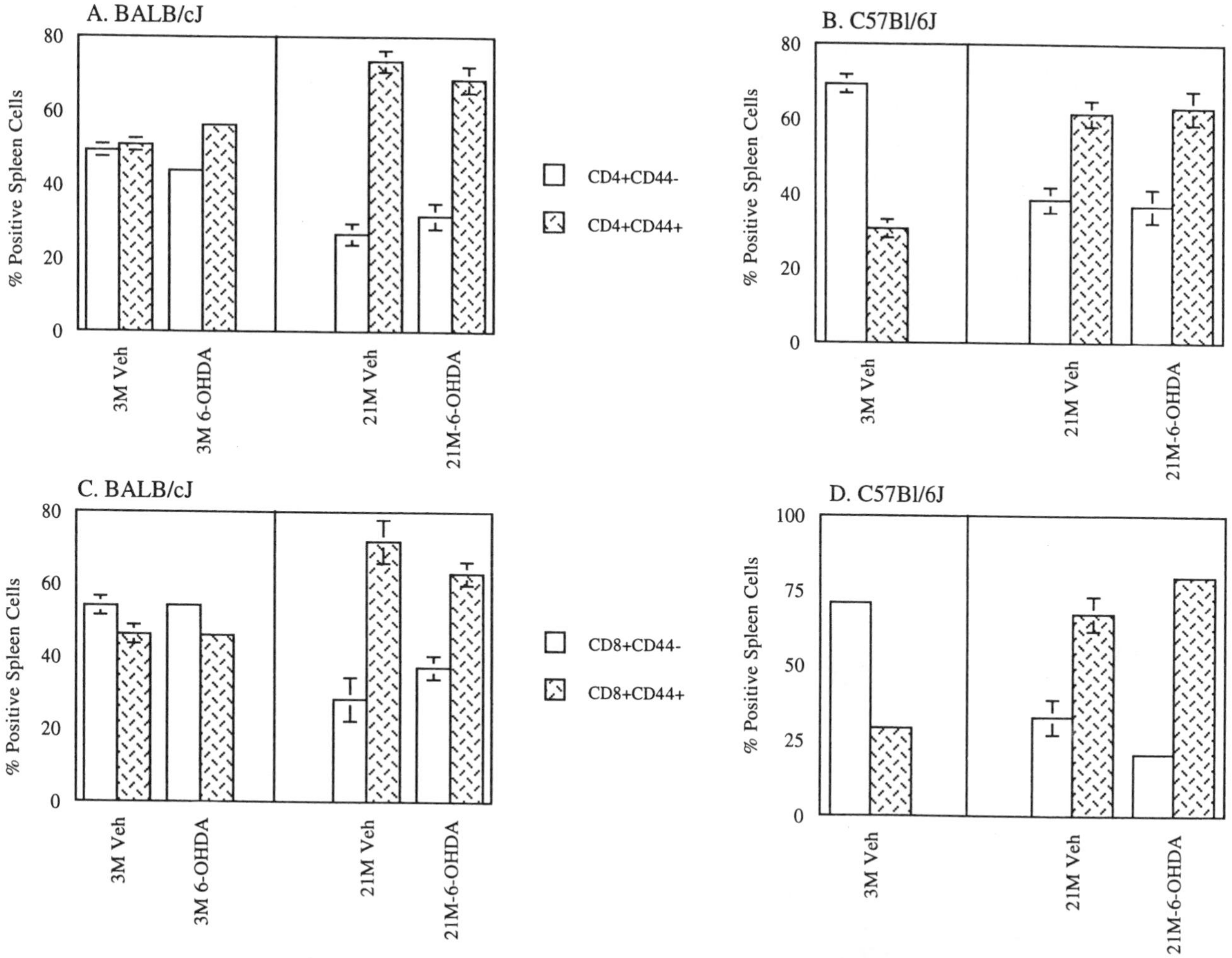

FIGURE 42 A and B. Percentage of $CD4^+$ naive and memory cells in young and old BALB/c (A) and C57Bl/8 (B) mice. C and D. Percentage of $CD8^+$ naive and memory cells in young and old BALB/c (C) and C57Bl/6 (D) mice. There was no effect of sympathectomy on the percentages of $CD4^+$ and $CD8^+$ naive or memory T cells, but there was and age-related difference in the percentages of naive and memory cells of both the CD4 and CD8 phenotype.

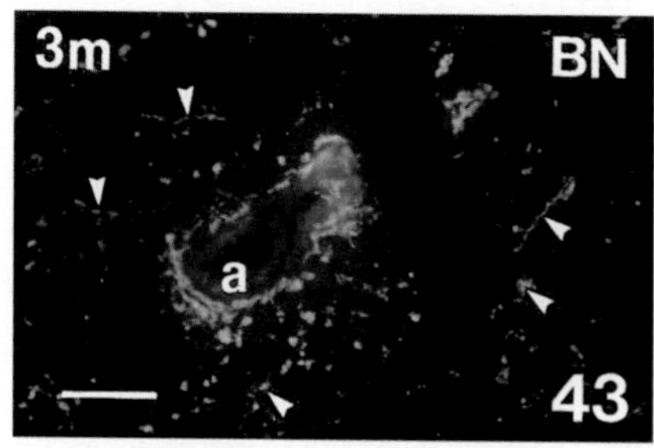

FIGURE 43 In the spleen of a 3-month-old (3m) Brown-Norway (BN) rat, a dense vascular plexus travels along the central arteriole (a), and NA nerve fibers (arrowheads) are present in the periarteriolar lymphatic sheath. The density of NA nerve fibers is similar to that seen in other rat strains of similar age. Glyoxylic acid-induced HF for CAs. X43. Calibration bar = 100 μm.

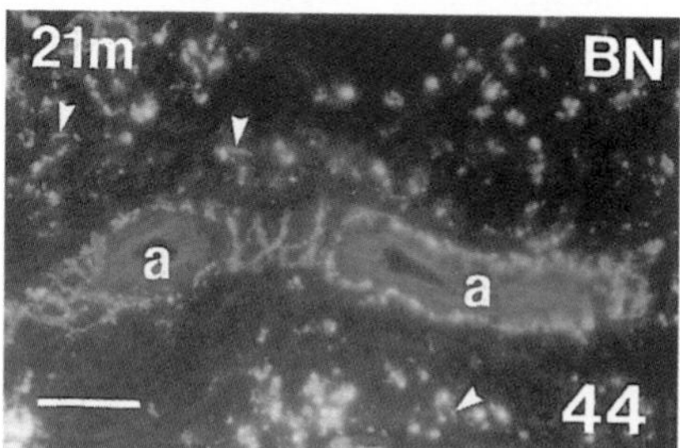

FIGURE 44 At 21-months of age (21m), NA innervation of the white pulp of spleens from Brown-Norway (BN) rats in this photomicrograph is similar in the density of nerve fibers, the intensity of fluorescence in the nerve profiles, and in their pattern of distribution along the central arteriole (a) and the surrounding periarteriolar lymphatic sheath (arrowheads) to that seen in 3-month-old rats. Glyoxylic acid-induced HF for CAs. X43. Calibration bar = 100 μm.

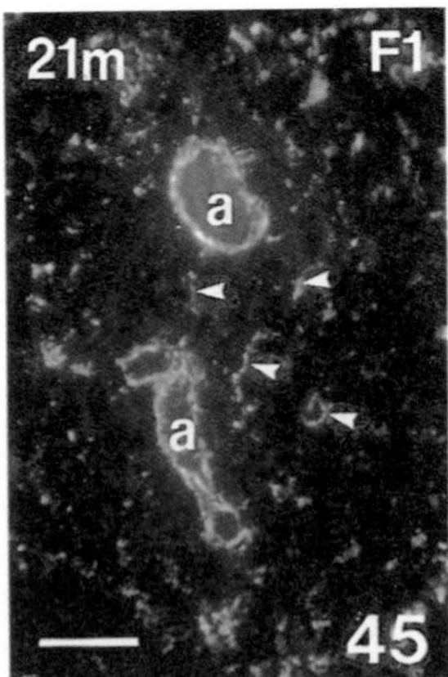

FIGURE 45 In 21-month-old (21m) Brown-Norway X F344 (F1) rats, a dense tangle of NA nerve fibers forms a vascular plexus around the central arteriole (a), with fibers exiting this plexus to enter the adjacent periarteriolar lymphatic sheath (arrowheads). Glyoxylic acid-induced HF for CAs. X85. Calibration bar = 100 μm.

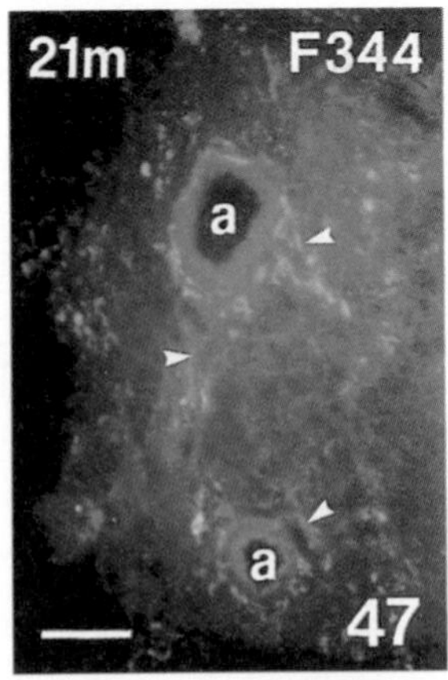

FIGURE 47 NA sympathetic innervation of spleens from old F344 rats (21 months of age, 21m) is greatly diminished along the central arteriole (a) and in the surrounding white pulp, and the intensity of fluorescence in age-resistant profiles is reduced compared with that seen in young adult animals. Glyoxylic acid-induced HF for CAs. X85. Calibration bar = 100 μm.

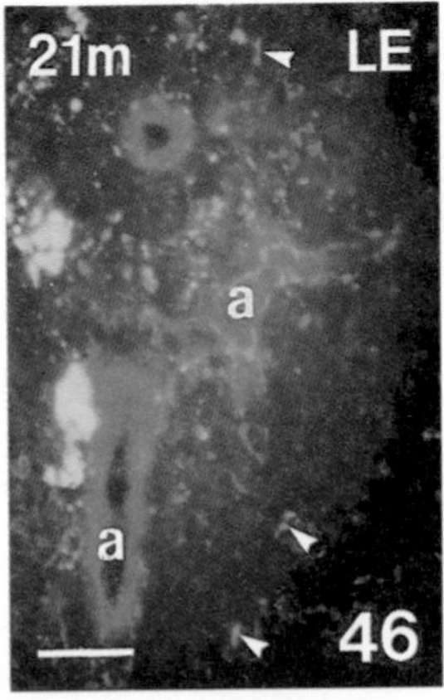

FIGURE 46 In old Lewis rats (21 months of age; 21m), there is a progressive loss on NA sympathetic nerve fibers along the central arteriole (a), and in the periarteriolar lymphatic sheath. Also the age-resistant NA nerve fibers lose some of the intensity in staining that is seen in 3-month-old rats (see Figure 43 for comparison). Glyoxylic acid-induced HF for CAs. X85. Calibration bar = 100 μm.

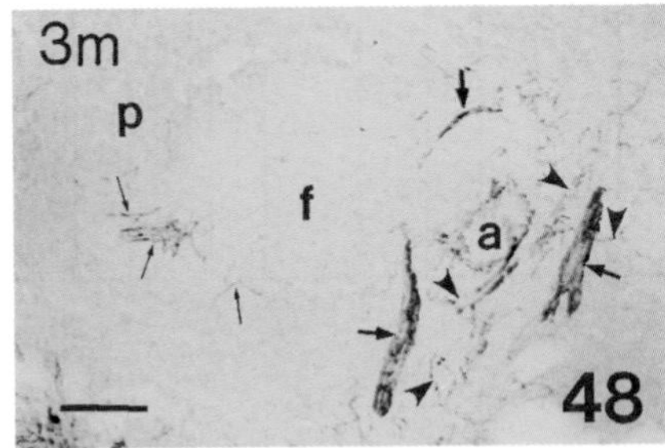

FIGURE 48 NPY$^+$ nerve fibers (black) course along the central arteriole (a) and extend into the surrounding periarteriolar lymphatic sheath (arrowheads). In the white pulp, NPY$^+$ nerve bundles (large arrows) are commonly found. Nerves immunoreactive for NPY also are abundant in the marginal zone and the parafollicular zone (p) (small arrows), and are sometimes present in the follicle (f). 3 months of age (3m). Single-label ICC for NPY. X43. Calibration bar = 200 μm.

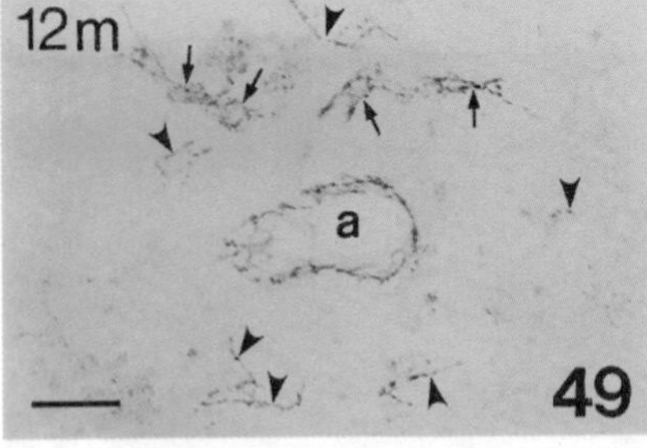

FIGURE 49 The density of NPY$^+$ nerve fibers (black) in the white pulp of the spleen from a 12-month-old (12m) F344 rats demonstrates robust innervation in the same compartments as seen in spleens from 3-month-old animals. a, central arteriole; arrowheads, individual NPY$^+$ profiles in the white pulp; arrows, NPY$^+$ nerves in vascular plexuses of the white pulp. Single-label ICC for NPY. X85. Calibration bar = 100 μm.

chromaffin cells, and higher plasma catecholamine levels in 6-OHDA-treated animals (De Champlain & van Ameringen, 1972; Gauthier, Nadeau, & De Champlain, 1972; Mueller, Thoenen, & Axelrod, 1969). Adrenal compensation resulting in an increased availability of NE for uptake into nerves in the spleen may explain the discrepancy between histochemical and neurochemical data; however, hyperinnervation of the hilar region also may explain these differences.

Similar discrepancies in the timing of nerve recovery, NE concentration, and return of effector function have been reported in other peripheral tissues after denervation with 6-OHDA. Recovery of peripheral sympathetic effector function precedes

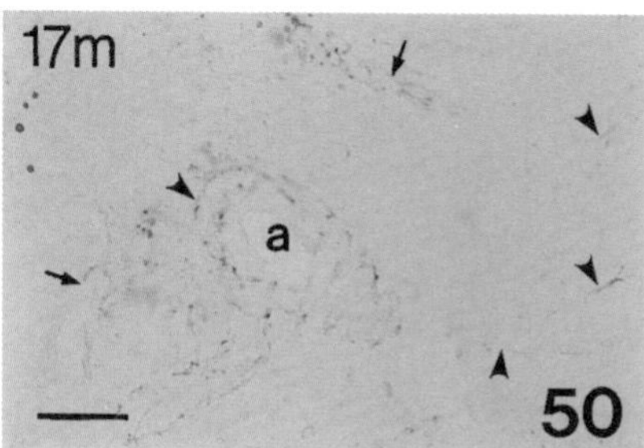

FIGURE 50 By 17 months of age (17m), the density of NPY$^+$ nerve fibers (black) in the white pulp is greatly diminished, especially distal from the hilus as seen in this photomicrograph. A few faintly immunoreactive profiles can be seen around the central arteriole (a) and in the adjacent white pulp, either as individual fibers (arrowheads) or in association with the vasculature (arrows). Single-label ICC for NPY. X85. Calibration bar = 100 μm.

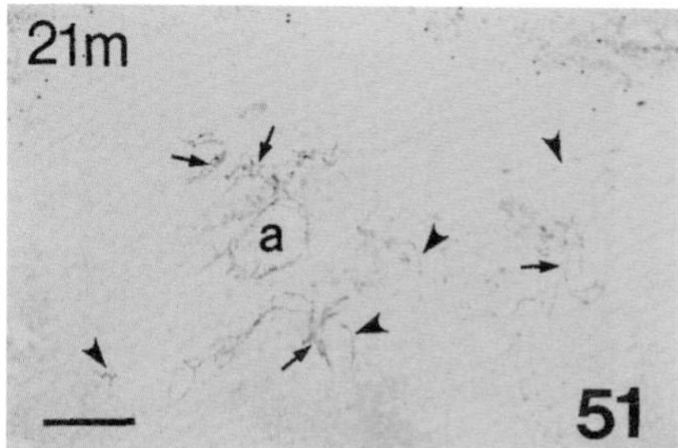

FIGURE 51 The loss of NPY-immunoreactive nerve fibers (black) in the white pulp of the spleen is still apparent at 21 months of age (21m). a, central arteriole; arrowheads, singly traveling NPY$^+$ nerve fibers in the white pulp; arrows, NPY$^+$ nerves in small vascular plexuses in the white pulp. Single-label ICC for NPY. X43. Calibration bar = 200 μm.

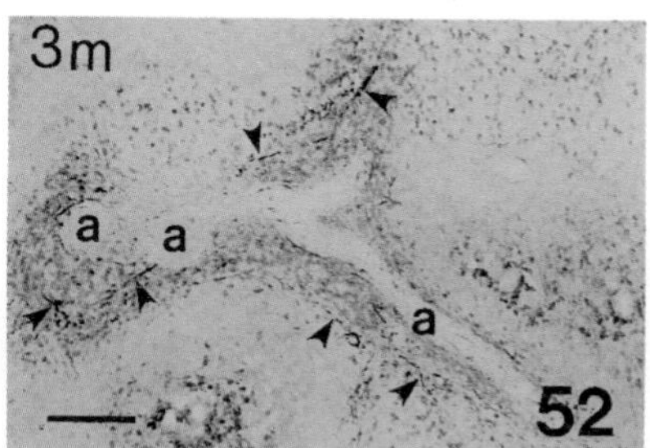

FIGURE 52 With double-label ICC, NPY$^+$ nerve fibers (black) (arrowheads) are found among OX19$^+$ T lymphocytes (brown) which form the periarteriolar lymphatic sheath around the central arteriole (a) in the spleen from a 3-month-old (3m) F344 rat. Double-label ICC for NPY and OX19, a pan T lymphocyte marker. X43. Calibration bar = 200 μm.

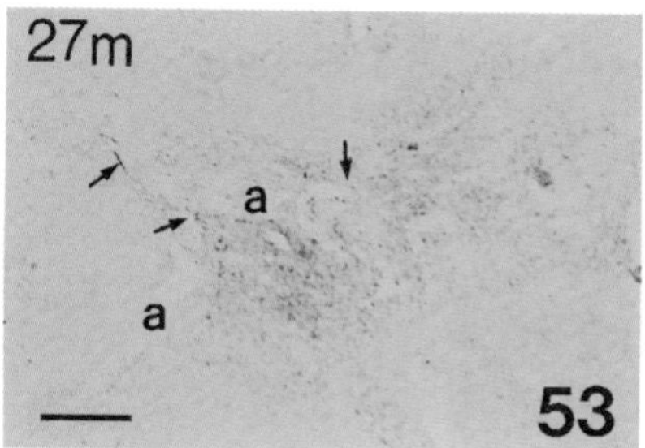

FIGURE 53 At 27 months of age (27m), NPY$^+$ nerve fibers (black) (arrows) are only occasionally found around the central arteriole (a). The density of OX19$^+$ T lymphocytes (brown) that form the periarteriolar lymphatic sheath is greatly reduced, and few NPY$^+$ nerve fibers are present among these lymphocytes. Double-label ICC for NPY and OX19, a pan T lymphocyte marker. X43. Calibration bar = 200 μm.

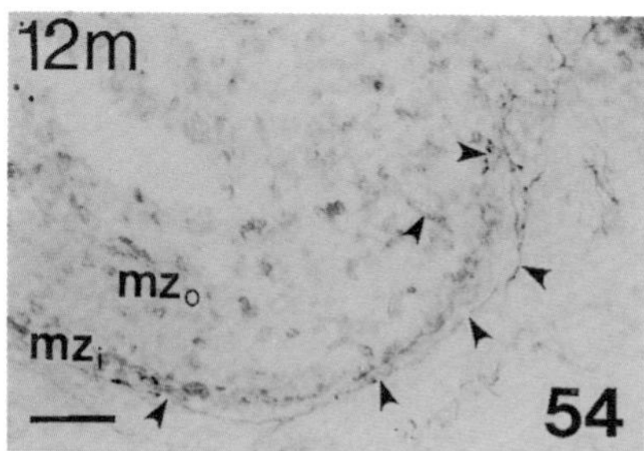

FIGURE 54 In the inner (mz_i) and outer (mz_o) marginal zone from a 12-month-old (12m) rat, a reduction in the density of the ED3$^+$ macrophages (brown) is apparent. NPY$^+$ nerve fibers (black), however, can still be found in both regions of the marginal zone among age-resistance macrophages. Double-label ICC for NPY and ED3. X170. Calibration bar = 50 μm.

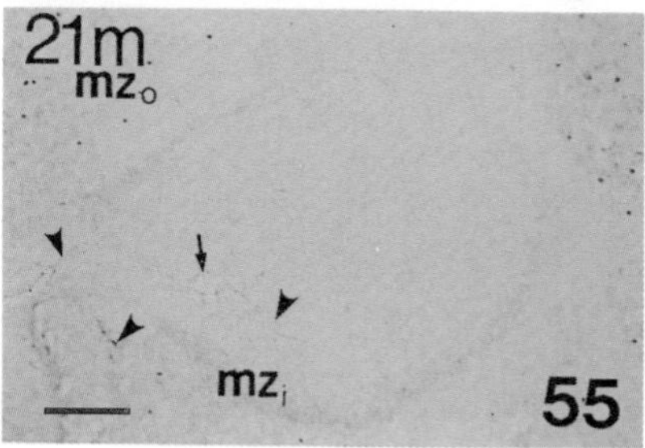

FIGURE 55 ED3$^+$ macrophages (brown) are greatly depleted from the inner (mz_i) and outer (mz_o) marginal zone from 21-month-old (21m) rats. Similarly, only an occasional, faintly, NPY-immunoreactive nerve fiber (black) (arrowheads) can be seen in the marginal zone among age-resistant ED3$^+$ cells, or around the central arteriole (arrow). Double-label ICC for NPY and ED3. X43. Calibration bar = 200 μm.

both NA nerve regeneration (Gauthier et al., 1972; Finch, Haeusler, Kuhn, & Thoenen, 1973) and recovery of NE content in the heart (Nadeau, De Champlain, & Tremblay, 1971). These reports support our hypothesis that recovery of effector function occurs before complete restoration of nerves and NE concentration, with compensatory mechanisms of enhanced synthesis and release of NE by regenerating nerves into the spleen, and adrenoceptor up-regulation in target cells that occurs following denervation. A large body of

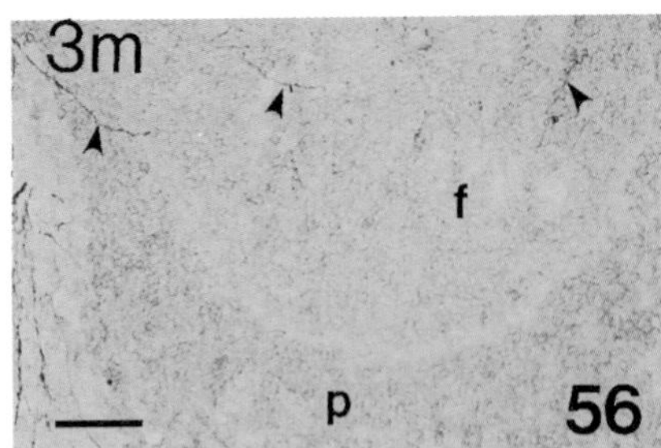

FIGURE 56 sIgM+ B lymphocytes (brown) are abundant in the marginal zone (not shown), parafollicular zone (p), and follicle (f). NPY$^+$ nerve fibers (black) (arrowheads) are commonly found in the marginal and parafollicular zones, and to a lesser extent in the follicles. 3m, 3-month-old rats. Double-label ICC for NPY and IgM. X170. Calibration bar = 50 μm.

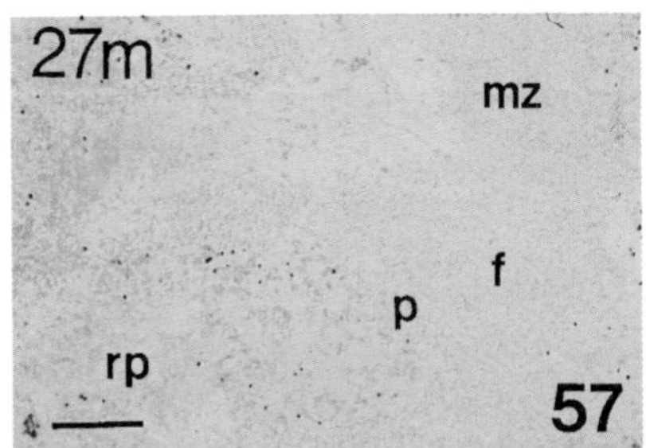

FIGURE 57 The density of sIgM+ B lymphocytes (brown) remains relatively stable in spleens from 27-month-old (27m) rats, even though NPY$^+$ nerve fibers are lost from compartments in which these cells reside. mz, marginal zone; p, parafollicular zone; f, follicle; rp, red pulp. Double-label ICC for NPY and IgM. X43. Calibration bar = 200 μm.

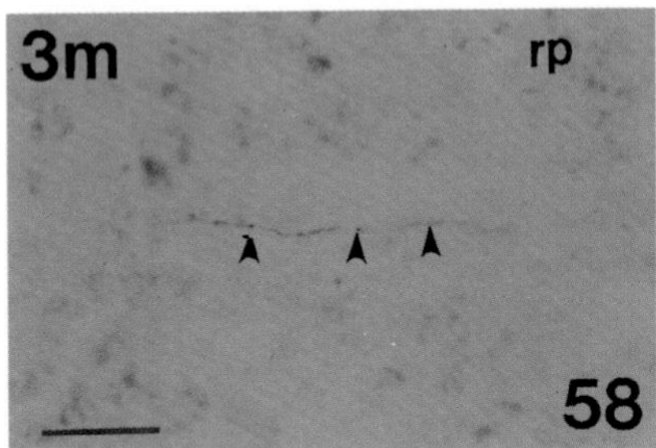

FIGURE 58 SP$^+$ nerve fibers (black) (arrowheads) are present as linear profiles in the red pulp (rp) of the 3-month-old (3m) rat spleen. Single-label ICC for SP. X218. Calibration bar = 50 μm.

literature indicates that sympathetic denervation in young adult rodents alters immune function (Madden & Livnat, 1991) (reviewed in chapter 5, volume 1, this book).

B. Ontogeny

Neonatal administration of 6-OHDA produces profound central and peripheral loss of catechola-

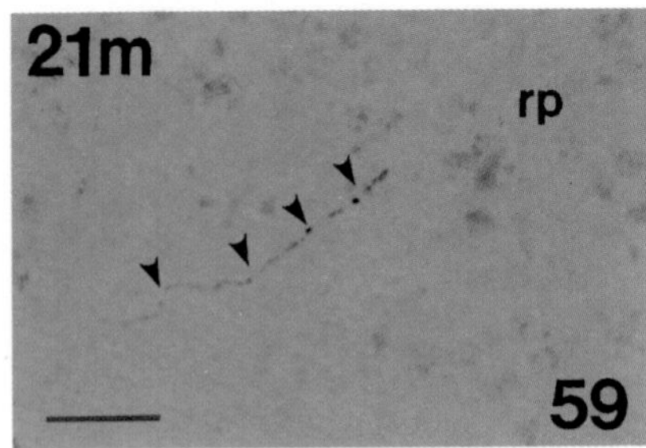

FIGURE 59 SP$^+$ nerve fibers (black) (arrowheads) course as linear profiles in the red pulp (rp) of the 21-month-old (21m) rat spleen with a similar frequency and staining intensity as seen in young adult rats. Single-label ICC for SP. X218. Calibration bar = 50 μm.

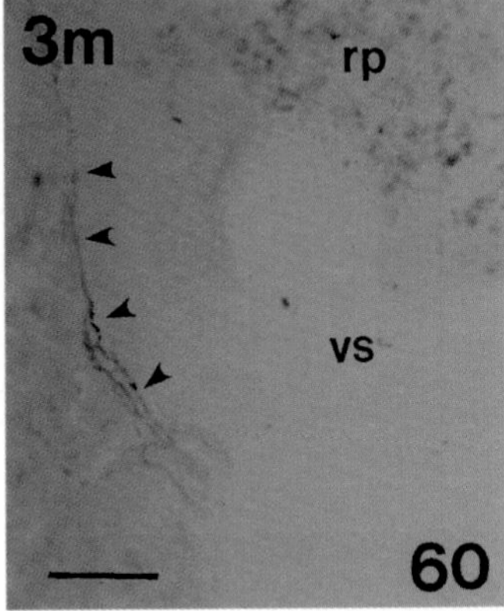

FIGURE 60 A plexus of SP$^+$ nerve fibers (black) (arrowheads) travels along a venous sinus (vs) in the spleen from a 3-month-old (3m) rat. Long, linear, varicose fibers can be seen exiting this venous plexus into the adjacent red pulp (rp) Single-label ICC for SP. X110. Calibration bar = 100 μm.

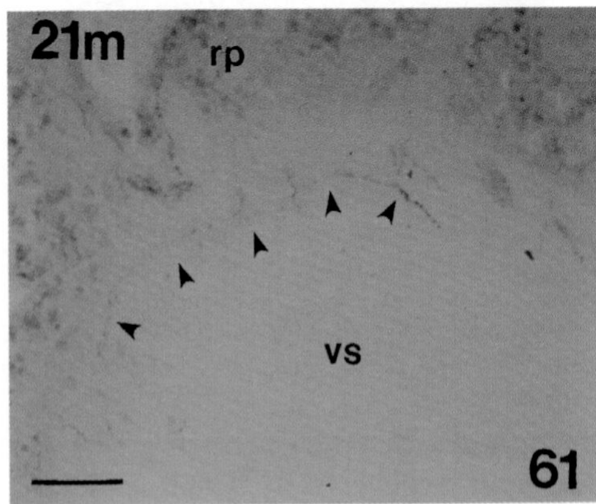

FIGURE 61 A density of SP$^+$ nerve fibers (black) (arrowheads) can be found along the venous sinuses (vs) of 21-month-old (21m) rats. rp, red pulp. Single-label ICC for SP. X110. Calibration bar = 100 μm.

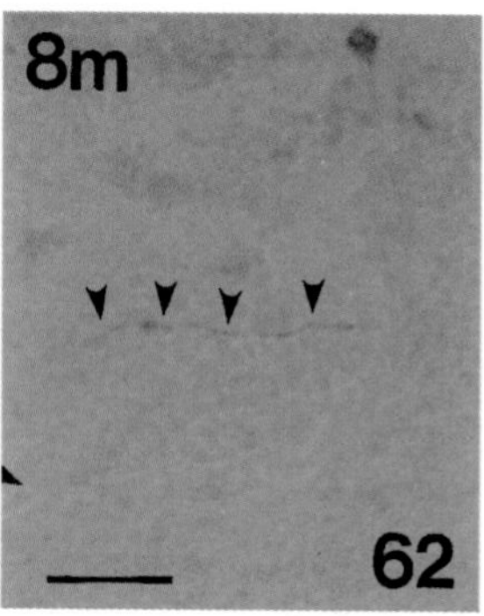

FIGURE 62 Occasionally, SP^+ nerve fibers (black) (arrowheads) course as individual, linear, and varicose profiles in the outer white pulp of spleens from young adult (8m) rats. Single-label ICC for SP. X218. Calibration bar = 50 μm.

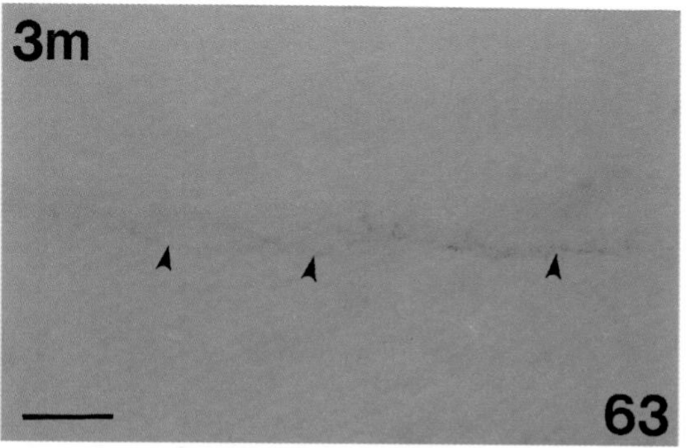

FIGURE 63 In the outer portion of the white pulp from a 3-month-old (3m) rat, a faint SP^+ nerve plexus (black) (arrowheads) is seen along a blood vessel. Single-label ICC for SP. X218. Calibration bar = 50 μm.

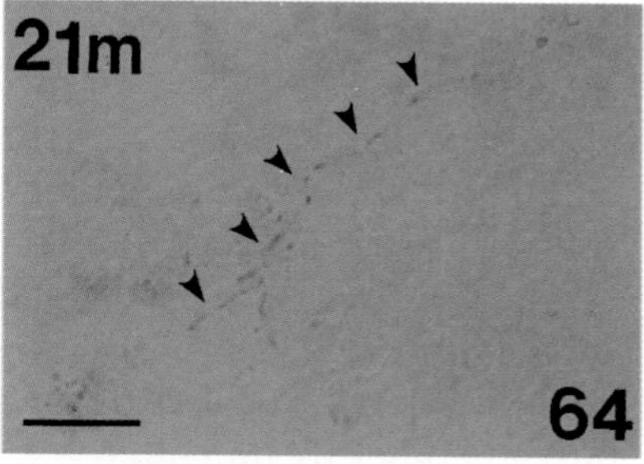

FIGURE 64 Individual SP^+ nerve fibers (black) (arrowheads) course in the outer portion of the white pulp in the spleen of a 21-month-old (21m) rat. The frequency, as well as the staining intensity, of individual fibers in this part of the white pulp appear to be increase with advancing age. Single-label ICC for SP. X218. Calibration bar = 50 μm.

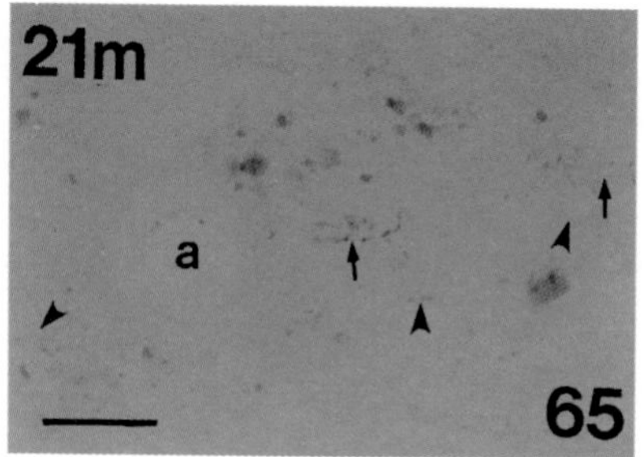

FIGURE 65 SP^+ nerves fibers (black) (arrows) course along blood vessels and as individual profiles (arrowheads) in the periarteriolar lymphatic sheath, but not along the central arteriole (a) in a spleen from a 21-month-old (21m) rat. However, an occasional SP^+ nerve fiber have been found associated with the central arteriole in the white pulp from old rats. This distribution pattern of SP^+ nerves was not seen in young adult rats. Single-label ICC for SP. X110. Calibration bar = 100 μm.

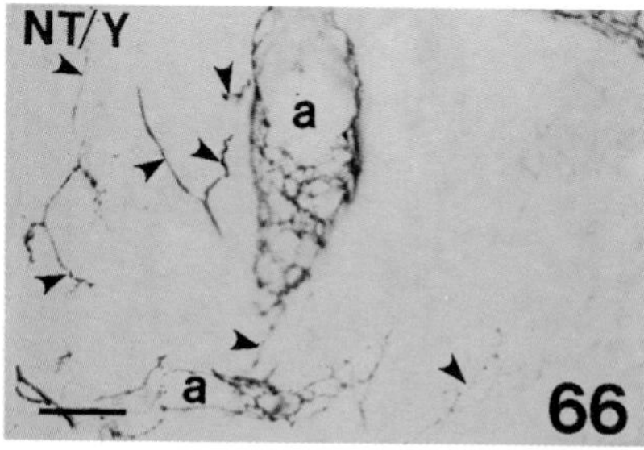

FIGURE 66 White pulp from the spleen of an untreated young adult (NT/Y) F344 rat immunocytochemically stained for TH demonstrates a dense plexus of TH^+ nerve fibers (brown) associated with the central arteriole (a), and individual TH^+ nerve fibers (arrowheads) in the surrounding periarteriolar lymphatic sheath. Single-label ICC for TH. X85. Calibration bar = 100 μm.

mines. Chemical sympathectomy by treatment with 6-OHDA at 1, 2, and 3 postnatal days of age results in virtual depletion of NE content in the thymus from denervated rats examined at 7 days of age (greater than 95% compared with vehicle-treated controls) (Ackerman, 1989). Between 7 and 56 days of age, thymic NE concentration progressively increases. At postnatal day 14, NE content in the thymus from denervated rats is greater than 60% of vehicle control values, and from 21 to 56 days of age, NE concentration in the thymus of 6-OHDA-treated rats is not significantly different from controls. These findings suggest full neurochemical recovery in the thymus after neonatal chemical sympathectomy.

Measurement of splenic NE after neonatal 6-OHDA administration reveals a more pronounced and longer-lasting denervation than in the thymus (Ackerman, 1989; Ackerman, Madden, Livnat, Felten, & Felten, 1991) Acute injection of young adult rats with 6-OHDA results in a 70% reduction of thymic NE content relative to vehicle controls, whereas splenic NE content in acutely sympathectomized rats is virtually absent through day 28 postnatally, and by 56 days of age still is depleted by greater than 80% of vehicle control values. A slight but consistent increase in splenic NE content occurs between 28 and 56 days of age. Although this increase may result from

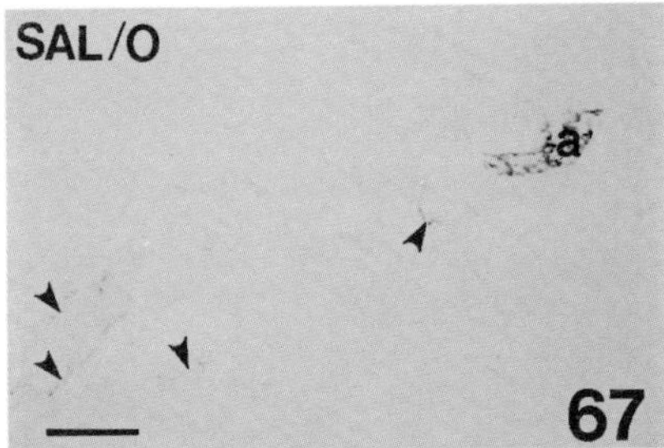

FIGURE 67 White pulp from the spleen of a saline-treated, old (SAL/O) rat immunocytochemically stained for TH reveals a loss of TH^+ nerve fibers (brown) in the white pulp of the aged rat spleen. Twenty-one-month-old F344 rats were treated daily with L-deprenyl or saline for 10 weeks followed by a 9-day drug wash-out period. arrowheads, individual TH^+ nerve fibers in the periarteriolar lymphatic sheath. Single-label ICC for TH. X85. Calibration bar = 100 μm.

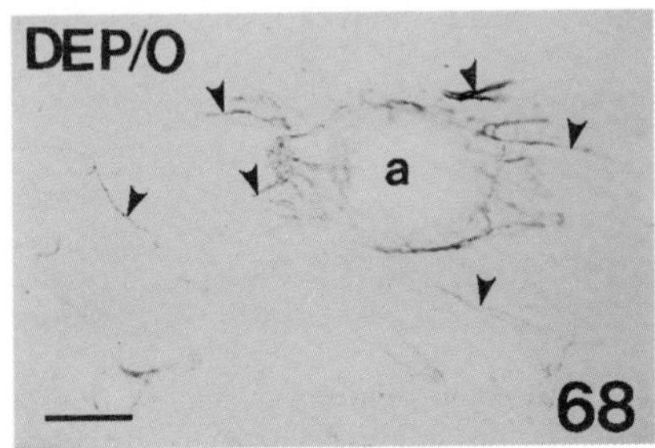

FIGURE 68 Treatment with L-deprenyl (1.0 mg/kg, i.p.) results in an increase in the density of TH^+ nerve fibers (brown) around the central arteriole (a) and as linear profiles (arrowheads) in the periarteriolar lymphatic sheath in spleens from old F344 rats (DEP/O). Twenty-one-month-old F344 rats were treated daily with L-deprenyl or saline for 10 weeks followed by a 9-day drug wash-out period. Single-label ICC for TH. X85. Calibration bar = 100 μm.

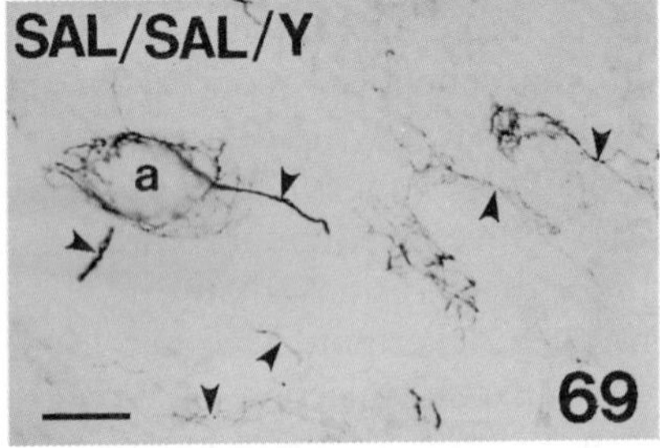

FIGURE 69 Nondenervated, saline-treated, young adult control spleen (SAL/SAL/Y) demonstrates the distribution of TH^+ nerve fibers (brown) associated with the central arteriole (a) or in the surrounding white pulp (arrowheads) of the spleen. F344 rats were treated daily with L-deprenyl or saline for a 30 days after 6-OHDA or saline treatment. central arteriole; arrowheads, individual TH^+ nerve fibers in the periarteriolar lymphatic sheath. Single-label ICC for TH. X85. Calibration bar = 100 μm.

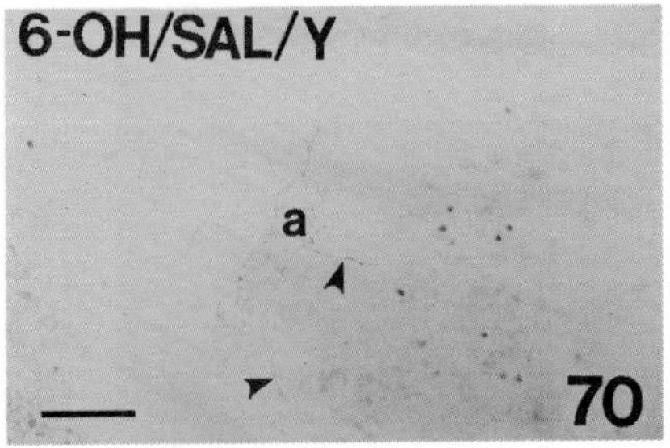

FIGURE 70 In young adult rats treated with 6-OHDA to destroy NA sympathetic nerve terminals (6-OH/SAL/Y), administration of the deprenyl vehicle, saline, does not alter the density of TH^+ nerves (brown) that regrow into the spleen. Arrowheads indicate faint TH^+ nerve fibers in the white pulp of the spleen. F344 rats were treated daily with L-deprenyl or saline for a 30 days after 6-OHDA or saline treatment. a, central arteriole (a). Single-label ICC for TH. X85. Calibration bar = 100 μm.

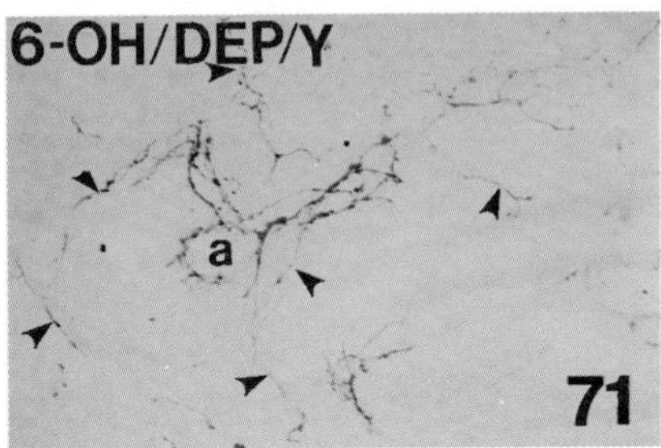

FIGURE 71 Administration of L-deprenyl (1.0 mg/kg, i.p.) causes an increase in the density of TH^+ nerve fibers (brown) along the central arterioles (a) and in the white pulp (arrowheads) from young adult rats previously treated with 6-OHDA (6-OH/DEP/Y). F344 rats were treated daily with L-deprenyl or saline for a 30 days after 6-OHDA or saline treatment. Single-label ICC for TH. X85. Calibration bar = 100 μm.

reinnervation by NA fibers, reinjection of neonatally sympathectomized rats with 6-OHDA on days 3 and 5 before sacrifice at 56 days of age does not alter the splenic NE concentration. Further, this slight rise in splenic NE concentration is not statistically significant compared with any other treatment group.

The ontogeny of in vitro spleen cell proliferation to T- and B-cell mitogens (Con A and a mixture of equal concentrations of *Salmonella typhimurium* and DxS [STM/DxS]), respectively) and immunoglobulin secretion was examined in neonatal F344 rats after treatment with 6-OHDA on days 1 through 3 (Ackerman, 1989; Ackerman, Madden et al., 1991). A shift in the proliferative response to Con A has been observed in splenocytes from sympathectomized rats sacrificed between postnatal day 7 and 14 compared with age-matched controls, with reduced responsiveness to low levels of Con A and increased responsiveness with higher doses. Between postnatal days 7 and

Morphometric analysis in adult and aged F344 rats. *Journal of Neuroscience Research, 18*, 55–63.

Bellinger, D. L., Felten, S. Y., & Felten, D. L. (1988). Maintenance of noradrenergic sympathetic innervation in the involuted thymus of the aged Fischer 344 rat. *Brain, Behavior, and Immunity, 2*, 133–150.

Bellinger, D. L., Felten, S. Y., & Felten, D. L. (1992). Noradrenergic sympathetic innervation of lymphoid organs during development, aging, and autoimmunity. In F. Amenta (Ed.), *Aging of the autonomic nervous system* (pp. 243–284). Boca Raton, Florida: CRC Press.

Bellinger, D. L., Felten, S. Y., Lorton, D., & Felten, D. L. (1989). Origin of noradrenergic innervation of the spleen in rats. *Brain, Behavior, and Immunity, 3*, 291–311.

Bellinger, D. L., Lorton, D., Felten, S. Y., & Felten, D. L. (1989). Effects of age on substance P (SP)+ nerve fibers in the spleen of Fischer 344 rats. *Society for Neuroscience Abstract, 15*, 714.

Bellinger, D. L., Lorton, D., Horn, L., Felten, S. Y., & Felten, D. L. (1997). Vasoactive intestinal polypeptide (VIP) innervation of rat spleen, thymus, and lymph nodes. *Peptides, 18*, 1139–1149.

Bellinger, D. L., Lorton, D., Romano, T., Olschowka, J. A., Felten, S. Y., & Felten, D. L. (1990). Neuropeptide innervation of lymphoid organs. *Annals of New York Academy of Science, 594*, 17–33.

Benedetti, A., Ferretti, G., Curatola, G., Jezequel, A. M., & Orlandi, F. (1988). Age and sex related changes of plasma membrane fluidity in isolated rat hepatocytes. *Biochemical and Biophysical Research Community, 156*, 840–845.

Bernard, J. T., Ameriso, S., Kempf, R. A., Rosen, P., Mitchell, M. S., & Fisher, M. (1990). Transient focal neurologic deficits complicating interleukin-2 therapy. *Neurology, 40*, 154–155.

Berquist, J., Josefsson, E., Tarkowski, A., Ekman, R., & Ewing, A. (1997). Measurements of catecholamine-mediated apoptosis of immunocompetent cells by capillary electrophoresis. *Electrophoresis, 18*, 1760–1766.

Besedovsky, H. O., del Rey, A., Sorkin, E., Da Prada, M., & Keller, H. H. (1979). Immunoregulation mediated by the sympathetic nervous system. *Cellular Immunology, 48*, 346–355.

Besedovsky, H. O., del Rey, A. E., Sorkin, E., Burri, R., Honegger, C. G., Schlumpf, M., & Lichtensteiger, W. (1987). T lymphocytes affect the development of sympathetic innervation of mouse spleen. *Brain, Behavior, and Immunity, 1*, 185–193.

Boyd, E. (1932). The weight of the thymus gland in health and in disease. *American Journal of Diseases in Children, 43*, 1162–1214.

Breneman, S. M., Moynihan, J. A., Grota, L. J., Felten, D. L., & Felten, S. Y. (1993). Splenic norepinephrine is decreased in MRL-lpr/lpr mice. *Brain, Behavior, and Immunity, 7*, 135–143.

Brenneman, D. E., Schultzberg, M., Bartfai, T., & Gozes, I. (1992). Cytokine regulation of neuronal survival. *Journal of Neurochemistry, 58*, 454–460.

Briggs, M. M., & Lefkowitz, R. J. (1980). Parallel modulation of catecholamine activation of adenylate cyclase and formation of high-affinity agonist-receptor complex in turkey erythrocyte membranes by temperature and cis-vaccenic acid. *Biochemistry, 19*, 4461–4466.

Bulloch, K., Cullen, M. R., Schwartz, R. H., & Longo, D. L. (1987). Development of innervation within syngeneic thymus tissue transplanted under the kidney capsule of the nude mouse: A light and ultrastructural microscope study. *Journal of Neuroscience Research, 18*, 16–27.

Bulloch, K., Hausman, J., Radojcic, T., & Short, S. (1991). Calcitonin gene-related peptide in the developing and aging thymus. An immunocytochemical study. *Annals of the New York Academy of Science, 621*, 218–228.

Bulloch, K., & Pomerantz, W. (1984). Autonomic nervous system innervation of thymic related lymphoid tissue in wild-type and nude mice. *Journal of Comparative Neurology, 228*, 57–68.

Burns, E. A., Lum, L. G., L'Hommedieu, G., & Goodwin, J. S. (1993). Specific humoral immunity in the elderly: In vivo response to vaccination. *Journal of Gerontology, 48*, B231–B236.

Caldirini, G., Bonetti, A. C., Battistella, A., Crews, F. T., & Toffano, G. (1983). Biochemical changes of rat brain membranes with aging. *Neurochemical Research, 8*, 483–492.

Calvo, W., & Forteza-Vila, J. (1969). On the development of bone marrow innervation in new-born rats as studied with silver impregnation and electron microscopy. *American Journal of Anatomy, 126*, 355–359.

Calvo, W., & Haas, R. J. (1969). Die Histogenese des Knochemarks der Ratte. *Zeitschrift fur Zellforschung und Mikroskopische Anatomie, 95*, 377–395.

Carlson, S. L., Felten, D. L., Livnat, S., & Felten, S. Y. (1987). Noradrenergic sympathetic innervation of the spleen: V. Acute drug-induced depletion of lymphocytes in the target fields of innervation results in redistribution of noradrenergic fibers but maintenance of compartmentation. *Journal of Neuroscience Research, 18*, 64–69.

Carlson, S. L., Johnson, S., Parrish, M. E., & Cass, W. A. (1998). Development of immune hyperinnervation in NGF-transgenic mice. *Experimental Neurology, 149*, 209–220.

Carnahan, J. F., Patel, D. R., & Miller, J. A. (1994). Stem cell factor is a neurotrophic factor for neural crest-derived chick sensory neurons. *Journal of Neuroscience, 14*, 1433–1440.

Chelmicka-Schorr, E., Kwasniewski, M. N., Thomas, B. E., & Arnason, B. G. W. (1989). The β-adrenergic agonist isoproterenol suppresses experimental allergic encephalomyelitis in Lewis rats. *Journal of Neuroimmunology, 25*, 203–207.

Ciriaco, E., Ricci, A., Bronzetti, E., Mammola, C. L., Germana, G., & Vega, J. A. (1995). Age-related changes of the noradrenergic and acetylcholinesterase reactive nerve fibres innervating the pigeon bursa of Fabricius. *Anatomischer Anzeiger, 177*, 237–242.

Clerici, M., DePalma, L., Roilides, E., Baker, R., & Shearer, G. M. (1993). Analysis of T helper and antigen-presenting cell functions in cord blood and peripheral blood leukocytes from healthy children of different ages. *Journal of Clinical Investigation, 91*, 2829–2836.

Colburn, K., Boucek, R., Gusewitch, G., Wong, A., Wat, P., & Weeks, D. (1990). β-adrenergic receptor stimulation increases anti-DNA antibody production in MRL/1pr mice. *Journal of Rheumatology, 17*, 138–141.

Collins, S. (1993). Recent perspectives on the molecular structure and regulation of the β_2-adrenoceptor. *Life Sciences, 52*, 2083–2091.

Consolo, S., Garattini, S., Ladinsky, H., & Thoenen, H. (1972). Effect of chemical sympathectomy on the content of acetylcholine, choline and choline acetyltransferase activity in the cat spleen and iris. *Journal of Physiology, 220*, 639–646.

Cosentino, M., Marino, F., Bombelli, R., Ferrari, M., Maestroni, G. J., Conti, A., Rasini, E., Lecchini, S., & Frigo, G. (1998). Association between the circadian course of endogenous noradrenaline and the hematopoietic cell cycle in mouse bone marrow. *Journal of Chemotherapy, 10*, 179–181.

De Blasi, A., Lipartiti, M., Algeri, S., Sacchetti, G., Costantini, C., Fratelli, M., & Cotecchia, S. (1986). Stress induced desensitization of lymphocyte β-adrenoceptors in young and aged rats. *Pharmacology, Biochemistry, and Behavior, 24*, 991–998.

De Champlain, J., & van Ameringen, M. R. (1972). Regulation of blood pressure by sympathetic nerve fibers and adrenal medulla in normotensive and hypertensive rats. *Circulation Research, 31*, 617–628.

del Rey, A., Besedovsky, H. O., Sorkin, E., Da Prada, M., & Arrenbrecht, S. (1981). Immunoregulation mediated by the sympathetic nervous system. *Cellular Immunology, 63*, 329–334.

del Rey, A., Besedovsky, H. O., Sorkin, E., Da Prada, M., & Bondiolotti, G. P. (1982). Sympathetic immunoregulation: Difference between high- and low-responder animals. *American Journal of Physiology, 242*, R30–R33.

DePace, D. M., & Webber, R. H. (1975). Electrostimulation and morphologic study of the nerves to the bone marrow of the albino rat. *Acta Anatomica, 93*, 1–18.

Dominguez-Gerpe, L., & Rey-Mendez, M. (1998a). Modulation of stress-induced murine lymphoid tissue involution by age, sex and strain: Role of bone marrow. *Mechanisms of Ageing and Development, 104*, 195–205.

Dominguez-Gerpe, L., & Rey-Mendez, M. (1998b). Age-related changes in primary and secondary immune organs of the mouse. *Immunology Investigation, 27*, 153–165.

El-Salhy, M., & Sandstrom, O. (1999). How age changes the content of neuroendocrine peptides in the murine gastrointestinal tract. *Gerontology, 45*, 17–22.

El-Salhy, M., Sandstrom, O., & Holmlund, F. (1999). Age-induced changes in the enteric nervous system in the mouse. *Mechanisms of Ageing and Development, 107*, 93–103.

Engwerda, C. R., Fox, B. S., & Handwerger, B. S. (1996). Cytokine production by T lymphocytes from young and aged mice. *Journal of Immunology, 156*, 3621–3630.

Ericsson, A., Schalling, M., McIntyre, K. R., Lundberg, J. M., Larhammar, D., Seroogy, K., Hokfelt, T., & Persson, H. (1987). Detection of neuropeptide Y and its mRNA in megakaryocytes: Enhanced levels in certain autoimmune mice. *Proceedings of the National Academy of Science of the United States of America, 84*, 5585–5589.

Ernström, U., & Sandberg, G. (1974). Stimulation of lymphocyte release from the spleen by theophylline and isoproterenol. *Acta Physiological Scandinavica, 90*, 202–209.

Ernström, U., & Söder, O. (1975). Influence of adrenaline on the dissemination of antibody-producing cells from the spleen. *Clinical and Experimental Immunology, 21*, 131–140.

Esler, M., Skews, H., Leonard, P., Jackman, G., Bobik, A., & Korner, P. (1981). Age dependence of noradrenaline kinetics in normal subjects. *Clinical Science, 60*, 217–219.

Feldman, R. D., Limbird, L. E., Nadeau, J., Robertson, D., & Wood, A. J. J. (1984). Alterations in leukocyte β-receptor affinity with aging. A potential explanation for altered β-adrenergic sensitivity in the elderly. *New England Journal of Medicine, 310*, 815–819.

Felten, D. L., Bellinger, D. L., & Felten, S. Y. (1989). Age-related alterations in the distribution of neuropeptide Y (NPY)-positive nerve fibers in the rat spleen. *Society for Neuroscience Abstracts, 15*, 714.

Felten, D. L., & Felten, S. Y. (1989). Innervation of the thymus. In M. D. Kendall & M. A. Ritter (Eds.), *Thymus update* (pp. 73–88). London: Harwood Academic Publishers.

Felten, D. L., Felten, S. Y., Bellinger, D. L., Carlson, S. L., Ackerman, K. D., Madden, K. S., Olschowka, J. A., & Livnat, S. (1987). Noradrenergic sympathetic neural interactions with the immune system: Structure and function. *Immunological Review, 100*, 225–260.

Felten, D. L., Felten, S. Y., Carlson, S. L., Bellinger, D. L., Ackerman, K. D., Romano, T. A., & Livnat, S. (1988). Development, aging, and plasticity of noradrenergic sympathetic innervation of secondary lymphoid organs: Implications for neural-immune interactions. In A. Dahlstrom, R. M. Belmaker, & M. Sandler (Eds.), *Progress in catecholamine research part A: Basic aspects and peripheral mechanisms* (pp. 517–524). New York: Alan R. Liss.

Felten, D. L., Felten, S. Y., Carlson, S. L., Olschowka, J. A., & Livnat, S. (1985). Noradrenergic and peptidergic innervation of lymphoid tissue. *Journal of Immunology, 135*, 755s–765s.

Felten, D. L., Felten, S. Y., Fuller, R. W., Romano, T. D., Smalstig, E. B., Wong, D. T., & Clemens, J. A. (1991). Chronic dietary pergolide preserves nigrostriatal neuronal integrity in aged Fischer 344 rats. *Neurobiology of Aging, 13*, 339–351.

Felten, D. L., Felten, S. Y., Madden, K. S., Ackerman, K. D., & Bellinger, D. L. (1989). Development, maturation, and senescence of sympathetic innervation of secondary immune organs. In M. P. Schreibman & C. G. Scanes, (Eds.), *Development, maturation, and senescence of neuroendocrine systems* (pp. 381–396). San Diego: Academic Press.

Felten, D. L., Felten, S. Y., Steece-Collier, K., Date, I., & Clemens, J. A. (1992). Age-related decline in the dopaminergic nigrostriatal system: The oxidative hypothesis and protective strategies. *Annals of Neurology, 32*, S133–S136.

Felten, D. L., Gibson-Berry, K., & Wu, J. H. D. (1996). Innervation of bone marrow by tyrosine hydroxylase-immunoreactive nerve fibers and hemopoiesis-modulating activity of a β-adrenergic agonist in mouse. *Molecular Biology of Hematopoiesis, 5*, 627–636.

Felten, D. L., Livnat, S., Felten, S. Y., Carlson, S. L., Bellinger, D. L., & Yeh, P. (1984). Sympathetic innervation of lymph nodes in mice. *Brain Research Bulletin, 13*, 693–699.

Felten, S. Y., Bellinger, D. L., Collier, T. J., Coleman, P. D., & Felten, D. L. (1987). Decreased sympathetic innervation of spleen in aged Fischer 344 rats. *Neurobiology of Aging, 8*, 159–165.

Felten, S. Y., & Felten, D. L. (1989). Are lymphocytes targets of noradrenergic innervation? In H. Weiner, D. Helhammer, R. Murison, & I. Florin (Eds.), *Frontiers of stress research* (pp. 56–71). Toronto: Hans Huber.

Felten, S. Y., & Felten, D. L. (1991). The innervation of lymphoid tissue. In R. Ader, D. L. Felten, & N. Cohen (Eds.), *Psychoneuroimmunology*, (2nd ed., pp. 27–69). New York: Academic Press.

Felten, S. Y., Felten, D. L., Bellinger, D. L., Carlson, S. L., Ackerman, K. D., Madden, K. S., Olschowka, J. A., & Livnat, S. (1988). Noradrenergic sympathetic innervation of lymphoid organs. *Progress in Allergy, 43*, 14–36.

Felten, S. Y., & Olschowka, J. A. (1987). Noradrenergic sympathetic innervation of the spleen: II. Tyrosine hydroxylase (TH)-positive nerve terminals form synaptic-like contacts on lymphocytes in the splenic white pulp. *Journal of Neuroscience Research, 18*, 37–48.

Felten, S. Y., Olschowka, J. A., Ackerman, K. D., & Felten, D. L. (1988). Catecholaminergic innervation of the spleen: Are lymphocytes targets of noradrenergic nerves? In A. Dahlström, R. H. Belmaker, & M. Sandler (Eds.), *Progress in catecholamine research, part A: Basic aspects and peripheral mechanisms* (pp. 525–531). New York: Alan R. Liss.

Fillenz, M., & Pollard, R. M. (1976). Quantitative differences between sympathetic nerve terminals. *Brain Research, 109*, 443–454.

Finch, C. E. (1973). Catecholamine metabolism in the brains of ageing mice. *Brain Research, 52*, 261–276.

Finch, L., Haeusler, G., Kuhn, H., & Thoenen, H. (1973). Rapid recovery of vascular adrenergic nerves in the rat after chemical sympathectomy with 6-hydroxydopamine. *British Journal of Pharmacology, 48*, 59–72.

Fink, T., & Weihe, E. (1988). Multiple neuropeptides in nerves supplying mammalian lymph nodes: Messenger candidates for sensory and autonomic neuroimmunomodulation? *Neuroscience Letters, 90*, 39–44.

Flurkey, K., Stadecker, M., & Miller, R. A. (1992). Memory T lymphocyte hyporesponsiveness to non-cognate stimuli: A key factor in age related immunodeficiency. *European Journal of Immunology, 22*, 931–935.

Forsthumber, T., Hualin, C. Y., & Lehmann, P. V. (1996). Induction of Th1 and Th2 immunity in neonatal mice. *Science, 271*, 1728–1730.

Franklin, R. A., Arkins, S., Li, Y. M., & Kelley, K. W. (1993). Macrophages suppress lectin-induced proliferation of lymphocytes from aged rats. *Mechanisms of Ageing and Development, 67*, 33–46.

Fried, G., Terenius, L., Brodin, E., Efendic, S., Dockray, G., Fahrenkrug, J., Goldstein, M., & Hökfelt, T. (1986). Neuropeptide Y, enkephalin and noradrenaline coexist in sympathetic neurons innervating the bovine spleen. Biochemical and immunohistochemical evidence. *Cell and Tissue Research, 243*, 495–508.

Fuchs, B. A., Albright, J. W., & Albright, J. F. (1988). β-Adrenergic receptors on murine lymphocytes: density varies with cell maturity and lymphocyte subtype and is decreased after antigen administration. *Cellular Immunology, 114*, 231–245.

Gauthier, P., Nadeau, R., & De Champlain, J. (1972). Acute and chronic cardiovascular effects of 6-hydroxydopamine in dogs. *Circulation Research, 31*, 207–217.

Geppetti, P., Frilli, S., Renzi, D., Santicioli, P., Maggi, C. A., Theodorsson, E., & Fanciullacci, M. (1988). Distribution of calcitonin gene-related peptide-like immunoreactivity in various rat tissues: Correlation with substance P and other tachykinins and sensitivity to capsaicin. *Regulatory Peptides, 23*, 289–298.

Geppetti, P., Maggi, C. A., Zecchi-Orlandini, S., Santicioli, P., Meli, A., Frilli, S., Spillantini, M. G., & Amenta, F. (1987). Substance P-like immunoreactivity in capsaicin-sensitive structures of the rat thymus. *Regulatory Peptides, 18*, 321–329.

Giron, L. T., Crutcher, K. A., & Davis, J. N. (1980). Lymph nodes—a possible site for sympathetic neuronal regulation of immune responses. *Annals of Neurology, 8*, 520–525.

Grossmann, A., Rabinovitch, P. S., Kavanagh, T. J., Jinneman, J. C., Gilliland, L. K., Ledbetter, J. A., & Kanner, S. B. (1995). Activation of murine T-cells via phospholipase-Cg1-associated protein tyrosine phosphorylation is reduced with aging. *Journal of Gerontology, 50A*, B205–B212.

Hall, N. R. S., O'Grady, M. P., & Farah, J. R., Jr. (1991). Thymic hormones and immune function: mediation via neuroendocrine circuits. In R. Ader, N. Cohen, & D. L. Felten (Eds.), *Psychoneuroimmunology* (2nd ed., pp. 515–528). New York: Academic Press.

Haugen, P. K., & Letourneau, P. C. (1990). Interleukin-2 enhances chick and rat sympathetic, but not sensory, neurite outgrowth. *Journal of Neuroscience Research, 532*, 323.

Hausdorff, W. P., Caron, M. G., & Lefkowitz, R. J. (1990). Turning off the signal: Desensitization of β-adrenergic receptor function. *FASEB Journal, 4*, 2881–2889.

Hobbs, M. V., Ernst, D. N., Torbett, B. E., Glasebrook, A. L., Rehse, M. A., McQuitty, D. N., Thoman, M. L., Bottomly, K., Rothermal, A. L., Noonan, D. J., & Weigle, W. O. (1991). Cell proliferation and cytokine production by $CD4^+$ cells from old mice. *Journal of Cellular Biochemistry, 46*, 312–320.

Hobbs, M. V., Weigle, W. O., Noonan, D. J., Torbett, B. E., McEvilly, R. J., Koch, R. J., Cardenas, G. J., & Ernst, D. N. (1993). Patterns of cytokine gene expression by $CD4^+$ cells from old mice. *Journal of Immunology, 150*, 3602–3614.

Irwin, M., Hauger, R., & Brown, M. (1992). Central corticotropin-releasing hormone activates the sympathetic nervous system and reduces immune function: Increased responsivity of the aged rat. *Endocrinology, 131*, 1047–1053.

Jagadeesh, G., Tian, W. N., Gupta, S., & Deth, R. C. (1990). Developmental changes in a1-adrenoceptor coupling to G-protein in bovine aorta. *European Journal of Pharmacology, 189*, 11–21.

Josefsson, E., Bergquist, J., Ekman, R., & Tarkowski, A. (1996). Catecholamines are synthesized by mouse lymphocytes and regulate function of these cells by induction of apoptosis. *Immunology, 88*, 140–146.

Kannan, Y., Bienenstock, J., Ohta, M., Stanisz, A. M., & Stead, R. H. (1996). Nerve growth factor and cytokines mediate lymphoid tissue-induced neurite outgrowth from mouse superior cervical ganglia in vitro. *Journal of Immunology, 156*, 313–320.

Kostrouch, Z., Raska, I., Felt, V., Nedvídková, J., & Holecková, E. (1987). Internalization of triiodothyronine-bovine serum albumin-colloidal gold complexes in human peripheral leukocytes. *Experientia, 43*, 1119–1120.

Kostrzewa, R. M., & Jacobwitz, D. M. (1974). Pharmacological actions of 6-hydroxydopamine. *Pharmacological Reviews, 26*, 199–288.

Krall, J. F., Connelly, M., Weisbart, R., & Tuck, M. L. (1981). Age-related elevation of plasma catecholamine concentration and reduced responsiveness of lymphocyte adenylatecyclase. *Journal of Clinical Endocrinology and Metabolism, 52*, 863–867.

Kranz, A., Kendall, M. D., & von Gaudecker, B. (1997). Studies on rat and human thymus to demonstrate immunoreactivity of calcitonin gene-related peptide, tyrosine hydroxylase and neuropeptide Y. *Journal of Anatomy, 191*, 441–450.

Kruszewska, B., Felten, S. Y., & Moynihan, J. A. (1995). Alterations in cytokine and antibody production following chemical sympathectomy in two strains of mice. *Journal of Immunology, 155*, 4613–4620.

Kruszewska, B., Felten, D. L., Stevens, S. Y., & Moynihan, J. A. (1998). Sympathectomy-induced immune changes are not abrogated by the glucocorticoid receptor blocker RU-486. *Brain, Behavior, & Immunity, 12*, 181–200.

Kuchroo, V. K., Das, M. D., Brown, J. A., Ranger, A. M., Zamvil, S. S., Sobel, R. A., Weiner, H. L., Nabavi, N., & Glimcher, L. H. (1995). B7-1 and B7-2 costimulatory molecules activate differentially the Th1/Th2 development pathways: application to autoimmune disease therapy. *Cell, 80*, 707–718.

Kushima, Y., Hama, T., & Hatanaka, H. (1992). Interleukin-6 as a neurotrophic factor for promoting the survival of cultured catecholaminergic neurons in a chemically defined medium from fetal and postnatal rat midbrains. *Journal of Neuroscience Research, 13*, 267–280.

Kusiak, J. W., & Pitha, J. (1983). Decreased response with age of the cardiac catecholamine sensitive adenylate cyclase system. *Life Sciences, 33*, 1679–1686.

Lake, C. R., Zeigler, M. G., Coleman, M. D., & Kopin, I. J. (1977). Age related norepinephrine levels are similar in normotensive and hypertensive subjects. *New England Journal of Medicine, 296*, 208–209.

Laverty, R., Sharman, D. F., & Vogt, M. (1965). Action of 2,4,5-trihydroxyphenylethylamine on the storage and release of noradrenaline. *British Journal of Pharmacology, 24*, 549–560.

Lerner, A., Yamada, T., & Miller, R. A. (1989). Pgp-1^{hi} T lymphocytes accumulate with age in mice and respond poorly to concanavalin A. *European Journal of Immunology, 19*, 977–982.

Levine, J. D., Coderre, T. J., Helms, C., & Basbaum, A. I. (1988). β_2-adrenergic mechanisms in experimental arthritis. *Proceedings of the National Academy of Sciences of the United States of America, 85*, 4553–4556.

Levine, J. D., Dardick, S. J., Basbaum, A. I., & Scipio, E. (1985). Reflex neurogenic inflammation. I. Contribution of the peripheral nervous system to spatially remote inflammatory responses that follow injury. *Journal of Neuroscience, 5*, 1380–1386.

Livnat, S., Felten, S. Y., Carlson, S. L., Bellinger, D. L., & Felten, D. L. (1985). Involvement of peripheral and central catecholamine systems in neural-immune interactions. *Journal of Neuroimmunology, 10*, 5–30.

Lorton, D., Bellinger, D. L., Duclos, M., Felten, S. Y., & Felten, D. L. (1996). Application of 6-hydroxydopamine into the fatpads surrounding the draining lymph nodes exacerbates adjuvant-induced arthritis. *Journal of Neuroimmunology, 64*, 103–113.

Lorton, D., Bellinger, D. L., Felten, S. Y., & Felten, D. L. (1989). Substance P (SP) and calcitonin gene-related peptide (CGRP) innervation of the rat spleen. *Society for Neuroscience Abstracts, 15*, 714.

Lorton, D., Bellinger, D. L., Felten, S. Y., & Felten, D. L. (1990a). Substance P innervation of the rat thymus. *Peptides, 11*, 1269–1275.

Lorton, D., Bellinger, D. L., Felten, S. Y., & Felten, D. L. (1991). Substance P innervation of spleen in rats: Nerve fibers associate with lymphocytes and macrophages in specific compartments of the spleen. *Brain, Behavior, and Immunity, 5*, 29–40.

Lorton, D., Hewitt, D., Bellinger, D. L., Felten, S. Y., & Felten, D. L. (1990). Noradrenergic reinnervation of the rat spleen following chemical sympathectomy with 6-hydroxydopamine: Pattern and time course of reinnervation. *Brain, Behavior, and Immunity, 4*, 198–222.

Lorton, D., Lubahn, C., Felten, S. Y., & Bellinger, D. L. (1997). Norepinephrine content in primary and secondary lymphoid organs is altered in rats with adjuvant-induced arthritis. *Mechanisms of Ageing and Development, 94*, 145–63.

Lundberg, J. M., Änggård, A., Pernow, J., & Hökfelt, T. (1985). Neuropeptide Y-, substance P- and VIP-immunoreactive nerves in cat spleen in relation to autonomic vascular and volume control. *Cell and Tissue Research, 239*, 9–18.

MacKay, I. R. (1972). Ageing and immunological function in man. *Gerontologia, 18*, 285–304.

Madden, K. S., Ackerman, K. D., Livnat, S., Felten, S. Y., & Felten, D. L. (1993). Neonatal sympathetic denervation alters development of natural killer (NK) cell activity in F344 rats. *Brain, Behavior, and Immunity, 7*, 344–351.

Madden, K. S., Bellinger, D. L., Felten, S. Y., Synder, E., Maida, M. E., & Felten, D. L. (1997). Alterations in sympathetic innervation of thymus and spleen in aged mice. *Mechanisms of Ageing and Development, 94*, 165–175.

Madden, K. S., Bellinger, D. L., Tong, A., Housel, J., Costello, N., & Richardson, C. (1992). Plasticity of noradrenergic nerves in spleens from aged F344 rats following chemical sympathectomy. *Society for Neuroscience Abstracts, 18*, 1009.

Madden, K. S., Felten, S. Y., Felten, D. L., & Bellinger, D. L. (2000). Alterations in T lymphocyte activity following chemical sympathectomy in young and old Fischer 344 rats. *Journal of Neuroimmunology, 103*, 131–145.

Madden, K. S., Felten, S. Y., Felten, D. L.,, & Bellinger, D. L. (1995). Sympathetic nervous system-immune system interactions in young and old Fischer 344 (F344) rats. *Annals of the New York Academy of Science, 771*, 523–534.

Madden, K. S., & Livnat, S. (1991). Catecholaminergic action on immunologic reactivity. In R. Ader, D. L. Felten, & N. Cohen (Eds.), *Psychoneuroimmunology* (2nd ed., pp. 283–310). New York: Academic Press.

Maestroni, G. J., & Conti, A. (1994). Modulation of hematopoiesis via alpha 1-adrenergic receptors on bone marrow cells. *Experimental Hematology, 22*, 313–320.

Maestroni, G. J., Conti, A., & Pedrinis, E. (1992). Effect of adrenergic agents on hematopoiesis after syngeneic bone marrow transplantation in mice. *Blood, 80*, 1178–1182.

Maestroni, G. J. M., Cosentino, M., Marino, F., Togni, M., Conti, A., Lecchini, S., & Frigo, G. (1998). Neural and endogenous catecholamines in the bone marrow. Circadian association of norepinephrine with hematopoiesis. *Experimental Hematology, 26*, 1172–1177.

Makinodan, T. (1976). Immunology of aging. *Journal of the American Geriatric Society, 24*, 249–252.

Makinodan, T., & Adler, W. H. (1975). Effects of aging on the differentiation and proliferation potentials of the immune system. *Federation Proceedings, 34*, 153–158.

Makinodan, T., Perkins, E. H., & Chen, M. G. (1971). Immunological activity of the aged. *Advances in Gerontological Research, 3*, 171–198.

Malmfors, T., & Sachs, C. (1968). Degeneration of adrenergic nerves produced by 6-hydroxydopamine. *European Journal of Pharmacology, 3*, 89–92.

Marchetti, B., Morale, M. C., & Pelletier, G. (1990). Sympathetic nervous system control of rat thymus gland maturation: Autoradiographic localization of the β_2-adrenergic receptor in the thymus and presence of sexual dimorphism during ontogeny. *Progress in NeuroEndocrinImmunology, 3*, 103–115.

McArthur, J. G., & Raulet, D. H. (1993). CD28-induced costimulation of T helper type 2 cells mediated by induction of responsiveness to interleukin-4. *Journal of Experimental Medicine, 178*, 1645–1653.

McElhaney, J. E., Meneilly, G. S., Lechelt, K. E., Beattie, B. L., & Bleackley, R. C. (1993). Antibody response to whole-virus and split-virus influenza vaccines in successful ageing. *Vaccine, 11*, 1055–1066.

McGeer, P. L., McGeer, E. G., & Suzuki, J. A. (1977). Aging and extrapyramidal function. *Archives of Neurology, 34*, 33–35.

Mehler, M. F., Rozental, R., Dougherty, M., Spray, D. C., & Kessler, J. A. (1993). Cytokine regulation of neuronal differentiation of hippocampal progenitor cells. *Nature, 362*, 62–65.

Miller, M. L., & McCuskey, R. S. (1973). Innervation of bone marrow in the rabbit. *Scandinavian Journal of Haematology, 10*, 17–23.

Miller, R., Jacobson, B., Weil, G., & Simons, E. (1987). Diminished calcium influx in lectin-stimulated T cells from old mice. *Journal of Cellular Physiology, 132*, 337–342.

Miller, R. A. (1989). The cell biology of aging: Immunological models. *Journal of Gerontology, 44*, B4–B8.

Mitchell, B., Kendall, M., Adam, E., & Schumacher, U. (1997). Innervation of the thymus in normal and bone marrow reconstituted severe combined immunodeficient (SCID) mice. *Journal of Neuroimmunology, 75*, 19–27.

Miyamato, A., Kowatch, M. A., & Roth, G. S. (1993). Similar effects of saponin treatment and aging on coupling of a_1-adrenergic receptor-G-protein. *Experimental Gerontology, 28*, 349–359.

Miyamoto, A., Kawana, S., Kimura, H., & Ohskika, H. (1994). Impaired expression of G_{sa} protein mRNA in rat ventricular myocardium with aging. *European Journal of Pharmacology, 266*, 147–154.

Montamant, S. C., & Davies, A. O. (1989). Physiological response to isoproterenol and coupling of beta-adrenergic receptors in young and elderly human subjects. *Journal of Gerontology, 44*, M100–M105.

Mueller, R. A., Thoenen, H., & Axelrod, J. (1969). Adrenal tyrosine hydroxylase: Compensatory increase in activity after chemical sympathectomy. *Science, 163*, 468–469.

Murphy, M., Reid, K., Brown, M. A., & Bartlett, P. F. (1993). Involvement of leukaemia inhibitory factor and nerve growth factor in the development of dorsal root ganglion neurons. *Development, 117*, 1173–1182.

Müller, S., & Weihe, E. (1991). Interrelation of peptidergic innervation with mast cells and ED1-positive cells in rat thymus. *Brain, Behavior, & Immunity, 5*, 55–72.

Nadeau, R. A., De Champlain, J., & Tremblay, G. M. (1971). Supersensitivity of the isolated rat heart after chemical sympathectomy with 6-hydroxydopamine. *Canadian Journal of Physiological Pharmacology, 49*, 36–44.

Nance, D. M., Hopkins, D. A., & Bieger, D. (1987). Re-investigation of the innervation of the thymus gland in mice and rats. *Brain, Behavior, and Immunity, 1*, 134–147.

O'Connor, S. W., Scarpace, P. J., & Abrass, I. B. (1983). Age-associated decrease in the catalytic unit activity of rat myocardial adenylate cyclase. *Mechanisms of Ageing and Development, 21*, 357–363.

O'Hara, N., Daul, A. E., Fesel, R., Siekmann, U., & Brodde, O.-E. (1985). Different mechanisms underlying reduced β_2-adrenoceptor responsiveness in lymphocytes from neonates and old subjects. *Mechanisms of Ageing and Development, 31*, 115–122.

Orly, J., & Schramm, M. (1975). Fatty acids as modulators of membrane functions: Catecholamine-activated adenylate cyclase of the turkey erythrocyte. *Biochemistry, 9*, 3433–3437.

Paparelli, A., Soldani, P., Breschi, M. C., Ricciardi, M. P., & Pellegrini, A. (1988). Age-related changes in the recovery of noradrenaline content in sympathetic fibres after reserpine treatment. *Acta Histochemica, 84*, 121–125.

Patel, H. R., & Miller, R. A. (1992). Age-associated changes in mitogen-induced protein phosphorylation in murine T lymphocytes. *European Journal of Immunology, 146*, 3332–3339.

Petkova, D. H., Momchilova, A. B., & Koumanov, K. S. (1986). Age-related changes in rat liver plasma membrane phospholipase A2 activity. *Experimental Gerontology, 21*, 187–193.

Popper, P., Mantyh, C. R., Vigna, S. R., Magioos, J. E., & Mantyh, P. W. (1988). The localization of sensory nerve fibers and receptor binding sites for sensory neuropeptides in canine mesenteric lymph nodes. *Peptides, 9*, 257–267.

Proust, J. J., Filburn, C. R., Harrison, S. A., Buchholz, M. A,. & Nordin, A. A. (1987). Age-related defect in signal transduction during lectin activation of murine T lymphocytes. *Journal of Immunology, 139*, 1472–1478.

Radojcic, T., Baird, S., Darko, D., Smith, D. & Bulloch, K. (1991). Changes in β-adrenergic receptor distribution on immunocytes during differentiation: An analysis of T cells and macrophages. *Journal of Neuroscience Research, 30*, 328–335.

Rasenick, M. M., Stein, P. J., & Bitensky, M. W. (1981). The regulatory subunit of adenylate cyclase interacts with cytoskeletal components. *Nature (London), 294*, 560–562.

Ridge, J. P., Fuchs, E. J., & Matzinger, P. (1996). Neonatal tolerance revisited: Turning on newborn T cells with dendritic cells. *Science, 271*, 1723–1726.

Rimon, G., Hanski, E., Braun, S., & Levitzki, A. (1978). Mode of coupling between hormone receptors and adenylate cyclase elucidated by modulation of membrane fluidity. *Nature (London), 276*, 394–396.

Romano, T., Felten, S. Y., Olschowka, J. A., & Felten, D. L. (1994). Noradrenergic and peptidergic innervation of lymphoid organs in the beluga, *Delphinapterus leucas*: An anatomical link between the nervous and immune systems. *Journal of Morphology, 221*, 243–259.

Romano, T. A., Felten, S. Y., Felten, D. L., & Olschowka, J. A. (1991). Neuropeptide-Y innervation of the rat spleen: Another potential immunomodulatory neuropeptide. *Brain, Behavior, and Immunity, 5*, 116–131.

Santambrogio, L., Benedetti, M., Chao, M.V., Muzaffar, R., Kulig, K., Gabellini, N., & Hochwald, G. (1994). Nerve growth factor production by lymphocytes. *Journal of Immunology, 153*, 4488–4495.

Sarzotti, M., Robbins, D. S., & Hoffman, P. M. (1996). Induction of protective CTL responses in newborn mice by a murine retrovirus. *Science, 271*, 1726–1728.

Scarpace, P. J. (1986). Decreased β-adrenergic responsiveness during senescence. *Federation Proceedings, 45*, 51–54.

Scarpace, P. J., & Abrass, I. B. (1983). Decreased beta-adrenergic agonist affinity and adenylate cyclase activity in senescent rat lung. *Journal of Gerontology, 38*, 143–147.

Scarpace, P. J., & Abrass, I. B. (1986). Beta-adrenergic agonist-mediated desensitization in senescent rats. *Mechanisms of Ageing and Development, 35*, 255–264.

Schultzberg, M., Svenson, S. B., Unden, A., & Bartfai, T. (1987). Interleukin-1-like immunoreactivity in peripheral tissues. *Journal of Neuroscience Research, 18*, 184–189.

Seder, R. A., Germain, R. N., Linsley, P. S., & Paul, W. E. (1994). CD28-mediated costimulation of interleukin-2 (IL-2) production plays a critical role in T cell priming for IL-4 and interferon-g production. *Journal of Experimental Medicine, 179*, 299–304.

Sergeeva, V. E. (1974). Histotopography of catecholamines in the mammalian thymus. *Bulletin of Experimental Biology and Medicine, 77*, 456–458.

Singh, U. (1979a). Effect of catecholamines on lymphopoiesis in fetal mouse thymic explants. *European Journal of Immunology, 14*, 757–759.

Singh, U. (1979b). Effect of catecholamines on lymphopoiesis in fetal mouse thymic explants. *Journal of Anatomy, 129*, 279–292.

Singh, U. (1985). Lymphopoiesis in the nude fetal mouse thymus following sympathectomy. *Cellular Immunology, 93*, 222–228.

Singh, U. (1984). Sympathetic innervation of fetal mouse thymus. *European Journal of Immunology, 14*, 757–759.

Singh, U., & Owen, J. J. T. (1976). Studies on the maturation of thymus stem cells. The effects of catecholamines, histamine, and peptide hormones on the expression of T alloantigens. *European Journal of Immunology, 6*, 59–62.

Stein, B. E. (1994). Vaccinating elderly people. Protecting from avoidable disease. *Drugs and Aging, 5*, 242–253.

Stephan, R. P., Lill-Elghanian, D. A., & Witte, P. L. (1997). Development of B cells in aged mice: decline in the ability of pro-B cells to respond to IL-7 but not to other growth factors. *Journal of Immunology, 158*, 1598–1609.

Stephan, R. P., Sanders, V. M., & Witte, P. L. (1996). Stage-specific alterations in murine B lymphopoiesis with age. *International Immunology, 8*, 509–518.

Sung, C. P., Arleth, A. J., & Feuerstein, G. Z. (1991). Neuropeptide Y upregulates the adhesiveness of human endothelial cells for leukocytes. *Circulation Research, 68*, 314–318.

Szewczuk, M. R., & Wade, A. W. (1983). Aging and the mucosal-associated lymphoid system. *Annals of the New York Academy of Science, 409*, 333–344.

Tabarowski, Z., Gibson-Berry, K., & Felten, S. Y. (1996). Noradrenergic and peptidergic innervation of the mouse femur. *Acta Histochemica, 98*, 453–457.

Theofilopoulos, A. N., & Dixon, F. J. (1985). Murine models of systemic lupus erythematosus. *Advances in Immunology, 37*, 269–390.

Thoman, M. L., & Weigle, O. (1989). The cellular and subcellular bases of immunosenescence. *Advances in Immunology, 46*, 221–261.

Thompson, C. B. (1995). Distinct roles for the costimulatory ligands B7-1 and B7-2 in T helper cell differentiation. *Cell, 80*, 979–982.

ThyagaRajan, S., Felten, S. Y., & Felten, D. L. (1998). Restoration of sympathetic noradrenergic nerve fibers in the spleen by low doses of L-deprenyl treatment in young sympathectomized and old Fischer 344 rats. *Journal of Neuroimmunology, 81*, 144–157.

ThyagaRajan, S., Madden, K. S., Kalvas, J. C., Dimitrova, S. S., Felten, S. Y., & Felten, D. L. (1998). L-deprenyl-induced increase in IL-2 and NK cell activity accompanies restoration of noradrenergic nerve fibers in the spleens of old F344 rats. *Journal of Neuroimmunology, 92*, 9–21.

Torii, H., Yan, Z., Hosoi, J., & Granstein, R. D. (1997). Expression of neurotrophic factors and neuropeptide receptors by Langerhans cells and the Langerhans cell-like cell line XS52: Further support for a functional relationship between Langerhans cells and epidermal nerves. *Journal of Investigative Dermatology, 109*, 586–591.

Tsujimoto, G., Lee, C., & Hoffman, B. B. (1986). Age-related decrease in beta adrenergic receptor-mediated vascular smooth muscle relaxation. *Journal of Pharmacology and Experimental Therapeutics, 239*, 411–415.

Vacca, A., Felli, M. P., Farina, A. R., Martinotti, S., Maroder, M., Screpanti, I., Meco, D., Petrangeli, E., Frati, L., & Gulino, A. (1992). Glucocorticoid receptor-mediated suppression of the interleukin 2 gene expression through impairment of the cooperativity between nuclear factor of activated T cells and AP-1 enhancer elements. *Journal of Experimental Medicine, 175*, 637–646.

van Coelln, R., Unsicker, K., & Krieglstein, K. (1995). Screening of interleukins for survival-promoting effects on cultured mesencephalic dopaminergic neurons from embryonic rat brain. *Developmental Brain Research, 89*, 150–154.

Walford, R. L. 1969. *The immunologic theory of aging*. Copenhagen: Manksgaard.

Wang, C. Q., Udupa, K. B., Xiao, H., & Lipschitz, D. A. (1995). Effect of age on marrow macrophage number and function. *Aging, 7*, 379–384.

Weihe, E., Müller, S., Fink, T., & Zentel, H. J. (1989). Tachykinins, calcitonin gene-related peptide and neuropeptide Y in nerves of the mammalian thymus: Interactions with mast cells in autonomic and sensory neuroimmunomodulation. *Neuroscience Letters, 100*, 77–82.

Weksler, M. E. (1982). Age-associated changes in the immune response. *Journal of the American Geriatric Society, 30*, 718–723.

Wiedmeier, S. E., Burnham, D. K., Singh, U., & Daynes, R. A. (1987). Implantation of thymic epithelial grafts into the anterior chamber of the murine eye: An experimental model for analyzing T-cell ontogeny. *Thymus, 9*, 25–44.

Williams, J. M., & Felten, D. L. (1981). Sympathetic innervation of murine thymus and spleen: A comparative histofluorescence study. *Anatomical Records, 199*, 531–542.

Williams, J. M., Peterson, R. G., Shea, P. A., Schmedtje, J. F., Bauer, D. C., & Felten, D. L. (1981). Sympathetic innervation of murine thymus and spleen: Evidence for a functional link between the nervous and immune systems. *Brain Research Bulletin, 6*, 83–94.

Zentel, H. J., & Weihe, E. (1991). The neuro-B cell link of peptidergic innervation in the bursa Fabricii. *Brain, Behavior, and Immunity, 5*, 132–147.

Ziegler, M. G., Lake, C. R., & Kopin, I. J. (1976). Plasma noradrenaline increases with age. *Nature (London), 261*, 333–335.

PART

II

NEUROENDOCRINE EFFECTS ON IMMUNITY

CHAPTER

9

Neuroendocrine Regulation of Macrophage and Neutrophil Function

CHAD S. BOOMERSHINE, TIANYI WANG, BRUCE S. ZWILLING

I. INTRODUCTION

A. The Macrophage

The mononuclear phagocyte is derived from bone marrow progenitor cells of the myeloid series. These cells enter the circulation as monocytes and are targeted to various tissues where they mature into macrophages. The macrophage traditionally has been thought of as a scavenger cell that removes tissue debris, foreign particles, and bacteria from the compromised host. However, more recent work has demonstrated that the macrophage plays a pivotal role in immunity and disease resistance (Stewart, Riedy, & Stewart, 1994; Van Furth, 1992). Macrophages are important phagocytic cells that can control the growth of microorganisms. Phagocytosis results in activation of the respiratory burst and production of reactive oxygen intermediates and hydrogen peroxide that have important antimicrobial activities (Robinson & Badway, 1994; Roos, Bolscher, & deBoer, 1992). The killed microorganisms are digested by enzymes in the phagolysosome and selected peptides become associated with major histocompatibility complex (MHC) class II glycoproteins (Safley & Ziegler, 1994). These peptides, together with MHC class II, are cycled to the cell surface where they serve as the basis for antigen recognition by $CD4^+$ T-helper cells. This is an important mechanism in controlling the immune response, as binding of antigen associated with MHC class II to the T-cell receptor (TCR) results in T cell activation. Thus, macrophages serve as important cells in controlling microbial growth and in presenting "processed" antigens to T cells and initiating the immune response.

Interactions with microorganisms and T cells stimulate macrophages to produce a variety of inflammatory cytokines including Interleukin (IL)-1, IL-6, and tumor necrosis factor (TNF)-α (Dinarello, 1992; Dinarello et al., 1991), and these cytokines can also affect macrophage and T cell function. Production of interferon-gamma (IFN-γ) by antigen-stimulated T cells and natural killer (NK) cells can result in macrophage activation. This activation results in enhanced cytotoxic activity including production of reactive nitrogen intermediates (RNIs) (Hibbs, Taintor, Vavrin, & Rachlin, 1988). RNIs are required for the control of many intracellular pathogens (Fortier et al., 1994; Green et al., 1994; Liew, Wei, & Proudfoot, 1997; Pope et al., 1998), and are particularly important in macrophage antimycobacterial activity (Bonecini-Almeida et al., 1998; Britton, Meadows, Rathjen, Roach, & Briscoe, 1998; Doi et al., 1993; Flesch & Kaufmann, 1991).

B. Pathogenesis of Tuberculosis

The initial step in the pathogenesis of tuberculosis depends on the establishment of a primary lesion. This begins with the inhalation of droplet nuclei generated by a patient with active tuberculosis (Wiegeshaus, Balasubramanian, & Smith, 1989). Although less than 10% of inhaled *Mycobacterium tuberculosis* organisms reach the respiratory bronchioles and alveoli—most will settle in the upper respiratory epithelium and be expelled by the mucociliary escalator (Nardell, 1993)—the infectious dose in tuberculosis is extremely low. A single droplet nucleus containing one-to-three tubercle bacilli is usually sufficient to initiate the development of a primary lesion in the lung (Dannenberg, 1993; O'Grady & Riley, 1963). Bacteria that reach the deep lung are phagocytized by alveolar macrophages. Phagocytosis can result in killing of the bacilli or the tubercle bacilli can survive to initiate an infection. Over a period of 2 to 3 weeks, the surviving bacilli replicate intracellularly, eventually resulting in lysis of their host macrophage (Kaplan et al., 1988; Wiegeshaus et al., 1989). The released mycobacteria are then ingested by newly arrived macrophages and, as this cycle is repeated, a primary lesion forms. Tubercle-laden macrophages travel to draining lymph nodes and eventually into the bloodstream.

This asymptomatic bacteremia coincides with the appearance of enhanced reactivity to the purified protein derivatives (PPD) of *M. tuberculosis* and the onset of cell-mediated immunity (Weigeshaus et al., 1989). As the tubercle-laden macrophages disperse the bacilli into the body, the bacilli are effectively trapped in the tissues and recreate metastatic foci. These granulomatous focal lesions are composed of macrophage-derived epithelioid giant cells and lymphocytes. T lymphocytes activated by macrophage-derived cytokines migrate to the foci, resulting in the further local activation of macrophages. This leads to caseaous necrosis resulting in the gradual sterilization of most metastatic lesions, with the exception of those lesions in the apical to subapical regions of the lung. Within the lung, the numbers of bacilli are reduced and a steady-state or latent infection becomes established. In most healthy individuals with intact immune function, organisms contained within these foci can remain dormant for decades. The relative strength of the host's cell-mediated immunity ultimately determines whether reactivation of the disease will occur. In 5 to 10% of infected individuals, a temporary suppression of the cellular arm of the immune system allows reactivation of the disease. The consequence of a resumption in multiplication of the bacilli leads to tissue destruction, systemic dissemination of disease, and, when left untreated, death.

II. EFFECT OF STRESS ON MACROPHAGE FUNCTION

The macrophage is an important effector cell in controlling mycobacterial growth. The susceptibility of humans to mycobacterial disease is determined, in part, by genetic differences (Crowle & Elkins, 1990; Stead, 1992; Stead, Lofgren, Sinner, & Riddick, 1990), but is also affected by socioeconomic factors such as homelessness, protein malnutrition associated with chronic alcoholism, immunoscenescence associated with aging, and stress. One of the first observations that stressful life events can affect the pathogenesis of disease was made by Ishigami (Ishigami, 1919). This landmark study looked at the opsonization of tubercle bacilli among chronically ill, tuberculous school children, and their teachers during both active and inactive phases of tuberculosis. During periods of emotional stress, Ishigami found decreased phagocytic cell activity and postulated that the stressful school environment led to the children's immunodepressed state and increased susceptibility to tuberculosis. It is now widely accepted that physical and psychological stress can modulate susceptibility to tuberculosis (Collins, 1989; Wiegeshaus et al., 1989), as well as immune function in general (Berkenbosch, Wolvers, & Derijk, 1991; Khansari, Murgo, & Faith, 1990; Kiecolt-Glaser and Glaser, 1995; Sheridan et al., 1998).

Physiologic responses to stressors are mediated by the sympathetic nervous system (SNS) and the hypothalamic-pituitary-adrenal (HPA) axis (Ader, Felten, & Cohen, 1991; Johnson, Kamilares, Chrousos, & Gold, 1992; Solomon, 1987). SNS activation results in the production of epinephrine by the adrenal medulla and the release of norepinephrine from sympathetic neurons innervating the secondary lymphoid organs (Felten et al., 1987). The SNS can directly modify immune function through adrenergic receptors, which have been characterized on macrophages (Abrass, O'Connor, Scarpace, & Abrass, 1985; Liggett, 1989), T cells (Sanders, 1995), and many other cells of the immune system (reviewed in Madden & Felten, 1995). Catecholamines alter many macrophage functions including cytokine production (Shen, Sha,

Kennedy, & Ou, 1994), antiviral activity (Kohut et al., 1998), and cytoplasmic motility (Fukushima et al., 1993; Petty & Martin, 1989) via changes in the concentration of cAMP.

The HPA axis regulates macrophage function by producing a cascade of hormones in response to a variety of stimuli that ultimately results in an increase in the production of glucocorticoids by the adrenals. Glucocorticoid effects are produced when the hormone binds to its cytoplasmic receptor. This results in internalization of the glucocorticoid-receptor complex and subsequent translocation into the nucleus. The glucocorticoid-receptor complex then binds to regulatory elements associated with certain genes resulting in their transcription (Payvar et al., 1981). Mononuclear cells represent one of the best studied primary target cells for glucocorticoids, as they possess high-affinity (type II) receptors for glucocorticoids (Crabtree, Munck, & Smith, 1980; Miesfeld, 1990; Munck, Mendel, Smith, & Ortl, 1990; Werb, Foley, & Munck, 1978). Many elements of the cellular immune response are altered by glucocorticoids. Glucocorticoids inhibit antigen processing and the presentation of antigen via expression of antigen in association with MHC class II by macrophages (Zwilling, Brown, & Pearl, 1991). Production of the proinflammatory cytokines IL-1, IL-6, and TNF-α by activated macrophages are blocked at the transcriptional and post-transcriptional level by glucocorticoids (Kern, Lamb, Reed, Daniele, & Nowell, 1988; Lee et al., 1988; Northrop, Crabtree, & Mattila, 1992). The down regulation of these potent mediators of inflammation underlies the immunosuppressive and antiinflammatory actions of the glucocorticoids.

A. HPA-Axis Mediated Immunomodulation

1. MHC Class II Expression

MHC class II glycoproteins serve as important restriction elements for antigen stimulation of $CD4^+$ T cells. Mice have two class II MHC haplotypes, I-A and I-E, whereas humans have three (HLA-DR, -DP, and -DQ). In humans, HLA-DR is constitutively expressed by monocytes whereas the expression of HLA-DP and HLA-DQ is lower (Beller & Unanue, 1981; Nunez et al., 1984; Smith & Ault, 1981; Sztein, Steeg, Johnson, & Oppenheim, 1984). In mice, neither I-A nor I-E is constitutively expressed, but are induced in vivo following injection of antigen or microorganisms or in vitro by treatment of macrophages with recombinant interferon (rIFN)-γ. Studies by our laboratory and others have shown that stress suppresses MCH class II expression (Jiang, Morrow-Tesch, Beller, Levy, & Black, 1990; Sonnenfeld, Cunnick, Armfield, Wood, & Ravin, 1992; Zwilling, Dinkins et al., 1990). Our work demonstrated that activation of the HPA axis by restraint stress suppressed MHC class II expression by murine peritoneal macrophages, and that this suppression coincided with peak levels of corticosterone in plasma.

Interestingly, subsequent work in our laboratory showed that the stress-induced suppression of MHC class II expression was limited to certain strains of mice (Zwilling, Brown et al., 1990). Mouse strains can be divided into two groups based on their ability to control the growth of mycobacteria in the spleen following intravenous injection of 10^4 CFU of *Mycobacterium bovis* BCG (Gros, Skamene, & Forget, 1981). Mice that are resistant to mycobacterial growth are termed Bcg^r, and this resistance is mediated by the *Nramp1* gene (formerly *Bcg*), which has been cloned in mice and humans (Barton, White, Roach, & Blackwell, 1994; Cellier et al., 1994; Vidal, Malo, Vogan, Skamene, & Gros, 1993). *Nramp1* codes for a phagolysosomal membrane product termed natural resistance associated macrophage protein that is expressed in macrophages (Cellier et al., 1994; Gros, Skamene, & Forget, 1983). Susceptible mice, termed Bcg^s, differ from Bcg^r mice in a nonconservative glycine to aspartic acid substitution within a predicted transmembrane domain of Nramp1 (Malo et al., 1994). *Nramp1* also mediates resistance to other mycobacterial species as well as other intracellular pathogens (Blackwell, Roach, Kiderlen, & Kaye, 1989; Stokes, Orme, & Collins, 1986; Taylor & O'Brian, 1982).

The presence of Nramp1 in Bcg^r mice results in a resistance of macrophages to the stress-induced decrease in MHC class II glycoprotein expression observed in Bcg^s mice. This difference is not due to a difference in susceptibility to stress, as corticosterone suppresses the induction of MHC class II by macrophages from both resistant and susceptible mice (Zwilling, Brown, & Pearl, 1992). Recently, we have shown that the difference in class II expression between resistant and susceptible mice is due to a difference in MHC class II mRNA stability (Figure 1, Brown, Lafuse, & Zwilling, 1997). Corticosterone decreases the stability of MHC class II mRNA in macrophages from Bcg^s mice but not from Bcg^r mice. The stability of mRNA of other IFN-γ-induced genes is similarly affected, thus accounting for the pleiotrophic effects that have been reported to be under the control of *Nramp1* (Formica, Roach, & Blackwell, 1994; Gazzinelli, Eltoum, Wynn, & Sher, 1993; Hilburger & Zwilling, 1994; Roach, Charterjee, & Blackwell, 1994). In support of this, our laboratory and others have

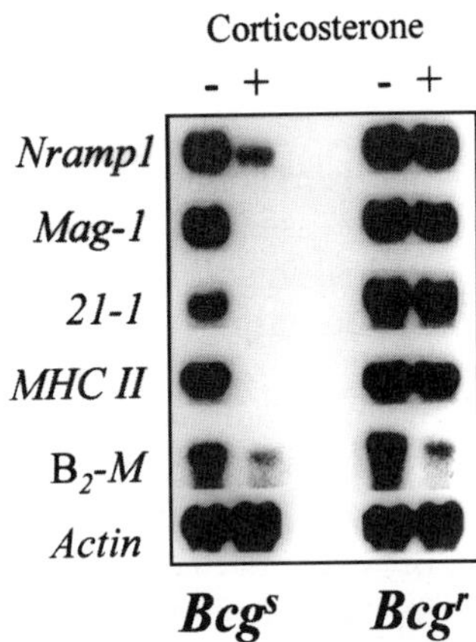

FIGURE 1 Differential effect of corticosterone on rIFN-γ-induced genes by macrophages from Bcg^r and Bcg^{s}mice. Splenic macrophages from Bcg^r and Bcg^s mice were stimulated with rIFN-γ for 24 h followed by treatment with corticosterone. After 20 h, total RNA was extracted, and the effect of corticosterone on the expression of rIFN-γ-induced genes was determined by Northern analysis. Copyright 1997 by the American Society for Microbiology, reprinted by permission from Brown et al., 1997.

shown that increasing rIFN-γ levels decreases the effect of restraint (Dunham, Arkins, Edwards, Dantzer, & Kelley, 1990; Szefler, Norton, Ball, Gross, Aida, & Pabst, 1989; Zwilling et al., 1992).

2. *Mycobacterial Resistance*

Our previous work on the differential expression of MHC class II glycoprotein in resistant and susceptible mice suggested that mycobacterial growth that is under *Nramp1* control also may be differentially affected by HPA axis activation. This led us to conduct a series of studies to determine the role of the HPA axis in regulating the growth of *M. avium* in congenic Bcg^s and Bcg^r mice. We found that activation of the HPA axis increased the susceptibility of Bcg^s mice to mycobacterial growth but did not affect the ability of Bcg^r mice to limit the growth of mycobacteria (Brown, Sheridan, Pearl, & Zwilling, 1993). As before, the failure of HPA axis activation to increase the susceptibility of Bcg^r mice was not due to unresponsiveness of the strain to HPA axis activation as evidenced by equal plasma corticosterone and adrenocortiotropic hormone levels produced in the two strains of mice in response to restraint. This, along with our previous work, suggested that HPA axis activation could account for the increased susceptibility of individuals to mycobacterial growth via increased levels of corticosterone. A series of experiments which demonstrated that corticosterone mediates the effects of restraint reinforced this hypothesis. Adrenalectomy of Bcg^s mice prevented the HPA axis-mediated increase in plasma corticosterone and abrogated the effect of HPA axis activation on mycobacterial growth. Artificially increasing plasma corticosterone levels to those attained during HPA axis activation by implantation of timed-release pellets resulted in an increased susceptibility of the adrenalectomized Bcg^s mice to mycobacterial growth. Finally, treatment of the Bcg^s mice with the glucocorticoid-receptor antagonist RU486 abrogated the effects of HPA axis activation.

The role of HPA axis activation in the control of the growth of tuberculosis in humans has been the subject of some discussion (Collins, 1989; Ishigami, 1919; Wiegeshaus et al., 1989). It has been shown that glucocorticoid treatment of human blood-derived macrophages and alveolar macrophages markedly suppressed antimicrobial activity (Schaffner, 1985). Rook et al. reported that dexamethasone increased the susceptibility of monocytes from some human donors to mycobacterial growth, but dexamethasone treatment of monocytes from other donors had no effect on the growth of bacilli (Rook, Steele, Ainsworth, & Leveton, 1987). These studies reinforce our observation on the differential effect of glucocorticoids on mycobacterial resistance in mice and suggest that similar mechanisms also control *M. tuberculosis* growth in humans.

B. SNS Influence on Macrophages

1. *Activation*

Numerous studies have reported that macrophage function can be suppressed or stimulated by catecholamines (reviewed in Zwilling, 1994). Generally, α-adrenergic receptor agonists enhance whereas β-adrenoceptor agonists decrease macrophage function. Catecholamines have been shown to stimulate macrophage function. Treatment of *M. avium*-infected macrophages with epinephrine or norepinephrine inhibited intracellular bacterial growth (Miles, Lafuse, & Zwilling, 1996). That is, the functional capacity of the macrophages was stimulated. The effect of the catecholamines was mediated by the α2-adrenergic receptor (Figure 2). Other laboratories also have shown that α-adrenoceptor stimulation can result in macrophage activation. Lappin and Whaley (1982) showed that treatment of monocytes with either epinephrine or norepinephrine enhanced the synthesis of complement components and this effect was mediated by the α1-adrenergic receptor. Epinephrine also has been shown to increase the production of hydrogen peroxide in activated macrophages (Costa Rosa, Safi, Cury, & Curi, 1992), and

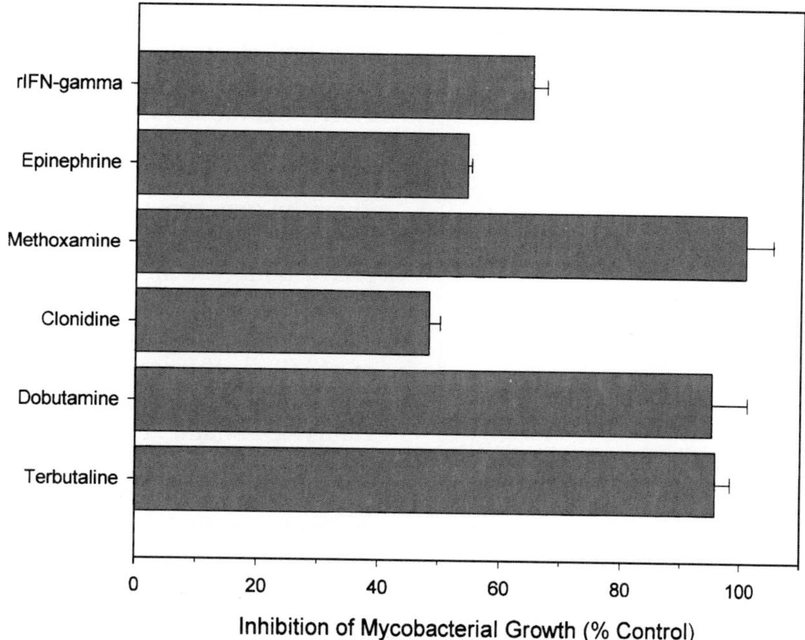

FIGURE 2 Effect of adrenergic receptor agonists on the antimycobacterial activity of peritoneal macrophages. Macrophages were infected with *Mycobaterium avium* during overnight culture. After washing to remove unphagocytized bacteria, the cultures were treated with adrenergic receptor agonists: epinephrine (mixed α and β), methoxamine (α1-specific), clonidine (α2-specific), dobutamine (β1-specific), and terbutaline (β2-specific). Cultures were incubated for 5 days prior to lysis of macrophages and ^{3}H-uracil labeling of bacteria overnight. The data represents the mean $\pm$ SD of three separate experiments.

Spengler et al. showed that norepinephrine increased TNF-α production by lipopolysaccharide (LPS) stimulated macrophages via α2-adrenergic receptor stimulation (Spengler, Allen, Remick, Strieter, & Kunkel, 1990; Spengler, Chensue, Giacherio, Blenk, & Kunkel, 1994).

2. *Inhibition*

Catecholamines can also inhibit macrophage activity. Epinephrine treatment of thioglycollate-elicited peritoneal macrophages decreased I-A expression induced by rIFN-γ (Zwilling, Brown, Feng, Sheridan, & Pearl, 1993). Koff and Dunegan have demonstrated that norepinephrine decreases macrophage phagocytosis and tumoricidal activity (Koff & Dunegan, 1985). Epinephrine and norepinephrine inhibited the capacity of rIFN-γ activated macrophages to kill herpes simplex virus-infected cells. Treating macrophages with cyclic adenosine monophosphate (cAMP) mimicked the effects of epinephrine (Koff & Dunegan, 1986; Koff, Fann, Dunegan, & Lachman, 1986). In contrast to the findings reported by Spengler et al. (1990, 1994), both α2- and β-adrenergic receptor agonists have been shown to inhibit TNF-α production in vivo (Elenkov, Haskó, Kovács, & Vizi, 1995). TNF-α synthesis by rat splenic macrophages was inhibited by norepinephrine (Hu, Goldmuntz, & Brosnan, 1991). Epinephrine has also been shown to modulate TNF-α production in human blood. Severn et al. (Severn, Rapson, Hunter, & Liew, 1992) demonstrated that epinephrine and isoproterenol, a specific β-adrenergic agonist, inhibited TNF-α production elicited by LPS in both whole blood and a human-macrophage cell line. This inhibition was dependent on increased cAMP levels. The observation that epinephrine decreased TNF-α production by human monocytes has been reported following both in vitro and in vivo treatment with LPS (Guirao et al., 1997 and Van der Poll, Coyle, Barbosa, Braxton, & Lowry, 1996, respectively). Our own experiments have confirmed the suppressive effect of epinephrine on TNF-α production in rIFN-γ primed, thioglycollate-elicited macrophages infected with *M. avium*. We went on to show that this inhibition is mediated through the β2-adrenergic receptor (Figure 3).

Van der Poll et al. (1996) also showed that, in addition to the decrease in TNF-α, epinephrine mediated an increase in the production of IL-10. IL-10 down-regulates the production IFN-γ, IL-2, granulocyte monocyte colony-stimulating factor (GM-CSF), and TNF-β by Th1-cells responding to antigen presenting cells (Fiorentino, Bond, & Mosmann, 1989; Fiorentino, Zlotnik, Vieira et al., 1991). Subsequent

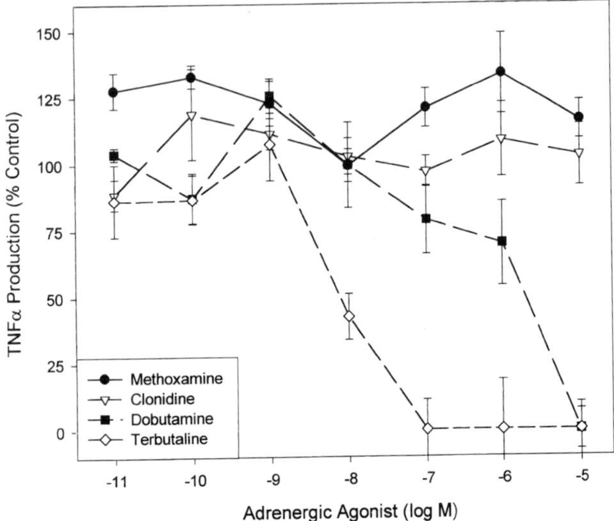

FIGURE 3 Effect of adrenergic receptor agonists on the production of TNF-α by peritoneal macrophages. Thioglycolate-elicited macrophages were treated with rIFN-γ overnight. Macrophages were then washed and infected with *Mycobacterium avium* and simultaneously treated with adrenergic-receptor agonists: methoxamine (α1-specific), clonidine (α2-specific), dobutamine (β1-specific), and terbutaline (β2-specific). Cultures were incubated for 48 h prior to determination of TNF-α in supernatants by ELISA. Values represent the mean percent of control (approximately 1000 pg/mL/2×10^5 cells) $\pm$ SE of three separate experiments.

studies showed that IL-10 inhibited Th1 activation through a suppression of antigen presentation by down-regulating MHC class II, ICAM-1, B7-1 and B7-2 expression on monocytes (Ding, Linsley, Huang, Germain, & Shevach, 1993; Kubin, Kamoun, & Trinchieri, 1994; Malefyt, Haanen et al., 1991; Willems et al., 1994). IL-10 has been shown to inhibit macrophage function directly by decreasing macrophage production of IL-8, GM-CSF, granulocyte colony-stimulating factor (G-CSF), as well as the proinflammatory cytokines TNF-α, IL-1α and β, and IL-6 (Bogdan, Vodovotz, & Nathan, 1991; Fiorentino, Zlotnik, Mosmann, Howard, & O'Garra, 1991; Malefyt, Abrams, Bennett, Figdor, & Devries, 1991). In addition to the decrease in cytokine production, IL-10 has also been shown to inhibit the killing of intracellular parasites by macrophages (Gazzinelli, Oswald, James, & Sher, 1992; Liew, 1993; Silva et al., 1992).

β-adrenergic agonists can increase IL-10 production by activated macrophages. Szabo et al. have shown that in vivo administration of isoproterenol to mice reduces LPS-induced plasma TNF-α and nitric oxide levels, along with a simultaneous increase in IL-10 (Szabo et al., 1997). Isoproterenol also has been shown to increase IL-10 levels in vitro by LPS-activated mouse peritoneal macrophages (Suberville et al., 1996). Siegmund et al. (Siegmund, Eigler, Hartmann, Hacker, & Endres, 1998) showed that epinephrine treatment enhanced the LPS-induced synthesis of IL-10 while at the same time suppressing TNF-α synthesis. The inhibitory effect was at both the protein and mRNA level and mediated through the cAMP-induced activation of protein kinase A. Recently, we reported that epinephrine treatment of *M. avium* infected macrophages increased IL-10 production (Chen, Boomershine, Wang, Lafuse, & Zwilling, 1999). This effect was mediated by the β2-adrenoceptor and could be mimicked by the addition of cAMP. IL-10 release is induced by *M. avium* infection of human monocytes (Muller, Aukrust, Lien, Haug, & Froland, 1998), and neutralization of IL-10 has been shown to increase resistance to *M. avium* infection in mice (Bermudez & Champsi, 1993; Denis & Ghadirian, 1993). These results suggest that catecholamine release, following sympathetic nervous system activation, may enhance mycobacterial growth.

Acquired resistance against organisms of the *Miavium* complex depends on the production of reactive nitrogen intermediates by macrophages (Denis, 1991). Nitric oxide production in macrophages occurs following induction of the nitric oxide synthase 2 (*NOS2*) gene (Mannick, Asano, Izumi, Kieff, & Stamler, 1994; Xie et al., 1992). *NOS2* has been dubbed iNOS for its unique ability to irreversibly bind calmodulin independent of intracellular calcium concentrations (Moncada & Higgs, 1993; Nathan & Xie, 1994). This ability allows iNOS to produce vast quantities of NO over extended time periods. The toxicity of NO requires tight regulation of *NOS2* expression at the transcriptional level to prevent damage to normal host cells (Lorsbach, Murphy, Lowenstein, Snyder, & Russell, 1993). Our laboratory recently investigated the catecholamine regulation of NO production by IFNγ-primed macrophages infected with *M. avium* (Boomershine, Lafuse, & Zwilling, 1999). We showed epinephrine treatment, at the time of infection, inhibited macrophage anti-mycobacterial activity by inhibiting NO production. This inhibition was mediated via the β2-adrenergic receptor by elevating cAMP and the subsequent activation of protein kinase A resulting in decreased iNOS mRNA. Although catecholamine treatment has been shown to decrease NO production and iNOS mRNA (Haskó, Németh, Szabo', Zsilla, Salzman, & Vizi, 1998), other studies have shown catecholamines increased or did not affect NO production in macrophages (Schena et al., 1999 and Feinstein, Galea, & Reis, 1993, respectively). To resolve these discrepancies, we are currently investigating the mechanism of β2-adrenoceptor-mediated inhibition of iNOS mRNA production.

III. NEUTROPHILS

A. Catecholamine Effects

Neutrophils make up 70% of the circulating white blood cells. Neutrophils migrate through the vascular endothelium when responding to inflammatory stimuli. The function of neutrophils can be altered by bacterial LPS, cytokines such as TNF-α, IFN-γ, and GM-CSF, and by chemokines and other chemotactic factors such as opsonized zymosan, N-formylated peptides (fMLP), and cleaved complement fragments.

The functional capacity of neutrophils can be modulated by the central nervous system. Neutrophils express both α- and β-adrenergic receptors (Galant, Durisetti, Underwood, & Insel, 1978; Motulsky & Insel, 1982; Panosian & Marinetti, 1983). The effect of catecholamines on the functional capacity of the cells appears to be concentration dependent. Thus, treatment of cells with low levels (10^{-10} M) of epinephrine has been reported to stimulate the production of reactive oxygen species, whereas higher levels of catecholamine hormones (10^{-5} M) suppressed the respiratory burst (Potselueva, Marinov, Pustovidko, Kudzina, & Evtodienko, 1997). Generally neutrophils require a chemotactic or phagocytic stimulus to activate the respiratory burst. The different effects of catecholamine hormones may be due to different responses initiated by these stimuli and the binding of the hormones to different receptors. The inhibitory effect of catecholamine stimulation appears to be mediated via the β-2 adrenergic receptor by increasing the concentration of intracellular cAMP (Mitsuyama, Tanaka, Hidaka, Abe, & Hara, 1995; Weiss et al., 1996). The addition of dibutryl cAMP mimics the effects of epinephrine in inhibiting the respiratory burst stimulated by fMLP (Bazzoni, Dejana, & Del Maschio, 1991). The effect of fMLP also was inhibited by the addition of isoproternol, a β-adrenergic agonist.

Interestingly, when the respiratory burst was induced by treating the cells with a calcium ionophore or with phorbol 12-myristate 13-acetate, a protein kinase C activator, isoproternol failed to inhibit the response (Mueller & Sklar, 1989). This has been interpreted as indicating that the increase in cAMP, which results in the activation of a cAMP dependent kinase, inhibits the interaction of the agonist with its G-protein. Treatment of animals with LPS results in an increase in circulating neutrophils (Altenburg, Martins, Silva, Cordeiro, & Castro-Faria-Neto, 1997). Depleting catecholamine stores with reserpine can reverse the effect of LPS. Additionally, injection of the rats with a selective α-1-adrenergic antagonist, but not α-2 or β antagonists, reversed the LPS effect. Indeed, infusion of human subjects with epinephrine also has been shown to result in an increase in circulating neutrophils (Davis et al., 1991). Epinephrine mobilized the entire marginated pool of neutrophils. Reduced neutrophil chemotaxis was observed as a consequence of catecholamine infusion. Thus, the LPS-induced neutrophilia appears to be mediated by catecholamines via an α-1 adrenergic receptor.

B. Glucocorticoid Effects

The effects of glucocorticoids on inflammatory cell function have been the subject of numerous reviews (Goldstein, Paul, Metcalfe, Busse, & Reece, 1994; Konstan, 1996; Miller & Levy, 1997) and will not be discussed here. Instead, we will focus our discussion on the effects of physiological concentrations of adrenal steroids. The extent to which endogenous glucocorticoids influence neutrophil migration and activation is not clear. Generally, glucocorticoids promote neutrophil survival. Indeed, catecholamines appear to act in concert with glucocorticoids; the catecholamine causes neutrophilia and glucocorticoids promote survival by inhibiting apoptotic mechanisms (Cox, 1995; Meagher, Cousin, Seckl, & Haslett, 1996). The antiinflammatory effects of glucocorticoids may be the result of an inhibition of neutrophil accumulation at inflammatory sites (Cronstein, Kimmel, Levin, Martiniuk, & Weissmann, 1992). The mechanism may involve the down-regulation of L-selection and CD18 (Burton and Kehrli, 1995; Burton, Kehrli, Kapil, & Horst, 1995).

IV. SUMMARY

The macrophage is an important cell in mediating host inflammatory responses and resistance to intracellular pathogens. Both glucocorticoids and catecholamine hormones affect the functional capacity of the macrophage. Although corticosteroids generally suppress macrophage function by down-regulating the production of inflammatory cytokines and MHC class II glycoprotein, this capacity is influenced by the expression of a macrophage resistance gene that controls the growth of some intracellular pathogens. The functional expression of the gene, termed *Nramp1*, results in resistance to corticosteroids indirectly by increasing the mRNA stability of a variety of macrophage activation genes. *Nramp1* may be an important genetic determinant in the susceptibility of individuals to stress-induced suppression of the immune system.

Neurotransmitters, such as catecholamine hormones produced by the SNS, also affect macrophage activity. The hormones will stimulate or inhibit macrophages depending on the activation state of the mononuclear phagocyte. Catecholamines enhance the functional capacity of resting macrophages through the α2-adrenergic receptor while inhibiting activated macrophages via the β2-adrenergic receptor. Catecholamine hormones also affect neutrophil function. The number of neutrophils in the circulation increases and glucocorticoids inhibit apoptosis of neutrophils, thus extending their functional life span.

References

Abrass, C. K., O'Connor, S. W., Scarpace, P. J., & Abrass, I. B. (1985). Characterization of the β-adrenergic receptor of the rat peritoneal macrophage. *Journal of Immunology, 135*, 1338–1341.

Ader, R., Felten, D. L., & Cohen, N. (Eds.) (1991). *Psychoneuroimmunology* (2nd ed.). New York: Academic Press.

Altenburg, S. P., Martins, M. A., Silva, A. R., Cordeiro, R. S., & Castro-Faria-Neto, H. C. (1997). LPS-induced blood neutrophilia is inhibited by alpha 1-adrenoceptor antagonists: a role for catecholamines. *Journal of Leukocyte Biology, 61*, 689–694.

Barton, C. H., White, J. K., Roach, T. I. A., & Blackwell, J. M. (1994). NH_2-terminal sequences of macrophage expressed natural resistance associated macrophage protein (Nramp) encodes a proline/serine rich putative Src homology 3 binding domain. *Journal of Experimental Medicine, 179*, 1683–1687.

Bazzoni, G., Dejana, E., & Del Maschio, A. (1991). Adrenergic modulation of human polymorphonuclear leukocyte activation, potentiating effect of adenosine. *Blood, 77*, 2042–2048.

Beller, D. I., & Unanue, E. R. (1981). Regulation of macrophage populations II. Synthesis and expression of Ia antigen by peritoneal exudate macrophages is a transient event. *Journal of Immunology, 126*, 263–269.

Berkenbosch, F., Wolvers, D. A. W., & Derijk, R. (1991). Neuroendocrine and immunological mechanisms in stress-induced immunomodulation. *Journal of Steroid Biochemistry, 40*, 639–647.

Bermudez, L. E., & Champsi, J. (1993). Infection with *Mycobacterium avium* induces production of IL-10, and administration of anti-IL-10 antibody is associated with enhanced resistance to infection in mice. *Infection and Immunity, 61*, 3093–3097.

Blackwell, J. M., Roach, T. I. A., Kiderlen, A., & Kaye, P. M. (1989). Role of Lsh in regulating macrophage priming/activation. *Research in Immunology, 140*, 798–805.

Bogdan, C., Vodovotz, Y., & Nathan, C. (1991). Macrophage deactivation by interleukin 10. *Journal of Experimental Medicine, 174*, 1549–1555.

Bonecini-Almeida M. G., Chitale, S., Boutsikakis, I., Geng J. Y., Doo, H., He., S. H., & Ho, J. L. (1998). Induction of in vitro human macrophage anti-Mycobacterium tuberculosis activity: Requirement for IFN-gamma and primed lymphocytes. *Journal of Immunology, 160*, 4490–4499.

Boomershine, C. S., Lafuse, W. P., & Zwilling, B. S. (1999). β2-adrenergic receptor stimulation inhibits nitric oxide generation by *Mycobacterium avium* infected macrophages. *Journal of Neuroimmunology, 101*, 68–75.

Britton, W. J., Meadows, N., Rathjen, D. A., Roach, D. R., & Briscoe, H. (1998). A tumor necrosis factor mimetic peptide activates a murine macrophage cell line to inhibit mycobacterial growth in a nitric oxide-dependent fashion. *Infection and Immunity, 66*, 2122–2127.

Brown, D. H., Lafuse, W. P., & Zwilling, B. S. (1997). Stabilized expression of mRNA is associated with mycobacterial resistance controlled by Nramp1. *Infection and Immunity, 65*, 597–603.

Brown, D. H., Sheridan, J., Pearl, D., & Zwilling, B. S. (1993). Regulation of mycobacterial growth by the hypothalamus-pituitary-adrenal axis: Differential responses of *Mycobacterium bovis* BCG-resistant and -susceptible mice. *Infection and Immunity, 61*, 4793–4800.

Burton, J. L., & Kehrli, M. E. Jr. (1995). Regulation of neutrophil adhesion molecules and shedding of *Staphylococcus aureus* in milk of cortisol- and dexamethasone-treated cows. *American Journal of Veterinary Research, 56*, 997–1006.

Burton, J. L., Kehrli, M. E. Jr., Kapil, S., & Horst, R. L. (1995). Regulation of L-selectin and CD18 on bovine neutrophils by glucocorticoids: Effects of cortisol and dexamethasone. *Journal of Leukocyte Biology, 57*, 317–325.

Cellier, M., Govoni, G., Vidal, S., Kwan, T., Groulx, N., Liu, J., Sanchez, F., Skamene, E., Schurr, E., & Gros, P. (1994). Human natural resistance associated macrophage protein: cDNA cloning, chromosomal mapping, genomic organization and tissue specific expression. *Journal of Experimental Medicine, 180*, 1741–1752.

Chen, L., Boomershine C. S., Wang, T., Lafuse, W. P., & Zwilling, B. S. (1999). Synergistic interaction of catecholamine hormones and *Mycobacterium avium* results in the induction of interleukin-10 mRNA expression by murine peritoneal macrophages. *Journal of Neuroimmunology, 93*, 149–155.

Collins, F. M. (1989). Mycobacterial disease: Immunosuppression and acquired immunodeficiency syndrome. *Clinical Microbiology Review, 2*, 360–377.

Costa Rosa, L. F., Safi, D. A., Cury, Y., & Curi, R. (1992). Effect of epinephrine on glucose metabolism and hydrogen peroxide content in incubated rat macrophages. *Biochemical Pharmacology, 44*, 2235–2241.

Cox, G. (1995). Glucocorticoid treatment inhibits apoptosis in human neutrophils. Separation of survival and activation outcomes. *Journal of Immunology, 154*, 4719–4725.

Crabtree, G. R., Munck, A., & Smith, K. A. (1980) Glucocorticoids and lymphocytes: Increased glucocorticoid receptor levels in antigen stimulated lymphocytes. *Journal of Immunology, 124*, 2430–2435.

Cronstein, B. N., Kimmel, S. C., Levin, R. I., Martiniuk, F., & Weissmann, G. A. (1992). Mechanism for the anti-inflammatory effects of corticosteroids- the glucocorticoid receptor regulates leukocyte adhesion to endothelial-cells and expression of endothelial leukocyte adhesion molecule-1 and intercellular-adhesion molecule-1. *Proceedings of the National Academy of Sciences USA, 89*, 9991–9995.

Crowle, A. J., & Elkins, N. (1990). Relative permissiveness of macrophages from black and white people for virulent tubercle bacilli. *Inflammation and Immunity, 58*, 632–638.

Dannenberg, A. M. (1993). Immunopathogenesis of pulmonary tuberculosis. *Hospital Practices, 1*(15), 51–58.

Davis, J. M., Albert, J. D., Tracy, K. J., Calvano, S. E., Lowry, S. F., Shires, G. T., & Yurt, R. W. (1991). Increased neutrophil mobilization and decreased chemotaxis during cortisol and epinephrine infusions. *Journal of Trauma-Injury and Infection in Critical Care, 31*, 725–732.

Denis, M. (1991). Tumor necrosis factor and granulocyte-macrophage colony-stimulating factor stimulate human macrophages to restrict growth of virulent *Mycobacterium avium* and to kill *M. avium*: Killing effect mechanism depends on the generation of reactive nitrogen intermediates. *Journal of Leukocyte Biology, 49,* 380–387.

Denis, M., & Ghadirian, E. (1993). IL-10 neutralization augments mouse resistance to systemic *Mycobacterium avium* infections. *Journal of Immunology, 151,* 5425–5430.

Dinarello, C. A. (1992). Role of interleukin-1 and tumor necrosis factor in systemic responses to infection and inflammation. In J. I. Gallin, I. M. Goldstein, & R. Snyderman (Eds.), *Inflammation: Basic principles and clinical correlates* (2nd ed., pp. 211–232). New York: Raven Press.

Dinarello, C. A., Cannon, J. C., Mancella, J., Bishai, I., Leis, J., & Coceani, F (1991). Interleukin 6 as an endogenous pyrogen: Induction of prostaglandin E2 in brain but not in peripheral mononuclear cells. *Brain Research, 562,* 199–206.

Ding, L., Linsley, P., Huang, L., Germain, R. N., & Shevach, E. M. (1993). IL-10 inhibits macrophage co-stimulatory activity by selectively inhibiting the up regulation of B7 expression. *Journal of Immunology, 151,* 1224–1234.

Doi, T., Ando, M., Akaike, T., Suga, M., Sato, K., & Maeda, H. (1993). Resistance to nitric oxide in *Mycobacterium avium* complex and its implication in pathogenesis. *Infection and Immunity, 61,* 1980–1989.

Dunham, D. M., Arkins, S., Edwards, C. K. III, Dantzer, R., & Kelley, K. W. (1990). Role of interferon-gamma in counteracting the suppressive effects of transforming growth factor beta-2 and glucocorticoids on the production of tumor necrosis factor. *Journal of Leukocyte Biology, 48,* 473–481.

Elenkov, I. J., Haskó, G., Kovács, K. J., & Vizi, E. S. (1995). Modulation of lipopolysaccharide-induced tumor necrosis factor-α production by selective α- and β-adrenergic drugs in mice. *Journal of Neuroimmunology, 61,* 123–131.

Feinstein, D. L., Galea, E., & Reis, D. J. (1993). Norepinephrine suppresses inducible nitric oxide synthase activity in rat astroglial cultures. *Journal of Neurochemistry, 60,* 1945–1948.

Felten, D. L., Felten, S. Y., Bellinger, D. L., Carlson, S. L., Ackerman, K. D., Madden, K. S., Olschowski, J. A., & Livnat, S. (1987). Noradrenergic sympathetic neural interactions with the immune system: Structure and function. *Immunology Review, 100,* 225–260.

Fiorentino, D. F., Bond, M. W., & Mosmann, T. R. (1989). Two types of mouse T helper cell. IV. Th2 clones secrete a factor that inhibits cytokine production by Th1 clones. *Journal of Experimental Medicine, 170,* 2081–2095.

Fiorentino, D. F., Zlotnik, A., Mosmann, T. R., Howard, M., & O'Garra, A. (1991). IL-10 inhibits cytokine production by activated macrophages. *Journal of Immunology, 147,* 3815–3822.

Fiorentino, D. F., Zlotnik, A., Vieira, P., Mosmann, T. R., Howard, M., Moore, K. W., & O'Garra, A. (1991). IL-10 acts on the antigen-presenting cell to inhibit cytokine production by Th1 cells. *Journal of Immunology, 146,* 3444–3451.

Flesch, I. E. A. and Kaufmann, S. H. E. (1991). Mechanisms involved in mycobacterial growth inhibition by gamma interferon-activated bone marrow macrophages: Role of Reactive Nitrogen Intermediates. *Infection and Immunity, 59,* 3213–3218.

Formica, S., Roach, T. I. A., & Blackwell, J. M. (1994). Interaction with extracellular matrix proteins influences *Lsh/Ity/Bcg* (candidate *Nramp*) gene regulation of macrophage priming/activation for tumor necrosis factor-α and nitrate release. *Immunology, 82,* 42–50.

Fortier, A. H., Green, S. J., Polsinelli, T., Jones, T. R., Crawford, R. M., Leiby, D. A., Elkins, K. L., & Meltzer, M. S. (1994). Life and death of an intracellular pathogen: Francisella tularensis and the macrophage. In B. S. Zwilling & T. K. Eisenstein (Eds.), *Macrophage-pathogen interactions* (pp. 349–361). New York: Dekker.

Fukushima, T., Sekizawa, K., Jin, Y., Yamaya, M., Sasaki, H., & Takishima, T. (1993). Effects of beta-adrenergic receptor activation on alveolar macrophage cytoplasmic motility. *American Journal of Physiology, 265,* L67–L72.

Galant, S. P., Durisetti, L., Underwood, S., & Insel, P. A. (1978). Beta-adrenergic receptors on polymorphonuclear leukocyes. *New England Journal of Medicine, 299,* 933–936.

Gazzinelli, R. T., Eltoum, I., Wynn, T. A., & Sher, A. (1993). Acute cerebral toxoplasmosis is induced by the *in vivo* neutralization of TNF-α and correlates with the downregulated expression of inducible nitric oxide synthase and other markers of macrophage activation. *Journal of Immunology, 151,* 3672–3681.

Gazzinelli, R. T., Oswald, I. P., James, S. L., & Sher, A. (1992) IL-10 inhibits parasite killing and nitric oxide production by IFN-γ activated macrophages. *Journal of Immunology, 148,* 1792–1796.

Goldstein, R. A., Paul, W. E., Metcalfe, D. D., Busse, W. W., & Reece, E. R. (1994). Asthma. *Annals of Internal Medicine, 121,* 698–708.

Green, S. J., Scheller, L. F., Marletta, M. A., Seguin, M. C., Klotz, F. W., Slayter, M., Nelson, B. J., & Nacy, C. A. (1994). Nitric oxide: Cytokine-regulation of nitric oxide in host resistance to intracellular pathogens. *Immunology Letters, 43*(1–2), 87–94.

Gros, P., Skamene, E., & Forget, A. (1981). Genetic control of natural resistance to *Mycobacterium bovis* (BCG) in mice. *Journal of Immunology,* 127, 2417–2421.

Gros, P., Skamene, E., & Forget, A. (1983). Cellular mechanisms of genetically controlled host resistance to *Mycobacterium bovis* (BCG). *Journal of Immunology, 131,* 1966–1972.

Guirao, X., Kumar, A., Katz, J., Smith, M., Lin, E., Keogh, C., Calvano, S. E., & Lowry, S. F. (1997). Catecholamines increase monocyte TNF receptors and inhibit TNF through β2-adrenoreceptor activation. *American Journal of Physiology, 273,* E1203–1208.

Haskó, G., Németh, Z. H., Szabó, C., Zsilla, G., Salzman AL., & Vizi, E. S. (1998). Isoproterenol inhibits IL-10, TNF-α, and nitric oxide production in RAW 264. 7 macrophages. *Brain Research Bulletin 45,* 183–187.

Hibbs, Jr., J. B., Taintor, R. R., Vavrin, Z., & Rachlin, E. M. (1988). Nitric oxide: A cytotoxic activated macrophage effector molecule. *Biochemical and Biophysical Research Communications, 157,* 87–94.

Hilburger, M., & Zwillling, B. S. (1994). Macrophage resistance genes: *Bcg/Ity/Lsh.* In T. K. Eisenstein & B. S. Zwilling (Eds.), *Macrophage-pathogen interactions* (pp. 233–245). New York: Marcel Dekker.

Hu, X. X., Goldmuntz, E. A., & Brosnan, C. F. (1991). The effect of norepinephrine on endotoxin-mediated macrophage activation. *Journal of Neuroimmunology, 31*(1), 35–42.

Ishigami, T. (1919). The influence of psychic acts on the progress of pulmonary tuberculosis. *American Review of Tuberculosis, 2,* 470–484.

Jiang, C. G., Morrow-Tesch, J. L., Beller, D. I., Levy, E., & Black, P. H. (1990). Immunosuppression in mice induced by cold water stress. *Brain, Behavior, and Immunity, 4,* 278–291.

Johnson, E. O., Kamilares, T. C., Chrousos, G. P., & Gold, P. W. (1992). Mechanisms of stress: A dynamic overview of hormonal and behavioral homeostasis. *Neuroscience Biobehavioral Review, 16,* 115–130.

Kaplan, G., Laal, S., Sheffel, G., Nusrat, A., Nath, I., Mathur, N. K., Mishra, R. S., & Cohn, Z. A. (1988). The nature and kinetics of delay-immune response to purified protein derivative of tuberculosis in the skin of lepromatous leprosy patients. *Journal of Experimental Medicine, 168*(5), 1811–1824.

Kern, J. A., Lamb, R. J., Reed, J. C., Daniele, R. P., & Nowell, P. C. (1988). Dexamethasone inhibition of interleukin-1beta production by human monocytes. *Journal of Clinical Investigation, 81*, 237–244.

Khansari, D. N., Murgo, A. J., & Faith, R. E. (1990). Effect of stress on the immune system. *Immunology Today, 11*, 170–175.

Kiecolt-Glaser, J. K. and Glaser, R. (1995). Psychoneuroimmunology and health consequences: data and shared mechanisms. *Psychosomatic Medicine, 57*, 269–274.

Koff, W. C., & Dunegan, M. A. (1985). Modulation of macrophage-mediated tumoricidal activity by neuropeptides and neurohormones. *Journal of Immunology, 135*(1), 350–354.

Koff, W. C. & Dunegan, M. A. (1986). Neuroendocrine hormones suppress macrophage mediated lysis of herpes virus infected cells. *Journal of Immunology, 136*(2), 705–709.

Koff, W. C., Fann, A. V., Dunegan, M. A., & Lachman, L. B. (1986). Catecholamine-induced suppression of interleukin-1 production. *Lymphokine Research, 5*, 239–247.

Kohut, M. L., Davis, J. M., Jackson, D. A., Colbert, L. H., Strasner, A., Essig, D. A., Pate, R. R., Ghaffar, A., & Mayer, E. P. (1998). The role of stress hormones in exercise-induced suppression of alveolar macrophage antiviral function. *Journal of Neuroimmunology, 81*, 193–200.

Konstan, M. W. (1996). Treatment of airway inflammation in cystic fibrosis. *Current Opinion in Pulmonary Medicine, 2*, 452–456.

Kubin, M., Kamoun, M., Trinchieri, G. (1994). TL-12 synergizes with B7/CD28 interaction in inducing efficient proliferation and cytokine production of human T cells. *Journal of Experimental Medicine, 180*, 211–222.

Lappin D., & Whaley K. (1982). Adrenergic receptors on monocytes modulate complement component synthesis. *Clinical Experimental Immunology, 47*, 606–612.

Lee, S. W., Tso, A. P., Chan, H., Thomas, J., Petrie, K., Eugui, E. M., & Allison, A. C. (1988). Glucocorticoids selectively inhibit the transcription of the interleukin 1-β gene and decrease the stability of interleukin 1-β mRNA. *Proceedings of the National Academy of Sciences USA, 85*, 1204–1208.

Liew, F. Y. (1993). The role of nitric oxide in parasitic diseases. *Annals of Tropical Medicine and Parasitology, 87*, 637–642.

Liew, F. Y., Wei, X. Q., Proudfoot, L. (1997). Cytokines and nitric oxide as effector molecules against parasitic infections. *Philosophical Transactions of the Royal Society of London—Series B: Biological Sciences, 352*, 1311–1315.

Liggett, S. B. (1989). Identification and characterization of a homogeneous population of beta 2-adrenergic receptors on human alveolar macrophages. *American Review of Respiratory Disease, 139*, 552–555.

Lorsbach, R. B., Murphy, W. J., Lowenstein, C. J., Snyder, S. H., & Russell, S. W. (1993). Expression of the nitric oxide synthase gene in mouse macrophages activated for tumor cell killing. Molecular basis for the synergy between interferon-gamma and lipopolysaccharide. *Journal of Biological Chemistry, 268*, 1908–1913.

Madden, K. S., & Felten, D. L. (1995). Experimental basis for neural-immune interactions. *Physiology Review, 75*, 77–106.

Malefyt, R. D., Abrams, J., Bennett, B., Figdor, C. G., & Devries, J. E. (1991). Interleukin-10 (IL-10) inhibits cytokine synthesis by human monocytes-an autoregulatory role of IL-10 producted by monocytes. *Journal of Experimental Medicine, 174*, 1209–1220.

Malefyt, R. D., Haanen, J., Spits, H., Roncarolo, M. G., Tevelde, A., Figdor, C., Johnson, K., Kastelein, R., Yssel, H, & Devries, J. E. (1991). IL-10 and viral IL-10 strongly reduced antigenic specific T cell proliferation by diminishing the antigen presenting capacity of monocytes via down regulation of class II MHC expression. *Journal of Experimental Medicine, 174*, 915–924.

Malo, D., Vogan, K., Vidal, S., Hu, J., Cellier, M., Schurr, E., Fuks, A., Bumstead, N., Morgan, K., & Gros, P. (1994). Haplotype mapping and sequence analysis of the mouse Nramp gene predict susceptibility to infection with intracellular parasites. *Genomics, 23*, 51–61.

Mannick, J. B., Asano, K., Izumi, K., Kieff, E., & Stamler, J. S. (1994). Nitric oxide produced by human B-lymphocytes inhibits apoptosis and Epstein-Barr virus reactivation. *Cell, 79*, 1137–1146.

Meagher, L. C., Cousin, J. M., Seckl, J. R., & Haslett, C. (1996). Opposing effects of glucocorticoids on the rate of apoptosis in neutrophilic and eosinophilic granulocytes. *Journal of Immunology, 156*, 4422–4428.

Miesfeld, R. L. (1990). Molecular genetics of corticosteroid action. *American Review of Respiratory Disease, 141*, S11–S17.

Miles, B. A., Lafuse, W. P., & Zwilling, B. S. (1996). Binding of alpha-adrenergic receptors stimulates the anti-mycobacterial activity of murine peritoneal macrophages. *Journal of Neuroimmunology, 71*, 19–24.

Miller, B. E., and Levy, J. H. (1997). The inflammatory response to cardiopulmonary bypass. *Journal of Cardiothoracic and Vascular Anesthesia, 11*, 355–366.

Mitsuyama, T., Tanaka, T., Hidaka, K., Abe, M., & Hara, N. (1995). Inhibition by erythromycin of superoxide anion production by human polymorphonuclear leukocytes through the action of cyclic AMP-dependent protein kinase. *Respiration, 62*, 269–273.

Moncada, S., & Higgs, A. (1993). The L-arginine-nitric oxide pathway. *New England Journal of Medicine, 329*, 2002–2012.

Motulsky, H. J., & Insel, P. A. (1982). Adrenergic receptors in man. *New England Journal of Medicine, 307*, 18–29.

Mueller, H., & Sklar, L. A. (1989). Coupling of antagonistic signalling pathways in modulation of neutrophil function. *Journal of Cellular Biochemistry, 40*, 287–294.

Muller, F., Aukrust, P., Lien, E., Haug, C. J., & Froland, S. S. (1998). Enhanced IL-10 production in response to *Mycobacterium avium* products in mononuclear cells from patients with human immunodeficiency virus infection. *Journal of Infectious Disease, 177*(3), 586–594.

Munck, A., Mendel, D. B., Smith, L. I., & Ortl, E. (1990). Glucocorticoid receptors and actions. *American Review of Respiratory Disease, 141*, S2–S10.

Nardell, E. (1993). Pathogenesis of tuberculosis. In L. B. Reichman and E. Hirschfield (Eds.), *Lung Biology in Health and Disease* (pp. 103–123). New York: Marcel Dekker.

Nathan, C., & Xie, Q.-W. (1994). Regulation of biosynthesis of nitric oxide. *Journal of Biological Chemistry, 269*, 13725–13728.

Northrop, J. P., Crabtree, G. R., & Mattila, P. S. (1992). Negative regulation of interleukin-2 transcription by the glucocorticoid receptor. *Journal of Experimental Medicine, 175*, 1235–1245.

Nunez, G., Giles, R. C., Ball, E. J., Hurley, C. K., Capra, J. D., & Stastny, P. (1984). Expression of HLA-DR, MB, MT, and SB antigens on human mononuclear cells: Identification of two phenotypically distinct monocyte populations. *Journal of Immunology, 133*, 1300–1306.

O'Grady, F., & Riley, R. L. (1963). Experimental airborne tuberculosis. *Advances in Tuberculosis Research, 12*, 150–190.

Panosian, J. O., & Marinetti, G. V. (1983). Alpha 2-adrenergic receptors in human polymorphonuclear leukocyte membranes. *Biochemical Pharmacology, 32*, 2243–2247.

Payvar, F., Wrange, O., Carlstedt-Duke, J., Okret, S., Gustafsson, J. A., & Yamamoto, K. R. (1981). Purified glucocorticoid receptors bind selectively in vitro to a cloned DNA fragment whose

Gawkrodger, 1994; Amkraut, Solomon, & Kraemer, 1971; Mei-Tal, Meyerowitz, & Engel, 1970; Pawlak et al., 1999; Solomon & Moos, 1964; Thomason, Brantley, Jones, Dyer, & Morris, 1992).

- Third, stress is known to exacerbate autoimmune and inflammatory diseases (Mei-Tal et al., 1970; Solomon & Moos, 1964; Thomason et al., 1992); however, stress hormones (glucocorticoids) are used clinically to treat these diseases (Schleimer et al., 1989).

In this chapter we present data and propose a model to describe interactions between stress, stress hormones, and immune function, which provides possible explanations for these paradoxical observations. In terms of stress hormones, this chapter will mainly focus on glucocorticoids since the immunomodulatory effects of catecholamines and other stress-responsive hormones are covered elsewhere is this volume.

We propose that four key parameters may influence the direction (enhancing versus suppressive) of the effects of stress or glucocorticoid hormones on a given immune measure: (1) the effects of stress or glucocorticoid hormones on leukocyte distribution in the body; (2) the differential effects of acute versus chronic stress (or acute versus chronic exposure to glucocorticoids) on immune function; (3) the differential effects of physiologic versus pharmacologic doses of glucocorticoids, and the differential effects of endogenous (e.g., cortisol, corticosterone) vs. synthetic (e.g., dexamethasone) glucocorticoids; and (4) the timing of stressor or glucocorticoid hormone exposure relative to the timecourse of the immune response. It is important to recognize that factors such as gender, genetics, age, route of administration, nature, and dose of the immunizing antigen, and time of day, may also significantly affect the relationship between stress and immune function.

IV. STRESS-INDUCED REDISTRIBUTION OF IMMUNE CELLS WITHIN THE BODY

The data presented below show that stress and stress hormones induce significant changes in the distribution of leukocytes within the body. It has been suggested that an important function of endocrine mediators released under conditions of acute stress may be to ensure that appropriate leukocytes are present in the right place and at the right time to respond to an immune challenge that might be initiated by the stress-inducing agent (e.g., attack by a predator, invasion by a pathogen, etc.) (Dhabhar et al., 1994, 1995b, 1996). Thus, the modulation of immune cell distribution by acute stress may be an adaptive response designed to enhance immune surveillance and increase immune preparedness for potential (or ongoing) immune challenge. Such changes in immune cell distribution may also have significant implications for the way in which data regarding the effects of stress on immune function in a specific body compartment are interpreted.

A. Effects of Stress on Blood Leukocytes

Immune cells or leukocytes circulate continuously from the blood, into various organs, and back into the blood. This circulation is essential for the maintenance of an effective immune defense network (Sprent & Tough, 1994). The numbers and proportions of leukocytes in the blood provide an important representation of the state of distribution of leukocytes in the body and of the state of activation of the immune system. Numerous studies have shown that stress and stress hormones induce significant changes in absolute numbers and relative proportions of leukocytes in the blood. In fact, decreases in blood leukocyte numbers were used as an indirect measure for increases in plasma corticosterone before methods were available to directly assay the hormone (Hoagland, Elmadjian, & Pincus, 1946). Stress-induced decreases in blood leukocyte numbers have been reported in fish (Pickford, Srivastava, Slicher, & Pang, 1971), mice (Jensen, 1969), rats (Dhabhar et al., 1994, 1995b; Johns, 1967; Rinner, Schauenstein, Mangge, Porta, & Kvetnansky 1992; Stefanski, Solomon, Kling, Thomas, & Plaeger, 1996), rabbits (Toft, Svendsen, Tonnesen, Rasmussen, & Christensen, 1993), horses (Snow, Ricketts, & Mason, 1983), nonhuman primates (Morrow-Tesch, McGlone, & Norman, 1993), and humans (Herbert & Cohen 1993; Schedlowski, Jacobs et al., 1993). This suggests that the phenomenon of stress-induced leukocyte distribution has been conserved through evolution, and that perhaps this redistribution has an important adaptive and functional significance.

Studies have shown that stress-induced increases in plasma corticosterone are accompanied by a significant decrease in numbers and percentages of lymphocytes, and by an increase in numbers and percentages of neutrophils in the blood. Stress-induced changes in blood leukocyte distribution are apparent within 30 min of applying the stressor (Dhabhar et al., 1995b). Thus, acute stress induces a large decrease (45–60% lower than baseline) in total blood leukocyte numbers. Flow cytometric analyses has revealed that absolute numbers of peripheral

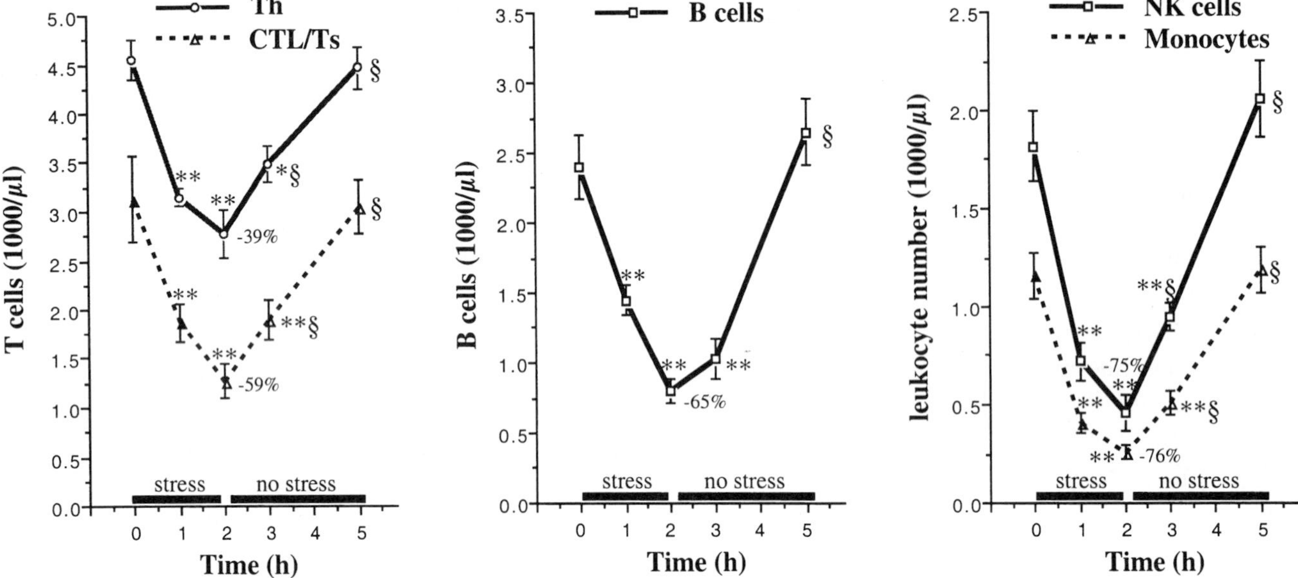

FIGURE 1 Stress-induced changes in peripheral blood leukocyte numbers, and recovery after cessation of stress (Dhabhar et al., 1995b). Changes in numbers of T cells, B cells, NK cells, and monocytes during a 2 h stress session, and a 3 h recovery session are shown. The percent decrease in leukocyte numbers after 2 h stress relative to baseline (0 h), is indicated for each subpopulation in each panel. Data are expressed as mean ± SEM (n=6). Statistically significant differences are indicated: $^{*}p<0.05$; $^{**}p<0.005$, significantly different from 0 h baseline (paired *t*-test). § $p<0.05$, significantly different from 2 h stress timepoint (paired *t*-test). (Adapted from Dhabhar, F. S. et al., J. Immunol. 1995, Vol 154, P 5511–5527. Copyright ©1995 The American Association of Immunologists.)

blood helper T cells (Th), cytolytic T cells (CTL), B cells, natural killer (NK) cells, and monocytes all show a rapid and significant decrease (40 to 70% lower than baseline) during stress (Dhabhar et al., 1995b) (Figure 1). Further experiments have revealed that stress-induced decreases in blood leukocyte numbers are rapidly reversed with leukocyte numbers returning to prestress baseline levels within 3 hours after the cessation of stress (Figure 1) (Dhabhar et al., 1995b).

B. Adrenal Stress Hormones Mediate Stress-Induced Changes in Blood Leukocyte Numbers

Dhabhar et al. have shown that the stress-induced changes in leukocyte distribution are mediated by hormones released by the adrenal gland (Dhabhar et al., 1996; Dhabhar & McEwen, 1999a). Thus, the magnitude of the stress-induced changes in blood leukocyte numbers is significantly reduced in adrenalectomized animals (Dhabhar et al., 1995b, 1996). Cyanoketone treatment, which virtually eliminates the corticosterone stress response, also virtually eliminates the stress-induced decrease in blood lymphocyte numbers, and significantly enhances the stress-induced increase in blood neutrophil numbers (Dhabhar et al., 1996).

Several studies have shown that glucocorticoid treatment induces changes in leukocyte distribution in mice (Cohen, 1972; Dougherty & White, 1945; Spain & Thalhimer, 1951; Zatz, 1975), guinea pigs (Fauci, 1975), rats (Dhabhar et al., 1996; Miller et al., 1994; Ulich, Keys, Ni, del Castillo, & Dakay, 1988), rabbits (Van Den Broek, Keuning, Soeharto, & Prop, 1983), and humans (Fauci, 1976; Fauci & Dale, 1974; Onsrud & Thorsby, 1981). It has been shown in rats that both adrenalectomy (which eliminates the corticosterone and epinephrine stress response) (Dhabhar et al., 1995b, 1996; Jensen, 1969; Keller, Weiss, Schleifer, Miller, & Stein, 1983), or cyanoketone treatment (which eliminates only the corticosterone stress reponse) virtually eliminate the stress-induced redistribution of blood leukocytes (Dhabhar et al., 1996).

Since adrenal steroids act at two distinct receptor subtypes that show a heterogeneity of expression in immune cells and tissues (Dhabhar, McEwen, & Spencer, 1993; Dhabhar, Miller, McEwen, & Spencer, 1995a; Miller et al., 1998; Spencer et al., 1999), Dhabhar et al., investigated the role played by each receptor subtype in mediating changes in leukocyte distribution (Dhabhar et al., 1996). Acute administration of aldosterone (a specific type I adrenal steroid receptor agonist) to adrenalectomized animals did not have a significant effect on blood leukocyte numbers. In contrast, acute administration of corticosterone (the endogenous type I and type II receptor agonist), or RU28362 (a specific type II receptor agonist) to adrenalectomized animals induced changes in leukocyte distribution similar to those observed in intact animals during stress. These results suggest that corticosterone, acting at the type II adrenal steroid receptor, is a major mediator of the stress-induced decreases in blood lymphocyte and monocyte number. Taken together, these studies show that stress and glucocorticoid hormones induce a significant decrease in blood lymphocyte numbers when administered under acute or chronic conditions.

In apparent contrast to glucocorticoid hormones, catecholamine hormones have been shown to increase blood leukocyte numbers in rats (Harris, Waltman, Carter, & Maisel, 1995) and humans (Landmann et al., 1984). On closer examination it was observed that following adrenaline or noradrenaline administration, neutrophil and NK cell numbers increase rapidly and dramatically whereas T and B cell numbers decrease (Benschop, Rodriguez-Feuerhahn, & Schedlowski, 1996; Landmann, 1992; Schedlowski, Falk et al., 1993; Tonnesen, Christensen, & Brinklov, 1987). Carlson et al., have shown that catecholamine pretreatment results in increased accumulation of lymphocytes in the spleen and lymph nodes (Carlson, Fox, & Abell, 1997), which would be in agreement with a catecholamine-induced decrease in lymphocytes in the blood. By acutely administering epinephrine, norepinephrine, selective α and β adrenergic receptor agonists, or corticosterone to adrenalectomized animals, Dhabhar and McEwen have shown that increases in blood granulocyte numbers may be mediated by the $\alpha 1$ and β adrenergic receptors and are counteracted by corticosterone acting at the type II adrenal steroid receptor (Dhabhar & McEwen, 1999a). Increases in lymphocytes may be mediated by the $\alpha 2$ receptor while decreases in lymphocytes may be mediated by β adrenergic and Type II adrenal steroid receptors (Dhabhar & McEwen, 1999a; Dhabhar et al., 1996).

Therefore, the absolute number of specific blood leukocyte subpopulations may be significantly affected by the ambient concentrations of epinephrine, norepinephrine, and corticosterone. Differences in concentrations and combinations of these hormones may explain reported differences in blood leukocyte numbers during different stress conditions (e.g., short- versus long-duration acute stress, acute versus chronic stress) and during exercise.

C. A Stress-Induced Decrease in Blood Leukocyte Numbers Represents a Redistribution rather than a Destruction or Net Loss of Blood Leukocytes

From the above discussion it is clear that stress and glucocorticoid hormones induce a rapid and significant decrease in blood lymphocyte, monocyte, and NK cell numbers. This decrease in blood leukocyte numbers may be interpreted in two possible ways. The decrease in cell numbers could reflect a large-scale destruction of circulating leukocytes. Alternatively, it could reflect a redistribution of leukocytes from the blood to other organs in the body. Several studies have shown that glucocorticoid-induced decrease in blood leukocytes reflects a redistribution rather than a destruction of immune cells (Cohen, 1972; Cox & Ford, 1982; Dougherty & White, 1945; Lundin & Hedman, 1978; Spain & Thalhimer, 1951; Zatz, 1975).

Dhabhar et al., conducted experiments to test the hypothesis that acute stress induces a redistribution of leukocytes from the blood to other compartments in the body (Dhabhar et al., 1995b; Dhabhar, 1998). The first series of experiments examined the kinetics of recovery of the stress-induced reduction in blood leukocyte numbers. It was hypothesized that if the observed effects of stress represented a redistribution rather than a destruction of leukocytes, one would see a relatively rapid return of leukocyte numbers back to baseline upon the cessation of stress. Results showed that all leukocyte subpopulations that showed a decrease in absolute numbers during stress showed a complete recovery, with numbers reaching prestress baseline levels within 3 h after the cessation of stress (Figure 1) (Dhabhar et al., 1995b). Plasma levels of lactate dehydrogenase (LDH), which is a marker for cell damage, also were monitored in the same experiment. If the stress-induced decrease in leukocyte numbers were the result of a destruction of leukocytes, one would expect to observe an increase in plasma levels of LDH during or following stress. However, no significant changes in plasma LDH were observed, further suggesting that a redistribution rather than a destruction of leukocytes was primarily responsible for the stress-induced decrease in blood leukocyte numbers (Dhabhar et al., 1995b).

It is important to bear in mind that glucocorticoids induce changes in various immune parameters (Callewaert, Moudgil, Radcliff, & Waite 1991; Munck et al., 1984), and in immune cell distribution (Cohen, 1972; Dhabhar et al., 1994, 1995b; Fauci, 1975; Fauci & Dale, 1974; Lundin & Hedman, 1978; Spry, 1972; Zatz, 1975), in the absence of cell death, even though these hormones are known to induce leukocyte apoptosis (Cohen, 1992). It has been suggested that some species may be "steroid-resistant" and others may be "steroid-sensitive," and that glucocorticoid-induced changes in blood leukocyte numbers represent changes in leukocyte redistribution in steroid-resistant species (humans & guinea pig), and leukocyte lysis in steroid-sensitive species (mouse & rat) (Claman, 1972). However, a large body of evidence now indicates that even in species previously thought to be steroid-sensitive, adrenal steroids induce leukocyte redistribution rather than leukocyte destruction (Cohen, 1972; Hedman & Lundin, 1977; Moorhead & Claman, 1972; Thompson & Van Furth, 1973).

D. Target Organs of a Stress-Induced Redistribution of Blood Leukocytes

Based on the above discussion, the obvious question one might ask is: "Where do blood leukocytes go during stress?" Numerous studies using stress or stress hormone treatments have investigated this issue. Using gamma imaging to follow the distribution of adoptively transferred radiolabeled leukocytes in rabbits, Toft et al. have shown that stress induces a redistribution of leukocytes from the blood to lymphatic tissues (Toft et al., 1993). It has been reported that anesthesia stress, as well as the infusion of adrenocorticotropic hormone (ACTH) and prednisolone, in rats results in decreased numbers of labeled lymphocytes in the thoracic duct, whereas the cessation of drug infusion results in normal circulation of labeled lymphocytes (Spry, 1972). This suggests that hormonal changes similar to those observed during stress induce the retention of circulating lymphocytes in different body compartments thus resulting in a decrease in lymphocyte numbers in the thoracic duct and a concomitant decrease in numbers in the peripheral blood (Spry, 1972). Fleshner et al. have shown that acute stress results in an increase in CD4 percentage and a decrease in CD8 percentage in the mesenteric lymph nodes and suggested that these changes in lymphocyte composition may mediate changes in antibody production by the affected lymph nodes (Fleshner, Watkins, Lockwood, Laudenslager, & Maier, 1992). It also has been reported that a single injecton of hydrocortisone, prednisolone, or ACTH results in increased numbers of lymphocytes in the bone marrow of mice (Cohen, 1972), guinea pigs (Fauci, 1975), and rats (Cox & Ford, 1982). Fauci et al. suggested that glucocorticoid-induced decreases in blood leukocyte numbers in humans also may reflect a redistribution of immune cells to other organs in the body (Fauci & Dale, 1974, 1975; Yu, Clements, Paulus, Peter, Levy & Barnett, 1974). Finally, corticosteroids have been shown to induce the accumulation of lymphocytes in mucosal sites (Walzer, LaBine, Redington, & Cushion, 1984), and the skin has been identified as a target organ to which leukocytes traffic during stress (Dhabhar & McEwen, 1996).

It is important to note that in these studies, a return to basal glucocorticoid levels is almost always followed by a rapid return to baseline numbers of blood lymphocytes, further supporting the hypothesis that the decrease in blood leukocyte numbers is the result of a glucocorticoid-induced redistribution rather than a glucocorticoid-induced destruction of blood leukocytes.

E. Stress-Induced Changes in Blood Leukocyte Numbers: Contradicting Results or a Biphasic Response?

As stated above, stress has been shown to induce a significant decrease in blood leukocyte numbers in fish (Pickford et al., 1971), mice (Jensen, 1969), rats (Dhabhar et al., 1994, 1995; Rinner et al., 1992), rabbits (Toft et al., 1993), horses (Snow et al., 1983), nonhuman primates (Morrow-Tesch et al., 1993), and humans (Herbert & Cohen, 1993; Schedlowski et al., 1993). However, studies have also shown that stress can increase rather than decrease blood leukocyte numbers in humans (Brosschot et al., 1994; Mills et al., 1995; Naliboff et al., 1991; Schedlowski et al., 1993). This apparent contradiction is resolved when three important factors are taken into account: First, stress-induced increases in blood leukocyte numbers are observed following stress conditions that primarily result in the activation of the sympathetic nervous system. These stressors are often of a very short duration (order of a few minutes) or are relatively mild (e.g., public speaking) (Brosschot et al., 1994; Mills et al., 1995; Naliboff et al., 1991; Schedlowski et al., 1993). Second, the increase in leukocyte numbers may be accounted for by stress- or catecholamine-induced increases in granulocytes and NK cells (Benschop et al., 1996; Brosschot et al., 1994; Mills et al., 1995; Naliboff et al., 1991; Schedlowski et al., 1993). Since granulocytes form a large proportion of circulating leukocytes in humans (60–80% granulocytes) an increase in granulocyte numbers is reflected as an increase in total leukocyte numbers in contrast to rats and mice (10–20% granulocytes). Third, stress or pharmacologically induced increases in glucocorticoid hormones induce a significant decrease in blood lymphocyte and monocyte numbers (Dhabhar et al., 1995b, 1996; Hoagland et al., 1946; Schedlowski et al.,

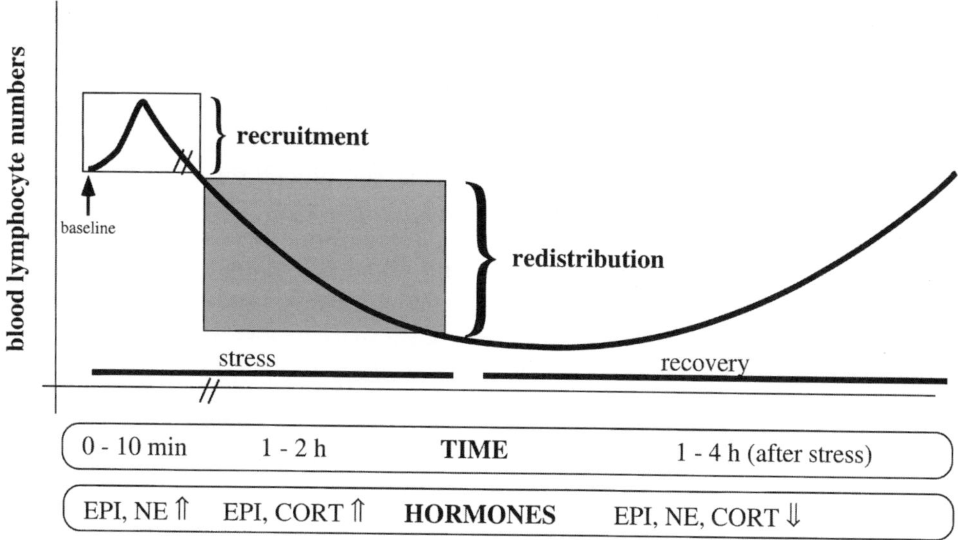

FIGURE 2 Biphasic stress-induced changes in blood leukocyte numbers. Acute stress may induce an initial increase followed by a decrease in blood leukocyte numbers according to the following pattern: Stress conditions which result in activation of the sympathetic (especially noradrenergic) nervous system, may induce an increase in circulating leukocyte numbers. These conditions may occur during the very beginning of a stress response, short duration stress (order of minutes), mild psychological stress, or during exercise. Under these conditions, catecholamine hormones and neurotransmitters induce the body's "soldiers" (leukocytes), to exit their "barracks" (spleen, lung, bone marrow) and enter the "boulevards" (blood vessels). This results in an increase in blood leukocyte numbers. In contrast, stress conditions which result in the activation of the hypothalamic-pituitary-adrenal (HPA) axis induce a decrease in circulating leukocyte numbers. These conditions often occur during the later stages of a stress response, long duration stressors (order of hours), or during severe psychological, physical or physiological stress. Under these conditions, glucocorticoid hormones induce leukocytes to exit the blood and take position at potential "battle stations" (skin, mucosal lining of gastro-intestinal and urinary-genital tracts, lung, liver, and lymph nodes) in preparation for immune challenges which may be imposed by the actions of the stressor (Dhabhar et al., 1994; Dhabhar et al., 1995b; Dhabhar & McEwen 1996; Dhabhar et al., 1996; Dhabhar & McEwen 1997).

1993; Stein, Ronzoni, & Gildea, 1951). Thus, stress conditions that result in a significant and sustained activation of the hypothalamic-pituitary-adrenal (HPA) axis will result in a decrease in blood leukocyte numbers.

We propose that acute stress induces an initial increase followed by a decrease in blood leukocyte numbers according to the following pattern (Figure 2): Stress conditions that result in activation of the sympathetic nervous system, especially conditions that induce high levels of norepinephrine, may induce an increase in circulating leukocyte numbers. These conditions may occur during the very beginning of a stress response, very short duration stress (order of minutes), mild psychological stress, or during exercise. In contrast, stress conditions that result in the activation of the HPA axis induce a decrease in circulating leukocyte numbers. These conditions often occur during the later stages of a stress response, long duration acute stressors (order of hours), or during severe psychological, physical, or physiological stress. An elegant and interesting example in support of this hypothesis comes from Schedlowski et al., who measured changes in blood T cell and NK cell numbers as well as plasma catecholamine and cortisol levels in parachutists (Schedlowski et al., 1993). Measurements were made 2 h before, immediately after, and 1 h after the jump. Results showed a significant increase in T cell and NK cell numbers immediately (minutes) after the jump, which was followed by a significant decrease 1 h after the jump. An early increase in plasma catecholamines preceeded early increases in lymphocyte numbers, whereas the more delayed rise in plasma cortisol preceeded the late decrease in lymphocyte numbers (Schedlowski et al., 1993). More important, changes in NK cell activity and antibody-dependent cell-mediated cytotoxicity (ADCC) closely paralleled changes in blood NK cell numbers, thus suggesting that changes in leukocyte numbers may be an important mediator of apparent changes in leukocyte "activity." Similarly, Rinner et al., have shown that a short stressor (1 min handling) induced an increase in mitogen-induced proliferation of T and B cells obtained from peripheral blood, whereas a longer stressor (2 h immobilization) induced a decrease in the same proliferative responses (Rinner et al., 1992). In another example, Manuck et al. showed that acute psychological stress induced a signifcant increase in blood CTL numbers only in those subjects who showed hightened catecholamine and cardiovascular reactions to stress (Manuck, Cohen, Rabin, Muldoon, & Bachen, 1991).

Thus, we propose that an acute stress response induces biphasic changes in blood leukocyte numbers (Figure 2). Soon after the beginning of stress (order of minutes) or during mild acute stress, or exercise, catecholamine hormones and neurotransmitters induce the body's "soldiers" (leukocytes), to exit their "barracks" (spleen, lung, marginated pool, and other organs) and enter the "boulevards" (blood vessels and lymphatics) (Figures 2 and 3). This results in an increase in blood leukocyte numbers, the effect being most prominent for NK cells and granulocytes. As the stress response continues, activation of the HPA axis results in the release of glucocorticoid hormones, which induce leukocytes to exit the blood and take position at potential "battle stations" (skin, mucosal lining of gastrointestinal and urinary-genital tracts, lung, liver, and lymph nodes) (Figures 2 and 3) in preparation for immune challenges that may be imposed by the actions of the stressor (Dhabhar et al., 1994, 1995b, 1996; Dhabhar & McEwen, 1996, 1997). Such a redistribution of leukocytes results in a decrease in blood leukocyte numbers, the effect being most prominent for T & B lymphocytes, NK cells, and monocytes. Thus, acute stress may result in a redistribution of leukocytes from the barracks, through the boulevards, and to potential battle stations within the body (Figure 3).

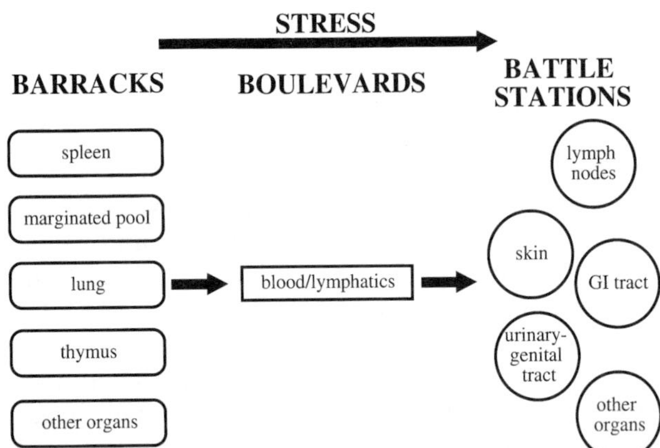

FIGURE 3 Proposed model describing stress-induced changes in leukocyte distribution within different body compartments. Acute stress initially results in recruitment of leukocytes from the spleen, marginated leukocyte pool, lung, thymus, and other organs, into the blood and lymphatic circulation. This is registered as an increase in blood leukocyte numbers. As the stress response progresses, blood leukocyte numbers decrease, as leukocytes leave the bloodstream and marginate within the vasculature of the skin, lymph nodes, gastro-intestinal tract (GI-tract), urinary-genital tract, and other organs which may serve as potential battle stations should the body's defenses be breached as a result of the actions of the stress-inducing agent. This redistribution is registered as a decrease in blood leukocyte numbers. Thus, changes in blood leukocyte numbers observed during acute stress represent a redeployment of leukocytes within the body.

F. Stress-Induced Redistribution of Blood Leukocytes—Mechanisms

It is likely that stress-induced changes in leukocyte distribution are mediated by changes in either the expression, or affinity, of adhesion molecules on leukocytes and/or endothelial cells. It has been suggested that following stress or glucocorticoid-treatment, specific leukocyte subpopulations (being transported by blood and lymph through different body compartments) may be selectively retained in those compartments in which they encounter a stress- or glucocorticoid- induced "adhesion match" (Dhabhar et al., 1995b). As a result of this selective retention, the proportion of some leukocyte subpopulations would decrease in the blood while it increases in the organ in which the leukocytes are retained (e.g., the skin) (Dhabhar & McEwen, 1996). We propose that adhesion molecules such as the selectins and their ligands, which mediate early adhesion events such as leukocyte rolling (McEver, 1994), are likely mediators of a stress-induced retention of blood leukocytes within the vasculature of target organs such as the skin and lymph nodes.

Support for the "selective retention" hypothesis comes from studies showing that prednisolone induces the retention of circulating lymphocytes within the bone marrow, spleen, and some lymph nodes, thus resulting in a decrease in lymphocyte numbers in the thoracic duct and a concomitant decrease in peripheral blood (Cox & Ford, 1982; Spry, 1972). Moreover, glucocorticoid hormones also influence the production of cytokines (Danes & Araneo, 1989; Munck & Guyre, 1989) and lipocortins (Hirata, 1989), which in turn can affect the surface adhesion properties of leukocytes and endothelial cells (Issekutz, 1990). Further investigation of the effects of endogenous glucocorticoids (administered in physiologic doses and examined under physiologic kinetic conditions) on changes in expression/activity of cell surface adhesion molecules and on leukocyte-endothelial cell adhesion is necessary.

G. Stress-Induced Redistribution of Blood Leukocytes — Functional Consequences

Dhabhar et al., were the first to propose that a stress-induced decrease in blood leukocyte numbers represents an adaptive response (Dhabhar et al., 1994, 1995b, 1996; Dhabhar & McEwen, 1996, 1997, 1999c). These authors have suggested that such a decrease in blood leukocyte numbers represents a redistribution of leukocytes from the blood to other organs such as the skin, mucosal lining of gastrointestinal and urinary-genital tracts, lung, liver, and lymph nodes, which may serve as battle stations should the body's defenses be breached. They also have suggested that such a leukocyte redistribution may enhance immune function in compartments into which leukocytes traffic during stress (Dhabhar et al., 1994, 1995b, 1996; Dhabhar & McEwen, 1996, 1997, 1999c).

Thus, an acute stress response may direct the body's soldiers (leukocytes) to exit their barracks (spleen and bone marrow), travel the boulevards (blood vessels), and take position at potential battle stations (skin, lining of gastrointestinal and urinary-genital tracts, lung, liver, and lymph nodes) in preparation for immune challenge (Dhabhar et al., 1994, 1995b, 1996; Dhabhar & McEwen, 1996, 1997). In addition to redeploying leukocytes to potential battle stations, stress hormones also may better equip them for battle by enhancing processes like antigen presentation, phagocytosis, and antibody production. Thus, a hormonal alarm signal released by the brain on detecting a stressor, may prepare the immune system for potential challenges (wounding or infection), which may arise due to the actions of the stress-inducing agent (e.g., a predator or attacker).

An important but under appreciated function of endocrine mediators released under conditions of acute stress may be to ensure that appropriate leukocytes are present in the right place and at the right time to respond to an immune challenge that might be initiated by the stress-inducing agent (e.g., attack by a predator, invasion by a pathogen, etc.). The modulation of immune cell distribution by acute stress may be an adaptive response designed to enhance immune surveillance and increase the capacity of the immune system to respond to challenge in immune compartments (such as the skin, and epithelia of lung, gastrointestinal, and urinary-genital tracts), which serve as major defense barriers for the body. Thus, endocrine mediators released during stress may serve to enhance immune preparedness for potential (or ongoing) immune challenge.

V. STRESS-INDUCED ENHANCEMENT OF IMMUNE FUNCTION

Although a majority of studies in the field of psychoneuroimmunology have focused on the immunosuppressive effects of stress, several studies have also revealed that stress can be immunoenhancing. In general, acute stress is found to be immunoenhancing whereas chronic stress is found to be immunosuppressive (as discussed in the previous section, in some instances the effects of stress on leukocyte numbers and proportions in the compartment being assayed need to be taken into consideration). Dhabhar et al. have suggested that a stress-induced enhancement of immune function may be an important adaptive response that prepares an organism for potential immunologic challenges (e.g., a wound or infection inflicted by an attacker) for which stress perception by the brain, and subsequent stress hormone and neurotransmitter release, may serve as an early warning (Dhabhar et al., 1995b; Dhabhar & McEwen, 1996, 1997, 1999c; Dhabhar, Satoskar, Bluethmann, David, & McEwen, 2000). Studies showing stress-induced enhancements in immune parameters in vivo and in vitro are reviewed in following sections.

A. Stress-Induced Enhancement of Cell-Mediated Immunity

As already discussed, acute stress induces a significant redistribution of leukocytes from the blood to other organs (e.g., skin and lymph nodes) in the body (Figures 2 and 3) (Dhabhar et al., 1995b; Dhabhar, 1998), and adrenal stress hormones are major mediators of this leukocyte redistribution (Dhabhar et al., 1996). Since the skin is one of the targets to which leukocytes traffic during stress, Dhabhar and McEwen (1996) hypothesized that a stress-induced leukocyte redistribution may increase immune surveillance in the skin and consequently enhance immune function should the skin be exposed to antigen following acute stress.

To test this hypothesis, they examined the effects of acute stress on skin immunity, using a rodent model for a skin delayed type hypersensitivity (DTH) response (Dhabhar & McEwen, 1996). To induce DTH, animals initially were sensitized to 2,4-dinitro-1-fluorobenzene (DNFB) by administering the chemical antigen to the skin of the dorsum. During the sensitization phase of a DTH reaction the organism develops an immunologic memory (through the generation of memory T cells) for the antigen with which it is immunized. Following sensitization, the ability of the animals to mount a DTH response against DNFB was examined by administering DNFB to the dorsal aspect of the pinna. The DTH response was subsequently measured as an increase in pinna thickness, which is proportional to the intensity of the ongoing immune reaction (Kimber & Dearman, 1993; Phanuphak, Moorhead, & Claman, 1974). This phase, also known as the elicitation phase, involves recruitment of memory T cells and effector cells such as neutrophils, macrophages, CTLs, and NK cells, which mount an immune response against the antigen to which the animal was previously sensitized. Acute restraint stress administered immediately before the challenge with antigen, resulted in a large and long-lasting enhancement of skin DTH (Figure 4) (Dhabhar & McEwen, 1996). Histological analysis identified significantly larger numbers of leukocytes in the skin of stressed animals both before and after exposure to antigen, and suggested that a stress-induced redistribution of leukocytes was one of the factors mediating the stress-induced enhancement of skin immunity (Dhabhar & McEwen 1996). Acute stress has similarly been shown to enhance skin DTH in mice (Blecha, Barry, & Kelley, 1982).

It was subsequently shown that acute stress administered at the time of sensitization also significantly enhances a skin DTH response following challenge (Dhabhar & McEwen 1999b). In these studies animals were stressed acutely (2 h restraint) before the administration of the sensitizing antigen. Compared with control animals, stressed animals showed a significantly larger DTH response following challenge, although no stress was applied at the time of challenge. These results showed that acute stress administered either during sensitization or challenge can significantly enhance a skin DTH response (Dhabhar & McEwen, 1999b, 1999c, 2000).

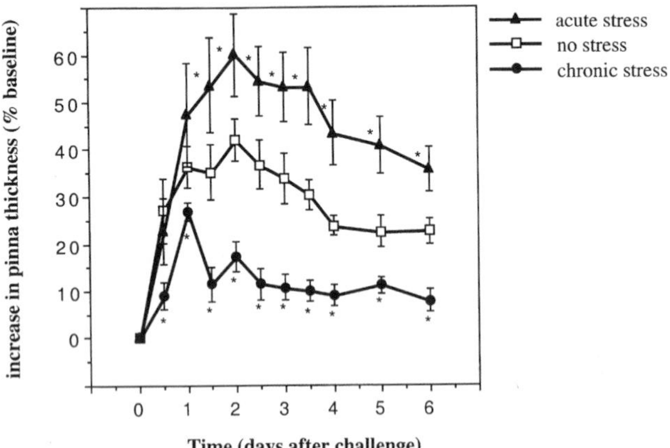

FIGURE 4 Acute stress enhances while chronic stress suppress a skin DTH response (Dhabhar & McEwen 1996; Dhabhar & McEwen 1997). A six day timecourse of changes in the thickness of right pinnae of previously sensitized animals challenged with DFNB is shown. Acute stress (restraint) was administered for 2 h before challenge with DNFB. Chronic stress was administered for 21 days before challenge. The DTH response of acutely stressed animals was significantly higher than that of controls, while that of chronically stressed animals was significantly lower ($p<0.05$, independent *t*-test). Data are expressed as mean ± SEM (n=5).

B. Stress-Induced Enhancement of Humoral Immunity

Wood et al. have shown that exposure to footshock stress enhances humoral as well as cell-mediated immunity to keyhole limpet hemocyanin (KLH) (Wood, Karol, Kusnecov, & Rabin, 1993). These investigators administered a single acute footshock session on days -1, 0, 1, and 3 relative to sensitization (day 0). They observed that, compared with non-stressed controls, animals stressed on days 0 or 1 showed enhanced immune responses with respect to serum anti-KLH IgG levels, splenocyte proliferation, and skin cell-mediated immunity to KLH antigen. Interestingly, nonstressed animals failed to show a significant increase in serum antibody titers and in KLH-stimulated splenocyte proliferation relative to nonimmunized animals (Wood et al., 1993). Similarly, Persoons et al., have shown that acute stress administered prior to intrathecal immunization with trinitrophenyl (TNP) KLH significantly enhanced the primary humoral response in rats (Persoons, Berkenbosch, Schornagel, Thepen, & Kraal 1995). They also showed that acute stress administered prior to antigen administration to previously immunized animals resulted in a significant enhancement of a secondary humoral response (Persoons et al.). In another study, Carr et al., reported that cold stress enhanced IgG and IgM production by splenocytes and that this enhancement was mediated by the alpha adrenergic receptor (Carr, Woolley, & Blalock, 1992).

Several other studies have reported stress-induced enhancement of humoral immune responses. For example, cold stress has been shown to accelerate antigen removal in mice (Sabiston, Ste Rose, & Cinader 1978). Other stressors have been shown to increase antigen-specific antibody titres in rats, mice, and pigs (Berkenbosch, Wolvers, & Derijk, 1991; Blecha & Kelley, 1981; Cocke, Moynihan, Cohen, Grota, & Ader, 1993; Persoons et al., 1995; Solomon, 1969; Wood et al., 1993). It has also been proposed that glucocorticoids may shift the balance of an ongoing immune response in favor of humoral immunity (Danes & Araneo, 1989; Gajewski, Schell, Nau, & Fitch, 1989; Mason, 1991; Mosmann & Coffman, 1989), and physiological doses of glucocorticoids have been shown to enhance immunoglobulin production by mitogen (Grayson, Dooley, Koski, & Blaese, 1981) and IL-4-stimulated (Wu et al., 1991) human lymphocytes in culture.

C. Stress-Induced Enhancement of in Vitro Immune Parameters

Acute stressors such as handling (Rinner et al., 1992), restraint (Jain & Stevenson, 1991), and footshock (Lysle, Cunnick, & Rabin, 1990; Shurin, Zhou, Kusnecov, Rassnick, & Rabin, 1994) have been shown to enhance mitogen-induced proliferation of blood and spleen leukocytes. Acute stress also has been shown to enhance spleen macrophage phagocytic function (Lyte, Nelson, & Baissa, 1990; Lyte, Nelson, & Thompson, 1990), blood polymorphonuclear leukocyte phagocytosis (Shurin, Kusnecov, Hamill, Kaplan, & Rabin 1994), and blood NK cell activity (Jain & Stevenson, 1991; Millar, Thomas, Pacheco, & Rollwagen, 1993). Several studies have shown that in vitro administration of stress hormones to immune cells can enhance different aspects of immune function. Low physiological concentrations of corticosterone have been shown to stimulate mitogen (Wiegers, Reul, Holsboer, & De Kloet, 1994) and anti-T cell receptor-induced (Wiegers et al., 1995) proliferation of splenocytes. Similarly, glucocorticoid hormones have been shown to enhance nitric oxide and IL-1β (Broug-Holub & Kraal, 1996) and tumor necrosis factor (TNF-α) secretion by macrophages (Renz et al., 1992).

D. Stress-Induced Enhancement of Immune Function: Implications for Disease

In view of the above discussion, one would hypothesize that a stress-induced enhancement of immune function may be beneficial in case of infections or cancer, but could also be harmful in case of autoimmune or inflammatory disorders. The phenomenon of a stress-induced increase in resistance to infections or cancer needs to be rigorously investigated. However, numerous studies have reported stress-induced exacerbation of autoimmune and inflammatory diseases. More than 30 years ago, Solomon & Moos (1964) described an association between stress and autoimmune disorders. Rimon & Laakso have classified two categories of rheumatoid arthritis, a disease form more associated with genetic factors, and another more associated with psychodynamic factors such as stress (Rimon & Laakso, 1985). Thomason et al. found that minor stress events such as day-to-day irritants were associated with exacerbations of rheumatoid arthritis (Thomason et al., 1992). Similarly, stress has been shown to be related to the onset and exacerbation of psoriasis (Al'Abadie et al., 1994). Stress also has been reported to precede the onset and exacerbation of multiple sclerosis (Mei-Tal et al., 1970); in some cases, however, it was chronic but not acute stress that was reported to precipitate disease (Philippopoulos, Wittkower, & Cousineau, 1958). It must be mentioned here that studies have also failed to discover consistent relationships between life stress and autoimmune disease (Hendrie, Parasekvas, Baragar, & Adamson, 1971; Zautra, Okun, Robinson, Lee, Roth, & Emmanual, 1989).

We suggest that certain stress conditions, mainly acute stress, may enhance immune function and increase resistance to infections and cancer, but may also predispose an individual toward developing autoimmune or inflammatory disorders. In contrast, as discussed in the following section, chronic stress may suppress immune function and increase susceptibility to infections and cancer, but ameliorate autoimmune and inflammatory disorders. It is clear that further studies are needed to rigorously examine both, stress-induced enhancement of resistance to infections and cancer, and stress-induced exacerbation of autoimmune and inflammatory disorders.

VI. STRESS-INDUCED SUPPRESSION OF IMMUNE FUNCTION

Numerous studies have shown that stress can be immunosuppressive and hence may be detrimental to health (for review see Black, 1994; Borysenko & Borysenko, 1982; Khansari et al., 1990; Kort, 1994; Sklar & Anisman, 1981; Zwilling, 1992; Irwin 1994). Since these studies have been reviewed and discussed extensively, here we present only a few relevant examples of a stress-induced suppression of immune function and refer the reader to these excellent reviews and other chapters in this volume for a more detailed account of the subject. It may be worth noting here that most stress conditions found to be immunoenhancing involve acute stress, and those found to be immunosuppressive involve chronic stress (with the effects of stress on leukocyte distribution being an important factor to be taken into account as discussed in this chapter).

It has been shown that in contrast to acute stress, chronic stress suppresses the skin DTH response (Figure 4) (Basso, Depiante-Depaoli, Cancela, & Molina 1993; Dhabhar & McEwen, 1997). A chronic stress-induced decrease in leukocyte mobilization from the blood to other body compartments is thought to be one of the mediators of this stress-induced suppression of skin DTH (Dhabhar & McEwen, 1997). Similarly in human and animal studies, chronic stress also has been shown to suppress different immune parameters, examples of which include delayed type hypersensitivity (Basso et al., 1993; Kelley, Greenfield, Evermann, Parish, & Perryman 1982), antibody production (Edwards & Dean, 1977; Fleshner, Laudenslager, Simons, & Maier, 1989), NK activity (Bartrop, Lazarus, Luckhurst, Kiloh, & Penny, 1977; Cheng, Morrow-Tesch, Beller, Levy, & Black, 1990; Kiecolt-Glaser et al., 1984; Irwin et al., 1990), leukocyte proliferation (Bartrop et al., 1977; Cheng et al., 1990; Regnier & Kelley, 1981), skin homograft rejection (Wistar & Hildemann 1960), virus-specific T cell and NK cell activity (Bonneau, Sheridan, Feng & Glaser, 1991), and antimycobacterial activity of macrophages from susceptible mouse strains (Brown & Zwilling, 1994).

A. Stress-Induced Increase in Susceptibility to Infections or Cancer

In addition to suppressing different immune parameters, human as well as animal studies have shown that chronic stress increases susceptibility to the common cold (Cohen et al., 1991), and to infection with viruses such as influenza (Sheridan, 1998) and bacteria such as *Toxoplasma* (Chao, Peterson, Filice, Pomeroy, & Sharp, 1990), and *Salmonella* (Edwards & Dean, 1977). Stress also has been shown to increase susceptibility to cancer (Andersen et al., 1998; Ben-Eliyahu et al., 1991; Brenner, Cohen, Ader, & Moynihan 1990). Similarly, chronic stress has been shown to delay wound healing in mice (Padgett et al., 1998) and humans (Marucha et al., 1998), and to impair the immune response to vaccination in human subjects (Glaser, Kiecolt-Glaser, Bonneau, Malarkey, Kennedy, & Hughes, 1991; Kiecolt-Glaser et al., 1996).

B. Stress-Induced Amelioration of Autoimmune Disease

Thus, if chronic stress suppresses immune function and increases susceptibility to infectious disease and cancer, it also may be hypothesized that under these conditions, stress should ameliorate autoimmune or inflammatory diseases. Numerous studies have investigated the effects of environmental or psychological stress on autoimmune reactions. Levine et al. (1962) have demonstrated that the administration of prolonged restraint stress to rats before the induction of experimental allergic encephalomyelitis (EAE) resulted in a suppression of the incidence and severity of disease (Levine & Saltzman, 1987). Rogers et al. (1980) have shown that exposure of rats to a variety of stressors results in a marked suppression of the clinical and histological manifestations of type II collagen-induced arthritis. Similarly, Griffin et al. have demonstrated suppression of EAE by chronic stress (Griffin, Warren, Wolny, & Whitacre, 1993).

Thus, it is evident that under certain conditions, stress suppresses different immune parameters. Although this increases susceptibility to infectious disease and cancer, it also may confer protection against autoimmune and proinflammatory diseases.

VII. THE STRESS SPECTRUM HYPOTHESIS

Dhabhar and McEwen have proposed that a stress response and its consequent effects on immune function may be viewed in the context of a Stress Spectrum (Figure 5) (Dhabhar & McEwen, 1997). One region of the stress spectrum is characterized by Eustress, i.e., conditions of acute, short-duration, or physiologically manageable stress that may result in immunopreparatory or immunoenhancing physiological conditions. An important characteristic of eustress is a rapid physiologic stress response mounted in the presence of the stressor, followed by a rapid shut-off of the response once the stressor has subsided. The other end of the stress spectrum is characterized by Distress, i.e., chronic, repeated, or physiologically exhausting stress that may result in immunosuppression. An important characteristic of distress is that the physiologic response either persists long after the stressor has subsided or is activated repeatedly to result in an overall integrated increase in exposure of the organism to stress hormones. Recently, the concept of allostatic load has been proposed to define the constant wear and tear that takes place while different physiologic systems respond to the exhausting demands placed by internal and external stressors under conditions of distress (for review see McEwen, 1998). We suggest that conditions of high allostatic load would result in deleterious immunosuppression. Importantly, a disruption of the circadian corticosterone rhythm may be an indicator and/or mediator of distress or high allostatic load (Dhabhar & McEwen, 1997; Sephton, Sapolsky, Kraemer, & Spiegel, 1998). The stress spectrum model also proposes that between eustress and distress is an area that represents Resilience, which we define as the ability of physiologic systems

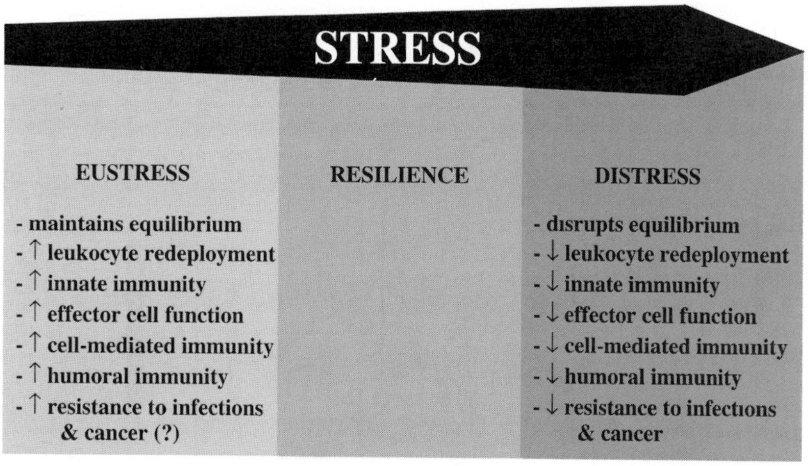

FIGURE 5 Hypothetical model representing the stress spectrum and its relationship to immune function (Dhabhar & McEwen 1997). One region of the stress spectrum is characterized by eustress, i.e., conditions of acute or circumscribed amounts of stress which may result in immuno-preparatory, or immunoenhancing conditions. The other end of the stress spectrum is characterized by distress, i.e., chronic, repeated, or physiologically exhausting stress which may result in immunosuppressive conditions. Between eustress and distress is an area which represents resilience, i.e., the ability of physiologic systems to enable survival for extended periods of time under increasingly demanding conditions.

to enable survival for extended periods of time under increasingly challenging conditions.

VIII. IMMUNOENHANCING EFFECTS OF GLUCOCORTICOID HORMONES

In contrast to the well-known immunosuppressive effects of glucocorticoids, several studies have revealed that glucocorticoid hormones also exert immunomodulating (for review see Wilckens, 1995; Wilckens & DeRijk, 1997) and immunoenhancing effects (for review see Jefferies, 1991; Spencer, Kalman, & Dhabhar, in press). In general, pharmacological concentrations of glucocorticoids exert immunosuppressive effects, whereas under different conditions, physiologic concentrations may exert immunomodulatory, immunoenhancing, or immunosuppressive effects. It is important to recognize that the source (natural versus synthetic) and concentration (physiologic versus pharmacologic) of glucocorticoid hormones, the effects of other physiologic factors (hormones, cytokines, and neurotransmitters), and the state of activation of an immune parameter (naive vs. activated leukocyte, early vs. late activation, etc.), are all important factors that ultimately determine the nature of the effects of glucocorticoids on a given immune response. Immunoenhancing effects of glucocorticoids are discussed in the following, whereas immunosuppressive effects are discussed in Section IX.

A. Glucocorticoid-Induced Enhancement of Cell-Mediated Immunity

An acute stress-induced enhancement of skin DTH has been shown to be mediated by adrenal stress hormones (Dhabhar & McEwen, 1999c). Adrenalectomy, which eliminates the glucocorticoid and epinephrine stress response, eliminated the stress-induced enhancement of skin DTH. Low-dose corticosterone (Figure 6) or epinephrine administration significantly enhanced skin DTH and produced a significant increase in T cell numbers in lymph nodes draining the site of the DTH reaction (Dhabhar & McEwen, 1999c). Moreover, simultaneous administration of these two stress hormones produced an additive increase in the skin DTH response. These results showed that hormones released during an acute stress response may help prepare the immune system for potential challenges (e.g., wounding or infection) for which stress perception by the brain may serve as an early warning signal (Dhabhar & McEwen, 1999c).

B. Glucocorticoid-Induced Enhancement of Humoral Immunity

A permissive role for glucocorticoids in antibody production was described more than 30 years ago. Several investigators reported that low levels of cortisol were a necessary factor in cell culture media to obtain in vitro antibody production (Ambrose,

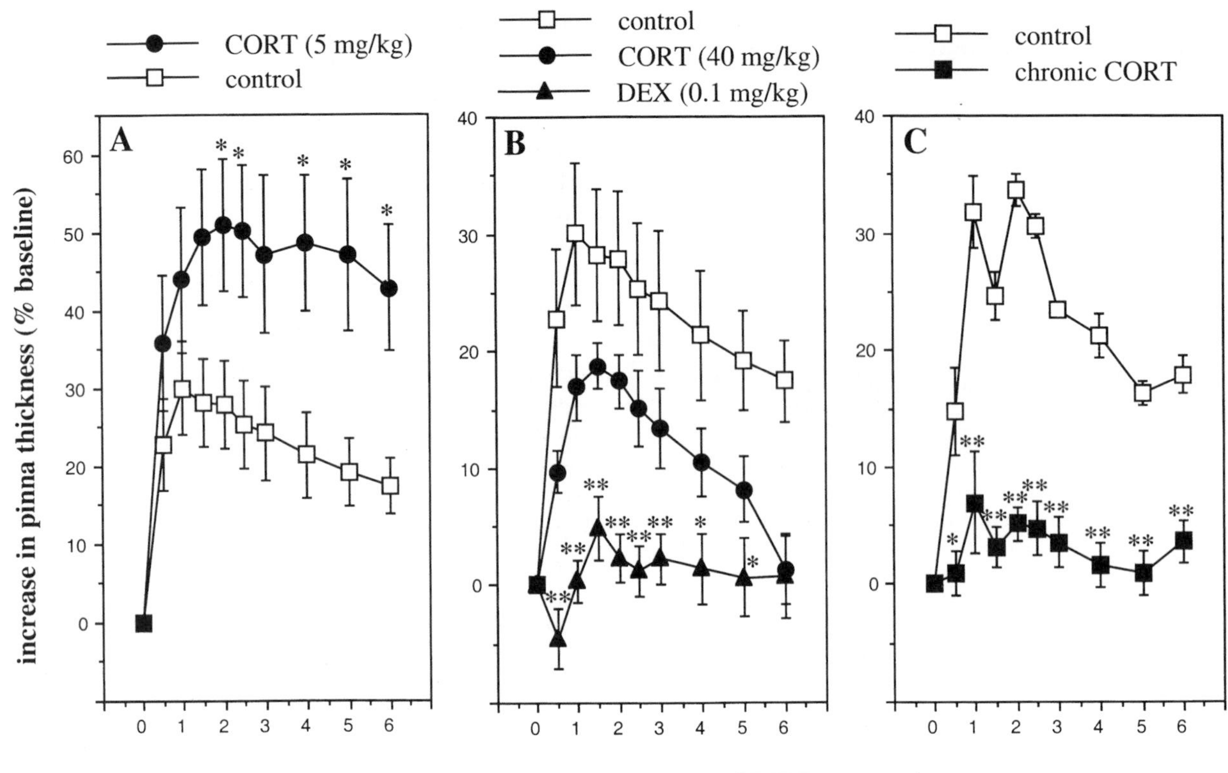

FIGURE 6 Biphasic effects of glucocorticoid hormones on skin DTH (Dhabhar & McEwen 1999). A six day timecourse of changes in the thickness of right pinnae of previously sensitized animals challenged with DNFB (0.5% w/v) is shown. Compared to vehicle treated control animals: Acute administration of a physiologic dose of corticosterone (CORT, 5 mg/kg) significantly enhances the skin DTH response (A). Acute administration of a pharmacologic dose of corticosterone, or of a low dose of the synthetic steroid, dexamethasone, significantly suppresses the skin DTH response (B). Chronic administration of corticosterone also supresses the DTH response (C). Data are expressed as means ± SEM (n=5 per treatment group). Statistically significant differences are indicated: *$p<0.05$, independent *t*-test.

1964; Halliday & Garvey, 1964). Moreover, glucocorticoids were determined to be the critical permissive component present in serum supplements of culture media, and it was suggested that variability in antibody production assays may be the result of variability of glucocorticoid content in different batches of serum (Halliday & Garvey, 1964).

Under some conditions, glucocorticoids have been shown to shift the balance of an immune response toward humoral immunity (Danes & Araneo, 1989; Gajewski et al., 1989; Mason, 1991; Mosmann & Coffman, 1989). Physiological doses of glucocorticoids have been shown to enhance immunoglobulin production by mitogen- (Grayson et al., 1981) and IL-4- (Wu et al., 1991) stimulated human lymphocytes in culture, and glucocorticoids have been shown to stimulate B cell number and antibody production in vitro and in vivo (Fauci, Pratt & Whalen, 1977; Rusu & Cooper, 1975; Tuchinda, Newcomb & DeVald, 1972; for review see Plaut, (1987)).

One possible mechanism by which glucocorticoids may enhance humoral immunity is by shifting the balance of an ongoing immune response toward a Th2 cytokine profile. Dexamethasone has been found to reduce IL-2 production and increase IL 4 production by mouse T cells both in vitro and in vivo (Daynes & Araneo, 1989; Daynes, Dudley, & Araneo, 1990). Low doses of cortisol also have been shown to stimulate IL-4 production by human peripheral blood mononuclear cells and human T cell lines (Snijdewint, Kapsenberg, Wauben-Penris, & Bos, 1995). Interestingly, the ubiquitous transcription factor Oct-1 and the B cell-selective transcription factor Oct-2 are thought to be important for immunoglobulin gene expression, and activated glucocorticoid receptors have been found to interact with both of these factors in vitro (Wieland, Dobbeling, & Rusconi, 1991). It is possible that glucocorticoids enhance antibody production by selectively inhibiting B cells that are less efficient at producing antibody. Thus, high concentrations of glucocorticoids present in vitro during the early stages of B cell stimulation can significantly suppress antibody production, however, even extremely high concentrations of glucocorticoids are not able to suppress antibody production once it has begun (Fauci et al., 1977). Similarly, B cells that differentiate to produce antibody following in vitro mitogenic stimulation are more resistant to the lethal effects of high levels of glucocorticoids than are B cells that do not produce antibody (Roess, Bellone, Ruh, Nadel, & Ruh, 1982). It also has been proposed that glucocorticoid-induced enhancement of humoral immunity may be induced by glucocorticoid actions on monocytes and subsequently on T cells, rather than a direct effect on B cells (Orson, Grayson, Pike, de Seau, & Blaese, 1983).

C. Glucocorticoid-Induced Enhancement of Innate Immunity

As will be described later, glucocorticoids can increase the expression of receptors for the proinflammatory cytokines, IL-1, TNF, IL-6, and MIF, and this may be a mechanism by which glucocorticoids potentiate cytokine induction of acute phase proteins. In the case of the acute phase protein, α1-acid glycoprotein, a glucocorticoid response element (GRE) has been localized within the gene's promoter region, thus suggesting a direct enhancer effect of glucocorticoids on the induction of this acute phase protein (Baumann, Jahreis, & Morella, 1990; Kulkarni, Reinke, & Feigelson, 1985). Glucocorticoids also have been found to increase the expression of serum amyloid A-3 mRNA levels in a macrophage cell line (Ishida, Matsuura, Setoguchi, Higuchi, & Yamamoto, 1994). Interestingly, although glucocorticoids inhibit the synthesis of the complement factor, C3, in human monocytes, they increase levels of factor B, C2, and C1 inhibitor by stabilizing their mRNA levels (Lappin & Whaley, 1991), and in endothelial cells glucocorticoids have been shown to potentiate the induction of both C3 and factor B by IL-1 (Coulpier et al., 1995). Immunoenhancing effects of glucocorticoids may also be mediated through a decrease the synthesis of the endogenous IL-1 receptor antagonist (Arzt et al., 1994).

Several in vivo studies have found a positive relationship between glucocorticoids and certain acute phase proteins. Treatment with glucocorticoids increases acute phase protein production and potentiates acute phase protein induction elicited by inflammatory stimuli (Baumann et al., 1983; Pos et al., 1988). In addition, combined glucocorticoid and catecholamine treatment acts synergistically to induce acute phase proteins (van Gool, Boers, Sala, & Ladiges 1984). The induction of acute phase proteins can be attenuated by adrenalectomy, hypophysectomy, or treatment with the corticosteroid synthesis inhibitor, metyrapone (Silveira & Limaos, 1990; Thompson, Abeles, Beall, Dinterman, & Wannemacher, 1976). Furthermore, the suppressive effect of adrenalectomy and hypophysectomy on acute phase protein induction is reversed by cortisol treatment (Thompson et al., 1976).

Clinical evidence for a facilitatory role of cortisol on acute phase activity comes from some cases of major depression. Maes et al. (Maes et al., 1995) have reported an association between depression and an acute phase response. Hypercortisolemia or nonsuppression to dexamethasone has been reported in some subsets of depressives (Gold, Goodwin, & Chrousos, 1988). Thus, it is conceivable that HPA axis hyperactivity in these patients may contribute to an upregulation of components of the acute phase response. Maes et al. (1993) have reported higher IL-6 levels in some subsets of depressed individuals and these levels were positively correlated with postdexamethasone challenge cortisol levels. These authors also have reported a significantly higher percentage of the acute phase protein α-2 globulin in depressed patients, which was positively correlated with basal cortisol levels (Maes et al., 1995).

D. Glucocorticoid-Induced Enhancement of T Cell Activation

Studies examining the effects of corticosterone on T lymphocyte proliferation in vitro, demonstrate an important mechanism by which corticosterone may mediate the enhancement of immune function (Wiegers et al., 1995). These studies have shown that during the early stages of T cell activation, low levels of corticosterone potently enhance anti-T cell receptor (TCR)- induced lymphocyte proliferation. Furthermore, they showed that corticosterone had to be present during the process of TCR activation to enhance the proliferative response. Other studies have suggested that low concentration, corticosterone-induced enhancement of concanavalin A-stimulated mitogenesis of splenocytes from adrenalectomy (ADX) animals may be mediated by the type 1 or mineralocorticoid receptor (Wiegers et al., 1994). It also has been shown that low doses of corticosterone stimulate DNA synthesis in thymic lymphoblasts (Whitfield, MacManus, & Gillan, 1973). Thus, these in vitro studies indicate a possible mechanism by which stress and stress hormones may enhance immune function in vivo.

E. Glucocorticoid-Induced Potentiation of Cytokine Function

Several lines of evidence indicate that glucocorticoid stress hormones may act synergistically with cytokines to enhance specific immune reactions. Thus, although glucocorticoids inhibit the synthesis of cytokines under some conditions, they also have been shown to induce release and potentiate the actions of cytokines under other conditions. For example, stress has been shown to induce increases in plasma levels of IL-1 and IL-6 (Mekaouche et al., 1994; Takaki, Huang, Somogyvari-Vigh, & Arimura, 1994) and glucocorticoids to induce the production of migration inhibitory factor (MIF) (Calandra et al., 1995). Acute stress has also been shown to induce IL-18 mRNA (Conti, Jahng, Tinti, Son, & Joh, 1997). Moreover, glucocorticoids synergistically enhance the induction of acute phase proteins by IL-1 and IL-6 (Baumann & Gauldie, 1994). Glucocorticoids similarly enhance the biological responses of other cytokines such as IL-2, gamma-interferon (IFN-γ), granulocyte colony-stimulating factor (G-CSF), granulocyte macrophage colony-stimulating factor (GM-CSF), and oncostatin M (for review see Wiegers & Reul, 1998). Using a liver perfusion model, Liao et al. have shown that direct administration of corticosterone at physiological doses stimulates the production of IL-6 and TNF-α (Liao, Keiser, Scales, Kunkel, & Kluger, 1995).

Synergistic interactions between glucocorticoids and cytokines may be mediated by glucocorticoid-induced upregulation of cytokine receptors on target cells as determined by increased cytokine binding or cytokine receptor mRNA expression. For example, glucocorticoids increase IL-1 binding to human peripheral blood B cells (Akahoshi, Oppenheim, & Matsushima, 1988) and to a glioblastoma cell line (Gottschall, Koves, Mizuno, Tatsuno, & Arimura, 1991). Glucocorticoids have also been shown to increase TNF receptor levels in airway epithelial cells (Levine, Logun, Chopra, Rhim, & Shelhamer, 1996). Glucocorticoids also act synergistically with IFN-γ to induce high affinity Fcγ receptors on human monocytic cell lines (Girard, Hjaltadottir, Fejes-Toth, & Guyre, 1987; Warren & Vogel, 1985) and stress-induced increases in endogenous glucocorticoids also appear to facilitate the expression of low affinity Fcγ receptors on peritoneal macrophages (Kizaki et al., 1996). Similarly, glucocorticoids potentiate granulocyte macrophage-colony stimulating factor-induced expression of MHC class II molecules on human monocytes (Sadeghi, Hawrylowicz, Chernajovsky, & Feldmann, 1992). Glucocorticoids also increase GM-CSF binding to human monocytes (Hawrylowicz, Guida, & Paleolog, 1994). This increased cytokine binding may mediate the potentiation of GM-CSF-induced expression of MHC class II molecules on human monocytes (Sadeghi et al., 1992). Although some studies have reported that glucocorticoids inhibit IL-2 receptor expression in leukocytes (Arya, Wong, & Gallo, 1984; Reed et al., 1986) a recent study indicates that the reduced IL-2 receptor expression is secondary to glucocorticoid suppression of IL-2 (Boumpas et al., 1991). In contrast, studies have found a stimulating effect of glucocorticoids on IL-2 induction of IL-2 receptor mRNA levels in several T cell lines (Lamas et al., 1993). Glucocorticoids have also been shown to upregulate IL-6 receptor binding and mRNA levels in epithelial and hepatoma cell lines (Snyers, DeWit, & Content, 1990) and this may be a mechanism for the glucocorticoid potentiation of IL-6 induction of acute phase proteins in liver (Baumann & Gauldie, 1994). Interestingly, glucocorticoids have recently been found to facilitate the actions of the cytokine responsive transcription factor, Stat5, via direct protein-protein interactions between activated glucocorticoid receptors and Stat5 (Stocklin, Wissler, Gouilleux, & Groner, 1996).

F. Glucocorticoid-Induced Increase in Resistance to Infection

Administration of physiologic doses of glucocorticoids has been reported to enhance immunity and reduce the number of respiratory infections observed in patients with adrenocortical insufficiency (Jefferies, 1981). Interestingly, an increase in glucocorticoid dosage at the onset of symptoms of respiratory illness induced a disappearance of symptoms that did not reappear on return to normal maintenance doses (Jefferies, 1981). It also has been reported that resistance to infection with influenza virus was lower in patients with adrenal insufficiency and that glucocorticoid replacement increased resistance to disease (Skanse & Miorner, 1959). A similar increase in resistance to influenza also has been reported in patients without adrenal insufficiency (Jefferies, 1981; Mickerson, 1959), and it has been suggested that viral infection might temporarily impair ACTH secretion and thus necessitate glucocorticoid replacement (Mickerson, 1959). Beneficial effects of cortisone replacement in cases of mononucleosis also have been reported (Bender, 1967; Chappel, 1962). These studies show that in addition to enhancing specific immune parameters, glucocorticoid hormones may also enhance resistance to infectious agents in vivo.

It is significant that there are numerous reports of local (Alani & Alani, 1972; Reitamo et al., 1986;

Wilkinson, 1994) or systemic (Murrieta-Aguttes et al., 1991; Peller & Bardana, 1985; Rosenblum, 1982; Vidal, Tome, Fernandex-Redondo, & Tato, 1994; Whitmore, 1995) reactions to corticosteroids. Given the above discussion, it is tempting to speculate that cases of exacerbation of inflammatory responses following glucocorticoid administration, which are often characterized as "corticosteroid hypersensitivity" (Wilkinson, 1994) or "pseudoallergic reactions" (Peller & Bardana, 1985), may occur because the ambient conditions (dosage and timing) favor a glucocorticoid-induced immunoenhancement rather than the desired immunosuppression.

The studies described in this section support a role for adrenal stress hormones as endogenous immunoenhancing agents. They also suggest that hormones released during an acute stress response may help prepare the immune system for potential challenges (e.g., wounding or infection) for which stress perception by the brain may serve as an early warning signal (Dhabhar & McEwen, 1999b, 1999c).

IX. IMMUNOSUPPRESSIVE EFFECTS OF GLUCOCORTICOID HORMONES

It was the immunosuppressive effects of glucocorticoid hormones that led Philip Hench and Edward Kendall to the Nobel Prize in 1950, which was awarded for their discovery of the use of corticosteroids in the treatment of autoimmune disease (Hench; 1952; Hench, Kendall, Slocumb, & Polley, 1949). Hench observed that patients suffering from autoimmune diseases showed recovery from these diseases during periods of other illnesses such as hepatitis. He postulated that the inflammatory response accompanying the other disease was stimulating the production of an endogenous immunosuppressive mediator that was responsible for inhibiting the autoimmune disease. Together with Kendall he determined that the cortisol was that endogenous mediator, and their finding revolutionized the treatment of autoimmune disease and a host of other inflammatory disorders. Since that time, glucocorticoid hormones have been widely used as immunosuppressive agents in various clinical and experimental situations (for review see (Fauci, 1979; Goldstein, Bowen, & Fauci, 1992; Marx, 1995; Schleimer et al., 1989)).

As stated previously, pharmacological concentrations of glucocorticoids exert immunosuppressive effects, whereas under different conditions, physiologic concentrations may exert modulatory, enhancing, or suppressive effects on immune function. It is important to recognize that the source (natural vs. synthetic) and concentration (physiologic vs. pharmacologic) of glucocorticoid hormones, the effects of other physiologic factors (hormones, cytokines, and neurotransmitters), and the state of activation of an immune parameter (naive vs. activated leukocyte, early vs. late activation, etc.), are all important factors that may ultimately determine the nature of the effects of glucocorticoids on a given immune response. For example, as discussed previously, it has been shown that ADX eliminated the stress-induced enhancement of skin DTH (Dhabhar & McEwen, 1999c). Low-dose corticosterone (Figure 6) or epinephrine administration to ADX animals at the time of antigenic challenge significantly enhanced a skin DTH reaction to the antigen and produced a significant increase in T cell numbers in lymph nodes draining the site of the DTH reaction. In contrast, high dose corticosterone, chronic corticosterone, or low-dose dexamethasone administration significantly suppressed skin DTH (Figure 6) (Dhabhar & McEwen, 1999c).

A. Immunosuppression by Pharmacologic Doses of Glucocorticoids

Several books and articles have extensively reviewed the anti-inflammatory or immunosupressive effects of glucocorticoid hormones (Cupps & Fauci, 1982; Fauci, 1979; Goldstein et al., 1992; Haynes, 1990; Marx, 1995; Munck & Guyre, 1989; Munck et al., 1984; Schleimer et al., 1989). It is apparent from these reviews that, under specific conditions, glucocorticoids have been shown to suppress immunoglobulin, prostaglandin, leukotriene, histamine, and cytokine production; neutrophil superoxide production; macrophage function; mitogen- and antigen-induced lymphocyte proliferation; lymphocyte differentiation; NK cell activity; and leukocyte migration and activation. In view of these potently immunosuppressive actions, glucorticoids are widely used in the clinic as antiinflammatory agents (Haynes, 1990; Schleimer et al., 1989). Given that the immunosuppressive actions of pharmacologic treatments with glucocorticoids have been reviewed extensively in the literature, here we focus mainly on immunosuppressive actions of physiologic changes in glucocorticoid hormones.

B. Physiological Changes in Glucocorticoid Levels have Protective Immunosuppressive Effects

It has been hypothesized that an important physiologic role of endogenous glucocorticoids might be to suppress an ongoing immune response so as to prevent it from reaching levels of reactivitiy that might cause damage (Munck et al., 1984). Strong support for this hypothesis comes from studies showing that adrenalectomized rats die within 24–48 h after being immunized with horse serum or Freund's complete adjuvant, but they can be rescued by corticosterone replacement therapy (Dougherty, 1949, 1950). A number of studies involving animal models of inflammatory disorders and autoimmune disease also lend support for this hypothesis (Mason, 1991). These studies have demonstrated the existence of a negative feedback loop between the immune system and the HPA axis, such that proinflammatory mediators arising from an ongoing immune reaction stimulate the HPA axis (Besedovsky, Del Ray, Sorkin, & Dinarello, 1986; Kroemer, Brezinschek, Faessler, Schauenstein, & Wick, 1988; Munck et al., 1984; Sapolsky, Rivier, Yamamoto, Plotsky, & Vale, 1987), which in turn results in the secretion of corticosterone that suppresses the immune response and prevents it from potentially damaging the host. The protective effects of immunosuppression by endogenous glucocorticoids are discussed in the following sections.

C. Glucocorticoid-Induced Immunosuppression: Protection against Sepsis

Studies have shown that endogenous glucocorticoids play a crucial role in containing an inflammatory response and preventing it from becoming systemic and leading to septic shock. It has been known for over 75 years that adrenalectomized animals are extremely sensitive to the lethal effects of various inflammatory agents, such as diphtheria toxin, typhoid vaccine, bacterial infection, foreign cells, and foreign serum (for review see Swingle & Remington, 1944). Moreover, it has been shown that the protective factor present in the adrenals is corticosterone. Thus, glucocorticoid administration to adrenalectomized animals protects them from inflammatory shock induced by endotoxin (LPS), cytokines such as IL-1 and TNF, carrageenin, superantigen (SEB), or cobra venom factor (Bertini, Bianchi, & Ghezzi, 1988; Gonzalo, Gonzalez-Garcia, Martinez, & Kroemer, 1993; Nakano, Suzuki, & Oh, 1987; Nakano, Suzuki, Oh, & Yamashita, 1986). Moreover, treatment of animals with the glucocorticoid receptor antagonist RU486 induces susceptibility to these inflammatory agents to nearly the same extent as adrenalectomy (Fan, Gong, Wu, Zhang, & Xu 1994; Gonzalo et al., 1993; Laue et al., 1988; Lazar Jr., Duda, & Lazar, 1992). Importantly, high doses of glucocorticoids are used to treat septic shock in humans, although their beneficial effects are controversial since sepsis may require glucocorticoid administration too early in the disease process to be practically useful (Cohen & Glauser, 1991). Glucocorticoids are thought to protect against sepsis by inhibiting toxin-induced increases in cytokines such as IL-1 and TNF (Beutler, Krochin, Milsark, Luedke, & Cerami, 1986; Lee et al., 1988), which are known to mediate early events leading to sepsis (Dinarello & Wolff, 1993). Interestingly, endotoxin treatment also induces a rise in plasma corticosterone (Nakano et al., 1987) which coincides with a decrease in plasma TNF (Zuckerman, Shelhaas, & Butler, 1989). Since glucocorticoids are known to supress the synthesis of IL-1 and TNF (Beutler et al., 1986; Lee et al., 1988), it is possible that the endotoxin-induced increase in corticosterone mediates the observed decrease in TNF levels. Moreover, adrenalectomy or RU486 treatment increases the amount and duration of TNF induction in response to LPS, further supporting a role for corticosterone in suppressing the endogenous production of proinflammatory cytokines following endotoxin exposure (Zuckerman et al., 1989; Lazar Jr. et al., 1992). In addition to suppressing the production of proinflammatory cytokines, glucocorticoids are also thought to protect against septic shock by inhibiting the actions of these cytokines by inhibitting the production of factors such as eicosanoids, histamine, platelet activating factor, and nitric oxide (Bertini et al., 1988; Radomski, Palmer, & Moncada, 1990; Williams & Yarwood, 1990).

D. Glucocorticoid-Induced Immunosuppression: Protection against Autoimmune Disease

Current evidence suggests that three contributing factors result in susceptibility to inflammatory and autoimmune disorders (Mason, 1991; Sternberg, 1995; Tsigos & Chrousos, 1994; Wick, Sgonc, & Lechner, 1998): (1) the presence of host immune response genes that carry the potential for contributing to autoimmunity; (2) exposure to a proinflammatory or antigenic challenge that initiates the cascade of immune reactions that ultimately result in autoimmunity; and (3) a deficiency in the HPA axis such that it is not capable of mounting an appropriate immunosuppressive corticosterone response in reaction to an ongoing immune reaction. Numerous studies have elegantly investigated the role played by the HPA axis in protecting the host from autoimmune reactions, and some of these studies are discussed in the following paragraph.

Sternberg et al. investigated the influence of the HPA axis on the development of streptococcal cell wall (SCW)-induced arthritis in female rats belonging to the genetically related Lewis/N (LEW/N) and Fischer 344/N (F344/N) strains (Sternberg & Wilder, 1989). The F344/N strain is resistant to the development of SCW-induced arthritis whereas the LEW/N strain is susceptible. Interestingly, the F344/N strain mounts a significantly higher corticosterone and ACTH response than the LEW/N strain when challenged with a variety of stressors or with inflammatory mediators like SCW peptidoglycan polysaccharide, or IL-1α (Sternberg, Hill et al., 1989; Sternberg, Young et al., 1989; Dhabhar et al., 1993, 1995a). Compared with the F344 strain, the Lewis strain shows a significantly greater habituation or adaptation to an acute or chronic stressor (Dhabhar, McEwen, & Spencer, 1997). F344/N rats treated with the glucocorticoid receptor antagonist RU486 are rendered susceptible to SCW-induced arthritis indicating that they do carry the immune response genes with potential for triggering autoimmunity (Sternberg, Hill et al., 1989; Sternberg, Young et al., 1989). Conversely, LEW rats treated with pharmacologic doses of dexamethasone, become completely resistant to the development of SCW-induced arthritis (Sternberg, Hill et al., 1989; Sternberg, Young et al., 1989). Furthermore, compared with Fischer 344 (F344 rats), adrenal steroid receptors in neural and immune tissues of LEW rats show a significantly lower magnitude of activation in response to stress-induced increases in plasma corticosterone (Dhabhar et al., 1993, 1995a). Thus, strain differences in plasma corticosterone levels are also manifest as significant differences in the extent of activation of corticosterone receptors in target tissues.

In view of the observations described above, it has been hypothesized that the robust corticosterone response mounted by the F344/N strain (in response to inflammatory mediators released by the SCW-induced immune reaction) suppresses the acute inflammatory response and prevents it from becoming self-reactive. In contrast, the weaker corticosterone response mounted by the LEW/N strain is thought to be insufficient to suppress the initiation and progression of an autoimmune response (Sternberg, Hill et al., 1989; Sternberg, Young et al., 1989).

EAE is another animal model of an autoimmune disease in which a similar immunosuppressive role for the HPA axis has been proposed (for review see Mason, MacPhee, & Antoni, 1990; Mason, 1991). The Lewis strain shows the greatest susceptibility to EAE (Mason, 1991). MacKenzie, Leonard, and Cuzner (1989) suggested that during the preclinical phase of EAE, elevations in plasma corticosterone may regulate the lymphoproliferative stage of the disease, and that during the clinical phase of the disease elevations in plasma corticosterone as well as splenic norepinephrine may regulate other recovery-oriented immune mechanisms (MacKenzie et al., 1989).

Although two rat models of HPA axis regulation of autoimmune diseases are discussed above, similar correlations between HPA axis hyporeactivity and susceptibility to autoimmune disease have been observed for autoimmune conditions in chickens (Wick et al., 1998), and mice (Lechner et al., 1996). Morever, hypoactivity of the HPA axis has also been associated with some types of autoimmune and inflammatory diseases in humans (Torpy & Chrousos, 1996). However, it is important to note that the generalizability of the above findings, namely that HPA axis hypoactivity predicts susceptibility to autoimmune disease, also has been questioned by studies showing that differential HPA axis responsivity does not necessarily predict differential susceptibility to adjuvant-induced arthritis (Chover-Gonzalez et al., 1998; Grasser, Moller, Backmund, Yassouridis, & Holsboer, 1996).

E. Glucocorticoid-Induced Suppression of Autoimmune Reactions — Potential Mechanisms

Glucocorticoid hormones may exert their protective immunosuppressive effects by inhibiting the production or actions of various proinflammatory molecules as discussed previously. In addition, it has been hypothesized that glucocorticoids may suppress certain autoimmune reactions by inducing a shift toward a Th2 or humoral immune response (Mason, 1991; Mason et al., 1990). For example, stimulation of the HPA axis by inflammatory mediators released during the initiation of an autoimmune response results in increased plasma corticosterone. Increased corticosterone levels may shift the balance of the ongoing immune reaction from a T_H1-directed (cell-mediated) response toward a T_H2-directed (antibody-mediated) response, by promoting the production of IL-4 and suppressing the production of IL-2 (Danes & Araneo, 1989). Since the pathology associated with EAE is thought to be the result of activation of T cells autoreactive with peptide fragments of myelin basic protein (Steinman, 1991), the net result of this shift from cell-mediated to humoral immunity could be the suppression EAE.

Griffin et al. showed that chronic stress administered to Lewis rats before myelin basic protein (MBP) challenge resulted in suppression of the clinical and histopathologic changes associated with EAE. However, the same stress regimen had no effect on the clinical course of EAE in rats challenged with MBP peptide fragment 68-88 (MBP 68-88), suggesting that the stress-induced increase in corticosterone could be affecting mechanisms involved in processing and/or presentation of the encephalitogen. It is significant that a decrease in frequency of MBP-reactive cells and a decrease in production of IL-2 and IFN-γ (i.e., a condition that would favor a humoral immune response) was observed in stressed animals relative to controls.

Antibodies directed against the encephalitogen MBP may be involved in the suppression of EAE since it has been reported that anti-MBP antibodies are first detected at the beginning of the refractory phase after plasma corticosterone levels rise in response to the initial phase of EAE (MacPhee, Day, & Mason, 1990). Further, it has been observed that symptoms in the initial phase of the disease are minimal if an animal makes an antipeptide antibody response during the early stages of EAE. If Lewis rats are immunized with different doses of MBP peptide linked to bovine serum albumin, recipients of low doses make fewer antipeptide antibodies and show severe clinical symptoms, the converse being true for recipients of high doses (Mason, 1991). It is also possible that part of the mechanism of suppression may involve the generation of antiidiotypic antibodies directed against variable regions of autoreactive T cell receptors.

Interestingly, in the case of myasthenia gravis, an autoantibody-mediated disease in humans, early investigators found that intensive treatment of patients with steroids exacerbated the symptoms. Therefore, the current treatment regimen involves a short initial intensive treatment followed by alternate-day steroid therapy. Improvement is observed 10–15 days after the beginning of therapy (Claman, 1989). It may be hypothesized that during the initial period of steroid treatment, the promotion of an antibody-biased response by steroid treatment might exacerbate the disease by stimulating autoantibody production. However later during steroid treatment, the production of inhibitory antibodies or the activation of other immunosuppressive mechanisms might result in suppression of the disease. Alternatively, as discussed earlier in this chapter, glucocorticoid treatment may under certain conditions stimulate other immune parameters such as innate immunity, antigen presentation, cell-mediated immunity, or effector cell function. This may in turn exacerbate an autoimmune disease if the enhanced response were directed against self antigens.

Wilder, Allen, and Hansen (1986) demonstrated an increase in expression of class II major histocompatibility antigen (Ia) in synovial tissues that parallels the development of SCW-induced arthritis. This increase is observed in the susceptible Lewis strain, but not in the resistant F344 strain. Doeberitz et al. showed that long-term treatment with dexamethasone reduces surface expression, membrane bound protein, and mRNA of class I major histicompatibility antigen on human epithelial cells (Doeberitz, Koch, Drzonek, & Hausen, 1990). Since strain differences in the ability to mount a corticosterone response to immune challenge are thought to be responsible for the strain differences in resistance to SCW-induced arthritis, it may be hypothesized that glucocorticoids may play a role in preventing the immunostimulatory upregulation of Ia expression. A role for HPA axis interactions with macrophage differentiation also has been proposed as a mediator of susceptibility to autoimmune disease (Damoiseaux, Huitinga, Dopp, & Dijkstra, 1992).

Recent evidence suggests that corticotropin-releasing hormone (CRH) produced in peripheral inflammatory sites might stimulate inflammatory reactions at these sites (Karalis et al., 1991). CRH has been shown to stimulate numerous immune functions. Stephanou et al., (1990) demonstrated CRH mRNA and immunoreactivity in human leukocytes, and CRH binding sites also have been observed on leukocytes (Stephanou, Jessop, Knight, & Lightman 1990). Importantly, Karalis et al. showed that administration of antiserum to CRH significantly suppresses inflammatory exudate volume and cell concentration in a model involving carrageenin-induced aseptic inflammation. Further, the same authors showed that glucocorticoids inhibit the production of immune CRH. Thus, it might be hypothesized that part of the immunosuppressive actions of glucocorticoids may involve suppression of CRH production at sites of inflammation.

One of the best known effects of glucocorticoids on the immune system is their ability to kill leukocytes. Glucocorticoids have been shown to mediate this effect through two mechanisms: apoptosis or programmed cell death, and cell lysis. Although there is a considerable amount of evidence showing that apoptosis is induced by physiological concentrations of glucocortcoids in vivo, nonspecific leukocyte lysis is thought to be the result of exposure to pharmacologic concentrations of glucocorticoids (Godlowski, 1952; Muehrcke, Lewis & Kark, 1952; Padawer & Gordon, 1952). Glucocorticoid-induced apoptosis of immune cells is thought to occur through the activation of genes that specifically regulate programmed cell death. It has been shown that mRNA and protein synthesis are both required for the apoptotic program to be executed, since agents like actinomycin D, emetine, and cyclohexamide significantly inhibit glucocorticoid-induced apoptosis (Cohen & Duke,

1984; Thomas, Edwards, & Bell, 1981; Wyllie, Morris, Smith, & Dunlop, 1984). It is believed that glucocorticoids stimulate the expression of a protein or a group of proteins, which in turn execute the apoptotic program (Cohen, 1989). The proteins induced by glucocortcoids are not thought to be directly lethal to the cell, but are thought to act through other intermediaries to effect cell death (Cohen, 1989).

Several other molecular mechanisms have been proposed for glucocorticoid-mediated immunosuppression (Barnes & Adcock, 1993). Glucocorticoids are thought to inhibit the actions of nuclear factor kappa B (NF-κB), a transcription factor that activates a number of genes coding for various immunoregulatory molecules, cytokines, and adhesion molecules (May & Ghosh, 1998). Glucocorticoid inhibition of NF-κB is achieved through glucocorticoid-induction of a negative regulator of NF-κB, IκBα, which by binding NF-κB prevents the induction of genes for proinflammatory molecules (Auphan, DiDonato, Rosette, Helmberg, & Karin, 1995; Scheinman, Cogswell, Lofquist, & Baldwin, 1995). AP-1 (e.g., Fos-Jun heterodimer) is another transcription factor that stimulates a variety of proinflammatory molecules (Park, Kaushansky, & Levitt, 1993; Serfling et al., 1989). Activated glucocorticoid receptors have been shown to directly bind and interfere with the function of both AP-1 (Schule & Evans, 1991) and NF-κB (Caldenhoven et al., 1995; Mukaida et al., 1994; Scheinman et al., 1995). Thus, glucocorticoids may exert their immunosuppressive effects by directly inhibiting the actions of activational transcription factors and by indirect inhibition through the induction of negative modulators of these transcription factors. Glucocorticoids may also directly regulate genes for certain immune mediators. For example, DNA regions with moderate homology to the consensus GRE have been identified in the promoter region of the IL-6 gene, and footprinting studies suggest that activated glucocorticoid receptors bind to regulatory regions of this gene (Ray, LaForge, & Seghal, 1990). Glucocorticoids may also inhibit certain immune molecules by reducing mRNA stability. This has been demonstrated for IL-1β mRNA levels following in vitro dexamethasone administration (Amano, Lee, & Allison, 1993; Lee et al., 1988).

X. INDIVIDUAL DIFFERENCES IN HPA AXIS RESPONSIVITY: EFFECTS ON RESISTANCE TO AUTOIMMUNE DISEASE, INFECTION, AND CANCER

The discussion above illustrates that HPA axis-induced immunosuppression can provide benefical protection from autoimmune reactions. Strains of animals that show a robust HPA axis response to environmental stress and immune challenge are relatively resistant to autoimmune disease even if they carry potentially autoreactive immune response genes and even if they have been exposed to antigens capable of inducing an autoimmune reaction. However, one might hypothesize that a robust HPA axis response that confers protection against autoimmune disease via immunosuppression might result in greater susceptibility to infectious diseases and cancer, which require a robust immune response for their elimination.

The significantly lower corticosterone response to stress and immune challenge observed in LEW rats compared with F344 rats (Dhabhar et al., 1993; Sternberg, Chrousos, Wilder & Gold 1992; Sternberg, HIll et al., 1989; Sternberg & Wilder, 1989), the significantly greater adaptation to acute or chronic stress observed in LEW rats (Dhabhar et al., 1997), and the significantly lower activation of adrenal steroid receptors seen in immune tissues of Lew rats (Dhabhar et al., 1995a), may contribute to the increased susceptibility of the Lew strain to autoimmune diseases. However, these conditions might also serve to protect this strain from diseases like viral or bacterial infections and cancer that require a robust immune response for their elimination. In contrast, the substantially higher levels of corticosterone (which result in greater activation of adrenal steroid receptors in immune tissues) of F344 rats may protect them from autoimmune diseases, but may also be responsible for the reported susceptibility of this strain to diseases like cancer.

A similar example is seen in differences between BALB/c and C57/BL mice in their ability to resist infection with *Leishmania major* (Mason, 1991). The BALB/c strain is susceptible to infection whereas the C57/BL strain is resistant. Compared with C57/BL mice, BALB/c mice show a more robust corticosterone response to stress. It has been hypothesized that the stronger corticosterone response induced by infection in BALB/c mice results in a bias toward a T_H2-directed, humoral immune response that results in susceptibility to infection (Mason, 1991). In contrast, the lower corticosterone response of C57/BL mice favors a T_H1-directed, cell-mediated response that confers resistance to the parasite. It is significant that administration of anti-IL-4 antibody to *L. major* - infected BALB/c mice confers resistance to further infection, suggesting that IL-4 mediated suppression may be responsible for susceptibility of BALB/c strain to the parasite.

Thus, intrinsic differences in the ability of the HPA axis to respond to stressful stimuli and immunologic challenge may translate into differences in the ability to resist autoimmune or infectious diseases and cancer. These differences are clearly observed as species or strain differences, but they may also contribute significantly to individual differences within strains in relative susceptibility or resistance to disease. Such individual differences are especially relevant for extensively outbred populations like those of humans. It may be hypothesized that individuals who show a low HPA axis responsivity may be relatively more susceptible to autoimmune diseases, but resistant to infectious diseases and cancer. For example, Buske-Kirschbaum et al. demonstrated that atopic children show an attenuated cortisol response to a laboratory stressor (Buske-Kirschbaum et al., 1997). Similarly, individuals who show a high HPA axis responsivity may be relatively resistant to autoimmune diseases, but susceptible to infectious diseases and cancer. Thus, although genetic factors acting at the level of the immune system may render an individual susceptible to a certain disease, genetic and/or environmental factors acting at the level of the neuroendocrine system may be able to compensate and confer protection on susceptible individuals.

XI. PARADOXICAL OBSERVATIONS REGARDING STRESS AND IMMUNE FUNCTION: AN ATTEMPT AT RESOLUTION

Based on the above discussion, we suggest that four key parameters may influence the direction (enhancing versus suppressive) of the effects of stress or glucocorticoid hormones on a given immune parameter (Figure 7): (1) the effects of stress or glucocorticoids on leukocyte distribution in the body; (2) the differential effects of acute versus chronic stress (or acute versus chronic exposure to glucocorticoids) on immune function; (3) the differential effects of physiologic versus pharmacologic doses of glucocorticoids, and the differential effects of endogenous (e.g., cortisol, corticosterone) vs. synthetic (e.g., dexamethasone) glucocorticoids; and (4) the timing of stressor or glucocorticoid hormone exposure relative to the timecourse of the immune response. It is important to recognize that factors such as gender, genetics, age, the route of administration and nature of the immunizing antigen, and time of day also may affect the relationship between stress and immune function.

A. A Stress or Glucocorticoid-Induced Redistribution of Leukocytes May Determine Immunoenhancement vs. Immunosuppression

Numerous studies examining the effects of stress or glucocorticoid hormones on immune function have focused on the effects of these factors on ex vivo measures of immune function as determined by in vitro cytotoxicity and proliferation assays. However, one of the most underappreciated aspects of the interaction between stress, glucocorticoid hormones, and the immune system is the effect of glucocorticoids on leukocyte distribution. It is important to note that such changes in leukocyte distribution may mediate many of the effects of stress and glucocorticoids on immune function.

1. A Redistribution of Blood Leukocytes May Represent an Adaptive Response

Dhabhar et al. were the first to propose that a stress-induced decrease in blood leukocyte numbers may represent an adaptive response (Dhabhar, 1998; Dhabhar et al., 1994, 1995b, 1996; Dhabhar & McEwen, 1996, 1997, 1999c). These authors suggested that such a decrease in blood leukocyte numbers may represent a redistribution of leukocytes from the blood to other organs such as the skin, mucosal lining of gastrointestinal and urinary-genital tracts, lung, liver, and lymph nodes, which may serve as potential battle stations should the body's defenses be breached (Figure 3). They also suggested that such a leukocyte redistribution may enhance immune function in those compartments to which leukocytes traffic during stress (Dhabhar et al., 1994, 1995b, 1996; Dhabhar & McEwen, 1996, 1997, 1999c).

Thus, an acute stress response may direct the body's soldiers (leukocytes) to exit their barracks (spleen, lung, other organs), travel the boulevards (blood vessels), and take position at potential battle stations (skin, lining of gastrointestinal and urinary-genital tracts, lymph nodes) in preparation for immune challenge (Figure 3) (Dhabhar et al., 1994, 1995b, 1996; Dhabhar & McEwen, 1996, 1997). In addition to redeploying leukocytes to potential battle stations, stress hormones also may better equip them for battle by enhancing processes like antigen presentation, phagocytosis, and antibody production. Thus, a hormonal alarm signal released by the brain on detecting a stressor may prepare the immune system for potential challenges (wounding or infection) that may arise due to the actions of the stress-inducing agent (e.g., a predator or attacker). The cellular and molecular mechanisms mediating these

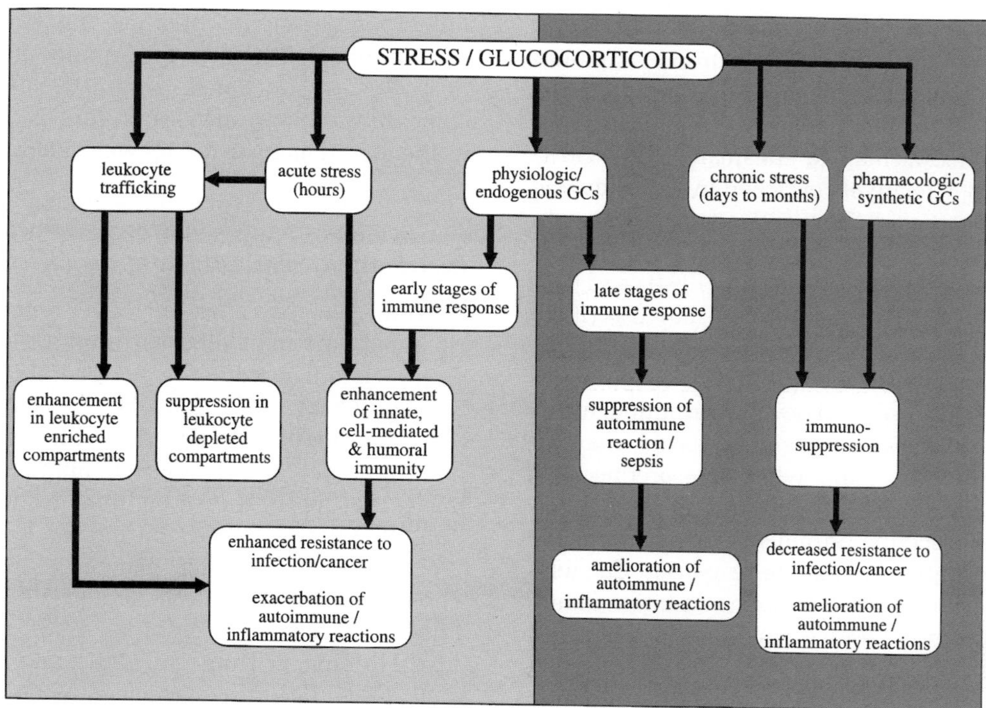

FIGURE 7 Proposed model for the relationship between different parameters of stress and glucocorticoid hormones, and their bidirectional effects on immune function. Immunoenhancement: A stress-induced redistribution of leukocytes within the body may result in enhanced immune function within compartments to which leukocytes traffic during stress and suppressed immune function in compartments which are relatively depleted of leukocytes. Acute stress, or physiological levels of glucocorticoid hormones acting during the early phase of an immune response may also enhance immune function. Immunoenhancement may be mediated by an increase in innate, cell-mediated, or humoral immunity. The beneficial effects of such immunoenhancement may include increased resistance to infections or cancer. The harmful effects of such immunoenhancement may include exacerbation of autoimmune or inflammatory disorders. Immunosupression: Chronic stress, pharmacological doses of glucocorticoid hormones, or synthetic glucocorticoids such as dexamethasone all suppress immune function. Physiological changes in glucocorticoid hormones acting at later stages during an immune response may also suppress immune function. Stress- or glucocorticoid- mediated immunosuppression may increase susceptibility to infections or cancer, but may also protect against autoimmune or inflammatory reactions.

effects of stress and stress hormones on immune function merit further investigation.

2. *Leukocyte Redistribution and the Interpretation of Experimental Data*

When interpreting data showing stress-induced changes in functional assays such as lymphocyte proliferation or NK activity it may be important to bear in mind the effects of stress on the leukocyte composition of the compartment in which an immune parameter is being measured. For example, it has been shown that acute stress induces a redistribution of leukocytes from the blood to the skin and that this redistribution is accompanied by a significant enhancement of a skin DTH response (Dhabhar & McEwen, 1996). In what might appear to be contradicting results, acute stress has been shown to suppress splenic and peripheral blood responses to T cell mitogens (Cunnick, Lysle, Kucinski, & Rabin, 1990; Monjan & Collector, 1977; Shurin et al., 1994; Weiss, Schleifer, Miller, & Stein, 1981) and splenic IgM production (Zalcman & Anisman, 1993). However, it is important to note that in contrast to the skin, which is enriched in leukocytes during acute stress, peripheral blood and spleen are relatively depleted of leukocytes during acute stress (Dhabhar, 1998; Keller et al., 1988). This stress-induced decrease in blood and spleen leukocyte numbers may contribute to the acute stress-induced suppression of immune function in these compartments.

In contrast to acute stress, chronic stress has been shown to suppress skin DTH and a chronic stress-induced suppression of blood leukocyte redistribution is thought to be one of the factors mediating the immunosuppressive effect of chronic stress (Figure 4)

(Dhabhar & McEwen, 1997). Again, in what might appear to be contradicting results, chronic stress has been shown to enhance mitogen induced proliferation of splenocytes (Monjan & Collector, 1977) and splenic IgM production (Zalcman & Anisman, 1993). However, the spleen is relatively enriched in T cells during chronic glucocorticoid administration, suggesting that it may also be relatively enriched in T cells during chronic stress (Miller et al., 1994), and this increase in spleen leukocyte numbers may contribute to the chronic stress-induced enhancement of immune parameters measured in the spleen.

Similarly, the issue of leukocyte distribution and of the immune compartment being assayed may be important to bear in mind while interpreting data from other experimental or pharmacological treatments, such as nicotine administration, which have been shown to suppress immune responses. Caggiula et al. have shown that nicotine administration supresses blood proliferative responses (Caggiula et al., 1992). An examination of their data reveals that nicotine administration induces a large magnitude corticosterone response (Caggiula et al.). Thus, it is possible that the observed immunosuppressive effects of nicotine administration are mediated through a nicotine-induced rise in corticosterone, which induces a significant decrease in blood leukocyte numbers.

3. *Leukocyte Redistribution: Functional Consequences*

It is also important to bear in mind that the heterogeneity of the stress-induced changes in leukocyte distribution (Dhabhar et al., 1995b) implies that using equal numbers of leukocytes in a functional assay may not account for stress-induced changes in relative percentages of different leukocyte subpopulations in the cell suspension being assayed. For example, samples that have been equalized for absolute numbers of total blood leukocytes from control vs. stressed animals may still contain drastically different numbers of specific leukocyte subpopulations (e.g., stress may alter the ratio between antigen presenting cells or helper T cells and effector T, B, and NK cells). Such changes in leukocyte composition may mediate the effects of stress even in functional assays using equalized numbers of leukocytes from different treatment groups. This possibility needs to be taken into account before concluding that a given treatment changes an immune parameter on a per cell rather than a per population basis.

Moreover, as discussed previously, a stress-induced redistribution of leukocytes from the blood to other compartments such as the skin may have significant consequences for immune function with a decrease in functional parameters in the blood coinciding with an increase in functional parameters in the skin (Dhabhar & McEwen, 1996, 1997).

4. *Circadian Changes in Blood Leukocyte Distribution: Similarity with the Effects of Stress*

Numerous investigators have reported that the circadian peak in blood corticosterone levels coincides with a circadian trough in peripheral blood lymphocyte numbers, and that the circadian trough in corticosterone levels coincides with a circadian peak in peripheral blood lymphocyte numbers. This rhythmicity has been shown in humans (Abo, Kawate, Itoh, & Kumagai, 1981; Bartter, Delea, & Halberg, 1962; Tavadia, Fleming, Hume, & Simpson 1975; Thompson, McMahon, & Nugent 1980), nonhuman primates (Morrow-Tesch et al., 1993), mice (Kawate, Abo, Hinuma, & Kumagai, 1981), and rats (Dhabhar et al., 1994; Griffin & Whitacre, 1991). Furthermore, Thompson et al. (1980) reported circadian variations in peripheral blood lymphocytes in healthy adults and showed that patients with adrenal insufficiency lack this circadian pattern, and that administration of cortisol to these patients causes a dose-dependent lowering of lymphocyte levels in the blood (Thompson et al., 1980). In addition, Kawate et al., (1981) demonstrated in mice that adrenalectomy abolishes the circadian rhythm in lymphocyte numbers, and that a single injection of prednisolone produces a reversible depression of circulating lymphocyte number soon after drug administration (Kawate et al., 1981).

Circadian changes in blood leukocyte distribution are similar in magnitude and in leukocyte subpopulation specificity to stress-induced changes and they may have similar functional consequences (Dhabhar et al., 1994). For example, a study examining human T lymphocyte antigen responsivity to tetanus toxoid found that the T cell proliferative response was lowest when corticosterone levels were at their circadian peak (Hiemke et al., 1995). These authors concluded that their studies, as well as other studies showing similar results (Eskola, Frey, Molnar, & Soppi, 1976; Kaplan et al., 1976), reflected a corticosteroid-induced circadian suppression of blood T lymphocytes. However, an alternate interpretation of their results could be proposed: the decrease in antigen-stimulated blood T cell proliferation at the beginning of the active phase of the human circadian cycle may reflect the fact that those T cells most capable of responding to the antigen had migrated from the bloodstream, redistributed to other compartments in the body, and hence were not available for assay. Normalizing total leukocyte numbers from different timepoints in such a study still would not account for heterogeneity in the subpopulation composition of blood samples from different timepoints. Thus, although leukocyte emigration from the blood might result in an apparent immunosuppression in the blood, its overall effects might in fact be immunoenhancing, because the T cells may have relocated to organs in the body where they might be more likely to encounter, and effectively deal with, the injected antigen.

Moreover, as with stress, the organs to which leukocytes traffic at the beginning of the active period (glucocorticoid peak) may be areas such as the skin, certain lymph nodes, and the lining of the urinary-genital and gastrointestinal tracts, organs that may serve as potential battle stations should the body's defenses be breached.

5. *Stress or Glucocorticoid-Induced Redistribution of Leukocytes: An Important Mediator of Neuroendocrine–Immune Effects*

The above discussion is not intended to discount the fact that stress and stress hormones may affect different immune parameters or susceptibility to infections and cancer independently of leukocyte trafficking. In fact, such effects of stress and glucocorticoids are discussed in the following section. However, the aim of the preceeding discussion is to highlight the role of stress-, and glucocorticoid-induced changes in leukocyte distribution as being important and underappreciated factors mediating the effects of stress on immune function and on the overall health of an organism. We also wish to emphasize that before final conclusions are made regarding the mechanisms by which a particular experimental manipulation or pharmacological treatment affects immunity, care must be taken to examine how the manipulation may induce changes in absolute numbers and relative proportions of leukocytes within different body compartments even if the assay being utilized "equalizes" total leukocyte numbers before sample addition to assay wells.

B. Acute Stress Enhances Whereas Chronic Stress Suppresses Immune Function (in Some Instances Stress-Induced Changes in Leukocyte Distribution Need to be Taken into Consideration)

The studies described in this chapter show that acute stress can be immunoenhancing whereas chronic stress can be immunosuppressive. These studies may help reconcile the apparent contradiction between reports showing that, on the one hand, stress suppresses immunity and increases susceptibility to infections and cancer (Borysenko & Borysenko, 1982; Cohen et al., 1991; Khansari et al., 1990; Kort, 1994; Maier et al., 1994), whereas on the other it exacerbates autoimmune diseases that should be ameliorated by a suppression of immune function (Al'Abadie et al., 1994; Mei-Tal et al., 1970; Rimon & Laakso, 1985; Solomon & Moos, 1964; Thomason et al., 1992).

Under normal conditions, acute stress may serve a protective role by enhancing an immune response directed toward a wound, infection, or cancer. For example, acute stress significantly enhances a skin immune response (Dhabhar & McEwen, 1996, 1997, 1999c). Moreover, administration of physiologic doses of glucocorticoids has been reported to enhance immunity and reduce the number of respiratory infections observed in patients with adrenocortical insufficiency (Skanse & Miorner, 1959; Jefferies, 1981). Interestingly, an increase in glucocorticoid dosage at the onset of symptoms of respiratory illness induced a disappearance of symptoms, which did not reappear on return to normal maintenance doses (Jefferies, 1981). It is important to note that although a stress-induced enhancement of immune function is beneficial in the case of an infectious or neoplastic challenge to the host, such an enhancement could also be detrimental if the immune response were directed against an innocuous (poison ivy, nickel in jewellery, latex, etc.) or autoimmunogenic antigen, and this could explain the well-known stress-induced exacerbations of autoimmune and inflammatory disorders (Al'Abadie et al., 1994; Mei-Tal et al., 1970; Rimon & Laakso, 1985; Solomon & Moos, 1964; Thomason et al., 1992). In contrast to acute stress, chronic stress suppresses immune function. This may explain stress-induced exacerbations of infections and cancer (Ben-Eliyahu et al., 1991; Cohen et al., 1991; Glaser et al., 1994; Sheridan, 1998) and stress-induced suppression of wound healing (Marucha et al., 1998; Padgett et al., 1998) and autoimmune reactions (Griffin et al., 1993; Levine, Strebel, Wenk, & Harman, 1962; Rogers et al., 1979).

C. Bidirectional Effects of Glucocorticoid Hormones on Immune Function

Studies of several physiologic systems have revealed a bidirectional regulatory role for glucocorticoids that consists of enhancing versus suppressive effects on key physiologic parameters. Low levels of glucocorticoids are generally permissive or stimulatory for a physiological process, whereas higher levels of glucocorticoids are inhibitory. For example, low concentrations of glucocorticoids are permissive for normal growth and body weight gain, whereas high levels of glucocorticoids are catabolic and suppress feeding (Devenport, Thomas, Knehans, & Sundstrom, 1990). In the central nervous system low glucocorticoid levels positively regulate tryptophan hydroxylase function and thereby are a necessary permissive factor for the synthesis of serotonin (for review see McEwen, de Kloet, & Rostene, 1986). However, high levels of glucocorticoids suppress tryptophan hydroxylase function and may dampen the effects of serotonin secretion by down-regulating serotonin receptor levels (Mendelson & McEwen, 1992). Similarly, low levels of glucocorticoids increase hippocampal neuronal excitability and enhance long-term potentiation, whereas higher levels of glucocorticoids inhibit these electrophysiological measures (Diamond, Bennett, Fleshner, & Rose 1992; Joels & de Kloet, 1992; Pavlides, Watanabe, Magarinos, & McEwen, 1995). Low levels of glucocorticoids are also required for the survival of granule cell neurons in the adult rat dentate gyrus (Sloviter et al., 1989; Woolley, Gould, Sakai, Spencer, & McEwen, 1991); however, high levels of glucocorticoids can lead to atrophy and neuronal loss of nearby hippocampal pyramidal neurons (Sapolsky, 1987; Woolley, Gould, & McEwen, 1990).

A modulatory role for glucocorticoid hormones with respect to immune system function has been suggested (for review see Jefferies, 1991; McEwen, 1998; McEwen et al., 1997; Munck & Naray-Fejes-Toth, 1992; Spencer et al., in press; Wilckens, 1995; Wilckens & DeRijk, 1997). This chapter has specifically discussed the bidirectional effects of glucocorticoid hormones on different immune parameters. For example, studies described in this chapter suggest that acute administration of physiologic doses of endogenous glucocorticoids can significantly enhance certain immune parameters (Figure 6) (Dhabhar & McEwen, 1999c). They also show that acute administration of high doses (Dhabhar & McEwen, 1999c; Fauci & Dale, 1974) and chronic administration of physiologic doses of endogenous glucocorticoids are immunosuppressive (Figure 6) (Dhabhar & McEwen, 1999c). Moreover, large differences are observed in the immunosuppressive potency of endogenous vs. synthetic glucocorticoids (Figure 6) with the immunosuppressive effects of glucocorticoid analogs such as dexamethasone being significantly more potent (Dhabhar & McEwen, 1999c; Fauci, 1976). In another example, glucocorticoids have been shown to potentiate the cytokine induction of acute phase proteins (Pos et al., 1988); however, glucocorticoids are also protective against the lethal effects of septic shock that can be triggered by a full blown acute phase response (Gonzalo et al., 1993). Another bidirectional effect of glucocorticoids that could affect a number of immune parameters may be the inhibitory and stimulatory effects of glucocorticoids on cytokine and cytokine receptor expression, respectively (Wiegers & Reul, 1998).

We suggest that the stimulatory effects of glucocorticoids occur with relatively low levels of circulating hormone as is seen with other physiological systems, whereas the inhibitory effects predominate in the presence of high glucocorticoid levels. Such dose-response relationships have been described for bidirectional effects of corticosterone on skin DTH responses in vivo (Dhabhar & McEwen, 1999c), for bidirectional effects of glucocorticoids on immunoglobulin synthesis and secretion by human peripheral lymphoyctes (Levo, Harbeck, & Kirkpatrick, 1985; Smith, Sherman, & Middleton, 1972), for the effects of hydrocortisone on human peripheral blood B cell activation (Fauci et al., 1977), for glucocorticoid-induced proliferation vs. apoptosis of thymocytes (Whitfield, MacManus, & Rixon 1970), and for bidirectional effects of corticosterone on T cell mitogenesis (Wiegers et al., 1994) and macrophage phagocytosis (Forner, Barriga, Rodriquez, & Ortega, 1995; Rhinehart, Sagone, Balcerzak, Ackerman, & LoBuglio, 1975). We suggest that in general, physiological changes in endogenous glucocorticoid hormones may help to enhance immune function and prepare the immune system to deal with challenges that may arise under conditions of stress (Dhabhar et al., 1995b; Dhabhar & McEwen, 1996, 1997, 1999c). In contrast, physiological changes in glucocorticoids that involve prolonged HPA axis activation by an immune response may lead to prolonged exposure to endogenous glucocorticoids and exert an inhibitory effect on immune function, and even in those cases counter-regulation may preferentially spare the effector phase of specific immune responses.

Of note, there are numerous reports of local (Alani & Alani, 1972; Reitamo et al., 1986; Wilkinson, 1994) or systemic (Murrieta-Aguttes et al., 1991; Peller & Bardana, 1985; Rosenblum, 1982; Vidal et al., 1994; Whitmore, 1995) reactions to corticosteroids. Given the above discussion, one might hypothesize that cases of exacerbation of inflammatory responses following glucocorticoid administration may occur because the ambient conditions (dosage and timing) favor a glucocorticoid-induced immunoenhancement rather than the desired immunosuppression.

The preceding discussion explains how under certain conditions glucocorticoids exert immunoenhancing effects, whereas under other conditions they are potently immunosuppressive. In general, glucocorticoids released during acute stress or endogenous glucocorticoids administered in physiologic concentrations have immunoenhancing effects. In contrast, glucocorticoids released during chronic stress, endogenous glucocorticoids administered chronically or in high doses, and synthetic glucocorticoids are all immunosuppressive. As described previously, the immunosuppressive effects of these hormones are well known, and these hormones (particularly their synthetic analogs) are widely used in the clinic as antiinflammatory agents.

D. Immunomodulatory Effects of Timing of Stress or Stress Hormone Administration Relative to the Course of an Immune Response

The preceding discussion suggests that under certain conditions physiological levels of endogenous glucocorticoids have immunoenhancing effects and under other conditions similar hormone levels suppress autoimmune and inflammatory reactions. We hypothesize that these differential effects may be achieved by differences in the glucocorticoid sensitivity or receptivity of the immune response being affected. At the very beginning of an immune response, certain components of the response such as leukocyte trafficking, antigen presentation, helper T cell function, leukocyte proliferation, cytokine and chemokine function, and effector cell function may all be receptive to glucocorticoid-mediated immunoenhancement. In contrast, at a later, more advanced stage of an immune response these components may be more receptive to glucocorticoid-mediated immunosuppression. Although this hypothesis needs to be tested through further experiments, examples from studies showing temporal differences in the sensitivity of immune reactions to the effects of physiologic concentrations of glucocorticoid hormones are presented in the following section.

1. Bidirectional Effects of Glucocorticoids on Early vs. Late Stages of T Lymphocyte Proliferation

Studies examining the effects of corticosterone on T lymphocyte proliferation in vitro support the hypothesis that there may be temporal differences in the receptivity of an immune response to the enhancing vs. suppressive effects of endogenous glucocorticoid hormones (Wiegers et al., 1995). These studies have shown that during the early stages of T cell activation, low levels of corticosterone potently enhance anti-TCR-induced lymphocyte proliferation. However, during later stages of culture the same levels of corticosterone suppress T lymphocyte proliferation (Wiegers et al., 1995). Furthermore, Wiegers et al. showed that corticosterone had to be present during the process of TCR activation to enhance the proliferative response. If corticosterone was added to the culture system more than 2 h after the initiation of TCR activation, the enhancement of lymphoproliferation was not observed.

Interestingly, Weigers et al., have shown that these bidirectional effects of corticosterone on different stages of T lymphocyte proliferation are mediated by opposing effects of corticosterone on IL-2 receptor (IL-2R) vs. the cytokine itself (for review see Wiegers & Reul, 1998). Thus, during the early stages of lymphocyte proliferation, corticosterone induces an increase in IL-2Rα expression. This increases the IL-2 receptivity of lymphocytes and is reflected by an increase in lymphocyte proliferation (Wiegers et al., 1995). Although corticosterone reduces the production of IL-2 under these conditions, this decrease is not rate limiting at this stage since exogenously added IL-2 fails to increase proliferation. However, if corticosterone is administered at later stages, the enhancement in IL-2R expression is absent, whereas the suppression of IL-2 production is still present. Under these conditions, the availability of IL-2 does become rate-limiting and hence corticosterone suppress the lymphoproliferative response. Thus, these studies indicate an important mechanism mediating an endogenous glucocorticoid-induced immunoenhancement during the early stages and an endogenous glucocorticoid-induced immunosuppression during the later stages of an immune response.

2. The Immune Response, Corticosteroid-Binding Globulin, and Ambient Glucocorticoid Levels

Corticosteroid-binding globulin (CBG) is a plasma binding protein to which both cortisol and corticosterone bind with a high affinity. In humans and rats, under basal conditions, the majority of circulating glucocorticoid hormone (greater than 80%) is bound by CBG (Brien, 1980; Henning, 1978; Siiteri et al., 1982). Only stress or peak circadian levels of glucocorticoids saturate the binding capacity of CBG enough to result in a significant proportion (greater than 50%) of free hormone in the bloodstream. Most studies of glucocorticoid action suggest that only the free hormone is capable of producing a cellular effect (Mendel, 1989). Thus, regulation of CBG levels, which in turn regulate the level of free glucocorticoid hormones, is critical in terms of the hormones being able to exert their cellular effects.

An ongoing immune response may help increase free circulating levels of glucocorticoid hormones by three main mechanisms by (1) stimulating HPA axis activity and resulting in greater adrenal secretion of glucocorticoids (discussed previously, for review see Munck et al., 1984; Munck & Guyre, 1989); (2) inducing a decrease in circulating CBG levels, presumably by decreasing CBG production in the liver (Savu, Lombart, & Nunez, 1980); (3) decreasing CBG levels locally at the site of an immune reaction (Hammond, Smith, Paterson, & Sibbald, 1990). For example, it has been determined that the CBG molecule can be cleaved by elastase, a serine protease, thus resulting in the release of bound corticosterone (Hammond, 1990). High levels of elastase secreted by activated neutrophils have been shown to induce the cleavage of CBG molecules and release high levels of free glucocorticoids in close proximity to the site of the inflammatory reaction (Hammond, Smith, Underhill, & Nguyen, 1990). This immune response-induced increase in availability of free systemic or local glucocorticoid hormones may occur toward the later stages of an immune response. The resultant increased levels of endogenous glucocorticoids may mediate the protective immunosuppression that prevents the ongoing immune response from going out of control and damaging self.

XII. CONCLUSIONS

Stress has long been suspected of playing a role in the etiology of many diseases, and numerous studies have shown that stress can be immunosuppressive and hence may be detrimental to health. Moreover, glucocorticoid stress hormones are widely regarded as being immunosuppressive and are used clinically as antiinflammatory agents. However, this chapter shows that under certain conditions stress and glucocorticoid hormones exert immunoenhancing effects. Dhabhar et al., have suggested that the physiologic stress response may play a critical evolutionarily adaptive role, with stress hormones and neurotransmitters serving as messengers that prepare the immune system for potential immunologic challenges (e.g., wounding or infection) perceived by the brain (e.g., the detection of predator or attacker) (Dhabhar et al., 1994, 1995b; Dhabhar & McEwen, 1996, 1997, 1999c, 2000). However, it is important to recognize that although a stress-induced enhancement of immune function may increase resistance to infections or cancer, it also may exacerbate autoimmune and inflammatory disease. In contrast, a stress- or glucocorticoid-induced suppression of immune function may increase susceptibility to infections or cancer, but may ameliorate autoimmune and inflammatory disorders. Therefore, there exists a yin-yang principle with respect to the effects of stress on immune function, and perhaps on most physiological parameters. Since these effects may potently influence the overall health of an organism, one might hypothesize that a physiologic equilibrium among these different systems would be most favorable for the maintenance of health.

It is also important to recognize that humans as well as animals experience stress as an intrinsic part of life, and in conjunction with many standard diagnostic, clinical, and experimental manipulations. Unintended stressors may significantly affect these diagnostic and clinical measures and overall health outcomes. Thus, when conducting clinical, diagnostic, or experimental manipulations, it may be important to account for the effects of stress on the specific physiologic parameter or health outcome being measured.

The above discussion and the summary presented in Figure 7 illustrate the complex role that stress and glucocorticoid hormones play as modulators and regulators of an immune response. Clearly, there is evidence to show that under certain conditions stress and/or glucocorticoids are immunoenhancing, whereas under other conditions they are immunosuppressive. We have proposed a few defining characteristics for these conditions. For example, important factors that distinguish between the immunoenhancing versus immunosuppressive effects of stress or glucocorticoid hormones include (1) changes in leukocyte distribution within the body; (2) The duration (acute vs. chronic) of stress; (3) the dose (physiologic vs. pharmacologic), duration (acute vs. chronic), and nature (endogenous vs. synthetic) of glucocorticoid hormone exposure; and (4) the timing of stress or glucocorticoid administration relative to the stage (early vs. late) of an immune response. However, the precise characteristics of these different conditions and interactions between these conditions and other genetic and physiological factors that lead to these bidirectional effects need to be further investigated and defined.

A determination of the physiologic mechanisms through which stress and stress hormones enhance or suppress immune responses may help our understanding and treatment of diseases thought to be affected by stress. The cellular and molecular mechanisms by which stress and stress hormones up- or down-regulate an immune response merit further investigation. A greater understanding of these mechanisms would help in the development of biomedical treatments that could harness an individual's physiology to selectively enhance (during vaccination, wounding, infections, or cancer) or suppress (during autoimmune or inflammatory disorders) the immune response depending on what would be most beneficial for the patient.

Acknowledgments

Portions of the work described in this chapter were supported by a grant from the John D. & Catherine T. MacArthur Foundation, and by a DeWitt Wallace Foundation Fellowship (F.S.D.).

References

Abo, T., Kawate, T., Itoh, K., & Kumagai, K. (1981). Studies on the bioperiodicity of the immune response I. Circadian rhythms of human T, B, and K cell traffic in the peripheral blood. *Journal of Immunology, 126*, 1360–1363.

Ader, R., & Cohen, N. (1993). Psychoneuroimmunology: Conditioning and stress. *Annual Reviews Psychology, 44*, 53–85.

Ader, R., Cohen, N., & Felten, D. L. (1995). Psychoneuroimmunology: Interactions between the nervous system and the immune system. *Lancet, 435*, 99–103.

Ader, R., Felten, D. L., & Cohen, N. (1991). Psychoneuroimmunology. San Diego: Academic Press.

Akahoshi, T., Oppenheim, J. J., & Matsushima, K. (1988). Induction of high-affinity interleukin 1 receptor on human peripheral blood lymphocytes by glucocorticoid hormones. *Journal of Experimental Medicine, 167*, 924–936.

Al'Abadie, M. S., Kent, G. G., & Gawkrodger, D. J. (1994). The relationship between stress and the onset and exacerbation of psoriasis and other skin conditions. *British Journal of Dermatology, 130*, 199–203.

Alani, M. D. Alani, S. D. (1972). Allergic contact dermatitis to corticosteroids. *Annals of Allergy, 30*, 181–185.

Amano, Y., Lee, S. W., & Allison, A. C. (1993). Inhibition by glucocorticoids of the formation of interleukin-1α, interleukin-1β, and interleukin-6: Mediation by decreased mRNA stability. *Molecular Pharmacology, 43*, 176–182.

Ambrose, C. T. (1964). The requirement for hydrocortisone in antibody-forming tissue cultivated in serum-free medium. *Journal of Experimental Medicine, 119*, 1027–1049.

Amkraut, A. A., Solomon, C. F., & Kraemer, H. C. (1971). Stress, early experience and adjuvant-induced arthritis in the rat. *Psychosomatic Medicine, 33*, 203–214.

Andersen, B. L., Farrar, W. B., Golden-Kreutz, D., Kutz, L. A., MacCallum, R., Courtney, M. E., & Glaser, R. (1998). Stress and immune responses after surgical treatment for regional breast cancer. *Journal of the National Cancer Institute, 90*, 30–36.

Arya, S. K., Wong-Stal, F., & Gallo, R. C. (1984). Dexamethasone-mediaed inhibition of human T cell growth factor and γ-interferon messenger RNA. *Journal of Immunology, 133*, 273–276.

Arzt, E., Sauer, J., Pollmacher, T., Labeur, M., Holsboer, F., Reul, J. M., & Stalla, G. K. (1994). Glucocorticoids suppress interleukin-1 receptor antagonist synthesis following induction by endotoxin. *Endocrinology, 134*, 672–677.

Auphan, N., DiDonato, J. A., Rosette, C., Helmberg, A., & Karin, M. (1995). Immunosuppression by glucocorticoids: Inhibition of NF-κB activity through induction of IκB synthesis. *Science, 270*, 286–290.

Barnes, P. J.Adcock, I. (1993). Anti-inflammatory actions of steroids: Molecular mechanisms. *Trends in Pharmacological Sciences, 14*, 436–441.

Bartrop, R., Lazarus, L., Luckhurst, E., Kiloh, L. G., & Penny, R. (1977). Depressed lymphocyte function after bereavement. *Lancet, 8016*, 834–836.

Bartter, F. C., Delea, C. S., & Halberg, F. (1962). A map of blood and urinary changes related to circadian variations in adrenal cortical function in normal subjects. *Annals of the New York Academy of Sciences, 98*, 969–983.

Basso, A. M., Depiante-Depaoli, M., Cancela, L., & Molina, V. (1993). Seven-day variable-stress regime alters cortical β-adrenoreceptor binding and immunologic responses: Reversal by imipramine. *Pharmacology, Biochemistry & Behavior, 45*, 665–672.

Baumann, H., Firestone, G. L., Burgess, T. L., Gross, K. W., Yamamoto, K. R., & Held, W. A. (1983). Dexamethasone regulation of a1-acid glycoprotein and other acute phase reactants in rat liver and hepatoma cells. *Journal of Biological Chemistry, 10*, 563–570.

Baumann, H., & Gauldie, J. (1994). The acute phase response. *Immunology Today, 15*, 74–80.

Baumann, H., Jahreis, G. P., & Morella, K. K. (1990). Interaction of cytokine- and glucocorticoid-response elements of acute-phase plasma protein genes. *Journal of Biological Chemistry, 265*, 22275–22281.

Ben-Eliyahu, S., Yirmiya, R., Liebeskind, J. C., Taylor, A. N., & Gale, R. P. (1991). Stress increases metastatic spread of a mammary tumor in rats: Evidence for mediation by the immune system. *Brain, Behavior, & Immunity, 5*, 193–205.

Bender, C. E. (1967). The value of corticosteroids in the treatment of infectious mononucleosis. *Journal of the American Medical Association, 199*, 529–532.

Benschop, R. J., Rodriguez-Feuerhahn, M., & Schedlowski, M. (1996). Catecholamine-induced leukocytosis: Early observations, current research, and future directions. *Brain, Behavior, & Immunity, 10*, 77–91.

Berkenbosch, F., Wolvers, D. A., & Derijk, R. (1991). Neuroendocrine and immunological mechanisms in stress-induced immunomodulation. *Journal of Steroid Biochemistry & Molecular Biology, 40*, 639–647.

Bertini, R., Bianchi, M., & Ghezzi, P. (1988). Adrenalectomy sensitizes mice to the lethal effects of interleukin 1 and tumor necrosis factor. *Journal of Experimental Medicine, 167*, 1708–1712.

Besedovsky, H., Del Ray, A., Sorkin, E., & Dinarello, C. A. (1986). Immunoregulatory feedback between interleukin-1 and glucocorticoid hormones. *Science, 233*, 652–655.

Beutler, B., Krochin, N., Milsark, I. W., Luedke, C., & Cerami, A. (1986). Control of cachectin (tumor necrosis factor) synthesis: Mechanisms of endotoxin resistance. *Science, 232*, 977–980.

Black, P. H. (1994). Immune system-central nervous system interactions: Effect and immunomodulatory consequences of immune system mediators on the brain. *Antimicrobial Agents & Chemotherapy, 38*, 7–12.

Blecha, F., Barry, R. A., & Kelley, K. W. (1982). Stress-induced alterations in delayed-type hypersensitivity to SRBC and contact sensitivity to DNFB in mice. *Proceedings of the Society for Experimental Biology, 169*, 239–246.

Blecha, F., & Kelley, K. W. (1981). Effects of cold and weaning stressors on the antibody-mediated immune response of pigs. *Journal of Animal Science, 53*, 439–447.

Bonneau, R. H., Sheridan, J. F., Feng, N., & Glaser, R. (1991). Stress-induced effects on cell-mediated innate and adaptive memory components of the murine immune response to herpes simplex virus infection. *Brain, Behavior, & Immunity, 5*, 274–295.

Borysenko, M., & Borysenko, J. (1982). Stress, behavior, and immunity: Animal models and mediating mechanisms. *General Hospital Psychiatry, 4*, 59–67.

Boumpas, D. T., Paliogianni, F., Anastassiou, E. D., & Balow, J. E. (1991). Glucocorticosteroid action on the immune system: Molecular and cellular aspects. *Clinical & Experimental Rheumatism, 9*, 413–423.

Brenner, G. J., Cohen, N., Ader, R., & Moynihan, J. A. (1990). Increased pulmonary metastases and natural killer cell activity in mice following handling. *Life Sciences, 47*, 1813–1819.

Brien, T. G. (1980). Free cortisol in human plasma. *Hormone & Metabolic Research, 12*, 643–650.

Brosschot, J. F., Benschop, R. J., Godaert, G. L., Olff, M., De Smet, M., Heijnen, C. J., & Ballieux, R. E. (1994). Influence of life stress on immunological reactivity to mild psychological stress. *Psychosomatic Medicine, 56*, 216–224.

Broug-Holub, E.Kraal, G. (1996). Dose- and time-dependent activation of rat alveolar macrophages by glucocorticoids. *Clinical & Experimental Immunology, 104*, 332–336.

Brown, D. H., & Zwilling, B. S. (1994). Activation of the hypothalamic-pituitary-adrenal axis differentially affects the anti-mycobacterial activity of macrophages from BCG-resistant and susceptible mice. *Journal of Neuroimmunology, 53*, 181–187.

Buske-Kirschbaum, A., Jobst, S., Psych, D., Wustmans, A., Kirschbaum, C., Rauh, W., & Hellhammer, D. (1997). Attenuated free cortisol response to psychosocial stress in children with atopic dermatitis. *Psychosomatic Medicine, 59*, 419–426.

Caggiula, A. R., McAllister, C. G., Epstein, L. H., Antelman, S. M., Knopf, S., Saylor, S., & Perkins, K. (1992). Nicotine suppresses the proliferative response of peripheral blood lymphocytes in rats. *Drug Development Research, 26*, 473–479.

Calandra, T., Bernhagen, J., Metz, C. N., Spiegel, L. A., Bacher, M., Donnelley, T., Cerami, A., & Bucala, R. (1995). MIF as a glucocorticoid-induced modulator of cytokine production. *Nature, 377*, 68–71.

Caldenhoven, E., Liden, J., Wissink, S., Van de Stolpe, A., Raaijmakers, J., Koenderman, L., Okret, S., Gustafsson, J.-A., & Van der Saag, P. T. (1995). Negative cross-talk between RelA and the glucocorticoid receptor: A possible mechanism for the antiinflammatory action of glucocorticoids. *Molecular Endocrinology, 9*, 401–412.

Callewaert, D. M., Moudgil, V. K., Radcliff, G., & Waite, R. (1991). Hormone specific regulation of natural killer cells by cortisol — Direct inactivation of the cytotoxic function of cloned human NK cells without an effect on cellular proliferation. *FEBS Letters, 285*, 108–110.

Carlson, S. L., Fox, S., & Abell, K. M. (1997). Catecholamine modulation of lymphocyte homing to lymphoid tissues. *Brain, Behavior, & Immunity, 11*, 307–320.

Carr, D. J., Woolley, T. W., & Blalock, J. E. (1992). Phentolamine but not propranolol blocks the immunopotentiating effect of cold stress on antigen-specific IgM production in mice orally immunized with sheep red blood cells. *Brain, Behavior, & Immunity, 6*, 50–63.

Chao, C. C., Peterson, P. K., Filice, G. A., Pomeroy, C., & Sharp, B. M. (1990). Effects of immobilization stress on the pathogenesis of acute murine toxoplasmosis. *Brain, Behavior, & Immunity, 4*, 162–169.

Chappel, M. R. (1962). Infectious mononucleosis. *Southwest Med, 43*, 253–256.

Cheng, G. J., Morrow-Tesch, J. L., Beller, D. I., Levy, E. M., & Black, P. H. (1990). Immunosuppression in mice induced by cold water stress. *Brain, Behavior, & Immunity, 4*, 278–291.

Chover-Gonzalez, A. J., Tejedor-Real, P., Harbuz, M. S., Gibert-Rahola, J., Larsen, P. J., & Jessop, D. S. (1998). A differential response to stress is not a prediction of susceptibility or severity in adjuvant-induced arthritis. *Stress, 2*, 221–226.

Claman, H. N. (1972). Corticosteroids and lymphoid cells. *New England Journal of Medicine, 287*, 388–397.

Claman, H. N. (1989). Glucocorticoids and autoimmune disorders. In R. P. Schleimer, H. N. Claman & A. Oronsky. (Eds.), *Anti-inflammatory steroid action: Basic and clinical aspects* (pp. 409–422). Academic Press: San Diego.

Cocke, R., Moynihan, J. A., Cohen, N., Grota, L. J., & Ader, R. (1993). Exposure to conspecific alarm chemosignals alters immune responses in BALB/c mice. *Brain, Behavior, & Immunity, 7*, 36–46.

Cohen, J.Glauser, M. P. (1991). Septic shock: Treatment. *Lancet, 338*, 736–739.

Cohen, J. J. (1992). Glucocorticoid-induced apoptosis in the thymus. *Seminars in Immunology, 4*, 363–369.

Cohen, J. J. (1989). Lymphocyte death induced by glucocorticoids. In R. P. Schleimer, H. N. Claman, & A. Oronsky (Eds.), *Anti-inflammatory steroid action: Basic and clinical aspects* (pp. 110–131). Academic Press: San Diego.

Cohen, J. J. (1972). Thymus-derived lymphocytes sequestered in the bone marrow of hydrocortisone-treated mice. *Journal of Immunology, 108*, 841–844.

Cohen, J. J., & Duke, R. C. (1984). Glucocorticoid activation of a calcium-dependent endonuclease in thymocyte nuclei leads to cell death. *Journal of Immunology, 132*, 38–42.

Cohen, S., & Herbert, R. B. (1996). Health psychology: Psychological factors and physical disease from the perspective of human psychoneuroimmunology. *Annual Reviews Psychology, 47*, 113–142.

Cohen, S., Tyrrell, D. A. J., & Smith, A. P. (1991). Psychological stress and susceptibility to the common cold. *New England Journal of Medicine, 325*, 606–612.

Conti, B., Jahng, J. W., Tinti, C., Son, J. H., & Joh, T. H. (1997). Induction of Interferon-γ inducing factor in the adrenal cortex. *Journal of Biological Chemistry, 272*, 2035–2037.

Coulpier, M., Andreev, S., Lemercier, C., Dauchel, H., Lees, O., Fontaine, M., & Ripoche, J. (1995). Activation of the endothelium by IL-1a and glucocorticoids results in major increase of complement C3 and factor B production and generation of C3a. *Clinical & Experimental Immunology, 101*, 142–149.

Cox, J. H., & Ford, W. L. (1982). The migration of lymphocytes across specialized vascular endothelium. IV. Prednisolone acts at several points on the recirculation pathway of lymphocytes. *Cellular Immunology, 66*, 407–422.

Cunnick, J. E., Lysle, D. T., Kucinski, B. J., & Rabin, B. S. (1990). Evidence that shock-induced immune suppression is mediated by adrenal hormones and peripheral beta-adrenergic receptors. *Pharmacology, Biochemistry & Behavior, 36*, 645–651.

Cupps, T. R., & Fauci, A. S. (1982). Corticosteroid-mediated immunoregulation in man. *Immunological Reviews, 65*, 133–155.

Damoiseaux, J. G., Huitinga, I., Dopp, E. A., & Dijkstra, C. D. (1992). Expression of the ED3 antigen on rat macrophages in relation to experimental autoimmune diseases. *Immunobiology, 184*, 311–320.

Daynes, R. A., & Araneo, B. A. (1989). Contrasting effects of glucocorticoids on the capacity of T cells to produce the growth factors interleukin 2 and interleukin 4. *European Journal of Immunology, 19*, 2319–2325.

Daynes, R. A., Dudley, D. J., & Araneo, B. A. (1990). Regulation of murine lymphokine production in vivo. II. Dehydroepiandrosterone is a natural enhancer of interleukin 2 synthesis by helper T cells. *European Journal of Immunology, 20*, 793–802.

Deak, T., Meriwether, J. L., Fleshner, M., Spencer, R. L., Abouhamze, A., Moldawer, L. L., Grahn, R. E., Watkins, L. R., & Maier, S. F. (1997). Evidence that brief stress may induce the acute phase response in rats. *American Journal of Physiology, 273*, R1998–2004.

Devenport, L., Thomas, T., Knehans, A., & Sundstrom, A. (1990). Acute, chronic, and interactive effects of type I and II corticosteroid receptor stimulation on feeding and weight gain. *Physiology & Behavior, 47*, 1221–1228.

Dhabhar, F. S. (1998). Stress-induced enhancement of cell-mediated immunity. In S. M. McCann, J. M. Lipton, E. M. Sternberg, G. P. Chrousos, P. W. Gold, & C. C. Smith (Eds.), *Neuroimmunomodulation: Molecular, integrative systems, and clinical advances* (pp. 359–372). New York: New York Academy of Sciences.

Dhabhar, F. S., & McEwen, B. S. (1997). Acute stress enhances while chronic stress suppresses immune function in vivo: A potential role for leukocyte trafficking. *Brain, Behavior, & Immunity, 11*, 286–306.

Dhabhar, F. S., & McEwen, B. S. (1999a). Changes in blood leukocyte distribution: Interactions between catecholamine & glucocorticoid hormones. *Neuroimmunomodulation, 6*, 213.

Dhabhar, F. S., & McEwen, B. S. (1999b). Enhancement of the immunization/sensitization phase of cell-mediated immunity: The role of acute stress & adrenal stress hormones. *Neuroimmunomodulation, 6*, 213.

Dhabhar, F. S., & McEwen, B. S. (1999c). Enhancing versus suppressive effects of stress hormones on skin immune function. *Proceedings of the National Academy of Sciences USA, 96*, 1059–1064.

Dhabhar, F. S., & McEwen, B. S. (1996). Stress-induced enhancement of antigen-specific cell-mediated immunity. *Journal of Immunology, 156*, 2608–2615.

Dhabhar, F. S., McEwen, B. S., & Spencer, R. L. (1997). Adaptation to prolonged or repeated stress—Comparison between rat strains showing intrinsic differences in reactivity to acute stress. *Neuroendocrinology, 65*, 360–368.

Dhabhar, F. S., McEwen, B. S., & Spencer, R. L. (1993). Stress response, adrenal steroid receptor levels, and corticosteroid-binding globulin levels—a comparison between Sprague Dawley, Fischer 344, and Lewis rats. *Brain Research, 616*, 89–98.

Dhabhar, F. S., Miller, A. H., McEwen, B. S., & Spencer, R. L. (1995a). Differential activation of adrenal steroid receptors in neural and immune tissues of Sprague Dawley, Fischer 344, and Lewis rats. *Journal of Neuroimmunology, 56*, 77–90.

Dhabhar, F. S., Miller, A. H., McEwen, B. S., & Spencer, R. L. (1995b). Effects of stress on immune cell distribution—dynamics and hormonal mechanisms. *Journal of Immunology, 154*, 5511–5527.

Dhabhar, F. S., Miller, A. H., McEwen, B. S., & Spencer, R. L. (1996). Stress-induced changes in blood leukocyte distribution—role of adrenal steroid hormones. *Journal of Immunology, 157*, 1638–1644.

Dhabhar, F. S., Miller, A. H., Stein, M., McEwen, B. S., & Spencer, R. L. (1994). Diurnal and stress-induced changes in distribution of peripheral blood leukocyte subpopulations. *Brain, Behavior, & Immunity, 8*, 66–79.

Dhabhar, F. S., Satoskar, A. R., Bluethmann, H., David, J. R., & McEwen, B. S. (2000). Stress-induced enhancement of skin immune function: A role for IFNγ. *PNAS, USA, 97*, 2846.

Diamond, D. M., Bennett, M. C., Fleshner, M., & Rose, G. M. (1992). Inverted-U relationship between the level of peripheral corticosterone and the magnitude of hippocampal primed burst potentiation. *Hippocampus, 2*, 421–430.

Dinarello, C. A., & Wolff, S. M. (1993). The role of interleukin-1 in disease. *New England Journal of Medicine, 328*, 106–113.

Doeberitz, M. V. K., Koch, S., Drzonek, H., & Hausen, H. Z. (1990). Glucocorticoid hormones reduce the expression of major histocompatibility class I antigen on human epithelial cells. *European Journal of Immunology, 20*, 35–40.

Dougherty, R. F., & White, A. (1945). Functional alterations in lymphoid tissue induced by adrenal cortical secretion. *American Journal of Anatomy, 77*, 81–116.

Dougherty, T. F. (1952). Effect of hormones on lymphatic tissue. *Physiological Review, 32*, 379–401.

Dougherty, T. F. (1949). Role of the adrenal gland in the protection against anaphylactic shock. *Anatomical Records, 103*, 24.

Dougherty, T. F. (1950). The protective role of adrenal cortical secretion in the hypersensitive state. In R. C. Christman (Ed.), *Pituitary-adrenal function* (pp. 79–87). Washington DC: American Association for the Advancement of Science.

Edwards, E. A., & Dean, L. M. (1977). Effects of crowding of mice on humoral antibody formation and protection to lethal antigenic challenge. *Psychosomatic Medicine, 39*, 19–24.

Eskola, J., Frey, H., Molnar, G., & Soppi, E. (1976). Biological rhythm of cell-mediated immunity in man. *Clinical & Experimental Immunology, 26*, 253–257.

Fan, J., Gong, X.-Q., Wu, J., Zhang, Y.-F., & Xu, R.-B. (1994). Effect of glucocorticoid receptor (GR) blockage on endotoxemia in rats. *Circulatory Shock, 42*, 76–82.

Fauci, A. S. (1979). Immunosuppressive and anti-inflammatory effects of glucocorticoids. In J. D. Baxter & G. G. Rousseau (Eds.), *Glucocorticoid Hormone Action* (pp. 449–465). Berlin: Springer-Verlag.

Fauci, A. S. (1975). Mechanisms of corticosteroid action on lymphocyte subpopulations. I. Redistribution of circulating T and B lymphocytes to the bone marrow. *Immunology, 28*, 669–680.

Fauci, A. S. (1976). Mechanisms of corticosteroid action on lymphocyte subpopulations. II. Differential effects of in vivo hydrocortisone, prednisone, and dexamethasone on in vitro expression of lymphocyte function. *Clinical & Experimental Immunology, 24*, 54–62.

Fauci, A. S., & Dale, D. C. (1975). Alternate-day prednisone therapy and human lymphocyte subpopulations. *Journal of Clinical Investigation, 55*, 22–32.

Fauci, A. S., & Dale, D. C. (1974). The effect of in vivo hydrocortisone on subpopulations of human lymphocytes. *Journal of Clinical Investigation, 53*, 240–246.

Fauci, A. S., Pratt, K. R., & Whalen, G. (1977). Activation of human B lymphocytes. IV. Regulatory effects of corticosteroids on the triggering signal in the plaque-forming cell response of human peripheral blood B lymphocytes to polyclonal activation. *Journal of Immunology, 119*, 598–603.

Felten, D. L., Felten, S. Y., Bellinger, D. L., & Madden, K. S. (1993). Fundamental aspects of neural-immune signaling. *Psychotherapy & Psychosomatics, 60*, 46–56.

Fleshner, M., Laudenslager, M. L., Simons, L., & Maier, S. F. (1989). Reduced serum antibodies associated with social defeat in rats. *Physiology & Behavior, 45*, 1183–1187.

Fleshner, M., Watkins, L. R., Lockwood, L. L., Laudenslager, M. L., & Maier, S. F. (1992). Specific changes in lymphocyte subpopulations: A potential mechanism for stress-induced immunomodulation. *Journal of Neuroimmunology, 41*, 131–142.

Forner, M. A., Barriga, C., Rodriquez, A. B., & Ortega, E. (1995). A study of the role of corticosterone as a mediator in exercise-induced stimulation of murine macrophage phagocytosis. *Journal of Physiology, 488,* 789–794.

Gajewski, T. F., Schell, S. R., Nau, G., & Fitch, F. W. (1989). Regulation of T-cell activation: Differences among T-cell subsets. *Immunological Reviews, 111,* 79–110.

Girard, M. T., Hjaltadottir, S., Fejes-Toth, A. N., & Guyre, P. M. (1987). Glucocorticoids enhance the γ-interferon augmentation of human monocyte IgG Fc receptor expression. *Journal of Immunology, 138,* 3235–3241.

Glaser, R., Kiecolt-Glaser, J. K., Bonneau, R. H., Malarkey, W., Kennedy, S., & Hughes, J. (1991). Stress-induced modulation of the immune response to recombinant hepatitis B vaccine. *Psychosomatic Medicine, 54,* 22–29.

Glaser, R., Pearl, D. K., Kiecolt-Glaser, J. K., & Malarkey, W. B. (1994). Plasma cortisol levels and reactivation of latent Epstein-Barr virus in response to examination stress. *Psychoneuroendocrinology, 19,* 765–772.

Godlowski, Z. Z. (1952). The fate of eosinophils in hormonally induced eosinopenia and its significance. *Journal of Endocrinology, 8,* 102–125.

Gold, P. W., Goodwin, F. K., & Chrousos, G. P. (1988). Clinical and biochemical manifestations of depression — relation to the neurobiology of stress (Part 2). *New England Journal of Medicine, 319,* 413–420.

Goldstein, R. A., Bowen, D. L., & Fauci, A. S. (1992). Adrenal Corticosteroids. In J. I. Gallin, I. M. Goldstein & R. Snyderman (Eds.), *Inflammation: Basic principles and clinical correlates* (pp. 1061–1081). New York: Raven Press.

Gonzalo, J. A., Gonzalez-Garcia, A., Martinez, A. C., & Kroemer, G. (1993). Glucocorticoid-mediated control of the activation and clonal deletion of peripheral T cells in vivo. *Journal of Experimental Medicine, 177,* 1239–1246.

Gottschall, P. E., Koves, K., Mizuno, K., Tatsuno, I., & Arimura, A. (1991). Glucocorticoid upregulation of interleukin 1 receptor expression in a glioblastoma cell line. *American Journal of Physiology, 261,* E362–E368.

Grasser, A., Moller, A., Backmund, H., Yassouridis, A., & Holsboer, F. (1996). Heterogeneity of hypothalamic-pituitary-adrenal system response to a combined dexamethasone-CRH test in multiple sclerosis. *Experimental & Clinical Endocrinology & Diabetes, 104,* 31–37.

Grayson, J., Dooley, N. J., Koski, I. R., & Blaese, R. M. (1981). Immunoglobulin production induced in vitro by glucocorticoid hormones: T cell-dependent stimulation of immunoglobulin production without B cell proliferation in cultures of human peripheral blood lymphocytes. *Journal of Clinical Investigation, 68,* 1539–1547.

Griffin, A. C., Warren, D. L., Wolny, A. C., & Whitacre, C. C. (1993). Suppression of experimental autoimmune encephalomyelitis by restraint stress. *Journal of Neuroimmunology, 44,* 103–116.

Griffin, A. C., & Whitacre, C. C. (1991). Sex and strain differences in the circadian rhythm fluctuation of endocrine and immune function in the rat: Implications for rodent models of autoimmune disease. *Journal of Neuroimmunology, 35,* 53–64.

Halliday, W. J., & Garvey, J. S. (1964). Some factors affecting the secondary immune response in tissue cultures containing hydrocortisone. *Journal of Immunology, 93,* 757–762.

Hammond, G. L. (1990). Molecular properties of corticosteroid binding globulin and the sex-steroid binding proteins. *Endocrine Reviews, 11,* 65–79.

Hammond, G. L., Smith, C. L., Paterson, N. A. M., & Sibbald, W. J. (1990). A role for corticosteroid-binding globulin in delivery of cortisol to activated neutrophils. *Journal of Clinical Endocrinology & Metabolism, 71,* 34–39.

Hammond, G. L., Smith, C. L., Underhill, C. M., & Nguyen, V. T. (1990). Interaction between corticosteroid binding globulin and activated leukocytes in vitro. *Biochemical & Biophysical Research Communications, 172,* 172–177.

Harris, T. J., Waltman, T. J., Carter, S. M., & Maisel, A. S. (1995). Effect of prolonged catecholamine infusion on immunoregulatory function: Implications in congestive heart failure. *Journal of the American College of Cardiology, 26,* 102–109.

Hawrylowicz, C. M., Guida, L., & Paleolog, E. (1994). Dexamethasone up-regulates granulocyte-macrophage colony-stimulating factor receptor expression on human monocytes. *Immunology, 83,* 274–280.

Haynes, R. C. J. (1990). Adrenocorticotropic hormone; adrenocortical steroids and their structural analogs; inhibitors of the synthesis and actions of adrenocortical hormones. In A. G. Gilman, T. W. Rall, A. S. Nies, & P. Taylor (Eds.), *The pharmacological basis of experimental therapeutics* (pp. 1431–1462). New York: Pergamon.

Hedman, L. A., & Lundin, P. M. (1977). The effect of steroids on the circulating lymphocyte population. II. Studies of the thoracic duct lymphocyte population of the guinea pig after neonatal thymectomy and prednisolone treatment. *Lymphology, 10,* 192–198.

Hench, P. S. (1952). The reversibility of certain rheumatic and nonrheumatic conditions by the use of cortisone or of the pituitary adrenocorticotropic hormone. *Annals of Internal Medicine, 36,* 1–25.

Hench, P. S., Kendall, E. C., Slocumb, C. H., & Polley, H. (1949). The effect of a hormone of the adrenal cortex (17-hydroxy-11-dehydrocorticosterone: Compound E) and of pituitary adrenocorticotropic hormone on rheumatoid arthritis. *Proceedings Staff Meeting Mayo Clinic, 24,* 181–197.

Hendrie, H. C., Parasekvas, R., Baragar, F. D., & Adamson, J. D. (1971). Stress, immunoglobulin levels, and early polyarthritis. *Journal of Psychosomatic Research, 15,* 337–342.

Henning, S. J. (1978). Plasma concentrations of total and free corticosterone during development in the rat. *American Journal of Physiology, 235,* E451–E456.

Herbert, T. B., & Cohen, S. (1993). Stress and immunity in humans: A meta-analytic review. *Psychosomatic Medicine, 55,* 364–379.

Hiemke, C., Brunner, R., Hammes, E., Müller, H., Meyer Zum Büschenfelde, K.-H., & Lohse, A. W. (1995). Circadian variations in antigenic-specific proliferation of human T lymphocytes and correlation to cortisol production. *Psychoneuroendocrinology, 20,* 335–342.

Hirata, F. (1989). The role of lipocortins in cellular function as a second messenger of glucocorticoids. In R. P. Schleimer, H. N. Claman, & A. Oronsky. (Eds.), *Anti-inflammatory steroid action — Basic and clinical aspects,* (pp. 67–95). San Diego, Academic Press.

Hoagland, H., Elmadjian, F., & Pincus, G. (1946). Stressful psychomotor performance and adrenal cortical function as indicated by the lymphocyte reponse. *Journal of Clinical Endocrinology & Metabolism, 6,* 301–311.

Irwin, M. (1994). Stress-induced immune suppression: Role of brain corticotropin releasing hormone and autonomic nervous system mechanisms. *Advances in Neuroimmunology, 4,* 29–47.

Irwin, M., Patterson, T., Smith, T. L., Caldwell, C., Brown, S. A., Gillin, C. J., & Grant, I. (1990). Reduction of immune function in life stress and depression. *Biological Psychiatry, 27,* 22–30.

Ishida, T., Matsuura, K., Setoguchi, M., Higuchi, Y., & Yamamoto, S. (1994). Enhancement of muring serum amyloid A3 mRNA expression by glucocorticoids and its regulation by cytokines. *Journal of Leukocyte Biology, 56*, 797–806.

Issekutz, T. B. (1990). Effects of six different cytokines on lymphocyte adherence to microvascular endothelium and in vivo lymphocyte migration in the rat. *Journal of Immunology, 144*, 2140–2146.

Jain, S., & Stevenson, J. R. (1991). Enhancement by restraint stress of natural killer cell activity and splenocyte responsiveness to concanavalin A in Fischer 344 rats. *Immunological Investigations, 20*, 365–376.

Jefferies, W. M. (1991). Cortisol and immunity. *Medical Hypotheses, 34*, 198–208.

Jensen, M. M. (1969). Changes in leukocyte counts associated with various stressors. *Journal of the Reticuloendothelial Society, 8*, 457–465.

Joels, M., & de Kloet, E. R. (1992). Control of neuronal excitability by corticosteroid hormones. *Trends in Neuroscience, 15*, 25–30.

Johns, M. W. (1967). Leukocyte response to sound stress in rats: Role of the adrenal gland. *Journal of Pathology & Bacteriology, 93*, 681–685.

Kaplan, M. S., Byers, V. S., Levin, A. S., German, D. F., Fudenberg, H. H., & Lecam, L. N. (1976). Circadian rhythm of stimulated lymphocyte blastogenesis. *Journal of Allergy & Clinical Immunology, 58*, 180–189.

Karalis, K., Sano, H., Redwine, J., Listwak, S., Wilder, R. L., & Chrousos, G. P. (1991). Autocrine or paracrine inflammatory actions of corticotropin-releasing hormone in vivo. *Science, 254*, 421–423.

Kawate, T., Abo, T., Hinuma, S., & Kumagai, K. (1981). Studies on the bioperiodicity of the immune response II. Co-variations of murine T and B cells and a role for corticosteroid. *Journal of Immunology, 126*, 1364–1367.

Keller, S. E., Schleifer, S. J., Liotta, A. S., Bond, R. N., Farhoody, N., & Stein, M. (1988). Stress-induced alterations of immunity in hypophysectomized rats. *Proceedings of the National Academy of Sciences USA, 85*, 9297–9301.

Keller, S. E., Weiss, J. M., Schleifer, S. J., Miller, N. E., & Stein, M. (1983). Stress-induced suppression of immunity in adrenalectomized rats. *Science, 221*, 1301–1304.

Kelley, K. W., Greenfield, R. E., Evermann, J. F., Parish, S. M., & Perryman, L. E. (1982). Delayed-type hypersensitivity, contact sensitivity, and PHA skin-test responses of heat- and cold-stressed calves. *American Journal of Veterinary Research, 43*, 775–779.

Khansari, D. N., Murgo, A. J., & Faith, R. E. (1990). Effects of stress on the immune system. *Immunology Today, 11*, 170–175.

Kiecolt-Glaser, J. K., Garner, W., Speicher, C., Penn, G. M., Holliday, J., & Glaser, R. (1984). Psychosocial modifiers of immunocompetence in medical students. *Psychosomatic Medicine, 46*, 7–14.

Kiecolt-Glaser, J. K., Glaser, R., Gravenstein, S., Malarkey, W. B., & Sheridan, J. (1996). Chronic stress alters the immune response to influenza virus vaccine in older adults. *Proceedings of the National Academy of Sciences USA, 93*, 3043–3047.

Kimber, I., & Dearman, R. (1993). Approaches to the identification and classification of chemical allergens in mice. *Journal of Pharmacology & Toxicology Methods, 29*, 11–16.

Kizaki, T., Oh-Ishi, S., Ookawara, T., Yamamoto, M., Izawa, T., & Ohno, H. (1996). Glucocorticoid-mediated generation of suppressor macrophages with high density FcγRII during acute cold stress. *Endocrinology, 137*, 4260–4267.

Kort, W. J. (1994). The effect of chronic stress on the immune system. *Advances in Neuroimmunology, 4*, 1–11.

Kroemer, G., Brezinschek, H. P., Faessler, R., Schauenstein, K., & Wick, G. (1988). Physiology and pathology of an immunoendocrine feeback loop. *Immunology Today, 9*, 163–165.

Kulkarni, A. B., Reinke, R., & Feigelson, P. (1985). Acute phase mediators and glucocorticoids elevate α1-acid glycoprotein gene transcription. *Journal of Biological Chemistry, 260*, 15386–15389.

Lamas, M., Sanz, E., Martin-Parras, L., Espel, E., Sperisen, P., Collins, M., & Silva, A. G. (1993). Glucocorticoid hormones upregulate interleukin 2 receptor a gene expression. *Cellular Immunology, 151*, 437–450.

Landmann, R. (1992). Beta-adrenergic receptors in human leukocyte subpopulations. *European Journal of Clinical Investigation, 22* (Suppl. 1), 30–36.

Landmann, R., Muller, F. B., Perini, C. H., Wesp, M., Erne, P., & Buhler, F. R. (1984). Changes of immunoregulatory cells induced by psychological and physical stress: Relationship to plasma catecholamines. *Clinical & Experimental Immunology, 58*, 127–135.

Lappin, D. F., & Whaley, K. (1991). Modulation of complement gene expression by glucocorticoids. *Biochemical Journal, 280*, 117–123.

Laue, L., Kawai, S., Brandon, D. D., Brightwell, D., Barnes, K., Knazek, R. A., Loriaux, D. L., & Chrousos, G. P. (1988). Receptor-mediated effects of glucocorticoids on inflammation: Enhancement of the inflammatory response with a glucocorticoid antagonist. *Journal of Steroid Biochemistry, 29*, 591–598.

Lazar Jr., G., Duda, E., & Lazar, G. (1992). Effect of RU38486 on TNF production and toxicity. *FEBS Letters, 308*, 137–140.

Lechner, O., Hu, Y., Jafarian-Tehrani, M., Dietrich, H., Schwarz, S., Herold, M., Haour, F., & Wick, G. (1996). Disturbed immunoendocrine communication via the hypothalamo-pituitary-adrenal axis in murine lupus. *Brain, Behavior, & Immunity, 10*, 337–350.

Lee, S. W., Tsou, A.-P., Chan, H., Thomas, J., Petrie, K., Eugui, E. M., & Allison, A. C. (1988). Glucocorticoids selectively inhibit the transcription of the interleukin 1β gene and decrease the stability of interleukin 1β mRNA. *Proceedings of the National Academy of Sciences USA, 85*, 1204–1208.

Levine, S., & Saltzman, A. (1987). Nonspecific stress prevents relapses of experimental allergic encephalomyelitis in rats. *Brain, Behavior, & Immunity, 1*, 336–341.

Levine, S., Strebel, R., Wenk, E., & Harman, P. (1962). Suppression of experimental allergic encephalomyelitis by stress. *Proceedings of the Society for Experimental Biology, 109*, 294–298.

Levine, S. J., Logun, C., Chopra, D. P., Rhim, J. S., & Shelhamer, J. H. (1996). Protein kinase C, interleukin-1 beta, and corticosteroids regulate shedding of the type I, 55 kDa TNF receptor from human airway epithelial cells. *American Journal of Respiratory Cell & Molecular Biology, 14*, 254–261.

Levo, Y., Harbeck, R. J., & Kirkpatrick, C. H. (1985). Regulatory effect of hydrocortisone on the in vitro synthesis of IgE by human lymphocytes. *International Archives of Allergy & Applied Immunology, 77*, 413–424.

Liao, J., Keiser, J. A., Scales, W. E., Kunkel, S. L., & Kluger, M. J. (1995). Role of corticosterone in TNF and IL-6 production in isolated perfused rat liver. *American Journal of Physiology, 268*, R699–706.

Lundin, P. M., & Hedman, L. A. (1978). Influence of corticosterone on lymphocyte recirculation. *Lymphology, 11*, 216–221.

Lysle, D. T., Cunnick, J. E., & Rabin, B. S. (1990). Stressor-induced alteration of lymphocyte proliferation in mice: Evidence for enhancement of mitogenic responsiveness. *Brain, Behavior, & Immunity, 4*, 269–277.

Lyte, M., Nelson, S. G., & Baissa, B. (1990). Examination of the neuroendocrine basis for the social conflict-induced enhancement of immunity in mice. *Physiology & Behavior, 48*, 685–691.

Lyte, M., Nelson, S. G., & Thompson, M. L. (1990). Innate and adaptive immune responses in a social conflict paradigm. *Clinical Immunology & Immunopathology, 57*, 137–147.

MacKenzie, F. J., Leonard, J. P., & Cuzner, M. L. (1989). Changes in lymphocyte B-adrenergic receptor density and noradrenaline content of the spleen are early indicators of immune reactivity in acute experimental allergic encephalomyelitis in the Lewis rat. *Journal of Neuroimmunology, 23*, 93–100.

MacPhee, I. A. M., Day, M. J., & Mason, D. W. (1990). The role of serum factors in the suppression of experimental allergic encephalomyelitis: Evidence for immunoregulation by antibody to the encephalitogenic peptide. *Immunology, 70*, 527–534.

Madden, K. S., & Felten, D. L. (1995). Experimental basis for neural-immune interactions. *Physiological Review, 75*, 77–106.

Maes, M., Scharpe, S., Meltzer, H. Y., Bosmans, E., Suy, E., Calabrese, J., & Cosyns, P. (1993). Relationships between interleukin-6 activity, acute phase proteins, and function of the hypothalamic-pituitary-adrenal axis in severe depression. *Psychiatry Research, 49*, 11–27.

Maes, M., Wauters, A., Neels, H., Scharpe, S., Van Gastel, A., D'Hondt, P., Peeters, D., Cosyns, P., & Desnyder, R. (1995). Total serum protein and serum protein fractions in depression: Relationships to depressive symptoms and glucocorticoid activity. *Journal of Affective Disorders, 34*, 61–69.

Maes, M. A. (1993). A review on the acute phase response in major depression. *Reviews in Neuroscience, 4*, 407–416.

Maier, S. F., Watkins, L. R., & Fleshner, M. (1994). Psychoneuroimmunology — the interface between behavior, brain, and immunity. *American Psychologist, 49*, 1004–1017.

Manuck, S. B., Cohen, S., Rabin, B. S., Muldoon, M. F., & Bachen, E. A. (1991). Individual differences in cellular immune response to stress. *Psychological Science, 2*, 111–115.

Marucha, P. T., Kiecolt-Glaser, J. K., & Favagehi, M. (1998). Mucosal wound healing is impaired by examination stress. *Psychosomatic Medicine, 60*, 362–365.

Marx, J. (1995). How the glucocorticoids suppress immunity. *Science, 270*, 232–233.

Mason, D. (1991). Genetic variation in the stress response: Susceptibility to experimental allergic encephalomyelitis and implications for human inflammatory disease. *Immunology Today, 12*, 57–60.

Mason, D., MacPhee, I., & Antoni, F. (1990). The role of the neuroendocrine system in determining genetic susceptibility to experimental allergic encephalomyelitis in the rat. *Immunology, 70*, 1–5.

May, M. J., & Ghosh, S. (1998). Signal transduction through NF-kB. *Immunology Today, 19*, 80–88.

McEver, R. P. (1994). Selectins. *Current Opinions in Immunology, 6*, 75–84.

McEwen, B. S. (1998). Protective and damaging effects of stress mediators: Allostasis and allostatic load. *New England Journal of Medicine, 338*, 171–179.

McEwen, B. S., Biron, C. A., Brunson, K. W., Bulloch, K., Chambers, W. H., Dhabhar, F. S., Goldfarb, R. H., Kitson, R. P., Miller, A. H., Spencer, R. L., & Weiss, J. M. (1997). Neural-endocrine-immune interactions: The role of adrenalcorticoids as modulators of immune function in health and disease. *Brain Research Reviews, 23*, 79–133.

McEwen, B. S., de Kloet, E. R., & Rostene, W. (1986). Adrenal steroid receptors and actions in the nervous system. *Physiological Review, 66*, 1121–1188.

Mei-Tal, V., Meyerowitz, S., & Engel, G. (1970). Role of psychological process in a somatic disorder: Multiple sclerosis. *Psychosomatic Medicine, 32*, 67–86.

Mekaouche, M., Givalois, L., Barbanel, G., Siaud, P., Maurel, D., Malaval, F., Bristow, A. F., Boissin, J., Assenmacher, I., & Ixart, G. (1994). Chronic restraint enhances interleukin-1-beat release in the basal state and after endotoxin challenge, independently of adrenocorticotropin and corticosterone release. *Neuroimmunomodulation, 1*, 292–299.

Mendel, C. M. (1989). The free hormone hypothesis: A physiologically based mathematical model. *Endocrine Reviews, 10*, 232–274.

Mendelson, S. C., & McEwen, B. S. (1992). Autoradiographic analyses of the effects of adrenalectomy and corticosterone on 5-HT1A and 5-HT1B receptors in the dorsal hippocampus and cortex of the rat. *Neuroendocrinology, 55*, 444–450.

Mickerson, J. N. (1959). Influenzal pituitary suppression. *Lancet, 1*, 1118–1120.

Millar, D. B., Thomas, J. R., Pacheco, N. D., & Rollwagen, F. M. (1993). Natural killer cell cytotoxicity and T-cell proliferation is enhanced by avoidance behavior. *Brain, Behavior, & Immunity, 7*, 144–153.

Miller, A. H., Spencer, R. L., Hasset, J., Kim, C., Rhee, R., Cira, D., Dhabhar, F. S., McEwen, B. S., & Stein, M. (1994). Effects of selective Type I and Type II adrenal steroid receptor agonists on immune cell distribution. *Endocrinology, 135*, 1934–1944.

Miller, A. H., Spencer, R. L., Pearce, B. D., Pisell, T. L., Azrieli, Y., Tanapat, P., Moday, H., Rhee, R., & McEwen, B. S. (1998). Glucocorticoid receptors are differentially expressed in the cells and tissues of the immune system. *Cellular Immunology, 186*, 45–54.

Mills, P. J., Berry, C. C., Dimsdale, J. E., Ziegler, M. G., Nelesen, R. A., & Kennedy, B. P. (1995). Lymphocyte subset redistribution in response to acute experimental stress: Effects of gender, ethnicity, hypertension, and the sympathetic nervous system. *Brain, Behavior, & Immunity, 9*, 61–69.

Monjan, A. A., & Collector, M. I. (1977). Stress-induced modulation of the immune response. *Science, 196*, 307–308.

Moorhead, J. W., & Claman, H. N. (1972). Thymus-derived lymphocytes and hydrocortisone: Identification of subsets of theta-bearing cells and redistribution to bone marrow. *Cellular Immunology, 5*, 74–86.

Morrow-Tesch, J. L., McGlone, J. J., & Norman, R. L. (1993). Consequences of restraint stress on natural killer cell activity, behavior, and hormone levels in rhesus macaques (*Macaca mulatta,*). *Psychoneuroendocrinology, 18*, 383–395.

Mosmann, T. R., & Coffman, R. L. (1989). TH1 and TH2 cells: Different patterns of lymphokine secretion lead to different functional properties. *Annual Reviews Immunology, 7*, 145–173.

Muehrcke, R. C., Lewis, J. L., & Kark, R. M. (1952). The effects of cortisone and heparin on eosinophils in defibrinated human blood. *Science, 115*, 377–378.

Mukaida, N., Morita, M., Ishikawa, Y., Rice, N., Okamoto, S., Kasahara, T., & Matsushima, K. (1994). Novel mechanism of glucocorticoid-mediated gene repression. *Journal of Biological Chemistry, 269*, 13289–13295.

Munck, A., & Guyre, P. M. (1989). Glucocorticoid physiology and homeostasis in relation to anti-inflammatory actions. In R. P. Schleimer, H. N. Claman, & A. Oronsky (Eds.), *Anti-inflammatory steroid action — basic and clinical aspects* (pp. 30–47). San Diego: Academic Press.

Munck, A., Guyre, P. M., & Holbrook, N. J. (1984). Physiological functions of glucocorticoids in stress and their relation to pharmacological actions. *Endocrine Reviews, 5*, 25–44.

Munck, A., & Naray-Fejes-Toth, A. (1992). The ups and downs of glucocorticoid physiology. Permissive and suppressive effects revisited. *Molecular & Cellular Endocrinology, 90*, C1–C4.

Murrieta-Aguttes, M., Michelen, V., Leynadier, F., Duarte-Risselin, C., Halpern, G. M., & Dry, J. (1991). Systemic allergic reactions to corticosteroids. *Journal of Asthama, 28,* 329–339.

Nakano, K., Suzuki, S., & Oh, C. (1987). Significance of increased secretion of glucocorticoids in mice and rats injected with bacterial endotoxin. *Brain, Behavior, & Immunity, 1,* 159–172.

Nakano, K., Suzuki, S., Oh, C., & Yamashita, K. (1986). Possible role of glucocorticoids in a complement-activated state induced by cobra venom factor in rats. *Acta Endocrinologica, 112,* 122–129.

Naliboff, B. D., Benton, D., Solomon, G. F., Morley, J. E., Fahey, J. L., Bloom, E. T., Makinodan, T., & Gilmore, S. L. (1991). Immunological changes in young and old adults during brief laboratory stress. *Psychosomatic Medicine, 53,* 121–132.

Onsrud, M., & Thorsby, E. (1981). Influence of in vivo hydrocortisone on some human blood lymphocyte subpopulations. *Scandinavian Journal of Immunology, 13,* 573–579.

Orson, F. M., Grayson, J., Pike, S., de Seau, V., & Blaese, R. M. (1983). T cell-replacing factor for glucocorticosteroid-induded immunoglobulin production. A unique steroid-dependent cytokine. *Journal of Experimental Medicine, 158,* 1473–1482.

Padawer, J., & Gordon, A. S. (1952). A mechanism for the eosinopenia induced by cortisone and epinephrine. *Endocrinology, 51,* 52–88.

Padgett, D. A., Marucha, P. T., & Sheridan, J. F. (1998). Restraint stress slows cutaneous wound healing in mice. *Brain, Behavior, & Immunity, 12,* 64–73.

Parillo, J. E., & Fauci, A. S. (1979). Mechanisms of glucocorticoid action and immune processes. *Annual Review of Pharmacology & Toxicology, 19,* 179–201.

Park, J. H., Kaushansky, K., & Levitt, L. (1993). Transcriptional regulation of interleukin 3 (IL3) in primary human T lymphocytes. Role of AP-1- and octamer-binding proteins in control of IL3 gene expression. *Journal of Biological Chemistry, 268,* 6299–6308.

Pavlides, C., Watanabe, Y., Magarinos, A. M., & McEwen, B. S. (1995). Opposing roles of type I and type II adrenal steroid receptors in hippocampal long-term potentiation. *Neuroscience, 68,* 387–394.

Pawlak, C., Heiker, H., Witte, T., Wiese, B., Heijnen, C. J., Schmidt, R. E., & Schedlowski, M. (1999). A prospective study of daily stress and disease activity in patients with systemic lupus erythematosus. *Neuroimmunomodulation, 6,* 241.

Peller, J. S., & Bardana, E. J. J. (1985). Anaphylactoid reaction to corticosteroid: Case report and review of the literature. *Annals of Allergy, 54,* 302–305.

Persoons, J. H. A., Berkenbosch, F., Schornagel, K., Thepen, T., & Kraal, G. (1995). Increased specific IgE production in lungs after the induction of acute stress in rats. *Journal of Allergy & Clinical Immunology, 95,* 765–770.

Phanuphak, P., Moorhead, J. W., & Claman, H. N. (1974). Tolerance and contact sensitivity to DNFB in mice. I. In vivo detection by ear swelling and correlation with in vitro cell stimulation. *Journal of Immunology, 112,* 115–123.

Philippopoulos, G. S., Wittkower, E. D., & Cousineau, A. (1958). The etiologic significance of emotional factors in onset and exacerbation of multiple sclerosis. *Psychosomatic Medicine, 20,* 458–474.

Pickford, G. E., Srivastava, A. K., Slicher, A. M., & Pang, P. K. T. (1971). The stress response in the abundance of circulating leukocytes in the Killifish, Fundulus heteroclitus. I The cold-shock sequence and the effects of hypophysectomy. *Journal of Zoology, 177,* 89–96.

Plaut, M. (1987). Lymphocyte hormone receptors. *Annual Reviews Immunology, 5,* 621–669.

Pos, O., Van Dijk, W., Ladiges, N., Linthorst, C., Sala, M., Van Tiel, D., & Boers, W. (1988). Glycosylation of four acute-phase glycoproteins secreted by rat liver cells invivo and in vitro. Effects of inflammation and dexamethasone. *European Journal of Cell Biology, 46,* 121–128.

Radomski, M. W., Palmer, R. M. J., & Moncada, S. (1990). Glucocorticoids inhibit the expression of an inducible, but not the constitutive, nitric oxide synthase in vascular endothelial cells. *Proceedings of the National Academy of Sciences USA, 87,* 10043–10047.

Ray, A., LaForge, K. S., & Seghal, P. B. (1990). On the mechanism of efficient repression of the interleukin-6 promoter by glucocorticoids: Enhancer, TATA bod, and RNA start site (Inr Motif) occlusion. *Molecular & Cellular Biology, 10,* 5736–5746.

Reed, J., Abidi, A., Alpers, J., Hoover, R., Robb, R., & Nowell, P. (1986). Effect of cyclosporin A and dexamethasone on interleukin 2 receptor gene expression. *Journal of Immunology, 137,* 150–154.

Regnier, J. A., & Kelley, K. W. (1981). Heat- and cold-stress suppresses in vivo and in vitro cellular immune response of chickens. *American Journal of Veterinary Research, 42,* 294–299.

Reitamo, S., Lauerma, A., Stubb, S., Kayhko, K., Visa, K., & Forstrom, L. (1986). Delayed hypersensitivity to topical corticosteroids. *Journal of the American Academy of Dermatology, 14,* 582–589.

Renz, H., Henke, A., Hofmann, P., Wolff, L. J., Schmidt, A., Rüschoff, J., & Gemsa, D. (1992). Sensitization of rat alveolar macrophages to enhanced TNF-α release by in vivo treatment with dexamethasone. *Cellular Immunology, 144,* 249–257.

Rhinehart, J. J., Sagone, A. L., Balcerzak, S. P., Ackerman, G. A., & LoBuglio, A. F. (1975). Effects of corticosteroid therapy on human monocyte function. *New England Journal of Medicine, 292,* 236–241.

Riley, V. (1981). Psychoneuroendocrine influences on immunocompetence and neoplasia. *Science, 212,* 1100–1109.

Rimon, R., & Laakso, R.-L. (1985). Life stress and rheumatoid arthritis. *Psychotherapy & Psychosomatics, 43,* 38–43.

Rinner, I., Schauenstein, K., Mangge, H., Porta, S., & Kvetnansky, R. (1992). Opposite effects of mild and severe stress on in vitro activation of rat peripheral blood lymphocytes. *Brain, Behavior, & Immunity, 6,* 130–140.

Roess, D. A., Bellone, C. J., Ruh, M. F., Nadel, E. M., & Ruh, T. S. (1982). The effect of glucocorticoids on mitogen-stimulated B-lymphocytes: Thymidine incorporation and antibody secretion. *Endcrinology, 110,* 169–175.

Rogers, M. P., Trentham, D. E., McCune, W. J., Ginsberg, B. I., Reich, P., & David, J. R. (1979). Abrogation of type II collagen-induced arthritis in rats by psychological stress. *Transactions of the Association of American Physicians, 92,* 218–228.

Rosenblum, G. A. (1982). Selective allergy to systemic and topical corticosteroids. *Arizona Medicine, 39,* 780–781.

Rusu, V. M., & Cooper, M. D. (1975). In vivo effects of cortisone on the B cell line in chickens. *Journal of Immunology, 115,* 1370–1374.

Sabiston, B. H., Ste Rose, J. E. M., & Cinader, B. (1978). Temperature stress and immunity in mice. *Journal of Immunogenetics, 5,* 197–212.

Sadeghi, R., Hawrylowicz, C. M., Chernajovsky, Y., & Feldmann, M. (1992). Synergism of glucocorticoids with granulocyte macrophage colony stimulating factor (GM-CSF) but not interferon gamma or interleukin-4 on induction of HLA class II expression on human monocytes. *Cytokine, 4,* 287–297.

Sapolsky, R., Rivier, C., Yamamoto, G., Plotsky, P., & Vale, W. (1987). Interleukin-1 stimulates the secretion of hypothalamic corticotropin releasing factor. *Science, 238,* 522–525.

Sapolsky, R. M. (1987). Glucocorticoids and hippocampal damage. *Trends in Neuroscience, 10*, 346–349.

Savu, L., Lombart, C., & Nunez, E. A. (1980). Corticosterone binding globulin: An acute phase "negative" protein in the rat. *FEBS Letters, 113*, 102–106.

Schedlowski, M., Falk, A., Rohne, A., Wagner, T. O. F., Jacobs, R., Tewes, U., & Schmidt, R. E. (1993). Catecholamines induce alterations of distribution and activity of human natural killer (NK) cells. *Journal of Clinical Immunology, 13*, 344–351.

Schedlowski, M., Jacobs, R., Stratman, G., Richter, S., Hädike, A., Tewes, U., Wagner, T. O. F., & Schmidt, R. E. (1993). Changes of natural killer cells during acute psychological stress. *Journal of Clinical Immunology, 13*, 119–126.

Scheinman, R. I., Cogswell, P. C., Lofquist, A. K., & Baldwin, A. S. J. (1995). Role of transcriptional activation of IκBα in mediation of immunosuppression by glucocorticoids. *Science, 270*, 283–286.

Schleimer, R. P., Claman, H. N., & Oronsky, A. (Eds.). (1989). *Anti-inflammatory steroid action: Basic and clinical aspects*,. San Diego: Academic Press.

Schobitz, B., Reul, J. H. M., & Holsboer, F. (1994). The role of the hypothalamic-pituitary-adrenocortical system during inflammatory conditions. *Critical Reviews in Neurobiology, 8*, 263–291.

Schule, R., & Evans, R. M. (1991). Cross-coupling of signal transduction pathways: Zinc finger meets leucine zipper. *Trends in Genetics, 7*, 377/381.

Sephton, S. E., Sapolsky, R. M., Kraemer, H. C., & Spiegel, D. (1998). Absence of diurnal cortisol variation predicts early breast cancer mortality. *Neuroimmunomodulation, 5*, 45.

Sephton, S. E., Sapolsky, R. M., Kraemer, H. C., & Spiegel, D. (in press). Early mortaility in metastatic breast cancer patients with absent or abnormal diurnal cortisol rhythms. *Journal of the National Cancer Institute, 92*, (12).

Serfling, E., Barthelmas, R., Pfeuffer, I., Schenk, B., Zarius, S., Swoboda, R., Mercurio, F., & Karin, M. (1989). Ubiquitous and lymphocyte-specific factors are involved in the induction of the mouse interleukin 2 gene in T lymphocytes. *EMBO Journal, 8*, 465–473.

Sheridan, J. F. (1998). Stress-induced modulation of anti-viral immunity—Normal Cousins Memorial Lecture 1997. *Brain, Behavior, & Immunity, 12*, 1–6.

Shurin, M. R., Kusnecov, A., Hamill, E., Kaplan, S., & Rabin, B. S. (1994). Stress-induced alteration of polymorphonuclear leukocyte function in rats. *Brain, Behavior, & Immunity, 8*, 163–169.

Shurin, M. R., Zhou, D., Kusnecov, A., Rassnick, S., & Rabin, B. S. (1994). Effect of one or more footshocks on spleen and blood lymphocyte proliferation in rats. *Brain, Behavior, & Immunity, 8*, 57–65.

Siiteri, P. K., Murai, J. T., Hammond, G. L., Nisker, J. A., Raymoure, W. J., & Kuhn, R. W. (1982). The serum transport of steroid hormones. *Recent Progress In Hormone Research, 38*, 457–503.

Silveira, V. L., & Limaos, E. V. (1990). Effect of bacterial endotoxin on plasma concentration of haptoglobin and fibrinogen in rats treated with metyropone. *Agents & Actions, 31*, 143–147.

Skanse, B., & Miorner, G. (1959). Asian influenza with adrenocortical insufficiency. *Lancet, 1*, 1121–1123.

Sklar, L. S., & Anisman, H. (1981). Stress and cancer. *Psychology Bulletin, 89*, 369–406.

Sloviter, R. S., Valiquette, G., Abrams, G. M., Ronk, E. C., Sollas, A. I., Paul, L. A., & Nuebort, a. S. L. (1989). Selective loss of hippocampal granule cells in the mature rat brain after adrenalectomy. *Science, 243*, 535–538.

Smith, R. S., Sherman, N. A., & Middleton, E. (1972). Effect of hydrocortisone on immunoglobulin synthesis and secretion by human peripheral blood lymphocytes in vitro. *International Archives of Allergy, 43*, 859–870.

Snijdewint, F. G., Kapsenberg, M. L., Wauben-Penris, P. J. J., & Bos, J. D. (1995). Corticosteroids class-dependently inhibit in vitro Th1- and Th2-type cytokine production. *Immunopharmacology, 39*, 93–101.

Snow, D. H., Ricketts, S. W., & Mason, D. K. (1983). Hematological responses to racing and training exercise in Thoroughbred horses, with particular reference to the leukocyte response. *Equine Veterinary Journal, 15*, 149–154.

Snyers, L., DeWit, L., & Content, J. (1990). Glucocorticoid up-regulation of high-affinity IL-6 receptors on human epithelial cells. *Proceedings of the National Academy of Sciences USA, 87*, 2838–2842.

Solomon, G. F. (1969). Stress and antibody response in rats. *International Archives of Allergy, 35*, 97–104.

Solomon, G. F., & Moos, R. H. (1964). Emotions, immunity and disease. *Archives of General Psychiatry, 11*, 657–669.

Spain, D. M., & Thalhimer, W. (1951). Temporary accumulation of eosinophilic leucocytes in spleen on mice following administration of cortisone. *Proceedings of the Society for Experimental Biology, 76*, 320–322.

Spencer, R. L., Kalman, B. A., & Dhabhar, F. S. (in press). Role of endogenous glucocorticoids in immune system function: Regulation and counterregulation. In B. S. McEwen (Ed.), *Handbook of Physiology*.

Spencer, R. L., Kalman, B. A., & Dhabhar, F. S. (in press). Role of endogenous glucocorticoids in immune system function: Regulation and counterregulation. In B. S. McEwen (Ed.), *Handbook of Physiology: Coping with the environment*. New York: Oxford University Press.

Sprent, J., & Tough, D. F. (1994). Lymphocyte life-span and memory. *Science, 265*, 1395–1400.

Spry, C. J. F. (1972). Inhibition of lymphocyte recirculation by stress and corticotropin. *Cellular Immunology, 4*, 86–92.

Stefanski, V., Solomon, G. F., Kling, A. S., Thomas, J., & Plaeger, S. (1996). Impact of social confrontation on rat CD4 T cells bearing different CD45R isoforms. *Brain, Behavior, & Immunity, 10*, 364–379.

Stein, M., Ronzoni, E., & Gildea, E. F. (1951). Physiological responses to heat stress and ACTH of normal and schizophrenic subjects. *American Journal of Psychiatry, 6*, 450–455.

Steinman, L. (1991). The development of rational strategies for selective immunotherapy against autoimmune demyelinating disease. *Advances in Immunology, 49*, 357–379.

Stephanou, A., Jessop, D. S., Knight, R. A., & Lightman, S. L. (1990). Corticotropin-releasing factor-like immunoreactivity and mRNA in human leukocytes. *Brain, Behavior, & Immunity, 4*, 67–73.

Sternberg, E. M. (1995). Neuroendocrine factors in susceptibility to inflammatory disease: Focus on the hypothalamic-pituitary-adrenal axis. *Hormone Research, 43*, 159–161.

Sternberg, E. M., Chrousos, G. P., Wilder, R. L., & Gold, P. W. (1992). The stress response and the regulation of inflammatory disease. *Annals of Internal Medicine, 117*, 854–866.

Sternberg, E. M., Hill, J. M., Chrousos, G. P., Kamilaris, T., Listwak, S. J., Gold, P. W., & Wilder, R. L. (1989). Inflammatory mediator-induced hypothalamic-pituitary-adrenal axis activation is defective in streptococcal cell wall arthritis-susceptible Lewis rats. *Proceedings of the National Academy of Sciences USA, 86*, 2374–2378.

Sternberg, E. M., & Wilder, R. L. (1989). The role of the hypothalamic-pituitary-adrenal axis in an experimental model of arthritis. *Progress in NeuroEndocrinImmunology, 2*, 102–108.

Sternberg, E. M., Young, W. S., Bernadini, R., Calogero, A. E., Chrousos, G. P., Gold, P. W., & Wilder, R. L. (1989). A central nervous system defect in biosynthesis of corticotropin releasing hormone is associated with susceptibility to streptococcal cell wall-induced arthritis in Lewis rats. *Proceedings of the National Academy of Sciences USA, 86*, 4771–4775.

Stocklin, E., Wissler, M., Gouilleux, F., & Groner, B. (1996). Functional interactions between Stat5 and the glucocorticoid receptor. *Nature, 383*, 726–728.

Swingle, W. W., & Remington, J. W. (1944). The role of the adrenal cortex in physiological processes. *Physiological Review, 24*, 89–127.

Takaki, A., Huang, Q.-H., Somogyvari-Vigh, A., & Arimura, A. (1994). Immobilization stress may increase plasma interleukin-6 via central and peripheral catecholamines. *Neuroimmunomodulation, 1*, 335–342.

Tavadia, H. B., Fleming, K. A., Hume, P. D., & Simpson, H. W. (1975). Circadian rhythmicity of human plasma cortisol and PHA-induced lymphocyte transformation. *Clinical & Experimental Immunology, 22*, 190–193.

Thomas, N., Edwards, J. L., & Bell, P. A. (1981). Studies of the mechanism of glucocorticoid-induced pyknosis in isolated rat thymocytes. *Journal of Steroid Biochemistry, 18*, 519–524.

Thomason, B. T., Brantley, P. J., Jones, G. N., Dyer, H. R., & Morris, J. L. (1992). The relations between stress and disease activity in rheumatoid arthritis. *Journal of Behavioral Medicine, 15*, 215–220.

Thompson, J., & Van Furth, R. (1973). The effect of glucocorticoids on the kinetics of promonocytes and monocytes of the bone marrow. *Journal of Experimental Medicine, 137*, 10–21.

Thompson, S. P., McMahon, L. J., & Nugent, C. C. (1980). Endogenous cortisol: A regulator of the number of lymphocytes in peripheral blood. *Clinical Immunology & Immunopathology, 17*, 506–514.

Thompson, W. L., Abeles, F. B., Beall, F. A., Dinterman, R. E., & Wannemacher, J. R.W. (1976). Influence of the adrenal glucocorticoids on the stimulation of synthesis of hepatic ribonucleic acid and plasma acute-phase globulins by leukocytic endogenous mediator. *Biochemical Journal, 156*, 25–32.

Toft, P., Svendsen, P., Tonnesen, E., Rasmussen, J. W., & Christensen, N. J. (1993). Redistribution of lymphocytes after major surgical stress. *Acta Anesthesiologica Scandinavica, 37*, 245–249.

Tonnesen, E., Christensen, N. J., & Brinklov, M. M. (1987). Natural killer cell activity during cortisol and adrenaline infusion in healthy volunteers. *European Journal of Clinical Investigation, 17*, 497–503.

Torpy, D. J., & Chrousos, G. P. (1996). The three-way interactions between the hypothalamic-pituitary-adrenal and gonadal axes and the immune system. *Baillieres Clinical Rheumatology, 10*, 181–198.

Tsigos, C., & Chrousos, G. P. (1994). Physiology of the hypothalamic-pituitary-adrenal axis in health and dysregulation in psychiatric and autoimmune disorders. *Endocrinology & Metabolism Clinics of North America, 23*, 451–466.

Tuchinda, M., Newcomb, R. W., & DeVald, B. L. (1972). Effect of prednisone treatment on the human immune response to keyhole limpet hemocyanin. *International Archives of Allergy, 42*, 533–544.

Ulich, T. R., Keys, M., Ni, R. X., del Castillo, J., & Dakay, E. B. (1988). The contributions of adrenal hormones, hemodynamic factors, and the endotoxin-related stress reaction to stable prostaglandin analog-induced peripheral lymphopenia and neutrophilia. *Journal of Leukocyte Biology, 43*, 5–10.

Van Den Broek, A. A., Keuning, F. J., Soeharto, R., & Prop, N. (1983). Immune suppression and histophysiology of the immune response I. Cortisone acetate and lymphoid cell migration. *Virchows Archiv [Archives], 43*, 43–54.

van Gool, J., Boers, W., Sala, M., & Ladiges, N. C. J. J. (1984). Glucocorticoids and catecholamines as mediators of acute-phase proteins, especially rat α-macrofoetoprotein. *Biochemical Journal, 220*, 125–132.

Vidal, C., Tome, S., Fernandex-Redondo, V., & Tato, F. (1994). Systemic allergic reaction to corticosteroids. *Contact Dermatitis, 31*, 273–274.

Walzer, P. D., LaBine, M., Redington, T. J., & Cushion, M. T. (1984). Lymphocyte changes during chronic administration of and withdrawal from corticosteroids: Relation to *Pneumocystis carinii* pneumonia. *Journal of Immunology, 133*, 2502–2508.

Warren, M. K., & Vogel, S. N. (1985). Opposing effects of glucocorticoids on interferon-γ-induced murine macrophage Fc receptor and Ia antigen expression. *Journal of Immunology, 134*, 2462–2469.

Weiss, J. M., Schleifer, S. J., Miller, N. E., & Stein, M. (1981). Suppression of immunity by stress: Effect of a graded series of stressors. *Science, 213*, 1397–1400.

Whitfield, J. F., MacManus, J. P., & Gillan, D. J. (1973). The calcium-dependent stimulation of thymic lymphoblast DNA synthesis and proliferation by a low concentration of cortisol. *Hormone & Metabolic Research, 5*, 200–204.

Whitfield, J. F., MacManus, J. P., & Rixon, R. H. (1970). Cyclic AMP-mediated stimulation of thymocyte proliferation by low concentrations of cortisol. *Proceedings of the Society For Experimental Biology, 134*, 1170–1174.

Whitmore, S. E. (1995). Delayed systemic allergic reactions to corticosteroids. *Contact Dermatitis, 32*, 193–198.

Wick, G., Sgonc, R., & Lechner, O. (1998). Neuroendocrine-immune disturbances in animal models with spontaneous autoimmune diseases. *Annals of the New York Academy of Sciences, 840*, 591–598.

Wiegers, G. J., Labeur, M. S., Stec, I. E., Klinkert, W. E., Holsboe, R. F., & Reul, J. M. (1995). Glucocorticoids accelerate anti-T cell receptor-induced T cell growth. *Journal of Immunology, 155*, 1893–1902.

Wiegers, G. J., & Reul, J. M. H. M. (1998). Induction of cytokine receptors by glucocorticoids: Functional and pathological significance. *Trends In Pharmacological Sciences, 19*, 317–321.

Wiegers, J. G., & Reul, J. M. H. M., Holsboer, F., & De Kloet, E. R. (1994). Enhancement of rat splenic lymphocyte mitogenesis after short term exposure to corticosteroids in vitro. *Endocrinology, 135*, 2351–2357.

Wieland, S., Dobbeling, U., & Rusconi, S. (1991). Interference and synergism of glucocorticoid receptor and octamer factors. *EMBO Journal, 10*, 2513–2521.

Wilckens, T. (1995). Glucocorticoids and immune function: Physiological relevance and pathogenic potential of hormonal dysfunction. *Trends In Pharmacological Sciences, 16*, 193–197.

Wilckens, T., & DeRijk, R. (1997). Glucocorticoids and immune function: Unknown dimensions and new frontiers. *Immunology Today, 18*, 418–424.

Wilder, R. L., Allen, J. B., & Hansen, C. (1986). Thymus-dependent and -independent regulation of Ia antigen expression in situ by cells in the synovium of rats with streptococcal cell wall-induced arthritis. *Journal of Clinical Investigation, 79*, 1160–1171.

Wilkinson, S. M. (1994). Hypersensitivity to topical corticosteroids. *Clinical & Experimental Dermatology, 19*, 1–11.

Williams, T. J., & Yarwood, H. (1990). Effect of glucocorticoids on microvascular permeability. *American Review of Respiratory Diseases, 141*, S39–S43.

Wistar, R., & Hildemann, W. H. (1960). Effect of stress on skin transplantation immunity in mice. *Science, 131*, 159–160.

Wood, P. G., Karol, M. H., Kusnecov, A. W., & Rabin, B. S. (1993). Enhancement of antigen-specific humoral and cell-mediated immunity by electric footshock stress in rats. *Brain, Behavior, & Immunity, 7*, 121–134.

Woolley, C. S., Gould, E., & McEwen, B. S. (1990). Exposure to excess glucocorticoids alters dendritic morphology of adult hippocampal pyramidal neurons. *Brain Research, 531*, 225–231.

Woolley, C. S., Gould, E., Sakai, R. R., Spencer, R. L., & McEwen, B. S. (1991). Effets of aldosterone or RU28362 treatment on adrenalectomy-induced cell death in the dentate gyrus of the adult rat. *Brain Research, 554*, 312–315.

Wu, C. Y., Sarfati, M., Heusser, C., Forunier, S., Rubio-Trujillo, M., Peleman, R., & Delespesse, G. (1991). Glucocorticoids increase the synthesis of immunoglobulin E by interleukin 4-stimulated human lymphocytes. *Journal of Clinical Investigation, 87*, 870–877.

Wyllie, A. H., Morris, R. G., Smith, A. L., & Dunlop, D. (1984). Chromatin cleavage in apoptosis: Association with condensed chromatin morphology and dependence on macromolecular synthesis. *Journal of Pathology, 142*, 67–77.

Yu, D. T. Y., Clements, P. J., Paulus, H. E., Peter, J. B., Levy, J., & Barnett, E. V. (1974). Human lymphocyte subpopulations. Effects of corticosteroids. *Journal of Clinical Investigation, 53*, 565–571.

Zalcman, S., & Anisman, H. (1993). Acute and chronic stressor effects on the antibody response to sheep red blood cells. *Pharmacology, Biochemistry & Behavior, 46*, 445–452.

Zatz, M. M. (1975). Effects of cortisone on lymphocyte homing. *Israel Journal of Medical Sciences, 11*, 1368–1372.

Zautra, A. J., Okun, M. A., Robinson, S. E., Lee, D., Roth, S. H., & Emmanual, J. (1989). Life stress and lymphocyte alterations among patients with rheumatoid arthritis. *Health Psychology, 8*, 1–14.

Zuckerman, S. H., Shelhaas, J., & Butler, L. D. (1989). Differential regulation of lipopolysaccharide-induced interleukin 1 and tumor necrosis factor synthesis: Effects of endogenous and exogenous glucocortcioids and the role of the pituitary-adrenal axis. *European Journal of Immunology, 19*, 301–305.

Zwilling, B. (1992). Stress affects disease outcomes. Confronted with infectious disease agents, the nervous and immune systems interact in complex ways. *ASM News, 58*, 23–25.

C H A P T E R

11

Growth Hormone and Insulin-like Growth Factor as Cytokines in the Immune System

HOMER D. VENTERS, ROBERT DANTZER, GREGORY G. FREUND, SUZANNE R. BROUSSARD, KEITH W. KELLEY

I. INTRODUCTION

Two mediators of several functional properties of the immune system are growth hormone and insulin-like growth-factor-I (IGF-I). In addition to the classical endocrine response mode of growth hormone and IGF-I, cells and tissues of the immune system synthesize and respond to these hormones in both an autocrine and paracrine fashion (Arkins, Dantzer, & Kelley, 1993; Arkins, Rebeiz, Brunke-Reese, Biragyn, & Kelley, 1995; Weigent & Blalock, 1995, 1997). The fact that lymphoid and myeloid cells produce growth hormone, the IGF-I peptide, and some of the IGF binding proteins (IGFBP; Li et al., 1996) points to both endocrine and paracrine elements of immune regulation. Consequently, growth hormone, the closely related molecule PRL, and IGF-I are likely to be key players in this communication network by regulating diverse physiological responses during inflammation as well as controlling the growth and differentiation of hematopoietic elements.

This article summarizes recent developments in our understanding of the growth hormone–IGF-I–immune system axis, focusing in particular on the role of these proteins during hematopoiesis. Readers are referred to our original review on this topic (Kelley, 1989), as well as more recent considerations for an overview of the literature on the role of growth hormone in immunity (Burgess et al., 1999; Johnson, Arkins, Dantzer, & Kelley, 1997; Kelley, Arkins, Minshall, Liu, & Dantzer, 1996). We also explore and elaborate on the original concept that neuro-endocrine–immune interaction is bidirectional (Besedovsky, del Rey, & Sorkin, 1985; Blalock, 1984; Blalock, Harbour-McMenamin, & Smith, 1985) with cytokine products modulating pituitary growth hormone and hepatic and extra-hepatic IGF-I production as well as an array of host metabolic responses. This interaction between proinflammatory cytokines and hormone action has a significant impact on metabolism and growth and affects homeostatic defense mechanisms.

II. GROWTH HORMONE AND IGF-I: THE LIGANDS

Native human growth hormone is a protein consisting of 191 amino acids and is secreted primarily by somatotrophs in the adenohypophysis, although leukocytes are now known to synthesize this protein (Weigent & Blalock, 1995). Growth hormone indirectly mediates growth of peripheral tissues by inducing hepatic synthesis of the growth-promoting peptide, IGF-I. The latter is a single-chain nonglycosylated 70-amino acid polypeptide that is extremely well conserved across species, with no more than 4 amino acid substitutions in all mammals investigated (reviewed by LeRoith, Kavsan, Koval, & Roberts, 1993). Structurally related to insulin and IGF-II, plasma IGF-I is primarily derived from hepatic secretion in response to growth hormone and mediates the anabolic effects of the latter hormone in many tissues. Unlike insulin, however, which is expressed only in β cells in the islets of the pancreas, the IGFs are produced by a variety of tissues in the body. Both in the general circulation and in extracellular tissue compartments, IGF-I is not found as the free peptide but, instead, is closely associated with one of six binding proteins (Jones & Clemmons, 1995). The level of sophistication in the regulation of the biological activities of growth hormone and IGF-I is comparable to that evidenced in the cytokine system with its network of soluble receptors, shared ligands, and common second signaling mechanisms (Kishimoto, Taga, & Akira, 1994).

III. THE GROWTH HORMONE RECEPTOR

The growth hormone, prolactin, and placental lactogen receptors belong to the cytokine receptor superfamily of receptors (Sato & Miyajima, 1994). Members of this receptor superfamily share homology in their extracellular binding domains and tertiary structure and include the receptors for interleukin (IL)-2-7, 9, 11, 13, granulocyte-colony stimulating factor (G-CSF), granulocyte-macrophage (GM)-CSF, ciliary neurotrophic factor (CNTF), leukemia inhibition factor (LIF), erythropoietin (EPO), oncostatin M (OSM), and interferon (IFN)-α, β, and γ. Receptors in this superfamily have limited extracellular homology but share conserved motifs such as four positionally conserved cysteine pairs in one extracellular domain and a conserved WSXWS motif in the second juxtamembrane domain (Ronco, Doyle, Raines, Park, & Gasson, 1995). There is also limited homology in the intracellular domain of the receptors. A membrane proximal region of the cytoplasmic domain of one or more of the receptors, known as the box 1 and box 2 motifs, is required for mitogenesis (Avalos et al., 1995). The intracellular domains of these receptors lack intrinsic kinase activity. Instead, binding of growth hormone, as well as prolactin, to its receptor produces a complex consisting of one molecule of hormone and two molecules of receptor, which in turn recruits intracellular nonreceptor protein tyrosine kinases. Signaling by the cytokine receptor superfamily is mediated by members of the Janus kinase (JAK) family (Yamauchi et al., 1998). Following dimerization, JAK-2 and JAK-1 are recruited to the proline rich box 1/box 2 motif of the growth hormone receptor and phosphorylate STAT (signal transducer and activator of transcription) proteins, which subsequently translocate to the nucleus where they form transcription complexes that interact with DNA. Identification of JAK-2 as a growth hormone receptor-associated tyrosine kinase established tyrosyl phosphorylation as being critical for growth hormone signaling (Wang & Wong, 1998). In addition to the growth hormone receptor, other receptors in the cytokine/hemopoietin receptor superfamily activate JAK-2 in response to ligand binding. However, pathways other than the JAK-STAT activation sequence may also operate in growth hormone signaling since this hormone has been shown to share with insulin, IFN-γ and LIF the ability to induce tyrosine phosphorylation of insulin-receptor substrate-1 (IRS-1; Argetsinger et al., 1995). This suggests that there may be common signaling pathways for the many members of the cytokine receptor superfamily and that specificity of signaling may be due to regulation of receptor expression or differential expression and activation of intracellular signaling molecules.

IV. THE IGF-I RECEPTOR

The physiological actions of IGF-I on cellular growth, metabolism, and differentiation are mediated via activation of the IGF-I receptor, which is expressed by many normal and transformed cells. This receptor has a high affinity for IGF-I (1×10^{-10} M), an approximately 10-fold lower affinity for IGF-II and an approximately 100- to 1,000-fold lower affinity for insulin (Werner & LeRoith, 1995). IGF-I mediates its effects by signaling through a transmembrane disulfide linked heterotetramer ($\beta\alpha\alpha\beta$) that shares a high degree of homology to the closely related insulin receptor. The ligand-binding β chains are extracellular and transmembrane β chains are intracellular and are essentially protein tyrosine kinases. As with insulin, the receptor for IGF-I undergoes ligand-induced autophosphorylation on three clustered tyrosine residues in the kinase domain of the intracellular β chain. The best characterized and predominant tyrosine-containing substrates of the IGF-I receptor, IRS-1 and IRS-2, are also the major substrates of the insulin receptor (LeRoith, Werner, Beitner-Johnson, & Roberts, 1995; Uddin et al., 1997). These cytosolic substrates have multiple tyrosine residues located in YMXM or YXXM motifs and act as docking proteins that associate with and regulate the activities of other intracellular proteins containing the src homology 2 (SH2) domains (Valverde, Lorenzo, Pons, White, & Benito, 1998).

The phosphorylation of IRS proteins on tyrosine residues leads to their association with the 85 Kda regulatory subunit of phosphatidylinositol-3′ kinase (PI 3-kinase). PI 3-kinase is a lipid and serine kinase consisting of an 85 Kda regulatory subunit containing two SH2 domains and a catalytic subunit of 110 Kda that catalyzes the phosphorylation of membrane bound PI, PI 4-phosphate, and PI 4,5-biphosphate on the 3′ position of the inositol ring. Products of the PI 3-kinase reaction are D-3 phosphorylated phosphoinositides that signal downstream events involved in regulating cell growth and metabolism (Toker & Cantley, 1997). Other responses to IGF-I receptor activation include *c-myc*, *c-jun*, and *c-fos* gene expression and MAP-2 kinase activation (Downard, 1995; LeRoith et al., 1995; Richards, Walker, Sebastian, & DiAugustine, 1998).

V. CYTOKINES AFFECT THE GROWTH HORMONE-IGF-I AXIS

A. General Considerations

There is ample evidence that cytokines affect the neuroendocrine system. The novel finding that leukocytes express receptors for pituitary peptides, in addition to having the capacity to synthesize and secrete those same peptides, indicated the presence of a highly integrated, well-developed system for conveying information from the brain to the immune system. The idea that the immune system may somehow act on the neuroendocrine system was suggested by observations from Wexler, Dolgin, and Tryczynski (1957a, 1957b) indicating that administration of bacterial endotoxin increased plasma concentrations of corticosterone. Increases in corticosterone paralleled the immune response (Besedovsky, Sorkin, Keller, & Muller, 1975). When Besedovsky, Del Rey, and Sorkin (1981) subsequently reported that supernatants from concanavalin A-stimulated rat spleen cells administered into rats increased plasma corticosterone, it became clear that activation of the neuroendocrine system was due to an immunogenic mechanism rather than a pathogenic mechanism. The bioactive product in conditioned supernatants was later described as IL-1 (Berkenbosch, van Oers, Del Rey, Tilders, & Besedovsky, 1987; Bernton, Beach, Holaday, Smallridge, & Fein, 1987; Besedovsky, del Rey, Sorkin, & Dinarello, 1986; Sapolsky, Rivier, Yamamoto, Plotsky, & Vale, 1987).

Bacterial infection and trauma induce mononuclear myeloid cells to synthesize and secrete at least three proinflammatory cytokines that are now known to have profound effects on the hypothalamic-pituitary axis. These include, but are certainly not limited to, IL-1, IL-6, and tumor necrosis factor-α (TNF-α). There now exists a large body of evidence suggesting IL-1 acts directly in the central nervous system (CNS) to stimulate the hypothalmic-pituitary-adrenal (HPA) axis. Administration of nanogram-levels of IL-1 directly into a lateral cerebral ventricle of the brain rapidly increases plasma ACTH (Rivier, Vale, & Brown, 1989). Immunoneutralization of CRH markedly reduces the increase in plasma ACTH caused by IL-1 (Berkenbosch et al., 1987), whereas IL-1 receptor antibodies inhibit the lipopolysaccaride (LPS)-induced increase in ACTH (Rivier, Chizzonite, & Vale, 1989). Furthermore, peripheral administration of LPS increases the expression of mRNA encoding for CRH in the hypothalamic paraventricular nucleus (PVN) (Kakucska, Qi, Clark, & Lechan, 1993). The increase in CRH mRNA is dependent on IL-1 in the CNS because central but not peripheral administration of the IL-1 receptor antagonist (IL-1ra) blocks entirely the expression of CRH transcripts in the PVN following peripheral LPS (Kakucska, Qi, Clark, & Lechan, 1993). These data demonstrate the ability of IL-1 to alter the neuroendocrine system by acting directly within the CNS. Of course, this does not preclude the important possibility that IL-1 acts directly on corticotrophs to induce ACTH (Fukata, Usui, Nakai, & Imura, 1989; Johnson, Blalock, & Smith, 1988; Lee & Rivier, 1994; Woloski, Smith, Meyer, Fuller, & Blalock, 1985). Indeed the traditional debate whether IL-1 causes the release of pituitary ACTH indirectly via induction of CRH in the hypothalamus or through a direct effect on the pituitary appears to have been resolved by the important observation that hypothalamic CRH, released in response to IL-1, not only stimulates the pituitary to release ACTH, but also sensitizes the pituitary to the direct ACTH-releasing effects of IL-1 (Payne, Weigent, & Blalock, 1994).

B. Growth Hormone and IGF-I Endocrine Responses Following Activation of the Immune System

In addition to the development of an immune response, the host responds to infectious challenge with many changes in intermediary metabolism (Mulligan & Bloch, 1998). We have shown that type I IL-1 receptors are present in the adenohypophysis (Parnet et al., 1993), and we subsequently used an immunohistochemical approach with specific monoclonal antibodies to demonstrate that both the p80 and p68 isoforms of IL-1 receptors are located primarily on somatotrophs (French et al., 1996). Administration of LPS elicits a growth hormone endocrine response that appears to be species-specific, resulting in increases in growth hormone secretion in humans and in sheep but a reduction in cattle, chickens, and rats (reviewed by Sartin, Elsasser, Gunter, & McMahon, 1998). The increase in growth hormone secretion in humans extends to another cytokine, IL-6, which substantially increases plasma growth hormone within a few hours following subcutaneous administration of recombinant IL-6 (Tsigos et al., 1997). The LPS-induced increase in growth hormone secretion in sheep (Briard et al., 1998) is associated with an inability of TNF to inhibit growth hormone secretion in this species (Fry, Gunter, McMahon, Steele, & Sartin, 1998), which contrasts with the rat (Walton & Cronin, 1989). Indeed, injection of rats with endotoxin (Soto, Martin, Millan, Vara, & Lopez-Calderon, 1998) or IL-1α or IL-1β (but not IL-2 or IL-6; Wada et al., 1995) causes an immediate decrease in circulating growth hormone levels, which return to normal after 24 h. However, there is also a diminished plasma concentration of IGF-I, which remains 35–45% of control animals after 24 h (Fan, Molina, Gelato, & Lang, 1994). In critically ill rats with LPS-mediated kidney damage, IGF-I can partially restore kidney function (Manzo, Dickerson, Settle, & Rajter, 1993). In mice given intraperitoneal injections of LPS, pretreatment with growth hormone or IGF-I significantly reduces bacterial counts in peritoneal lavage fluid and increases peritoneal neutrophil numbers (Inoue, Saito, Tsuno, et al., 1998), phagocytosis, and respiratory burst activity (Balteskard, Unneberg, Halvorsen, Hansen, & Revhaug, 1998).

Similar to growth hormone, IGF-I administration promotes wound healing (Bitar, 1997) and lessens harmful events following wounding, such as intestinal translocation of LPS (Sugiura et al., 1997). Although injection of LPS to human subjects and sheep results in transient elevations of growth hormone, there is no detectable increase in free IGF-I levels and generally a significant decrease in plasma IGF-I (Sartin et al., 1998; Lang et al., 1997). IGF binding protein (IGFBP)-1 and -2 are significantly elevated under these circumstances (Lang et al., 1997). This supports recent studies in humans, showing decreases in plasma IGF-I levels in patients with sepsis (Dahn & Lange, 1998). The reduction in plasma IGF-I levels cannot be ascribed to changes in growth hormone, which increases in the short term following administration of LPS into humans. The increase in proinflammatory cytokines caused by endotoxin also appears to inhibit the biological activity of IGF-I (Lazarus, Moldawer, & Lowry, 1993). This finding suggests the existence of both pituitary and hepatic regulation of the growth hormone/IGF-I axis by inflammatory mediators. These observations are supported by the recent demonstration that endotoxin-induced suppression of the somatotropic axis is mediated by IL-1β and corticotropin-releasing factor which, in turn, suppresses the release of growth hormone releasing hormone (Peisen, McDonnell, Mulroney, & Lumpkin, 1995). Indeed, a generalized suppression of somatolactogen release from the anterior pituitary by LPS is suggested by the demonstration that subcutaneous administration of endotoxin results in decreased levels of circulating PRL in postpartum pigs (Smith & Wagner, 1984), leading to a reduction in milk production during lactation. The mechanism of growth attenuation following infectious challenge may not be limited to gram negative bacteria since swine infected with the protozoan parasite *Sarcocystis miescheriana* also have reduced serum IGF-I and elevated IGFBP levels (Prickett, Latimer, McCusker, Hausman, & Prestwood, 1992). These data demonstrate that cytokines can serve as potent regulators of pituitary growth hormone and hepatic IGF-I and IGFBP secretion. Indeed, following endotoxin exposure, or sepsis, it appears that hepatic IGF-I secretion becomes refractory to growth hormone stimulation (Fan et al., 1994), suggesting that there may be direct effects of LPS or proinflammatory cytokines on hepatic IGF-I and IGFBP synthesis, as has already been demonstrated in extra-hepatic sites (Arkins, Rebeiz, Brunke-Reese, Biragyn, et al., 1995; Lin, Wang, Nagpal, Chang, & Calkins, 1992).

VI. GROWTH HORMONE AND INSULIN-LIKE GROWTH FACTOR-I IN THE IMMUNE SYSTEM: RECENT FINDINGS

A. Growth Hormone

Both growth hormone and IGF-I have been shown to affect a variety of immune events, and these data were recently reviewed by us (Arkins, Johnson, Minshall, Dantzer, & Kelley, 2000; Burgess et al., 1999; Johnson et al., 1997) and others (Clark, 1997; Fabris, Mocchegiani, & Provinciali, 1997; Foster, Montecino-Rodriguez, Clark, & Dorshkind, 1998; Geffner, 1997; Koojiman, Hooghe-Peters, & Hooghe, 1996; Van Buul-Offers & Kooijman, 1998). Perhaps the earliest and most consistent observation is that both growth hormone and IGF-I increase the size and cellularity of both primary (e.g., thymus) and secondary (e.g., spleen) lymphoid organs, particularly in hormone-deficient animals. This biological effect occurs throughout life, from the fetus (Tarantal, Hunter, & Gargosky, 1997) to the very aged animal (Kelley et al., 1986). Several years ago we demonstrated that growth hormone greatly improves the survival of rats infected with *Salmonella typhimurium* (Edwards, Yunger, Lorence, Dantzer, & Kelley, 1991), and these results have been extended to the protective effects of growth hormone on the survival of mice infected with *Escherichia coli* (Inoue, Saito, Matsuda, et al., 1998). These protective effects of growth hormone are likely to be mediated by directed effects on macrophages and polymorphonuclear cells because incubation of neutrophils in vitro with growth hormone increases their ability to kill *E. coli* (Edwards, Ghiasuddin, Schepper, Yunger, & Kelley, 1988; Fu, Arkins, Li, Dantzer, & Kelley, 1994; Inoue et al., 1998a, 1998b). Similar bactericidal promoting activity of neutrophils has now been demonstrated for IGF-I (Inoue). One likely mechanism for these effects is the finding by us and others that growth hormone and IGF-I increase the production of oxygen free radicals by both mononuclear (Edwards et al., 1988) and polymorphonuclear (Bjerknes & Aarskog, 1995; Fu, Arkins, Wang, & Kelley, 1991; Warwick-Davies, Lowrie, & Cole, 1995) myeloid cells and by promoting phagocytosis by these same cells (Edwards et al., 1992). For example, we demonstrated that growth hormone is nearly as effective as IFN-γ in promoting killing of *Escherichia coli* by neutrophils in vitro, and this functional activity correlates very well with the ability of growth hormone and IFN-γ to increase the secretion of superoxide anion (Figure 1; Fu et al., 1994). The fact that killing of *E. coli* by neutrophils is blocked by pretreatment with scavengers of oxygen metabolites (superoxide dismutase and catalase) offers strong support for the idea that secretion of superoxide anion is responsible for the bactericidal activity. Indeed, phagocytosis of both monocytes and neutrophils has been reported to be reduced in children with idiopathic growth hormone

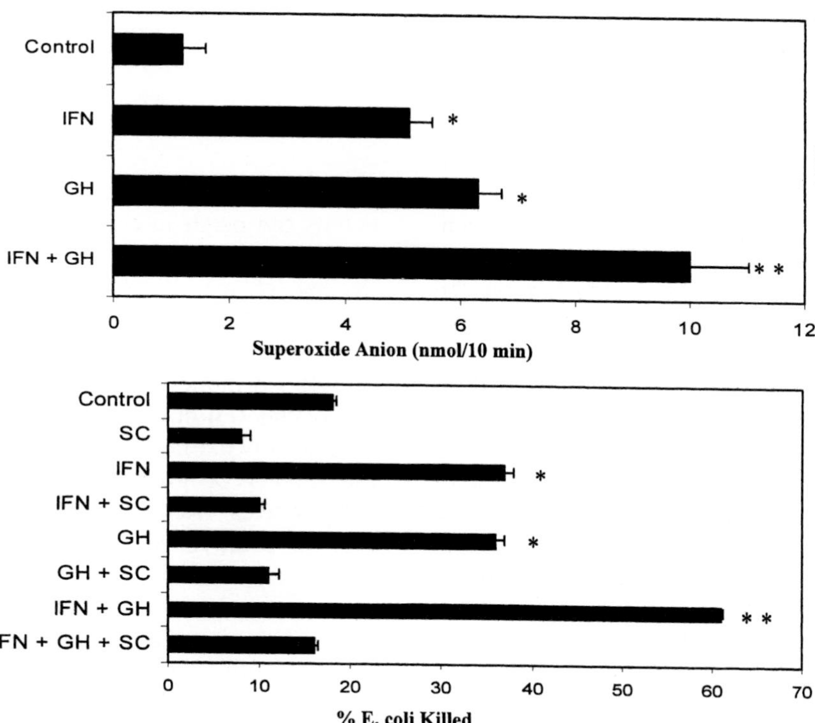

FIGURE 1 Treatment of bone marrow-derived polymorphonuclear neutrophils from rats with either IFN-γ (IFN) or growth hormone (GH) augments the secretion of superoxide anion and promotes neutrophil killing of *E. coli*. Bacterial killing was blocked by pretreatment of cells with the scavengers or oxygen metabolites (SC; superoxide dismutase and catalase). * indicates $P < 0.05$;** indicates $P < 0.01$) (Data from Fu et al., 1994. Used with permission from the American Society for Microbiology.)

deficiency, and this defect is restored by exogenous treatment with growth hormone (Manfredi et al., 1994). Similar results were obtained in growth hormone-deficient adults, who have a 40% reduction in the ability of neutrophils to produce superoxide anion, and this defect was reversed by a 6-month treatment regimen with recombinant human growth hormone (Reinisch, Schratzberger, Finkenstedt, Kahler, & Wiedermann, 1996). The macrophage-activating activity of growth hormone extends to osteoclasts, in which case the downstream activation may be osteoblast-derived IGF-I (Guicheux, et al., 1998). However, although several endocrine actions of growth hormone are achieved by induction of IGF-I, many others in the immune system are not (Kelley et al., 1996; Minshall, Liu, Arkins, & Kelley, 1996). Given the ability of each factor to often exert similar cellular responses, identification of growth hormone-specific actions has often been difficult when tested in vivo, particularly in humans.

Growth hormone receptors are expressed by many types of leukocytes, including thymocytes, splenocytes, B lymphocytes, and T lymphocytes. In the human thymus, the growth hormone receptor is expressed primarily on immature hematopoietic cells that do not express CD4 or CD8 antigens but do express CD34 (de Mello-Coelho, Gagnerault, et al., 1998). Both human thymocytes and thymic epithelial cells have recently been confirmed to express growth hormone mRNA (de Mello-Coelho, Savino, Postel-Vinay, & Dardenne, 1998), and it has been proposed that this is a self-contained growth hormone secreting unit that functions separately from pituitary-derived growth hormone (Hull & Harvey, 1998). In humans, this thymus-derived growth hormone has been reported to augment thymocyte proliferation by inducing the synthesis of IGF-I (Sabharwal & Varma, 1996). Expression of the growth hormone receptor is evident in the thymus early in fetal development, at least in the bovine species (Chen, Schuler, & Schultz, 1998). Outside of the thymus, a greater proportion of B cells and macrophages express the growth hormone receptor than T cells, and approximately 20% of lymph node cells are growth hormone receptor positive (Dardenne, Mello-Coelho, Gagnerault, & Postel-Vinay, 1998). Expression of growth hormone receptors on leukocytes may be inversely related to linear growth (Valerio et al., 1997). Interestingly, the prolactin receptor is expressed on all peripheral T cells that express the growth hormone receptor (Dardenne et al., 1998).

Contemporary understanding of growth hormone action includes activity far outside the realm of the traditional endocrine system. Growth hormone augments cellular proliferation in both T and B lymphocytes, even in aged primates (Postel-Vinay, de Mello Coelho, Gagnerault, & Dardenne, 1997; LeRoith et al., 1996). An interesting and potentially important recent observation is that administration of growth hormone in vivo or in vitro, but not IGF-I, increases the synthesis of IFN-γ (Liao, Rudling, & Angelin, 1997; Mustafa et al., 1997). This finding is entirely consistent with the promotion of a Th1 immune response in mice subjected to burns (Takagi, Suzuki, Barrow, Wolf, & Herndon, 1998) or injected with an HIV antigen (Mellado et al., 1998) and the lack of an effective Th2 response in mice that overexpress growth hormone (Gonzalo et al., 1996). Similarly, both basal and stimulated natural killer activity is lower in growth hormone-deficient humans, and this is reversed with either growth hormone (Bidlingmaier, Auernhammer, Feldmeier, & Strasburger, 1997) or IGF-I (Auernhammer, Feldmeier, Nass, Pachman, & Strasburger, 1996). Growth hormone administration has recently been shown to promote the regeneration of hematopoietic cells following syngeneic bone marrow transplantation in mice, suggesting that growth hormone may be useful clinically for enhancing bone marrow grafting (Tian et al., 1998). In the specific case of the thymus, growth hormone also increases expression of extracellular matrix ligands and receptors, resulting in an increase in thymocyte adhesion to epithelial cells and thymocyte release from thymic nurse cells (de Mello-Coelho, Villa-Verde, Dardenne, & Savino, 1997).

B. IGF-I

The ability of growth hormone to regulate immune events can occur in either a direct or IGF-I-mediated manner, but these effects are not necessarily related (Kelley et al., 1996). For example, both growth hormone and IGF-I promote the activation of neutrophils and monocytes, but this does not occur by growth hormone inducing the synthesis of IGF-I by leukocytes (Fu et al., 1991; Warwick-Davies, Lowrie, & Cole, 1995). Similar results have been reported for the effects of growth hormone and IGF-I on B lymphocytes (Kelley et al., 1996), the survival of murine promyeloid progenitors (Minshall, Arkins, Dantzer, Freund, & Kelley, 1999), and differentiation of human promyeloid cells into macrophages (Liu, Ning, Dantzer, Freund, & Kelley, 1998). Indeed, although the synthesis of IGF-I by murine bone marrow cells is dramatically increased by CSF-I and IL-3 (Arkins, Dantzer, et al., 1993; Arkins, Rebeiz, et al., 1993; Arkins, Rebeiz, Brunke-Reese, Minshall, et al., 1995; Arkins, Rebeiz, Brunke-Reese, Biragyn, & Kelley, 1995), we have not be able to detect an up-regulation of either leukocyte-derived IGF-I mRNA or peptide by treatment with growth hormone. Even at early stages of fetal development, growth hormone receptor expression occurs in areas in which IGF-I transcripts are both present and absent (Edmondson et al., 1995), suggesting that these two factors exert independent as well as coordinate influences. These and other data (e.g., Liao et al., 1997) establish that the effects of growth hormone and IGF-I on the immune system can be distinct.

Plasma levels of IGF-I and a variety of immune events are jointly reduced by many factors, including aging (Ceda et al., 1998; Lamberts, van den Beld, & van der Lely, 1997), alcoholism (Breese et al., 1995; Mendenhall et al., 1989), and caloric restriction (Mendenhall, Roselle, Gartside, & Grossman, 1997; Mendenhall, Roselle, Grossman, & Gartside, 1997; Savendahl & Underwood, 1997), and exogenous IGF-I is able to reverse many of these immunological abnormalities. IGF-I promotes hematopoiesis, lymphopoiesis, and erythropoiesis (Burgess et al., 1999), consistent with the observation of abundant receptors for IGF-I on hematopoietic progenitors as well as mature monocytes, B lymphocytes and T lymphocytes (Xu, Mardell, Xian, Zola, & Read, 1995). Administration of growth hormone-releasing hormone to aged humans not only increases plasma growth hormone and IGF-I but augments a number of immune responses as well (Khorram, Yeung, Vu, & Yen, 1997). Interestingly, dehydroepiandrosterone also reverses a number of immunological changes that occur in aged men, including a significant elevation in plasma levels of IGF-I (Khorram et al., 1997). Investigation of bone marrow recovery in mice has shown that IGF-I administration increases thymopoiesis during aging (Montecino-Rodriguez, Clark, & Dorshkind, 1998) as well as B cell lymphopoiesis (Jardieu, Clark, Mortensen, & Dorshkind, 1994). Similar increases in B and T lymphocyte survival and proliferation are observed in thymus and spleen in vivo even after treatment with the immunosuppressive synthetic glucocorticoid, dexamethasone (Hinton, Peterson, Dahly, & Ney, 1998).

Bone marrow stromal cells synthesize both IGF-I and IL-7 (Dong & Wortis, 1994), and IGF-I induces the differentiation of pro-B cells (Landreth, Narayanan, & Dorshkind, 1992). Furthermore, pro-B cells proliferate in response to IL-7, and this event is potentiated by IGF-I (Gibson, Piktel, & Landreth 1993; Landreth et al., 1992). The dramatic decrease in pro-B cell proliferation in aged mice correlates with a loss of B cell sensitivity to the cytokine IL-7 but not IGF-I (Stephan, Lill-Elghanian, & Witte, 1997). Subsequent investigations have shown that contact between lymphoid and primary stromal cells is required for B cell proliferation, suggesting that cell contact is required for the release of IL-7 (Stephan, Reilly, & Witte, 1998). IGF-I and insulin increase proliferation of a variety of B cell lines. Cell adhesion is also a critical factor in IGF-I expression by mononuclear cells. Monocyte adhesion has been shown to selectively regulate expression of several factors, including IGF-I mRNA (Jendraschak, Kaminski, Kiefl, & von Schacky, 1998).

Traditional characterizations of IGF-I as an important growth factor for hematopoietic cells (Tsarfaty, Longo, & Murphy, 1994) have been broadened with recent discoveries of the potent apoptosis-reducing properties of IGF-I. Numerous cell types, including hematopoietic (Minshall, Arkins, Freund, & Kelley, 1996; Minshall et al., 1997) and neuronal (D'Mello, Galli, Ciotti, & Calissano, 1993) cells, have been shown to respond to the antiapoptotic actions of IGF-I. The oncogene properties of *c-myc*, which promotes apoptosis through the CD95 (also known as FAS or APO-1) receptor-ligand pathway, are inhibited by IGF-I. IGF-I signaling is able to act on the *c-myc* pathway downstream of CD95 in reducing apoptosis (Hueber et al., 1997). This antagonism of apoptosis is observed in neonatal rat islets of Langerhans where treatment with TNF-α and IFN-γ augmented CD95-mediated apoptosis. Pretreatment with IGF-I eliminated CD95-mediated killing (Harrison et al., 1998). Similar results were observed in glomerular mesangial cells (Mooney, Jobson, Bacon, Kitamura, & Savill, 1997).

In contrast, both growth hormone and IGF-I have been observed to amplify DNA damage and p53 protein expression when human blood peripheral lymphocytes were exposed to the radiomimetic agent bleomycin (Cianfarani et al., 1998). Confirmation of these results may support theories of a dual role for both growth hormone and IGF-I with regard to apoptosis, which leads to the promotion of cell survival and also the loss of postapoptotic cells that may have unstable genomes.

VII. IGF-I PROMOTES SURVIVAL AND DEVELOPMENT OF HEMATOPOIETIC PROGENITORS

A. IGF-I Increases Mitogenesis of Myeloid Progenitor Cells

When administered in vivo, neuroendocrine hormones such as growth hormone and IGF-I have dramatic effects on the formation of new blood cells, and these effects have been reviewed (Berczi, 1997;

Woody et al., 1999). For example, transgenic mice overexpressing bovine growth hormone display augmented splenic hematopoietic colony formation (Blazar, Brennan, Broxmeyer, Shultz, & Vallera, 1995). Similarly, in vivo administration of IGF-I increases hematopoietic progenitor cells in the bone marrow of mice (Tsarfaty et al., 1994). Administration of either growth hormone or IGF-I increases the number of B lineage cells in both the bone marrow and spleen of mice, even though growth hormone-deficient and IGF-I knockout mice appear to have normal B cell lymphopoiesis (Montecino-Rodriguez, Clark, & Dorshkind, 1998).

We have reported that IGF-I treatment in vitro, at concentrations of <5 ng/mL, significantly augments the proliferation of myeloid progenitor cells of both human (Li et al., 1997) and murine (Minshall et al., 1996) origin. The human promyelocytic cell line (HL-60) can be induced to differentiate into monocytes or granulocytes, whereas the murine factor dependent cell progenitor cell line (FDC-P1/MAC) relies on IL-3 for survival. In each case, low concentrations of IGF-I significantly increase proliferation of these cells, as well as murine primary bone marrow cells (Minshall, Arkins, Freund, & Kelley, 1996) (Figure 2). The importance of the IGF-I receptor in the control of cellular proliferation in mammalian cells has been linked to expression of the proliferating cell nuclear antigen (PCNA) (Miura, Li, Dumenil, & Baserga, 1994), and preliminary results in our laboratory have confirmed this finding (Liu and colleagues, unpublished observations).

B. IGF-I Promotes Survival of Myeloid Progenitor Cells

Insulin and IGF-I have also been recently shown to increase the survival of human CD34 positive cells, but not their proliferation (Ratajczak et al., 1998). In our experiments with primary murine bone marrow cells, we easily detected an augmentation in cell survival in response to increasing amounts of IGF-I (Figure 2). The increase in survival of these cells was caused by IGF-I inhibiting their apoptotic death, as revealed by flow cytometric analysis (Minshall and colleagues, 1996). IL-3 and IGF-I inhibited apoptosis in primary progenitor-enriched bone marrow cells, as well as in FDC-P1/MAC myeloid progenitors, even in the presence of inhibitors of RNA synthesis (actinomycin D) or mitosis (mitomycin C). These results suggested that the early actions of both ligands involved specific postreceptor, cell signaling mechanisms. We then showed that both IL-3 and IGF-I induced heightened activation of the enzyme PI 3-kinase in FDC-P1/MAC cells, lending credence to the suspicion that PI 3-kinase is an essential and global mediator of survival promotion in myeloid progenitors. However, addition of the PI 3-kinase inhibitor wortmannin revealed that IGF-I, but not IL-3, required PI 3-kinase to prevent apoptosis (Minshall, Arkins, Freund, & Kelley, 1996) (Figure 3). These were some of the first data to establish that the survival of hematopoietic progenitors is maintained by at least two distinct intracellular signaling pathways, one requiring PI 3-kinase and one that does not. In related experiments, similar analysis of human HL-60 promyeloid cell populations revealed that IGF-I rescues cells from apoptosis following treatment with vitamin A and that blockage of the enzyme PI 3-kinase dramatically inhibits the ability of IGF-I to prevent apoptosis (Liu et al., 1997).

A critical and previously unrecognized link suggesting that IL-4 also might affect the survival of

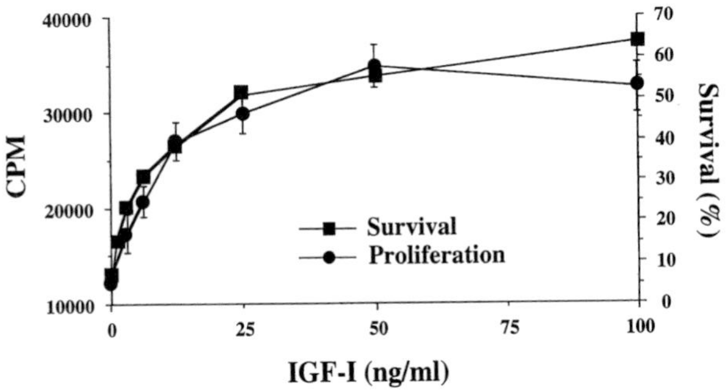

FIGURE 2 IGF-I stimulates proliferation (CPM of [^{3}H]-TdR) and survival (the vital dye MTT in presence of actinomycin D) of primary murine progenitor-enriched bone marrow cells. IGF-I increased proliferation by four fold at 6 ng/mL ($P<0.01$) and promoted cell survival by 50% at 12 ng/mL ($P<0.05$). (Data from Minshall, Arkins, Freund, & Kelley, 1996.)

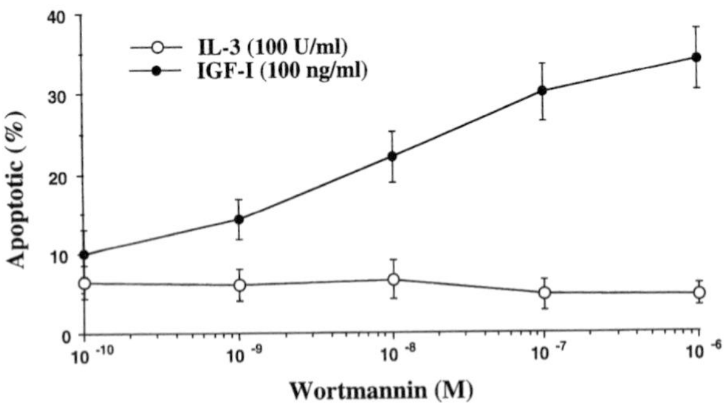

FIGURE 3 IL-3 and IGF-I prevent apoptosis via different signaling pathways. FDCP-1/Mac-1 cells were treated with increasing concentrations of wortmannin, an inhibitor of PI 3-kinase, in the presence of IGF-I or IL-3. Wortmannin at 1 nM inhibited ($P<0.05$) the protective effect of IGF-I but did not affect the apoptotic population of IL-3-treated cells. (Data from Minshall, Arkins, Freund, & Kelley, 1996.)

promyeloid cells, much like IGF-I, came from the original finding that the IL-4 receptor tyrosine phosphorylates a high molecular weight substrate originally known as 4PS (IL-4 Phosphorylated Substrate). This novel molecule was cloned by Morris White's group in 1995 (Sun et al., 1995) and renamed Insulin Receptor Substrate-2 (IRS-2) because of its extensive homology with the originally defined substrate that is utilized by both insulin and IGF-I receptors, IRS-1. Both the IRS proteins contain inducible phosphotyrosine residues and two IRS homology domains. Similarly, both IRS proteins act by linking their cytokine receptors to signaling molecules with Src homology domains (Sun et al., 1997), like the p85 subunit of PI 3-kinase. We determined that IL-4, like IGF-I, inhibited the apoptotic death of growth-factor-deprived FDC-P1/MAC cells (Minshall et al., 1997).

The protooncogene product Bcl-2 is known to regulate cell survival in both the immune and central nervous systems (reviewed by Adams & Cory, 1998). We next established that induction of apoptosis is associated with a dramatic decrease in Bcl-2 expression and that IL-4, as well as IL-3 and IGF-I, exhibited the ability to maintain levels of intact Bcl-2 protein and prevent apoptosis (Figure 4). This effect on up-regulation of Bcl-2 was specific because IL-3, IL-4, or IGF-I did not change expression of the apoptotic inducer, Bax. We have very recently shown that inhibition of PI 3-kinase blocks the ability of IGF-I as well as IL-4, but not IL-3, to increase expression of Bcl-2 and to protect promyeloid cells from apoptosis (Minshall et al., 1999). These experiments established that the signaling pathways of IGF-I and IL-4 converge at the point of Bcl-2 and probably downstream of IRS-activation of PI 3-kinase.

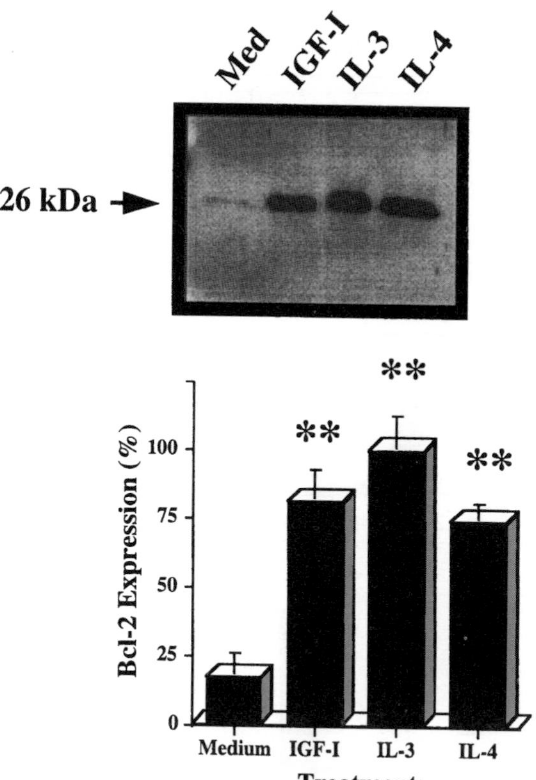

FIGURE 4 IGF-I and IL-4 prevent the decline of Bcl-2 protein following withdrawal of IL-3. Pretreatment with IGF-I or IL-4 maintains the amount of Bcl-2 protein at 85 and 90%, respectively, of those treated with IL-3 (* indicates $P < 0.01$). (Data from Minshall et al., 1997.)

C. IGF-I Promotes Differentiation of Promyeloid Cells

Although IGF-I is well known to promote the growth of many cell types, recent investigations have suggested that IGF-I may also promote differentiation of cells such as adipocytes (Valverde et al., 1998). We tested this hypothesis in human promyeloid cells by adding vitamin D_3 to induce their differentiation toward the macrophage lineage (Liu et al., 1998). As a positive control, we cultured HL-60 cells in 10% fetal bovine serum (FBS) and measured the expression of a myeloid lineage marker, the α subunit of the β_2 integrin CD11b, following addition of vitamin D_3 (Figure 5 and Table I). As expected, vitamin D_3 increased the proportion of Cd11b-expressing cells from 9 to 72%. When FBS was removed and the HL-60 cells were cultured in serum-free medium, only 21% of the progenitors differentiated into macrophages. This was not caused by serum withdrawal inducing cell death, because the proportion of apoptotic cells cultured with vitamin D_3 in the presence or absence of FBS was similar (~6%) (Table I). However, when IGF-I was added to cells treated with vitamin D_3, the proportion of cells differentiating into macrophages in serum-free medium increased from 21 to 72%. It is important that IGF-I alone did not cause myeloid progenitor cells to differentiate into macrophages (Figure 5). IGF-I-promoted macrophage differentiation was specifically blocked by preincubation of HL-60 cells with either an anti-IGF-I receptor antibody or IGFBP-3. These results established that IGF-I, a classic growth factor, is also able to promote the differentiation of myeloid progenitors into macrophages.

In similar experiments we examined the ability of vitamin A (retinoic acid) to promote the differentiation of HL-60 cells along the granulocyte lineage (Liu et al., 1997a). Once again, expression of the mature myeloid cell surface marker, CD11b, was measured. In the presence of 10% FBS, 45% of the cells developed

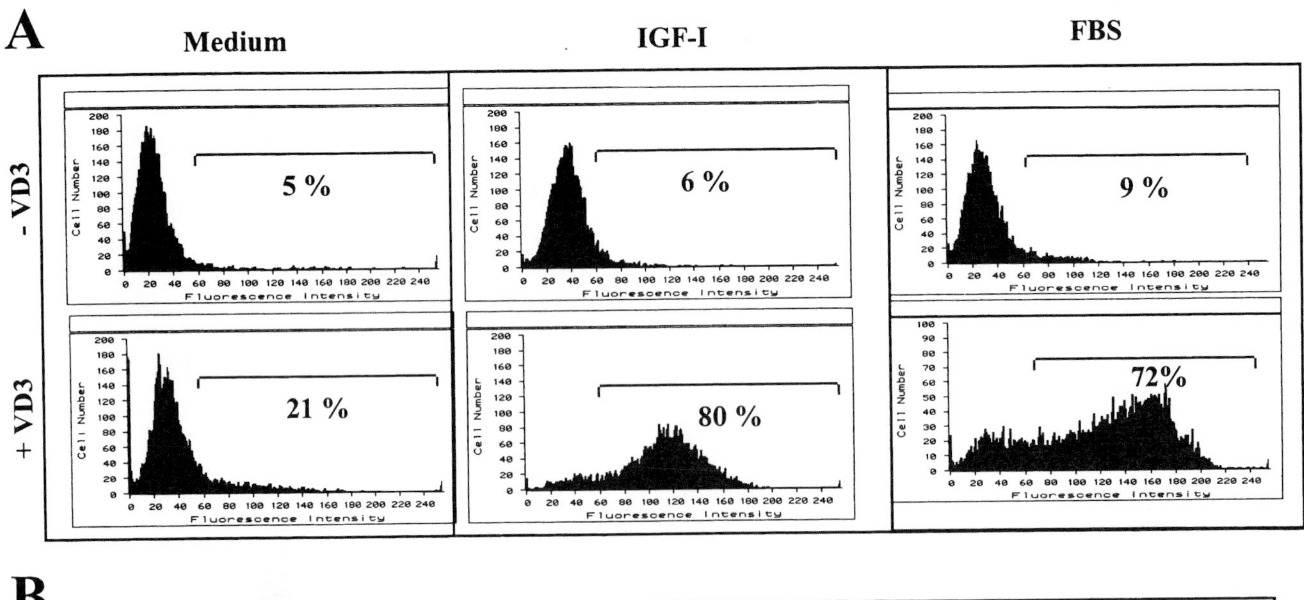

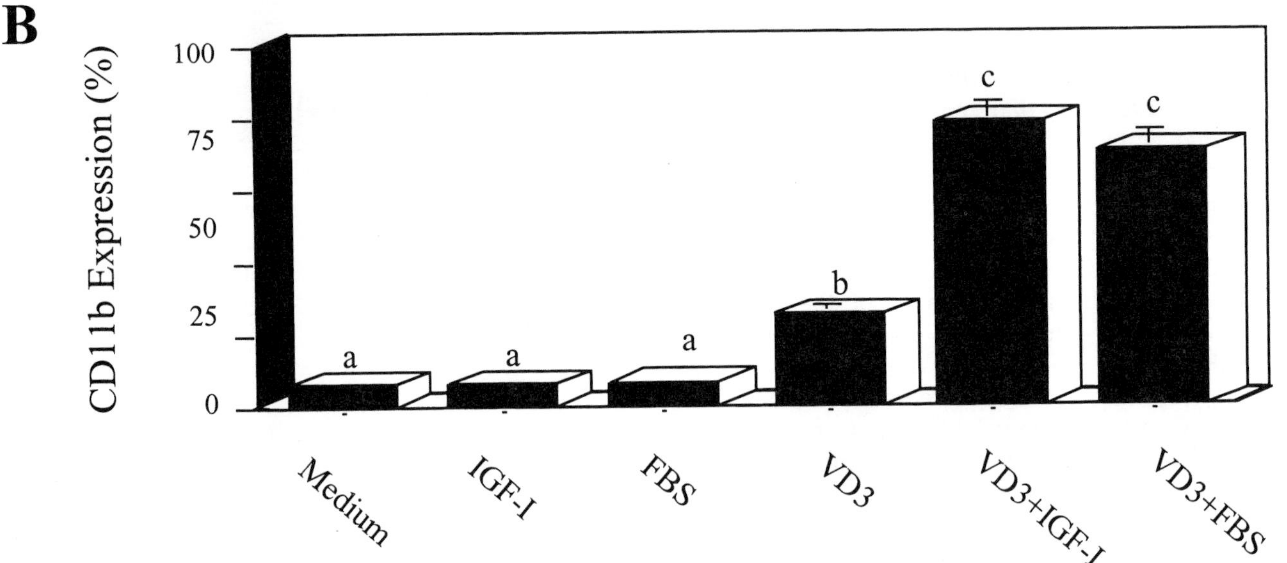

FIGURE 5 IGF-I increases vitamin D_3-induced CD11b expression in promyeloid cells. Vitamin D_3 (VD3) alone increased expression of CD11b when cultured in 10% fetal bovine serum (FBS) or in serum-free conditions. In the absence of vitamin D_3, neither IGF-I nor serum affected CD11b expression. However, when IGF-I was added to vitamin D_3-treated cells, CD11b expression increased to 80%, which was similar to the percentage of CD11b expression in vitamin D_3-treated cells cultured in 10% FBS. Columns with different superscripts are different ($P<0.01$) (Data from Liu et al., 1998.)

into granulocytes following addition of vitamin A (Table I). When serum was removed, vitamin A promoted the development of only 22% of these cells into granulocytes. This reduction was accompanied by an increase in the amount of apoptotic cells in the presence of vitamin A, from 6 to 31% (Table I). Addition of IGF-I to cells treated with vitamin A under serum-free conditions increased the proportion of CD11b-positive cells to a level that was similar to that of vitamin A-treated cells cultured in serum-containing medium. Furthermore, IGF-I prevented the increase in apoptotic cells caused by vitamin A. Blocking the IGF-I-induced activation of PI 3-kinase inhibited the ability of IGF-I to prevent apoptosis and to promote granulocyte differentiation in the presence of vitamin A. These data demonstrate that IGF-I acts on vitamin A-treated progenitors to promote their differentiation along the granulocytic lineage and on vitamin D_3-treated progenitors to increase differentiation toward the macrophage lineage, although the mechanisms of action differ according the cell lineage.

TABLE I IGF-I Promotes the Differentiation of HL-60 Promyeloid Cells along the Macrophage (Treatment with Vitamin D_3; VD3) and Granulocyte (Treatment with Retinoic Acid; RA) Lineages

Treatment	CD11b-Positive cells (%) Serum-free	CD11b-Positive cells (%) FBS	Apoptotic cells (%) Serum-free	Apoptotic cells (%) FBS
Medium	6 ± 2	7 ± 2	6 ± 3	4 ± 2
IGF-I	5 ± 2	ND	5 ± 2	ND
VD3	24 ± 3^a	70 ± 5^a	6 ± 2	6 ± 3
VD3 + IGF-I	73 ± 4^b	76 ± 3	5 ± 2	4 ± 2
RA	22 ± 2^a	45 ± 4^a	31 ± 3^c	5 ± 2
RA + IGF-I	50 ± 4^b	52 ± 5	6 ± 3	4 ± 2

Note: Data from Liu et al., (1998). HL-60 cells were incubated for 48 h in serum-free medium or 10% fetal bovine serum (FBS) plus vitamin D_3 (VD3; 1 μM), retinoic acid (RA, 1 μM) or IGF-I (100 ng/mL). ND = Not done.

[a]Indicates that vitamin D_3 and retinoic acid increased ($p < 0.01$) expression of CD11b in both serum-free medium and FBS compared with medium alone. However, expression of CD11b was consistently greater ($p < 0.01$) in the presence of FBS than in serum-free medium.

[b]Indicates that IGF-I, in the presence of either vitamin D_3 or retinoic acid, increased ($p < 0.01$) expression of CD11b in serum-free medium only when compared with vitamin D_3 or retinoic acid alone.

[c]Indicates that retinoic acid caused an increase ($p < 0.01$) in the proportion of the apoptotic cells compared with those in serum-free medium alone. This increase in apoptotic cells was totally blocked by the addition of IGF-I or FBS.

VIII. CLINICAL CONSIDERATIONS

Although growth hormone has been utilized extensively in both children and adults with growth hormone deficiency, long-term studies with humans using recombinant growth hormone are not yet available (Marcus & Hoffman, 1998). For this and other reasons, the use of growth hormone in healthy adults, other than in approved clinical trials, is not currently recommended. Following the discovery of the apparent transmission of Crutzfield-Jacob disease in preparations of human pituitary-derived growth hormone, the recombinant form of human growth hormone has become a preferred alternative in growth hormone-deficient children (Grumbach, Bin-Abbas, & Kaplan, 1998). Growth hormone affects a variety of physiologic processes, and the immune system is now recognized as one of the targeted physiologic systems. The following paragraphs summarize new results that are likely to affect the clinical application of growth hormone and IGF-I in humans.

A. Infectious Disease

Growth hormone improves host resistance to both *Salmonella typhimurium* and *E. coli* infections, as described above, likely via a direct effect on phagocytic cells. These protective effects of both growth hormone and IGF-I on gram-negative infections have now been extended to pigs (Balteskard, Unneberg, Halvorsen, Hansen, & Revhaug, 1998; Balteskard, Unneberg, Mjaaland, Jenssen, & Revhaug, 1998) and cattle (Sartin et al., 1998). However, no evidence exists that these hormones exert similar influences over recovery from parasitic infections. During the human parasitic infection of Leishmaniasis, IGF-I directly promotes growth of Leishmania parasites (Goto, Gomes, Corbett, Monteiro, & Gidlund, 1998). IGF-I is present in skin where cutaneous Leishmaniasis lesions develop and is able to bind to a receptor that is expressed on both the free (promastigotes) and phagocytized (amastigotes) forms of this parasite. IGF-I subsequently induces a rapid tyrosine phosphorylation of parasitic proteins that are unique to each form of Leishmania. IGF-I is also known to stimulate growth of the intestinal parasite *Giardia lamblia* (Lujan, Mowatt, Helman, & Nash, 1994). In parasite-infected swine, serum IGF-I levels are dramatically reduced. It is possible that decreases in growth and immune status associated with parasitic infection may be due to reduced synthesis of IGF-I in both the liver and at the inflammatory site as well as parasitic utilization of local IGF-I.

Numerous reports have noted the ability of growth hormone and IGF-I to ameliorate wasting and muscle loss associated with human immunodeficiency virus (HIV) infection (Nguyen et al., 1998). Recent reports have identified the ability of growth hormone to promote bone collagen formation in HIV-infected patients regardless of weight loss. With respect to albumin synthesis, however, the effectiveness of growth hormone therapy diminishes with the severity of disease (McNurlan et al., 1998). In the later stages of HIV infection, both lean body mass and body weight of patients are largely unresponsive to growth hormone and IGF-I treatment (McNurlan et al., 1997). It is thought that responsiveness of both growth hormone and IGF-I receptor signaling pathways is reduced as part of HIV pathology (Grinspoon, Corcoran, Stanley, Katznelson, & Klibanski, 1998), but the intracellular signals that may responsible for this receptor resistance are only beginning to be explored.

Conflicting evidence has been reported with regard to the ability of IGF-I to inhibit HIV replication in vitro. An early report of IGF-I inhibition of HIV-1 replication in cultured umbilical blood mononuclear cells and HIV-infected U937 cells (Germinario, DeSantis, & Wainberg, 1995) has been contradicted by a more recent series of experiments showing the failure of IGF-I to inhibit HIV-1 replication in these and other cells (Sharma, Song, Casella, & Schwartz, 1997).

Infection of mice with HIV-1-gp120 results in selective activation of Th2 lymphocytes, an event characterized by IL-4 production. Simultaneous administration of gp120 and growth hormone results in switching of Th2 to Th1 response (Mellado et al., 1998). This subset switch is accompanied by an increase in IFN-γ and IL-2 production and a reduction in IL-4 secretion. The ability of IGF-I to increase IL-2 production has been observed in response to several HIV envelope proteins (Nguyen et al., 1998) and may provide insight into initiation of a more robust HIV-specific immune response.

B. Prostate Cancer

The potential role of IGF-I in the etiology and progression of a variety of cancers has been recently reviewed (Baserga, Resnicoff, & Dews, 1997; Blakesley, Stannard, Kalebic, Helman, & LeRoith, 1997), so only selected recent results will be presented here. For example, Butler and colleagues, (Butler et al., 1998) showed that IGF-I promotion of cancer cell growth is largely dependent on IGF-I receptor expression. In these studies, systemic IGF-I stimulated the growth of fibrosarcoma cells derived from fibroblasts of athymic nude mice by directly stimulating mitosis. Furthermore, the tumorigenic properties of IGF-I relied on the level of IGF-I receptor expression. However, it is important to recognize that malignant prostate epithelial cells proliferate slowly, which renders metastasis to distant organs, such as bones, the clinically relevant therapeutic target of this disease.

Epidemiologic studies have correlated high levels of serum IGF-I with increased incidence of prostate cancer in older men (Chan et al., 1998; Wolk et al., 1998), resulting in four times greater risk of dying from prostate cancer if subjects were in the upper quartile of plasma IGF-I (294 to 500 ng/mL). Additionally, sex hormone-induced prostate cell carcinogenesis has been reported to depend on IGF-I, an effect that is coregulated by vascular endothelial cell growth factor (Wang & Wong, 1998). It is now appreciated that prostate specific antigen (PSA), the most commonly used clinical blood marker for prostate cancer, is in reality a protease for the IGFBP-3. PSA can reduce the interaction of IGFBP-3 with IGF-I and therefore has been reported to potentiate some of the biological effects of IGF-I (Cohen, Peehl, Graves, & Rosenfeld, 1994). We have shown that another IGF binding protein, known as IGFBP-4, is synthesized by macrophages (Li et al., 1996). Overexpression of this binding protein in an immortalized human prostate epithelial cell line (M12) retards the formation of prostate tumors in nude mice (Damon, Maddison, Ware, & Plymate, 1998). Paradoxically, expression of the IGF-I receptor on human prostate epithelial cells declines during transformation to the malignant phenotype, and reexpression of the IGF-I receptor on malignant M12 prostate epithelial cells decreases tumor growth and colony formation (Plymate, Bae, Maddison, Quinn, & Ware, 1997). In rats, however, antisense RNA directed toward the IGF-I receptor suppresses the growth of prostate cancer epithelial cells (Burfeind, Chernicky, Rininsland, Ilan, & Ilan, 1996) and glioblastomas (Trojan et al., 1993). This finding is consistent with the observation that overexpression of the p53 tumor suppressor gene reduces expression of the IGF-I receptor, which in turn promotes apoptosis (Prisco, Hongo, Rizzo, Sacchi, & Baserga, 1997). However, several other important paradoxes remain, such as the newly described ability of IGF-I to promote multidrug resistance in colon cancer cells (Guo, Jin, Houston, Thompson, & Townsend, 1998) and the ability of both IGF-I and growth hormone to promote drug (bleomycin)-induced DNA damage in human lymphocytes (Cianfarani et al., 1998). Molecular explanations for these disparate observations are not yet apparent. However, the positive correlation between high IGF-I levels in plasma and deaths attributed to prostate cancer demands that cause-and-effect experiments be conducted to answer these important questions.

C. Breast Cancer

Factors that affect the incidence and development of breast cancer are of tremendous importance since the 5-year survival rate for women with metastatic breast cancer is currently only 25–30%. Preliminary investigations of the role of IGF-I and growth hormone in breast cancer cell survival have revealed that IGF-I is mitogenic for several types of breast cancer cells (Surmacz, Guvakova, Nolan, Nicosia, & Sciacca, 1998) as well as normal, differentiated human mammary epithelial cells (Ng et al., 1997). Recently, a positive correlation was found between high plasma IGF-I and the relative risk of breast cancer, but this occurred only in a small subset of women who were premenopausal and less than 50 years of age (Hankinson et al., 1998). A potential causal relation between IGF-I and breast cancer was established by showing that the proliferation of breast cancer cells is associated with IGF-I recruitment of IRS-1 and activation of PI 3-kinase (Jackson, White, & Yee, 1998).

An important development in breast cancer research is the observation that breast cancer cells resistant to IGF-I are less likely to metastasize. Mutation of MDA-MB-435 metastatic breast cancer cells by transfection of a dominant negative form of the IGF-I receptor leads to decreased metastasis to the lung, liver, lymph nodes, and lymph vessels (Dunn et al., 1998). However, elimination of the IGF-I receptor in these cells does not significantly suppress growth of the primary tumor. In related experiments, vitamin D derivatives have been observed to limit breast cancer cell responsiveness to IGF-I, likely through inhibition of IGF-I receptor expression (Rozen, Yang, Huynh, & Pollak, 1997) or induction of IGFBP-3 (Colston, Perks, Xie, & Holly, 1998; Gill, Perks, Newcomb, & Holly, 1997).

Favorable prognosis of breast cancer patients is associated with expression of the estrogen receptor, and these estrogen receptor positive mammary adenocarcinomas often coexpress the IGF-I receptor (Papa et al., 1993). These patients may benefit from treatment with the antiestrogen tamoxifen, but this drug often leads to an increased incidence of endometrial cancer (Kleinman et al., 1996). Although estrogens are known as major growth stimulators of endometrial tumors, tamoxifen may have a similar influence by causing a sharp reduction in IGF-I binding protein levels. These results are inconsistent with findings showing that reduced IGF-I levels are one mechanism by which tamoxifen inhibits breast neoplasm proliferation (Kleinman et al., 1996). The previously mentioned FAS/CD95 apoptotic pathway has recently been shown to reduce IGF-I promotion of breast cancer cell growth when FAS/CD95 is overexpressed (Freiss, Puech, & Vignon, 1998).

D. Stroke and Demyelinating Diseases of the Nervous Systems

As a well-documented trophic factor in numerous systems, IGF-I is known to promote the growth and differentiation of many CNS cell types. IGF-I is expressed in neural tissue late in neural development and is pervasive in neurons of the thalamus, cerebellum, retina, and olfactory bulb (de Pablo & de la Rosa, 1995). In contrast to expression of the peptide, the IGF-I receptor is distributed widely throughout the brain and most predominantly during development. Although IGFBP expression is varied throughout the CNS, there is a clear increase in basal concentrations of IGFBP-3, concomitant with the increase in IGF-I, that occurs during the onset puberty in response to sex hormone secretion (Belgorosky & Rivarola, 1998). All of the IGFBPs are found in the nervous system and up-regulation of each type occurs selectively, based on location and nature of CNS insult (Hammarberg, Risling, Hokfelt, Cullheim, & Piehl, 1998).

The ability of IGF-I to inhibit normal neuronal death and to increase axonal regeneration following nerve cell injury has led to the widespread investigation of potential therapeutic applications for IGF-I in CNS disorders. In addition to neurons, glial cells are known to both express and respond to IGF-I. The rapid infiltration of astrocytes to sites of nerve damage has led to numerous investigations of a role for IGF-I in astroglial scarring. One recent report indicates that continuous infusion of IGF-I to the cerebellum decreases this type of reactive astrogliosis (Fernandez, Garcia-Estrada, Garcia-Segura, & Torres-Aleman, 1997). Similarly, overexpression of IGFBP-1 in mice results in decreased astrogliosis in response to mechanical lesion (Ni, Rajkumar, Nagy, & Murphy, 1997). Overexpression of IGF-I has also been shown to enhance myelination and overall brain size in developing mice (Carson, Behringer, Brinster, & McMorris, 1993). Clearly, more research is warranted into the nature of IGF-I interaction with various cell types in the CNS.

Preliminary results suggest that the IGF-I peptide is beneficial in treatment of several neurodegenerative diseases, including multiple sclerosis (MS) and amyotrophic lateral sclerosis (ALS) reviewed in (Dore, Kar, & Quirion 1997; McMorris & McKinnon, 1996). IGF-I is well known to promote oligodendrocyte development, myelin production, and survival via a PI 3-kinase dependent pathway (Vemuri & McMorris, 1996). Investigations into both MS and ALS have examined serum levels of IGF-I for correlation with these disorders. Patients suffering from ALS exhibited decreased IGF-I levels in conjunction with increased amounts of several circulating IGFBPs (Torres-Aleman, Barrios, Lledo, & Berciano, 1996; Torres-Aleman, Barrios, Lledo, & Berciano, 1998). On the contrary, MS patients did not display significant differences in either IGF-I or IGFBP plasma levels. In addition, IGF-I receptor density in chronic plaques of MS patient brains appears unchanged as compared with normal white matter (Wilczak & De Keyser, 1997).

In animal models of experimental autoimmune encephalomyelitis (EAE), treatment with IGF-I reduces both clinical and pathological deficits (Yao, Liu, Hudson, & Webster, 1995; Liu 1997b; Li et al., 1998). Similarly, treatment with an IGF-I/IGFBP-3 conjugate delayed onset of inflammatory cells entering the central nervous system during EAE (Lovett-Racke, Bittner, Cross, Carlino, & Racke, 1998). However, the conjugate also resulted in more severe disease, perhaps by causing proliferation of encephalitogenic T cells. Use of IGF-I as a therapeutic intervention for ALS has shown promise with respect to slowing of disease progression (Lai et al., 1997). Although the quality of life of these patients treated with IGF-I is clearly improved, the incidence of mortality is not (Borasio et al., 1998). The use of IGF-I in these cases was reported to be safe and well-tolerated, but separate clinical trials of IGF-I in type II diabetic patients have noted potential adverse effects including edema, tachycardia, and muscle and joint pain (Jabri et al., 1994).

IGF-I attenuates neuronal damage that occurs as a result of ischemia. Stroke patients exhibit an immediate decrease in plasma IGF-I and IGFBP-3 levels, which is sustained throughout 10 days postinfarct (Schwab, Spranger, Krempien, Hacke, & Bettendorf, 1997). A similar observation has been made with regard to IGF-I and IGFBP mRNA expression after hypoxic-ischemic injury in rat brain (Lee, Wang, Seaman, & Vannucci, 1996). An immediate (1 h of recovery) decrease in gene expression of all IGF-I system components becomes more pronounced at 24 h of recovery. Although IGF-I and IGFBP levels in the CNS remain low at 72 h of recovery, reactive astrocytes produce IGF-I and IGFBP-5 by this time. A more recent report (Beilharz et al., 1998) indicates that under similar conditions, IGF-I accumulates in blood vessels of the damaged area within 5 h. By 3 days of recovery, IGF-I and IGFBP-2 mRNA are strongly induced in astrocytes and microglia around the area of injury whereas IGFBP-3 and 5 are moderately induced. These same investigations failed to observe any change in IGF-I receptor expression at any time during injury or immediately following recovery. Administration of IGF-I both before (Tagami et al., 1997) and after (Guan, William, Skinner, Mallard, & Gluckman, 1996) hypoxic-ischemic injury reduces neuronal death. Use of IGF-I recombinant analogs to occupy IGFBPs, thereby releasing more IGF-I for neuroprotection, has also been shown to provide assistance in treatment of stroke (Loddick et al., 1998). Clearly, the availability of IGF-I to ischemic brain tissue, and the coordinate presence of regulatory IGFBPs, offers an important opportunity for therapeutic intervention in cases of stroke.

E. General Vascular Disease

Analysis of human vascular disease specimens consisting of atherosclerotic and restenotic lesions display increased expression of IGF-I receptors (Balaram, Agrawal, Allen, Kuszynski, & Edwards, 1997). These studies using human umbilical cord cells revealed that IGF-I increases monocyte-endothelial cell adhesion by up-regulation of specific cell adhesion molecules, including P- and E-selectin. The stimulation and adhesion of endothelial cells to leukocytes via P- and E-selectin expression is known to play an important role in the development of vascular disease (Dong et al., 1998). It is also known that growth hormone increases chemotactic responses of both human monocytes (Wiedermann, Reinisch, & Braunsteiner, 1993), and T lymphocytes (Taub et al., 1994). Finally, uptake of cholesterol by macrophages occurs early in atherosclerosis, and both growth hormone and IGF-I increase the degradation of low density lipoproteins in human monocytes (Hochberg, Aviram, Rubin, & Pollack, 1997).

IX. GROWTH HORMONE AND IGF-I: ARE THEY CYTOKINES?

A. Hormone vs. Cytokine: Generic Considerations

Both growth hormone and IGF-I are synthesized by leukocytes and affect various components of the immune system, which leads one to consider the possibility that both of these proteins are, in effect, cytokines. First, however, it is instructive to consider the general properties of both hormones and cytokines. The immune and endocrine systems are jointly involved in the maintenance of metabolic and physiologic activities as well as protection against infection and disease. Hormones and cytokines serve the joint function as primary humoral signaling molecules in this dynamic integration. In the immune system, cytokines are the major mediators of communication between T cells, B cells, macrophages and other cells of the hematopoietic lineage (Janeway & Travers, 1997). Within this array of cytokines exists a byzantine assortment of pro- and antiinflammatory agents. Likewise, in the endocrine system, hormones mediate either promotion or suppression of the immune responses. Cytokines are well known to act in both paracrine, autocrine and even endocrine (e.g., IL-6, IL-1) fashions. Similarly, hormones such as corticotropin-releasing hormone (Giraldi & Cavagnini, 1998), parathyroid hormone (Iezzoni, Bruns, Frierson, Scott, Pence, Deftos, & Bruns, 1998), and IGF-I (Walter, Berry, Hill, & Logan, 1997) are now known to act both in paracrine and autocrine modes.

Contemporary observations of hormone and cytokine action have blurred the distinctions between these two classes of compounds. The separate classification of cytokines from hormones might be considered as a useful tool for teaching medical students, whereby hormones can be dealt with in an endocrinology course and cytokines can be taught in an immunology course. This artificial separation of hormones and cytokines is even convenient for creating panels of either endocrinologists or immunologists to review research grants. Although this approach may be convenient for teaching, an arbitrary separation of hormones and cytokines into disparate physiologic systems is likely to impair progress toward understanding how the body mobilizes all of its resources to resist and recover from infectious, autoimmune, and neoplastic insults. In reality, it appears that hormones and cytokines share a number of general similarities, as outlined in Table II.

Hormones of the endocrine system were classically defined as chemicals that are synthesized in ductless glands and that are transported by the circulatory system to another region of the body. Both the tissues of hormone secretion as well as those acted on by a hormone are specific, so that one hormone is generally synthesized and secreted from a particular endocrine gland and evokes a response in one corresponding type of tissue. The rich vascularization of endocrine glands allows for rapid communication of hormones to their target organs, even at great distances (Turner & Bagnara, 1971), albeit less quickly than signals relayed by the nervous system. Exocrine tissues, such as those of the pancreatic acinar, secrete substances such as digestive enzymes through the pancreatic duct directly into the duodenum of the small intestine. In contrast, it is well known that leukocytes, cytokines and extracellular fluids find their way into the circulation via the lymph, which is collected by the thoracic duct and empties into the bloodstream via the left subclavian vein. However, it is also clear that both circulating blood lymphocytes and monocytes can also synthesize and secrete cytokines, which could be considered to be a form of direct secretion into the bloodstream, not unlike what ultimately occurs with anterior pituitary hormone secretion directly into capillary sinuses. Viewed in this way, cytokines could be considered to be of both endocrine (circulating blood leukocytes) and exocrine (through ducts of the lymphatic system) origin and to be capable of acting on distant targets. The original concept that each cytokine would have a single target cell has proven to be wrong for almost every cytokine that has been investigated.

TABLE II General Properties of Hormones and Cytokines

Characteristic	Protein hormone	Steroid hormone	Cytokine
Endocrine	✓	✓	✓
Exocrine	✓		✓
Paracrine	✓	✓	✓
Ductless glands	✓	✓	✓
Ducted glands	✓		✓
Found in circulation	✓	✓	✓
Epithelial cells	✓	✓	✓
Connective cells	✓	✓	✓
Neuronal cells	✓		✓
Cytoplasmic/nuclear receptor		✓	
Surface receptor	✓		✓
Tyrosine kinase receptor	✓		✓
Nonreceptor tyrosine kinases	✓		✓

Originally, all cytokines were measured by relatively insensitive, functional biological assays, which made it difficult to detect cytokines in the circulation. However, with the production of recombinant cytokines and technical advances that have occurred in antibody production and ELISA assays, several cytokines such as IL-1, TNF, and IL-6 (Haveman, Geerdink, & Rodermond, 1998) can now be readily detected in blood. In this general way, cytokines could be considered as both endocrine and exocrine secretions, being carried by the blood and lymph to act on distant targets. Several years ago we demonstrated how cytokines in the periphery can act as communication molecules to the brain (Kent, Bluthé, Kelley, & Dantzer, 1992). We had previously established that an intraperitoneal injection of IL-1 induces symptoms of sickness in rats, as assessed by reductions in food-motivated behavior and in social investigation. To test the hypothesis that peripheral cytokines can communicate with the brain in a biologically important manner, rats were pretreated with the IL-1 receptor antagonist in the ventricles of the brain, which was followed by an intraperitoneal injection of IL-1. As expected, peripheral injection of IL-1 caused an 86% reduction in food-motivation. However, if the rats were first pretreated in the central nervous system with the IL-1 receptor antagonist prior to the injection of peripheral IL-1, the animals showed only a 39% decrease in food motivation. Similarly, social investigation was reduced by 85% by an intraperitoneal injection of IL-1, but this decline was totally prevented by pretreatment with the IL-1 receptor antagonist into the ventricles of the brain. These data clearly established that a recombinant cytokine injected peripherally can have important biological effects that are mediated by the CNS. It therefore seems reasonable to conclude that cytokines, like hormones, can act as messengers to convey information to distant targets.

Little distinction can be made between cell types secreting hormones and cytokines. Among the four basic types of cells, consisting of epithelial, connective, muscle, and nervous cells, the profile of steroid hormone, peptide hormone, and cytokine expression is remarkably similar (Table II). For example, epithelial cells are boundary tissues that cover surfaces of organs and the body and line the lumen of organs (Alberts, Bray, Lewis, Raff, Roberts, & Watson, 1994). They are categorized by the shape (squamous, columnar) and arrangement (simple, stratified) of cells. Connective tissues support and essentially bind to tissues and organs. Connective tissues are characterized by cell matrix and type (vascular, cartilage, connective proper, bone). Muscle provides for movement of the organs, the body being composed of contractile cells (skeletal, cardiac, visceral) and fibers. Neuronal tissue is fundamental to components of the nervous system such as the brain, spinal cord, and nerves.

Steroid hormones, and notably the sex hormones, are secreted by numerous types of epithelial cells. For example, granulosa cells of the ovary synthesize and secrete progesterone (Breard, Benhaim, Feral, & Leymarie, 1998). In addition, interstitial cells of the testis, which secrete testosterone, are of connective tissue origin (Wilson, Foster, & Kronenberg, 1998). Other hormones secreted by epithelial cells include the chromaffin cells of the adrenal medulla (epinephrine/norepinephrine). Peptide hormones are produced by epithelial cells, the classic example being all of the hormone-secreting cells of the adenohypophysis as well as principal cells of the thyroid gland (thyroxine). Peptide hormones are also synthesized by neuronal cells, such as hypothalamic neurons that secrete releasing and inhibiting factors and neurons in the neurohypophysis that secrete vasopressin and oxytocin. In contrast to most cytokines, many protein hormones are stored intracellularly and released on appropriate stimulation. However, it is noteworthy that several protein hormones (e.g., ACTH, growth hormone, prolactin) and neuropeptides (e.g., corticotrophin releasing hormone, leutinizing hormone releasing hormone) are synthesized by leukocytes (Weigent & Ballock, 1995), a connective tissue. Cytokines can also be secreted by epithelial cells, such as folliculo-stellate cells of the hypophysis, which produce IL-6 (Allearts et al., 1997). However, most cytokines are a product of many cell types rather than a single organ, including cells as diverse as connective tissue (leukocytes and fibroblasts) and neurons (e.g., TNF).

Although steroid hormone receptors are detected in the cytoplasm/nucleus of target cells, receptors for both cytokines and protein hormones are expressed on the cell surface (Wilson et al., 1998). Some of these receptors for hormones (e.g., insulin) and cytokines (e.g, stem cell factor, macrophage colony-stimulating factor) contain intracellular chains that are tyrosine kinases, whereas others use intracellular nonreceptor protein tyrosine kinases in their signaling pathway (e.g., growth hormone, prolactin, IL-3). Indeed, the large number of general similarities between hormones and cytokines suggest that there is little a priori reason to consider them as two distinct groups of proteins that are involved only in the functioning of the endocrine and immune systems, respectively.

B. Growth Hormone and IGF-I as Cytokines?

Both growth hormone and IGF-I exhibit characteristics classically reserved for cytokines. Although growth hormone-deficient children generally are not predisposed to an overabundance of clinical infections or tumors (Auernhammer et al., 1996; Bidlingmaier et al., 1997; Kelley, 1989; Velkeniers, Dogusan, Naessens, Hoogh, & Hooghe-Peters, 1998), neither are a number of animals that have a genetic deletion in a number of cytokine genes, including the first two cytokines that were discovered (IL-1 and IL-2). Like recombinant cytokines, this finding does not diminish the potential usefulness of hormones and cytokines to improve immunological defense systems. It would therefore seem that the classic cytokine properties of pleiotropy and redundancy apply to the immunological effects of growth hormone and IGF-I. A variety of mononuclear and polymorphonuclear myeloid cells, as well as lymphocytes, express surface receptors for both these hormones. Although most of the circulating growth hormone is derived from the adenohypophysis and that of IGF-I from the liver, the role of locally synthesized and released IGF-I is key to the promotion and maintenance of neuronal survival in the CNS (Dudek et al., 1997). Several years ago we proposed a model for the autocrine and paracrine immunological effects of IGF-I in the bone marrow, thymus, and lymph nodes (Kelley, Arkins, & Li, 1992). We have updated this model by showing that growth hormone and IGF-I are very similar to hematopoietic cytokines because both affect three general properties of myeloid and lymphoid cells and their progenitors: (a) promoting cell survival and differentiation, (b) increasing DNA synthesis, and (c) enhancing effector functions (Arkins et al., in press). The fact that growth hormone-secreting cells of the adenohypophysis express abundant receptors for the cytokine IL-1, and that myeloid cells that synthesize abundant IL-1 express receptors for both growth hormone and IGF-I, provides a structural basis for reciprocal regulation of the immune and endocrine systems. Expression of IGF-I in leukocytes is increased by cytokines other than growth hormone, including CSF-1, IL-3, IL-1, and TNF-α, whereas IFN-γ inhibits expression of IGF-I (Arkins et al., in press). In the central nervous system, IGF-I promotes the survival of neurons (Dudek et al., 1997) as well as hematopoietic progenitors (Minshall et al., 1997).

Taken collectively, these facts support the view that two hormones that were originally discovered as major players in growth physiology are also very actively involved in immunophysiology. As such, growth hormone and IGF-I should be considered as both hormones and cytokines. It is likely that other cytokines that have already been discovered will prove to be hormones, and vice versa. Trying to understand these evolving concepts is what makes research in the fast-moving area of immunophysiology, and the broader area of psychoneuroimmunology, so much fun.

Acknowledgments

This work was supported by grants to K.W.K from the National Institutes of Health (AG-06246, DK-49311 and MH-51569) and the Pioneering Research Project in Biotechnology financed by the Japanese Ministry of Agriculture, Forestry and Fisheries.

References

Adams, J. M., & Cory, S. (1998). The Bcl-2 protein family: Arbiters of cell survival. *Science, 281*, 1322–1326.

Alberts, B., Bray, D., Lewis, J., Raff, M., & Roberts, K., Watson, J., (1994). *Molecular biology of the cell* New York: Garland Publishing.

Allaerts, W., Jeucken, P. H., Debets, R., Hoefakker, S., Claassen, E., & Drexhage, H. A. (1997). Heterogeneity of pituitary folliculo-stellate cells: Implications for interleukin-6 production and accessory function in vitro. *Journal of Neuroendocrinology*, 9, 43–53.

Argetsinger, L. S., Hsu, G. W., Myers, M. G. Jr., Billestrup, N., White, M. F., & Carter-Su, C. (1995). Growth hormone, interferon-γ, and leukemia inhibitory factor promoted tyrosyl phosphorylation of insulin receptor substrate-1. *Journal of Biological Chemistry, 270*, 14685–14692.

Arkins, S., Dantzer, R., & Kelley, K. W. (1993). Somatolactogens, somatomedins and immunity. *Journal of Dairy Science, 76*, 2437–2450.

Arkins, S., Johnson, R. W., Minshall, C., Dantzer, R., & Kelley, K. W. (in press). Immunophysiology: The interaction of hormones, lymphohemopoietic cytokines and the neuroimmune axis. In B. S. McEwen (Ed.), *Coping with the environment: Neural and endocrine mechanisms, handbook of physiology*, Section 7: *Endocrinology*, vol. 4. New York: Oxford University Press.

Arkins, S., Rebeiz, N., Biragyn, A., Reese, D. L., & Kelley, K. W. (1993). Murine macrophages express abundant IGF-I class I, Ea and Eb transcripts. *Endocrinology, 133*, 2334–2343.

Arkins, S., Rebeiz, N., Brunke-Reese, D. L., Biragyn, A., & Kelley, K. W. (1995). Interferon-gamma inhibits macrophage insulin-like growth factor-I synthesis at the transcriptional level. *Molecular Endocrinology, 9*, 350–360.

Arkins, S., Rebeiz, N., Brunke-Reese, D. L., Minshall, C., & Kelley, K. W. (1995). The colony stimulating factors induce expression of insulin-like growth factor-I messenger ribonucleic acid during hematopoiesis. *Endocrinology, 136*, 1153–1160.

Auernhammer, C. J., Feldmeier, H., Nass, R., Pachmann, K., & Strasburger, C. J. (1996). Insulin-like growth factor I is an independent coregulatory modulator of natural killer (NK) cell activity. *Endocrinology, 137*, 5332–5336.

Avalos, B. R., Hunter, M. G., Parker, J. M., Ceselski, S. K., Druker, B. J., Corey, S. J., & Mehta, V. B. (1995). Point mutations in the conserved box 1 region inactivate the human granulocyte colony-stimulating factor receptor for growth signal transduction and tyrosine phosphorylation of p75c-rel. *Blood, 85*, 3117–3126.

Balaram, S. K., Agrawal, D. K., Allen, R. T., Kuszynski, C. A., & Edwards, J. D. (1997). Cell adhesion molecules and insulin-like growth factor-1 in vascular disease *Journal of Vascular Surgeryy, 25*, 866–876.

Balteskard, L., Unneberg, K., Mjaaland, M., Jenssen, T. G., & Revhaug, A. (1998). Growth hormone and insulin-like growth factor 1 promote intestinal uptake and hepatic release of glutamine in sepsis. *Annals of Surgery, 228*, 131–139.

Balteskard, L., Unneberg, K., Halvorsen, D., Hansen, J. B., & Revhaug, A. (1998). Effects of insulin-like growth factor 1 on neutrophil and monocyte functions in normal and septic states. *Journal of Parenteral and Enteral Nutrition, 22*, 127–135.

Baserga, R. (1994). Oncogenes and the strategy of growth factors. *Cell, 79*, 927–930.

Baserga, R., Resnicoff, M., & Dews, M. (1997). The IGF-I receptor and cancer. *Endocrine, 7*, 99–102.

Beilharz, E. J., Russo, V. C., Butler, G., Baker, N. L., Connor, B., Sirimanne, E. S., Dragunow, M., Werther, G. A., Gluckman, P. D., Williams, C. E., & Scheepens, A. (1998). Co-ordinated and cellular specific induction of the components of the IGF/IGFBP axis in the rat brain following hypoxic-ischemic injury. *Brain Research Molecular Brain Research, 31*, 119–134.

Belgorosky, A., & Rivarola, M. A. (1998). Irreversible increase of serum IGF-1 and IGFBP-3 levels in GnRH-dependent precocious puberty of different etiologies: Implications for the onset of puberty. *Hormone Research, 49*, 226–232.

Benveniste, E. N. (1992). Inflammatory cytokines within the central nervous system: Sources, function, and mechanism of action. *American Journal Physiology, 263*, C1-C16.

Berkenbosch, F., van Oers, J., Del Rey, A., Tilders, F., & Besedovsky, H. (1987). Corticotropin-releasing factor-producing neurons in the rat activated by interleukin-1. *Science, 238*, 524–526.

Berczi, I. (1997). Pituitary hormones and immune function. *Acta Paediatrica, 423* (suppl.), 70–75.

Bernton, E. W., Beach, J. E., Holaday, J. W., Smallridge, R. C., & Fein, H. G. (1987). Release of multiple hormones by a direct action of interleukin-1 on pituitary cells. *Science, 238*, 519–521.

Bernton, E. W., Meltzer, M. S., & Holaday, J. W. (1988). Suppression of macrophage activation and T-lymphocyte function in hypoprolactinemic mice. *Science, 239*, 401–404.

Besedovsky, H. O., del Rey, A. E., & Sorkin, E. (1985). Immune-neuroendocrine interactions. *Journal of Immunology, 135*, 750s–754s.

Besedovsky, H. O., del Rey, A. E., Sorkin, E., & Dinarello, C. A. (1986). Immunoregulatory feedback between interleukin-1 and glucocorticoid hormones. *Science, 233*, 652–654.

Besedovsky, H. O., del Rey, A. E., & Sorkin, E. (1981). Lymphokine-containing supernatants from Con A-stimulated cells increase corticosterone blood levels. *Journal of Immunology, 126*, 385–387.

Besedovsky, H. O., Sorkin, E., Keller, M., & Muller, J. (1975). Changes in blood hormone levels during the immune response. *Proceedings of the Society of Experimental Biological Medicine, 150,* 466–470.

Bidlingmaier, M., Auernhammer, C. J., Feldmeier, H., & Strasburger, C. J. (1997). Effects of growth hormone and insulin-like growth factor I binding to natural killer cells. *Acta Paediatrica, 423* (suppl.), 80–81.

Bitar, M. S. (1997). Insulin-like growth factor-1 reverses diabetes-induced wound healing impairment in rats. *Hormone Metabolism Research, 29,* 383–386.

Bjerknes, R., & Aarskog, D. (1995). Priming of human polymorphonuclear neutrophilic leukocytes by insulin-like growth factor I: Increased phagocytic capacity, complement receptor expression, degranulation, and oxidative burst. *Journal of Clinical Endocrinolgy Metabolism, 80,* 1948–1955.

Blakesley, V. A., Stannard, B. S., Kalebic, T., Helman, L. J., & LeRoith, D. (1997). Role of the IGF-I receptor in mutagenesis and tumor promotion. *Journal of Endocrinology, 152,* 339–344.

Blalock, J. E. (1984). The immune system as a sensory organ. *Journal of Immunology, 132,* 1067–1070.

Blalock, J. E. (1994b). The immune system. Our sixth sense. *Immunologist, 2,* 8–15.

Blalock, J. E. (1994a). The syntax of immune-neuroendocrine communication. *Immunology Today, 15,* 504–511.

Blalock, J. E., Harbour-McMenamin, D., & Smith, E. M. (1985). Peptide hormones shared by the neuroendocrine and immunologic systems. *Journal of Immunology, 135,* 858s–861s.

Blazar, B. R., Brennan, C. A., Broxmeyer, H. E., Shultz, L. D., & Vallera, D. A. (1995). Transgenic mice expressing either bovine growth hormone (bGH) or human GH releasing hormone (hGRH) have increased splenic progenitor cell colony formation and DNA synthesis in vitro and in vivo. *Experimental Hematology, 23,* 1397–1406.

Borasio, G. D., Robberecht, W., Leigh, P. N., Emile, J., Guiloff, R. J., Jerusalem, F., Silani, V., Vos, P. E., Wokke, J. H., & Dobbins, T. (1998). A placebo-controlled trial of insulin-like growth factor-I in amyotrophic lateral sclerosis. *Neurology, 51,* 583–586.

Breard, E., Benhaim, A., Feral, C., & Leymarie, P. (1998). Rabbit ovarian production of interleukin-6 and its potential effects on gonadotropin-induced progesterone secretion in granulosa and theca cells. *J Endocrinology, 159,* 479–487.

Breese, C. R., D'Costa, A., Rollins, Y. D., Adams, C., Booze, R. M., Sonntag, W. E., & Leonard, S. (1996). Expression of insulin-like growth factor-1 (IGF-1) and IGF-binding protein 2 (IGF-BP2) in the hippocampus following cytotoxic lesion of the dentate gyrus. *Journal Comparative Neurology, 369,* 388–404.

Briard, N., Guillaume, V., Frachebois, C., Rico-Gomez, M., Sauze, N., Oliver, C., & Dutour, A. (1998). Endotoxin injection increases growth hormone and somatostatin secretion in sheep. *Endocrinology, 139,* 2662–2669.

Burfeind, P., Chernicky, C. L., Rininsland, F., Ilan, J., & Ilan, J. (1996). Antisense RNA to the type I insulin-like growth factor receptor suppresses tumor growth and prevents invasion by rat prostate cancer cells in vivo. *Proceedings of the National Academy of Sciences of the United States of America, 93,* 7263–7268.

Burgess, W., Liu, Q., Zhou, J., Tang, Q., Ozawa, A., VanHoy, R., Arkins, S., Dantzer, R., & Kelley, K. W. (1999). The immune-endocrine loop during aging: Role of growth hormone and insulin-like growth factor-I. *Neuroimmunomodulation, 6,* 56–68.

Butler, A. A., Blakesley, V. A., Tsokos, M., Wood, T. L., LeRoith, D., Pouliki, V. (1998). Stimulation of tumor growth by recombinant human insulin-like growth factor-I (IGF-I) is dependent on the dose and the level of IGF-I receptor expression. *Cancer Research, 58,* 3021–3027.

Carson, M. J., Behringer, R. R., Brinster, R. L., & McMorris, F. A. (1993). Insulin-like growth factor I increases brain growth and central nervous system myelination in transgenic mice. *Neuron, 10,* 729–740.

Ceda, G. P., Dall'Aglio, E., Magnacavallo, A., Vargas, N., Fontana, V., Maggio, M., Valenti, G., Lee, P. D., Hintz, R. L., & Hoffman, A. R. (1998). The insulin-like growth factor axis and plasma lipid levels in the elderly. *Journal of Clinical Endocrinology Metabolism, 83,* 499–502.

Chan, J. M., Stampfer, M. J., Giovannucci, E., Gann, P. H., Ma, J., Wilkinson, P., Hennekens, C. H., & Pollak, M. (1998). Plasma insulin-like growth factor-I and prostate cancer risk: A prospective study. *Science, 279,* 563–566.

Chen, H. T., Schuler, L. A., & Schultz, R. D. (1998). Growth hormone receptor and regulation of gene expression in fetal lymphoid cells. *Molecular and Cellular Endocrinology, 137,* 21–29.

Cianfarani, S., Tedeschi, B., Germani, D., Prete, S. P., Rossi, P., Vernole, P., Caporossi, D., & Boscherini, B. (1998). In vitro effects of growth hormone (GH) and insulin-like growth factor I and II (IGF-I and -II) on chromosome fragility and p53 protein expression in human lymphocytes. *European Journal of Clinical Investigation, 28,* 41–47.

Clark, R. (1997). The somatogenic hormones and insulin-like growth factor-1: Stimulators of lymphopoiesis and immune function. *Endocrinology Review, 18,* 157–179.

Cohen, P., Peehl, D. M., Graves, H. C., & Rosenfeld, R. G. (1994). Biological effects of prostate specific antigen as an insulin-like growth factor binding protein-3 protease. *Journal of Endocrinology,* 142, 407–415.

Colston, K. W., Perks, C. M., Xie, S. P., & Holly, J. M. (1998). Growth inhibition of both MCF-7 and Hs578T human breast cancer cell lines by vitamin D analogues is associated with increased expression of insulin-like growth factor binding protein-3. *Journal of Molecular Endocrinology, 20,* 157–162.

Dahn, M. S., & Lange, M. P. (1998). Systemic and splanchnic metabolic response to exogenous human growth hormone *Surgery, 123,* 528–538.

Damon, S. E., Maddison, L., Ware, J. L., & Plymate, S. R. (1998). Overexpression of an inhibitory insulin-like growth factor binding protein (IGFBP), IGFBP-4, delays onset of prostate tumor formation. *Endocrinology, 139,* 3456–3464.

Dardenne, M., Mello-Coelho, V., Gagnerault, M. C., & Postel-Vinay, M. C. (1998). Growth hormone receptors and immunocompetent cells. *Annals of the New York Academy of Science, 840,* 510–517.

D'Mello, S. R., Galli, C., Ciotti, T., & Calissano, P. (1993). Induction of apoptosis in cerebellar granule neurons by low potassium: Inhibition of death by insulin-like growth factor I and cAMP. *Proceedings of the National Academy of Sciences of the United States of America, 90,* 10989–10993.

de Mello-Coelho, V., Gagnerault, M. C., Saberbielle, J. C., Strasburger, C. J., Savino, W., Dardenne, M., & Postel-Vinay, M. C. (1998). Growth hormone and its receptor are expressed in human thymic cells. *Endocrinology, 139,* 3837–3842

de Mello-Coelho, V., Savino, W., Postel-Vinay, M. C., & Dardenne, M. (1998). Role of prolactin and growth hormone on thymus physiology. *Developmental Immunology, 6,* 317–323.

de Mello-Coelho, V., Villa-Verde, D. M., Dardenne, M., & Savino, W. (1997). Pituitary hormones modulate cell-cell interactions between thymocytes and thymic epithelial cells. *Journal of Neuroimmunology, 76,* 39–49.

de Pablo, F., & de la Rosa, E. J. (1995). The developing CNS: A scenario for the action of proinsulin, insulin and insulin-like growth factors. *Trends in Neuroscience, 18*, 143–150.

Dong, Z., & Wortis, H. H. (1994). Function of bone marrow stromal cell lines derived from nude mice. *Journal of Immunology, 153*, 1441–1448.

Dong, Z. M., Chapman, S. M., Brown, A. A., Frenette, P. S., Hynes, R. O., & Wagner D. D. (1998). The combined role of P- and E-selectins in atherosclerosis. *Journal of Clinical Investigation, 102* 145–152.

Dore, S., Kar, S., & Quirion, R. (1997). Rediscovering an old friend, IGF-I: Potential use in the treatment of neurodegenerative diseases. *Trends in Neuroscience, 20*, 326–331.

Downward, J. (1995). Signal transduction: A target for PI(3) kinase. *Nature, 376*, 553–554.

Dudek, H., Datta, S. R., Franke, T. F., Birnbaum, M. J., Yao, R., Cooper, G. M., Segal, R. A., Kaplan, D. R., & Greenberg, M. E. (1997). Regulation of neuronal survival by the serine-threonine protein kinase Akt. *Science, 275*, 661–665.

Dunn, S. E., Ehrlich, M., Sharp, N. J., Solomon, G., Hawkins, R., Baserga, R., & Barrett, J. C. (1998). A dominant negative mutant of the insulin-like growth factor-I receptor inhibits the adhesion, invasion, and metastasis of breast cancer. *Cancer Research, 58*, 3353–3361.

Edmondson, S. R., Werther, G. A., Russell, A., LeRoith, D., Roberts, C. T. Jr., & Beck, F. (1995). Localization of growth hormone receptor/binding protein messenger ribonucleic acid (mRNA) during rat fetal development: Relationship to insulin-like growth factor-I mRNA. *Endocrinology, 136*, 4602–4609.

Edwards, C. K. III, Ghiasuddin, S. M., Schepper, J. M., Yunger, L. M., & Kelley, K. W. (1988). A newly defined property of somatotropin: priming of macrophages for production of superoxide anion. *Science, 239*, 769–771.

Edwards, C. K. III, Ghiasuddin, S. M., Yunger, L. M., Lorence, R. M., Arkins, S., Dantzer, R., & Kelley, K. W. (1992). In vivo administration of recombinant growth hormone or interferon-γ activates macrophages: Enhanced resistance to experimental *Salmonella typhimurium* infection is correlated with the generation of reactive oxygen intermediates. *Infection and Immunity, 60*, 2514–2521.

Edwards, C. K. III, Lorence, R. M., Dunham, D. M., Arkins, S., Yunger, L. M., Greager, J. A., Walter, R. J., Dantzer, R., & Kelley, K. W. (1991). Hypophysectomy inhibits the synthesis of tumor necrosis factor γ by rat macrophages: Partial restoration by exogenous growth hormone or interferon γ. *Endocrinology, 128*, 989–996.

Edwards, C. K. III, Yunger, L. M., Lorence, R. M., Dantzer, R., & Kelley, K. W. (1991). The pituitary gland is required for protection against lethal effects of *Salmonella typhimurium*. *Proceedings of the National Academy of Sciences of the United States of America, 88*, 2274–2277.

Fabris, N., Mocchegiani, E., & Provinciali, M. (1997). Plasticity of neuroendocrine-thymus interactions during aging. *Experiments in Gerontology, 32*, 415–429.

Fan, J., Molina, P. E., Gelato, M. C., & Lang, C. H. (1994). Differential tissue regulation of insulin-like growth factor-I content and binding proteins after endotoxin. *Endocrinology, 134*, 1685–1692.

Fernandez, A. M., Garcia-Estrada, J., Garcia-Segura, L. M., & Torres-Aleman, I. (1997). Insulin-like growth factor I modulates c-Fos induction and astrocytosis in response to neurotoxic insult. *Neuroscience, 76*, 117–122.

Foster, M., Montecino-Rodriguez, E., Clark, R., & Dorshkind, K. (1998). Regulation of B and T cell development by anterior pituitary hormones. *Cellular Molecular Life Science, 54*, 1076–1082.

Freiss, G., Puech, C., & Vignon, F. (1998). Extinction of insulin-like growth factor-I mitogenic signaling by antiestrogen-stimulated Fas-associated protein tyrosine phosphatase-1 in human breast cancer cells. *Molecular Endocrinology, 12*, 568–579.

French, R. A., Zachary, J., Dantzer, R., Frawley, S., Chizzonite, R., Parnet, P.,& Kelley, K. W. (1996). Dual expression of p80 type I and p68 type II interleukin-1 receptors on anterior pituitary cells synthesizing growth hormone. *Endocrinology, 137*, 4027–4036.

Fry, C., Gunter, D. R., McMahon, C. D., Steele, B., & Sartin, J. L. (1998). Cytokine-mediated growth hormone release from cultured ovine pituitary cells. *Neuroendocrinology, 68*, 192–200.

Fu, Y. K., Arkins, S., Fuh, G., Cunningham, B. C., Wells, J. A., Fong, S., Cronin, M. J., Dantzer, R., & Kelley, K. W. (1992). Growth hormone augments superoxide anion secretion of human neutrophils by binding to the prolactin receptor. *Journal of Clinical Investigation, 89*, 451–457.

Fu, Y. K., Arkins, S., Li, Y. M, Dantzer, R., & Kelley, K. W. (1994). Reduction in superoxide anion secretion and bactericidal activity of neutrophils from aged rats: Reversal by the combination of gamma interferon and growth hormone. *Infection and Immunity, 62*, 1–8.

Fu, Y. K., Arkins, S., Wang, B. S., & Kelley, K.W. (1991). A novel role of growth hormone and insulin-like growth factor-I, Priming neutrophils for superoxide anion secretion. *Journal of Immunology, 146*, 1602–1608.

Fukata, J., Usui, T., Nakai, Y., & Imura, H. (1989). Effects of recombinant human interleukin-1α, -1β, -2 and -6 on ACTH synthesis and release in the mouse pituitary tumor line AtT-20. *Journal of Endocrinology, 122*, 33–39.

Geffner, M. (1997). Effects of growth hormone and insulin-like growth factor I on T- and B-lymphocytes and immune function *Acta Paediatrica, 423*, (suppl.) 76–79.

Germinario, R. J., DeSantis, T., & Wainberg, M. A. (1995). Insulin-like growth factor 1 and insulin inhibit HIV type 1 replication in cultured cells *AIDS Research Human Retroviruses, 11*, 555–561.

Gibson, L. F., Piktel, D., & Landreth, K. S. (1993). Insulin-like growth factor-I potentiates expansion of interleukin-7 dependent pro-B cells. *Blood, 82*, 3005–3011.

Gill, Z. P., Perks, C. M., Newcomb, P. V., & Holly, J. M. (1997). Insulin-like growth factor-binding protein (IGFBP-3) predisposes breast cancer cells to programmed cell death in a non-IGF-dependent manner. *Journal of Biological Chemistry, 272*, 25602–25607.

Giraldi, F. P., & Cavagnini, F. (1998). Corticotropin-releasing hormone is produced by rat corticotropes and modulates ACTH secretion in a paracrine/autocrine fashion. *Journal of Clinical Investigation, 101*, 2478–2484.

Gonzalo, J. A., Mazuchelli, R., Mellado, M., Frade, J. M., Carrera, A. C., von Kobbe, C., Merida, I., & Martinez,- A. C. (1996). Enterotoxin septic shock protection and deficient T helper 2 cytokine production in growth hormone transgenic mice. *Journal of Immunology, 157*, 3298–3304.

Goto, H., Gomes, C. M., Corbett, C. E., Monteiro, H. P., & Gidlund, M. (1998). Insulin-like growth factor I is a growth-promoting factor for Leishmania promastigotes and amastigotes. *Proceedings of the National Academy of Sciences of the United States of America, 95*, 13211–13216

Grinspoon, S., Corcoran, C., Stanley, T., Katznelson, L., & Klibanski, A. (1998). Effects of androgen administration on the growth hormone-insulin-like growth factor I axis in men with acquired immunodeficiency syndrome wasting. *Journal of Clinical Endocrinology Metabolism, 83*, 4251–4256.

Grumbach, M. M., Bin-Abbas, B. S., & Kaplan, S. L. (1998). The growth hormone cascade: Progress and long-term results of growth hormone treatment in growth hormone deficiency. *Hormone Research, 49*, 41–57.

Guan, J., Williams, C. E., Skinner, S. J., Mallard, E. C., & Gluckman, P. D. (1996). The effects of insulin-like growth factor (IGF)-1, IGF-2, and des-IGF-1 on neuronal loss after hypoxic-ischemic brain injury in adult rats: Evidence for a role for IGF binding proteins. *Endocrinology, 137*, 893–898.

Guicheux, J., Heymann, D., Rousselle, A. V., Gouin, F., Pilet, P., Yamada, S., & Daculsi G. (1998). Growth hormone stimulatory effects on osteoclastic resorption are partly mediated by insulin-like growth facor I: An in vitro study. *Bone, 22*, 25–31.

Guo, Y. S., Jin, G. F., Houston, C. W., Thompson, J. C., & Townsend, C. M. Jr. (1998). Insulin-like growth factor-I promotes multidrug resistance in MCLM colon cancer cells. *Journal of Cell Physiology, 175*, 141–148.

Hammarberg, H., Risling, M., Hokfelt, T., Cullheim, S., & Piehl, F. (1998). Expression of insulin-like growth factors and corresponding binding proteins (IGFBP 1-6) in rat spinal cord and peripheral nerve after axonal injuries. *Journal of Comparative Neurology, 400*, 57–72.

Hankinson, S. E., Willett, W. C., Colditz, G. A., Hunter, D. J., Michaud, D. S., Deroo, B., Rosner, B., Speizer, F. E., & Pollak, M. (1998). Circulating concentrations of insulin-like growth factor-I and risk of breast cancer. *Lancet, 351*, 1393–1396.

Harrison, M., Dunger, A. M., Berg, S., Mabley, J., John, N., Green, M. H., & Green, I.C. (1998). Growth factor protection against cytokine-induced apoptosis in neonatal rat islets of Langerhans: Role of Fas. *FEBS Letters, 435*, 207–210.

Haveman, J., Geerdink, A. G., & Rodermond, H. M. (1998). TNF, IL-1 and IL-6 in circulating blood after total-body and localized irradiation in rats. *Oncology Reports, 5*, 679–683.

Hernandez-Sanchez, C., Lopez-Carranza, A., Alarcon, C., de La Rosa, E. J., & de Pablo, F. (1995). Autocrine/paracrine role of insulin-related growth factors in neurogenesis: Local expression and effects on cell proliferation and differentiation in retina. *Proceedings of the National Academy of Sciences of the United States of America, 92*, 9834–98348.

Hinton, P. S., Peterson, C. A., Dahly, E. M., & Ney, D. M. (1998). IGF-I alters lymphocyte survival and regeneration in thymus and spleen after dexamethasone treatment. *American Journal of Physiology, 274*, R912–R920.

Hochberg, Z., Aviram, M., Rubin, D., & Pollack, S. (1997). Decreased sensitivity to insulin-like growth factor I in Turner's syndrome: A study of monocytes and T lymphocytes. *European Journal of Clinical Investigation, 27*, 543–547.

Hooghe-Peters, E. L., & Hooghe, R. (1995). *Growth hormone, prolactin and IGF-I as lymphohemopoietic cytokines.* Austin: R. G. Landes.

Hueber, A. O., Zornig, M., Lyon, D., Suda, T., Nagata, S., & Evan, G.I. (1997). Requirement for the CD95 receptor-ligand pathway in c-Myc-induced apoptosis. *Science, 278*, 1305–1309.

Hull, K. L., & Harvey, S. (1998). Autoregulation of central and peripheral growth hormone receptor mRNA in domestic fowl. *Journal of Endocrinology, 156*, 323–329.

Iezzoni, J. C., Bruns, M. E., Frierson, H. F., Scott, M. G., Pence, R. A., Deftos, L. J., & Bruns, D. E. (1998). Coexpression of parathyroid hormone-related protein and its receptor in breast carcinoma: A potential autocrine effector system. *Modern Pathology, 11*, 265–270.

Inoue, T., Saito, H., Matsuda, T., Fukatsu, K., Han, I., Furukawa, S., Ikeda, S., & Muto, T. (1998a). Growth hormone and insulin-like growth factor I augment bactericidal capacity of human polymorphonuclear neutrophils. *Shock, 10*, 278–284.

Inoue, T., Saito, H., Tsuno, N., Fukatsu, K., Lin, M. T., Inaba, T., Han, I., Furukawa, S., Ikeda, S., Matsuda, T., & Muto, T. (1998b). Effects of growth hormone and insulin-like growth factor I on opsonin receptor expression on local and systemic phagocytes in a lethal peritonitis model. *Critical Care Medicine, 26*, 338–343.

Jabri, N., Schalch, D. S., Schwartz, S. L., Fischer, J. S., Kipnes, M. S., Radnik, B. J., Turman, N. J., Marcsisin, V. S., & Guler, H. P. (1994). Adverse effects of recombinant human insulin-like growth factor I in obese insulin-resistant type II diabetic patients. *Diabetes, 43*, 369–374.

Jackson, J. G., White, M. F., & Yee, D. (1998). Insulin receptor substrate-1 is the predominant signaling molecule activated by insulin-like growth factor-I, insulin, and interleukin-4 in estrogen receptor-positive human breast cancer cells. *Journal of Biological Chemistry, 273*, 9994–10003.

Janeway, C. & Travers, P., (1997). *Immunobiology* New York: Garland.

Jardieu, P., Clark, R., Mortensen, D., & Dorshkind K. (1994). In vivo administration of insulin-like growth factor-I stimulates primary B lymphopoiesis and enhances lymphocyte recovery after bone marrow transplantation. *Journal of Immunology, 152*, 4320–4327.

Jendraschak, E., Kaminski, W. E., Kiefl, R., & von Schacky C. (1998). IGF-1, PDGF and CD18 are adherence-responsive genes: Regulation during monocyte differentiation. *Biochimica Biophysica Acta, 1396*, 320–335.

Johnson, E. W., Blalock, J. E., & Smith, E. M. (1988). ACTH receptor-mediated induction of leukocyte cyclic AMP. *Biochemistry Biophysics Research Communications, 157*, 1205–1211.

Johnson, R. W., Arkins, S., Dantzer, R., & Kelley, K. W. (1997). Hormones, lymphohemopoietic cytokines and the neuroimmune axis. *Comparative Biochemistry and Physiology, 116*, 183–201.

Jones, J. I., & Clemmons, D. R. (1995). Insulin-like growth factors and their binding proteins: Biological actions. *Endocrinology Review, 16*, 3–34.

Kakucska, I., Qi, Y., Clark, B. D., & Lechan, R. M. (1993). Endotoxin-induced corticortropin-releasing hormone gene expression in the hypothalamic paraventricular nucleus is mediated centrally by interleukin-1. *Endocrinology, 133*, 815–821.

Kelley, K. W. (1989). Growth hormone, lymphocytes and macrophages. *Biochemical Pharmacology, 38*, 705–713.

Kelley, K. W., Arkins, S., & Li, Y. M. (1992). Growth hormone, prolactin, and insulin-like growth factors: New jobs for old players. *Brain, Behavior, and Immunology, 6*, 317–326.

Kelley, K. W., Arkins, S., Minshall, C., Liu, Q., & Dantzer, R., (1996). Growth hormone, growth factors and hematopoiesis. *Hormone Research, 45*, 38–45.

Kelley, K. W., Brief, S., Westly, H. J., Novakofski, J., Bechtel, P. J., Simon, J., & Walker, E. B. (1986). Growth hormone$_3$ pituitary adenoma implants can reverse thymic aging in rats. *Proceedings of the National Academy of Sciences of the United States of America, 83*, 5663–5667.

Kent, S., Bluthé, R. M., Dantzer, R., Hardwick, A. J., Kelley, K. W., Rothwell, N. J., & Vannice, J. L. (1992). Different receptor mechanisms mediate the pyrogenic and behavioral effects of interleukin 1. *Proceedings of the National Academy of Sciences of the United States of America, 89*, 9117–9120.

Kent, S., Bluthé, R. M., Kelley, K. W., & Dantzer, R. (1992). Sickness behavior as a new target for drug development. *Trends in Pharmacological Science, 13*, 24–28.

Khorram, O., Yeung, M., Vu, L., & Yen, S. S. (1997). Effects of [norleucine27] growth hormone-releasing hormone (GHRH) (1-29)-NH2 administration on the immune system of aging men and women. *Journal of Clinical Endocrinological Metabolism, 82*, 3590–3596.

Kishimoto, T., Taga, T., & Akira, S. (1994). Cytokine signal transduction. *Cell, 76*, 253–262.

Kleinman, D., Karas, M., Danilenko, M., Arbell, A., Roberts, C. T., LeRoith, D., Levy, J., & Sharoni, Y. (1996). Stimulation of endometrial cancer cell growth by tamoxifen is associated with increased insulin-like growth factor (IGF)-I induced tyrosine phosphorylation and reduction in IGF binding proteins. *Endocrinology, 137*, 1089–1095.

Kooijman, R., Lauf, J. J., Kappers, A. C., & Rijkers, G. T. (1995). Insulin-like growth factor induces phosphorylation of immunoreactive insulin receptor substrate and its association with phosphatidylinositol-3 kinase in human thymocytes. *Journal of Experimental Medicine, 182*, 593–597.

Kooijman, R., Hooghe-Peters, E. L., & Hooghe, R. (1996). Prolactin, growth hormone, and insulin-like growth factor-I in the immune system. *Advances in Immunology, 63*, 377–454.

Lai, E. C., Felice, K. J., Festoff, B. W., Gawel, M. J., Gelinas, D. F., Kratz, R., Murphy, M. F., Natter, H. M., Norris, F. H., & Rudnicki, S. A. (1997). Effect of recombinant human insulin-like growth factor-I on progression of ALS. A placebo-controlled study of the North American ALS/IGF-I Study Group. *Neurology, 49*, 1621–1630.

Lamberts, S. W. J., van den Beld, A. W., & van der Lely, A. J. (1997). The endocrinology of aging. *Science, 278*, 419–424.

Landreth, K. S., Narayanan, R., & Dorshkind, K. (1992). Insulin-like growth factor-I regulates pro-B cell differentiation. *Blood, 80*, 1207–1212.

Lang, C. H., Pollard, V., Fan, J., Traber, L. D., Traber, D. L., Frost, R. A., Gelato, M. C., & Prough, D. S. (1997). Acute alterations in growth hormone-insulin-like growth factor axis in humans injected with endotoxin. *American Journal of Physiology, 273*, 371–378.

Lazarus, D. D., Moldawer, L. L., & Lowry, S. F. (1993). Insulin-like growth factor-I activity is inhibited by interleukin-1α, tumor necrosis factor-α, and interleukin-6. *Lymph Cyt Research, 12*, 219–223.

Lee, S., & Rivier, C. (1994). Hypophysiotropic role and hypothalamic gene expression of corticotropin-releasing factor and vasopressin in rats injected with interleukin-1 beta systemically or into the brain ventricles. *Journal of Neuroendocrinology, 6*, 217–224.

Lee, W. H., Wang, G. M., Seaman, L. B., & Vannucci, S. J. (1996). Coordinate IGF-I and IGFBP5 gene expression in perinatal rat brain after hypoxia-ischemia. *Journal of Cerebral Blood Flow Metabolism, 16*, 227–236.

LeRoith, D., Kavsan, V. M., Koval, A. P., & Roberts, C. T. Jr. (1993). Phylogeny of the insulin-like growth factors (IGFs) and receptors: A molecular approach. *Molecular Reproductive Development, 35*, 332–336.

LeRoith, D., Werner, H., Beitner-Johnson, D., & Roberts, C. T. Jr. (1995). Molecular and cellular aspects of the insulin-like growth factor I receptor. *Endocrinological Review, 16*, 143–163.

LeRoith, D., Yanowski, J., Kaldjian, E. P., Jaffe, E. S., LeRoith, T., Purdue, K., Cooper, B. D., Pyle, R., & Adler, W. (1996). The effects of growth hormone and insulin-like growth factor I on the immune system of aged female monkeys. *Endocrinology, 137*, 1071–1079.

Li, Y. M., Arkins, S., McCusker, R. H. Jr., Donovan, S. M., Liu, Q., Jayaraman, S., Dantzer, R., & Kelley, K. W. (1996). Macrophages synthesize and secrete a 25 KDa protein that binds insulin-like growth factor-I. *Journal of Immunology, 156*, 64–72.

Li, W., Quigley, L., Yao, D. L., Hudson, L. D., Brenner, M., Zhang, B. J., Brocke, S., McFarland, H. F., & Webster, H. D. (1998). Chronic relapsing experimental autoimmune encephalomyelitis: Effects of insulin-like growth factor-I treatment on clinical deficits, lesion severity, glial responses, and blood brain barrier defects. *Journal of Neuropathology and Experimental Neurology, 57*, 426–438.

Li, Y. M., Schacher, D. H., Liu, Q., Arkins, S., Rebeiz, N., McCusker, R. H. Jr., Dantzer, R., & Kelley K. W. (1997). Regulation of myeloid growth and differentiation by the insulin-like growth factor I receptor. *Endocrinology, 138*, 362–368.

Liao, W., Rudling, M., & Angelin, B. (1997). Contrasting effects of growth hormone and insulin-like growth factor I on the biological activities of endotoxin in the rat. *Endocrinology, 138*, 289–295.

Lin, T., Wang, D., Nagpal, M. L., Chang, W., & Calkins, J. H. (1992). Down-regulation of Leydig cell insulin-like growth factor-I gene expression by interleukin-I. *Endocrinology, 130*, 1217–1224.

Liu, Q., Arkins, S., Biragyn, A., Minshall, C., Parnet, P., Dantzer, R., & Kelley, K. W. (1994). Competitive reverse transcriptase-polymerase chain reaction using a synthetic internal RNA standard to quantitate transcripts for leukocyte-derived hormones. *Neuroimmunomodulation, 1*, 33–41.

Liu, Q., Ning, W., Dantzer, R., Freund, G. G., & Kelley, K. W. (1998). Activation of protein kinase C-zeta and phosphatidylinositol 3'-kinase and promotion of macrophage differentiation by insulin-like growth factor-I. *Journal of Immunology, 160*, 1393–1401.

Liu, Q., Schacher, D., Hurth, C., Freund, G. G., Dantzer, R., & Kelley, K. W. (1997a). Activation of phosphatidylinositol 3'-kinase by insulin-like growth factor-I rescues promyeloid cells from apoptosis and permits their differentiation into granulocytes. *Journal of Immunology, 159*, 829–837.

Liu, X., Linnington, C., Webster, H. D., Lassmann, S., Yao, D. L., Hudson, L. D., Wekerle, H., & Kreutzberg, G. W. (1997b). Insulin-like growth factor-I treatment reduces immune cell responses in acute non-demyelineative experimental autoimmune encephalomyelitis. *Journal of Neuroscience Research, 47*, 531–538.

Liu, X., Yao, D. L., & Webster, H. (1995). Insulin-like growth factor I treatment reduces clinical deficits and lesion severity in acute demyelinating experimental autoimmune encephalomyelitis. *Multiple Sclerosis, 11*, 2–9.

Loddick, S. A., Liu, X. J., Lu, Z. X., Liu, C., Behan, D. P., Chalmers, D. C., Foster, A. C., Vale, W. W., Ling, N., & De Souza, E. B. (1998). Displacement of insulin-like growth factors from their binding proteins as a potential treatment for stroke. *Proceedings of the National Academy of Sciences of the United States of America, 95*, 1894–1898.

Lovett-Racke, A. E., Bittner, P., Cross, A. H., Carlino, J. A., & Racke, M. K. (1998). Regulation of experimental autoimmune encephalomyelitis with insulin-like growth factor (IGF-1) and IGF-1/IGF-binding protein-3 complex (IGF-1/IGFBP3). *Journal of Clinical Investigation, 101*, 1797–1804.

Lujan, H. D., Mowatt, M. R., Helman, L. J., & Nash, T. E. (1994). Insulin-like growth factors stimulate growth and L-cysteine uptake by the intestinal parasite *Giardia lamblia*. *Journal of Biological Chemistry, 269*, 13069–13072.

Manfredi, R., Tumietto, F., Azzaroli, L., Zucchini, A., Chiodo, F., & Mandredi, G. (1994). Growth hormone (GH) and the immune system: Impaired phagocytic function in children with idiopathic GH deficiency is corrected by treatment with biosynthetic GH. *Journal of Pediatric Endocrinology, 7*, 245–251.

Manzo, C. B., Dickerson, R. N., Settle, R. G., & Rajter, J. J. (1993). Insulin-like growth factor 1 and endotoxin-mediated kidney dysfunction in critically ill, parenterally fed rats *Nutrition, 9*, 528–531.

Marcus, R., & Hoffman, A. R. (1998). Growth hormone as therapy for older men and women. *Annual Review of Pharmacological Toxicology, 38*, 45–61.

McMorris, F. A., & McKinnon, R. D. (1996). Regulation of oligodendrocyte development and CNS myelination by growth factors: Prospects for therapy of demyelinating disease. *Brain Pathology, 6*, 313-329.

McNurlan, M. A., Garlick, P. J., Frost, R. A., DeCristofaro, K. A., Lang, C. H., Steigbigel, R. T., Fuhrer, J., & Gelato, M. (1998). Albumin synthesis and bone collagen formation in human immunodeficiency virus-positive subjects: Differential effects of growth hormone administration. *Journal of Clinical Endocrinological Metabolism, 83*, 3050–3055.

McNurlan, M. A., Garlick, P. J., Steigbigel, R. T., DeCristofaro, K. A., Frost, R. A., Lang, C. H., Johnson, R. W., Santasier, A. M., Cabahug, C. J., Fuhrer, J., & Gelato, M. (1997). Responsiveness of muscle protein synthesis to growth hormone administration in HIV-infected individuals declines with severity of disease. *Journal of Clinical Investigations, 100*, 2125–2132.

Mellado, M., Llorente, M., Rodriguez-Frade, J. M., Lucas, P., Martinez, C., & del Real, G. (1998). HIV-1 envelope protein gp120 triggers a Th2 response in mice that shifts to Th1 in the presence of human growth hormone. *Vaccine, 16*, 1111–1115.

Mendenhall, C. L., Chernausek, S. D., Ray, M. B., Gartside, P. S., Roselle, G. A., Grossman, C. J., & Chedid, A. (1989). The interactions of insulin-like growth factor I(IGF-I) with protein-calorie malnutrition in patients with alcoholic liver disease: V.A. Cooperative Study on Alcoholic Hepatitis VI. *Alcohol, and Alcoholism, 24*, 319–329.

Mendenhall, C. L., Roselle, G. A, Gartside, P., & Grossman, C. J. (1997). Effects of recombinant human insulin-like growth factor-1 and recombinant human growth hormone on anabolism and immunity in calorie-restricted alcoholic rats. *Alcohol Clinical Experimental Research, 21*, 1–10.

Mendenhall, C. L., Roselle, G. A., Grossman, C. J., & Gartside, P. (1997). I: the effects of recombinant human insulin-like growth factor-1 on nutritional recovery in the malnourished alcoholic rat. *Alcohol Clinical Experimental Research, 21*, 1676–81.

Minshall, C., Arkins, S., Dantzer, R., Freund, G. G., & Kelley, K. W. (1999). Phosphatidylinositol 3′-kinase, but not S6-kinase, is required for IGF-I and IL-4 to maintain expression of Bcl-2 and promote survival of myeloid progenitors. *Journal of Immunology, 162*, 4542–4549.

Minshall, C., Arkins, S., Freund, G. G., & Kelley, K. W. (1996). Requirement for phosphatidylinositol 3′-kinase to protect hemopoietic progenitors against apoptosis depends upon the extracellular survival factor. *Journal of Immunology, 156*, 939–947.

Minshall, C., Arkins, S., Straza, J., Conners, J., Dantzer, R., Freund, G. G., & Kelley, K. W. (1997). IL-4 and insulin-like growth factor-I inhibit the decline in Bcl-2 and promote the survival of IL-3-deprived myeloid progenitors. *Journal of Immunology, 159*, 1225–1232.

Minshall, C., Liu, Q., Arkins, S., & Kelley, K. W. (1996). Growth hormone and immunology. In M.H. Torosian (Ed.), *Growth hormone in critical illness—research and clinical studies*. (pp. 161–186). Austin, TX: R. G. Landes.

Miura, M., Li, S. W., Dumenil, G., & Baserga, R. (1994). Platelet-derived growth factor-induced expression of messenger RNA for the proliferating cell nuclear antigen requires a functional receptor for the insulin-like growth factor I. *Cancer Research, 54*, 2472–2477.

Montecino-Rodriguez, E., Clark, R., & Dorshkind, K. (1998). Effects of insulin-like growth factor administration and bone marrow transplantation on thymopoiesis in aged mice. *Endocrinology, 139*, 4120–4126.

Mooney, A., Jobson, T., Bacon, R., Kitamura, M., & Savill, J. (1997). Cytokines promote glomerular mesangial cell survival in vitro by stimulus-dependent inhibition of apoptosis. *Journal of Immunology, 159*, 3949–3960.

Mulligan, K., & Bloch, A. S. (1998). Energy expenditure and protein metabolism in human immunodeficiency virus infection and cancer cachexia. *Seminars in Oncology, 25*, 82–91.

Mustafa, A., Nyberg, F., Mustafa, M., Bakhiet, M., Mustafa, E., Winblad, B., & Adem, A. (1997). Growth hormone stimulates production of interferon-gamma by human peripheral mononuclear cells. *Hormone Research, 48*, 11–15.

Ng, S. T., Zhou, J., Adesanya, O. O., Wang, J., LeRoith, D., & Bondy, C. A. (1997). Growth hormone treatment induces mammary gland hyperplasia in aging primates. *Nature Medicine, 3*, 1141–1144.

Nguyen, B. Y., Clerici, M., Venzon, D. J., Bauza, S., Murphy, W. J., Longo, D. L., Baseler, M., Gesundheit, N., Broder, S., Shearer, G. & Yarchoan, R. (1998). Pilot study of the immunologic effects of recombinant human growth hormone and recombinant insulin-like growth factor in HIV-infected patients. *HIV Infection, 12*, 895–904.

Ni, W., Rajkumar, K., Nagy, J. I., & Murphy, L. J. (1997). Impaired brain development and reduced astrocyte response to injury in transgenic mice expressing IGF binding protein-1. *Brain Research, 769*, 97–107.

Papa, V., Gliozzo, B., Clark, G. M., McGuire, W. L., Moore, D., Fujita-Yamaguchi, Y., Vigneri, R., Goldfine, I. D., & Pezzino, V. (1993). Insulin-like growth factor-I receptors are overexpressed and predict a low risk in human breast cancer. *Cancer Research, 53*, 3736–3740.

Parnet, P., Brunke, D. L., Goujon, E., Mainard, J. D., Biragyn, A., Arkins, S., Dantzer, R., & Kelley, K. W. (1993). Molecular identification of two types of interleukin-1 receptors in the murine pituitary gland. *Journal of Neuroendocrinology, 5*, 213–219.

Payne, L. C., Weigent, D. A., & Blalock, J. E. (1994). Induction of pituitary sensitivity to interleukin-1β: A new function for corticotropin releasing hormone. *Biochemistry Biophysics Research Communications, 198*, 480–484.

Peisen, J. N., McDonnell, K. J., Mulroney, S. E., & Lumpkin, M. D. (1995). Endotoxin-induced suppression of the somatotropic axis is mediated by interleukin-1? and corticotropin-releasing factor in the juvenile rat. *Endocrinology, 136*, 3378–3390.

Plymate, S. S., Bae, V. L., Maddison, L., Quinn, L. S., & Ware, J. L. (1997). Type-1 insulin-like growth factor receptor reexpression in the malignant phenotype of SV40-T-immortalized human prostate epithelial cells enhances apoptosis. *Endocrine, 7*, 119–124.

Postel-Vinay, M. C., de Mello Coelho, V., Gagnerault, M. C., & Dardenne, M. (1997). Growth hormone stimulates the proliferation of activated mouse T lymphocytes. *Endocrinology, 138*, 1816–1820.

Prickett, M. D., Latimer, A. M., McCusker, R. H., Hausman, G. J., & Prestwood, A. K. (1992). Alterations of serum insulin-like growth factor-I (IGF-I) and IGF-binding proteins (IGFBPS) in swine infected with the protozoan parasite *Sarcocystis Miescheriana. Domestic Animal Endocrinology, 9*, 285–296.

Prisco, M., Hongo, A., Rizzo, M. G., Sacchi, A., & Baserga, R. (1997). The insulin-like growth factor I receptor as a physiologically relevant target of p53 in apoptosis caused by interleukin-3 withdrawal. *Molecular Cellular Biology, 17*, 1084–1092.

Ratajczak, J., Zhang, Q., Pertusini, E., Wojczyk, B. S., Wasik, M. A., & Ratajczak, M. Z. (1998). The role of insulin (INS) and insulin-like growth factor-I (IGF-I) in regulating human erythropoiesis. Studies in vitro under serum-free conditions—comparison to other cytokines and growth factors. *Leukemia, 12*, 371–381.

Reinisch, N., Schratzberger, P., Finkenstedt, G., Kahler, C. M., & Wiedermann, C. J. (1996). Superoxide anion release from neutrophils in growth hormone deficient adults before and after replacement therapy with recombinant human growth hormone. *Archives of Pharmacology, 354*, 369–373.

Richards, R. G., Walker, M. P., Sebastian, J., & DiAugustine, R. P. (1998). Insulin-like growth factor-1 (IGF-1) receptor-insulin receptor substrate complexes in the uterus. Altered signaling response to estradiol in the IGF-1(m/m) mouse. *Journal of Biological Chemistry, 273*, 11962–11969.

Rivier, C., Chizzonite, R., & Vale, W. (1989). In the mouse, the activation of the hypothalamic-pituitary-adrenal axis by a lipopolysaccharide (endotoxin) is mediated through interleukin-1. *Endocrinology, 125*, 2800–2805.

Rivier, C., Vale, W., & Brown, M. (1989). In the rat, interleukin-1α and -β stimulate adrenocorticotropin and catecholamine release. *Endocrinology, 125*, 3096–3102.

Rodriguez-Tarduchy, G., Collins, M. K., Garcia, I., & Lopez-Rivas, A. (1992). Insulin-like growth factor-I inhibits apoptosis in IL-3 dependent hemopoietic cells. *Journal of Immunology, 149*, 535–540.

Ronco, L. V., Doyle, S. E., Raines, M., Park, L. S., & Gasson, J. C. (1995). Conserved amino acids in the human granulocyte-macrophage colony-stimulating factor receptor-binding subunit essential for tyrosine phosphorylation and proliferation. *Journal of Immunology, 154*, 3444–3453.

Rozen, F., Yang, X. F., Huynh, H., & Pollak, M. (1997). Antiproliferative action of vitamin D-related compounds and insulin-like growth factor-binding protein 5 accumulation. *Journal of the National Cancer Institute, 89*, 652–656.

Rozen, F., Zhang, J., & Pollak, M. (1998). Antiproliferative action of tumor necrosis factor-alpha on MCF-7 breast cancer cells is associated with increased insulin-like growth factor binding protein-3 accumulation. *International Journal of Oncology, 13*, 865–869.

Sabharwal, P., & Varma, S. (1996). Growth hormone synthesized and secreted by human thymocytes acts via insulin-like growth factor I as an autocrine and paracrine growth factor. *Journal of Clinical Endocrinol Metab, 81*, 2663–2669.

Sapolsky, R., Rivier, C., Yamamoto, G., Plotsky, P., & Vale, W. (1987). Interleukin-1 stimulates the secretion of hypothalamic corticotropin-releasing factor. *Science, 238*, 522–524.

Sartin, J. L., Elsasser, T. H., Gunter, D. R., & McMahon, C. D. (1998). Endocrine modulation of physiological responses to catabolic disease. *Domestic Animal Endocrinology, 15*, 423–429.

Sato, N., & Miyajima, A. (1994). Multimeric cytokine receptors: Common versus specific functions. *Current Opinion in Cellular Biology, 6*, 174–179.

Savendahl, L., & Underwood, L. E. (1997). Decreased interleukin-2 production from cultured peripheral blood mononuclear cells in human acute starvation. *Journal of Clinical Endocrinolgy Metabolism, 82*, 1177–1180.

Schwab, S., Spranger, M., Krempien, S., Hacke, W., & Bettendorf, M. (1997). Plasma insulin-like growth factor I and IGF binding protein 3 levels in patients with acute cerebral ischemic injury. *Stroke, 28*, 1744–1748.

Sharma, U. K., Song, H., Casella, S. J., & Schwartz, D. H. (1997). Failure of insulin-like growth factor type I to suppress HIV type 1 in adult or umbilical cord mononuclear blood cells. *AIDS Research Human Retroviruses, 13*, 105–110.

Smith, B. B., & Wagner, W. C. (1984). Suppression of prolactin in pigs by *Escherichia coli* endotoxin. *Science, 224*, 605–607.

Soto, L., Martin, A. I., Millan, S., Vara, E., & Lopez-Calderon, A. (1998). Effects of endotoxin lipopolysaccharide administration on the somatotropic axis. *Journal of Endocrinology, 159*, 239–246.

Stephan, R. P., Lill-Elghanian, D. A., & Witte, P. L. (1997). Development of B cells in aged mice: Decline in the ability of pro-B cells to respond to IL-7 but not to other growth factors. *Journal of Immunology, 158*, 1598–1609.

Stephan, R. P., Reilly, C. R., & Witte, P. L. (1998). Impaired ability of bone marrow stromal cells to support B-lymphopoiesis with age. *Blood, 91*, 75–88.

Sugiura, T., Tashiro, T., Yamamori, H., Morishima, Y., Otsubo, Y., Hayashi, N., Furukawa, K., Nitta, H., Nakajima, N., Ishizuka, T., Tatibana, M., Ino, H., & Ito, I. (1997). Effects of insulin-like growth factor-1 on endotoxin translocation in burned rats receiving total parenteral nutrition. *Nutrition, 13*, 783–787.

Sun, X. J., Pons, S., Wang, L. M., Zhang, Y., Yenush, L., Burks, D., Meyers, M. G. Jr., Glasheen, E., Copeland, N. G., Jenkins, N. A., Pierce, J. H., & White, M. F. (1997). The IRS-2 gene on murine chromosome 8 encodes a unique signaling adapter for insulin and cytokine action. *Molecular Endocrinology, 11*, 251–262.

Sun, X. J., Wang, L. M., Zhang, Y., Yenush, L., Myers, M. G. Jr., Glasheen, E., Lane, W. S., Pierce, J. H., & White, M. F. (1995). Role of IRS-2 in insulin and cytokine signaling. *Nature, 377*, 173–177.

Surmacz, E., Guvakova, M. A., Nolan, M. K., Nicosia, R. F. & Sciacca, L. (1998). Type I insulin-like growth factor receptor function in breast cancer. *Breast Cancer Research and Treatment, 47*, 255–267.

Tagami, M., Ikeda, K., Nara, Y., Fugino, H., Kubota, A., Numano, F., & Yamori, Y. (1997). Insulin-like growth factor-1 attenuates apoptosis in hippocampal neurons caused by cerebral ischemia and reperfusion in stroke-prone spontaneously hypertensive rats. *Laboratory Investigation, 76*, 613–617.

Takagi, K., Suzuki, F., Barrow, R. E., Wolf, S. E., & Herndon, D. N. (1998). Recombinant human growth hormone modulates Th1 and Th2 cytokine response in burned mice. *Annals of Surgery, 228*, 106–111.

Tarantal, A. F., Hunter, M. K., & Gargosky, S. E. (1997). Direct administration of insulin-like growth factor to fetal rhesus monkeys (*Macaca mulatta*). *Endocrinology, 138*, 3349–3358.

Taub, D. D., Tsarfaty, G., Lloyd, A. R., Durum, S. K., Longo, D. L., & Murphy, W. J. (1994). Growth hormone promotes human T cell adhesion and migration to both human and murine matrix proteins in vitro and directly promotes xenogenic engraftment. *Journal of Clinical Investigation, 94*, 293–300.

Tian, Z. G., Woody, M. A., Sun, R., Welniak, L. A., Raziuddin, A., Funakoshi, S., Tsarfaty, G., Longo, D. L., & Murphy, W. J. (1998). Recombinant human growth hormone promotes hematopoietic reconstitution after syngeneic bone marrow transplantation in mice. *Stem Cells, 16*, 193–199.

Toker, A., & Cantley, L. C. (1997). Signalling through the lipid products of phosphoinositide-3-OH kinase. *Nature, 387*, 673–676.

Torres-Aleman, I., Barrios, V., & Berciano, J. (1998). The peripheral insulin-like growth factor system in amyotrophic lateral sclerosis and in multiple sclerosis. *Neurology, 50*, 772–776.

Torres-Aleman, I., Barrios, V., Lledo, A., & Berciano, J. (1996). The insulin-like growth factor I system in cerebellar degeneration. *Annual Neurology, 39*, 335–342.

Trojan, J., Johnson, T. R., Rudin, S. D., Ilan, J., Tykocinski, M. L., & Ilan, J. (1993). Treatment and prevention of rat glioblastoma by immunogenic C6 cells expressing antisense insulin-like growth factor I RNA. *Science, 259*, 94–97.

Tsarfaty, G., Longo, D. L., & Murphy, W. J. (1994). Human insulin-like growth factor I exerts hematopoietic growth-promoting effects after in vivo administration. *Experimental Hematology, 22*, 1273–1277.

Tsigos, C., Papanicolaou, D. A., Defensor, R., Mitsiadis, C. S., Kyrou, I., & Chrousos, G. P. (1997). Dose effects of recombinant human interleukin-6 on pituitary hormone secretion and energy expenditure. *Neuroendocrinology, 66*, 54–62.

Turner, C. & Bagnara, J. (1971). *General endocrinology*. Philadelphia: W. B. Saunders.

Uddin, S., Fish, E. N., Sher, D., Gardziola, C., Colamonici, O. R., Kellum, M., Pitha, P. M., White, M. F., & Platanias, L. C. (1997). The IRS-pathway operates distinctively from the Stat-pathway in hematopoietic cells and transduces common and distinct signals during engagement of the insulin or interferon-alpha receptors. *Blood, 90*, 2574–2582.

Valverde, A. M., Lorenzo, M., Pons, S., White, M. F., & Benito, M. (1998). Insulin receptor substrate (IRS) proteins IRS-1 and IRS-2 differential signaling in the insulin/insulin-like growth factor-I pathways in fetal brown adipocytes. *Molecular Endocrinology, 12*, 688–697.

van Buul-Offers, S. C., & Kooijman, R. (1998). The role of growth hormone and insulin-like growth factors in the immune system. *Cellular Molecular Life Science, 54*, 1083–1094.

Valerio, G., Bond, H. M., Badolato, R., Petrella, A., Di Maio, S., Salerno, M., Waters, M. J., Venuta, S., & Tenore, A. (1997). Expression of growth hormone receptor by peripheral blood lymphocytes in children: Evaluation in clinical conditions of impaired growth. *Clinical Endocrinology, 47*, 329–335.

Velkeniers, B., Dogusan, Z., Naessens, F., Hooghe, R., & Hooghe-Peters E. L. (1998). Prolactin, growth hormone and the immune system in humans. *Cellular Molecular Life Science, 54*, 1102–1108.

Vemuri, G. S., & McMorris, F. A. (1996). Oligodendrocytes and their precursors require phosphatidylinositol 3-kinase signaling for survival. *Development, 122*, 2529–2537.

Wada, Y., Sato, M., Niimi, M., Tamaki, M., Ishida, T., & Takaha, J. (1995). Inhibitory effects of interleukin-1 growth hormone secretion in conscious male rats. *Endocrinology, 136*, 3936–3941.

Walter, H. J., Berry, M., Hill, D. J., & Logan, A. (1997). Spatial and temporal changes in the insulin-like growth factor (IGF) axis indicate autocrine/paracrine actions of IGF-I within wounds of the rat brain. *Endocrinology, 138*, 3024–3034.

Walton, P. E., & Cronin, M. J. (1989). Tumor necrosis factor-α inhibits growth hormone secretion from cultured anterior pituitary cells. *Endocrinology, 125*, 925–929.

Wang, L.-M., Myers, M. G., Sun, X.-J., & Aaronson, S. A., White, M. and Pierce, J. H. (1993). IRS-1: Essential for IL-4 stimulated mitogenesis in hematopoietic cells. *Science, 261*, 1591–1594.

Wang, Y. Z., & Wong, Y. C. (1998). Sex hormone-induced prostatic carcinogenesis in the noble rat: The role of insulin-like growth factor-I (IGF-I) and vascular endothelial growth factor (VEGF) in the development of prostate cancer. *Prostate, 35*, 165–177.

Warwick-Davies, J., Lowrie, D. B., & Cole, P. J. (1995). Growth hormone is a human macrophage activating factor. Priming of human monocytes for enhanced release of H_2O_2. *Journal of Immunology, 154*, 1909–1918.

Wiedermann, C. J., Reinisch, N., & Braunsteiner, H. (1993). Stimulation of monocyte chemotaxis by human growth hormone and its deactivation by somatostatin. *Blood, 82*, 954–960.

Weigent, D. A., & Blalock, J. E. (1995). Associations between the neuroendocrine and immune systems. *Journal of Leukocyte Biology, 57*, 137–150.

Weigent, D. A., & Blalock, J. E. (1997). Production of peptide hormones and neurotransmitters by the immune system. *Chemical Immunology, 69*, 1–30.

Werner, H., & LeRoith, D. (1995). Insulin-like growth factor I receptor: structure, signal transduction and function. *Diabetes Review, 3*, 28–37.

Wexler, B. C., Dolgin, A. E., & Tryczynski, E. W. (1957a). Effects of bacterial polysaccharide (piromen) on the pituitary-adrenal axis: adrenal ascorbic acid, cholesterol and histologic alterations. *Endocrinology, 61*, 300–308.

Wexler, B. C., Dolgin, A. E., & Tryczynski, E. W. (1957b). Effects of bacterial polysaccharide (piromen) on the pituitary-adrenal axis: Further aspects of hypophyseal-mediated control of response. *Endocrinology, 61*, 488–499.

Wilczak, N., & De Keyser, J. (1997). Insulin-like growth factor-I receptors in normal appearing white matter and chronic plaques in multiple sclerosis. *Journal of Brain Research, 772*, 243–246.

Wilson, J., Foster, D., & Kronenberg, H. (1998). *Williams textbook of endocrinology*. Philadelphia: W. B. Saunders.

Wolk, A., Mantzoros, C. S., Andersson, S. O., Bergstrom, R., Signorello, L. B., Lagiou P., Adami H. O., & Trichopoulos, D. (1998). Insulin-like growth factor 1 and prostate cancer risk: A population-based, case-control study. *Journal of the National Cancer Institute, 90*, 911–915.

Woloski, B. M., Smith, E. M., Meyer, W. J., Fuller, G. M., & Blalock, J. E. (1985). Corticotropin-releasing activity of monokines. *Science, 230*, 1035–1037.

Woody, M. A., Welniak, L. A., Richards, S., Taub, D. D., Tian, Z., Sun, R., Longo, D. L., & Murphy, W. J. (1999). Use of neuroendocrine hormones to promote reconstitution after bone marrow transplantation. *Neuroimmunomodulation, 6*, 69–80.

Xu, X., Mardell, C., Xian, C. J., Zola, H., & Read, L. C. (1995). Expression of functional insulin-like growth factor-1 receptor on lymphoid cell subsets of rats. *Immunology, 85*, 394–399.

Yamauchi, T., Kaburagi, Y., Ueki, K., Tsuji, Y., Stark, G. R., Kerr, I. M., Tsushima, T., Akanuma, Y., Komuro, I., Tobe, K., Yazaki, Y., & Kadowaki, T. (1998). Growth hormone and prolactin stimulate tyrosine phosphorylation of insulin receptor substrate-1, -2, and -3, their association with p85 phosphatidylinositol 3-kinase (PI3-kinase), and concomitantly PI3-kinase activation via JAK2 kinase. *Journal of Biological Chemistry, 273*, 157190–15726.

Yao, D. L., Liu, X., Hudson, L. D., & Webster, H. D. (1995). Insulin-like growth factor I treatment reduces demyelination and up-regulates gene expression of myelin-related proteins in experimental autoimmune encephalomyelitis. *Proceedings of the National Academy of Sciences of the United States of America, 92*, 6190–6194.

Zellweger, R., Zhu, X. -H., Wichmann, M. W., Ayala, A., DeMaso, C. M., & Chaudry, I. H. (1996). Prolactin administration following hemorrhagic shock improves macrophage cytokine release capacity and decreases mortality from subsequent sepsis. *Journal of Immunology, 157*, 5748–5754.

CHAPTER

12

The Hypothalamo-Pituitary-Gonadal Axis and the Immune System

BIANCA MARCHETTI, MARIA C. MORALE, FRANCESCO GALLO, EMILIO LOMEO, NUCCIO TESTA, CATALDO TIROLO, SALVATORE CANIGLIA, GAETANO GAROZZO

I. INTRODUCTION

A cardinal physiological feature of a living organism, its reproductive capacity, requires precisely modulated communications among the immune, nervous, and endocrine systems. This concept of integrated bidirectionally regulated neuroendocrine–immune (NEI) axes has received strong experimental support in the last decade (see Blalock, 1992, 1994; McCann, 1993, 1994; Pierpaoli & Spector, 1994). One of the best examples of an NEI axis is the hypothalamo-pituitary-gonadal (HPG) axis whose signals, generated within the brain and peripheral target organs, symbiotically interact to finely orchestrate every aspect of reproduction (Besedovsky & Sorkin, 1974; Calzolari, 1988; Marchetti, 1989; Marchetti, Moral, et al., 1990; Pierpaoli, 1975). Luteinizing hormone-releasing hormone (LHRH), a hypothalamic decapeptide, is defined classically as the neuroendocrinological trigger and essential pacemaker of mammalian reproduction. LHRH acts not only at the level of the brain-pituitary-gonadal unit, but also is recognized now to directly influence immune organs and cells. As such, it finely regulates reproductive homeostasis (Marchetti et al., 1998). Further appreciation of the integration of the reproductive and immune systems comes from the realization that the "quality" and "intensity" of a coordinated NEI response strictly depends on gender (i.e., the reproductive status) and the integrity of another NEI axis, the hypothalamo-pituitary-adrenocortical (HPA) axis (McEwen, this volume) as well as on other variables including age, genetic vulnerability, or pathologic conditions. Indeed, the neurophysiological and biochemical events that are set into motion following stress-activation of the HPA all interact with the specific sex-steroid and immunological background.

A complex interplay among genotype, circulating gonadal and adrenal hormones, and the intrinsic capability to respond to stressful (including inflammatory) and immunological stimuli, may then determine individual, susceptibility to diseases of psychiatric, neurologic, or immunological etiologies (Chrousos, 1995; Holsboer & Barden, 1996; Marchetti, Gallo, et al., 1997; Sternberg, 1989; Wick, Hu, Schwarz & Kroemer, 1993). In medicine, especially in psychiatry, gender-differentiated predisposition to a number of illnesses is historically exemplified by sex differences in the prevalence of depression in women. Here, vulnerability is associated with oral contraceptives, abortion, the premenstrual period, the puerpuerium, and menopause (reviewed by Parry, 1995). By acting on the neuroendocrine and immune systems during the stress response, life events may greatly affect homeostasis and favor the appearance of disease. Perhaps the best example of such a psychoimmune–endocrine circuit was described by Galen, in approximately 200 AD, when he observed an increased susceptibility to breast cancer of melancholic women compared with sanguine women. If women are currently thought of as having a higher risk than men for developing certain psychiatric and most autoimmune disorders, they also seem more resistant to the development of a number of neurological diseases including Alzheimer's disease (Schneider & Finch, 1997). Much experimental literature has established that the major signals of the HPG axis, the gonadal hormones, are responsible not only for the sexual differentiation of neural circuitry, which mediates a variety of reproductive behaviors and physiological mechanism(s), but also for the generation of the sexually driven immunological dimorphisms as well as the sex-linked differential response of the HPA axis. Interestingly, the female hormones, estrogens, have received increased attention and consideration thanks to the appreciation of their "beneficial/buffering" (in a word, neuroprotective) properties (Behl et al., 1997; Dubal, Kashon, Pettigrew, Ren, Finklensten, Rau, & Wise, 1998; Patchev & Ameida, 1996; Schneider & Finch, 1997). The precise underlying biochemical and molecular mechanism(s), however, are far from being completely disclosed. Besides others, the crucial interaction of this class of hormones at the neuroendocrine–immune interface can be easily anticipated, and future studies will verify such potential modulation. Another player, the brain astrocytic compartment (Barres, 1989; Attwell, 1994) must be added to this scenario. Indeed, astrocytes are elements of the central nervous system (CNS) that share receptors and transduction mechanisms with neuronal, endocrine, and immune cells. Astrocytes represent key entities not only during development of the CNS, but also in the mature brain and during neurodegenerative events (see Benveniste, 1995; Giulian, 1990). Thus, it is not surprising that the HPG axis (and especially estrogens and LHRH) powerfully and dynamically interact with the astroglial cell compartment (Garcia-Segura, Chowen, Duenas, Torres-Aleman & Naftolin 1994; Marchetti, 1996, 1997) to achieve a further level of NEI integration.

This chapter deals with the actions and interactions of the neuroendocrine–immune network of signaling systems in relation to reproductive homeostasis, with a particular focus on the LHRH-immune dialogue and interacting cascades. The various components of the HPG axis and the different mechanism(s) of communication with the immune system are presented. Advances in the LHRH-immune field are summarized, and a number of experimental approaches to analyzing the ongoing NEI dialogue are described. Emphasis is given to HPG–HPA interactions in mediating gender differences in immunological responses. The impact of a dysfunctional HPA system in a transgenic mouse model expressing a glucocorticoid receptor (GR) antisense RNA for the programming of NEI functions is summarized briefly.

II. LHRH: THE PRIME MOVER ORCHESTRATING REPRODUCTION

The control mechanisms subserving the reproductive capacity of mammals represent an extraordinarily complex relationship, in time and function, among a number of anatomically distant structures. The changes in the activity of the trophic structures in the brain and pituitary that control gonadotropin secretion, the maturation of an ovum and ovulation, and the associated changes in the sex steroid background, all periodically prepare the endometrium for implantation of an embryo (Knobil & Hotchkiss, 1988). There are also specific mechanisms responsible for protecting the mammalian embryo against the potentially immunologically hostile maternal environment (Vinatier & Monier, 1993; Sargent, 1993). Interestingly, these mechanisms appear to vary according to the different stages of reproduction from fertilization to implantation to full development of the fetus. They are also unique since they vary from species to species and result from exceptional genetic and immunological processes (Sargent, 1993; Ussa, Cadavid, & Maldonadao, 1994). Indeed, pregnancy constitutes the most incredibly complex and fascinating achievement of mammalian evolution, where both developmental time and physiological processes are

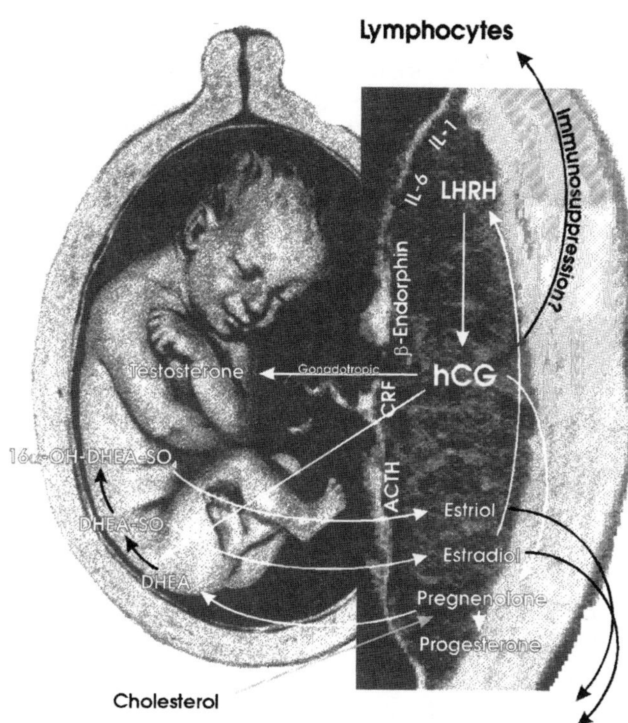

FIGURE 1 Neuroendocrine–immune interactions at the fetoplacental interphase. Some of the hormonal interactions among the three compartments (the mother, the placenta, and the fetus) are depicted. Human chorionic gonadotropin (hCG) is involved in fetal development, maintenance of pregnancy, including intrauterne immune privilege, placental metabolism, and fetal gonadal development (see Marchetti et al., 1996a). The fetal source of estrogens is also indicated, together with the steps involved in maternal sex steroid synthesis. Placental luteinizing hormone-releasing hormone (LHRH) may regulate hCG expression and action. Potential intraplacental modulatory events include the possible interaction between neuropeptides (LHRH, adrenocorticotropin hormone (ACTH), corticotropin-releasing factor [CRF], and beta endorphin) and different cytokines (IL- 6, IL-1).

indispensably fused for weeks or months (Marchetti, Gallo, Farinella, et al., 1996) (Figure 1). The principal coordinator of each of these activities is the hypothalamic decapeptide, LHRH; the mechanisms by which LHRH may have a direct regulatory impact will now be presented.

III. LHRH IS A NEUROTRANSMITTER AND NEUROMODULATOR WITHIN THE CENTRAL FRAMEWORK OF HUMORAL AND IMMUNE SIGNALING SYSTEMS

In the adult rodent, LHRH is synthesized by diffusely organized forebrain neurons, which are scattered over a continuum extending from the septal region anteriorly to the premamillary area posteriorly (Silverman, 1988). LHRH, LHRH-like peptides, and LHRH receptors have been found in numerous extrahypothalamic regions including the olfactory and limbic systems (see Badr, Marchetti, & Pelletier, 1988; Choi et al., 1994; Silverman, 1988). It is now well documented that LHRH serves as a neurotransmitter and/or neuromodulator in a variety of neural and peripheral tissues. Since LHRH fibers and nerve terminals are located in the olfactory cortex, LHRH is involved in the modulation of hormonal and behavioral events stimulated by olfaction (Choi et al., 1994). For example, a pheromone in the male urine induces females to begin estrous and effects maturation of immature female animals. Moreover, urinary chemosignals from male cause accumulation of LHRH and norepinephrine in the olfactory bulb as well as growth of the ovaries and uterus (Dluzen & Ramirez, 1987; Lepri & Wysoski, 1987).

Different lines of evidence point to an interaction between LHRH and a central immune network. In the medial habenula of the ring dove, Silverman and collaborators (Silverman, Millar, King, Zhuang, & Silver, 1994) have identified a population of non-neuronal cells, presenting all the features of mast cells, which exhibit LHRH-like immunoreactivity. These authors have suggested that mast cell secretions into the brain may represent an additional delivery system for biologically active substances such as LHRH. In many regions, including the CNS, mast cells are either innervated or in close proximity to nerve terminals, and can be stimulated to release their granular content by neuropeptides (Silverman et al., 1994). Of particular interest is the clinical observation that histamine secretion from mast cells and cutaneous anaphylaxis can be induced with LHRH and LHRH-agonists (LHRH-A) and antagonists. Moreover, LHRH-A binding sites are present in mast cells (Sundaram, Didolkar, Thau, Chandhuri, & Schmidt, 1988). Mast cells respond not only to LHRH and its analogs, but also to gonadal steroids. Amine release can be triggered directly by progesterone (Silverman et al., 1996) in the rodent, and induced release can be augmented by estradiol. Moreover, estrogen receptors have been demonstrated in mast cells (Vliagoftis et al., 1990).

Communication between the hypothalamus and the pituitary–ovarian axis occurs via LHRH. Hypothalamic LHRH, released into portal capillaries that perfuse the anterior pituitary, drives the menstrual cycle by stimulating pituitary luteinizing hormone (LH) and follicle-stimulating hormone (FSH) (Knobil & Hotchkiss, 1988). There is a growing recognition that a network of neurons that elaborate three classes of messenger molecules, the classical aminergic neurotransmitters, the amino acids, and the neuropeptides, regulate the secretion of the trigger for the preovulatory surge of pituitary LH secretion in proestrus (see Kalra, 1993). A discussion of the intricate interplay between each of these neural components in the control of LHRH release is beyond the scope of this review. However, it is apparent that peptidergic signaling is crucial for the accelerated discharge of LHRH into the hypophyseal portal system in proestrus. Moreover, metabolic signals and interactive pathways related to the hypothalamic control of appetite impinge on the LHRH neuronal machinery. A local hypothalamic network composed of diverse peptidergic signals regulates episodic LHRH secretion and is directly subject to regulation by gonadal steroids (Kalra, 1993). The primary action of steroids is to facilitate the output of peptide signals and to amplify or adjust their postsynaptic response in a timely fashion. Centrally, sex steroids interact with both aminergic and peptidergic signals, resulting in appropriate and timely coordinated release of pulses of LHRH. The effect of sex steroids and of other modulators such as prolactin and opioids also may occur at the level of the anterior pituitary via action on the pituitary LHRH receptor system (Marchetti & Labrie, 1982; Marchetti, Reeves, Pelletier, & Labrie, 1982; Marchetti & Scapagnini, 1985) (Figure 2).

As will be reviewed later, we expect that, besides the regulation of LHRH secretion at the level of LHRH cell bodies or terminals at the median eminence (ME), LHRH may be modulated locally by dynamic relationships among neuron terminals, glia, and basal lamina, as demonstrated for oxytocin and vasopressin (Hatton, Perlmutter, Salra, & Tweedle, 1984). Accordingly, different interplays between products of the astroglial cell compartment, the neuronal terminals, and the hormonal background may be envisaged according to the particular reproductive (i.e., specific sex steroid background) condition (see Marchetti, 1996, 1997, for reviews; Figure 2).

The similarity of signaling systems used by immune and neuroendocrine cells is well illustrated by the powerful interaction between the cytokines and the LHRH system, at both the central and peripheral levels (see Rettori, Gimeno, Karara, Gonzalez, & McCann, 1991; Rivest, Lee, Attardi, & Rivier, 1993; Rivier & Erickson, 1993; Rivier & Vale, 1989). At the CNS level, acute administration of interleukin (IL)-1 decreases plasma LH levels, a phenomenon attributed to the inhibition of hypothalamic secretion of LHRH and LHRH gene expression (Rivest et al., 1993). That IL-1β represents an extremely potent factor that inhibits the activity of the HPG axis is supported by findings showing the ability of this cytokine to inhibit the physiological or experimentally induced afternoon proestrous LH surge in female rats (Rivest et al., 1993). Accordingly, expression of the early *c-fos* gene, which occurs within the LHRH cell nuclei during this same period of the cycle, is concomitantly inhibited. In addition, the chronic intracerebroventricular (icv) infusion of IL-1β results in a complete disruption of the estrous cycle, decreased release of hypothalamic LHRH and pituitary gonadotropins, and a block in luteolysis of newly formed corpora lutea (Rivier & Erickson, 1993; Rivest et al., 1993). The effect of immune and metabolic challenges on LHRH neuronal system in cycling female rats was recently evaluated at a transcriptional level (Nappi & Rivest, 1997). After induction of an acute phase response via an i.p. injection of lipopolysaccharide (LPS), the number of LHRH-immunoreactive and LHRH-expressing neurons displaying c-Fos-immunoreactive (ir) nuclei during the aftemoon of proestrus was significantly inhibited 3 h after endotoxin administration. This effect was accompanied by attenuation of the physiological increase of LHRH primary transcript in the organum vasculosum laminae terminalis/medial preoptic area structure at 15.00 h of proestrus (Nappi and Rivest, 1997).

It would appear, therefore, that according to the stage of the estrous cycle, the peptidergic and aminergic background, and the local dialogue between neuronal and glial cells, that a number of

FIGURE 2 Schematic representation of hypothalamic peptidergic and aminergic signals, environmental factors, and hypophyseal-mediated mechanisms in the control of the episodic discharge of LHRH. The model includes the LHRH pulse generator, the neural elements (the clock) regulating directly the activity of this generator, and those elements involved in its indirect regulation via the negative feedback action of gonadal steroids, as reviewed by Kalra (1993). Around this unit are also pictured a number of other important factors modulating the phasic LHRH discharge leading to the preovulatory LH surge and ovulation. These include a number of neuropeptides such as the opioids peptides, NPY, galanine, and neurotensin, with both positive and negative effects. A modulatory influence is represented by the action of sex steroids impinging in this circuitry at both central and peripheral (hypophyseal level) via estrogen receptors, as well as by modifications in the number of pituitary LHRH receptors responsible for alterations in the sensitivity of the gonadotropes to LHRH (Marchetti et al., 1982). Besides the classical aminergic and peptidergic regulation at the level of LHRH cell bodies/terminals, the dynamic interactions between LHRH neurons and astroglial cells, with possible interference of endogenously produced cytokines and growth factors, is also depicted. (β-END=β-endorphin; NPY=neuropeptide Y; NT=neurotensin; GAL=galanin.)

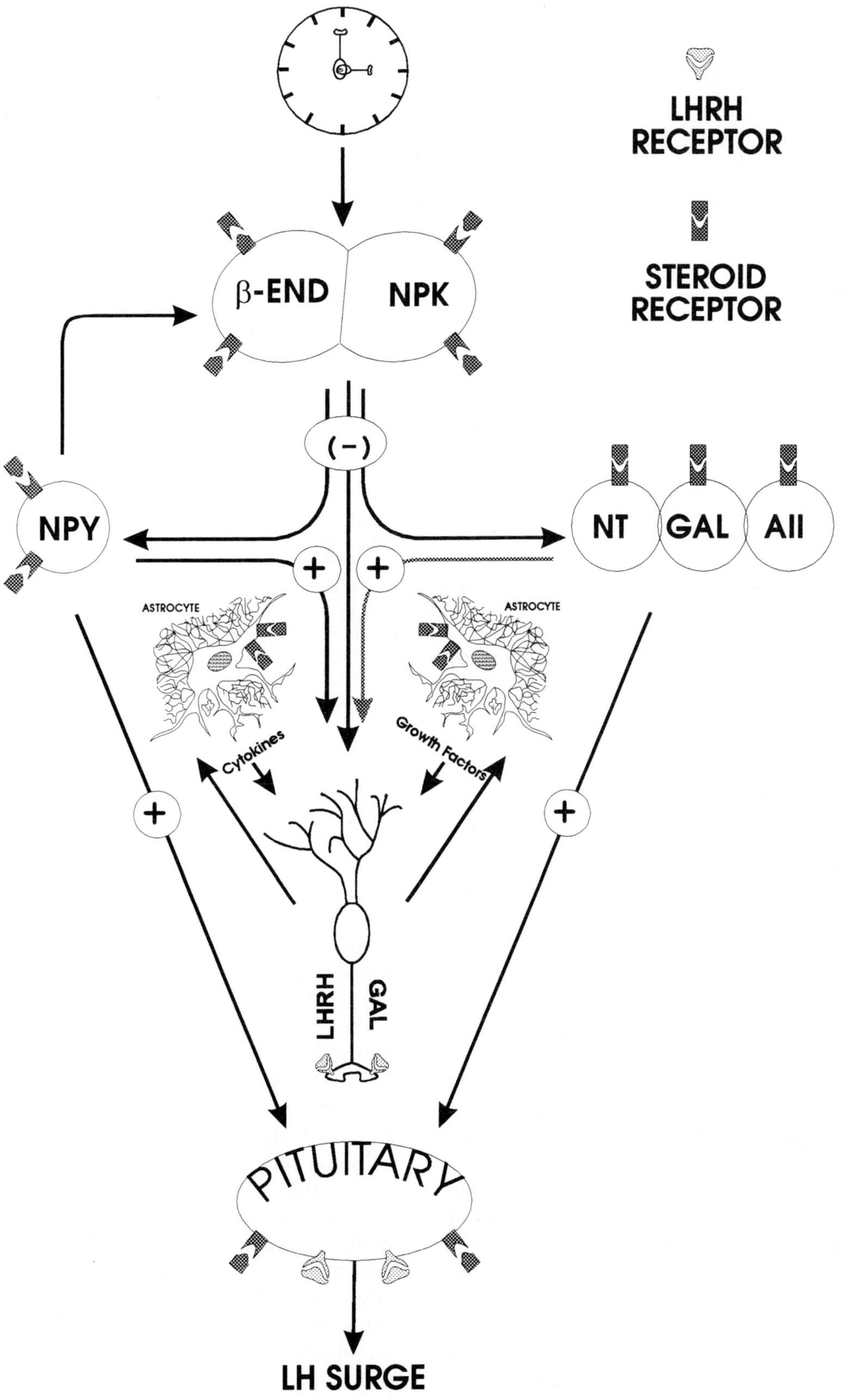
LHRH
RECEPTOR
STEROID
RECEPTOR
β-END
NPK
(−)
NPY
NT
GAL
AII
+
+
ASTROCYTE
ASTROCYTE
Cytokines
Growth Factors
+
+
LHRH
GAL
PITUITARY
LH SURGE

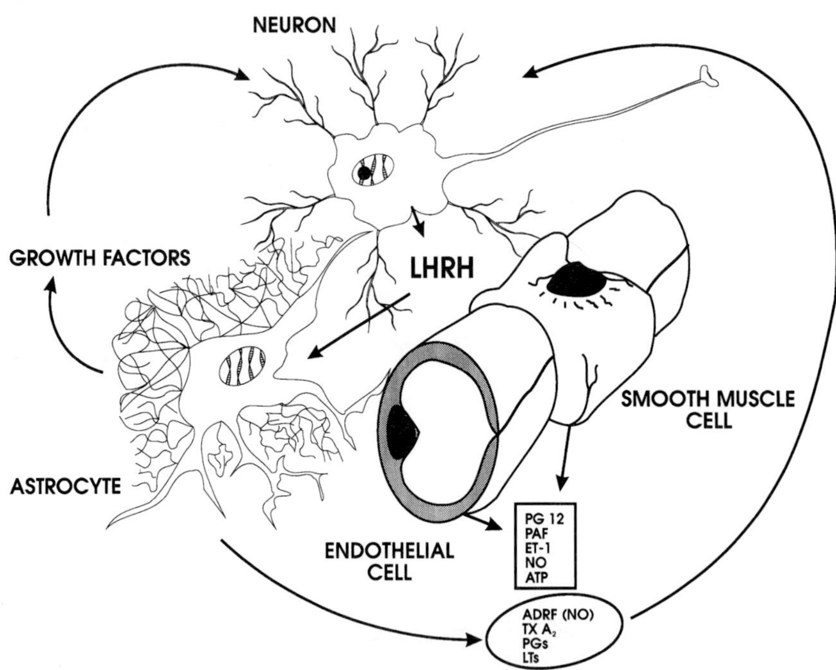

FIGURE 3 Dynamic interaction between the astroglial cell compartment and the endothelial and the LHRH neurons. On selective stimulation, astrocytes may release products able to alter the vascular endothelium. The expression of receptors on astrocytes, their ability to synthesize vasoactive products, and the close spatial relationships of these cells both with neurons and cells of the vasculature implicate astroglial cells in bidirectional signaling processes in the CNS. PG: prostaglandin, PAF: platelet activating factor, TXA_2: thromboxane, NO: nitric oxide, ATP: adenosine triphosphate, ADRF (NO): astrocyte-derived (vaso)-relaxing factor (nitric oxide).

potential interactions between the cytokines and the LHRH system may be envisaged (Figure 3). Indeed, in this context it is noteworthy that one major brain compartment that serves as a source of cytokines is represented by astroglial and microglial cells (for reviews, see Benveniste, 1995; Marchetti, 1997).

The neurosecretory LHRH system is very diffuse. LHRH neurons are scattered along the basal forebrain, their heaviest concentration being found in the anterior hypothalamus, the preoptic area, and the septum. Fibers project not only to the median eminence, but also through the hypothalamus and midbrain (Silverman, 1988). During this passage, LHRH neurons interact with many types of neurons and glia. Indeed, the architecture of the arcuate nucleus of the hypothalamus is unique because of the arrangement of glial cells within it. Tanicytes, specialized ependymal cells, line the ventricular walls and send their processes in an arching trajectory toward the surface of the brain (Basco, Woodhams, Haljos, & Balasz, 1981). Astrocytes of varying morphologies also are located in this region (Millhouse, 1972). Interestingly, LHRH neurons migrate from the epithelium of the medial olfactory pit into the developing basal forebrain (Schwanzel-Fukuda & Pfaff, 1989). Failure of LHRH neuronal migration, as seen in Kallman's syndrome (Kallman, Schoenfeld & Barrera, 1944), results in suppression of the pituitary-gonadal axis (Crawley & Jameson, 1992; Schwanzel-Fukuda, Jorgenson, Bergen, Weesner, & Pfaff, 1992) and a number of immunological disturbances (unpublished observation). Studies of the molecular basis of LHRH-guided migration suggest a crucial participation of the neural cell adhesion molecule, N-CAM (Schwanzel-Fukuda et al., 1992). The contribution of glial elements to LHRH axonal targeting was suggested by the early experiments of Kozlowski & Coates (1985), who demonstrated the existence of ependymal tunnels and their association with LHRH axons. More recently, relationships of glia to LHRH axonal outgrowth from third ventricular grafts in hypogonadal mice have been described by Silverman and colleagues (Silverman, Gibson, & Silverman, 1991). Owing to the absence of a functional gene for LHRH, the hypogonadal (hpg) mice have infantile reproductive tracts in adulthood, a condition that can be reversed by the implantation of normal fetal preoptic area tissue that contains LHRH neurons. It is noteworthy that hpg mice show severe immunological defects ranging from cell-mediated and

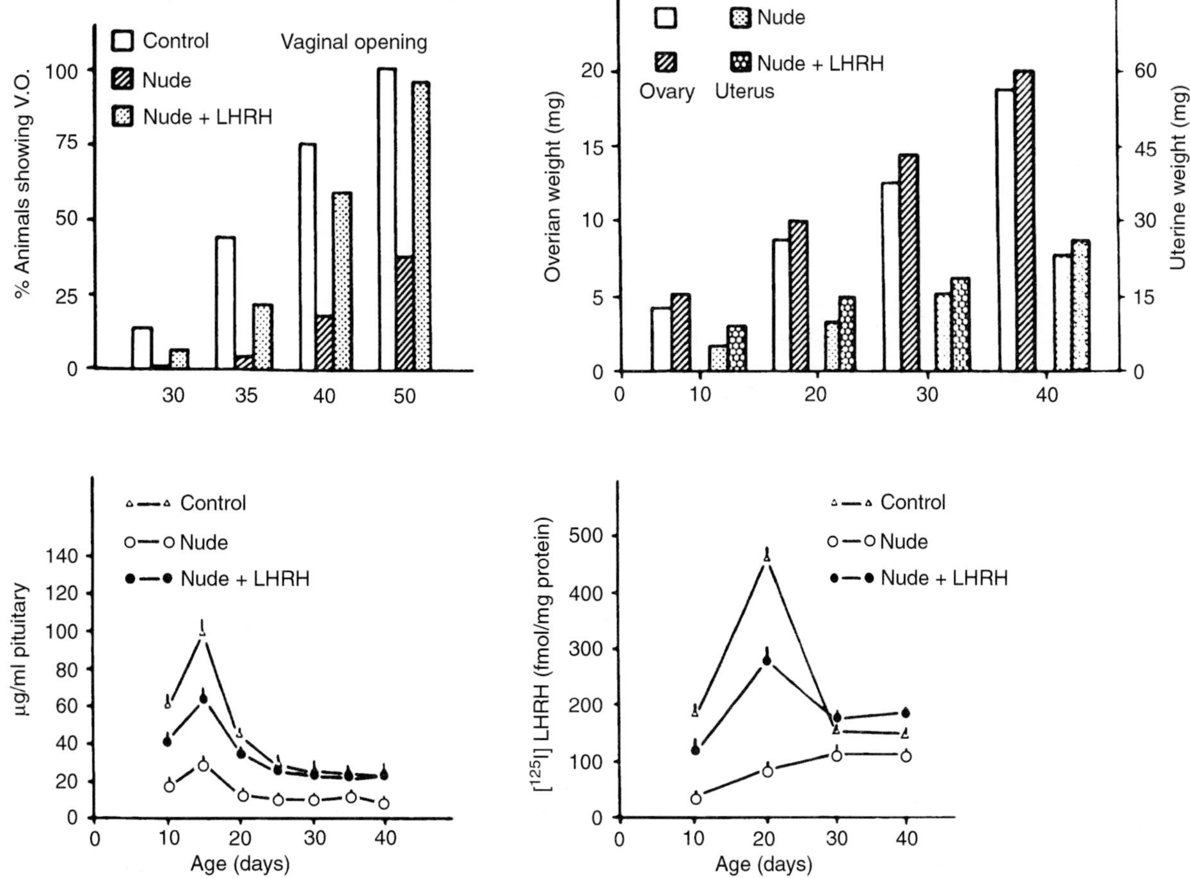

FIGURE 6 Effect of LHRH neonatal treatment in the onset of puberty in nude mice. Different parameters (vaginal opening, ovarian and uterine weights, pituitary LH concentration, pituitary LHRH receptors) of sexual maturation were analyzed in control intact female mice and nude mice without and during a treatment with LHRH. Upper panels: note that in nude mice, only 25–45% of animals show vaginal opening at 50 days of age. Intact mice or nude mice treated with LHRH started to show vaginal opening at around 35 days (25–35%), and the totality of mice exhibited vaginal opening at 50 days (left panel). Ovarian and uterine weights increase progressively in control mice, with highest weights measured around puberty (right panel). Pituitary LH and LHRH receptors (lower panels) do not show the physiological prepuberal and puberal modifications in nude mice, whereas treatment with LHRH significantly increased both parameters.

LHRH agonists might act on the immune system by directly affecting B and/or T lymphocytes. Alternatively, its effects might be indirect, through a reduction in gonadotropins or alterations in cytokine production by immune cells. The fact that LHRH analogs can modulate murine lupus independently of effects on sex hormone production is of special interest, since it raises the possibility that hormones other than gonadal steroids might contribute to the well-known gender differences in expression of autoimmune diseases (Jacobson et al., 1994).

More recently, the effect of neonatal treatment with an LHRH antagonist on developmental changes in circulating lymphocyte subsets of rhesus monkeys were analyzed by Gould and co-workers (Gould, Akinbami, & Mann, 1998). By analogy with what has been observed in rodents (Morale et al., 1991), the overall data provide further evidence that neonatal treatment of male rhesus monkeys with LHRH-antagonists may alter the early programming of the immune system. The effects of treatment with LHRH-A or antagonists in pathophysiological human states is now being evaluated by a number of laboratories, including our own. Our results suggest a potential immunological influence of these peptides in a number of endocrine disorders (i.e., endometriosis, hypogonadal hypogonadism, precocious puberty), and cancer states (postmenopausal breast cancer, prostate cancer).

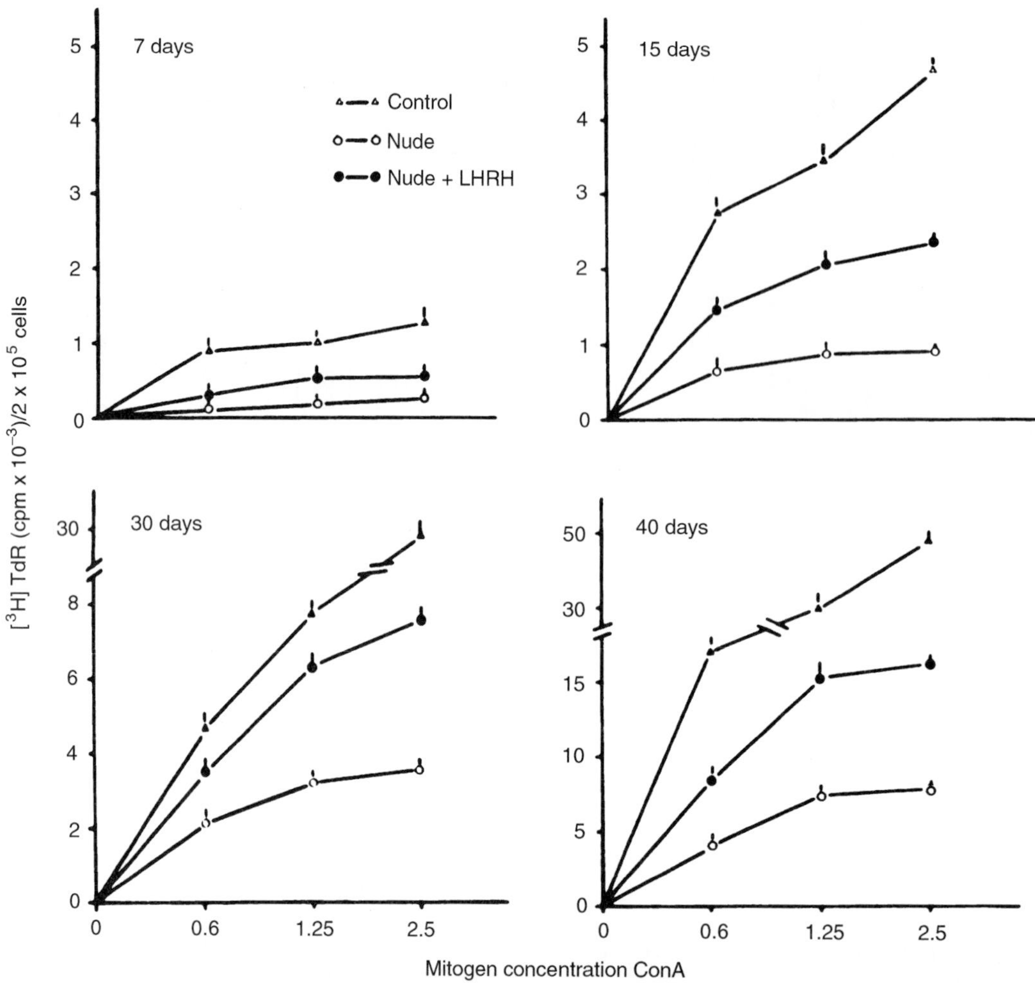

FIGURE 7 Effect of LHRH neonatal treatment in the maturation cell-mediated immune response in spleen of nude mice. The development of blastogenic potential in intact and nude mice, without and during a treatment with LHRH, is illustrated. Animals treated or not treated with LHRH were sacrificed at different time intervals (7–40 days after birth), and the organs were carefully removed and processed for preparation of cellular cultures. [^{3}H]thymidine incorporation (TdR) was measured before and after application of the T-dependent mitogen, concanavalin-A (Con A, 0.5-2.5 μg/mL) (Morale et al., 1991). Note the failure of splenocytes from nude mice to efficiently respond to Con A during postnatal development, whereas treatment with LHRH almost completely restored splenocyte proliferative response.

V. LHRH IN THE HYPOTHALAMO-PITUITARY-GONADAL-THYMIC AXIS

The fundamental importance of the thymus in the regulation of reproductive processes is reflected by the fact that the physiological development of an operative HPG axis requires the presence of an intact immune system. In fact, immunosuppressed animals show numerous reproductive disorders (see Grossman, 1984, 1990; Marchetti, 1989). Moreover, inflammatory and infectious diseases often coincide with changes in reproductive functions that include a decline in fertility, an increased incidence of spontaneous abortion, and full-term birth of abnormal progeny (see Marchetti, Morale, & Pelletier, 1990a, for review). Conversely, hypogonadic patients with Klinefelter's syndrome appear to have very high rates of lupus erythematosus.

Since the primary communication between the immune and the reproductive systems is known to involve the thymus and its peptide secretion, it seems important to place LHRH within the context of a hypothalamo-pituitary-gonadal-thymic (HPGT) axis. Communication between the gonadal axis and lymphoid organs has been proposed for over a century, and the studies of Grossman and co-workers (see Grossman, 1990) have even emphasized the existence of such a reciprocal relationship between the HPG

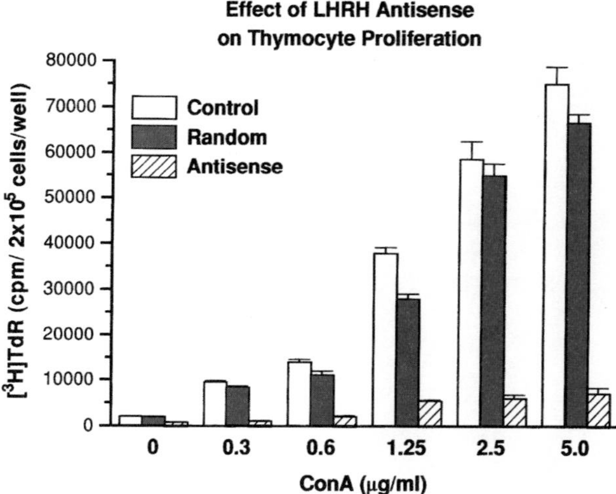

FIGURE 8 Effect of a synthetic antisence oligodeoxynucleotide to the hypothalamic neuropeptide LHRH on Con- A-induced thymocyte proliferation. Thymocyte cultures prepared from proestrus female rats were pretreated with an LHRH antisense or the random oligonucleotide in the absence (0) or the presence of increasing concentrations of Con A (0–3.5 μg/mL). The cultures were then processed as previously described (Batticane et al., 1991). Results represent the mean ±SEM of quadruplicate wells, and of three individual determinations.

axis and the brain thymus-lymphoid axis. A schematic representation of the possible interactions between the HPG and the thymus, with LHRH serving as a primary channel for communication, is presented in Figure 9. This illustration shows a bidirectional network carrying information to both the immune and the reproductive systems via LHRH, as well as direct aminergic and peptidergic innervation of both the gonads and immune organs. Circulating hypophyseal and gonadal hormones exert a regulatory feedback mechanism at the level of the thymus gland and provide a potential modulatory system regulating thymic cell function and thymic peptide production. The thymus and its peptide secretion (thymosin fraction 5 and one of its peptidic constituent, thymosin beta -4) can exert a modulation of gonadotropin secretion via a direct action at the hypothalamic LHRH neuronal level.

A. Thymic LHRH during the Estrous Cycle and Pregnancy

It is important to emphasize that activity of the intrathymic LHRH system varies according to the phases of the estrous cycle. Interestingly, a sex dimorphic pattern of LHRH synthesis accompanies the sexually dimorphic immune response during ontogeny and the estrous cycle (Figure 10). Surprisingly, LHRH mRNA concentration exhibits clear sex-dependent fluctuations during the rat estrous cycle, which are accompanied by a change in thymocyte responsiveness to LHRH; a maximal response to the natural decapeptide occurs in proestrus (Figures 10, 11). Such an increase in thymocyte responsiveness to LHRH during the proestrus phase of the cycle is analogous to the known increased responsiveness of the pituitary gonadotrope to LHRH that is responsible for the gonadotropin surge and ovulation. This finding suggests that the sex-steroid priming effect at the level of the pituitary gland also might be operative within the thymus. On the other hand, after ovulation (i.e., the estrous phase of the cycle in rodents) the reduced thymocyte response to T-cell mitogens and to LHRH is markedly reduced (Figure 11), suggesting the possible participation of LHRH and sex steroids in these events. Such mechanism(s), therefore, might participate in the reduction of immune responsiveness observed during pregnancy. It is tempting to speculate that by altering the expression of target genes within the thymus, sex steroids may modify the responsiveness of immune cells to hormones, neuropeptides, or neurotransmitters (see following sections). Indeed, the ability of estrogens to directly alter LHRH gene expression has been demonstrated in the placenta (Radvick et al., 1991).

VI. GENDER DIFFERENCES IN NEUROENDOCRINE AND IMMUNE AXES: PATHOPHYSIOLOGICAL IMPLICATIONS

Gonadal steroids are critically involved in several aspects of brain development and in the maintenance of brain function. Indeed, it has been suggested that the loss of sex hormones at menopause may be critical with respect to the cognitive decline associated with degenerative brain pathologies, such as Alzheimer's disease (see Schneider & Finch, 1997; Cummings, Vinters, Cole, & Khachatunian, 1998). In recent years, considerable interest has been generated by the role of gender in the development of psychiatric, neurodegenerative, or autoimmune diseases (Bebo, Schuster, Derback, & Offlier, 1998; Kritzer & Kohama, 1998; Parry, 1995; Schultz, Braak & Braak, 1996). The impact of gender in the response of different neuroendocrine axes is well known. For example, a key role for gonadal hormones in the control of the HPA axis is indicated in a number of studies over the last 30 years. In particular, the neuroendocrine response to stress has been shown to display a profound gender-specific

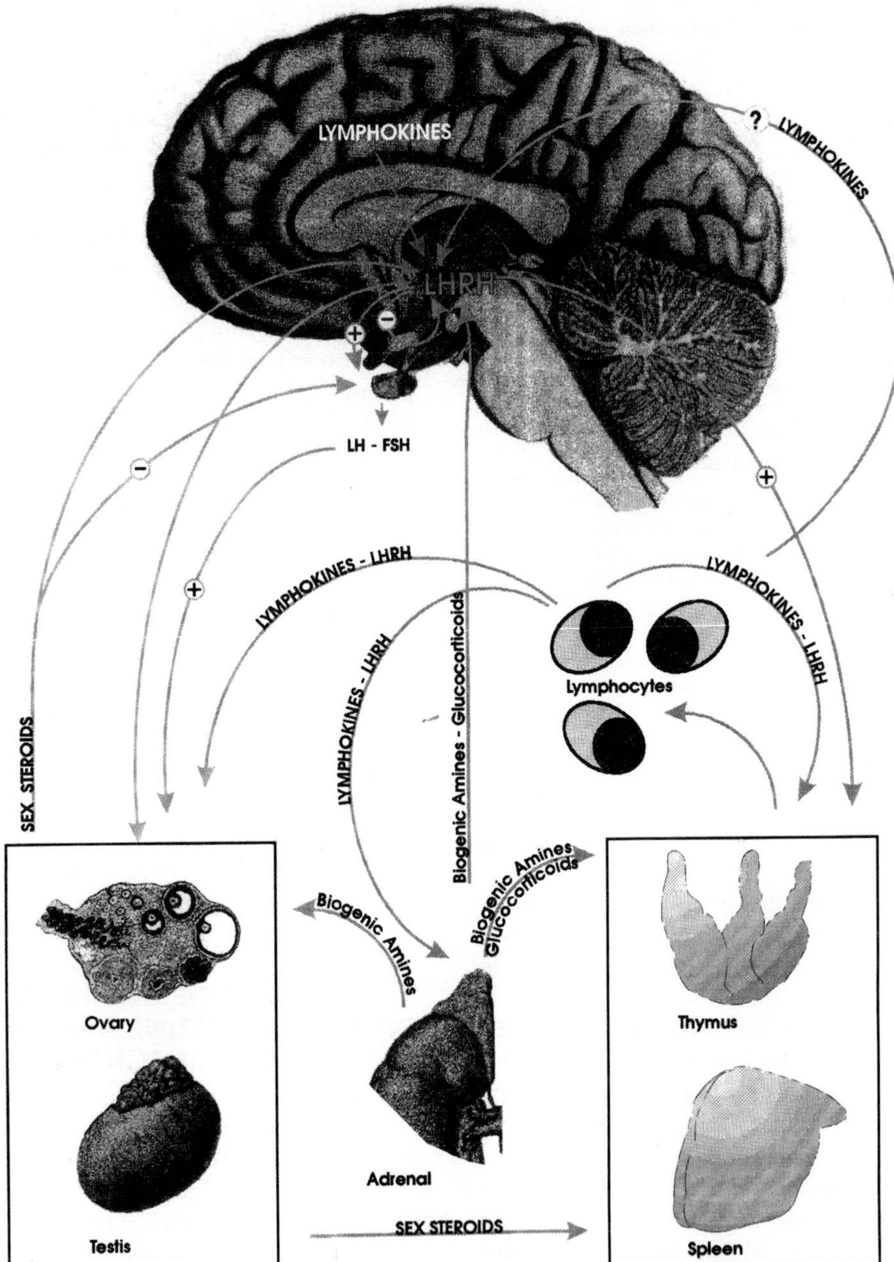

FIGURE 9 Schematic representation of the possible interactions between the hypothalamus-hypophyseal-gonadal axis and the thymus, with LHRH serving as a major channel of communication. Hypothalamic LHRH governs the release of the pituitary gonadotropins LH and FSH, responsible for gonadal production of the sex steroids. The gonadal hormones in turn feed back information to the thymus and hypothalamus. At the thymus level, sex steroids act on specific receptors present on the reticuloepithelial matrix and induce both up- and down-regulation of target genes involved in the control of T-cell responses. On the other hand, the sex steroid background alters the production of thymic peptides (thymosins) and neuropeptides such as LHRH, with autocrine/paracrine regulatory influence within the thymic microenvironment. The direct neural pathways innervating immune and endocrine organs together the modulatory influence of glucocorticoids and catecholamines are also indicated.

difference, the manifestation of which largely depends on the presence of gonadal steroids (Chisari, Perone, Giovanbattista, & Spinedi, 1998; Spinedi, Suescun, Hadid, Deneva, & Gaillard, 1992). Higher circulating levels of corticosterone are found in females, and greater variations in plasma corticosterone both diurnally and in response to stress have been described in female animals (Critclow, Liebelt, Bar-

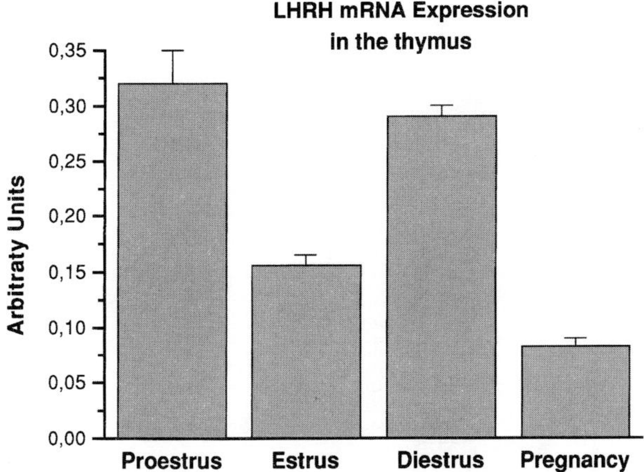

FIGURE 10 Expression of LHRH mRNA within the rat thymus gland as a function of the estrous cycle and pregnancy. Poly(A) mRNAs isolated from female rat thymuses at the indicated reproductive phases, were reverse-transcribed to cDNA and amplified by polymerase chain reaction (PCR) after addition of specific primers, electrophoresed on 2% agarose gel, prepared for transfer, and blotted onto nitrocellulose, as described in Maier et al. (1992). After hybridization and the washing of filters at high stringency conditions, dry filters were exposed to X-ray film at −70°C with enhancing screens. For quantitative PCR determinations, β-actin was used as internal control. Results represent the mean ± SEM of 2–3 thymic samples, and are expressed in arbitrary optical density units.

Sela, Mountcastle, & Lipcomb, 1963). Plasma concentrations of transcortin in female rats are at least double those found in males (Gala & Westphal, 1965). Sex-related differences also have been found for GR affinity, binding capacity, and nuclear translocation in rat brain (Turner & Weaver, 1985). On the other hand, estrogens have been shown to powerfully modulate GR gene expression in the brain and pituitary (Peiffer & Barden, 1987; Peiffer, Lapointe, & Barden, 1991). The sex steroid hormone-dependence of the brain during early postnatal development also may result in gender-specific patterns in the neural mechanisms controlling HPA axis activity (Patchev & Almeida, 1996). Indeed, distinct sex differences in the genes encoding corticotropin-releasing hormone (CRH) in the hypothalamus and GR in the hippocampus have been identified. Recent studies (Patchev & Almeida, 1996) demonstrate that gonadal steroids exert facilitating effects on glucocorticoid-mediated transcriptional regulation of CRH and GR genes in the rat brain. These and other data suggest that when the HPA axis is activated and responds to stressful stimuli, including infectious diseases, the sex steroid hormone milieu may qualitatively and qualitatively influence such responses. Such marked sensitivity of the HPA axis to the sex steroid background is reflected at the level of the immune system by the known immunological sex-dimorphisms and increased vulnerability of females to autoimmune diseases. The impact of the circulating gonadal hormones in immune homeostasis via its interaction with the HPA system may represent another aspect of NEI regulation. The pathophysiological implications of such regulatory network include the susceptibility to develop inflammatory/autoimmune diseases. The biochemical and molecular mechanism(s), or the exact timing of these interactions, are not completely known.

Steroid hormones mediate physiological and developmental effects in higher eukaryotes by interaction with their intracellular receptors in target cells (Burnstein & Cidlowski, 1989). A likely way for these hormones to modulate immune system function might involve the regulation of receptor expression within the thymus. Gonadal hormones influence mammalian reproductive function through their action during the perinatal period. The expression of sex-dimorphic functions in the adult is maintained by adequate levels of circulating hormones. Immunological dimorphism might depend on two fundamental influences of gonadal steroid hormones. The first occurs during the perinatal period when these hormones may permanently alter the developmental pattern of thymocyte selection and turnover with the establishment of a specific (male vs. female) T-cell repertoire. In this way, sex steroids may have permanent effects on a particular subset of T cells. For instance, the development of the medullary epithelium that occurs early in ontogeny may be irreversibly modulated by the sex steroid hormone milieu, giving rise to a population of progenitor cells. The second influence of gonadal hormones may be exerted during adulthood by maintaining the sex dimorphic immune function through the production of adequate levels of circulating gonadal hormones.

A. Molecular Mechanism of Sex Steroid Action within the Thymus in the Regulation of Immune Responsiveness: Up- and Down-Regulation of Receptor Gene Expression

One way to decipher the mechanism of steroid action at a molecular level is to study whether physiological changes in sex steroid levels occurring during the estrous cycle and pregnancy would alter the expression of specific genes coding for neuroendocrine hormones and their receptors. Besides LHRH-R, we have been interested in GR and β-adrenergic receptor (BAR) gene expression in the thymus. Glucocorticoid hormones are crucial hormones in the control of immunity. They are the most potent

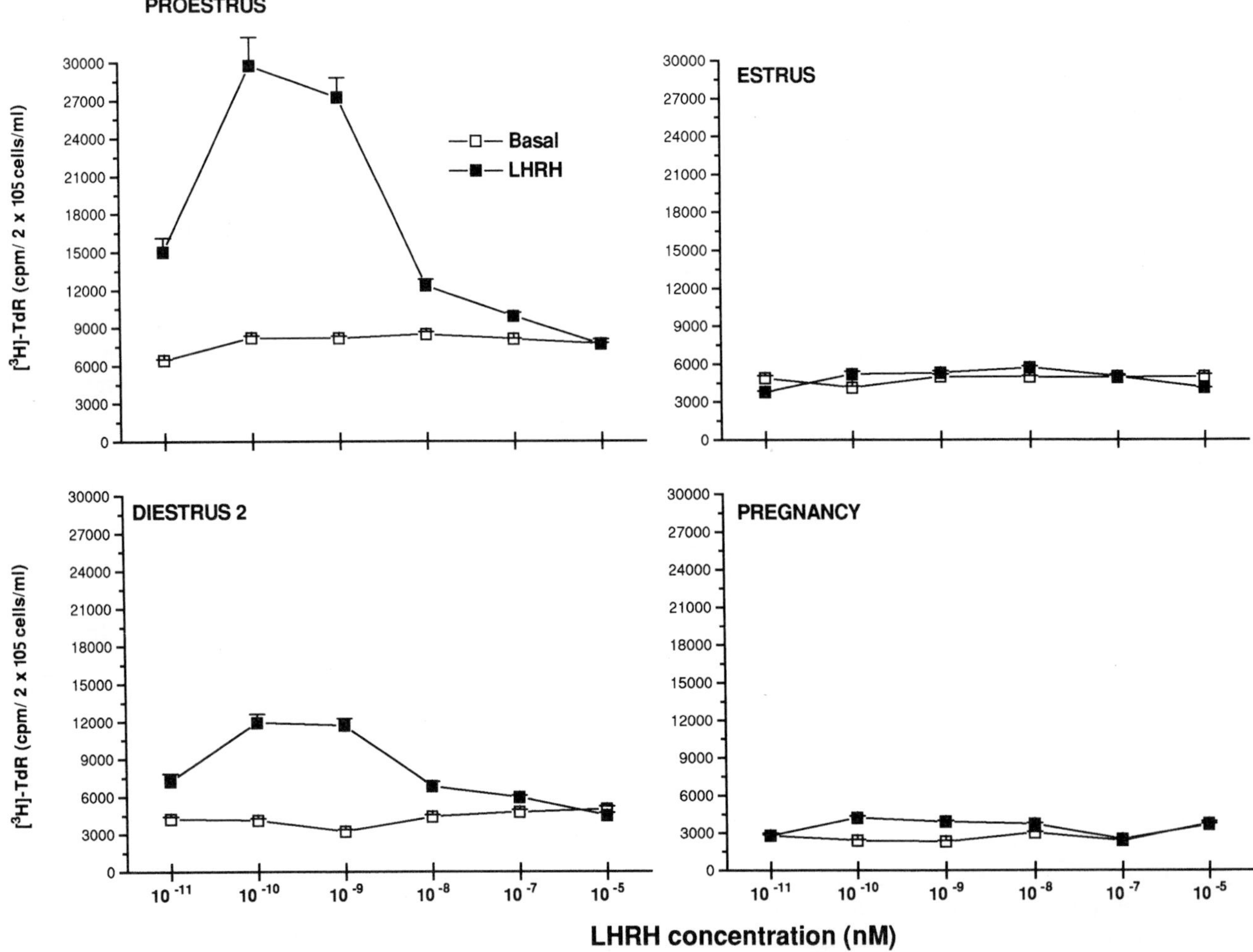

FIGURE 11 LHRH regulation of thymic cell proliferation under different hormonal conditions. The ability of the natural decapeptide LHRH to influence thymocyte proliferation under the different hormonal conditions studied was assessed in thymocyte cell preparations by the incorporation of [^{3}H]-thymidine under both basal and stimulated conditions (Con A, 2.5 mg/mL) conditions (panels B and D). Thymic cells from the indicated hormonal conditions were prepared as described elsewhere (Morale et al., 1991), and LHRH (10^{-11} to 10^{-5}M) was added to the cultures in the absence or presence of Con A. Results represent the mean ± SEM of quadruplicate wells, and of three individual determinations. Note the significant increase of proliferative capacity induced by LHRH on proestrus, whereas a marked drop of proliferative capacity was observed in estrus and pregnant thymic cell preparations.

antiinflammatory, antiallergic, and immunosuppressive agents known, and they act in a very complex way at various steps of the immune response (see Wick et al., 1993). The effects of corticosteroids on cells of the immune system, as on other corticosteroid responsive cells, are mediated through both soluble and nuclear GRs (McEwen, 1990). Estrogens and glucocorticoids influence GR mRNA concentrations in rat brain and pituitary (Peiffer et al., 1991; Peiffer & Barden, 1988). Similar control mechanisms in the thymus could have important implications on the regulatory influence of glucocorticoids on immune functions (see Machetti, Peiffer, et al., 1994; Peiffer, Morale, Barden, & Marchetti, 1994). One major immune compartment where glucocorticoids exert their effects is the thymus (Wick et al., 1993). Since the observation that glucocorticoids induce atrophy of the cortical area of the thymus, there have been many studies on the morphologic changes and both cellular and biochemical events that lead to loss of cell viability (see Troiano et al., 1995; Wick et al., 1993). The dramatic alterations of thymus architecture and function that accompany sexual maturation (see Marchetti et al., 1989, 1990) clearly indicate a possible role of sex steroids in the processes of thymic programmed cell death.

One way to clarify estrogens-glucocorticoid interactions is to study possible changes in GR gene expression under physiological as well as pharmacological conditions that are accompanied by marked variations of the sex steroid hormonal milieu, and to then correlate such changes with alterations in immune responsiveness. Our studies have clearly shown that thymic GR mRNA concentration is under the control of gonadal and adrenal hormones (Peiffer et al., 1994). We have observed up-regulation of GR mRNA content during the luteal (i.e., estrous) phase, and a down-modulation of GR transcript on proestrous, corresponding to the phase of maximal estrogenic stimulation (Peiffer et al., 1994). The hormonal sensitivity of type II GR in the thymus is further substantiated by the sharp decrease in GR transcript during pregnancy, whereas the hormonal milieu of lactation lead to a normalization of GR mRNA concentrations to those levels measured in diestrous rats. Plasma estradiol and progesterone levels are markedly elevated during pregnancy, thus representing factors that are potentially responsible for the observed inhibition of GR mRNA concentration. On the other hand, during lactation, although the plasma estrogen concentration is low, plasma progesterone and prolactin levels are markedly elevated. It is possible, therefore, that the hormonal milieu of lactation stimulates GR transcripts within the thymus, and that the estradiol-to-progesterone ratio may be critical in the regulation of GR mRNA. The powerful modulatory effect of gonadal hormones on thymic GR was further corroborated by the sharp increase in GR transcripts following removal of ovarian steroids by ovariectomy (OVX), and by the specific decrease of GR mRNA concentration induced by a concomitant treatment of ovariectomized rats with 17-beta estradiol (Figure 12).

In addition, the ability of corticosterone in vitro to influence a T cell-mediated response in the thymus (i.e., blastogenic transformation of thymocytes) depends on the sex steroid hormone milieu. Thus, the hormonal conditions accompanied by higher GR transcript levels in the thymus (i.e., OVX, estrus) are characterized by a high degree of corticosterone inhibition of T-cell proliferation (Figure 13). On the other hand, the endogenous levels of glucocorticoids are able to influence thymocyte proliferation, whereas exogenous corticosterone application to thymocyte cultures from adrenalectomized rats produced a sharp inhibition of thymocyte proliferation (Peiffer et al., 1994).

The observed cyclic changes in immune responsiveness could have a physiological implication. For example, the decrease or suppression in cell-mediated immunity observed in the postovulatory phase of the cycle and pregnancy might play a role during the implantation process and the establishment of pregnancy. In this context, the ability of corticosterone to directly inhibit both GR transcript levels and the cell-mediated immune response within the thymus, and the modulation of such inhibitory effect by the sex steroid hormonal milieu, may offer an explanation and a molecular mechanism whereby stress may have a negative influence on reproductive processes, also via immunomodulation. Hormonally mediated alterations in immunity might also have a pathological implication in sex-related immune diseases. For example, in mice and humans, lupus erythematosus is more prevalent in females, and estrogen accelerates the disease process. In contrast, menstruation is known to exacerbate idiopathic thrombocytopenia purpura (Grossman, 1990). The sex steroid hormone milieu might also have a role in immunomodulating the stress response. Estrogens inhibit IL-6 production by IL-1-stimulated cells (Tabibzadeh, Santharan, Sehgal, & May, 1989). Since IL-6, in turn, appears to enhance cortisol levels by activating the HPA axis, it would follow that estrogenic status might influence glucocorticoid-lymphokine interactions. It seems possible, therefore, that the degree of susceptibility to, or severity of, inflammatory diseases in response to a given proinflammatory trigger may well depend on the sex steroid modulation of the HPA activity, in addition to genetic factors. The tissue-specific sensitivity to estrogen of GR mRNA concentration ob-

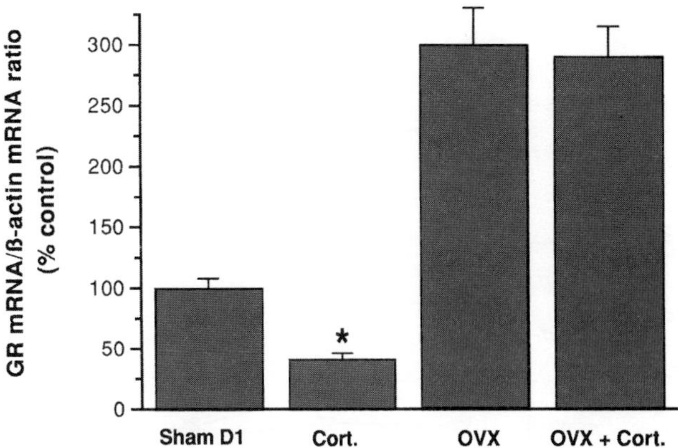

FIGURE 12 Alterations of GR mRNA transcript levels in female thymuses after castration and treatment with steroids. Total RNA was extracted from thymus of intact female rats on diestrous 1 (D1), 3 weeks after castration (OVX), and from OVX rats receiving a replacement with corticosterone (cort.) for 2 weeks. Total RNA was hybridized on Northern blots. Results are expressed as the mean ±SEM of individual determination in each thymic preparation (6 animals/group), expressed as percentages of GR mRNA/β-actin mRNA ratios relative to control values normalized to 100%. $*p < 0.01$ (by Dunkan-Kramer test).

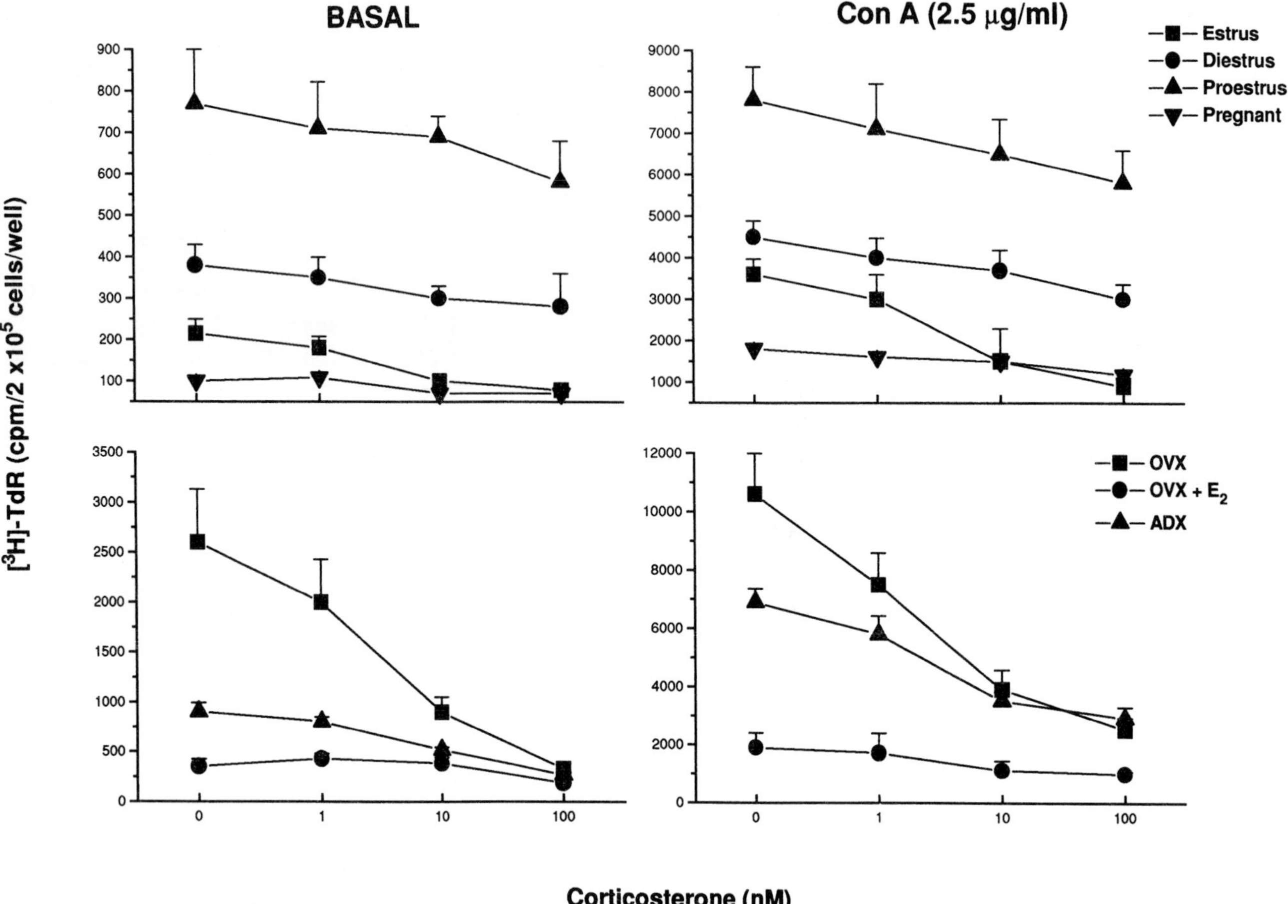

FIGURE 13 Glucocorticoid regulation of thymic cell proliferation under different hormonal conditions. The ability of corticosterone to influence thymocyte proliferation under the different hormonal conditions studied was assessed in thymocyte cell preparations by the incorporation of [^{3}H]thymidine incorporation both in basal (Panels A and C) and stimulated (Con A, 2.5 μg/mL) conditions (Panels B and D). Thymic cells from the hormonal conditions were prepared as described (see Peiffer et al., 1994), and corticosterone (1–100 nM) added to cultures in the absence or presence of Con A. Results represent the mean ±SEM of quadruplicate wells, and of three individual determinations. Note the significant inhibition of proliferative capacity induced by corticosterone in ovariectomized (OVX) and adrenalectomized (ADR) groups. On the other hand, the low proliferative capacity measured in estrus and pregnant rats was significantly reduced only at high doses of the steroid (Peiffer et al., 1994).

served in particular subsets of neurons such as the hypothalamic neurons, and at peripheral integration sites such as the pituitary gland and the thymus, point to their possible modulatory role in glucocorticoid feedback regulation and immune homeostasis.

Another potential molecular mechanism of estrogen regulation of sexual dimorphism of thymus-dependent immune functions might involve another receptor system in the thymus, the beta$_2$ adrenergic receptor (BAR). In studies using in vitro autoradiography, we demonstrated the presence of BAR in the rat thymus (Marchetti et al., 1990a, 1990b). Therefore, in the thymus, norepinephrine could act as an immunomodulator via the BAR, both as a paracrine hormone available to receptors on thymic cells, and as a localized transmitter in nerve terminals that directly contacts cortical thymocytes, mast cells, and eosinophils. Thymic BARs are preferentially found in the medullar compartment of the gland, and there is a clear sexual dimorphism in receptor organization during sexual maturation (Marchetti et al., 1990a, 1990b). A cyclic variation of receptor density accompanies the different phases of the estrous cycle with a significant increase in receptor density observed during the period of maximal estrogenic stimulation (Marchetti et al., 1990a, 1990b). The upregulation of thymic BARs induced by physiological changes in circulating sex steroid hormones is further supported by the sharp decrease in receptor density observed after castration, and by the dramatic stimulation of receptor levels accompanying the treatment of castrated rats with 17-beta estradiol. E expression of BARs in the rat thymus was further substantiated by the presence in thymic tissue of an mRNA species of 2.3 Kb that specifically hybridizes with a cDNA encoding the full coding sequence of the human BAR (Morale, Gallo, Batticane, & Marchetti, 1992; Marchetti, Morale, Paradis, & Bouvier, 1994a). The presence of BAR mRNA in cells of the immune system and the marked modulation exerted by sex steroids is intriguing in the light of the reported interactions between gonadal steroids and the immune system. The importance of such interactions seems underscored by the finding that the BAR-stimulated adenyl cyclase is markedly modulated by the sex steroid hormone background (Marchetti et al., 1994) (Figure 14). Indeed, BARs characterized in the thymic tissue preparations are functionally coupled to the adenyl cyclase system, with a sensitivity characteristic of a beta$_2$ subtype receptor. Both a high affinity state of the receptor for isoproterenol and an isoproterenol-stimulated adenyl cyclase activity could be detected in the thymus membrane preparations, with the guanine nucleotide converting all high affinity into low affinity receptors (Marchetti et al., 1994). Furthermore, an almost 70% loss of the enzyme response to GTP following castration suggests that ovarian steroids may exert potent effects on the BAR signaling pathway (Figure 14). In fact, parallel changes in both BAR density and BAR mRNA levels followed the hormonal changes associated with the rat estrous cycle, pregnancy, or castration. Such quantitative changes suggest a subtype-specific hormonal regulation of the BAR population (Marchetti et al., 1994). The effects of estrogen and progesterone on adrenergic responsiveness have been clearly established in numerous tissues; in some cases, the effects have been associated with alterations in the density of various adrenergic receptor subtypes. The regulatory effects of sex steroids on adrenergic functions include modulation of adrenergic receptor number and/or adenylate cyclase activity in the brain, uterus, ovary, prostate, mammary gland, and mammary tumors (Marchetti, Fortier, Poyet, Follea, Pelletier & Labrie, 1990d; Marchetti, & Labrie, 1990; Marchetti, Spinola, Plante, Poyet, Follea, Pelletier, & Labrie, 1987). Results of the sex steroid-dependent modulation of BAR-stimulated

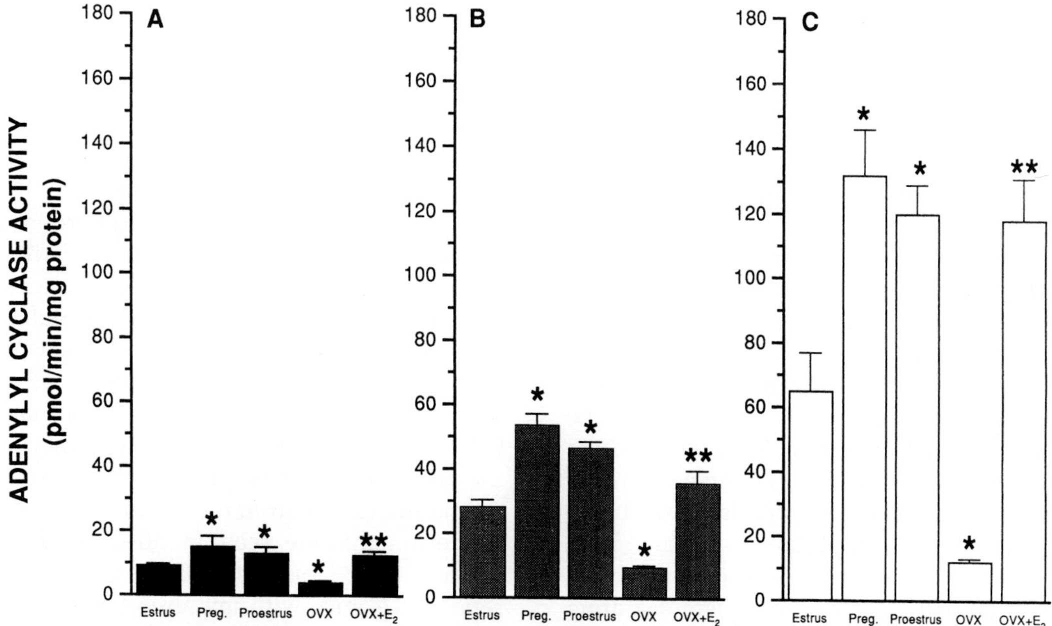

FIGURE 14 Hormonal modulation of adenylate cyclase activity. Effect of guanosine 5′-triphosphate (GTP, 10 μM) in the absence (Panel B) or presence of (−)isoproterenol (10 μM, Panel C), on adenylate cyclase activity in thymic membrane prepared from intact estrus, pregnant (Preg), or proestrus rats, as well as 3 weeks after ovariectomy (OVX) with or without concomitant treatment with 17-beta estradiol (E2, 1.125 μg twice daily for 3 weeks). Enzymatic activity was measured in the absence of GTP(A), the presence of GTP (B), or in the presence of GTP plus isoproterenol (C). Note the significant modulation of enzyme activity exerted by the different sex steroid milieu in basal conditions (A), and the sharp inhibition of the adenyl cyclase response to GTP after OVX. The stimulation of cAMP formation by isoproterenol is additive to the stimulatory effect of GTP in all the hormonal conditions studied, whereas OVX results in a complete loss of the enzyme response to isoproterenol.

cAMP accumulation in rat thymus are consistent with other data obtained in the mammary gland where the GTP-stimulated adenylate cyclase showed the highest activity during pregnancy (Marchetti et al., 1990). Of interest is that a major inhibition of thymic cell proliferation follows incubation with isoproterenol of thymocytes prepared from pregnant rats, the stage when BAR expression and both basal and GTP-stimulated adenylate cyclase activity are at their highest levels. Ovariectomy almost completely abolished the isoproterenol response in basal and activated conditions (Figure 14), a situation paralleled by a loss of BAR mRNA and adenyl cyclase activity (Marchetti et al., 1994). Moreover, treatment with estrogen and progesterone restored the isoproterenol inhibitory response and brought both receptor expression and cAMP formation back to normal levels. Although the mechanisms by which β-adrenergic stimulation alters thymocyte proliferation are unknown, one attractive possibility involves interaction at the level of second messengers. Simulation of adenyl cyclase provides inhibitory signals for T-cell proliferation. In mature T-cells, IL-2, induced by agonists of the phosphoinositide pathway, effects a series of cascading interactions that eventuate in cell proliferation (see Batticane et al., 1991). Since IL-2 activates PKC, which in turn inhibits adenyl cyclase activity, agents affecting either of these biochemical pathways may potentiate or inhibit T-cell proliferation.

On the other hand, we have provided evidence (Morale et al., 1992) that the immune system may provide signals that alter the BAR-adenyl cyclase signaling pathway within the thymus. Down- and up-regulation of BAR activity accompanies the ascending and the descending phases of the immune response elicited by an antigenic challenge, suggesting that an integrated network of hormones (steroid hormones, catecholamines) and soluble immune products might regulate immune functions also via modulation of the thymic BAR and coupled intracellular transduction mechanisms (Morale et al., 1992). The pathophysiological importance of the BAR system characterized in peripheral blood monocytes is further substantiated by findings demonstrating BAR overexpression in cytotoxic T lymphocytes and natural killer cells associated with marked disturbances of immune function in Down syndrome (Morale et al., 1992).

From the information presented, it is tempting to suggest that within the thymus, estrogen may induce, on the one hand, an increase in BAR and LHRH-R activities. These effects may then result in increased sensitivity of thymic cells to catecholamines (either circulating or locally released) and LHRH. On the other hand, a sharp decrease of both GR transcripts and thymocyte responses to corticosterone follows estrogen treatment/exposure. Such estrogen-induced up- or down-regulation of BAR, LHRH-R, and GR mRNA levels in the thymus may result in a complex control of lymphocyte sensitivity to physiological variation of endogenous hormones (Figure 15).

VII. IMPACT OF A DYSFUNCTIONAL HPA AXIS IN THE DEVELOPMENT OF IMMUNOLOGICAL SEX-DIMORPHISM AND T-CELL MATURATION IN TRANSGENIC MICE EXPRESSING GR ANTI-SENSE RNA

If the expression of genes coding for vital functions of lymphocytes are turned on and off by glucocorticoids, and if sex steroids are important in HPA axis modulation, what could be the effect of mutations of the GR gene on the immunoendocrine dialogue, as far as the maturation of thymus-dependent immune functions is concerned? To address this issue, we have used transgenic (Tg) mice that express a glucocorticoid receptor antisense RNA to study the maturation of the HPA-immune axis (Marchetti et al., 1994b; Morale, Batticane, Gallo, Barden, & Marchetti, 1995; Marchetti et al., 1997a, b; 1998; Sacedòn, Vicente, Varas, Morale, Barden, Marchetti, & Zapata, 1999). Through the expression of GR antisense RNA, Barden and associates (Pepin, Pothier and Barden, 1992) have produced Tg mice that have a hyperactive HPA axis similar to that seen in depressed patients (Barden, 1995; Holsboer, Bardelesben, Gerken, Stalla, & Muller, 1984; Hoelsboer & Barden, 1996). This model has supported the hypothesis that disturbed corticosteroid receptor regulation could be a primary factor in CRH and arginine vasopressin hyperdrive, leading to the increased activity of the HPA system and the premature escape from the cortisol suppressing action of dexamethasone seen in affective disorders (see Barden, 1995; Holsboer & Barden, 1996). In previous reports, Tg mice with impaired GR function showed decreased GR mRNA levels in brain, pituitary, and lymphoid organs, and reduced thymic and splenic GR binding capacities (Holsboer & Barden, 1996; Pepin et al., 1992, 1993; Morale et al., 1995). Moreover, Tg mice display reduced sensitivity to glucocorticoids, exaggerated adrenocorticotropic hormone (ACTH) responses to stress and exogenously administrated CRH, but maintain normal early morning levels of both ACTH and corticosterone in the face of reduced

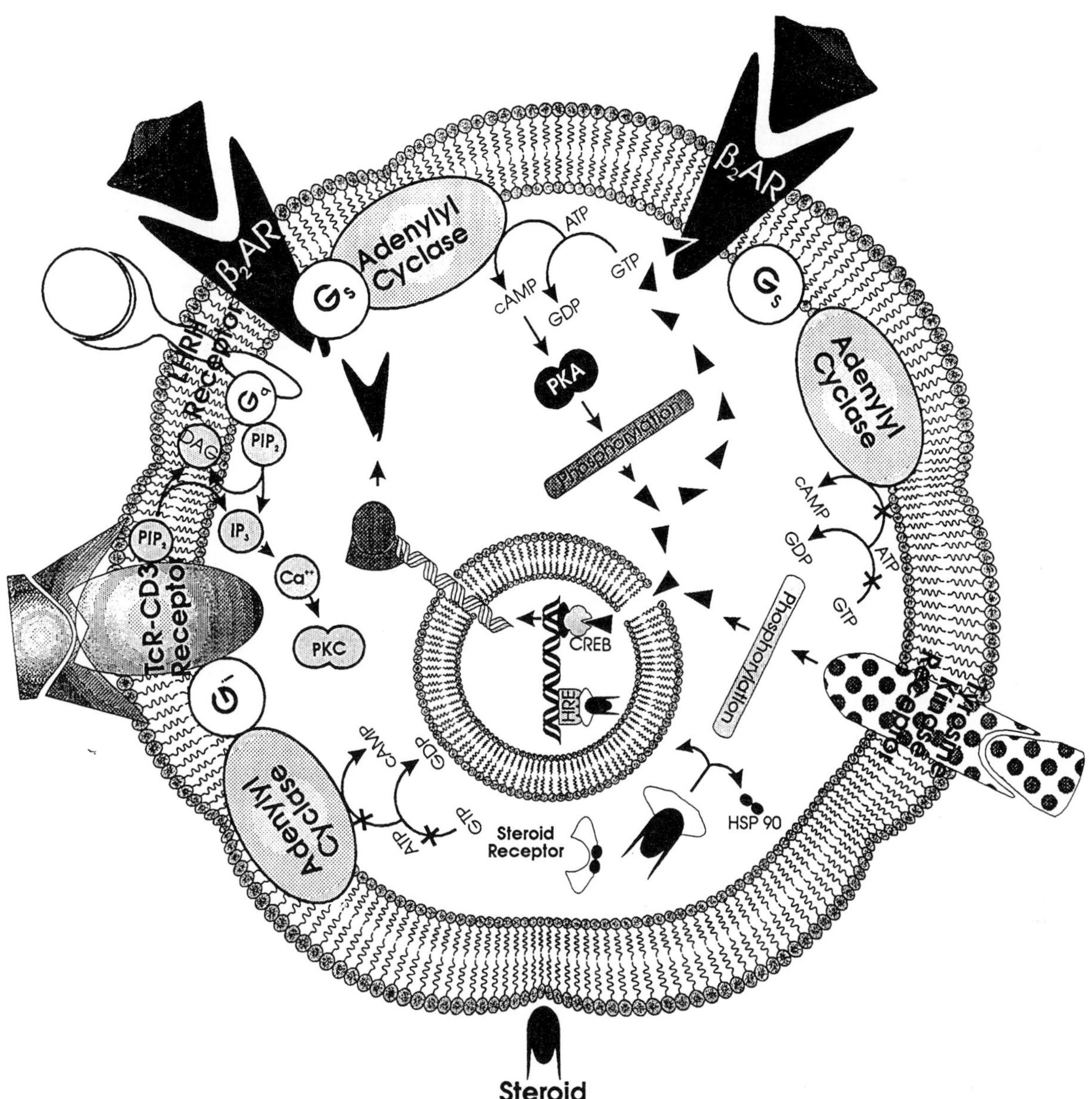

FIGURE 15 Receptors coupled to intracellular signaling systems in T-lymphocytes. Intracellular pathways elicited by the signaling through the T-cell CD3 receptor complex. The potential crosstalk between the beta$_2$ adrenergic receptor (BAR), the LHRH receptor, and steroid receptor signaling pathways, is illustrated. The stimulatory pathway (mobilizing membrane polyphosphoinositides) converging on T-cell proliferation may by activated via either LHRH-R or the TcR-CD3 complex. Crosstalk between second messenger systems (protein kinase C, PKC, protein kinase A, PKA) adjusts/downregulates the stimulatory signals. Estrogens modulate the amplitude/degree of T-cell activation by acting on LHRH-R, BAR and GR gene expression via hormone-responsive elements (HRE), resulting in amplification of either the stimulatory or inhibitory pathways. As an example, the effect of estrogens on BAR gene expression is illustrated together with interaction of cAMP responsive element (CREB) modulating the BAR cycle.

activity of hypothalamic CRH neurons (Barden, 1995; Dijkistra et al., 1998; Karanth et al., 1997; Stea, Barden, Reul, & Holsboer, 1994).

In studying the postnatal ontogeny of the HPA-immune axis loop in mice, a specific developmental pattern of GR mRNA concentration was observed in male and female mice (Morale et al., 1995). GR mRNA transcript levels were very low in 2-day-old mice and gradually increased to reach maximal levels by approximately 25 days in both males and females. However, a sexual dimorphism in the postnatal development of GR expression within the thymus was clearly observed during the course of maturation (Morale et al., 1995). At 25 days of age, GR mRNA concentration was approximately 2.5 times higher in males than in females, whereas the onset of puberty resulted in a general decline of GR mRNA levels in both male and female mice. In male mice, however, GR mRNA transcript levels were significantly greater than levels measured in female mice. On the other hand, Tg mice showed a significant loss of GR mRNA content, with levels being approximately 40 to 60% reduced compared with nontransgenic mice (Morale et al., 1995). Interestingly, GR gene expression in the thymus was low during the first 2 weeks of life, corresponding to the stress hyporesponsive period. This finding may indicate a reduced influence of corticosterone effects in the thymus. Glucocorticoids can decrease the number of receptors in both hippocampus and pituitary, and increases in corticosterone levels under stress situation may represent an additional factor in down-regulating postnatal maturation of GR within thymus gland. The significant inhibition of the age-dependent increase in GR transcript normally observed in intact mice (Morale et al., 1995), and the absence of a sexual dimorphism in mRNA concentration, underline a developmental disruption of the HPA-immune axis of Tg mice. Such effects were accompanied by a significant reduction of thymocyte responsiveness to either corticosterone or dexamethasone at physiological, but not pharmacological, concentrations (Morale et al., 1995). Of particular interest is that the phenotypic analysis of the lymphocyte subsets in Tg mice showed an imbalance in the T-cell compartment, with alterations in the distribution of the different T-cell subsets both in the thymus gland and the spleen, resulting in shifting the T-cell balance toward the CD4+ helper subset. Such phenotypic changes were reflected by functional alterations in T-cell proliferative capacity (Morale et al., 1995). The developmental pattern of T-cell responsiveness in Tg mice was characterized by loss of sex dimorphism and by a marked stimulation of blastogenesis that between 25 and 60 days (Morale et al., 1995). These Tg mice failed to show the physiological inhibition of immune responsiveness that normally occurs at the onset of puberty. In summary, it seems likely that the processes controlling T-cell trafficking/migration, as well as clonal deletion (programmed cell death) during ontogeny are disrupted in these transgenic mice.

More recently, we have studied the intrathymic differentiation during ontogeny in Tg and control mice and revealed a number of alterations (Sacedòn et al., 1999). The Tg mice exhibit a partial blockade of T-cell differentiation and a decreased percentage of apoptotic cells during fetal development but not in adult life. In contrast, thymic stroma is profoundly altered from early fetal stages, and large epithelium-free areas appear in the adult thymus (Sacedòn et al., 1999). Our study also revealed a reduction of the splenic TcRα/β population accompanied by an increase in the CD4/CD8 ratio. An analysis of different adhesion molecules and activation markers demonstrated that most of them were normally expressed in transgenic lymphocytes, whereas CD44 and CD62L expression was altered, indicating the existence of an increased proportion of primed T-cells in these animals. These data suggest a key role for glucocorticoids in coordinating the physiological dialogue between the developing thymocytes and their microenvironment (Sacedon et al., 1999). Since the fetal HPA axis is highly sensitive to events occurring early in life, and in the light of the bidirectional communication between the neuroendocrine and immune system, it seems highly important to clarify whether a disruption in the thymic developmental response early in fetal life might modulate the neuroendocrine–immune response of the adult animal to immunological and endocrinological challenges (Marchetti, Gallo, et al. 1997).

Neonatal exposure to either synthetic glucocorticoids or to stress situations has long-term effects on the responsivity of the HPA axis (Sapolsky, 1996; McEwen, 1998). Given the involvement of plasma corticosterone in the control of cellular and humoral immune responses, all conditions that affect the ontogeny of the HPA axis may have important ramifications for individual susceptibility to the development of different diseases (Chrousos, 1995; Marchetti et al., 1997; Marchetti, Morale, et al., 1997; Sternberg, 1989; Wick., 1993).

VIII. SUMMARY AND CONCLUSION

In this chapter we have attempted to describe some of the pathways responsible for the bidirectional communication between the brain-pituitary-reproductive axis and the brain-thymus-lymphoid axis. Indeed, these two systems are linked by an array of internal mechanisms of communication that use similar signals (neurotransmitters, peptides, and hormones) and act on similar recognition targets (the receptors). This communication network controls each step and every level of reproductive physiology. This chapter has focused primarily on the LHRH system as the primary channel of communication.

From the initiation of a sexually organized response, the detection of sex pheromones, and the induction of mating behavior, extra hypothalamic and hypothalamic LHRH orchestrate the psychoneuroendocrine modulation of reproductive events and the gonadotropin hormones release. On the other hand, the local expression of the neuropeptide within the ovary may directly control specific events such as follicular atresia. The presence of LHRH receptors in oocytes clearly anticipates a potential action of this decapeptide also during the process of fertilization and/or implantation.

From the bulk of the reviewed information on LHRH-astroglial interactions, it seems reasonable to hypothesize that the functional integration between the LHRH neuronal system and the astroglial cell compartment make this system suitable to study neuroimmune communications. The presence of this bidirectional informative network lends support to the concept that such crosstalk plays a major role in the integration of the multiplicity of brain signals participating in the pathophysiological control of LHRH function. Moreover, studying neuron–astroglia interactions at a cellular and molecular levels may further advance our knowledge on the specific signals and coupled mechanisms used in this crosstalk.

Within the thymus and other peripheral immune organs, LHRH plays a unique role of immunomodulator, contributing to the sex-dependent changes in immune responsiveness during the estrus/menstrual cycle as well as during pregnancy. Reciprocity of the neuroendocrine–immune signaling system is further supported by the ability of sex steroids to modulate thymus-dependent immune functions via direct effects on gene expression of specific receptor systems involved in the development of sex-dimorphism and sex dimorphic immune responses. The neuroendocrine and immunomodulatory role of LHRH continues well after parturition, since the presence of LHRH-like material within the mammary gland and milk participates in the physiological modulation of hypophyseal, gonadal, and immune functions of the pups. In fact, abolition of such influence during neonatal life sharply interferes with the programming of both neuroendocrine and immune functions. This significant role played by the hypothalamic peptide in the modulation of immune responsiveness suggests that LHRH is the signal that conveys information to both neuroendocrine and immune cells, with the role of informing and then transducing the messages into appropriate biological responses.

Cloning and sequencing lymphocyte LHRH suggests that it is identical to hypothalamic LHRH. Data on the expression of LHRH receptor mRNA in lymphocytes suggests these receptors are no different from those in the pituitary. These observations, plus the similarity of the transduction mechanisms and the sex steroid sensitivity of the pituitary and intralymphocytic LHRH system, suggest that in addition to its neuroendocrine role, LHRH acts as an immunological response modifier in the brain-pituitary-lymphoid-gonadal axis. The widespread therapeutic application of LHRH and its potent agonists and antagonistic analogs in a number of pathologies, in pediatric, gynecologic, urologic, and oncologic medicine underlines the potential clinical implications of the described experimental findings.

The section of this chapter dealing with HPA axis disruption in Tg mice with a dysfunctional GR illustrated abnormalities in the maturation of thymus gland function. Such effects may have potential pathological consequences and may influence the individual susceptibility to develop certain diseases. Disturbances of the mechanism described, on a systemic or localized basis, have significant potential for immunological dysfunctions. Characterization of the events and their underlying mechanisms that occur at different physiological glucocorticoid and sex steroid concentrations during immune reactions may aid understanding of the development of disease and generate new ideas for pharmacological strategies. The physiological role of steroid hormones is not merely immunosuppressive or immunoenhancing, but rather immunomodulatory. The central role of these hormones in the interactive communication between the neuroendocrine and immune systems requires that the mechanisms that determine efficacy in neuroimmunomodulation be further characterized at both biochemical and molecular levels. In particular, such studies will give us new insights not only into the problems of fertility regulation, but also into more general issues concerned with the pathological consequences resulting from the malfunction of a NEI axis. More importantly, we hope such studies will provide us with new tools that can be used to either reverse, minimize, or counteract some adverse events associated with dysfunctions of NEI communications.

References

Ataya, K. M., Sakr, W., Blacker, C. M., Mutchnick, M. A., & Latif, Z. A. (1989). Effect of GnRH agonists on the thymus in female rats. *Acta Endocrinologica, 121*, 833–836.

Atkinson, H. C., & Waddel, B. J. (1997). Circadian variations of corticosterone and adrenocoticotropin in the rat: sexual dimorphism and changes across the estrous cycle. *Endocrinology, 138*, 3842–3845.

Attwell, D. (1994). Glia and neurons in dialogue. *Nature, 369*, 707–708.

Azad, N., Emanuele, N. V., Halloran, M. M., 'I'entler, J., & Kelley, M. R. (1991). Presence of luteinizing hormone-releasing hormone (LHRH) mRNA in rat spleen lymphocytes. *Endocrinology, 128*, 1679–1685.

Azad, N., La Paglia, N., Abel, K., Jurgens, J., Kirsteins, L., Emanuele, N. V., Kelley, M., Lawrence, A. M., & Moaghepour, N. (1993). Immunoactivation enhances the concentration of luteinizing hormone-releasing hormone peptide and its gene expression in human peripheral T-lymphocytes. *Endocrinology, 133*, 215–222.

Badr, M., Marchetti, B., & Pelletier, G. (1988). Modulation of hippocampal LHPH receptors by sex steroids in the rat. *Peptides, 9*, 441–444.

Barden, N. (1995). Do antidepressant stabilize mood through actions on the hypothalamic-pituitary-adrenocortical system? *Trends in Neuroscience, 18*, 6–11.

Barres, A. B. (1989). A new form of transmission? *Nature, 339*, 343–344.

Basco, I., Woodhams, P. L., Halios, F., & Balasz, R. (1981). Immunocytochemical demonstration of glial fibrillary acidic protein in mouse tanycytes. *Anatomical Embryology, 162*, 217–222

Batticane, N., Morale, M. C., Gallo, F., Farinella, Z., & Marchetti, B. (1991). Luteinizing hormone-releasing hormone signaling at the lymphocyte involves stimulation of interleukin-2 receptor expression. *Endocrinology, 128*, 277–286.

Bebo, B. F., Schuster, J. C., Derback, A. A., & Offlier, H. (1998). Gender differences in experimental autoimmune encephalomyelitis develop during the induction of the immune response to enclephalitogenic peptides. *Journal of Neuroscience Research, 52*, 420–426.

Behl, C., Skutella, T., Lezoualc'h, F., Post A., Widmann, N., Newton, C. J., & Holsboer, F. (1997). Neuroprotection against oxidative stress by estrogens: Structure activity relationship. *Molecular Pharmacology, 110*, 535–541.

Benveniste, E. N. (1995). Cytokine production. In H. Kettenman & B. R. Ransom (Eds.), *Neuroglia* (pp. 700–716). New York: Oxford University Press.

Besedovsky, H. O., & Sorkin, E. (1974). Thymus involvement in sexual maturation. *Nature, 249*, 356–359

Blalock, J. E. (Ed.). (1992). *Neuroimmunoendocrinology (chemical immunology vol. 52)*, (2nd ed). Basel: Karger.

Blalock, J. E. (1994). Shared ligands and receptors as a molecular mechanism for communication between the immune and neuroendocrine systems. *Annals of the New York: Academy of Science, 741*, 292–298.

Brus, L., Lambalk, C. B., Helder, M. N., Janssens, R. M., & Shoemaker, J. (1997). Specific gonadotropin-releasing hormone binding predominantly in human luteinized follicular aspirates and not in human pre-ovulatory follicles. *Human Reproduction, 12*, 769–773.

Burnstein, K. L., & Cidlowski, J. A. (1989). Regulation of gene expression by glucocorticoids. *Annual Review of Physiology, 51*, 683–701.

Calzolari, A. (1989). Recherches experimentales sur un rapport probable entre la fonction du thymus et celle des testicules. *Archivi Italiani Biologia (Tor), 307*, 71–76.

Chisari, A. N., Perone, M. J., Giovanbattista, A., & Spinedi, E. (1998). Gender-dependent characteristics of the hypothalamo-corticotrope axis function in glucocorticoid-replete and glucocorticoid-depleted rats. *Journal of Endocrinological Investigation, 21*, 737–743.

Choi, W. S., Kim, M. O., Lee, B. J., Kim, J. H., Sun, W., Seong, J. Y., & Kim, K. (1994). Presence of gonadotropin-releasing hormone mRNA in the rat olfactory piriform cortex. *Brain Research, 648*, 148–152.

Chrousos, G. P. (1995). The hypothalamic-pituitary-adrenal axis and immune-mediated inflammation. *New England Journal of Medicine, 332*, 1351–1362.

Collado, P., Beyer, C., Utchison, J. B., & S. D. (1995). Holman: Hypothalamic distribution of astrocytes is gender-related in Mongolian gerbils. *Neuroscience Letters, 184*, 86–89.

Crawley, W. F., & Jameson, J. L. (1992). Clinical counterpoint: Gonadotropin-releasing hormone deficiency: Perspectives from clinical investigations. *Endocrine Review, 13*, 635–640.

Critchlow, V., Liebelt, R. A., Bar-Sela, M., Mountcastle, W., & Lipscomb, H. S. (1963). Sex differences in resting pituitary adrenal function in the rat. *American Journal of Physiology, 205*, 807–810.

Cummings, J. L., Vinters, H. V., Cole, G. M, & Khachaturian, Z. S. (1998). Alzheimer's disease: Etiologies, pathophysiology, cognitive reserve, and treatment opportunities. *Neurology, 5* (suppl.), S2–17.

Dijkistra, I., Tilders, F. J., Aguilera, G., Kiss, A, Rabadan-Diehl, C., Barden, N., Karanth, S., Hoelsboer, F, & Reul, J. M. (1998). Reduced activity of hypothalamic corticotropin-releasing hormone neurons in transgenic mice with impaired glucocorticoid receptor function. *Journal of Neuroscience, 18*, 3909–3918.

Dluzen, D. B., & Ramirez, V. D. (1987). Involvement of olfactory bulb catecholamines and luteinizing hormone-releasing hormone in response to social stimuli mediated reproductive functions. *Annals of the New York Academy of Science, 519*, 252–257.

Dubal, D. B., Kashon, M. L., Pettigrew, L. C., Ren, J. M., Finkelstein, S. P. O., Rau, S. W., & Wise, P. M. (1998). Estradiol protects against ischemic injury. *Journal of Cerebral Blood Flow Metabolism, 18*, 1253–1258.

Gala, R. R., & Westphal, U. (1965). Corticosteroid-binding globulin in the rat: Studies on the sex differences. *Endocrinology, 77*, 841–847.

Gallo, F., Morale, M. C., Spina-Parrello, V., Tirolo, C., Testa, N., Farinella, Z., Avola, R., Beaudet, A., & Marchetti, B. (2000). Basic fibroblast growth factor acts on both neurons and glia to mediate the neurotrophic effects of astrocytes on LHRH neurons in culture. *Synapse, 36*, 233–253.

Gallo, F., Morale, M. C., Avola, R., & Marchetti, B. (1995). Cross-talk between luteinizing hormone-releasing hormone (LHRH) neurons and astroglial cells: Developing glia release factors that accelerate neuronal differentiation and stimulate LHRH release from the GT1 cell line and LHRH neurons stimulate astroglia proliferation. *Endocrine Journal, 3*, 863–874.

Gallo, F., Morale, M. C., Farinella, Z., Avola, R., & Marchetti, B. (1996). Growth factors released from astroglial cells in primary culture participate in the crosstalk between luteinizing hormone-releasing hormone (LHRH) neurons and astrocytes: Effects on LHRH neuronal proliferation and secretion. *Annals of the New York Academy of Science, 784*, 513–516.

Garcia-Segura, L. M., Chowen, J. A., Duenas, M., Torres-Aleman, I., & Naftolin, F. (1994). Gonadal steroids as promoters of neuroglial plasticity. *Psychoneuroendocrinology, 19*, 445–453.

Giulian, D. (1990). Microglia, cytokines, and cytotoxins: Modulators of cellular responses after injury to the central nervous system. *Journal of Immunology and Immunopharmacology, 10*, 15–21.

Gould, K. G., Akinbami, M. A., & Mann, D. R. (1998). Effect of neonatal treatment with a gonadotropin-releasing hormone antagonist on developmental changes in circulating lymphocytes subsets: A longitudinal study in male rhesus monkeys. *Developmental Immunology, 22*, 456–467.

Greenstein, B. D., Fitzpatrick, F. T. A., Kendall, M. D., Wheeler, M. J. (1987). Regeneration of the thymus in old male rats treated with a stable analogue of LHRH. *Journal of Endocrinology, 112*, 345–348.

Grossman, C. J. (1984). Regulation of the immune system by sex steroids. *Endocrine Review, 5*, 435–445.

Grossman, C. J. (1990). Are there underlying immune-neuroendocrine interactions responsible for immunological sexual dimorphism? *Progress in Neuroendocrinology, 3*, 75–80.

Hatton, G. I., Perlmutter, L. S., Salm, A. K., & Tweedle, C. D. (1984). Dynamic neuronal-glial interactions in hypothalamus and pituitary: Implications for control of hormone synthesis and release, *Peptides, 5* (Suppl. 1), 121–124.

Holsboer, F., Bardelebe, U., Gerken, A., Stalla G. K., & Muller O. A. (1984). Blunted corticotropin releasing factor in depression. *New England Journal of Medicine, 311*, 112–119.

Holsboer, F., & Barden, N. (1996). Antidepressant and hypothalamic-pituitary-adrenocortical regulation. *Endocrine Review, 17*, 187–205.

Hugues, F. M., & Gorospe, W. C. (1991). Biochemical evidence of apoptosis (programmed cell death) in granulosa cells: Evidence for a potential mechanism underlying follicular atresia. *Endocrinology, 129*, 2415–2419.

Jacobson, J. D., Nisula, B. C., & Steinberg, A. D. (1994). Modulation of the expression of murine lupus by gonadotropin-releasing hormone analogs. *Endocrinology, 134*, 2516–2521.

Kallman, F. J., Schoenfeld, W. A., & Barrera, S. E. (1944). The genetic aspects of primary enucoidism. *American Journal of Mental Deficit, 48*, 203–236.

Kalra, S. P. (1993). Mandatory neuropeptide-steroid signaling for the preovulatory luteinizing hormone-releasing hormone discharge. *Endocrine Review, 14*, 507–538.

Karanth, S., Linthorst, A. C. E., Stalla, G. K., Barden, N., Holsboer, F., & Reul, J. M. (1997). Hypothalamic-pituitary adrenocortical axis changes in a transgenic mouse with impaired glucocorticoid receptor function. *Endocrinology, 138*, 3476–3485.

King, J. C., & Letourneau, R. J. (1994). Luteinizing hormone-releasing hormone terminals in the median eminence of rats undergo dramatic changes after gonadectomy, as revealed by electron microscopic image analysis. *Endocrinology 134*, 1340–1351.

Knobil, E., & Hotchkiss, J. (1988). The menstrual cycle and its neuroendocrine control. In E. Knobil & J. Neill (Eds.), *The physiology of reproduction* (pp. 1971–1994). New York: Raven Press.

Kohama, S. J., Goss, J. R., Finch, C. E., & McNeill, T. H. (1995). Increases of glial fibrillary acidic protein in the aging female mouse brain. *Neurobiology of Aging, 16*, 59–67.

Kohama, S. G., Goss, J. R., McNeill, T. H., & Finch, C. E. (1995). Glial fibrillary protein increases at proestrus in the arcutae nucleus of mice. *Neuroscience Letters, 183*, 164–166.

Kozlowski, G. P., & Coates, P. W. (1985). Ependymo-neuronal specializations between LHRH fibers and cells of the cerebroventricular system. *Cell and Tissue Research, 242*, 301–311.

Kritzer, M. F., & Kohama, S. G. (1998). Ovarian hormones influence the morphology, distribution and density of tyrosine hydroxylase immunoreactive axons in dorsolateral prefrontal cortex of adult rhesus monkeys. *Journal of Comparative Neurology, 395*, 1–17.

Labue, F., Séguin, G., LeFebvre, F. A., Reeves, S. S., Bélanger, A., Massicotte, J., Cusan, L., Kelley, P. A., & Marchetti, B. (1982). Gonadal LHRH receptors and direct gonadal effects of LHRH agonists. In G. Tolis and K. B. Ruf (Eds.), *Frontiers in hormone research (Advances in Neuroendocrine Physiology)*, (pp. 33–53). Basel : Karger.

Lepri, J. J., & Wysoski, C. J. (1987). Vomeronasal chemoreception may activate reproduction in reflex-ovulating prairie voles. *Taste and Olfaction, 510*, 449–452.

McCann, S. M., Milenkovic, L., Gonzalez, M. C., Lyson, K., Karnth, S., & Rettori, V. (1993). Endocrine aspects of neuroimmunomodulation: Methods and overview. In E. B. de Souza (Ed.), *Neurobiology of cytokines* (Part A, Vol 16, pp. 187–210). San Diego: Academic Press.

McCann, S. M., Karanth, S., Kamat, A., LesDees, W., Lyson, V., Gimeno, M., & Rettori, V. (1994). Induction by cytokines of the pattern of pituitary hormone secretion in infection. *Neuroimmunomodulation, 1*, 2–13.

McEwen, B. S. (1998). Protective and damaging effects of stress mediators. *New England Journal of Medicine, 238*, 171–179.

McQueen, M., & Wilson, H. (1994). The development of astrocytes immunoreactive for glial fibrillary acidic protein in the mediobasal hypothalamus of hypogonadal mice. *Molecular and Cellular Neuroscience, 5*, 623–631.

Maier, C. C., Marchetti, B., LeBoeuf, R. D., & Blalock, J. E. (1992). Thymocytes express a mRNA that is identical to hypothalamic luteinizing hormone-releasing hormone mRNA. *Cellular and Molecular Neurobiology, 12*, 447–454.

Marchetti, B. (1997). Cross-talk signals in the CNS: Role of neurotrophic and hormonal factors, adhesion molecules and intercellular signaling agents in luteinizing hormone-releasing hormone (LHRH) neuron-astroglia interactive network. *Trends in Bioscience, 2*, 1–32.

Marchetti, B. (1989). Involvement of the thymus in reproduction. *Progress in NeuroendocrinImmunology, 2*, 64–69.

Marchetti, B. (1996). The LHRH-astroglial network of signals as a model to study neuroimmune interaction: Assessment of messenger systems and transduction mechanisms at cellular and molecular levels. *Neuroimmunomodulation, 3*, 1–27.

Marchetti, B., Fortier, M., Poyet, P., Folléa, N., Pelletier, G., & Labrie, F. (1990). β_2-adrenergic receptor in the rat mammary gland during pregnancy and lactation: Characterization, distribution, and coupling to adenylate cyclase. *Endocrinology, 126*, 565–574.

Marchetti, B., Gallo, F., Farinella, Z., & Morale, M. C. (1995). Neuroendocrineimmunology (NEI) at the turn of the century: Towards a molecular understanding of basic mechanisms and implications for reproductive physiopathology. *Endocrine Journal, 3*, 845–861.

Marchetti, B., Gallo, F., Farinella, Z., & Morale, M. C. (1996). Unique neuroendocrine-immune (NEI) interactions during pregnancy. In M. Kendal & J. Marsh (Eds.), *The physiology of immunity* (pp. 297–328). London: CRC Press.

Marchetti, B., Gallo, F., Romeo, C., Farinella, Z., & Morale, M. C. (1996). The luteinizing hormone-releasing hormone (LHRH) receptors in the neuroendocrine immune network: Biochemical bases and implications for reproductive physiopathology. *Annals of the New York Academy of Science, 784*, 209–236.

Marchetti, B., Gallo, F., Tirolo, C., Sacedòn, R., Testa, N., Farinella, Z., Barden, N., Brouwer, J., Huitinga, I., Zapata, A., Dijkistra, C., & Morale, M. C. (1997). Developmental consequence of hypothalamic-pituitary-adrenocortical system disruption: Impact on thymus gland maturation and the susceptibility to develop neuroimmune diseases. *Developmental Brain Dysfunction, 10*, 503–527.

Marchetti, B., Gallo, F., Tirolo, C., Testa, N., Farinella, Z., & Morale, M. C. (1998). Luteinizing hormone-releasing hormone (LHRH) is a primary signaling molecule in the neuroimmune network of signals. *Annals of the New York Academy of Science, 840*, 205–248.

Marchetti, B., Guarcello, V., Morale, M. C., Bartoloni, G., Farinella, Z., Cordaro, S., & Scapagnini, U. (1989). Luteinizing hormone-releasing hormone (LHRH) binding sites in the rat thymus: Characteristic and biological function. *Endocrinology, 125*, 1025–1034.

Marchetti, B., Guarcello, V., Morale, M. C., Bartoloni, G., Raiti, F., Palumbo, Jr. G., Farinella, Z., Cordaro, S., & Scapagnini, U. (1989). Luteinizing hormone-releasing hormone (LHRH) agonist restoration of age associated decline of thymus weight, thymic LHRH receptors, and thymocyte proliferative capacity. *Endocrinology, 125*, 1037–1048.

Marchetti, B., Guarcello, V., & Scapagnini, U. (1988). Luteinizing hormone-releasing hormone agonist (LHRH-A) binds to lymphocytes and modulates the immune response. In L. Castagnetta & I. Nenci (Eds.), *Biology and biochemistry of normal and cancer cell growth* (pp. 149–152): London: Harwood Academic Press.

Marchetti, B., & Labrie, F. (1990). Hormonal regulation of beta-adrenergic receptors in the rat mammary gland during the estrous cycle and lactation: Role of sex steroid and prolactin. *Endocrinology, 125*, 575–588.

Marchetti, B., & Labrie, F. (1982). Prolactin inhibits pituitary LHRH receptors in the rat. *Endocrinology, 111*, 1209–1219.

Marchetti, B., Morale, M. C., Brouwer, J., Tirolo, C., Testa, N., Farinella, Z., Dijikistra, C., & Barden, N. (1997). Neurochemical, pharmacological and immunological assessments in a transgenic mouse model of neuroendocrine changes in depression. *Aging, Clinical and Experimental Research, 9*: 26–27.

Marchetti, B., Morale, M. C., Guarcello, Cutuli, V., Raiti, F., Batticane, N., Palumbo G. Jr., Farinella, Z., & Scapagnini, U. (1990). Crosstalk communication in the neuroendocrine-reproductive axis: Age-dependent alterations in the common communication networks. *Annals of the New York Academy of Science, 594*, 309–325.

Marchetti, B., Morale, M. C., Paradis, P., & Bouvier, M. (1994). Characterization, expression and hormonal control of a β_2-adrenergic receptor. *American Journal of Physiology, 267*, E718–E731.

Marchetti, B., Morale, M. C., & Pelletier, G. (1990a). Sympathetic nervous system control of thymus gland maturation: Autoradiographic characterization and localization of the beta$_2$-adrenergic receptor in the rat thymus gland and presence of a sexual dimorphism during ontogenic development. *Progress in. NeuroendocrinImmunology, 3*, 103–111.

Marchetti, B., Morale, M. C., & Pelletier, G. (1990b). The thymus gland as a major target for the central Nervous system and the neuroendocrine system: Neuroendocrine modulation of thymic beta$_2$-adrenergic receptor distribution as revealed by in vitro autoradiography. *Molecular and Cellular Neurosciences, 1*, 10–21.

Marchetti, B., Palumbo, G., Cittadini, E., Cianci, A., Palermo, R., Lomeo, E., Cianci, S., & Scapagnini, U. (1987). LHRH receptors in human ovary and corpus luteum: Possible role in the intragonadal regulation of human reproductive function. In E. S. Teoh, S. S. Ratman, & V. H. H. Goh (Eds.), *Releasing hormones and genetics and immunology in human reproduction (Advances in Fertility and Sterility)*, (pp. 43–55), Parthenon Publishing Groups, Casterton.

Marchetti, B., Peiffer, A., Morale, M. C., Batticane, N., Gallo, F., & Barden, N. (1994). Transgenic animals with impaired type II glucocorticoid receptor expression: A model to study aging of the neuroendocrine immune system. *Annals of the New York Academy of Science, 719*, 308–327.

Marchetti, B., Reeves, J. J., Pelletier, G., & Labrie, F. (1982). Modulation of pituitary luteinizing hormone-releasing hormone receptors by sex steroids and LHRH in the rat. *Biology of Reproduction, 27*, 133–144.

Marchetti, B., & Scapagnini, U. (1985). Modulation of opioid influence on pituitary luteinizing hormone-releasing hormone receptors in the female rat. *Neuroendocrinology Letters, 7*, 11–18.

Millhouse, O. E. (1972). Light and electron microscopic studies of the ventricular wall. *Zeitschrift für Zellforschung, 127*, 149–174.

Morale, M. C., Batticane, N., Bartoloni, G., Guarcello, V., Farinella, Z., Galasso, M. G., & Marchetti, B. (1991). Blockade of central and peripheral luteinizing hormone-releasing hormone (LHRH) receptors in neonatal rats with a potent LHRH-antagonist inhibits the morphofunctional development of the thymus and maturation of cell-mediated and humoral immune responses. *Endocrinology, 128*, 1073–1085.

Morale, M. C., Batticane, N., Cioni, M., & Marchetti, B. (1992). Upregulation of lymphocyte beta-adrenergic receptors in Down's syndrome: A biological marker of a neuroimmune deficit. *Journal of Neuroimmunology, 38*, 185–198.

Morale, M. C., Batticane, N., Gallo, F., Barden, N., & Marchetti, B. (1995). Disruption of hypothalamic-pituitary-adrenocortical system in transgenic mice expressing type glucocorticoid receptor antisense ribonucleic acid permanently impairs T-cell functions: Effects on T-cell trafficking and T-cell responsiveness during post-natal maturation. *Endocrinology, 136*, 3949–3960.

Morale, M. C., Gallo, F., Batticane, N., & Marchetti, B. (1992). The immune response evokes up- and down-modulation of a β_2-adrenergic receptor messenger RNA concentration in the male rat thymus. *Molecular Endocrinology, 6*, 1513–1522.

Naftolin, F., Leranth, C., Perez, J., & Garcia Segura, L. M. (1993). Estrogen induces synaptic plasticity in adult primate neurons. *Neuroendocrinology, 57*, 935–939.

Nappi, R. E., & Rivest, S. (1997). Effect of immune and metabolic challenges on the luteinizing hormone-releasing hormone neuronal system in cycling female rats: An evaluation at the transcriptional level. *Endocrinology, 138*, 1374–1384.

Nichols, C., Finch, C. E., & Nelson, J. F. (1995). Food restriction delays the age-related increase in GFAP mRNA in rat hypothalamus. *Neurobiology of Aging, 16*, 105–110.

Ojeda, G. A., Dissen, & Junier, M. P. (1993). Neurotrophic factors and female sexual development. *Front Neuroendocrinology , 13*, 120–162.

Parry, B. L. (1995). Mood disorders linked to the reproductive cycle in women. In F. E. Bloom & D. J. Kupfer (Eds.), *Psychopharmacology: The fourth generation of progress* (pp. 1029–1042). New York: Raven Press.

Patchev, V. K., & Almeida, O. F. X. (1996). Gonadal steroids exert facilitating "buffering" effects on glucocorticoid-mediated transcriptional regulation of corticotropin-releasing hormone and corticosteroid receptor genes in rat brain. *Journal of Neuroscience, 16*, 7077–7084.

Peiffer, A., & Barden, N. (1987). Estrogen-induced decrease of glucocorticoid receptor messenger ribonucleic acid concentration in rat anterior pituitary gland. *Molecular Endocrinology, 1*, 435–440.

Peiffer, A., Lapointe, B., & Barden, N. (1991). Hormonal regulation of Type II glucocorticoid receptor messenger ribonucleic acid in rat brain. *Endocrinology, 129*, 2166–2174.

Peiffer, A., Morale, M. C., Barden, N., & Marchetti, B. (1994). Modulation of glucocorticoid receptor gene expression in the thymus by the sex steroid hormone milieu and correlation with sexual dimorphism of immune response. *Endocrine Journal, 2*, 181–191.

Pepin, M. C., Pothier, F., & Barden, N. (1992). Impaired type II glucocorticoid-receptor function in mice bearing antisense RNA transgene. *Nature, 355*, 725–728.

Pierpaoli, W., & Besedovsky, H. O. (1975). Interdependence of the thymus in programming neuroendocrine functions. *Clinical and Experimental Immunology, 20*, 323–329.

Pierpaoli, W., & Spector, N. H. (Eds.). (1994). *Neuroimmunomodulation: Interventions in aging and cancer, Proceedings of New York Academy of Sciences (USA)*, 719.

Radvick, S,. Ticknor C. M., Nayakama, Y., Notides, A. C., Rahman, A., Weintraub, B. D., Cuttler, G. B., & Wondisford, F. E. (1991). Evidence for direct estrogen modulation of the human gonadotropin-releasing hormone gene. *Journal of Clinical Investigation, 88*, 1649–1653.

Rettori, V., Gimeno, M. F., Karara, A., Gonzalez, M., & McCann, S. M. (1991). Interleukin-1 alpha inhibits prostaglandin E2 release to suppress pulsatile release of luteinizing hormone but not follicle-stimulating hormone. *Proceedings of the National Academy of Sciences (USA), 88*, 2763–2767.

Rivest, S., Lee, S., Attardi, B., & Rivier, C. (1993). The chronic intracerebroventricular infusion of interleukin-1 beta alters the activity of the hypothalamic-pituitary-gonadal axis of cycling rats. *Endocrinology, 133*, 2424–2430.

Rivier, C., & Erickson, G. (1993). The chronic intracerebral infusion of interleukin 1-beta alters the activity of the hypothalamic-pituitary gonadal axis of cycling rats. Induction of pseudopregnant-like corpora lutea. *Endocrinology, 133*, 2431–2437.

Rivier, C., & Vale, W. (1989). In the rat interleukin acts at the level of the brain and gonads to interfere with gonadotropin and sex steroids secretion. *Endocrinology, 124*, 205–209.

Sacedòn, R., Vicente, A., Varas, A., Morale, M. C., Barden, N., Marchetti, B., & Zapata, A. (1999). Partial blockade of T-cell differentiation during ontogeny and marked alterations of the thymic microenvironment in transgenic mice with impaired glucocorticoid receptor function. *Journal of Neuroimmunology, 98*, 157–167.

Sapolsky, R. M. (1996). Stress, glucocorticoids and damage to the nervous system: The current state of confusion. *Stress, 1*, 1–19.

Schneider L. S., & Finch, C. E. (1997). Can estrogens prevent neurodegeneration? *Drugs Aging, 11*, 87–95.

Schultz, C., Braak, H., & Braak, E. (1996). A sex difference in the neurodegeneration of the human hypothalamus. *Neuroscience Letters, 212*, 103–106.

Shwanzel-Fukuda, M., & Pfaff, D. W. (1989). Origin of luteinizing hormone-releasing hormone neurons. *Nature, 338*, 161–164.

Schwanzel-Fukuda, M., Jorgeson, K. L., Bergen, H. T., Weesner, G. D., & Pfaff, S. W. (1992). Biology of normal luteinizing hormone-releasing neurons during and after their migration from olfactory placode. *Endocrine Review, 13*, 623–634.

Silveman, A. J. (1988). The gonadotropin-releasing hormone (GnRH) neuronal system: Immunocytochemistry. In E. Knobil & J. D. Neil (Eds.), *The physiology of reproduction* (pp. 3789–3831). New York: Raven Press.

Silverman, R. C., Gibson, M. J., & Silverman, A. J. (1991). Relationship of glia to GnRH axonal outgrowth from third ventricular grafts in hpg hosts. *Experimental Neurology, 114*, 259–274.

Silverman, A. J., Millar, R. P., King, J. A., Zhuang, X., & Silver, R. (1994). Mast-cells with gonadotropin-releasing hormone-like immunoreactivity in the brain of doves. *Proceeding of the National Academy of Sciences (USA), 91*, 3695–3699.

Spinedi, E., Suescun, M. O., Hadid, R., Daneva, T., Gaillard, R. C. (1992). Effects of gonadectomy on the endotoxin-stimulated hypothalamo-pituitary adrenal axis: Evidence for a neuroendocrine immunological sexual dimorphism. *Endocrinology, 131*, 2430.

Stea, I., Barden, N., Reul, J. M. H., & Holsborn, F. (1994). Dexamethasone nonsuppression in transgenic mice expressing antisense RNA to the glucocorticoid receptor. *Journal of Psychiatric Research, 28*, 1–5.

Sternberg, E. M. (1989). The role of the hypothalamic-pituitary-adrenal axis in an experimental model of arthritis. *Progress in Neuroendocrinimmunology, 2*, 103–108.

Stojikovic, S. S., Reinhart, J., & Catt, K. J. (1994). Gonadotropin-releasing hormone receptor: Structure and signal transduction pathways. *Endocrine Review, 15*, 462–498.

Sundaram, K., Didolkar, A., Thau, R., Chandhuri, M., & Schmidt, F. (1988). Antagonists of luteinizing hormone releasing hormone bind to rat mast cells and induce histamine release. *Agents Actions, 25*, 307–310.

Tabibzadeh, S. S., Santhanam, U., Sehgal, P. B., & May, L. T. (1989). Cytokine-induced production of IFN-beta$_2$/ IL-6 by freshly explanted human endometrial stromal cells. *Journal of Immunology, 42*, 3134–3139.

Tremblay, Y., Belanger, A., & Marchetti, B. (1985). Specificity of the direct effect on LHRH agonist on testicular 17-alpha hydroxylase but not 5-alpha reductase activity in hypophysectomized adult rats. *Molecular and Cellular Endocrinology, 40*, 33–43.

Troiano, L., Monti, D., Cossarizza, A., Lovato, E., Tropea, F., Barbieri, D., Morale, M. C., Gallo, F., Marchetti, B., & Franceschi, C. (1995). Involvement of CD45 in and heat-shock induced apoptosis of rat thymocytes. *Biochemical and Biophysical Research Communications, 214*, 941–948.

Turner, B. B., & Weaver, D. A. (1985). Sexual dimorphism of glucocorticoid in rat brain. *Brain. Research, 343*, 16–19.

Ussa, J. E., Cadavid, A. P., & Maldonado, J. G. (1994). Is the immune system necessary for placental reproduction? A hypothesis on the mechanisms of alloimmunotherapy in recurrent spontaneous abortion, *Medical Hypotheses*, 42, 193–197.

Wilson, T. M., Yu-Lee, L., & Kelly, M. R. (1995). Coordinate gene expression of luteinizing hormone-releasing hormone (LHRH) and the LHRH-receptor following prolactin stimulation in the rat Nb2 T cell line: Implications for a role in immunomodulation and cell-cycle gene expression. *Molecular Endocrinology, 110*, 134–141.

Wick, G., Hu. Y., Schwarz, S., & Kroemer, G. (1993). Immunoendocrine communication via the hypothalamo-pituitary-adrenal axis in autoimmune diseases. *Endocrine Reviews, 14*, 539–563.

CHAPTER

13

Preproenkephalin: An Unappreciated Neuroimmune Communicator

FREDRIK ERIKSSON, ANNEMIEKE KAVELAARS, COBI J. HEIJNEN

I. INTRODUCTION

Ever since Wybran and colleagues showed the existence of opioid receptors on T cells in 1979 (Wybran, Appelboom, Famaey, & Govaerts, 1979), the possible role of opioids in the immune system has been investigated. Although it has been shown in the last 20 years that opioids do play important roles in physiological systems other than the central nervous system (CNS), their role as neurotransmitters is often considered as their main function. This review focuses on the role of preproenkephalin (PPE) gene products in the immune system and argues that this role is important and compatible with PPE's role as a neurotransmitter.

The endogenous opioids all stem from one of three propeptides that are encoded by one of the three opioid genes. Proopiomelanocortin (POMC) was the first to be cloned, and it encodes several products such as adrenocorticotropic hormone (ACTH), β-lipotropin, α-melanocyte-stimulating hormone, and β-endorphin. So far POMC is the only opioid gene that has been shown to encode nonopioid bioactive peptides. Another endogenous opioid precursor is prodynorphin, which encodes dynorphin and Leu-enkephalin. The focus of this review is the PPE gene and its products. Its main products are considered to be the pentapeptides Met- and Leu-enkephalin. The PPE gene also encodes several larger products, many of which contain the enkephalin sequence, the so-called enkephalin-containing peptides (ECP).

II. STRUCTURE OF THE PPE GENE

Met- and Leu-enkephalin were the first endogenous opioids to be discovered. Hughes and colleagues identified them as natural ligands for the then newly isolated opioid receptor (Hughes, Smith, Kosterlitz, Fothergill, Morgan, & Morris, 1975). Pert and Snyder discovered the first opioid receptor in 1973 by observing binding of radiolabeled naloxone to rodent brain tissue (Pert & Snyder, 1973a, 1973b).

Enkephalins, with their five-amino-acid sequence, are generally regarded as the smallest peptides that can bind to and activate the opioid receptor. However, there are some reports that show an opioid receptor-mediated effect of a three-amino-acid part of enkephalin (Haberstock & Marotti, 1995; Haberstock, Marotti, & Banfic, 1996). The sequences for Met- and Leu-enkephalins differ by only one amino acid at the carboxy terminal end, Tyr-Gly-Gly-Phe-Xxx (Xxx=Met or Leu). Although the enkephalins were

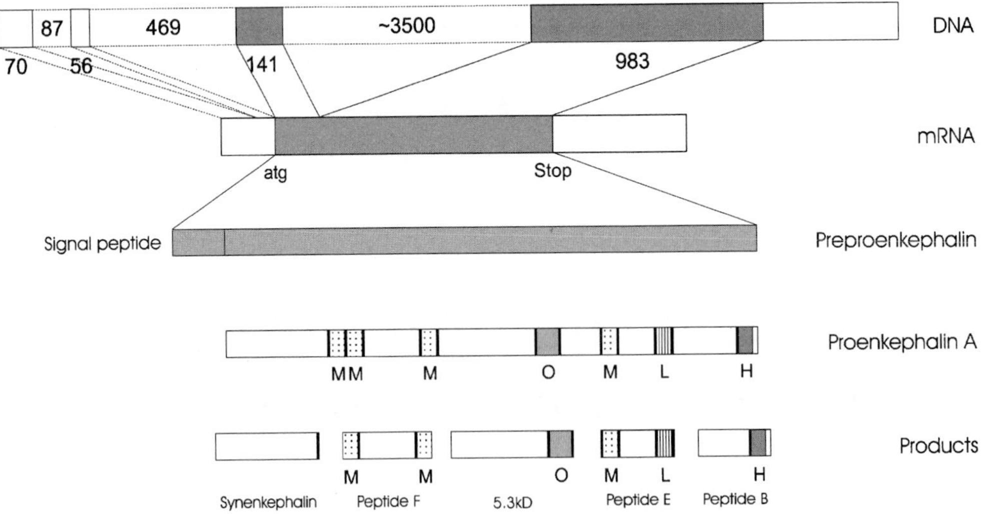

FIGURE 1 The structure of the PPE gene including its transcription, translation, and processing. The products shown are examples of some final PPE gene products. The number of base pairs are given in the gene map.

discovered in 1975, it took until 1982 before the PPE gene, which encodes the enkephalins, was cloned. Several groups worked on cloning parts of the PPE gene (Comb, Rosen, Seeburg, Adelman, & Herbert, 1983; Comb, Seeburg, Adelman, Eiden, & Herbert, 1982; Gubler, Seeburg, Hoffman, Gage, & Udenfreund, 1982; Legon et al., 1982; Noda et al., 1982). The structure of the gene is shown in Figure 1. It contains four exons and three introns. Only exon three and part of exon four are translated into the human 243-amino-acid propeptide, proenkephalin A (PEA). As shown in Figure 1, part of intron three of the PPE gene has not been sequenced yet.

III. PROCESSING OF THE PPE GENE PRODUCT

PEA contains four Met-enkephalin sequences, two C terminal extended Met-enkephalins, and one Leu-enkephalin sequence (Figure 1). Pairs of basic amino acids are flanking all the enkephalin sequences. PEA is processed in several steps by a number of endopeptidases. In this metabolic process a number of intermediate size peptides are created (Table I). Some intermediate size peptides, the ECP, contain one or more enkephalin sequences and therefore have potential opioid bioactivity. In certain opioid receptor assays some ECP (e.g., peptide E and BAM-20P) have been shown to be more potent than the free pentapeptide in stimulating the opioid receptor (Dillen, Miserez, Claeys, Aunis, & De Potter, 1993). The paired basic amino acids flanking the enkephalins determine where processing takes place. Two types of enzyme activity are necessary for PEA processing: a trypsin-like activity that recognizes and cuts di-basic amino acids, and a carboxypeptidase B-like activity that removes basic amino acids at the carboxy

TABLE I Bovine Adrenal Medulla PPE Gene Products, Including Their Positions and Calculated Molecular Weights

PPE fragment	Sequence in PPE	Molecular weight
Synenkephalin	1–72	7993
Proenkephalin 1–77	1–77	8549
Proenkephalin 1–239	1–239	27,262
Proenkephalin 1–206	1–206	23,338
Proenkephalin 1–165	1–165	18,224
Proenkephalin 1–113	1–113	12,660
Peptide F	80–113	3845
Amidorphin	80–106	3005
Amidorphin 8–26	87–106	2193
Proenkephalin 166–165	116–165	5325
Peptide I	168–206	4848
Proenkephalin 168–179	168–179	1426
Peptide E	182–206	3157
BAM 18P	182–199	2335
Methorphamide	182–190	1042
BAM 20P	182–201	2619
BAM 22P	182–203	2839
BAM 12P	182–193	1425
Peptide B	209–239	3657
Heptapeptide	233–239	877
Octapeptide	158–165	900
Leu-enkephalin	202–206	556
Met-enkephalin	73–77	574

Note: Table adapted from Dillen and colleagues (1993).

terminal of peptides (Wilson, 1991). Several trypsin-like enzymes, both membrane bound and soluble, have been shown to participate in the processing (Evangelista, Ray, & Lewis, 1982; Mizuno & Matsuo, 1985; Shen, Roberts, & Lindberg, 1989). A carboxypeptidase enzyme involved is carboxypeptidase H (enkephalin convertase) (Fricker & Snyder, 1982; Fricker, Supattapone, & Snyder, 1982).

Although the enkephalins were first discovered in brain tissue, they were soon shown to be expressed in other tissues as well. Schultzberg and colleagues showed a high expression in chromaffin cells of the adrenal medulla (Schultzberg, Hokfelt, et al., 1978; Schultzberg, Lundberg, et al., 1978). Chromaffin cells actually have a higher expression of enkephalins than brain tissue. Therefore, much of the work done on elucidating the processing steps of PEA has been done in chromaffin cells from bovine adrenal medulla. ECP also were first discovered in bovine adrenal medulla (Lewis, Stern, Rossier, Stein, & Udenfriend, 1979). When these ECP are treated with trypsin and carboxypeptidase B, enkephalin pentapeptides are detected (Kimura et al., 1980; Lewis et al., 1980; Lewis et al., 1979).

Wilson demonstrated in 1991 that the processing of PEA in chromaffin cells is completed within 2 h. The processing occurs before the PEA products are finally incorporated in the chromaffin storage vesicles. Although further processing in the vesicles has been shown to take place, it is at such a low rate compared with the initial processing that no significant change in the ratio of ECP and free enkephalin takes place (Fleminger, Ezra, Kilpatrick, & Udenfriend, 1983; Rossier, Trifaro, Lewis, Lee, Stern, Kimura, Stein, & Udenfriend, 1980; Wilson, 1991). This strongly suggests that the composition of PPE products normally found in chromaffin cells is representative of the full range of final products produced; i.e., the intermediate size PEA-derived peptides found are not mere processing intermediates but end products (Wilson, 1991). In accordance with this conclusion, when chromaffin cells are stimulated to release their vesicle content intermediate size PEA products can be shown to be in circulation.

Studies of processing in brain tissues revealed the interesting fact that PEA is processed differently in the various tissues. Liston and colleagues showed that the PPE products found in the supraoptic nucleus, the pituitary stalk, and the pituitary differed in their size profiles. They also made comparisons with the processing in chromaffin cells and found even more variety in the size profiles of the final products. So far, no alternative PPE mRNA species has been described, and it is therefore likely that the amount and regulation of processing enzymes differs between tissues. It appeared that in the CNS, PEA is initially cleaved at the amino terminal, whereas initial processing in chromaffin cells takes place at the carboxy terminal end (Dillen et al.,1993; Liston, Patey, & Rossier, 1984).

The difference in processing of PPE seen in the CNS and the adrenal medulla opens the possibility that PPE is processed in a unique fashion in the immune system as well. This processing may yield unique PPE products with previously unknown functions. Focusing on PPE gene products in general, rather than mainly at the enkephalins, may prove fruitful in the search for the role of PPE gene products within the immune system.

IV. CLASSICAL ROLE OF PPE

The classical role of PPE gene products is as neurotransmitters involved in pain relief. This is probably because the first studies on opioid receptors and enkephalins had neuropeptide function as the main focus. The motivation behind the research on receptor isolation was the identification of the mechanism via which exogenous opiates, such as opium and morphine, functioned. Endogenous opioids were later discovered to be the natural ligands for the opioid receptors.

Nociception, the sensing of pain, is a multistep process, and opioids have been shown to affect it at several levels. Figure 2 outlines, at a cellular level, the

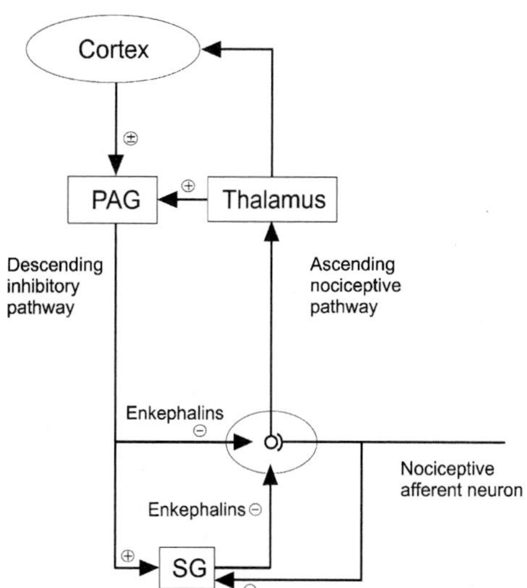

FIGURE 2 Schematic view of the nociceptive pathway, indicating were enkephalins act. Periaqueductal grey matter (PAG); substantia gelationsa (SG).

mechanism of nociception and the site where opioids act. At the molecular level, opioids bind to specific receptors on neurons and cause hyperpolarization via an increase in K^+ conductance. This process in turn decreases Ca^{2+} influx during action potential, which causes a decrease in firing rate and thus presynaptic inhibition of neurotransmitter release (Rang & Dale, 1991).

Early in opioid research it became clear that both the opioid peptides and their receptors were also expressed outside the CNS. From these data two interesting questions could be raised: where did the opioid signalling system originate from, and what function does it play in other organs?

V. ORIGIN OF THE PPE SIGNALING SYSTEM

When the opioid signaling system was first discovered, researchers assumed that it stemmed from the nervous system. Because opioid signaling was shown to play an integrated and important role in the nervous system, it seemed likely that it had evolved within that system. When opioids and other neuropeptides and their receptors were found in the endocrine system as well, it was suggested that the endocrine system might have originated from the nervous system. However, as opioids were discovered in more and more diverse physiological systems and also in other species, it became clear that this signaling system was much older than any single organ system. Many neuropeptides, including PPE products, are found in less complex organisms, such as invertebrates and unicellular organisms. Closely related molecules have even been found in plants. The latter suggests that the PPE signaling system developed in organisms whose ancestors diverged some 500 million years ago and that it has proven fundamental to the evolutionary survival of many organisms (Roth, 1982, 1985). As organs and physiological systems evolved in more complex multicellular organisms, they adopted and adapted the existing signaling systems. This elegantly explains why different organs and physiological systems in more complex organisms can use the same signaling system, without implying that one system necessarily originates from another. That the opioid signaling system is so highly conserved is not strange since it has been shown that the complexity of a system actually contributes to its conservation throughout evolutionary functional divergence (Suzuki, Funada, Narita, Misawa, & Nagase, 1991).

In the body, PPE products have been shown to have functions that vary widely from their classic role in nerves. Rosen and colleagues have performed interesting studies on the possible role of opioids in development. They showed that PPE mRNA is specifically expressed in several tissues outside the CNS during organogenesis. In addition, they found that as mesenchymal tissues differentiated into cartilage, bone, dermis, kidney tubules, and chorioid of the eyes, there was a transient expression of PPE mRNA that completely ceased once differentiation was complete (Keshet, Polakiewicz, Itin, Ornoy, & Rosen, 1989). These authors went on to show that PEA is processed differentially in different tissues. In heart and skin tissue, PPE gene products are present in the form of larger intermediate peptides, whereas in brain and kidney the pentapeptides are produced (Polakiewicz & Rosen, 1990). Their results suggest that, as with several other neuropeptides, PPE products may play an important role in controlling cell differentiation and proliferation.

VI. ROLE OF PPE IN THE IMMUNE SYSTEM

The opioid receptor was the first part of the opioid signaling system to be found in the immune system (Wybran et al., 1979). In a series of studies following the initial discovery, Wybran and colleagues demonstrated that opioids bind to leukocytes. In the initial experiment, enkephalin binding to leukocytes could be blocked with the opioid receptor antagonist naloxone. Several other laboratories confirmed the existence of classic opioid binding sites. However, later experiments revealed that the effects of enkephalin could be mediated via both the classic opioid receptor (naloxone reversible) and via a naloxone insensitive site.

It was discovered that the classic opioid binding site consisted of several receptor subtypes: μ, δ, κ, ϵ, and σ. The σ receptor binds only one synthetic opioid agonist and is no longer considered a true opioid receptor (Bhargava, 1991). The μ-, δ-, and κ-receptor subtypes have been shown to have effects in the immune system, although μ and δ are the most studied receptor subtypes. These three receptors are all G-protein coupled, and they regulate adenylate cyclase activity (Koski & Klee, 1981). Receptor-specific agonists and antagonists were developed and used to supply evidence for the presence of μ-, δ- and κ-type binding sites on leukocytes (Burke et al., 1984; De Montis, Devoto, Preti, & Tagliamonte, 1987; Dickenson, Sullivan, Knox, Zajac, & Roques, 1987;

Jacobson, Bajwa, Streaty, Klee, & Rice, 1983; Neil, Kayser, Gacel, Besson, & Guilbaud, 1986; Portoghese et al., 1986; Rice et al., 1983). With the cloning of the receptors in the early 1990s, it became possible to show their expression with more detail and certainty. Wick and colleagues showed that δ- and κ-receptor mRNA is expressed in peripheral blood lymphocytes as well as in a number of human and animal leukocyte cell lines (Wick, Minnerath, Roy, Ramakrishnan, & Loh, 1996). The functions in the immune system of the different opioid receptors are still debated (Plotnikoff, Faith, Murgo, Herberman, & Good, 1997).

The fact that opioid receptors were present in the immune system gave rise to the idea of direct CNS control of immune functions. This in itself was an extraordinary new idea. However, if leukocytes could also express opioid peptides themselves, a two-way communication between immune system and CNS would even be possible. This possibility was truly revolutionary (Blalock, 1994). Another aspect of the presence of both signaling peptide and receptor in the immune system would be the possibility that opioids could function in a paracrine way within the immune system.

The first indications that opioids were produced by leukocytes came from mouse studies in the mid-1980s (Smith, Morrill, Meyer, & Blalock, 1986). Immunoreactivity for enkephalins in leukocyte cultures was detected, as was PPE mRNA in mouse cell lines and isolated mast cells (Martin, Prystowsky, & Angeletti, 1987). PPE mRNA was also shown to be inducible in mouse T-helper cell lines (Zurawski et al., 1986). Another piece of evidence for leukocyte PPE expression is the observation that circulating Met-enkephalin may either come from or be stored in the white blood cell fraction of blood. Free pentapeptide has a very short half-life, about 90 s, due to degradation by enkephalinase and aminopeptidases (Roda, Venturelli, & Roscetti, 1986). Despite its short half-life, free Met-enkephalin is found in the circulation at a concentration of around 10^{-12} M (Clement-Jones, Lowry, Rees, & Besser, 1980; Plotnikoff et al., 1997). Enkephalins must therefore either both be produced and released at a high rate or the enkephalins must be protected in some way. If blood is separated into leukocytes, red blood cells, and platelets, it has been found that the leukocyte compartment contains about a 100-fold higher amount of Met-enkephalin than the other two compartments (Bhargava, 1991). Leukocytes also have been shown to adsorb Met-enkephalin better than the other compartments, although platelets have been shown to bind enkephalins as well.

Another interesting observation is that in mice, from which two major classical sources of enkephalin have been removed, the adrenal and pituitary gland, there is an increase rather than a decrease in circulating Met-enkephalin (Di Giulio, Picotti, Cesura, Panerai, & Mantegazza, 1982). These facts suggest that leukocytes may play an important role in the production and maintenance of circulating Met-enkephalin (Bhargava, 1991). Considering the circulatory nature of the cellular part of the immune system, it is an organ well suited for the production and maintenance of circulating unstable peptides. Evidence of this kind compelled people to look more in detail at opioids and their role within the immune system.

A. Expression of the PPE Gene in Leukocytes

The PPE gene has been shown to be translated in T cells and translated and processed in macrophages and activated monocytes (Kamphuis et al., 1997; Kuis, Villiger, Leser, & Lotz, 1991; Martin et al., 1987) but not in unactivated monocytes (LaMendola, Martin, & Steiner, 1997). LaMendola and colleagues showed that, together with two genes encoding peptide processing enzymes, the PPE gene is switched on as peripheral blood monocytes spontaneously differentiate into macrophages (LaMendola et al., 1997). Enkephalins have also been shown in CD68 positive monocytes from psoriatic lesions. For these monocytes enkephalin expression was shown to be independent of the activation state of the cell (Nissen, Lund, Stengaard-Pedersen, & Kragballe, 1997). Activated B cells also have been shown to express PPE mRNA. Stimulation with lipopolysaccharide (LPS) triggered B cells to express PPE mRNA with a peak production within 3 h. The expression is down to very low levels after 10 h (Rosen, Behar, Abramsky, & Ovadia, 1989). In these experiments only low levels of PPE products were secreted. Rosen and colleges speculated that PPE products might play an autocrine or paracrine role in early B cell activation.

B. The Influence of PPE Products on Leukocytes

The effects of PPE products on the immune system are now well documented by many groups. Proliferation, cytokine production, and cell-specific effects such as antibody production or respiratory burst are prominent examples of immune functions that can be regulated by enkephalins.

In T-cell proliferation Met-enkephalin works both by itself and in conjunction with other stimuli. When

Met-enkephalin acts in concert with other stimuli, it has been shown to modify the response in the target cell in a bimodal fashion, showing opposite effects when present at high vs. low concentrations. An example is the proliferative response of peripheral blood mononuclear cells to *Candida* antigens. If a high concentration of Met-enkephalin is added to such a culture, it enhances proliferation. Addition of a low concentration of Met-enkephalin inhibits proliferation (Roscetti, Ausiello, Palma, Gulla, & Roda, 1988). It also has been shown that Met-enkephalin alone can stimulate proliferation in lymphocytes in a concentration-dependent manner (Bajpai et al., 1995; Hucklebridge, Hudspith, Lydyard, & Brostoff, 1990). Hucklebridge and colleagues showed with the help of selective antagonists that this effect is mediated via the δ-opioid receptor (Hucklebridge et al., 1990).

In contrast to the effects of exogenously added enkephalins we demonstrated that autocrine PPE products from T cells could inhibit T-cell proliferation. When PPE translation was inhibited in T cells with a specific antisense oligonucleotide, an increase in proliferation could be seen (Kamphuis et al., 1998). Similarly, an increase in proinflammatory cytokines such as interferon-γ (INF-γ) and interleukin (IL)-6 was observed. The latter data indicate that the role of immune system-derived PPE gene products could be to control/down-regulate T-cell proliferation and cytokine production. Addition of Met-enkephalin pentapeptide to the antisense culture did not reverse the effects nor did the addition of a specific δ-opioid receptor agonist, deltorphin. The latter results show that the modulatory effect of endogenous PPE products is not mediated via the enkephalin pentapeptide or via the δ-opioid receptor. The conclusion must be that PPE products produced by the cell itself play an opposite role compared with exogenously added synthetic Met-enkephalin, via a nonclassical opioid–receptor interaction.

The antisense approach was also used in a setup where monocytes were stimulated by LPS, using IL-6 and IL-8 production as a read-out system. We demonstrated that monocytes showed a decrease in cytokine production when the specific antisense oligonucleotide probe was present in the culture. However, in contrast to T cells in monocytes this effect can be completely reversed by the addition of Met-enkephalin or deltorphin.

In experiments with T cells and monocytes, Kuis and colleagues shows that concanavalin A (Con A) stimulated T cells express the PPE gene. However, free enkephalins could not be detected in the supernatant. Moreover, treatment of the supernatant with processing enzymes leads to the detection of free enkephalin pentapeptides, indicating that the PPE gene is translated but that the processing of PEA does not go as far as to free enkephalin pentapeptide in T cells (Kuis et al., 1991). However, immunostaining of stimulated T cells with an antibody specific for met-enkephalin revealed that the pentapeptide is present in the cytoplasm. Therefore, we conclude that PEA can be processed intracellularly in T cells but that it is either not secreted at a detectable level or that it plays an intracellular role. This would be efficient since Met-enkephalins have a very short half-life outside the cell. Monocytes, on the other hand, did secrete free enkephalins when the PPE gene was expressed. In view of these data we would like to conclude that monocytes can be induced to secrete Met-enkephalin, which will be used by the monocyte to increase cytokine production. However, as stated above, T cells secrete only intermediate PPE products, which inhibit the proliferative capacity via nonopioid binding sites. T cells can be functionally subdivided into T helper 1 (Th1) and T helper 2 (Th2) cells. Current data indicate that Th2 cells are the main producers and secretors of opioids. This means that T cells will secrete only these PPE products at sites where Th2 cells are present. The latter hypothesis is confirmed by our recent results in the synovial fluid of patients with juvenile rheumatoid arthritis (JRA). We could demonstrate that JRA patients with a mild form of the disease showed higher expression of Th2 cytokines in the synovial fluid, such as IL-4 and IL-10, than did those patients with a more severe form of the disease. We found that high PPE gene expression in synovial cells was associated with the presence of Th2 cytokine mRNA in the synovial cells. In a recent article we also demonstrated that Th2 cytokines like IL-4 and IL-10, but not Th1 cytokines such as IFN-γ, can induce T cells to express PPE mRNA and to secrete ECP. The latter would implicate that PPE products will be used by the T cells where inflammatory processes are under control by the Th2 compartment (Kamphuis et al., 1997).

C. Antibody-Dependent Cell-Mediated Cytotoxicity

In monocytes, enkephalins also affect antibody-dependent cell-mediated cytotoxicity (ADCC) and production of reactive oxygen species. Moreover, enkephalins can also function as chemoattractants (Foris, Medgyesi, & Hauck, 1986; van Epps & Saland, 1984). Foris and colleagues showed that for some immunoglobulin G (IgG) subclasses enkephalins enhanced ADCC, whereas for other IgG subclasses it did not (Foris, Medgyesi, Gyimesi, & Hauck, 1984).

In a follow-up study they demonstrated that the cells involved increased their Na^+ and Ca^{2+} uptake and that levels of cAMP and cGMP increased on enkephalin stimulation (Foris et al., 1986). These intracellular effects were concentration dependent, and some effects did show opposite effects at low vs. high enkephalin concentrations.

D. Polymorphonuclear Leukocytes

Enkephalins also affect the production of reactive oxygen species in polymorphonuclear leukocytes (PMNs) (Marotti, Sverko, & Hrsak, 1990). As in monocytes, resting levels of reactive oxygen species are enhanced in PMNs by enkephalin, whereas during mitogen-triggered respiratory bursts levels are suppressed (Peterson, Sharp, Gekker, Brummitt, & Keane, 1987). It appeared that the response to enkephalin depended on the state of activation of the cell. Enkephalin suppresses superoxide anion release from mitogen-stimulated PMNs in individuals who show a high or medium baseline oxygen-radical response. In individuals with low baseline response to mitogen stimulation, enkephalins have an enhancing effect (Marotti et al., 1990). The concentration of the peptide also influences the final level of oxygen radicals. Low concentrations of enkephalins stimulate the respiratory burst, whereas high concentrations suppress this response (Marotti, Haberstok, Sverko, & Hrsak, 1992). The effect of enkephalins on PMNs also seems to depend on the hydroxylation of the enkephalins. If enkephalins are hydroxylated by exposure to oxygen radicals before they are added to PMN culture, they stimulate the respiratory burst. Unhydroxylated enkephalins have been reported to be inactive or even suppressive (Rabgaoui, Slaoui Hasnaoui, & Torreilles, 1993; Slaoui-Hasnaoui, Guerin, Le Doucen, Loubatiere, & Torreilles, 1992). The respiratory burst is the most common parameter measured in PMNs, but other aspects of immunological function such as adhesion, motility, and cell shape also have been shown to be modulated by enkephalins (Fischer & Falke, 1987; Stefano, Scharrer, & Cadet, 1989; Stefano, Shipp, & Scharrer, 1991; van Epps & Kutvirt, 1987).

E. Natural Killer Cells

Several reports show that enkephalins enhance natural killer cell (NK) activity in vitro as well as in vivo (Bajpai et al., 1995; Burger, Warren, Huffman, & Sidwell, 1995; Faith, Liang, Plotnikoff, Murgo, & Nimeh, 1987; Kawabata, Iwatsubo, Takaya, & Takagi, 1996; Kowalski, 1997; Kowalski, Belowski, & Wielgus, 1995). Faith and colleagues showed that the largest enhancement occurred in individuals with low baseline NK activity (Faith, Liang, Murgo, & Plotnikoff, 1984). This was confirmed by Oleson and Johnson, who in addition reported a suppressive effect of enkephalins in individuals with high baseline NK activity (Oleson & Johnson, 1988). In accordance, NK activity can be enhanced in patients with acquired immunodeficiency syndrome, who show characteristically low NK activity (Oleson, Grierson, Goldsmith, Purtilo, & Johnson, 1989). It has been suggested that the in vivo effects of enkephalins, such as suppression of tumor growth in mice, may be due to an increase in NK cell numbers rather than an enhanced activity per cell (Faith et al., 1987; Kowalski, 1997). The effect of enkephalin on NK cell activity in vitro also has been shown to change with time. At first enkephalin enhances NK activity. If, however, the cells are cultured for 4 days, enkephalin will suppress NK activity (Gabrilovac, Martin-Kleiner, Ikic-Sutlic, & Osmak, 1992; Kowalski et al., 1995).

F. B Cell

Antibody (Ab) production in B cells is inhibited by Met-enkephalin (Das, Hong, & Sanders, 1997; Hiddinga, Isaak, & Lewis, 1994; Morgan, 1996). Das and colleagues showed that production of most immunoglobulin (Ig) isotypes are down-regulated when Met-enkephalin is added to LPS/dextransulfate-stimulated splenic B cells. The effect is seen even at very low concentrations of Met-enkephalin, down to 10^{-16} M. They also studied the effects of unprocessed PEA in the same cultures, but could not demonstrate a detectable effect (Das et al., 1997). PEA and Met-enkephalin are the extremes of the PPE product spectrum and Hiddinga and colleagues made a perhaps more relevant choice when they studied the effects of peptide F, E, and B on Ab formation. They found that, in contrast to Met-enkephalin, the intermediate peptides stimulated Ab production in splenocytes stimulated with both T cell-dependent and T cell-independent antigen. They do, however, suggest that the effect may be mediated via T cells since the effect was not seen in cells from athymic animals (Hiddinga et al., 1994).

G. Opioid Receptor Expression

δ- and κ-opioid receptor mRNA has been shown in T cells, both in cell lines and in peripheral blood cells (Gaveriaux, Peluso, Simonin, Laforet, & Kieffer, 1995; Wick et al., 1996). Recently, Sharp and colleagues found that the T cell-enriched fraction in splenocyte cultures showed an up-regulation of δ- opioid receptor mRNA. This upregulation was, contrary to their assumptions, down-regulated in the presence of Con A (Sharp, Shahabi, McKean, Li, & McAllen, 1997).

Although in monocytes the δ-opioid receptor is the only one to have been detected on the level of mRNA, there is pharmacological evidence suggesting that monocytes express other receptor subtypes as well (Gaveriaux et al., 1995).

Both δ- and κ-opioid receptor mRNA is expressed in human B cell lines (Gaveriaux et al., 1995). Moreover, selective agonists have shown that in addition to these two receptors, the μ-opioid receptor may also be expressed (Morgan, 1996), although Gaveriaux and colleagues did not detect mRNA for the μ-receptor subtype in their system.

It is evident from the literature that there is a large variation in the abovementioned results. Some data seem to lead to contradictory conclusions about the role of enkephalins in the immune system. Donor variation can explain some of this, but widely varying differences in material and methods used by the various laboratories is perhaps the most important factor (Agro & Stanisz, 1995).

VII. THE EXTENDED ROLE OF THE PPE GENE

With a few exceptions (Hiddinga et al. and Wilson et al.) enkephalin pentapeptides have so far been the main focus of research. This preference may stem from the fact that the enkephalin pentapeptides have long been considered as the only active PPE product. The nonenkephalin part of ECP often has been regarded as a modulatory hang-on, perhaps important as an enhancer or stabilizer of the active enkephalin part of the peptide. There are, however, reasons to doubt the dominance of the enkephalin pentapeptide as the main PPE product of active importance to the immune system. Three crucial points in this respect: enkephalin pentapeptides have a relatively short half-life; in some cells ECP are the final product; and in some systems naloxone is a weak antagonist. Firstly, the enkephalins short half-life makes it difficult to see how they could have a sustained effect without enormous release. Of course, it is conceivable that local release rates may be high enough for sustained effects. Secondly, and perhaps more puzzling, some leukocytes such as T cells do express the PPE gene in specific conditions, but they do not secrete pentapeptide. In these cells the evidence points to ECP rather than pentapeptides as the final product. Finally, opioid receptor antagonists such as naloxone are not, even at high concentrations, able to inhibit all the effects of PPE gene products, which suggests that nonenkephalin-containing PPE products may be important. Taken together these assumptions suggest that the role of PPE gene products in the immune system needs to be extended.

A. The PPE Gene as a Fine-Tuner of the Immune System

The PPE gene has been conserved throughout evolution, and it has been shown to regulate cell activation, proliferation, and differentiation. These regulatory effects of PPE have also, in part, been shown in leukocytes (*vide supra*). The picture emerges that PPE products play a role as coregulators in an immune response. Often they have little or no effect by themselves, but the peptides can regulate a leukocyte response to another stimulus. This suggests a role for PPE products as fine-tuners of an immune response. The bidirectional effect that some PPE products show on leukocytes supports this concept, because it is conceivable that the bidirectional effect of PPE products is dependent on the activation state of the target cell. PPE products may support activation of low cellular activity and suppress the activity of an activated cell. Therefore, the peptides will help to keep the cell at a specific activation state. For example, IL-2 stimulates NK cells to change from a resting to an activated state. PPE products alone cannot drive this switch, but the peptides may play a role in determining the exact level of activation of the NK cell. The opioids also may be involved in keeping the active NK cell from becoming over- or underactive. The time and concentration dependence of the effects of PPE products shown in some cells can conceivably function as a self-limiting mechanism, first stimulating a response and then contributing to its down-regulation. Intermediate products, for example, can be produced at a lower ratio than free enkephalin and therefore reach their activity threshold concentration later than the enkephalin pentapeptides.

The activation state of the cell also may be reflected in varying levels of receptors for the PPE products on the target cell. In that case the mechanism of the bidirectional effect could be in the intracellular signaling of the target cell. The relatively weak signal caused by stimulation of a low number of receptors could activate sensitive genes causing, for example, activation of the cell and upregulation of receptors for PPE gene products. As the increased level of receptors are stimulated, they will confer a stronger signal to the nucleus, and other less sensitive down-regulatory genes may be activated, resulting in a dampening of the response. The receptors involved do not have to be the same since the PPE gene has many products, some of which do not contain the enkephalin pentapeptide. Interaction with the classic opioid receptors can play a role in reaction to enkephalins and ECP exposing enkephalins at their amino terminal. For ECP (with or without exposed enkephalin) and non-ECP other receptors, perhaps yet to be discovered, may interact with nonenkephalin parts of the peptides.

Stein and colleagues have done a number of elegant studies in which they demonstrate at several levels that immune system-derived opioids play an important role in peripheral analgesia. Their work was done in a rat model of acute inflammation caused by injection of Freund's complete adjuvant in the hind paw. μ- and δ-opioid receptor agonists were shown to induce naloxone reversible antinociception in inflamed limbs (Stein, Millan, Yassouridis, & Herz, 1988; Stein, Millan, Shippenberg, Peter, & Herz, 1989). They also demonstrated that μ- and δ-opioid receptors were axonaly transported toward the inflamed tissue, and that they were present at an increased concentration on neurons and in tissue at the inflamed site (Hassan, Ableitner, Stein, & Herz, 1993). In addition, they showed that cold water swimming (CWS) stress gave a naloxone reversible antinociception. This stress-induced effect was not totally dependent on centrally produced opioids, since removal of the adrenal glands and the pituitary did not completely abolish the effect (Parsons, Czlonkowski, Stein, & Herz, 1990; Stein, Gramsch, & Herz, 1990). These authors showed that a peripheral source of opioids was located in the infiltrating leukocytes, having increased levels of β-endorphin and Met-enkephalin peptide and of POMC and PPE mRNA. Experiments showing that immunosuppressive treatment with either whole-body irradiation or cyclosporine A abolished the CWS stress-induced analgesia lent further support to the idea that peripheral antinociception is based on immune-derived opioids (Przewlocki et al., 1992; Stein, Hassan, et al., 1990).

Similar results have been observed in a human study in which synovial fluid from patients undergoing knee surgery was studied. β-endorphin and Met-enkephalin were detected in the synovial fluid. In addition, patients receiving naloxone locally after surgery reported more pain than did control patients (Stein, Hassan, Lehrberger, Giefing, & Yassouridis, 1993). In another human study Hogeweg and colleagues reported that the pain threshold in inflamed joints of JRA patients was inversely related to the number of joints involved. Kamphuis and colleagues found a similar inverse relationship between the number of joints involved in JRA patients and Met-enkephalin containing PPE products in the synovial fluid (*vide supra*). In contrast to these findings, Elhassan and colleagues reported a decrease rather then an increase of Met-enkephalin in joints of arthritic rats (Elhassan, Adem, & Lindgren, 1998; Elhassan, Lindgren, Hultenby, Bergstrom, & Adem, 1998). However, Elhassan looked at free pentapeptide and Kamphuis looked at any enkephalin-containing PPE product. A likely reason for the low levels of pentapeptide is the increase of peptidases seen in inflammation. Appelboom and colleagues reported a specific inflammation-related increase in enkephalinase concentration in synovial fluid from patients with swollen joints (Appelboom, Maertelaer, Prez, Hauzeur, & Deshodt-Lanckman, 1991).

The innervation of secondary lymphoid organs like the spleen and lymph nodes gives the possibility of extensive neuroimmune interaction. Since important immunological decisions, such as activation of naive T cells via dendritic cells, are made in secondary lymph organs, direct interaction gives a potent possibility of two-way interaction. Here the nerves may detect levels of PPE products as a means for the CNS to gauge the state of the immune system. As a response, PPE products from nerves may then help to fine-tune an ongoing response.

With this in mind, it is tempting to speculate about the role of enkephalins in the inflamed joint. The infiltrating leukocytes increase their expression of the opioid genes PPE and POMC. This leads to an increase of opioid gene products in the synovial fluid. To control the effects of different signaling molecules, the concentrations of peptidases increase as well, among them enkephalinase. Part of the role of opioid peptides in the inflamed joint is to give peripheral analgesia and part is to serve as regulators of the inflammatory response. Met-enkephalin, which is coexpressed with Th2-type cytokines, may work to dampen the inflammatory response. PPE products other than enkephalin probably also play a role since they have been shown to be secreted by activated T cells. Since Met-enkephalin and other PPE products may have opposite effects on immune function it is conceivable that they may work antagonistically, or they may even have independent effects. The latter hypothesis leads to complex regulatory pathways in local joint inflammation in which PPE gene products and enkephalinase expression play an integral role.

It would be too simplistic to suggest that PPE gene products or any other single communication molecule would be the one important link between the CNS and the immune system. Rather, the PPE products can serve as a model for how communication in the body can be seen in a more holistic perspective. The fact that PPE products seem to fine-tune the immune system does not imply that the CNS influence therefore is unimportant. Instead it suggests that in the normal functioning of the healthy immune system, relatively weak signals regulate its everyday running. This everyday activity may take place in secondary lymphoid tissue such as lymph nodes, where it could regulate the initial responses to antigens. In case of disease the larger changes in immune status will require stronger signals, such as the classical cytokines. The fine-tuning signals may then play a role in maintaining the new equilibrium.

VIII. CONCLUSION

Considering that enkephalins and cytokines are both produced by the neuroendocrine system and the immune system leads to the following hypothesis. In the neuroendocrine system PPE products are used for both intra- and interorgan communication. We hypothesize that the main role of immune-derived enkephalins is not interorgan but rather intraorgan communication. The immune system's need for interorgan communication is fulfilled by the classical cytokines. Within the neuroendocrine system cytokines are recognized and produced but are used for intraorgan communication. In other words, the two organ systems speak the same language but they use different dialects (Figure 3).

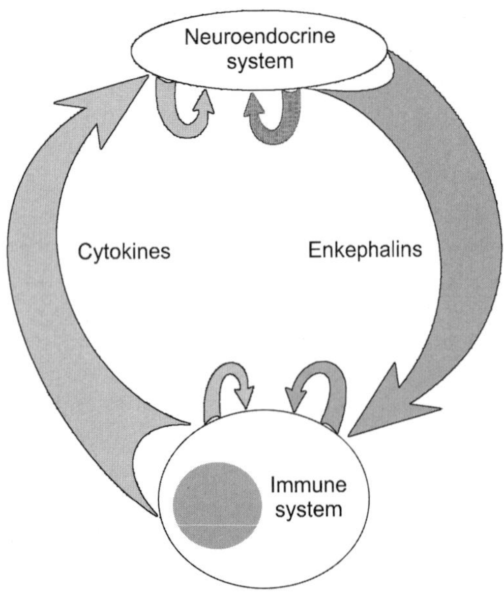

FIGURE 3 Immune–neuroendocrine communication.

The PPE gene has come a long way, in more then one sense. In the eyes of modern science its smallest product started as the natural ligand to the opioid receptor. It moved up to become an important molecule in its own right in neuroscience. It has now moved on to a stage in which many of its products show possible roles at diverse sites in the body. From its original analgesic effects in neuroscience it has moved into the fields of developmental biology and immunology, showing diverse effects on a wide variety of tissues. The PPE gene also has been with us since the earliest beginnings of life, serving, we believe, as a means for cells to communicate. Although the future is notoriously difficult to predict, it possible that the PPE gene may prove even more diverse than we already know it to be.

References

Agro, A., & Stanisz, A. M. (1995). Neuroimmunomodulation: Classical and non-classical cellular activation. *Advances in Neuroimmunology, 5*, 311–319.

Appelboom, T., Maertelaer, V., Prez, E., Hauzeur, J., & Deshodt-Lanckman, M. (1991). Enkephalinase: a physiologic neuroimmunomodulator detected in the synovial fluid. *Arthritis and Rheumatism, 34*, 1048–1051.

Bajpai, K., Singh, V. K., Agarwal, S. S., Dhawan, V. C., Naqvi, T., Haq, W., & Mathur, K. B. (1995). Immunomodulatory activity of met-enkephalin and its two potent analogs. *International Journal of Immunopharmacology, 17*, 207–212.

Bhargava, H. N. (1991). Opioid systems and immune functions. In N. Plotnikoff, A. Murgo, R. Faith, & J. Wybran, (Eds.), *Stress and immunity* (pp. 329–342). Boca Raton, FL: CRC Press.

Blalock, J. E. (1994). The syntax of immune–neuroendocrine communication. *Immunology Today, 15*, 504–511.

Burger, R. A., Warren, R. P., Huffman, J. H., & Sidwell, R. W. (1995). Effect of methionine enkephalin on natural killer cell and cytotoxic T lymphocyte activity in mice infected with influenza A virus. *Immunopharmacology and Immunotoxicology, 17*, 323–334.

Burke, T. R. J., Bajwa, B. S., Jacobson, A. E., Rice, K. C., Streaty, R. A., & Klee, W. A. (1984). Probes for narcotic receptor mediated phenomena. 7. Synthesis and pharmacological properties of irreversible ligands specific for mu or delta opiate receptors. *Journal of Medicinal Chemistry, 27*, 1570–1574.

Clement-Jones, V., Lowry, P. J., Rees, L. H., & Besser, G. M. (1980). Met-enkephalin circulates in human plasma. *Nature, 283*, 295–297.

Comb, M., Rosen, H., Seeburg, P., Adelman, J., & Herbert, E. (1983). Primary structure of the human proenkephalin gene. *DNA, 2*, 213–229.

Comb, M., Seeburg, P. H., Adelman, J., Eiden, L., & Herbert, E. (1982). Primary structure of human met-and leu-enkephalin precursor and its mRNA. *Nature, 295*, 663–666.

Das, K. P., Hong, J. S., & Sanders, V. M. (1997). Ultralow concentrations of proenkephalin and [met5]-enkephalin differentially affect IgM and IgG production by B cells. *Journal of Neruoimmunology, 73*, 37–46.

De Montis, G. M., Devoto, P., Preti, A., & Tagliamonte, A. (1987). Differential effect of mu, delta, and kappa opioid agonists on adenylate cyclase activity. *Journal of Neuroscience Research, 17*, 435–439.

Di Giulio, A. M., Picotti, G. B., Cesura, A. M., Panerai, A. E., & Mantegazza, P. (1982). Met-enkephalin immunoreactivity in blood platelets. *Life Sciences, 30*, 1605–1614.

Dickenson, A. H., Sullivan, A. F., Knox, R., Zajac, J. M., & Roques, B. P. (1987). Opioid receptor subtypes in the rat spinal cord: Electrophysiological studies with mu- and delta-opioid receptor agonists in the control of nociception. *Brain Research, 413*, 36–44.

Dillen, L., Miserez, B., Claeys, M., Aunis, D., & De Potter, W. (1993). Posttranslational processing of proenkephalins and chromogranins/secretogranins. *Neurochemistry International, 22*, 315–352.

Elhassan, A. M., Adem, A., & Lindgren, J. U. (1998). Met-enkephalin decreases in adjuvant arthritic ankles. *Journal of Rheumatology, 25*, 1953–1956.

Elhassan, A. M., Lindgren, J. U., Hultenby, K., Bergstrom, J., & Adem, A. (1998). Methionine-enkephalin in bone and joint tissues. *Journal of Bone and Mineral Research, 13*, 88–95.

Evangelista, R., Ray, P., & Lewis, R. V. (1982). A "trypsin-like" enzyme in adrenal chromaffin granules: A proenkephalin processing enzyme. *Biochemical and Biophysical Research Communications, 106*, 895–902.

Faith, R. E., Liang, H. J., Murgo, A. J., & Plotnikoff, N. P. (1984). Neuroimmunomodulation with enkephalins: Enhancement of human natural killer (NK) cell activity in vitro. *Clinical Immunology and Immunopathology, 31*, 412–418.

Faith, R. E., Liang, H. J., Plotnikoff, N. P., Murgo, A. J., & Nimeh, N. F. (1987). Neuroimmunomodulation with enkephalins: In vitro enhancement of natural killer cell activity in peripheral blood lymphocytes from cancer patients. *Natural Immunity and Cell Growth Regulation, 6*, 88–98.

Fischer, E. G., & Falke, N. E. (1987). Interaction of met-enkephalin with human granulocytes. *Annals of the New York Academy of Sciences, 496*, 146–150.

Fleminger, G., Ezra, E., Kilpatrick, D. L., & Udenfriend, S. (1983). Processing of enkephalin-containing peptides in isolated bovine adrenal chromaffin granules. *Proceedings of the National Academy of Sciences of the United States of America, 80*, 6418–6421.

Foris, G., Medgyesi, G. A., Gyimesi, E., & Hauck, M. (1984). Met-enkephalin induced alterations of macrophage functions. *Molecular Immunology, 21*, 747–750.

Foris, G., Medgyesi, G. A., & Hauck, M. (1986). Bidirectional effects of Met-enkephalin on macrophage effector functions. *Molecular and Cellular Biochemistry, 69*, 127–137.

Fricker, L. D., & Snyder, S. H. (1982). Enkephalin convertase: Purification and characterization of a specific enkephalin-synthesizing carboxypeptidase localized to adrenal chromaffin granules. *Proceedings of the National Academy of Sciences of the United States of America, 79*, 3886–3890.

Fricker, L. D., Supattapone, S., & Snyder, S. H. (1982). Enkephalin convertase: A specific enkephalin synthesizing carboxypeptidase in adrenal chromaffin granules, brain, and pituitary gland. *Life Sciences, 31*, 1841–1844.

Gabrilovac, J., Martin-Kleiner, I., Ikic-Sutlic, M., & Osmak, M. (1992). Interaction of Leu-enkephalin and alpha-interferon in modulation of NK activity of human peripheral blood lymphocytes. *Annals of the New York Academy of Sciences, 650*, 140–145.

Gaveriaux, C., Peluso, J., Simonin, F., Laforet, J., & Kieffer, B. (1995). Identification of kappa- and delta-opioid receptor transcripts in immune cells. *FEBS Letters, 369*, 272–276.

Gubler, U., Seeburg, P., Hoffman, B. J., Gage, L. P., & Udenfreund, S. (1982). Molecular cloning establishes proenkephalin precursor of enkephalin-containing peptides. *Nature, 295*, 206–208.

Haberstock, H., & Marotti, T. (1995). The relevance of intact enkephalin molecule in predominantly delta opioid receptor mediated superoxide anion release. *Neuropeptides, 29*, 357–365.

Haberstock, H., Marotti, T., & Banfic, H. (1996). Neutrophil signal transduction in Met-enkephalin modulated superoxide anion release. *Neuropeptides, 30*, 193–201.

Hassan, A. H., Ableitner, A., Stein, C., & Herz, A. (1993). Inflammation of the rat paw enhances axonal transport of opioid receptors in the sciatic nerve and increases their density in the inflamed tissue. *Neuroscience, 55*, 185–195.

Hiddinga, H. J., Isaak, D. D., & Lewis, R. V. (1994). Enkephalin-containing peptides processed from proenkephalin significantly enhance the antibody-forming cell responses to antigens. *Journal of Immunology, 152*, 3748–3759.

Hucklebridge, F. H., Hudspith, B. N., Lydyard, P. M., & Brostoff, J. (1990). Stimulation of human peripheral lymphocytes by methionine enkephalin and delta-selective opioid analogues. *Immunopharmacology, 19*, 87–91.

Hughes, J., Smith, T. W., Kosterlitz, H. W., Fothergill, L. A., Morgan, B. A., & Morris, H. R. (1975). Identification of two related pentapeptides from the brain with potent opiate agonist activity. *Nature, 258*, 577–579.

Jacobson, A. E., Bajwa, B. S., Streaty, R. A., Klee, W. A., & Rice, K. C. (1983). Probes for narcotic receptor mediated phenomena. 5. Narcotic antagonist irreversible ligands based on endoethenotetrahydrooripavine. *Life Sciences, 33* (suppl 1), 159–162.

Kamphuis, S., Eriksson, F., Kavelaars, A., Zijlstra, J., van-de, P. M., Kuis, W., & Heijnen, C. J. (1998). Role of endogenous pro-enkephalin A-derived peptides in human T cell proliferation and monocyte IL-6 production. *Journal of Neruoimmunology, 84*, 53–60.

Kamphuis, S., Kavelaars, A., Brooimans, R., Kuis, W., Zegers, B. J., & Heijnen, C. J. (1997). T helper 2 cytokines induce preproenkephalin mRNA expression and proenkephalin A in human peripheral blood mononuclear cells. *Journal of Neruoimmunology, 79*, 91–99.

Kawabata, A., Iwatsubo, K., Takaya, S., & Takagi, H. (1996). Central antinociceptive effect of L-ornithine, a metabolite of L-arginine, in rats and mice. *European Journal of Pharmacology, 296*, 23–31.

Keshet, E., Polakiewicz, R. D., Itin, A., Ornoy, A., & Rosen, H. (1989). Proenkephalin A is expressed in mesodermal lineages during organogenesis. *EMBO Journal, 8*, 2917–2923.

Kimura, S., Lewis, R. V., Stern, A. S., Rossier, J., Stein, S., & Udenfriend, S. (1980). Probable precursors of [Leu]enkephalin and [Met]enkephalin in adrenal medulla: peptides of 3–5 kilodaltons. *Proceedings of the National Academy of Sciences of the United States of America, 77*, 1681–1685.

Koski, G., & Klee, W. A. (1981). Opiates inhibit adenylate cyclase by stimulating GTP hydrolysis. *Proceedings of the National Academy of Sciences of the United States of America, 78*, 4185–4189.

Kowalski, J. (1997). Effect of enkephalins and endorphins on cytotoxic activity of natural killer cells and macrophages/monocytes in mice. *European Journal of Pharmacology, 326*, 251–255.

Kowalski, J., Belowski, D., & Wielgus, J. (1995). Bidirectional modulation of mouse natural killer cell and macrophage cytotoxic activities by enkephalins. *Polish Journal of Pharmacology, 47*, 327–331.

Kuis, W., Villiger, P. M., Leser, H. G., & Lotz, M. (1991). Differential processing of proenkephalin-A by human peripheral blood monocytes and T lymphocytes. *Journal of Clinical Investigation, 88*, 817–824.

LaMendola, J., Martin, S. K., & Steiner, D. F. (1997). Expression of PC3, carboxypeptidase E and enkephalin in human monocyte-derived macrophages as a tool for genetic studies. *FEBS Letters, 404*, 19–22.

Legon, S., Glover, D. M., Hughes, J., Lowry, P. J., Rigby, P. W., & Watson, C. J. (1982). The structure and expression of the preproenkephalin gene. *Nucleic Acids Research, 10*, 7905–7918.

Lewis, R. V., Stern, A. S., Kimura, S., Rossier, J., Stein, S., & Udenfriend, S. (1980). An about 50, 000-dalton protein in adrenal medulla: A common precursor of [Met]- and [Leu]enkephalin. *Science, 208*, 1459–1461.

Lewis, R. V., Stern, A. S., Rossier, J., Stein, S., & Udenfriend, S. (1979). Putative enkephalin precursors in bovine adrenal medulla. *Biochemical and Biophysical Research Communications, 89*, 822–829.

Liston, D., Patey, G., & Rossier, J. (1984). Processing of proenkephalin is tissue-specific. *Science, 225*, 734–737.

Marotti, T., Haberstok, H., Sverko, V., & Hrsak, I. (1992). Met- and Leu-enkephalin modulate superoxide anion release from human polymorphonuclear cells. *Annals of the New York Academy of Sciences, 650*, 146–153.

Marotti, T., Sverko, V., & Hrsak, I. (1990). Modulation of superoxide anion release from human polymorphonuclear cells by Met- and Leu-enkephalin. *Brain, Behavior, and Immunity, 4*, 13–22.

Martin, J., Prystowsky, M. B., & Angeletti, R. H. (1987). Preproenkephalin mRNA in T-cells, macrophages, and mast cells. *Journal of Neuroscience Research, 18*, 82–87.

Mizuno, K., & Matsuo, H. (1985). Proenkephalin processing enzyme with specificity toward paired basic residues purified from bovine adrenal chromaffin granules. *Neuropeptides, 5*, 489–492.

Morgan, E. L. (1996). Regulation of human B lymphocyte activation by opioid peptide hormones. Inhibition of IgG production by opioid receptor class (μ-, κ-, and δ-) selective agonists. *Journal of Neruoimmunology, 65*, 21–30.

Neil, A., Kayser, V., Gacel, G., Besson, J. M., & Guilbaud, G. (1986). Opioid receptor types and antinociceptive activity in chronic inflammation: Both kappa- and mu-opiate agonistic effects are enhanced in arthritic rats. *European Journal of Pharmacology, 130*, 203–208.

Nissen, J. B., Lund, M., Stengaard-Pedersen, K., & Kragballe, K. (1997). Enkephalin-like immunoreactivity in human skin is found selectively in a fraction of CD68-positive dermal cells: Increase in enkephalin-positive cells in lesional psoriasis. *Archives of Dermatological Research, 289*, 265–271.

Noda, M., Teranishi, Y., Takahashi, H., Toyosato, M., Notake, M., Nakanishi, S., & Numa, S. (1982). Isolation and structural organization of the human preproenkephalin gene. *Nature, 297*, 431–434.

Oleson, D., Grierson, H., Goldsmith, J., Purtilo, D. T., & Johnson, D. (1989). Augmentation of natural cytotoxicity by leucine enkephalin in cultured peripheral blood mononuclear cells from patients infected with human immunodeficiency virus. *Clinical Immunology and Immunopathology, 51*, 386–395.

Oleson, D. R., & Johnson, D. R. (1988). Regulation of human natural cytotoxicity by enkephalins and selective opiate agonists. *Brain, Behavior, and Immunity, 2*, 171–186.

Parsons, C. G., Czlonkowski, A., Stein, C., & Herz, A. (1990). Peripheral opioid receptors mediating antinociception in inflammation. Activation by endogenous opioids and role of the pituitary-adrenal axis. *Pain, 41*, 81–93.

Pert, C. B., & Snyder, S. H. (1973b). Opiate receptor: Demonstration in nervous tissue. *Science, 179*, 1011–1014.

Pert, C. B., & Snyder, S. H. (1973a). Properties of opiate-receptor binding in rat brain. *Proceedings of the National Academy of Sciences of the United States of America, 70*, 2243–2247.

Peterson, P. K., Sharp, B., Gekker, G., Brummitt, C., & Keane, W. F. (1987). Opioid-mediated suppression of cultured peripheral blood mononuclear cell respiratory burst activity. *Journal of Immunology, 138*, 3907–3912.

Plotnikoff, N. P., Faith, R. E., Murgo, A. J., Herberman, R. B., & Good, R. A. (1997). Methionine enkephalin: A new cytokine-human studies. *Clinical Immunology and Immunopathology, 82*, 93–101.

Polakiewicz, R. D., & Rosen, H. (1990). Regulated expression of proenkephalin A during ontogenic development of mesenchymal derivative tissues. *Molecular and Cellular Biology, 10*, 736–742.

Portoghese, P. S., Larson, D. L., Sayre, L. M., Yim, C. B., Ronsisvalle, G., Tam, S. W., & Takemori, A. E. (1986). Opioid agonist and antagonist bivalent ligands. The relationship between spacer length and selectivity at multiple opioid receptors. *Journal of Medicinal Chemistry, 29*, 1855–1861.

Przewlocki, R., Hassan, A. H., Lason, W., Epplen, C., Herz, A., & Stein, C. (1992). Gene expression and localization of opioid peptides in immune cells of inflamed tissue: functional role in antinociception. *Neuroscience, 48*, 491–500.

Rabgaoui, N., Slaoui Hasnaoui, A., & Torreilles, J. (1993). Boomerang effect between [Met]-enkephalin derivatives and human polymorphonuclear leukocytes. *Free Radical Biology and Medicine, 14*, 519–529.

Rang, H. P., & Dale, M. M. (1991). Analgesic drugs. In *Pharmacology* (pp. 706–732). Edinburgh: Churchill Livingstone.

Rice, K. C., Jacobson, A. E., Burke, T. R. J., Bajwa, B. S., Streaty, R. A., & Klee, W. A. (1983). Irreversible ligands with high selectivity toward delta and mu opiate receptors. *Science, 220*, 314–316.

Roda, L. G., Venturelli, F., & Roscetti, G. (1986). Hydrolysis and protection from hydrolysis of circulating enkephalins. *Comparative Biochemistry and Physiology, 85*, 449–454.

Roscetti, G., Ausiello, C. M., Palma, C., Gulla, P., & Roda, L. G. (1988). Enkephalin activity on antigen-induced proliferation of human peripheral blood mononucleate cells. *International Journal of Immunopharmacology, 10*, 819–823.

Rosen, H., Behar, O., Abramsky, O., & Ovadia, H. (1989). Regulated expression of proenkephalin A in normal lymphocytes. *Journal of Immunology, 143*, 3703–3707.

Rossier, J., Trifaro, J. M., Lewis, R. V., Lee, R. W., Stern, A., Kimura, S., Stein, S., & Udenfriend, S. (1980). Studies with [35S]methionine indicate that the 22, 000-dalton [Met]enkephalin-containing protein in chromaffin cells is a precursor of [Met]enkephalin. *Proceedings of the National Academy of Sciences of the United States of America, 77*, 6889–6891.

Roth, J., LeRoith, D., Collier, E. S., Weaver, N. R., Watkinson, A., Cleland, C. F., & Glick, S. M. (1985). Evolutionary origins of neuropeptides, hormones, and receptors: Possible applications to immunology. *Journal of Immunology, 135*, 816s–819s.

Roth, J., LeRoith, D., Shiloach, J., Rosenzweig, J. L., Lesniak, M. A., & Havrankova, J. (1982). The evolutionary origins of hormones, neurotransmitters, and other extracellular chemical messengers. *New England Journal of Medicine, 306*, 523–527.

Schultzberg, M., Hokfelt, T., Lundberg, J. M., Terenius, L., Elfvin, L. G., & Elde, R. (1978). Enkephalin-like immunoreactivity in nerve terminals in sympathetic ganglia and adrenal medulla and in adrenal medullary gland cells. *Acta Physiologica Scandinavica, 103*, 475–477.

Schultzberg, M., Lundberg, J. M., Hokfelt, T., Terenius, L., Brandt, J., Elde, R. P., & Goldstein, M. (1978). Enkephalin-like immunoreactivity in gland cells and nerve terminals of the adrenal medulla. *Neuroscience, 3*, 1169–1186.

Sharp, B. M., Shahabi, N., McKean, D., Li, M. D., & McAllen, K. (1997). Detection of basal levels and induction of delta opioid receptor mRNA in murine splenocytes. *Journal of Neruoimmunology, 78*, 198–202.

Shen, F. S., Roberts, S. F., & Lindberg, I. (1989). A putative processing enzyme for proenkephalin in bovine adrenal chromaffin granule membranes. Purification and properties. *Journal of Biological Chemistry, 264*, 15600–15605.

Slaoui-Hasnaoui, A., Guerin, M. C., Le Doucen, C., Loubatiere, J., & Torreilles, J. (1992). Reciprocal effects between opioid peptides and human polymorphonuclear leukocytes–II. Enhancement of phorbol myristate acetate-induced respiratory burst in human polymorphonuclear leukocyte by opioid peptides previously exposed to activated oxygen species. *Biochemical Pharmacology, 43*, 503–506.

Smith, E. M., Morrill, A. C., Meyer, W. J., & Blalock, J. E. (1986). Corticotropin releasing factor induction of leukocyte-derived immunoreactive ACTH and endorphins. *Nature, 321*, 881–882.

Stefano, G. B., Scharrer, B., & Cadet, P. (1989). Stimulatory effects of opioid neuropeptides on locomotary activity and conformational changes in invertebrate and human immunoytes: Evidence for a subtype of ð receptor. *Proceedings of the National Academy of Sciences of the United States of America, 86*, 6307–6311.

Stefano, G. B., Shipp, M. A., & Scharrer, B. (1991). A possible immunoregulatory function for [met]-enkephalin-arg6- phe7 involving human and invertebrate granulocytes. *Journal of Neruoimmunology, 31*, 97–103.

Stein, C., Gramsch, C., & Herz, A. (1990). Intrinsic mechanisms of antinociception in inflammation: Local opioid receptors and beta-endorphin. *Journal of Neuroscience, 10*, 1292–1298.

Stein, C., Hassan, A. H., Lehrberger, K., Giefing, J., & Yassouridis, A. (1993). Local analgesic effect of endogenous opioid peptides [see comments]. *Lancet, 342*, 321–324.

Stein, C., Hassan, A. H., Przewlocki, R., Gramsch, C., Peter, K., & Herz, A. (1990). Opioids from immunocytes interact with receptors on sensory nerves to inhibit nociception in inflammation. *Proceedings of the National Academy of Sciences of the United States of America, 87*, 5935–5939.

Stein, C., Millan, M., Yassouridis, A., & Herz, A. (1988). Antinociceptive effects of mu and kappa-agonists in inflammation are enhanced by a peripheral opioid receptor-specific mechanism. *European Journal of Pharmacology, 155*, 255–264.

Stein, C., Millan, M. J., Shippenberg, T. S., Peter, K., & Herz, A. (1989). Peripheral opioid receptors mediating antinociception in inflammation. Evidence for involvement of mu, delta and kappa receptors. *Journal of Pharmacology and Experimental Therapeutics, 248*, 1269–1275.

Suzuki, T., Funada, M., Narita, M., Misawa, M., & Nagase, H. (1991). Perussis toxin abolishes mu- and delta-opioid agonist-induced place preference. *European Journal of Pharmacology, 205*, 85–88.

van Epps, D. E., & Kutvirt, S. L. (1987). Modulation of human neutrophil adherence by beta-endorphin and met-enkephalin. *Journal of Neruoimmunology, 15*, 219–228.

van Epps, D. E., & Saland, L. (1984). Beta-endorphin and met-enkephalin stimulate human peripheral blood mononuclear cell chemotaxis. *Journal of Immunology, 132*, 3046–3053.

Wick, M. J., Minnerath, S. R., Roy, S., Ramakrishnan, S., & Loh, H. H. (1996). Differential expression of opioid receptor genes in human lymphoid cell lines and peripheral blood lymphocytes. *Journal of Neruoimmunology, 64*, 29–36.

Wilson, S. (1991). Processing of proenkephalin in adrenal chromaffin cells. *Journal of Neurochemistry, 57*, 876–881.

Wybran, J., Appelboom, T., Famaey, JP., & Govaerts, A. (1979). Suggestive evidence for receptors for morphine and methionine-enkephalin on normal human blood T lymphocytes. *Journal of Immunology, 123*, 1068–1070.

Zurawski, G., Benedik, M., Kamb, B. J., Abrams, J. S., Zurawski, S. M., & Lee, F. D. (1986). Activation of mouse T-helper cells induces abundant preproenkephalin mRNA synthesis. *Science, 232*, 772–775.

CHAPTER

14

Opioidergic Modulation of the Immune System

DANIEL J. J. CARR, RICHARD J. WEBER

I. INTRODUCTION

Both cognitive (e.g., behavior and environmental cues) and noncognitive (e.g., microbial pathogens and toxins) stimuli can elicit reactions from the immune and neuroendocrine systems including changes in neuronal firing rates, the release of neurotransmitters and neuroendocrine hormones, and the production of cytokines, chemokines, and antibodies. Coincidentally (or not), many of these secreted products are produced by both systems and interface in a specific and selective fashion with molecules (receptors) found on or in cells from the other system. As a result of the sharing of these chemical mediators it is possible for these two systems to communicate and respond to each other's molecules in an exquisitely sensitive and selective manner. One family of hormones shared between the central nervous system (CNS) and immune system (IS) are the opioid peptides. During periods of stress (which we define as perceived yet unfamiliar environmental cues), the brain releases a number of chemical mediators including opioid peptides that have been shown to alter a number of systems including the IS (Adler, Geller, & Rogers, 1993; Carr, Rogers, & Weber, 1996; Rouveix, 1992; Roy & Loh, 1996). Because of the chemical linguistics shared between the CNS and IS, it may be inferred that a drug acting on the CNS may affect immune cell functions, and vice versa.

Opioid action is known to mimic the effects of stress. Opioid agonists represent a group of natural, semisynthetic, or synthetic drugs with the ability to relieve pain, but with the potential risk to induce physical dependence, and additionally, alter immune function through specific types of opioid receptors classified as delta (δ), kappa (κ), and mu (μ). One means by which opioids have been found to modify the IS indirectly is by binding to μ opioid receptors (OR) within the CNS (Band et al., 1992; Shavit et al., 1986; Weber & Pert, 1989). Recent studies have determined the specific brain region(s) involved in opioid-induced immunoregulation. In this respect, the periaqueductal gray (PAG) matter of the mesencephalon has been identified as a site of morphine-mediated, naltrexone-sensitive suppression of rat splenic natural killer (NK) cell activity (Weber & Pert, 1989). Additional studies have found the in vivo administration of μ-OR selective agonists to suppress a variety of immune parameters including lymphocyte profileration, the production of cytokines, T-cell mediated cytotoxicity, and antibody formation (Band et al., 1992; Bussiere, Adler, Rogers, & Eisenstein,

1992; Carpenter & Carr, 1995; Fecho, Maslonek, Coussons-Read, Dykstra, & Lysle, 1994; Fecho, Maslonek, Dykstra, & Lysle, 1996; Gomez-Flores & Weber, 1999a, 1999b, 1999c; Rojavin et al., 1993; Weber & Pert, 1989). The activation of the CNS μ ORs can regulate immune function by activating the hypothalamo-pituitary-adrenal (HPA) axis and the sympathetic nervous system (SNS) (Carr & Serou, 1995). Morphine activation of the HPA axis elicits the production of steroid hormones including the immunosuppressive glucocorticoids (Freier & Fuchs, 1994), whereas the activation of the SNS, which innervates both primary and secondary lymphoid organs, elicits the release of catecholamines that also possess immunomodulatory characteristics (Carr, Gebhardt, & Paul, 1993; Fecho, Maslonek, Dykstra, & Lysle, 1994). Most of the immunomodulatory effects of μ opioid agonists have been attributed to receptors located in the CNS. However, evidence for the direct action of opioids on cells of the immune system was substantiated following early reports of opioid receptor expression by leukocytes (Falke, Fischer, & Martin, 1985; McDonough et al., 1980; Wybran, Appelboom, Famaey, & Govaerts, 1979). Recent studies showing molecular evidence for ORs in immunocytes (Belkowski et al., 1995; Chuang et al., 1994; Chuang, Chuang, et al., 1995; Chuang, Killam, et al., 1995; Sedqi, Roy, Ramakrishnan, Elde, & Loh, 1995), and evidence for endogenous opioid peptide production by lymphocytes (Harbour-McMenamin, Smith, & Blalock, 1985; Harbour, Smith, & Blalock, 1987) and macrophages (Lolait, Lim, Toh, & Funder, 1984) have strengthened the theory that these secretory peptides act as autocrine/paracrine regulators of leukocyte activation, proliferation, and differentiation. In fact, localized inflammation of a rat's hind paw has been found to elicit accumulation of β-endorphin from lymphocytes correlating with the nociceptive effect in this inflammatory model (Cabot et al., 1997). Within the immune system, a recent study has found that the synthesis of the endogenous opioid precursor proenkephalin A in human T cells and monocytes is induced through stimulation of CD2/CD28 receptors following lipopolysaccharide treatment (Kamphuis et al., 1998). Furthermore, the lack of enkephalin production resulted in inhibition of monocytic interleukin (IL)-6 production acting via membrane ORs (Kamphuis et al., 1998). Understanding the role these endogenous peptides and exogenous opioids play in the immune system may provide clinical and therapeutic benefits to patients suffering from infectious diseases such as acquired immunodeficency syndrome (AIDS) and hepatitis B, and to patients presenting with autoimmune disorders or cancer. In this chapter we review the literature with respect to ORs on cells of the immune system, regulation of immune function by opioids, signal transduction pathways activated by opioid action, and relevance of opioid action in autoimmunity, cancer, and infectious diseases.

II. OPIOID RECEPTORS ON CELLS OF THE IMMUNE SYSTEM

Exogenous administration and endogenous opioid action affect not only behavior and the neuroendocrine and autonomic systems, but also the IS. Opioid agonist activities depend on binding to high-affinity receptors on CNS tissue and on cells of the IS. These receptors exhibit different patterns of ligand selectivity, stereoselectivity, saturability, and nanomolar affinity for opioids (Carr, 1991; Sibinga & Goldstein, 1988; Weber & Pert, 1984). The prototypic ligands for the δ OR are the enkephalins, whereas the ligands associated with the κ OR are the dynorphins, and that for the μ receptor, morphine. A fourth related receptor or site was found to bind β-endorphin in a naloxone-insensitive manner but still possessed immunomodulatory effects in in vitro assays (Carr, 1991). Still another type of OR was reported to exist on granulocytes having specificity to alkaloid opiates (Makman, Bilfinger, & Stefano, 1995). The data showing the direct modulation of immune function by opioids and the capacity of opioid antagonists to block most of the effects elicited by opioid ligands in in vitro experiments strongly supported the idea that specific receptors for these ligands are present on immune cells.

The original observations hypothesizing ORs on cells of the IS (McDonough et al., 1980; Wybran et al., 1979) were substantiated by binding studies (Falke et al., 1985; Mehrishi & Mills, 1983; Ovadia, Nitsan, & Abramsky, 1989) and biochemical analysis of the binding sites using site-specific probes (Carr et al., 1989; Carr, Kim, et al., 1988; Radulescu et al., 1991). Likewise, antibodies to ORs and fluorescent labeled opioid ligands have been shown to selectively recognize sites on immune cells (Bidlack, Saripalli, & Lawrence, 1992; Buchner et al., 1997; Carr et al., 1989; Lawrence, El-Hamouly, Archer, Leary, & Bidlack, 1995; Madden, Donahoe, Zwemmer-Collins, Shafer, & Falek, 1987; Patrini et al., 1996; Stefano et al., 1993). However, it was not until the application of molecular techniques in cloning neuronal ORs that probes could be generated to prove the existence of these receptors within cells of the IS (Evans, Keith, Magendzo, Morrison, & Edwards, 1992; Kieffer,

Befort, Gaveriaux-Ruff, & Hirth, 1992; Thompson, Mansour, Akil, & Watson, 1993; Wang et al., 1993; Yasuda et al., 1993). κ (Belkowski et al., 1995), μ (Sedqi et al., 1995), and δ (Sedqi, Roy, Ramakrishnan, & Loh, 1996) ORs have now been cloned from immune cells. The expression of genes for κ and δ ORs has been demonstrated in human lymphocytes and monocytes (Chuang et al., 1994; Gaveriaux, Peluso, Simonin, Laforet, & Kieffer, 1995), human lymphoid cell lines (Gaveriaux et al., 1995), murine lymphocytes (Gaveriaux et al., 1995; Miller, 1996), and murine lymphoid cell lines (Gaveriaux et al., 1995), as well as μ ORs in rat macrophages (Sedqi et al., 1995) and δ ORs in monkey lymphocytes (Chuang et al., 1994). Recent reverse transcriptase-polymerase chain reaction (RT-PCR) assays were also utilized to obtain cDNA clones from human T lymphocytes, which are nearly identical to the δ and κ OR cDNA isolated from human brain and placenta, respectively (Wick, Minnerath, Roy, Ramakrishnan, & Loh, 1996). The κ receptor is present on immature mouse CD4+/CD8+ thymocytes (Ignatowski & Bidlack, 1999) and human fetal microglia (Chao et al., 1996). δ opioid receptors also have been found in quiescent murine thymocytes (Sedqi, Roy, Ramakrishnan, & Loh, 1996). Likewise, μ OR mRNA is reportedly constitutively expressed in human microglial cells (Chao et al., 1997).

Collectively, there is now molecular proof for the existence of ORs on cells of the IS complementing earlier pharmacological, biochemical, and immunological studies. However, the relevance of these receptors within the confines of immunophysiology (autocrine and paracrine regulation) have not been fully elucidated. However, one recent study using μ receptor knockout mice suggests that μ receptor deficient mice show no apparent change in the cellular immune parameters measured (Gaveriaux, Matthes, Peluso, & Kieffer, 1998).

III. MODULATION OF SIGNAL TRANSDUCTION PATHWAYS BY OPIOID ACTION

The ligation of opioid agonists with their receptors activates a number of intracellular transduction pathways including cAMP levels (Carpenter, Garza, Gebhardt, & Carr, 1994; Carr & France, 1993; Fulop, Kekessy, & Foris, 1987; Kavellars, Ballieux, & Heijnen, 1990; Lawrence & Bidlack, 1993), K^+ channel conductance (Carr, Bubien, Woods, & Blalock, 1988; Hough Halperin, Mazorow, Yeandle, & Millar, 1990), and levels of the AP-1 transcription factor complexes (Hedin et al., 1997). Additional intracellular events induced following leukocyte opioid receptor activation include changes in intracellular Ca^{2+} concentrations (Heagy, Shipp, & Finberg, 1992; Hough et al., 1990; Sharp et al., 1996; Sorensen & Claesson, 1998), increased Ca^{2+} influx and cGMP levels (Fóris, Medgyesi, & Hauck, 1986), inhibition in the production of phosphatidylinositol (Chiappelli, Nguyen, Bullington, & Fahey, 1992), alteration in the phosphorylation of the CD3 γ chain of (Kavelaars, Eggen, De Graan, Gispen, & Heijnen, 1990), and an increase in *c-myc* mRNA levels (Hough et al., 1990).

As one might expect, receptor-mediated changes in intracellular or stored levels of Ca^{2+} pools are translated into biological events at the cellular level. Recent studies have found that the release of free β/γ subunits of the G_I protein facilitates chemotaxis of HEK293 cells following OR activation (Neptune & Bourne, 1997). In another study, superoxide release from neutrophils correlated with a dose-dependent increase in diacylglycerol concentration and protein kinase C translocation to the neutrophil membrane, accompanied by increases in intracellular calcium concentrations following OR activation (Haberstock, Marotti, & Banfic, 1996). Collectively, these results reinforce the hypothesis of the existence of biologically relevant ORs on cells of the IS.

IV. STRUCTURE AND EXPRESSION OF OPIOID RECEPTORS AND GENES IN LEUKOCYTES

Neural and immune system ORs coupled to classical G proteins possessing an extracellular amino terminus, seven transmembrane domains connected by three extracellular and intracellular loops, and an intracellular carboxy terminus. Binding studies have determined the leukocyte-derived OR subtypes bind a wide range of agonists and antagonists with differences in specificity, affinity, and selectivity similar to their neuroendocrine counterparts. Studies have recently begun to focus on the regions of the receptors responsible for transducing agonist and antagonist signals. In one investigation, neutralizing antibodies specific for a portion of the N-terminal sequence of the human κ receptor [anti-kR-(33–52)] blocks κ OR (KOR) specific agonist U50,488H-mediated immunosuppression of (a) *Staphylococcus aureus* Cowen strain I-induced B and T lymphocyte proliferation, (b) PHA-induced T lymphocyte proliferation, and (c) *S. aureus* Cowen strain I-induced IgG synthesis (Buchner et al., 1997). The antibody acted as a noncompetitve antagonist, suggesting that a portion of the N-terminus of the KOR (amino acids 33–52) elicits antagonistic activity when occupied. Another study addressing the structural/function relationship of the OR found that the loss of the C-terminus of the δ OR transfected in CHO cells did not result in significant alteration of ligand specificity, targeting, and agonist-dependent activation (Zhu et al., 1997). These studies are essentially based on the "message-address" concept of ligand recognition. Using naltrexone-derived ligands, naltrindole (a δ OR-selective antagonist), and norbinaltorphimine (a κ OR-selective antagonist), binding and selectivity of ORs can be structurally rationalized. Specifically, the common naltrexone core of these ligands binds to the receptor and places key "address elements" in close proximity to selectivity-determining regions of the respective receptor. Amino acid sequence differences at these points determine selectivity (Paterlini, Portoghese, & Ferguson, 1997). Binding affinities to derivatives of naloxone benzoylhydrazone (NalBroH) show dramatic differences among various OR subtypes. Despite modest ranges of affinities for μ receptor types (i.e., μ_1 and μ_2), affinity ranges for the others (δ ORs and κ ORs) varies 30–100-fold (Ciszewska et al., 1996). To further follow this type of analysis, κ OR subtype chimeras were in which the first coding exon of the KOR-type 3 was replaced by the corresponding first coding exon of either mu OR (MOR)-1 or delta OR (DOR)-1. These constructs were transfected into CHO cells and binding profiles for various opioid ligands, and their functional activities in cyclase studies were characterized. NalBroH inhibited cAMP accumulation in the KOR-3 and the DOR-1/KOR-3 chimeras. Although NalBroH has higher affinity for the MOR-1/KOR-3 chimera in binding studies than KOR-3 alone, it was inactive in cyclase studies using the MOR-1/KOR-3 chimera, implying that the replacement of the first coding exon increases affinity while decreasing intrinsic activity (Pan et al., 1996).

Characterization of the genomic organization of OR in immunocytes has been pursued to elucidate the regulation, processing, and neuronal homology of these proteins. Analysis of the μ, κ, and δ amino acid sequences shows that they have a high degree of amino acid homology with each other. However, genetic differences have been revealed in which the μ and δ subtypes possess three exon coding regions whereas the κ receptor contains an additional exon 5′ of the translational start site (Carr et al., 1996). In a similar setting an "orphan" opioid-like receptor (ORL) cDNA originally described on murine lymphocytes (Halford, Gebhardt, & Carr, 1995) was cloned from a PHA (phytohemagglutinin)-activated human lymphocyte population and was found to have complete homology to the clone isolated from human brain but with divergence at the 5′ untranslated region (Wick, Minnerath, Roy, Ramakrishnan, & Loh, 1995). Distribution of the ORL transcript has been observed in normal circulating human T, B, and monocytic cell lines by RT-PCR and RNAse protection (Peluso et al., 1998). These transcripts were found to lack a 15 nucleotide stretch between exons 1 and 2 comprising the first intracellular loop but otherwise showed similar distribution to the brain transcripts of the cortical areas, striatum, thalamus, and hypothalamus (Perluso et al., 1998). In addition to the ORL, using very sensitive RT-PCR techniques, low levels of δ OR transcripts have been consistently detected from murine splenocytes with preferential expression in the T-cell fraction (Sharp, Shahabi, McKean, Li, & McAllen, 1997). In another study, the lymphocyte δ OR could be induced by the mitogen concanavalin A suggesting a potential role for the δ OR in lymphocyte activation (Miller, 1996). This notion is supported by the observation that the activation of the δ OR modulates calcium mobilization, IL-2 production, chemotaxis, and proliferation of T lymphocytes (Sorensen & Claesson, 1998). Taken together, selective, high-fidelity oligonucleotide probes derived from neural OR sequences have been used to specifically and reproducibly amplify products from leukocytes that are nearly identical to the "parent" neuroendocrine ORs.

V. OPIOIDS IN AUTOIMMUNITY, CANCER, AND INFECTIOUS DISEASES

An association between opioid levels or opioid exposure and the incidence of disease has been known for some time, but more rigorous and complete investigations seem warranted. For example, an association between β-endorphin levels and Crohn's disease (Wiedermann et al., 1994) and other autoimmune processes have been noted, but there are no definitive studies confirming more than a simple association (for review, Panerai & Sacerdote, 1997). In studies with narcotic opioids, morphine has been found to either enhance, suppress, or have no effect on tumor growth in vitro or in vivo depending on the dose and route of administration (Ishikawa, Tanno, Kamo, Takayanagi, & Sasaki, 1993; Maneckjee & Minna, 1990; Provinciali, Di Stefano, Raffaeli, Pari, Desiderio, & Fabris, 1991; Reubi, 1985; Simon & Arbo, 1986; Yeager & Colacchio, 1991). However, there is evidence to support the beneficial effects of morphine on tumor burden by reducing the stress associated consequences of neoplasia (Carr, Scott, Brockunier,

Bagley & France, 1995; Sklar & Anisman, 1981) or surgery (Page, Ben-Eliyahu, Yirimiya, & Liebeskind, 1993).

Perhaps the most convincing data associating opioids with disease pertains to microbial pathogens. Early observations with heroin addicts reported an increased incidence of protozoan, viral, and bacterial infections attributed to the use of non-sterile needles during mainline injection rather than immunosuppression (Briggs, McKerron, Souhami, Taylor, & Andrews, 1967; Hussey & Katz, 1950; Most, 1940). During the earlier years of the AIDS epidemic, there was a high incidence of human immunodeficiency virus (HIV) seroconversion among drug abusers, suggesting a readily accessible source to harbor and spread the virus (Curran et al., 1988). In vitro studies showed morphine or heroin facilitated the replication of HIV by an as yet ill-defined mechanism (Adler, Geller, Rogers, Henderson, & Eisenstein, 1993; Peterson et al., 1990). In addition, the recently defined endogenous morphine peptide, endomorphin, which has been found in a number of immune organs (David Jessop, personal communication), facilitates HIV-1 expression in human brain cell cultures (Peterson, Gekker, Hu, Lokensgard, Portoghese, & Chao, 1999). Although alkaloid opioids have been found to augment the pathogenesis of a number of microbial agents in animal models (Hilburger et al., 1997, for review, Risdahl, Khanna, Peterson, & Molitar, 1998) or increase the susceptibility to infection in humans (Haverkos & Lange, 1990), other studies have shown exposure to opioids (e.g., morphine) either has no effect or, reduces the pathological consequences of infection (Alonzo & Carr, 1999; Donahoe, 1992; Risdahl, Peterson, Chao, Pijoan, & Molitor, 1993; Starec, Rouveix, Sinet, Chau, Desforges, Pocidalo, & Lechat, 1991; Veyries, Sinet, Desforges, & Rouveix, 1995). Using HIV-1 transactivator of transcription (TAT) transgenic mice, which exhibit suppressed cellular immune responses including NK activity, cytotoxic T lymphocyte (CTL) activity, and IL-2 production (Garza, Prakash, & Carr, 1994, 1996), morphine was found to partially restore splenic NK (Figure 2) and CTL activity (Figure 3) as well as

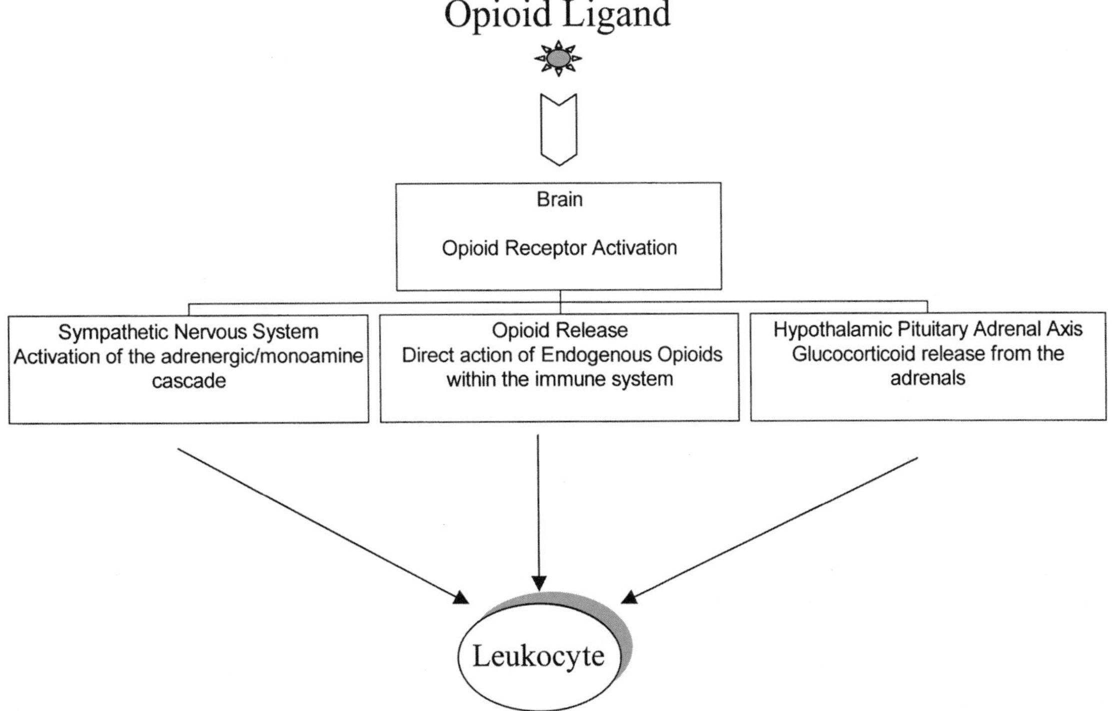

FIGURE 1 Opioid ligand activation of neuroendocrine pathways. The administration of exogenous opioids (primarily μ class alkaloids) seems to interact with brain opioid receptors located within in PAG of the mesencephalon. μ opioid receptor ligation results in (1) the activation of the sympathetic nervous system and the release of monoamines including catecholamines into the immune organ (e.g., lymph node or spleen) via "hard wiring" of this tissue with adrenergic/noradrenergic fibers; (2) the release of neuropeptides directly into the tissue (e.g., metenkephalin) through hard-wiring of immune organs with peptidergic fibers; or (3) the activation of the HPA axis, resulting in the release of steroids including corticosteroids that have potent immunomodulatory effects.

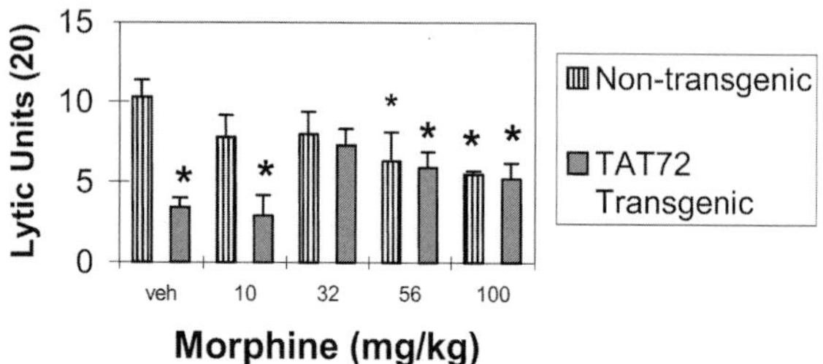

FIGURE 2 Morphine partially restores splenic NK activity in TAT_{72}-transgenic mice. Morphine (10–100 mg/kg, subcutaneous administration) was administered to alloimmunized (1×10^7 irradiated DBA/2 splenocytes) transgenic and wild type mice ($n = 5$/group) daily for 5 days. Splenic lymphocytes were subsequently harvested and assayed for NK activity using ^{51}chromium-labeled YAC-1 cells as targets in a 4-h microcytotoxicity assay. $^*p < 0.05$ comparing vehicle- and morphine-treated TAT_{72} transgenic mice with vehicle-treated, wild type mice as determined by analysis of variance and Tukey's post hoc *t*-test.

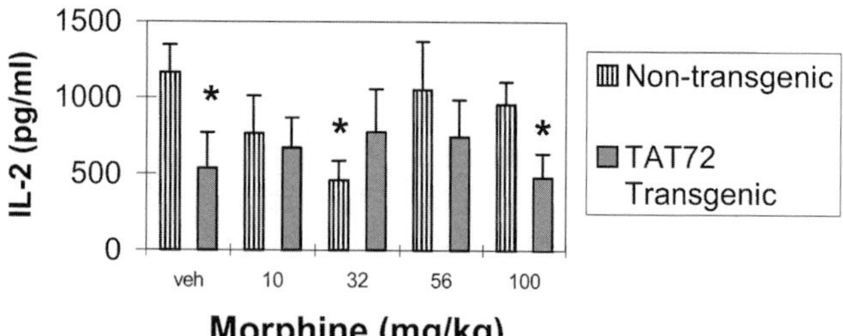

FIGURE 4 Morphine partially restores IL-2 production in concavalin A (Con A)-stimulated splenic lymphocytes from TAT_{72}-transgenic mice. Splenic lymphocytes (2×10^6 cells/culture) obtained from mice ($n = 4$/group) treated as described in the legend of Figure 1 were cultured in the presence of Con A (10 μg/mL, 2 mL culture) and screened for IL-2 production by enzyme-linked immunosorbent assay 24 h poststimulation. $^*p < .05$ comparing all groups with the vehicle-treated, wild type mice.

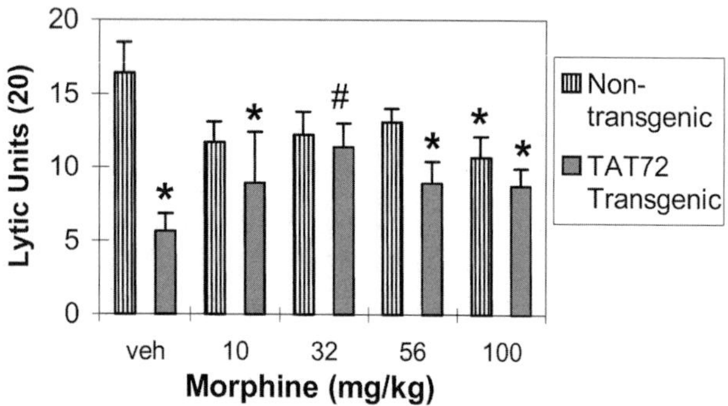

FIGURE 3 Morphine partially restores splenic CTL activity in TAT_{72}-transgenic mice. Mice ($n = 5$/group) treated as described in the legend of Figure 1 were sacrificed and the splenic lymphocytes were harvested and assayed for CTL activity using ^{51}chromium-labeled P815 cells as targets in a 4-h microcytotoxicity assay. $^*p < .05$ comparing all groups to the wild type, vehicle-treated group. $p < .05$ comparing the morphine (32.0 mg/kg)-treated, TAT_{72}-transgenic group with the vehicle-treated TAT_{72} transgenic animals.

augment IL-2 production in response to mitogen (Figure 4). Consistent with other studies (Carr et al., 1993; Scott & Carr, 1966), morphine was found to suppress splenic NK (Figure 2) and CTL (Figure 3) activity in wild type controls. Whether acute or chronic exposure to morphine modifies the production of exogenous opioid peptides or the expression of ORs on immune cells is not known. However, preliminary evidence suggests chronic morphine exposure does not alter the expression of the pro-opiomelanocortin transcript that encodes endorphins (Carpenter et al., 1994). Collectively, there is a continued need to determine the biological significance of both endogenous and exogenous opioid compounds as they relate to disease states. The results of such studies may provide additional insight into the regulation of the IS in the presence and absence of infection and neoplasia.

VI. DISCUSSION

Lymphocytes, NK cells, and macrophages are very sensitive to opioid action. The role of opioids in regulating immune responses has become more significant because of the implications of drug abuse on immunity against infectious diseases and cancer. Opioids may interact directly with ORs on cells of the IS or through receptors within the CNS. Since the peripheral or central administration of opioids appears to interact with brain ORs, the HPA axis, and the SNS are hypothesized to regulate immune function. The activation of the HPA axis elicits the production of adrenocorticotropin hormone from the pituitary, which in turn elicits the release of the immunosuppressive glucocorticoids. On the other hand, the activation of the SNS by opioids through innervation of primary and secondary lymphoid organs elicits the release of catecholamines, which have been demonstrated to regulate lymphocyte, NK cell, and macrophage functions. Numerous studies have provided evidence that the interactions between the immune, neuroendocrine, and nervous systems maintains homeostasis. Immune, endocrine, and neural cells express receptors for cytokines, hormones, neuropeptides, and transmitters. Moreover, these cells coexist in lymphoid, endocrine, and neural tissue. Investigating the cellular mechanisms of opioid action in regulating immune functions must be complemented by studying the molecular pathways of opioid-mediated immunosuppression through the CNS. Changes in intracellular signaling cascades with emphasis on cAMP and Ca^{2+}

have been associated with opioid-mediated immunoregulation. However, scarce information exists about the involvement of other signaling transduction cascades and transcriptional regulatory elements after ex vivo opioid action. From a systemic standpoint, it seems required that future studies provide concrete epidimiological data to support the observations on the effects of opioids on immune function using laboratory animals. Until such matters are addressed, based on the data at hand it is currently difficult to clearly resolve the impact opioids have on the human condition relative to immune homeostasis, immunocompetence, and adaptive immune responses to infectious pathogens and cancer.

Acknowledgments

Preparation of this manuscript was supported by a U.S. Public Health Service grant, NINDS 35470, to DJJC and NIDA/NIH Grants DA/AI08988, DA12095, and DA05865 to RJW.

References

Adler, M. W., Geller, E. B., Rogers, T. J., Hernderson, E. E., & Eisenstein, T. K. (1993). Opioids, receptors, and immunity. *Advances in Experimental Medicine and Biology, 335*, 13–20.

Alonzo, N. & Carr, D. J. J. (1999). Morphine reduces the incidence of HSV-1-mediated encephalitis. *Immunopharmacology, 41*, 187–197.

Band, L. C., Pert, A., Williams, W., de Costa, B. R., Rice, K. C., & Weber, R. J. (1992). Central μ-opioid receptors mediate suppression of natural killer activity in vivo. *Progress in Neuroendocrinimmunology, 5*, 95–101.

Belkowski, S. M., Zhu, J., Liu-Chen, L.-Y., Eisenstein, T. K., Adler, M. W., & Rogers, T. J. (1995). Sequence of κ-opioid receptor cDNA in the R1. 1 thymoma cell line. *Journal of Neuroimmunology, 62*, 113–117.

Bidlack, J. M., Saripalli, L. D., & Lawrence, D. M. P. (1992). κ-Opioid binding sites on a murine lymphoma cell line. *European Journal of Pharmacology, 227*, 257–265.

Briggs, J. H., McKerron, C. G., Souhami, R. L., Taylor, D. J. E., & Andrews, H. (1967). Severe systemic infections complicating in "mainline" heroin addiction. *Lancet ii*, 1227–1231.

Buchner, R. R., Vogen, S. M., Fischer, W., Thoman, M. L., Sanderson, S. D., & Morgan, E. L. (1997). Anti-human κ opioid receptor antibodies. Characterization of site-directed neutralizing antibodies specific for a peptide κR(33-52) derived from the predicted amino terminal region of the human κ receptor. *Journal of Immunology, 158*, 1670–1680.

Bussiere, J. L., Adler, M. W., Rogers, T. J., & Eisenstein, T. K. (1992). Differential effects of morphine and naltrexone on the antibody response in various mouse strains. *Immunopharmacology and Immunotoxicology, 14*, 657–673.

Cabot, P. J., Carter, L., Gaiddon, C., Zhang, Q., Schafer, M., Loeffler, J. P., & Stein, C. (1997). Immune cell-derived beta-endorphin. Production, release, and control of inflammatory pain in rats. *Journal of Clinical Investestigation, 100*, 142–148.

Carpenter, G. W., Garza, H. H. Jr., Gebhardt, B. M., & Carr, D. J. J. (1994). Chronic morphine treatment suppresses CTL-mediated cytolysis, granulation, and cAMP responses to alloantigen. *Brain Behavior and Immunity, 8*, 185–203.

Carr, D. J. J. (1991). The role of endogenous opioids and their receptors in the immune system. *Proceedings of the Society for Experimental Biology and Medicine, 198*, 710–720.

Carr, D. J. J., Bubien, J. K., Woods, W. T., & Blalock, J. E. (1988). Opioid receptors on murine splenocytes: Possible coupling to K^+ channels. *Annals of the New York Academy of Sciences, 540*, 694–697.

Carr, D. J. J., DeCosta, B. R., Kim, C.-H., Jacobson, A. E., Bost, K. B., Rice, K. C., & Blalock, J. E. (1990). Anti-opioid receptor antibody recognition of a binding site on brain and leukocyte opioid receptors. *Neuroendocrinology, 51*, 552–560.

Carr, D. J. J., DeCosta, B. R., Kim, C.-H., Jacobson, A. E., Guarcello, V., Rice, K. C., & Blalock, J. E. (1989). Opioid receptors on cells of the immune system: Evidence for δ- and κ-classes. *The Journal of Endocrinology, 122*, 161–168.

Carr, D. J. J., & France, C. P. (1993). Immune alterations in morphine-dependent rhesus monkeys. *Journal of Pharmacology and Experimental Therapeutics, 267*, 9–15.

Carr, D. J. J., Gebhardt, B. M., & Paul, D. (1993). α-Adrenergic and μ_2 opioid receptors are involved in morphine-induced suppression of splenocyte natural killer activity. *Journal of Pharmacology and Experimental Therapeutics, 264*, 1179–1186.

Carr, D. J. J., Kim, C.-H., DeCosta, B., Jacobson, A. E., Rice, K. C., & Blalock, J. E. (1988). Evidence for a δ-class opioid receptor on cells of the immune system. *Cellular Immunology, 116*, 44–51.

Carr, D. J. J., Rogers, T. J., & Weber, R. J. (1996). The relevance of ORs on immunocompetence and immune homeostasis. *Proceedings of the Society for Experimental Biology and Medicine, 213*, 248–257.

Carr, D. J. J., Scott, M., Brockunier, L. L., Bagley, J. R., & France, C. P. (1995). The effect of novel opioids on natural killer activity and tumor surveillance in vivo. *Advances in Experimental Biology and Medicine, 402*, 5–12.

Carr, D. J. J., & Serou, M. (1995). Exogenous and endogenous opioids as biological response modifiers. *Immunopharmacology, 31*, 59–71.

Chao, C. C., Gekker, G., Hu, S., Sheng, W. S., Shark, K. B., Bu, D. F., Archer, S., Bidlack, J. M., & Peterson, P. K. (1996). Kappa ORs in human microglia downregulate human immunodeficiency virus 1 expression. *Proceedings of the National Academy of Sciences USA, 93*, 8051–8056.

Chao, C. C., Hu, S., Shark, K. B., Sheng, W. S., Gekker, G., & Peterson, P. K. (1997) Activation of mu ORs inhibits microglial cell chemotaxis. *Journal of Pharmacology and Experimenal Therapeutics, 281*, 998–1004.

Chiappelli, F., Nguyen, L., Bullington, R., & Fahey, J. L. (1992). β-Endorphin blunts phosphatidylinositol formation during in vitro activation of isolated human lymphocytes: Preliminary report. *Brain, Behavior, and Immunity, 6*, 1–10.

Chuang, L. F., Chuang, T. K., Killam, K. F. Jr., Chuang, A. J., Kung, H. F., Yu, L., & Chuang, R. Y. (1994). Delta OR gene expression in lymphocytes. *Biochemical Biophysical Research Communication, 202*, 1291–1299.

Chuang, L. F., Chuang, T. K., Killam, K. F. Jr., Qiu, Q., Wang, X. R., Lin, J. J., Kung, H. F., Sheng, W., Chao, C., & Yu, L. (1995). Expression of kappa ORs in human and monkey lymphocytes. *Biochemical Biophysical Research Communication, 209*, 1003–1010.

Chuang, T. K., Killam, K. F. Jr., Chuang, L. F., Kung, H. F., Sheng, W. S., Chao, C. C., Yu, L., & Chuang, R. Y. (1995). Mu OR gene expression in immune cells. *Biochemical Biophysical Research Communication, 216*, 922–930.

Ciszewska, G. R., Ginos, J. A., Charton, M., Standifer, K. M., Brooks, A. I., Brown, G. P., Ryan-Moro, J. P., Berzetei-Gurske, I., Toll, L., & Pasternak, G. W. (1996). Synthesis and characterization of substituted benzoylhydrazones of naloxone. *Synapse, 24*, 193–201.

Curran, J. W., Jaffe, H. W., Hardy, A. M., Morgan, W. M., Selik, R. M., & Dondero, T. J. (1988). Epidemiology of HIV infection and AIDS in the United States. *Science, 239*, 610–616.

Donahoe, R. M. (1992). Neuroimmunomodulation by opiates: Relationship to HIV-1 and AIDS. *Advances in Neuroimmunology, 3*, 31–46.

Evans, C. J., Keith, D., Magendzo, K., Morrison, H., & Edwards, R. H. (1992). Cloning of a delta opioid receptor by functional expression. *Science, 258*, 1952–1955.

Falke, N. E., Fischer, E. G., & Martin, R. (1985). Stereospecific opiate binding in living human polymorphonuclear leukocytes. *Cellular Biology International Reports, 9*, 1041–1047.

Fecho, K., Maslonek, K. A., Dykstra, L. A., & Lysle, D. T. (1996). Evidence for sympathetic and adrenal involvement in the immunomodulatory effects of acute morphine treatment in rats. *Journal of Pharmacology and Experimental Therapeutics, 277*, 633–645.

Fecho, K., Maslonek, K. A., Coussons-Read, M. E., Dykstra, L. A., & Lysle, D. T. (1994). Macrophage-derived nitric oxide is involved in the depressed concanavalin A responsiveness of splenic lymphocytes from rats administered morphine in vivo. *Journal of Immunology, 152*, 5845–5852.

Fóris, G., Medgyesi, G. A., & Hauck, M. (1986). Bidirectional effect of met-enkephalin on macrophage effector functions. *Molecular and Cellular Biochemistry, 69*, 127–137.

Freier, D. O., & Fuchs, B. A. (1994). A mechanism of action for morphine-induced immunosuppression: corticosterone mediates morphine-induced suppression of natural killer cell activity. *Journal of Pharmacology and Experimental Therapeutics, 270*, 1127–1133.

Fulop, T. Jr., Kekessy, D., & Foris, G. (1987). Impaired coupling of naloxone sensitive opiate receptors for adenylate cyclase in PMNLs of aged male subjects. *International Journal of Immunopharmacology, 9*, 652–657.

Garza, H. H. Jr., Prakash, O., & Carr, D. J. J. (1994). Immunologic characterization of TAT_{72}-transgenic mice: Effects of morphine on cell-mediated immunity. *International Journal of Immunopharmacology, 12*, 1061–1070.

Garza, H. H. Jr., Prakash, O., & Carr, D. J. J. (1996). Aberrant regulation of cytokines in HIV-1 TAT_{72}-transgenic mice. *Journal of Immunology, 156*, 3631–3637.

Gaveriaux, C., Matthes, H. W. D., Peluso, J., & Kieffer, B. L. (1998). Abolition of morphine-immunosuppression in mice lacking μ-opioid receptor gene. *Proceedings of the National Academy of Sciences USA, 95*, 6326–6330.

Gaveriaux, C., Peluso, J., Simonin, F., Laforet, J., & Kieffer, B. (1995). Identification of kappa- and delta-OR transcripts in immune cells. *FEBS Letters, 369*, 272–276.

Gomez-Flores, R., & Weber, R. J. (1999a). Suppression of splenic macrophage functions after acute morphine action in the rat mesencephalon periaqueductal gray. *Brain, Behavior, and Immunity, 13*, 212–224.

Gomez-Flores, R., & Weber, R. J. (1999b). Inhibition of IL-2 production and downregulation of IL-2 and transferrin receptors on rat splenic lymphocytes following PAG morphine administration: A role in NK and T cell suppression. *Journal of Interferon and Cytokine Research, 19*, 625–630.

Gomez-Flores, R., & Weber, R. J. (1999c). Opioids, opioid receptors, and the immune system. In N. P. Plotnikoff, R. E. Faith, A. J. Murgo, & R. A. Good (Eds.), *Cytokines—stress and immunity*, (pp. 281–314), Boca Raton: CRC Press.

Haberstock, H., Marotti, T., & Banfic, H. (1996). Neutrophil signal transduction in Met-enkephalin modulated superoxide anion release. *Neuropeptides, 30*, 193–201.

Harbour-McMenamin, D., Smith, E. M., Blalock, J. E. (1985). Bacterial lipopolysaccharide induction of leukocyte-derived corticotropin and endorphins. *Infection and Immunity, 48*, 813–817.

Harbour, D. V., Smith, E. M., & Blalock, J. E. (1987). Splenic lymphocyte production of an endorphin during endotoxic shock. *Brain, Behavior, and Immunity, 1*, 123–133.

Haverkos, H. W. & Lange, W. R. (1990). Serious infections other than human immunodeficiency virus among intravenous drug abusers. *Journal of Infectious Diseases, 161*, 894–902.

Heagy, W., Shipp, M. A., & Finberg, R. W. (1992). Opioid receptor agonists and Ca^{2+} modulation in human B cell lines. *Journal of Immunology, 149*, 4074–4081.

Hedin, K. E., Bell, M. P., Kalli, K. R., Huntoon, C. J., Sharp, B. M., & McKean, D. J. (1997). δ-Opioid receptors expressed by Jurkat T cells enhance IL-2 secretion by increasing AP-1 complexes and activity of the NF-AT/AP-1 binding promoter element. *Journal of Immunology, 159*, 5431–5440.

Hilburger, M. E., Adler, M. W., Truant, A. L., Meissler, J. J. Jr., Satishchandran, V., Rogers, T. J., & Eisenstein, T. K. (1997). Morphine induces sepsis in mice. *Journal of Infectious Diseases, 176*, 183–188.

Hough, C. J., Halperin, J. I., Mazorow, D. L., Yeandle, S. L., & Millar, D. B. (1990). β-endorphin modulates T-cell intracellular calcium flux and *c-myc* expression via a potassium channel. *Journal of Neuroimmunology, 27*, 163–171.

Hucklebridge, F. H., Hudspith, B. N., Lydyard, P. M., & Brostoff, J. (1990). Stimulation of human peripheral lymphocytes by methionine enkephalin and δ-selective analogues. *Immunopharmacology, 19*, 87–91.

Hussey, H. H. & Katz, S. (1950). Infections resulting from narcotic addiction. *American Journal of Medicine, 9*, 186–193.

Ignatowski, T. A., & Bidlack, J. M. (1999). Differential kappa-opioid receptor expression on mouse lymphocytes at varying stages of maturation and on mouse macrophages after selective elicitation. *Journal of Pharmacology and Experimental Therapeutics, 290*, 863–870.

Ishikawa, M., Tanno, K., Kamo, A., Takayanagi, Y., & Sasaki, K.-I. (1993). Enhancement of tumor growth by morphine and its possible mechanism in mice. *Biology and Pharmacology Bulletin, 16*, 762–766.

Kamphuis, S., Eriksson, F., Kavelaars, A., Zijlstra, J., van de Pol, M., Kuis, W., & Heijnen, C. J. (1998). Role of endogenous pro-enkephalin A-derived peptides in human T cell proliferation and monocyte IL-6 production. *Journal of Neuroimmunology, 84*, 53–60.

Kavellars, A., Ballieux, R. E., & Heijnen, C. J. (1990). Differential effects of β-endorphin on cAMP levels in human peripheral blood mononuclear cells. *Brain, Behavior, and Immunity, 4*, 171–179.

Kavelaars, A., Eggen, B. J. L., De Graan, P. N. E., Gispen, W. H., & Heijnen, C. J. (1990). The phosphorylation of the CD3 γ chain of T lymphocytes is modulated by β-endorphin. *European Journal of Immunology, 20*, 943–945.

Kieffer, B. L., Befort, K., Gaveriaux-Ruff, C., & Hirth, C. G. (1992). The δ-opioid receptor: Isolation of a cDNA by expression cloning and pharmacological characterization. *Proceedings of the National Academy of Sciences USA, 89*, 12048–12052.

Lawrence, D. M. P., & Bidlack, J. M. (1993). The kappa opioid receptor expressed on the mouse R1. 1 thymoma cell line is coupled to adenylyl cyclase through a pertussis toxin-sensitive guanine nucleotide-binding protein. *Journal of Pharmacology and Experimental Therapeutics, 266*, 1678–1683.

Lawrence, D. M. P., El-Hamouly, W., Archer, S., Leary, J. F., & Bidlack, J. M. (1995). Identification of κ receptors in the immune system by indirect immunofluorescence. *Proceedings of the National Academy of Sciences USA, 92*, 1062–1066.

Lolait, S. J., Lim, A. T., Toh, B. H., & Funder, J. W. (1984). Immunoreactive beta-endorphin in a subpopulation of mouse spleen macrophages. *Journal of Clinical Investigation, 73*, 277–280.

Madden, J. J., Donahoe, R. M., Zwemer-Collins, J., Shafer, D. A., & Falek, A. (1987). Binding of naloxone to human T lymphocytes. *Biochemical Pharmacology, 36*, 4103–4109.

Makman, M. H., Bilfinger, T. V., & Stefano, G. B. (1995). Human granulocytes contain an opiate alkaloid-selective receptor mediating inhibition of cytokine-induced activation and chemotaxis. *Journal of Immunology, 154*, 1323–1330.

Manackjee, R. & Minna, J. D. (1992). Noncenventional opioid binding sites mediate growth inhibitory effects of methadone on human lung cancer cells. *Proceedings of the National Academy of Sciences USA, 89*, 1169–1173.

McDonough, R. J., Madden, J. J., Falek, A., Shafer, D., Pline, M., Gordon, D., Bokos, P., Kuehnle, J. C., & Mendelson, J. (1980). Alterations of T and null lymphocyte frequencies in the peripheral blood of opiate addicts: In vivo evidence of opiate receptor sites on T lymphocytes. *Journal of Immunology, 125*, 2539–2543.

Mehrishi, J. N. & Mills, I. H. (1983). Opiate receptors on lymphocytes and platelets in man. *Clinical Immunology and Immunopathology, 27*, 240–249.

Miller, B. (1996). δ opioid receptor expression is induced by concanavalin A in $CD4^+$ T cells. *Journal of Immunology, 157*, 5324–5328.

Most, H. (1940). Falciporum malaria among drug addicts. *American Journal of Public Health, 30*, 403–410.

Neptune, E. R., & Bourne, H. R. (1997). Receptors induce chemotaxis by releasing the betagamma subunit of Gi, not by activating Gq or Gs. *Proceedings of the National Academy of Sciences USA, 94*, 14489–14494.

Ovadia, H., Nitsan, P., & Abramsky, O. (1989). Characterization of opiate binding sites on membranes of rat lymphocytes. *Journal of Neuroimmunology, 21*, 93–102.

Page, G., Ben-Eliyahu, S., Yirmiya, R., & Liebeskind, J. (1993). Morphine attenuates surgery-induced enhancement of metastatic colonization in rats. *Pain, 54*, 21–28.

Pan, Y. X., Xu, J., Ryan-Moro, J., Mathis, J., Hom, J. S., Mei, J., & Pasternak, G. W. (1996). Dissociation of affinity and efficacy in KOR-3 chimeras. *FEBS Letters, 395*, 207–210.

Panerai, A. E., & Sacerdote, P. (1997). β-endorphin in the immune system: A role at last? *Immunology Today, 19*, 317–319.

Paterlini, G., Portoghese, P. S., & Ferguson, D. M. (1997). Molecular simulation of dynorphin A-(1-10) binding to extracellular loop 2 of the kappa-opioid receptor. A model for receptor activation. *Journal of Medicinal Chemistry, 40*, 3254–3262.

Patrini, G., Massi, P., Ricevuti, G., Mazzone, A., Fossati, G., Mazzucchelli, I., Gori, E., & Parolaro, D. (1996). Changes in opioid receptor density on murine splenocytes induced by in vivo teatment with morphine and methadone. *Journal of Pharmacology and Experimental Therapeutics, 279*, 172–176.

Peluso, J., Laforge, K. S., Matthes, H. W., Kreek, M. J., Kieffer, B. L., & Gaveriaux-Ruff, C. (1998). Distribution of nociceptin/orphanin FQ receptor transcript in human central nervous system and immune cells. *Journal of Neuroimmunology, 81*, 184–192.

Peterson, P. K., Gekker, G., Hu, S., Lokensgard, J., Portoghese, P. S., & Chao, C. C. (1999). Endomorphin-1 potentiates HIV-1 expression in human brain cell cultures: Implication of an atypical mu-opioid receptor. *Neuropharmacology, 38*, 273–278.

Peterson, P. K., Sharp, B. M., Gekker, G., Porteghese, P. S., Sannerud, K., & Balfour, H. H. Jr. (1990). Morphine promotes the growth of HIV-1 in human peripheral blood mononuclear cell cocultures. *AIDS, 4*, 869–873.

Provinciali, M., Di Stefano, G., Raffaeli, W., Pari, G., Desiderio, F., & Fabri, N. (1991). Evaluation of NK and LAK cell activities in neoplastic patients during treatment with morphine. *International Journal of Neuroscience, 59*, 127–133.

Radulescu, R. T., DeCosta, B. R., Jacobson, A. E., Rice, K. C., Blalock, J. E., & Carr, D. J. J. (1991). Biochemical and functional characterization of a μ-opioid receptor binding site on cells of the immune system. *Progress in Neuroendocrinimmunology, 4*, 166–179.

Reubi, J. C. (1985). Central nervous system-mediated growth inhibition of a rat prostate carcinoma by an opioid. *Journal of Endocrinology, 107*, 247–250.

Risdahl, J. M., Khanna, K. V., Peterson, P. K., & Molitor, T. W. (1998). Opiates and infection. *Journal of Neuroimmunology, 83*, 4–18.

Risdahl, J. M., Peterson, P. K., Chao, C. C., Pijoan, C., & Molitor, T. W. (1993). Effects of morphine dependence on the pathogenesis of swine herpesvirus infection. *Journal of Infectectious Diseases, 167*, 1281–1287.

Rojavin, M., Szabo, I., Bussiere, J. L., Rogers, T. J., Adler, M. W., & Eisenstein, T. K. (1993). Morphine treatment in vitro or in vivo decreases phagocytic functions of murine macrophages. *Life Sciences, 53*, 997–1006.

Rouveix, B. (1992). Opiates and immune function. Consequences on infectious diseases with special reference to AIDS. *Therapie, 47*, 503–512.

Roy, S., & Loh, H. H. (1996). Effects of opioids on the immune system. *Neurochemical Reseach, 21*, 1375–1386.

Scott, M. & Carr, D. J. J. (1996). Morphine suppresses the alloantigen-driven CTL response in a dose-dependent and naltrexone-reversible fashion. *Journal of Pharmacology and Experimental Therapeutics, 278*, 980–988.

Sedqi, M., Roy, S., Ramakrishnan, S., Elde, R., & Loh, H. H. (1995). Complementary DNA cloning of a μ-opioid receptor from rat peritoneal macrophages. *Biochemical Biophysics Research Communication, 209*, 1003–1010.

Sedqi, M., Roy, S., Ramakrishnan, S., & Loh, H. H. (1996). Expression cloning of a full-length cDNA encoding delta opioid receptor from mouse thymocytes. *Journal of Neuroimmunology, 65*, 167–170.

Sharp, B. M., Shahabi, N. A., Heagy, W., McAllen, K., Bell, M., Huntoon, C., & McKean, D. J. (1996). Dual signal transduction through delta opioid receptors in a transfected human T-cell line. *Proceedings of the National Academy of Sciences USA, 93*, 8294–8299.

Sharp, B. M., Shahabi, N., McKean, D., Li, M. D., & McAllen, K. (1997). Detection of basal levels and induction of delta OR mRNA in murine splenocytes. *Journal of Neuroimmunology, 78*, 198–202.

Shavit, Y., Depaulis, A., Martin, F. C., Terman, G. W., Pechnick, R. N., Zane, C. J., Gale, R. P., & Liebeskind, J. C. (1986). Involvement of brain opiate receptors in the immune-suppressive effect of morphine. *Proceedings of the National Academy of Sciences USA, 83*, 7114–7117.

Sibinga, N. E. S., & Goldstein, A. (1988). Opioid peptides and opioid receptors in cells of the immune system. *Annual Reviews of Immunology, 6*, 219–249.

Simon, R., & Arbo, T. (1986). Morphine increases metastatic tumor growth. *Brain Research Bulletin, 16*, 363–367.

Sklar, L., & Anisman, H. (1981). Stress and cancer. *Psychology Bulletin, 89*, 369–406.

Sorensen, A. N., & Claesson, M. H. (1998). Effect of the opioid methionine enkephalinamide on signal transduction in human T-lymphocytes. *Life Sciences, 62*, 1251–1259.

Stefano, G. B., Digenis, A., Spector, S., Leung, M. K., Bilfinger, T., Makman, M. H., Scharrer, B., & Abumrad, N. N. (1993). Opiate-like substances in an invertebrate, an opiate receptor on invertebrate and human immunocytes, and a role in immunosuppression. *Proceedings of the National Academy of Sciences USA, 90*, 11099–11103.

Starec, M., Rouveix, B., Sinet, M., Chau, F., Desforges, B., Pocidalo, J.-J., & Lechat, P. (1991). Immune status and survival of opiate- and cocaine-treated mice infected with Friend virus. *Journal of Pharmacology and Experimental Therapeutics, 259*, 745–750.

Thompson, R. C., Mansour, A., Akil, H., & Watson, S. J. (1993). Cloning and pharmacological characterization of a rat μ opioid receptor. *Neuron, 11*, 903–913.

Veyries, M.-L., Sinet, M., Desforges, B., & Rouveix, B. (1995). Effects of morphine on the pathogenesis of murine Friend retrovirus infection. *Journal of Pharmacology and Experimental Therapeutics, 272*, 498–504.

Wang, J. B., Imai, Y., Eppler, C. M., Gregor, P., Spivak, C. E., Uhl, G. R. (1993). μ opioid receptor: cDNA cloning and expression. *Proceedings of the National Academy of Sciences USA, 90*, 10230–10234.

Weber, R. J., & Pert, C. B. (1984). Opiatergic modulation of the immune system. In E. E. Muller & A. R. Genazzani (Eds.), *Central and peripheral endorphins: Basic and clinical aspects*. New York: Raven Press.

Weber, R. J., & Pert, A. (1989). The periaqueductal gray matter mediates opiate-induced immunosuppression. *Science, 245*, 188–190.

Wick, M. J., Minnerath, S. R., Roy, S., Ramakrishnan, S., & Loh, H. H. (1995). Expression of alternate forms of brain opioid 'orphan' receptor mRNA in activated human peripheral blood lymphocytes and lymphocytic cell lines. *Brain Research Molecular Brain Research, 32*, 342–347.

Wick, M. J., Minnerath, S. R., Roy, S., Ramakrishnan, S., & Loh, H. H. (1996). Differential expression of opioid receptor genes in human lymphoid cell lines and peripheral blood lymphocytes. *Journal of Neuroimmunology, 64*, 29–36.

Wiedermann, C. J., Sacerdote, P., Propst, A., Propst, T., Judmaier, G., Kathrein, H., Vogel, W., & Panerai, A. (1994). Decreased β-endorphin content in peripheral blood mononuclear leukocytes from patients with Crohn's disease. *Brain, Behavior, and Immunity, 8*, 261–269.

Wybran R. J., Appelboom, T., Famaey, J.-P., & Govaerts, A. (1979). Suggestive evidence for receptors for morphine and methionine-enkephalin on normal human blood T lymphocytes. *Journal of Immunology, 123*, 1068–1070.

Yasuda, K., Raynor, K., Kong, H., Breder, C. D., Takeda, J., Reisine, T., & Bell, G. I. (1993). Cloning and functional comparison of κ and δ opioid receptors from mouse brain. *Proceedings of the National Academy of Sciences USA, 90*, 6736–6740.

Yeager, M. P., & Colacchio, T. A. (1991). Effect of morphine on growth of metastatic colon cancer in vivo. *Archives of Surgeory, 126*, 454–456.

Zhu, X., Wang, C., Cheng, Z., Wu, Y., Zhou, D., & Pei, G. (1997). The carboxyl terminus of mouse delta-OR is not required for agonist-dependent activation. *Biochemical Biophysics Research Communication, 232*, 513–516.

CHAPTER

15

Marijuana, the Cannabinoid System, and Immunomodulation

THOMAS W. KLEIN, CATHY NEWTON, ELIZABETH SNELLA, HERMAN FRIEDMAN

I. INTRODUCTION

It now is clear that endogenous cannabinoid ligands and cannabinoid receptors (CBRs) are found in both the brain and the periphery, especially in cells of the immune system. Thus, the cannabinoid system appears to be another example of the brain-immune connection. Our chapter in the previous addition of this volume concluded that marijuana cannabinoids, especially Δ^9-tetrahydrocannabinol (THC), suppressed the function of a wide variety of immune cells from both humans and animals and that these effects were thought to be due primarily to "nonspecific" effects of the lipophilic drugs on plasma membranes and other hydrophobic structures of the cell (Friedman, Klein, & Specter, 1991). In addition, we concluded that the impact of this drug-induced immunomodulation on the ability of humans and animals to fight infections and tumors and thereby cause disease was unclear because few studies in this area had been reported. Since the last edition, research in the area of cannabinoids and immune function has changed dramatically with the cloning of CBRs, and today major emphasis in the field is on establishing the distribution and function of receptor subtypes in various cells of the immune system. Additionally, some work has been reported on the effects of marijuana cannabinoids in disease models, but the overall health impact of CBR ligands is far from settled, and it was recently concluded that, although marijuana smoking is harmful, more research is needed to define the potential therapeutic efficacy of cannabinoid substances (Joy, Watson, & Benson, 1999). In this chapter we will review the basic structure of CBRs, their possible immune function, and the potential role of these receptors and their ligands in disease. The reader is referred to previous recent reviews in this area (Abood & Martin, 1996; Cabral & Dove Pettit, 1998; Howlett, 1995; Kaminski, 1998; Klein, Friedman, & Specter, 1998; Klein, Newton, & Friedman, 1998).

II. CANNABINOID RECEPTORS

A. Structure

The existence of CBRs was initially suggested by pharmacological evidence. The development and use of cannabinoid analogues allowed for the demonstration of structure-activity relationships among these compounds and furthermore established a linkage between cannabimimetic activities and inhibition of adenylyl cyclase in cell lines of neural origin (Howlett, Johnson, Melvin, & Milne, 1988). In addition, using a radiolabeled, synthetic, bicyclic derivative of THC, CP55,940, specific equilibrium binding was demonstrated in membrane extracts from brain, and in addition competitive displacement studies with labeled CP55,940 and unlabeled cannabinoids of various structures showed a K_i profile consistent with the biological potency of various cannabinoid analogues (Devane, Dysarz, Johnson, Melvin, & Howlett, 1988). These and other studies supported the existence of specific cannabinoid receptors that are negatively coupled to adenylyl cyclase.

A large number of neurotransmitters, hormones, and autocrine/paracrine factors elicit cellular changes through receptors coupled to G proteins. Hundreds of these receptors have been cloned and shown to possess the common structure of a single polypeptide with seven membrane-spanning domains; an extracellular, glycosylated N terminus; and an intracellular C terminus (Gether & Kobilka, 1998; Ji, Grossmann, & Ji, 1998; see Fig. 1). In 1990, Matsuda et al. reported the cloning of a novel cDNA from a rat brain cDNA library that encoded a protein with the structural features of a G protein-coupled receptor (Matsuda, Lolait, Brownstein, Young, & Bonner, 1990). The cDNA, when expressed in CHO cells, mediated cannabinoid-induced inhibition of forskolin-stimulated adenylyl cyclase activity, and cannabinoid responsive cell lines and brain areas contained the corresponding mRNA (Matsuda et al., 1990). The human homologue of this gene product was cloned a year later from a human brain stem cDNA library and the translated sequence contained 472 amino acids that were 97% identical to Matsuda's protein (Gerard, Mollereau, Vassart, & Parmentier, 1991; see Fig. 1). This CBR was termed CB1 to distinguish it from a second gene product, CB2, cloned by Munro et al. (Munro, Thomas, & Abu-Shaar, 1993). This cDNA was cloned from a human HL60 promyelocytic cell line library and was both structurally similar to members of the G protein-coupled receptor family and 44% identical to CB1. The cDNA coded for a protein of only 360 amino acids and containing a much shorter extracellular N terminus than CB1 (Figure 1). This gene product also differed from CB1 in that the mRNA was found in peripheral tissues rather than brain and, therefore, it was called CB2 (Munro et al., 1993). It appears now that CB1 is expressed in brain and the periphery whereas CB2 is expressed mainly in the periphery.

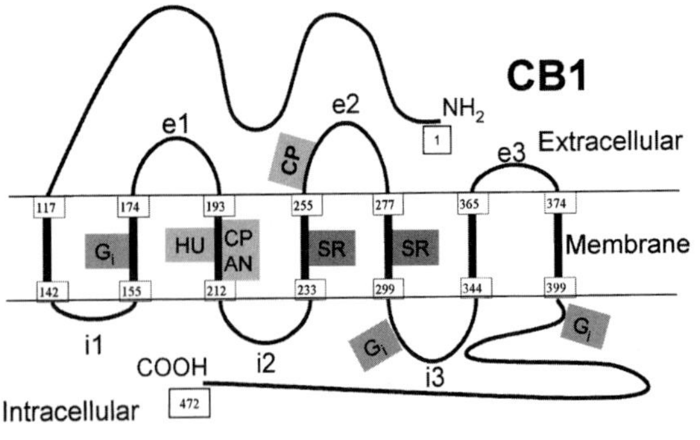

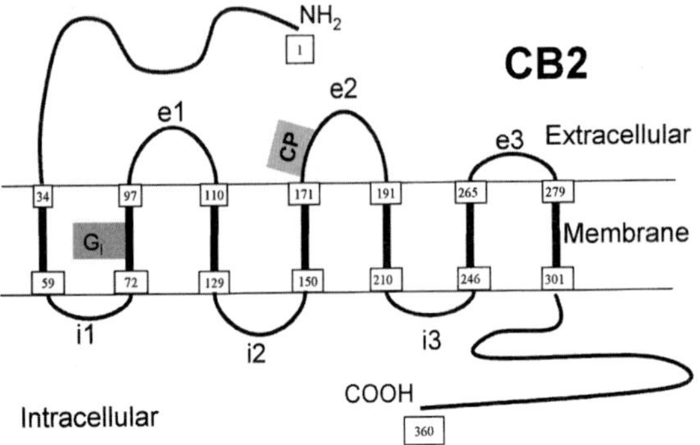

FIGURE 1 Cannabinoid receptors occur as two main subtypes, CB1 and CB2. CB1 is 472 amino acids (aa) in length, with an amino, extracellular end in excess of 100 aa and an intracellular carboxy end of approximately 70 aa. Various studies have shown that G proteins (G_i) bind at the second transmembrane region as well as the third intracellular loop (i3) and the carboxy tail. Furthermore, the receptor antagonist, SR141716A (SR) binds at the fourth and fifth transmembrane domains and the agonist CP55,940 (CP) binds to both the third transmembrane domain and the second extracellular loop. HU-210 (HU) and anandamide (AN) appear to bind the third transmembrane region. CB2 is 360 aa in length, with an amino, extracellular end of only about 35 aa and an intracellular carboxy end of approximately 60 aa. Studies have shown that G protein (G_i) binding occurs in the second transmembrane region and that CP55,940 (CP) binds in the second extracellular loop.

B. Interactions with Ligands and G Proteins

CB1 and CB2 bind various ligands in a defined rank order. For example, classical cannabinoids such as THC and cannabinol, and the fatty acid ethanolamide, anandamide, have a lower affinity than do nonclassical cannabinoids such as CP55,940, the aminoalkylindole WIN55212-2, and the dimethylheptyl derivative HU-210 (Slipetz et al., 1995; Thomas, Gilliam, Burch, Roche, & Seltzman, 1998). In addition, recent evidence suggests that CB2 has a higher affinity for WIN55212-2 and cannabinol as well as derivatives of HU210 (Felder et al., 1995; Huffman et al., 1996). Studies with other G protein-coupled receptors suggest that the ligand-binding domains are extremely diverse and range from the transmembrane regions and N terminus to the extracellular loops

factor-beta (TGF-β). Although no mechanisms were presented, the authors concluded that there was a potential health risk in using marijuana since production of protective inflammatory cytokines is suppressed whereas production of the immunosuppressive cytokines such as TGF-β is intact. This could result in a negative immune function status of marijuana users. Thus, it is likely that cannabinoids can modulate the cytokine activity of macrophages and, therefore, may induce immune depression; however, the role of CBRs in these findings is still unclear.

2. *Arachidonic Acid Release and Production of Anandamide*

Arachidonic acid (AA) metabolism and the cannabinoid system have had a close association for many years. In fact, at one time, both AA metabolites, such as prostaglandins, and cannabinoids were hypothesized to utilize the same receptor (Howlett, 1984). Furthermore, the endogenous ligands for CBR, anandamide (Devane et al., 1992), and 2-arachidonylglycerol (Mechoulam et al., 1995) are derivatives of AA. Macrophages, when perturbed by the environment, are known to be potent producers of AA metabolites (Dinarello & Wolff, 1993), and, therefore, it is not unreasonable to suspect that AA metabolism is a feature of cannabinoid treatment of macrophages, and that AA metabolites such as anandamide and 2-Ara-Gl might be produced by these cells. In support of this, several reports showed that THC treatment caused changes in cellular AA metabolism. For example, mouse peritoneal macrophage cultures readily release AA in response to incubation with THC (3 to 32 μM), and the mechanism of this effect involved phospholipase activity (Burstein, Budrow, Debatis, Hunter, & Subramanian, 1994) (see Table II). Human, PBMCs, and PBMC-derived adherent cells also release AA metabolites such as leukotrienes in response to THC (Diaz, Specter, Vanderhoek, & Coffey, 1994). Regarding CBR involvement, CB2 antisense treatment of RAW 264.7 cells attenuated the AA release in response to THC, suggesting these receptors, but not CB1, might play a role in this effect (Hunter & Burstein, 1997). Besides AA and leukotrienes, anandamide and related compounds also have been shown to be released from macrophage-like cells. Here, J774 cells, a macrophage-like cell line of mouse origin, were shown not only to produce anandamide constitutively but to produce more of it following stimulation with ionomycin (DiMarzo, DePetrocellis, Sepe, & Buono, 1996). It was speculated that these metabolites might be involved in modulating inflammatory cell function but no evidence for this was presented. From this, it appears that cannabinoid treatment of macrophages, like other environmental stimuli, affects AA metabolism, and that a portion of this metabolism produces cannabinoid ligands such as anandamide. Other ligands such as 2-Ara-Gl might also be produced as a consequence of CBR activation in these cells.

3. *Nitric Oxide Release*

THC and other cannabinoids have been shown to suppress the bactericidal and tumoricidal activity of macrophages (Klein, Friedman, et al., 1998). A portion of macrophage killing activity is contributed by reactive oxygen intermediates as well as nitrogen intermediates such as nitric oxide (NO; Moncada, Palmer, & Higgs, 1991), and it has been proposed that attenuation of killing by THC treatment of macrophages might involve effects on NO production (Coffey, Yamamoto, Snella, & Pross, 1996) (see Table II). Mouse peritoneal macrophage cultures were treated with LPS and IFN-γ to induce NO, and co-treated with THC and other cannabinoids. THC suppressed NO production at concentrations as low as 2 μM especially in cultures with less IFN-γ, and the drug effect appeared to be related to a suppression of NO synthase (NOS) cellular levels and enzyme activity. Regarding CBR involvement, Δ^8- and Δ^9-THC were more potent than other cannabinoids such as cannabidiol, cannabinol, and the (+) isomer of Δ^9-THC, and were more potent than anandamide. In addition, THC attenuated the cAMP response in the macrophage cultures, and the addition of 8-bromo-cAMP slightly, but significantly, restored NO levels following drug treatment. The authors concluded that only a portion of the cannabinoid suppressive effect was due to the CBR/cAMP pathway and that other molecular mechanisms were probably involved in this response (Coffey et al., 1996). Using a macrophage cell line, these findings were extended to show that THC inhibited NOS transcription by suppressing the activity of transcription factors such as NF-κB/RelA, the latter effect being linked to a THC-induced attenuation of the cAMP response (Jeon, Yang, Pulaski, & Kaminski, 1996). These studies suggest that cannabinoids can modulate the cAMP system of macrophages as well as associated downstream cellular functions such as NO production. Although not conclusive, a role for CBRs in these responses is suggested by these studies.

4. *Expression of CBR*

Antibodies to CBR proteins have not been readily forthcoming. Much of the evidence suggesting receptor expression in macrophages and other immune cells, therefore, derives from studies employing techniques other than the direct demonstration of receptor protein. For example, the use of quantitative RT-PCR on total RNA from human immune tissues and blood cell subpopulations first suggested that CB1 mRNA is expressed in differing amounts in different immune cell subpopulations (Bouaboula et al., 1993) (see Table II). Monocytes isolated from blood contained relatively little CB1 message in relation to natural killer (NK) cells or especially B cells, which had the highest level. Macrophage cell lines (e.g., U937) were positive for message but the amount was less than in B cell lines (Bouaboula et al., 1993). Similar results were obtained for CB2 wherein blood monocytes were mRNA positive but the level was lower than in NK and B cells; monocyte cell lines were also lower for CB2 message (Galieque et al., 1995). Polyclonal antibodies to CB2 reacted with tonsillar germinal center cells and the follicular mantle suggesting, but not proving, that receptor protein was expressed on macrophages in these anatomical areas. The initial report describing the cloning of CB2 also showed that immune subpopulations (purified from rat spleen) contained the CB2 mRNA (Munro et al., 1993). Specifically, $CD11b^+$ cells were strongly positive for CB2 whereas $CD5^+$ cells were negative. Because CD11b is on macrophages, NK cells, and neutrophils, these results suggested that all of these cells were CB2 positive whereas $CD5^+$ T cells (and subsets of B cells) were negative for CB2 mRNA under these conditions. Macrophages from mouse spleen were also shown to have relatively less CB1 message than B cells, but this message level could be increased in RAW264.7 cells following stimulation with LPS (Klein et al., 1995). Finally, a recent report using an affinity purified polyclonal antiserum to CB1 showed that MHC class II^+, macrophage-like, glial cells from the rat brain were positive for immunoreactive protein and also positive, by RT-PCR, for CB1 message (Sinha, Bonner, Bhat, & Matsuda, 1998). A glioma cell line and a B-lymphoblastoid cell line were also positive for this protein, which had an estimated molecular mass of 58 kDa. From the above evidence, it is clear that CBR message is readily detected in primary macrophages from different species and different macrophage cell lines. It is also clear that these cells appear to express less CBR mRNA than other immune cells such as B cells. However, further studies are needed to firmly establish to what extent and under what conditions CBRs are expressed and functional on macrophages and other cells of the mononuclear phagocyte lineage.

C. T Cells and B Cells

1. *T Cell Killing and Calcium Mobilization*

Previous studies had exhaustively established that THC suppressed the proliferation response to T cell mitogens using cells from a variety of sources (Friedman et al., 1991). However, mechanisms and CBR involvement in this inhibition was not reported. Yebra et al. examined the THC effect on one of the earliest events in T cell activation, i.e., the mobilization of cytosolic free calcium ([Ca^{2+}];Yebra, Klein, & Friedman, 1992) (see Table III). Mouse thymocytes were cultured with THC and concanavalin A (Con A) and the [Ca^{2+}] was measured by fluorescent Ca^{2+}-activated compounds. THC ($<10\,\mu M$) suppressed [Ca^{2+}] mobilization in response to Con A, blocking mobilization from both extracellular pools and intracellular stores (Yebra et al., 1992). The role of CBR was not examined. Besides proliferation, the effect of cannabinoids on other T cell functions such as cytolytic activity also was studied (Klein, Kawakami, Newton, & Friedman, 1991). Mouse splenocyte cytotoxic T cells (CTLs) were generated either in vitro or in vivo and exposed to THC and 11-hydroxy-THC. Both cannabinoids suppressed CTL killing activity by preventing the maturation and expansion of immature CTLs and by preventing the killing mechanisms of mature CTLs. THC, at a rather high dose of 50 mg/kg, also suppressed the splenic CTL activity when injected into mice undergoing sensitization and priming. Regarding the involvement of CBR, a very limited structure-activity study using only two cannabinoids showed that THC was more potent than 11-hydroxy-THC in suppressing the CTL response (Klein et al., 1991). It can be speculated that these effects on CTL killing are related to drug effects on both lymphocyte proliferation and early signaling mechanisms (see other sections of this chapter) which cause the suppression of functional maturation following CTL contact with the target cell.

2. *T Cell CBR Expression and cAMP*

As with the evidence for CBR expression on other immune cell subpopulations, the data for CBR expression on T cells is still preliminary and equivocal. By RT-PCR, mRNA for both receptors has been reported in human and mouse T cells (Bouaboula et al., 1993; Galieque et al., 1995; Klein et al., 1995) but, interestingly, the message for CB2 was not detected in T cells ($CD5^+$) from rat spleen (Munro et al., 1993) (see Table III). It is not clear if this is a true species difference or an artifact; T cells appear to express relatively lower amounts of CBR message

TABLE III Cannabinoid Effects on T Cells and B Cells

Function	Model	Drug used	Reference
T cell calcium mobilization			
	Mouse	THC[a]	Yebra '92
T cell cytolysis			
	Mouse	THC, 11-OH-THC[b]	Klein '91
T cell CBR expression			
	Human, cell line	N/A[c]	Bouaboula '93
	Human, cell line	N/A	Galieque '95
	Mouse, cell line	N/A	Klein '95
	Mouse, cell line	N/A	Schatz '97
	Cell line	N/A	Condie '96
	Cell line	N/A	Daaka '96
T cell cAMP			
	Cell line	THC	Schatz '97
	Cell line	THC, cannabinol	Condie '96
B cell proliferation			
	Mouse	THC, 11-OH-THC	Klein '85
	Mouse	2-Ara-G1[d], ANA[e]	Lee '95
	Human	THC, CP55, 940[f], WIN55212-2[g], SR141716A[h]	Derocq '95
B cell CBR expression			
	Human, cell line	N/A	Bouaboula '93
	Human, cell line	N/A	Galieque '95
	Mouse, cell line	N/A	Klein '95

[a] Δ^9-tetrahydrocannabibol.
[b] 11-hydroxy-Δ^9-tetrahydrocannabinol.
[c] Not applicable.
[d] 2-arachidonyl-glycerol.
[e] Anandamide.
[f] (*cis*)-3-[2-hydroxy-4-(1,1-dimethylheptyl)phenyl]-(*trans*)-4-(3-hydroxypropyl)cyclohexanol.
[g] (−)-3-(4-morpholinyemethyl)-S-methyl-6-(1-naphthylcarbonyl)-2,3-dihydropyrrolo[1,2,3-*de*]-1,4-benzoxazinemethanesulfonic acid.
[h] N-(Piperidin-1-yl)-5-(4-chlorophenyl)-1-(2,4-dichlorophenyl)-4-methyl-1H-pyrazole-3-carboxamide.

(Bouaboula et al., 1993; Galieque et al., 1995; Klein et al., 1995) and, therefore, the RT-PCR conditions in the rat studies may have been insufficient to detect the CB2 mRNA. Regarding T cell subsets such as CD 4 and 8, minor differences in both messages have been reported in human cells (Bouaboula et al., 1993; Galieque et al., 1995); similar reports have not appeared for rodent cells. The results to date suggest that rodent and human T cells express limited amounts of CBR mRNA that is generally less than that expressed by B cells; however, the demonstration of receptor proteins by specific antibodies on these cells has not been reported. This may be due to relatively low levels of expressed surface proteins as suggested by a report showing that purified mouse splenic T cells express only 100–300 receptors per cell (Schatz, Lee, Condie, Pulaski, & Kaminski, 1997). In contrast to primary T cells isolated from animals, T cell lines appear to express more CBR message and protein. For example, some, but not all, T cell lines expressed sufficient CB2 message to be detectable by Northern blotting whereas CB1 message was not detected (Condie, Herring, Koh, Lee, & Kaminski, 1996; Schatz et al., 1997). The detected transcripts were of different sizes depending on which T cell line was used. In addition to message, a human T cell line has been shown to express CB1 immunoreactive proteins; however, these were only expressed following cell activation by mitogen (Daaka, Friedman, & Klein, 1996). These findings that T cell lines express more CBR than primary cells coupled with the observation that activated cells might express more CBR than nonactivated, suggest that T cells may express a low basal level of receptors that can become activated following stimulation of the cells. Additional studies will be required to verify this possibility.

Other evidence that T cell lines express CBRs stems from studies demonstrating a disruption in the adenylyl cyclase/cAMP signaling system following treatment of these lines with cannabinol and THC. Human lines such as HPB-ALL were suppressed by

THC treatment only (Schatz et al., 1997) whereas mouse lines, such as EL4.IL-2, were suppressed by both cannabinoids (Condie et al., 1996). These studies provide indirect evidence of CBR-linked, G_i coupling in T cells.

3. *B Cell Proliferation and CBR Expression*

Many studies demonstrate that cannabinoids suppress the antibody response of humans and animals (Friedman et al., 1991; Klein, Friedman, et al., 1998; see other parts of this chapter). B cells, of course, are an essential component of the antibody response and several studies have attempted to test cannabinoid effects on this cell type. Initially, it was reported that THC suppressed the B cell proliferation response to LPS in mouse splenocyte cultures (Klein, Newton, Widen, & Friedman, 1985) (see Table III). Suppression of B cell proliferation appeared to be more sensitive to THC than the T cell proliferation response. Later studies with mouse spleen cultures could not establish a direct inhibitory effect of cannabinoids on B cells when measuring the in vitro antibody forming cell response to LPS stimulation (Schatz et al., 1993). However, in another study the cannabimimetic 2-Ara-Gl was shown to either increase or decrease LPS-induced, B cell proliferation of mouse splenocytes depending on the cell density of the cultures; interestingly, anandamide had no effect (Lee et al., 1995). Finally, human tonsillar B cells, stimulated in culture with anti-Ig or anti-CD40 antigen, were shown to express higher levels of proliferation when cocultured with various cannabinoids (Derocq, Segui, Marchand, LeFur, & Casellas, 1995). This cannabinoid effect appears to be mediated through a CB2 mechanism because it was not attenuated by the CB1 antagonist SR141716A but was attenuated by pertussis toxin, and the B cells expressed higher levels of CB2 mRNA than CB1. This study is remarkable because cannabinoids enhanced proliferation rather than suppressed it, and in addition, drug concentrations were in the nanomolar range rather than micromolar. However, it must be pointed out that the cell cultures in this study were performed in medium containing only 0.5% serum, and this low level may have contributed to the apparent drug potency of the system (Klein et al., 1985). Together, these results provide the strongest evidence to date that CBRs modulate B cell function. Perhaps the receptor signaling system in these cells is especially susceptible to regulation by the cannabinoid system, or B cells express an unusually high level of CBRs (Bouaboula et al., 1993; Galieque et al., 1995). Whatever the reason, B cells appear to provide a good model for studying the regulatory role of the cannabinoid system in immunity.

D. NK Cells

1. *CBR Expression and Gene Activation*

Previous studies suggested that THC and other cannabinoids suppressed the killing activity of mouse and human NK cells when tested in vitro and in vivo (Klein, Friedman, et al., 1998; Klein, Newton, et al., 1998). However, the role of CBRs in these effects was not clear because few structure/activity studies were done, the drug concentrations used were in the 10 μM range, and one study in humans reported that marijuana use had no effect on PBL NK activity (Dax, Pilotte, Adler, Nagel, & Lange, 1989). More recently, as with other immune subpopulations, CB1 and 2 mRNAs have been demonstrated by RT-PCR in human peripheral blood leukocyte (PBL) NK cells (Bouaboula et al., 1993; Galieque et al., 1995) and in a mouse NK-like cell line (Daaka et al., 1996) suggesting that the receptor might be expressed on these cells (see Table IV). Although receptor protein has not yet been demonstrated, indirect evidence suggests that CBRs are expressed and involved in signaling in NK cells. The NKB61A2 cell line is derived from mouse and contains many morphological and functional similarities to primary NK cells (Warner and Dennert, 1982). The IL-2-induced killing activity and proliferation of these cells was reported to be suppressed by THC and 11-hydroxy-THC with the ID_{50} for THC between 20 and 30 μM and significantly higher for 11-hydroxy-THC (Kawakami et al., 1988). The mechanism of this suppression was reported to stem partly from a drug-induced decrease in the number of high and intermediate affinity IL-2 binding sites, suggesting a suppression in the expression of IL-2 receptor (IL-2R) proteins (Zhu et al., 1993). Subsequent studies showed that THC treatment increased the cellular levels of IL-2R α and β proteins but decreased the γ protein and IL-2R function (Zhu, Igarashi, Friedman, & Klein, 1995). From this, it was concluded that drug treatment disturbed the relative expression of the various IL-2R chains resulting in overall receptor dysfunction and poor responsiveness to IL-2. Additional studies in this model linked CBR to these effects and also implicated the transcription factor, NF-κB, in these events (Daaka, Zhu, Friedman, & Klein, 1997). In these studies, THC increased the transcription of the α chain protein and increased the activity of NF-κB. In addition, through the use of antisense oligonucleotides to NF-κB protein, it was shown that the increase in α chain production by THC was linked to the increase in the transcription factor.

TABLE IV Cannabinoid Effects on Natural Killer Cells

Function	Model	Drug used	Reference
CBR expression			
	Human	N/A[a]	Bouaboula '93
	Human	N/A	Galieque '95
	Cell line	N/A	Daaka '96
Gene activation			
	Cell line	THC	Zhu '95
	Cell line	THC	Daaka '97

[a] Not applicable.

Furthermore, through the use of CB1 antisense, CBR was linked to the THC increase in α mRNA. It was concluded that in this NK-like cell line, a signaling pathway exists composed of CB1, NF-κB, and the IL-2Rα gene, thus providing indirect evidence of CBR coupling to gene activity in these cells. Other immune cell models have demonstrated linkage of CBR to NF-κB-mediated gene activity, but in these studies the drug effect was suppression rather than enhancement (Herring et al., 1998; Jeon et al., 1996). It is possible that CBR linkage to NF-κB varies depending on the type of immune cell or gene product involved, or that variations in CBR subtype or ligand used result in different molecular effects downstream of receptor binding. It is also possible, because cannabinoids do not appear, by themselves, to activate immune cells, that they function instead as secondary modulators as has been suggested for other neurotransmitters and hormones (Garza & Carr, 1997; Pennisi, 1997).

IV. CANNABINOIDS AND DISEASE

A. Health Status and Pulmonary Disease

The above data supporting cellular immune effects of cannabinoids suggest that the use of marijuana or exposure to cannabinoids should result in a higher incidence of health problems linked to altered immunity. For example, morbidity and mortality from infections should be higher in subjects abusing this drug. Few human studies addressing this issue have been reported. One of the largest and most recent was conducted in a large cohort of 65,000 members of a California health plan using questionnaires from 1979 to 1985 and following the subjects' health and mortality status through 1991. The study concluded that subjects using marijuana at the time they responded to the questionnaire (i.e., current users) had mortality rates similar to controls in the male, non-AIDS group, and in the total women's group (Sidney, Beck, Tekawa, Quesenberry, & Friedmen, 1997); however, there was an increased risk of mortality in the AIDS group using marijuana. The authors felt that marijuana use did not cause the mortality but that the increased risk reflected a strong association between marijuana use and homosexuality or bisexuality. However, this was not proven by the study and other explanations for the increased risk of mortality were discussed such as reduced defenses in the respiratory tract leading to infections, increased high-risk sexual behavior and intravenous drug abuse, and possible immunosuppressive properties of marijuana (Sidney et al., 1997). It is apparent from this study that moderate marijuana use did not increase the risk of death in the relatively healthy adult population that was followed for about 10 years. However, health factors other than mortality are currently being evaluated, such as the incidences of cancer and respiratory illness. It will be of interest to see if these are altered by marijuana smoking. Clearly, additional studies such as this are needed to assess the health impact of marijuana smoking.

Other health consequences of marijuana smoking involve alterations in bronchial epithelium, increased chronic bronchitis, and adverse effects on pulmonary macrophages. Bronchoscopy specimens from groups of smokers and nonsmokers were evaluated for the incidence of molecular markers that antedate the development of lung cancer (Barsky, Roth, Kleerup, Simmons, & Tashkin, 1998). Smokers of either marijuana, cocaine, or tobacco exhibited more molecular and histopathological alterations than did nonsmokers, and the smokers also reported a higher frequency of symptoms of chronic bronchitis. The authors concluded that marijuana and cocaine smoking, like tobacco smoking, places subjects at increased risk of developing lung cancer (Barsky et al., 1998). In another study from the same group, pulmonary alveolar macrophages were isolated from smokers and nonsmokers and functionally analyzed in vitro (Baldwin et al., 1997). It was reported that macrophages from marijuana smokers were deficient in the capacity to ingest and kill the bacterium, *Staphylococcus aureus*, to kill tumor cells, and were also deficient in NO formation and cytokine production (see section III, B, macrophages). Although the mechanisms of these inhibitory effects were not reported, these results clearly indicate a compromising of pulmonary resistance mechanisms by marijuana smoking suggesting that abusers may have enhanced susceptibility to pulmonary disease. Further studies of this type are needed to address this assertion more fully.

B. Infections and Cytokines

There is no direct evidence that marijuana smoking leads to an increased incidence of infectious diseases in humans. In fact, at least one study has suggested that marijuana use fails to promote the progression to AIDS in HIV positive individuals (Kaslow et al., 1989). However, animal studies dating back to the 1970s have shown drug effects on the progression of infections. Various models employing mice, rats, and guinea pigs infected with microbes ranging from herpes virus to spirochetes were examined. These showed that THC injection increased the morbidity and mortality of infected animals, and in many cases the drug compromised the functioning of the various immune cells, such as macrophages and T cells, that are responsible for host resistance (reviewed in Klein, Friedman, et al., 1998). More recently, cannabinoid-induced modulation of cytokine production has also been implicated in drug effects on host defenses. For example, IFN-α/β was reported to be suppressed by chronic treatment of mice with THC (Blanchard, Newton, Klein, Stewart III, & Friedman, 1986; Cabral, Lockmuller, & Mishkin, 1986) and the suppression of this antiviral cytokine might account for drug suppression of antiviral immunity. Likewise, TNF-α production by macrophages was also shown to be suppressed (Cabral & Vasquez, 1992; Zheng et al., 1992) perhaps accounting for reduced immunity to bacterial infections.

In contrast to suppression of cytokines, other studies showed that THC treatment increased cytokine production. For example, we reported that THC injection (8 mg/kg) 1 day before and 1 day after a sublethal infection with *Legionella pneumophila* resulted in animal mortality from what resembled septic shock (Klein, Newton, Widen, & Friedman, 1993). In support of this, acute phase cytokines such as TNF-α, IL-1, and IL-6, were shown to be elevated in the blood of treated animals and injection of antisera to these cytokines protected the mice from death. The mechanism of this drug effect was not fully elucidated. However, subsequent studies suggested that CBRs might be involved because the less potent cannabinoid, cannabinol, was less effective than either THC or CP55,940 in causing death (Smith, Yamamoto, Newton, Friedman, & Klein, 1996). The acute phase cytokine, IL-6, was also shown to be increased in a quite different model of infection and cytokine production (Molina-Holgado, Molina-Holgado, & Guaza, 1998). Here, mouse cortical astrocyte cultures were shown to increase the production of IL-6 if infected in vitro with Theiler"s murine encephalomyelitis virus. If the cultures were also treated with anandamide (1–25μM) the production of IL-6 was increased further. CBRs appeared to be involved because the enhancing effect was attenuated by the CB1 antagonist, SR141716A. Since IL-6 production may have a palliative effect in central nervous system diseases such as multiple sclerosis, it was speculated that this observation was in someway related to the protective effect of cannabinoids in diseases such as multiple sclerosis.

In another cytokine paradigm, mice given a single THC injection (4 mg/kg) one day before a sublethal infection with *Legionella* did not develop immunity when tested 3 weeks later (Newton, Klein, & Friedman, 1994). In other words, the drug prevented the mice from developing sufficient T cell immunity to defend against a second lethal infection with *Legionella*. Since T helper 1 (Th1) immunity must develop rather than T helper 2 (Th2) for protection against intracellular bacteria such as *Legionella* (Kaufmann, 1993), it was speculated that THC treatment suppressed the maturation and expansion of Th1 cells. Indeed, drug treatment of mice was shown to suppress Th1 anti-*Legionella* immunity as revealed by reduced production of IFN-γ and antibodies of the IgG_{2a} isotype (Newton et al., 1994). Other cytokines associated with the development of Th1 immunity such as IL-15 and IL-12 have also been observed to be depressed in this model (unpublished), and it appears from recent studies that CBRs might be involved. Th1 cells develop in a cytokine environment containing IL-12 and IFN-γ (O'Garra, 1998) and these cytokines can be detected in the serum of animals infected with microbes such as *Legionella* that induce the development of Th1 cells. We asked whether THC injection at the time of infection could reduce the level of serum IFN-γ, thus lessening the Th1 promoting environment, and further, if the cotreatment with CBR antagonists could inhibit the THC effect. Figure 2 shows the results of such a study. Four groups of mice were established. Group 1 was infected with *Legionella* only. A second group was injected with THC 18 hours prior to *Legionella* infection, and Groups 3 and 4 were injected with either the CB1 or CB2 antagonist 30 min prior to THC injection. As expected, *Legionella* infection resulted in a rise in the Th1-inducing cytokine, IFN-γ (Figure 2). Furthermore, THC treatment prior to infection suppressed the rise in IFN-γ. Of interest are the findings that both antagonists attenuated the drug effect and allowed for the *Legionella*-induced increase in IFN-γ. IL-12 also enhances Th1 subtypes, and this cytokine was likewise affected by the drugs in a similar manner (data not shown). Although it is not clear at this time exactly which cells in the body are responsible for the production of these cytokines, it is possible that the cells involved express both CB1 and CB2 receptors that are sensitive to modulation by cannabinoids. It is also possible that CBRs in the central nervous system as well as the periphery are participating in this response and that the regulation of Th cells, therefore, is a component of the neuroimmune axis.

C. Cytokine-Induced Cell Growth

As stated above, the physiological role of CBRs and their endogenous ligands such as anandamide and palmitylethanolamide is not known but several reports suggest that they may be involved in regulating cell proliferation and growth of not only immune cells but also hematopoietic cells and tumor cells. The first evidence for this stemmed from the finding that CBRs are linked to activating the MAP-kinase cascade associated with growth regulation of hematopoietic cells (Bouaboula et al., 1995). Anandamide was then reported to costimulate with other growth factors the proliferation of primary mouse bone marrow cells and hematopoietic growth factor dependent cell lines (Valk et al., 1997). Anandamide by itself was not a growth factor and the effect was not observed if the cells were cultured in serum-containing medium. Furthermore, although the anandamide concentrations used were quite low (i.e., 0.1 to 0.3 μM) and the effect was observed with established growth factors such as IL-3, GM-CSF, G-CSF, and erythropoietin, interestingly, other CBR ligands such as THC and CP55,940 had no effect. The mechanism of the growth-promoting effect was examined in a similar study using IL-3- and IL-6-dependent murine cell lines (Derocq et al., 1998). Here, several endogenous ligands including anandamide significantly enhanced cell growth in the presence of either IL-3 or IL-6, but as before, high-affinity cannabinoids such as CP55,940 were without effect. This suggested that CBRs were not involved in the growth-promoting effect, and other results employing receptor antagonists and the use of the G_i inhibitor, pertussis toxin, strongly supported this possibility (Derocq et al., 1998). These and other studies, including the observation of a growth promoting effect of arachidonic acid, lead to the hypothesis that endogenous fatty acids of this type can trigger signaling cascades in hematopoietic cells independent of the CBRs (Derocq et al., 1998). This novel idea warrants further study.

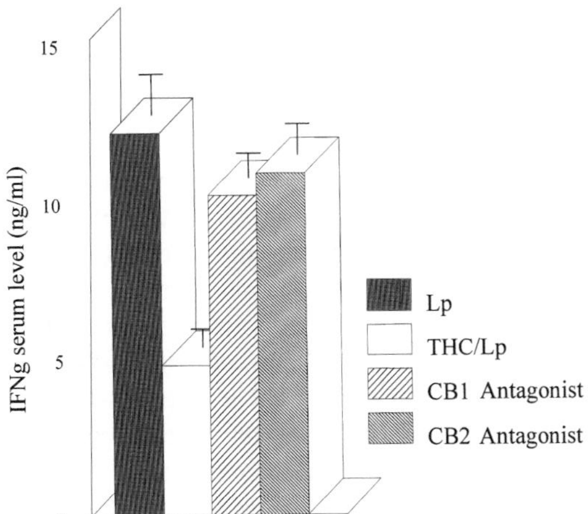

FIGURE 2 CBR antagonists attenuate the THC-induced increase in serum IFN-γ level. Mice were divided into four groups: (1) mice were iv infected with *Legionella pneumophila* (Lp); (2) mice were iv injected with THC (8 mg/kg) followed 18 h later with an Lp infection; (3) mice were iv injected with the CB1 antagonist (4 mg/kg), SR141716A, 30 min prior to THC, followed 18 h later with an Lp infection; and (4) mice were iv injected with the CB2 antagonist (4 mg/kg), SR144528, and then treated with THC and Lp. All mice were bled 8 h following Lp infection and the serum processed for IFN-γ analysis by enzyme-linked immunosorbent assay.

Anandamide also has been shown to suppress the proliferation of human breast cancer cell lines (De Petrocellis et al., 1998). In addition to anandamide, 2-Ara-Gly, HU-210, and arachidonic acid were also suppressive, but not palmitylethanolamide. However, with the exception of the arachidonic acid effect, the drug effects were blocked by pretreatment with the CB1 antagonist, SR141716A, suggesting that CB1 was involved. This antiproliferative effect appears to involve prolactin, which is a growth factor for these cells. Anandamide was shown to interfere with this prolactin pathway by suppressing the prolactin receptor system (De Petrocellis et al., 1998). These studies appear to be still other examples of how cannabimimetic substances can modulate the function of blood cells responding to environmental stimuli. As in the case of immune cells, the cannabinoids alone do not trigger the cells, but instead modify the cellular response once it has been triggered.

D. Therapeutic Uses of Cannabinoids

Many users of marijuana still advocate its use for ailments ranging from asthma and loss of appetite to pain and muscle spasticity (Joy et al., 1999); however, the scientific evidence to date does not, in a general sense, support their enthusiasm. One THC-containing formulation, Dronabinol, has been approved for use in loss of appetite in patients who are not responding to other agents, and it has proven to be of some value in this application (Adams & Martin, 1996). There has also been the suggestion that THC ameliorates the symptoms of multiple sclerosis and perhaps other brain–immune disorders (Mechoulam, Vogel, & Barg, 1994). However, all of these claims require more study and analysis.

Data from a few animal models have suggested that cannabinoid treatment can reduce immune-mediated diseases. For example, THC was shown to be of value in reducing disease in rat and guinea pig models of experimental autoimmune encephalomyelitis (EAE; Lyman, Sonett, Brosnan, Elkin, & Bornstein, 1989). EAE is an animal model for studying immune aspects of multiple sclerosis. The results were rather dramatic in that the drug (5 mg/kg/day, by gavage) almost completely reversed the clinical and histological evidence of disease and was effective when given either before or after the neural antigens. Similar results were obtained in a rat model of EAE using the Δ^8-THC analogue of THC along with daily oral administration of the drug (Wirguin et al., 1994). Here again, disease severity was significantly suppressed by the cannabinoid. Also of interest was the finding that the serum corticosterone level was doubled by the drug treatment leading to speculation that the elevated steroids were at least partly responsible for the lessening of the autoimmune response and EAE symptoms (MacPhee, Antoni, & Mason, 1989). Since THC injection markedly elevates corticosterone release in rats by a central mechanism (Weidenfeld, Feldman, & Mechoulam, 1994), it is possible that some of the immunosuppressive effects observed with cannabinoids are due to this hypothalamo-pituitary-adrenal input.

The attenuation of an inflammatory response also has been reported to occur following treatment with cannabimimetic agents such as WIN55,212-2, THC, and palmitylethanolamide (Berdyshev, Boichot, Corbel, Germain, & Lagente, 1998). Pulmonary inflammation, measured by the influx of polymorphonuclears (PMNs) and the rise in pulmonary TNF-α, was decreased by the intranasal administration of the these drugs, but anandamide had no effect, suggesting that CB2 might be involved. In contrast to this finding, however, suppression of inflammation was observed with the synthetic cannabinoid HU-211, which has low CBR affinity and therefore very little cannabimimetic activity. Two central nervous system models of inflammation were studied, one involving experimental pneumococcal meningitis (Bass, Engelhard, Trembovler, & Shohami, 1996), the other, closed head injury (Shohami, Gallily, Mechoulam, Bass, & Ben-Hur, 1997). In the meningitis model in rats, HU-211, in combination with the antibiotic, ceftriaxone, was significantly better than either agent alone in preventing the histopathological changes to the meninges. In the closed head injury model, the cannabinoid was as effective as other neural TNF-α inhibiting agents in shortening recovery time of rats. The cannabinoid also decreased the brain level of TNF-α after closed head injury (Shohami et al., 1997). Thus, these studies demonstrate that cannabinoids can modulate cytokines and inflammation in vivo just as they were shown to do in vitro. They also suggest that both CBR-mediated and nonreceptor mediated mechanisms might be involved.

V. CONCLUSION

The cannabinoid system of receptors and ligands is widely distributed throughout the body and probably plays a key role in the normal functioning of physiological systems including the central nervous system and the immune system. The receptors are G protein-coupled receptors and they appear to signal gene activity through known mediators such as cAMP. However, other mechanisms of signaling are possible, and the full extent of the genes activated by these receptors is not known. It is our feeling that CBRs are involved in a secondary level of immune cell regulation similar to other neuroimmune systems such as the opioid system. These secondary systems have a less pronounced functional role in regulating immune cell activity than do primary systems such as those directly stimulated by antigens, certain cell interaction molecules, and cytokine receptors. Because of the less prominent role in immune regulation, it is more difficult to demonstrate experimentally an involvement of CBRs using standard immune tests geared toward examining primary regulators. Therefore, new immune tests will be needed to reveal functions closely linked to and regulated by CBRs. The demonstration of receptor linkage to immune activity is also further complicated by the possibility that cannabimimetic agents might affect immune cell signaling through nonreceptor mechanisms. These nonreceptor effects will probably be much more difficult to define than the receptor effects. At this point, scientific evidence supports the hypothesis that marijuana smoking is harmful, and that THC suppresses numerous types of immune functions. However, it is counterintuitive to suspect that the cannabinoid system is inherently harmful; therefore, disease may come not only from exposure to cannabinoids but also from overexposure in much the same way that insulin shock can occur if too much insulin is administered. In our view, the key to understanding the negative consequences of cannabimimetics is to understand the role these agents play in the normal functioning of the brain, immune, and other physiological systems. Once we know the boundaries of normal, the limits of the abnormal will become clearer.

Acknowledgments

Our thanks to students and collaborators including Sasha Noe, Sumi Lee, & Liang Nong. This work was supported in part by grants #DA03646, DA10683, and DA07245 from the National Institute on Drug Abuse.

References

Abood, M. E., & Martin, B. R. (1996). Molecular neurobiology of the cannabinoid receptor. *International Review of Neurobiology, 39*, 197–221.

Adams, I. B., & Martin, B. R. (1996). Cannabis: pharmacology and toxicology in animals and humans. *Addiction, 91*, 1585–1614.

Baldwin, G. C., Tashkin, D. P., Buckley, D. M., Park, A. N., Dubinett, S. M., & Roth, M. D. (1997). Marijuana and cocaine impair alveolar macrophage function and cytokine production. *American Journal of Respiratory Critical Care Medicine, 156*, 1606–1613.

Barsky, S. H., Roth, M. D., Kleerup, E. C., Simmons, M., & Tashkin, D. P. (1998). Histopathologic and molecular alterations in bronchial epithelium in habitual smokers of marijuana, cocaine, and/or tobacco. *Journal of the National Cancer Institute, 90*, 1198–1204.

Bass, R., Engelhard, D., Trembovler, V., & Shohami, E. (1996). A novel nonpsychotropic cannabinoid, HU-211, in the treatment of experimental pneumococcal meningitis. *Journal of Infectious Diseases, 173*, 735–738.

Berdyshev, E., Boichot, E., Corbel, M., Germain, N., & Lagente, V. (1998). Effects of cannabinoid receptor ligands on LPS-induced pulmonary inflammation in mice. *Life Sciences, 63*, 125–129.

Blanchard, D. K., Newton, C., Klein, T. W., Stewart III, W. E., & Friedman, H. (1986). In vitro and in vivo suppressive effects of delta-9-tetrahydrocannabinol on interferon production by murine spleen cells. *International Journal of Immunopharmacology, 8*, 819–824.

Bouaboula, M., Poinot-Chazel, C., Bourrie, B., Canat, X., Calandra, B., Rinaldi-Carmona, M., Le Fur, G., & Casellas, P. (1995). Activation of mitogen-activated protein kinases by stimulation of the central cannabinoid receptor CB1. *Biochemical Journal, 312*, 637–641.

Bouaboula, M., Rinaldi, M., Carayon, P., Carillon, C., Delpech, B., Shire, D., LeFur, G., & Casellas, P. (1993). Cannabinoid-receptor expression in human leukocytes. *European Journal of Biochemistry, 214*, 173–180.

Burnette-Curley, D., & Cabral, G. A. (1995). Differential inhibition of RAW264.7 macrophage tumoricidal activity by Δ^9-tetrahydrocannabinol. *Proceedings of the Society for Experimental Biology and Medicine, 210*, 64–76.

Burstein, S., Budrow, J., Debatis, M., Hunter, S. A., & Subramanian, A. (1994). Phopholipase participation in cannabinoid-induced release of free arachidonic acid. *Biochemistry and Pharmacology, 48*, 1253–1264.

Cabral, G., & Dove Pettit, D. (1998). Drugs and immunity: Cannabinoids and their role in decreased resistance to infectious diseases. *Journal of Neuroimmunology, 83*, 116–123.

Cabral, G. A., Lockmuller, J. C., & Mishkin, E. M. (1986). Δ^9-tetrahydrocannabinol decreases alpha/beta interferon response to herpes simplex virus type 2 in the B6C3F1 mouse. *Proceedings of the Society for Experimental Biology and Medicine, 181*, 305–311.

Cabral, G. A., & Vasquez, R. (1992). Δ^9-tetrahydrocannabinol suppresses macrophage extrinsic antiherpesvirus activity. *Proceedings of the Society for Experimental Biology and Medicine, 199*, 255–263.

Coffey, R. G., Yamamoto, Y., Snella, E., & Pross, S. (1996). Tetrahydrocannabinol inhibition of macrophage nitric oxide production. *Biochemistry and Pharmacology, 52*, 743–751.

Condie, R., Herring, A., Koh, W. S., Lee, M., & Kaminski, N. E. (1996). Cannabinoid induction of adenylate cyclase-mediated signal transduction and interleukin 2 (IL-2) expression in the murine T-cell line, EL4.IL-2. *Journal of Biological Chemistry, 271*, 13175–13183.

Daaka, Y., Friedman, H., & Klein, T. W. (1996). Cannabinoid receptor proteins are increased in Jurkat, human T-cell line after mitogen activation. *Journal of Pharmacology and Experimental Therapeutics, 76*, 776–783.

Daaka, Y., Klein, T. W., & Friedman, H. (1995). Expression of cannabinoid receptor mRNA in murine and human leukocytes. In B. Sharp, T. K. Eisenstein, J. J. Madden, and H. Friedman (Eds.), *Advances in Experimental Medicine and Biology* (vol. 373, pp. 91–96). New York: Plenum Press.

Daaka, Y., Zhu, W., Friedman, H., & Klein, T. W. (1997). Induction of IL-2 receptor α gene by Δ^9-tetrahydrocannabinol is mediated by nuclear factor κB and CB1 cannabinoid receptor. *DNA Cell Biology, 16*, 301–309.

Dax, E. M., Pilotte, N. S., Adler, W. H., Nagel, J. E., & Lange, W. R. (1989). The effects of 9-ene-tetrahydrocannabinol on hormone release and immune function. *Journal of Steroid Biochemistry, 34*, 263–270.

De Petrocellis, L., Melck, D., Palmisano, A., Bisogno, T., Laezza, C., Bifulco, M., & Di Marzo, V. (1998). The endogenous cannabinoid anandamide inhibits human breast cancer cell proliferation. *Proceedings of the National Academy of Sciences of The United States of America, 95*, 8375–8380.

Derocq, J., Segui, M., Marchand, J., LeFur, G., & Casellas, P. (1995). Cannabinoids enhance human B-cell growth at low nanomolar concentrations. *FEBS Letters, 369*, 177–182.

Derocq, J. M., Bouaboula, M., Marchand, J., Rinaldi-Carmona, M., Segui, M., & Casellas, P. (1998). The endogenous cannabinoid anandamide is a lipid messenger activating cell growth via a cannabinoid receptor-independent pathway in hematopoietic cell lines. *FEBS Letters, 425*, 419–425.

Devane, W. A., Dysarz III, F. A., Johnson, M. R., Melvin, L. S., & Howlett, A. C. (1988). Determination and characterization of a cannabinoid receptor in rat brain. *Molecular Pharmacology, 34*, 605–613.

Devane, W. A., Hanus, L., Breuer, A., Pertwee, R. G., Stevenson, L. A., Griffin, G., Gibson, D., Mandelbaum, A., Etinger, A., & Mechoulam, R. (1992). Isolation and structure of a brain constituent that binds to the cannabinoid receptor. *Science, 258*, 1946–1949.

Diaz, S., Specter, S., & Coffey, R. G. (1993). Suppression of lymphocyte adenosine 3′:5′-cyclic monophosphate (cAMP) by delta-9-tetrahydrocannabinol. *International Journal of Immunopharmacology, 15*, 523–532.

Diaz, S., Specter, S., Vanderhoek, J. Y., & Coffey, R. G. (1994). The effect of delta-9-tetrahydrocannabinol on arachidonic acid metabolism in human peripheral blood mononuclear cells. *Journal of Pharmacology and Experimental Therapeutics, 268*, 1289–1296.

DiMarzo, V., DePetrocellis, L., Sepe, N., & Buono, A. (1996). Biosynthesis of anandamide and related acylethanolamides in mouse J774 macrophages and N18 neuroblastoma cells. *Biochemical Journal, 316*, 977–984.

Dinarello, C. A., & Wolff, S. M. (1993). The role of interleukin-1 in disease. *New England Journal of Medicine, 328*, 106–113.

Felder, C. C., Joyce, K. E., Briley, E. M., Mansouri, J., Mackie, K., Blond, O., Lai, Y., Ma, A. L., & Mitchell, R. L. (1995). Comparison of the pharmacology and signal transduction of the human cannabinoid CB1 and CB2 receptors. *Molecular Pharmacology, 48*, 443–450.

Fischer-Stenger, K., Dove Pettit, D. A., & Cabral, G. A. (1993). Δ^9-tetrahydrocannabinol inhibition of tumor necrosis factor-α: Suppression of post-translational events. *Journal of Pharmacology and Experimental Therapeutics, 267*, 1558–1565.

Friedman, H., Klein, T., & Specter, S. (1991). Immunosuppression by marijuana components. In A. R, F. DL, and C. N (Eds.), *Psychoneuroimmunology* (vol. 2, pp. 931–953). San Diego: Academic Press.

Galieque, S., Mary, S., Marchand, J., Dussossoy, D., Carriere, D., Carayon, P., Bouaboula, M., Shire, D., Le Fur, G., & Casellas, P. (1995). Expression of central and peripheral cannabinoid receptors in human immune tissues and leukocyte subpopulations. *European Journal of Biochemistry, 232*, 54–61.

Garza, H. H., & Carr, D. J. J. (1997). Neuroendocrine peptide receptors on cells of the immune system. *Chemical Immunology, 69*, 132–154.

Gerard, C. M., Mollereau, C., Vassart, G., & Parmentier, M. (1991). Molecular cloning of a human cannabinoid receptor which is also expressed in testis. *Biochemical Journal, 279*, 129–134.

Gether, U., & Kobilka, B. K. (1998). G protein-coupled receptors II. Mechanism of agonist activation. *Journal of Biological Chemistry, 273*, 17979–17982.

Herring, A. C., Koh, W. S., & Kaminski, N. E. (1998). Inhibition of the cyclic AMP signaling cascade and nuclear factor binding to CRE and κB elements by cannabinol, a minimally CNS-active cannabinoid. *Biochemistry and Pharmacology, 55*, 1013–1023.

Howlett, A. C. (1984). Inhibition of neuroblastoma adenylate cyclase by cannabinoid and nantradol compounds. *Life Sciences, 35*, 1803–1810.

Howlett, A. C. (1995). Pharmacology of cannabinoid receptors. *Annual Review of Pharmacology and Toxicology, 35*, 607–634.

Howlett, A. C., Johnson, M. R., Melvin, L. S., & Milne, G. M. (1988). Nonclassical cannabinoid analgetics inhibit adenylate cyclase: Development of a cannabinoid receptor model. *Molecular Pharmacology, 33*, 297–302.

Howlett, A. C., Song, C., Berglund, B. A., Wilken, G. H., & Pigg, J. J. (1998). Characterization of CB1 cannabinoid receptors using receptor peptide fragments and site-directed antibodies. *Molecular Pharmacology, 53*, 504–510.

Huffman, J. W., Yu, S., Showalter, V., Abood, M. E., Wiley, J. L., Compton, D. R., Martin, B. R., Bramblett, R. D., & Reggio, P. H. (1996). Synthesis and pharmacology of a very potent cannabinoid lacking a phenolic hydroxyl with high affinity for the CB2 receptor. *Journal of Medicinal Chemistry, 39*, 3875–3877.

Hunter, S. A., & Burstein, S. H. (1997). Receptor mediation in cannabinoid stimulated arachidonic acid mobilization and anandamide synthesis. *Life Sciences, 60*, 1563–1573.

Jeon, Y. J., Yang, K., Pulaski, J. T., Kaminski, N. E. (1996). Attenuation of inducible nitric oxide synthase gene expression by Δ^9-tetrahydrocannabinol is mediated through the inhibition of nuclear factor- κB/Rel activation. *Molecular Pharmacology, 50*, 334–341.

Ji, T. H., Grossmann, M., & Ji, I. (1998). G protein-coupled receptors I. Diversity of receptor-ligand interactions. *Journal of Biological Chemistry, 273*, 17299–17302.

Joy, J., Watson, S., & Benson, J. (1999). *Institute of medicine report on the medical use of marijuana*. Washington, DC: National Academy Press.

Kaminski, N. (1998). Regulation of the cAMP cascade, gene expression and immune function by cannabinoid receptors. *Journal of Neuroimmunology, 83*, 124–132.

Kaminski, N., Koh, W. S., Yang, K. H., Lee, M., & Kessler, F. K. (1994). Suppression of the humoral immune response by cannabinoids is partially mediated through inhibition of adenylate cyclase by a pertussis toxin-sensitive G-protein coupled mechanism. *Biochemistry and Pharmacology, 48*, 1899–1908.

Kaminski, N. E., Abood, M. E., Kessler, F. K., Martin, B. R., & Schatz, A. R. (1992). Identification of a functionally relevant cannabinoid receptor on mouse spleen cells that is involved in cannabinoid-mediated immune modulation. *Molecular Pharmacology, 42*, 736–742.

Kaslow, R. A., Blackwelder, W. C., Ostrow, D. G., Yerg, D., Palenicek, J., Coulson, A. H., & Valdiserri, R. O. (1989). No evidence for a role of alcohol or other psychoactive drugs in accelerating immunodeficiency in HIV-1 positive individuals: A report from the multicenter AIDS cohort study. *Journal of the American Medical Association, 261*, 3424–3429.

Kaufmann, S. H. E. (1993). Immunity to intracellular bacteria. *Annual Review of Immunology, 11*, 129–163.

Kawakami, Y., Klein, T. W., Newton, C., McCarthy, C. A., Djeu, J., Dennert, G., Specter, S., & Friedman, H. (1988). Suppression by cannabinoids of a cloned cell line with natural killer cell activity. *Proceedings of the Society for Experimental Biology and Medicine, 187*, 355–359.

Klein, T., Friedman, H., & Specter, S. (1998). Marijuana, immunity and infection. *Journal of Neuroimmunology, 83*, 102–115.

Klein, T., Newton, C., & Friedman, H. (1998). Cannabinoid receptors and immunity. *Immunology Today, 19*, 373–381.

Klein, T. W., & Friedman, H. (1990). Modulation of murine immune cell function by marijuana components. In R. Watson (Ed.), *Drugs of abuse and immune function* (pp. 87–111). Boca Raton, FL: CRC Press.

Klein, T. W., Kawakami, Y., Newton, C., & Friedman, H. (1991). Marijuana components suppress induction and cytolytic function of murine cytotoxic T cells in vitro and in vivo. *Journal of Toxicology and Environmental Health, 32*, 465–477.

Klein, T. W., Newton, C., Widen, R., & Friedman, H. (1993). Δ^9-tetrahydrocannabinol injection induces cytokine-mediated mortality of mice infected with *Legionella pneumophila*. *Journal of Pharmacology and Experimental Therapeutics, 267*, 635–640.

Klein, T. W., Newton, C., Zhu, W., Daaka, Y., & Friedman, H. (1995). Minireview: Δ^9-tetrahydrocannabinol, cytokines and immunity to *Legionella pneumophila*. *Proceedings of the Society for Experimental Biology and Medicine, 209*, 205–212.

Klein, T. W., Newton, C. A., Widen, R., & Friedman, H. (1985). The effect of delta-9-tetrahydrocannabinol and 11-hydroxy-delta-9-tetrahydrocannabinol on T lymphocyte and B lymphocyte mitogen responses. *Journal of Immunopharmacology, 7*, 451–466.

Lee, M., Yang, K. H., & Kaminski, N. E. (1995). Effects of putative cannabinoid receptor ligands, anandamide and 2-arachidonyl-glycerol, on immune function in B6C3F1 mouse splenocytes. *Journal of Pharmacology and Experimental Therapeutics, 275*, 529–536.

Luo, Y. D., Patel, M. K., Wiederhold, M. D., & Ou, D. W. (1992). Effects of cannabinoids and cocaine on the mitogen-induced transformations of lymphocytes of human and mouse origins. *International Journal of Immunopharmacology, 14*, 49–56.

Lyman, W. D., Sonett, J. R., Brosnan, C. F., Elkin, R., & Bornstein, M. B. (1989). Δ^9-tetrahydrocannabinol: a novel treatment for experimental autoimmune encephalomyelitis. *Journal of Neuroimmunology, 23*, 73–81.

Lynn, A. B., & Herkenham, M. (1994). Localization of cannabinoid receptors and nonsaturable high-density cannabinoid binding sites in peripheral tissues of the rat: Implications for receptor-mediated immune modulation in cannabinoids. *Journal of Pharmacology and Experimental Therapeutics, 268*, 1612–1623.

MacPhee, I. A. M., Antoni, F. A., & Mason, D. D. (1989). Spontaneous recovery of rats from experimental allergic encephalomyelitis is dependent on regulation of the immune system by endogenous adrenal corticosteroid. *Journal of Experimental Medicine, 169*, 431–445.

Matsuda, L. A., Lolait, S. J., Brownstein, M. J., Young, A. C., & Bonner, T. I. (1990). Structure of cannabinoid receptor and functional expression of the cloned cDNA. *Nature, 346*, 561–564.

Mechoulam, R., Ben-Shabat, S., Hanus, L., Ligumsky, M., Kaminski, N. E., Schatz, A. R., Gopher, A., Almog, S., Martin, B. R., Compton, D. R., Pertwee, R. G., Griffin, G., Bayewitch, M., Barg, J., & Vogel, Z. (1995). Identification of an endogenous 2-monoglyceride, present in canine gut, that binds to cannabinoid receptors. *Biochemistry and Pharmacology, 50*, 83–90.

Mechoulam, R., Hanus, L., & Martin, B. R. (1994). Search for endogenous ligands of the cannabinoid receptor. *Biochemistry and Pharmacology, 48*, 1537–1544.

Mechoulam, R., Vogel, Z., & Barg, J. (1994). CNS cannabinoid receptors: Role and therapeutic implications for CNS disorders. *CNS Drugs, 2*, 255–260.

Molina-Holgado, F., Molina-Holgado, E., & Guaza, C. (1998). The endogenous cannabinoid anandamide potentiates interleukin-6 production by astrocytes infected with Theiler's murine encephalomyelitis virus by a receptor-mediated pathway. *FEBS Letters, 433*, 139–142.

Moncada, S., Palmer, M., & Higgs, E. A. (1991). Nitric oxide: Physiology, pathophysiology, and pharmacology. *Pharmacology Reviews, 43*, 109–142.

Munro, S., Thomas, K. L., & Abu-Shaar, M. (1993). Molecular characterization of a peripheral receptor for cannabinoids. *Nature, 365*, 61–65.

Nakano, Y., Pross, S. H., & Friedman, H. (1992). Modulation of interleukin 2 activity by Δ^9-tetrahydrocannabinol after stimulation with concanavalin A, phytohemagglutinin, or anti-CD3 antibody. *Proceedings of the Society for Experimental Biology and Medicine, 201*, 165–168.

Newton, C. A., Klein, T. W., & Friedman, H. (1994). Secondary immunity to *Legionella pneumophila* and Th1 activity are suppressed by delta- 9-tetrahydrocannabinol injection. *Infection and Immunity, 62*, 4015–4020.

O'Garra, A. (1998). Cytokines induce the development of functionally heterogeneous T helper cell subsets. *Immunity, 8*, 275–283.

Pennisi, E. (1997). Tracing molecules that make the brain-body connection. *Science, 275*, 930–931.

Rhee, M. H., Bayewitch, M., Avidor-Reiss, T., Levy, R., & Vogel, Z. (1998). Cannabinoid receptor activation differentially regulates the various adenylyl cyclase isozymes. *Journal of Neurochemistry, 71*, 1525–1534.

Rinaldi-Carmona, M., Barth, F., Heaulme, M., Shire, D., Calandra, B., Congy, C., Martinez, S., Maruani, J., Neliat, G., Caput, D., Ferrara, P., Soubrie, P., Breliere, J. C., & LeFur, G. (1994). SR141716A, a potent and selective antagonist of the brain cannabinoid receptor. *FEBS Letters, 350*, 240–244.

Schatz, A. R., Kessler, F. K., & Kaminski, N. E. (1992). Inhibition of adenylate cyclase by Δ^9-tetrahydrocannabinol in mouse spleen cells: A potential mechanism for cannabinoid-mediated immunosuppression. *Life Sciences, 51*, PL 25–30.

Schatz, A. R., Koh, W. S., & Kaminski, N. E. (1993). Δ^9-tetrahydrocannabinol selectively inhibits T-cell dependent humoral immune responses through direct inhibition of accessory T-cell function. *Immunopharmacology, 26*, 129–137.

Schatz, A. R., Lee, M., Condie, R. B., Pulaski, J. T., & Kaminski, N. E. (1997). Cannabinoid receptors CB1 and CB2: A characterization of expression and adenylate cyclase modulation within the immune system. *Toxicology and Applied Pharmacology, 142*, 278–287.

Shire, D., Calandra, B., Delpech, M., Dumont, X., Kaghad, M., Le Fur, G., Caput, D., & Ferrara, P. (1996). Structural features of the central cannabinoid CB1 receptor involved in the binding of the specific CB1 antagonist SR 141716A. *Journal of Biological Chemistry, 271*, 6941–6946.

Shohami, E., Gallily, R., Mechoulam, R., Bass, R., & Ben-Hur, T. (1997). Cytokine production in the brain following closed head injury: Dexanabinol (HU-211) is a novel TNF-alpha inhibitor and an effective neuroprotectant. *Journal of Neuroimmunology, 72*, 169–177.

Sidney, S., Beck, J. E., Tekawa, I. S., Quesenberry, C. P., & Friedmen, G. D. (1997). Marijuana use and mortality. *American Journal of Public Health, 87*, 585–590.

Sinha, D., Bonner, T. I., Bhat, N. R., & Matsuda, L. A. (1998). Expression of the CB1 cannabinoid receptor in macrophage-like cells from brain tissue: Immunochemical characterization by fusion protein antibodies. *Journal of Neuroimmunology, 82*, 13–21.

Slipetz, D. M., O'Neill, G. P., Favreau, L., Dufresne, C., Gallant, M., Gareau, Y., Guay, D., Labelle, M., & Metters, K. M. (1995). Activation of the human peripheral cannabinoid receptor results in inhibition of adenylyl cyclase. *Molecular Pharmacology, 48*, 352–361.

Smith, M. S., Yamamoto, Y., Newton, C. A., Friedman, H., & Klein, T. W. (in press). Psychoactive cannabinoids increase mortality and alter acute phase cytokine responses in mice sublethally infected with *Legionella pneumophila. Proceedings of the Society for Experimental Biology and Medicine.*

Song, Z.-H., & Bonner, T. I. (1996). A lysine residue of the cannabinoid receptor is critical for receptor recognition by several agonists but not WIN55212-2. *Molecular Pharmacology, 49*, 891–896.

Sulcova, E., Mechoulam, R., & Fride, E. (1998). Biphasic effects of anandamide. *Pharmacology, Biochemistry and Behavior, 59*, 347–352.

Tao, Q., & Abood, M. E. (1998). Mutation of a highly conserved aspartate residue in the second transmembrane domain of the cannabinoid receptors, CB1 and CB2, disrupts G-protein coupling. *Journal of Pharmacology and Experimental Therapeutics, 285*, 651–658.

Thomas, B. F., Gilliam, A. F., Burch, D. F., Roche, M. J., & Seltzman, H. H. (1998). Comparative receptor binding analyses of cannabinoid agonists and antagonists. *Journal of Pharmacology and Experimental Therapeutics, 285*, 285–292.

Titishov, N., Mechoulam, R., & Zimmerman, A. M. (1989). Stereospecific effects of (−)- and (+)-7-hydroxy -delta-6-tetrahydrocannabinol-dimethylheptyl on the immune system of mice. *Pharmacology, 39*, 337–349.

Valk, P., Verbakel, S., Vankan, Y., Hol, S., Mancham, S., Ploemacher, R., Mayen, A., Lowenberg, B., & Delwel, R. (1997). Anandamide, a natural ligand for the peripheral cannabinoid receptor is a novel synergistic growth factor for hematopoietic cells. *Blood, 90,* 1448–1457.

Warner, J. F., & Dennert, G. (1982). Effect of a clonal cell line with NK activity on bone marrow transplants, tumor development and metastasis in vivo. *Nature* (Lond.), *300,* 31–34.

Watzl, B., Scuder, P., & Watson, R. R. (1991). Marijuana components stimulate human peripheral blood mononuclear cell secretion of interferon-gamma and suppress interleukin-1 alpha in vitro. *International Journal of Immunopharmacology, 13,* 1091–1097.

Weidenfeld, J., Feldman, S., & Mechoulam, R. (1994). Effect of brain constituent anandamide, a cannabinoid receptor agonist, on the hypothalamo-pituitary-adrenal axis in the rat. *Neuroendocrinology, 59,* 110–112.

Wirguin, I., Mechoulam, R., Breuer, A., Schezen, E., Weidenfeld, J., & Brenner, T. (1994). Suppression of experimental autoimmune encephalomyelitis by cannabinoids. *Immunopharmacology, 28,* 209–214.

Yebra, M., Klein, T. W., & Friedman, H. (1992). Δ^9-tetrahydrocannabinol suppresses concanavalin A induced increase in cytoplasmic free calcium in mouse thymocytes. *Life Sciences, 51,* 151–160.

Zheng, Z.-M., Specter, S., & Friedman, H. (1992). Inhibition by delta-9-tetrahydrocannabinol of tumor necrosis factor alpha production by mouse and human macrophages. *International Journal of Immunopharmacology, 14,* 1445–1452.

Zhu, W., Friedman, H., & Klein, T. W. (1998). Δ^9-tetrahydrocannabinol induces apoptosis in macrophages and lymphocytes: Involvement of Bcl-2 and caspase-1. *Journal of Pharmacology and Experimental Therapeutics, 286,* 1103–1109.

Zhu, W., Igarashi, T., Friedman, H., & Klein, T. W. (1995). Δ^9-Tetrahydrocannabinol (THC) causes the variable expression of IL2 receptor subunits. *Journal of Pharmacology and Experimental Therapeutics, 274,* 1001–1007.

Zhu, W., Igarashi, T., Qi, Z.-T., Newton, C., Widen, R. E., Friedman, H., & Klein, T. W. (1993). Delta-9-tetrahydrocannabinol (THC) decreases the number of high and intermediate affinity IL-2 receptors of the IL-2 dependent cell line NKB61A2. *International Journal of Immunopharmacology, 15,* 401–408.

Zhu, W., Newton, C., Daaka, Y., Friedman, H., & Klein, T. W. (1994). Δ^9-Tetrahydrocannabinol enhances the secretion of interleukin 1 from endotoxin-stimulated macrophages. *Journal of Pharmacology and Experimental Therapeutics, 270,* 1334–1339.

CHAPTER

16

Melatonin and Immune Function

GEORGES J. M. MAESTRONI

I. THE HORMONE OF DARKNESS

Melatonin (MLT), or N-acetyl-5-methoxytryptamine, is mainly secreted by the pineal gland into the blood circulation in most species studied. In the human brain, the pineal gland is located between the two cerebral hemispheres and in front of the cerebellum at the posterodorsal area of the diencephalon. A substance from pineal extracts that lightened the skin melanocytes of amphibians and fish was isolated in 1958 and called MLT (Lerner, Case, Takahashi, Lee, & Mori, 1958). In both diurnal and nocturnal species, the absence of light at night stimulates MLT biosynthesis. Electrical signals originating from the retina reach the suprachiasmatic nuclei, which, in turn, send inputs via the paraventricular nuclei to the spinal cord and then to the superior cervical ganglia of the sympathetic nervous system. The fibers terminate at the level of pinealocytes (Yu & Reiter, 1993). Absence of light results in an increased norepinephrine release and activation of $\alpha 1$ and β-adrenergic receptors on the pinealocyte. This triggers a series of intracellular responses resulting in activation of the enzymes N-acetyltransferase (EC 2.3.1.87), and hydroxyindole-O-methyl transferase (EC 2.1.1.4), which convert serotonin into MLT (Yu & Reiter, 1993). The circadian nocturnal release of MLT has a profound influence on the internal environment of the organism, with diverse physiological effects. Its main function seems to be that of synchronizing the organism in the photoperiod and may play a role in reproduction, metabolism, seasonality, thermoregulation, immunity, and possibly aging. MLT also has been pathophysiologically associated with cancer, sleep disorders, epilepsy, seasonal affective disorders, and ocular diseases (Feychting, Osterlund, & Ahlbom, 1998; Yu, Tsin, & Reiter, 1993).

II. MLT RECEPTORS

MLT effects seem mediated by specific high-affinity receptors on the plasma membrane and coupled to GTP-binding proteins. Two different G proteins coupled to MLT receptors have been described, one sensitive to pertussis toxin and the other sensitive to cholera toxin. Based on their molecular structure, three subtypes of receptors have been described: mt1 and mt2 in mammals and Mel1C in nonmammals (Reppert & Weaver, 1995; Vanecek, 1998). As far as concerns MLT receptors in immunocompetent cells, high affinity binding sites for MLT have been described in membrane homogenates of thymus, bursa of Fabricius, and spleen of a number of birds and mammals (Poon, Liu, Pang, Brown, & Pang, 1994). We have described a high-affinity binding site in bone marrow Th cells (Maestroni, 1995). Another study showed that MLT binds to human lymphoid cells modulating their proliferative response. Consistent with the finding that activated cells seem to be more responsive to MLT (Maestroni & Conti, 1990), T cell activation significantly increased MLT binding (Konakchieva, Kyurkchiev, Kehayov, Taushanova, & Kanchev, 1995). MLT binding sites and MLT receptor mRNA was mostly found in human Th cells, but also in CD8+ T and B cells (Garcia-Mauriño et al., 1997; Garcia-Perganeda, Pozo, Guerrero, & Calvo, 1997; Guerrero et al., 1996). Furthermore, human monocytes express MLT receptors depending on their state of maturation. Most interesting, it appears that in vitro monocyte differentiation negatively affects MLT receptor expression (Barjavel, Mamdouh, Raghbate, & Bakouche, 1998). Besides membrane receptors, nuclear receptors for MLT have been described in human and murine immunocompetent cells. Specific binding of MLT has been described in purified cell nuclei from spleen and thymus of the rat (Rafii-El-Idrissi, Calvo, Harmouch, Garcia-Maurino, & Guerrero, 1998). MLT seems to be the natural ligand for nuclear orphan receptors RZR/ROR. It appears that MLT down-regulates the expression of the RZR/ROR responsing gene, 5-lipoxygenase, a key enzyme in allergic and inflammatory disease (Carlberg & Wiesenberg, 1995). Most recently, it has been reported that the effect of MLT on cytokine production in human peripheral blood mononuclear cells seems to depend on activation of nuclear receptors rather than membrane receptors (Garcia-Maurino, Gonzales-Haba, Calvo, Goberna, & Guerrero, 1998). However, the specific and relative role of membrane and nuclear receptors is still obscure.

III. MLT AND CYTOKINES

Interleukin-2 (IL-2), interferon-gamma (IFN-γ), and opioid peptides released by activated Th cells seem to mediate, at least in part, the immunopharmacological action of MLT (Caroleo, Frasca, Nistico, & Doria, 1992; Colombo, Chen, Lopez, & Watson, 1992; Del Gobbo, Libri, Villani, Caliò, & Nistico, 1989; Garcia-Mauriño et al., 1997; Hofbauer & Heufelder, 1996; Maestroni & Conti, 1990; Pioli, Caroleo, Nistico, & Doria, 1993). Physiologically, the nocturnal MLT peak has been associated with high IFN-γ/IL-10 ratio, i.e., the MLT rhythm positively correlated with the rhythmicity of T-helper cell type 1/T-helper cell type 2 ratio (Petrovsky & Harrison, 1996). This implies that the nature of an immune response, for example, to vaccination, may be modified by the time of the day of antigen presentation, or be therapeutically manipulated by administration of MLT. Figure 1 (A & B) shows the effect of MLT on cytokine production in human mixed lymphocyte cultures: IL-2, IFN-γ, and IL-6 but not IL-4 production was stimulated by MLT at physiological concentration (10^{-9} M), (Garcia-Mauriño et al., 1997). Although MLT also seems to activate human monocytes and stimulate IL-1, IL-6, and IL-12 production (Garcia-Mauriño et al., 1997; Lissoni et al., 1997a; Morrey, McLachlan, Serkin, & Bakouche, 1994), T lymphocytes seem to be the main target of MLT in mice (Hofbauer & Heufelder 1996; Maestroni & Conti, 1990) and humans (Garcia-Mauriño et al., 1997; Guerrero et al., 1996). We have reported that the immunoenhancing and antistress effect of MLT is neutralized by the opioid antagonist naltrexone (Maestroni & Conti, 1990; 1991). Known opioid peptides could mimic the effects of MLT, with the kappa-agonist dynorphin being the most potent agent (Maestroni & Conti, 1989). Consistently, the hematopoietic protection involved the release of a Th cell factor constituted by two cytokines of 15 and 67 kDa MW with the common opioid sequence (Tyr-Gly-Gly-Phe) at their amino terminal and a carboxy-terminal extension, which resemble both IL-4 and dynorphin (Figure 2), (Maestroni, Hertens, Galli, Conti, & Pedrinis, 1996). Both activated lymph nodes Th cells and bone marrow Th cells released these opioid cytokines, which were named MLT-induced opioids, or MIO (Maestroni et al., 1996). Due to their size and unusual immunological characterization, the MIO might represent novel opioid cytokines. The lower molecular weight MIO (MIO-15) seems to mediate both the antistress and hematopoietic effects of MLT (Maestroni et al., 1996). Our data may reflect a physiological requirement for sustained MLT regulation of hematopoiesis.

IV. MLT AND NITRIC OXIDE IN SEPTIC SHOCK

Septic shock is characterized by hypotension, hyporeactivity to vasoconstrictor agents, inadequate tissue perfusion, vascular damage, and disseminated intravascular coagulation leading to multiple organ failure and death (Barron, 1993). Many of the pathological consequences of gram-negative shock are attributable to the bacterial membrane component lipopolysaccharide (LPS). Recent studies have linked the production of nitric oxide (NO) to LPS-induced hypotension, vascular hyporesponsiveness, and death, suggesting that excessive generation of NO plays an important role in septic shock (Beasley & Eldridge, 1994; Cunha et al., 1994). NO is generated from the oxidation of the terminal guanidino nitrogen

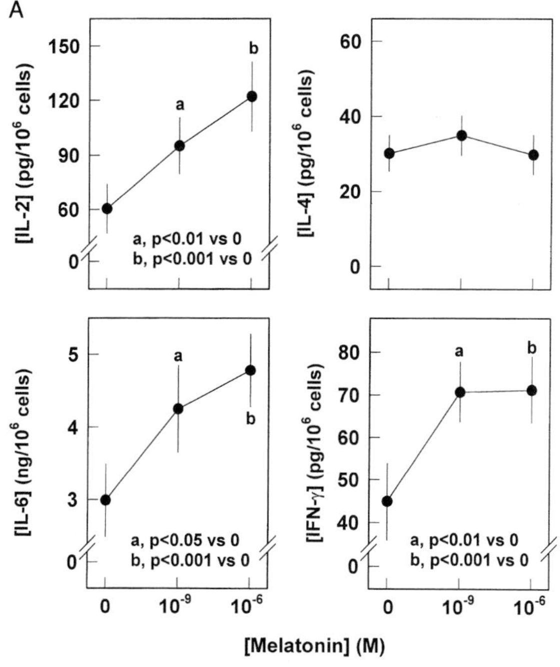

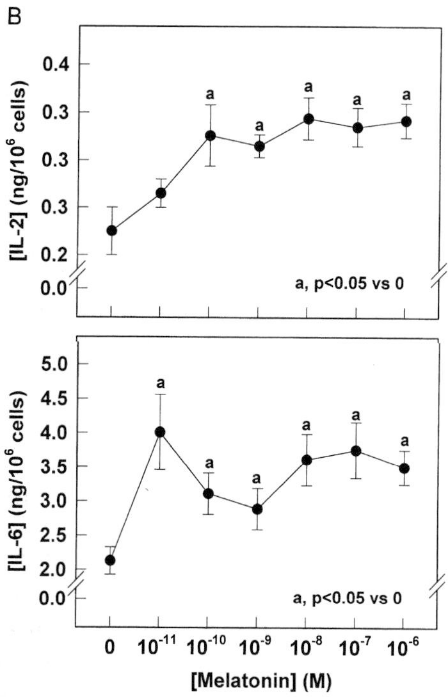

FIGURE 1 Effect of MLT on cytokine production by human PBMCs activated with irradiated allogeneic PBMCs (A) and dose response curve of the effect of MLT on IL-2 and IL-6 production in the same model (B). Cells were incubated for 72 h in the presence of irradiated PBMCs (0.5×10^6 cells/mL) and the indicated concentrations of MLT. At the end of the incubation period, the cell-free supernatants were used for cytokine determinations. Data are means ± SEM of 9 unrelated donors measured in triplicate. (From Garcia-Maurino et al., *Journal of Immunology*, 1997, 159:574–581, with permission. Copyright © 1997 The American Association of Immunologists.)

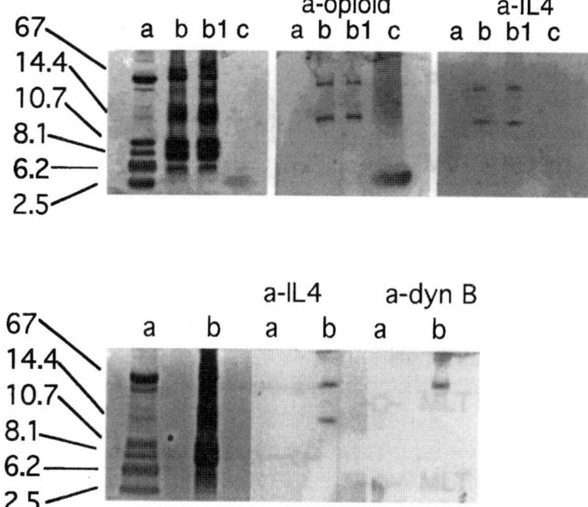

FIGURE 2 SDS-PAGE and immunoblotting of MIO. a: molecular weight markers; n,b1: supernatants from nonadherent bone marrow cells incubated with melatonin; c: β-endorphin; a-opioid: anti-Tyr-Gly-Gly-Phe amino terminal common opioid sequence; a-IL-4: anti-IL-4 mAb; a-dyn B: antidynophin B Ab. (From Maestroni et al., *Journal of Pineal Research*, 1996, 21: 131–139, with permission. Copyright © 1996 Munksgaard International Publishers Ltd. Copenhagen, Denmark.)

atom of L-arginine by NO synthase, of which an inducible type and a constitutive type have been identified (Hibbs et al., 1991). Antitumor necrosis factor-α and anti-IL-1-β antibodies markedly reduced LPS-induced shock and NO synthesis in vivo (Cunha et al., 1994). Other studies indicate, however, that at least part of the inflammatory response including NO synthesis might be beneficial in septic shock (Evans, Carpenter, Silva, & Cohen, 1994; Florquin, Amraoui, Dubois, Decuyper, & Goldman, 1994). As a matter of fact, septic shock is a major cause of death among patients in intensive care units and ranks high in the overall causes of death.

On this basis and taking in consideration the ability of MLT to affect cytokine production, we studied whether MLT could influence the pathophysiology of septic shock. We investigated the effect of MLT on survival of mice inoculated with a lethal dose of LPS. MLT was injected at various doses and at different times after LPS administration. MLT injected subcutaneously immediately after LPS at doses ranging from 1 to 10 mg/kg body weight improved the survival of mice, with a bell shaped dose-response curve (Figure 3). When injected 3 or 6 h after LPS administration, MLT was most effective. At 2 mg/kg body weight the percentage of mice that were protected ranged from 0% when MLT was injected

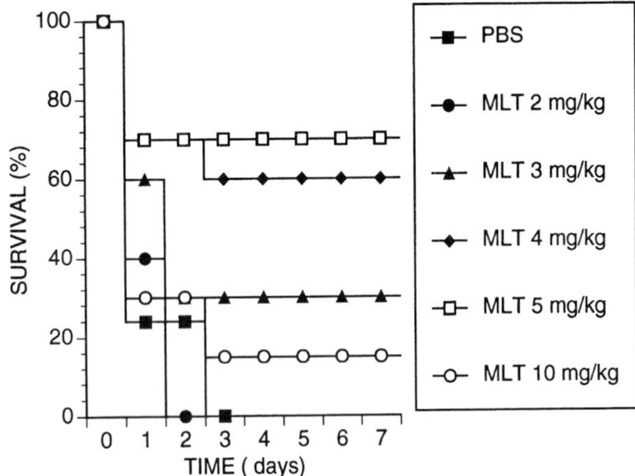

FIGURE 3 Dose-response curve of the protective effect of MLT in mice injected with a lethal dose of LPS: LPS (0127:B8, 25 mg/Kg body weight) was injected i.p. at 12 h, and MLT at the reported doses was injected s.c. just after LPS. Control mice were injected with phosphate buffered saline (PBS).

just after LPS, to 48 and 86% ($p = 0.0001$) when MLT was injected 3 and 6 h later, respectively (Maestroni, 1996). This effect apparently did not involve Th cells or inhibition of inflammatory cytokines. Nevertheless, plasma nitrate concentration, which reflects the rate of NO synthesis, showed a significant reduction at 18 and 24 h after LPS administration (Figure 4), (Maestroni, 1996). Consistent with our results, it recently has been reported that MLT inhibits expression of the inducible isoform of NO synthase in murine macrophages via inhibition of the transcription factor NFκB (Gilad et al., 1998). On the other hand, MLT has been reported to decrease NO synthase in rat cerebellum (Pozo, Reiter, Calvo, & Guerrero, 1994). These findings, together with the important clinical observation that MLT administration in cancer patients may counteract the severe hypotension that is a dose-limiting side effect of IL-2 therapy (Lissoni et al., 1990, 1992), directly support the use of MLT in septic shock. In fact, except for surgical and supportive care, no specific therapy is known. Unfortunately, selected new therapies for septic shock to inhibit bacterial toxins or endogenous mediators of inflammation have not shown any clinical efficacy. The strategy of breaking the inflammatory cytokine cascade may not be beneficial because immune cells and cytokines play both pathogenic and protective roles (Natanson, Hoffman, Suffredini, Eichacker, & Danner, 1994). The failure of MLT to inhibit inflammatory cytokines may thus be of further benefit in bacterial sepsis.

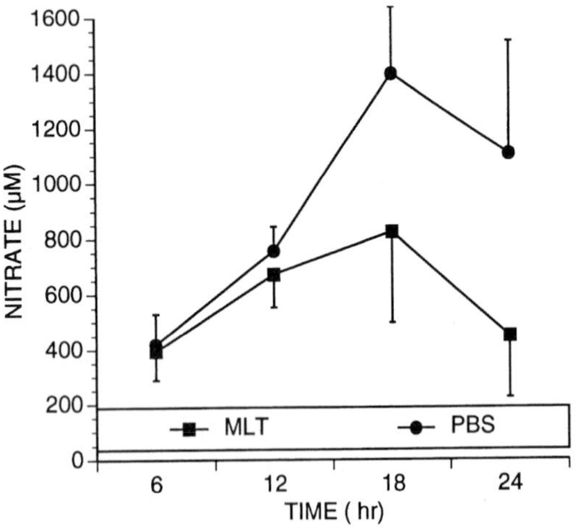

FIGURE 4 Effect of MLT on plasma nitrate concentration in LPS-injected mice. A sublethal dose of LPS (10 mg/Kg) was injected i.p. at 12 h, and MLT (5 mg/Kg) was injected s.c. 5 h later in normal C57BL/6 mice. The mice were bled at 6, 12, 18, and 24 h after LPS injection. The experiments were devised so that a mouse was bled (100–200 µL of blood) 6 and 18 h or at 12 and 24 h. The values represent the mean ± standard deviation of four experiments with 5 mice per group. a: $p < 0.005$; b :$p < 0.001$ analysis of variance. PBS = phosphate buffered saline.

V. MLT AND IMMUNE RESPONSE

Precocious involution and histological disorganization of the thymus due to putative changes in gonadal hormones was the effect of pinealectomy reported by most early studies (Barath & Csaba, 1974; Csaba & Barath, 1975; Csaba, Bodocky, Fischer, & Acs, 1965; Vaughan & Reiter, 1971). In 1981 we provided the first evidence of a possible involvement of endogenous MLT on humoral and T cell immune reactions, as well as on spleen and thymus cellularity in mice (Maestroni, Conti, & Pierpaoli, 1986; Maestroni and Pierpaoli, 1981). In another report, we showed that pinealectomy inhibits leukemogenesis in a radiation leukemia virus murine model, and that MLT has a promoting effect on the disease (Conti, Haran-Ghera, & Maestroni, 1992). Subsequently, a number of other authors further explored the effect of pinealectomy on the immune system (Becker et al., 1988; Champney & McMurray, 1991; Del Gobbo et al., 1989; Palermo, Vermeulen, & Giordano, 1994). Endogenous MLT also has been reported to influence the concentration of bone marrow granulocyte-macrophage colony-forming unity (GM-CFU) (Haldar, Haussler, & Gupta, 1992). From the pharmacological point of view, MLT can augment the immune response and correct immunodeficiency states that may follow acute stress, viral diseases, or drug treatment (Maestroni, 1993; Maestroni & Conti, 1989, 1990, 1993; Maestroni et al., 1986; Maestroni, Conti, & Pierpaoli, 1987; Maestroni, Covacci, & Conti, 1994b). This finding has been confirmed and extended, either in mice or in humans, to a variety of immune parameters (Caroleo et al., 1992; Champney & McMurray, 1991; Del Gobbo et al., 1989; Giordano & Palermo, 1991; Lissoni et al., 1992; Morrey, McLachlan, Serkin, & Bakouche, 1994; Palermo et al., 1994; Pioli et al., 1993). Similarly, a very significant biological effect of MLT is the protection of mice against encephalitis viruses and lethal bacterial infections (Ben-Nathan, Maestroni, & Conti, 1995, 1997; Bonilla, Valerofuenmajor, Pons, & Chacin-Bonilla, 1997). In general, the immunoenhancing action of MLT seems restricted to T-dependent antigens and to be most pronounced in immunodepressed situations. For example, MLT may completely counteract thymus involution and the immunological depression induced by stress events or glucocorticoid treatment (Maestroni & Conti, 1990). MLT is active only when injected in the afternoon or in the evening, i.e., with a schedule consonant with its physiological rhythm (Maestroni et al., 1986, 1987). In addition, MLT seems most active on antigen- or cytokine-activated immunocompetent cells (Maestroni et al., 1986, 1987). Consistently with these requirements, a recent report shows that MLT may also restore depressed immunological functions after soft-tissue trauma and hemorrhagic shock (Wichmann, Zellweger, DeMaso, Ayala, & Chaudry, 1996a). Beside acquired immunity, natural immune parameters also seem influenced by MLT (Angeli, Gatti, Sartori, Del Ponte, & Cerignola, 1988; Del Gobbo et al., 1989; Lewinsky, Zelazowsky, Sewerynek, Zerek-Melen, and Szudlinsky, 1989).

VI. MLT IN ONCOLOGY

An interesting finding, which might be associated with, and/or explained by, the immunoenhancing action of MLT, is the widely documented oncostatic role of the pineal gland and of MLT (Blask, 1993). In a tumor model of established lung metastases, we found that MLT could synergize with the anticancer effect of IL-2 (Figure 5). Based on these observations, over 200 advanced solid tumor patients for whom the standard anti-cancer chemotherapy was either not tolerated or ineffective, were treated with IL-2 and MLT. The results obtained show that this neuroimmunotherapeutic strategy may amplify the antitumoral activity of low dose IL-2; induce objective tumor regression; prolong progression-free time and overall survival; and, is a very well-tolerated treatment. It should be stressed that MLT seems to be required for the effectiveness of low dose IL-2 in those neoplasias that are generally resistant to IL-2 alone

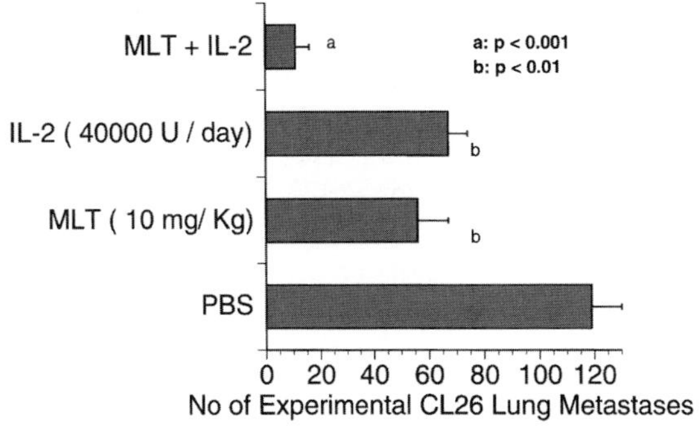

FIGURE 5 Effect of a combined MLT + IL-2 immunotherapy on established lung metastases in mice. Balb/c mice were injected i.v. with 105 CL26 cells on Day 0. Starting on Day 3 and for 15 consecutive days the mice were treated either with IL-2, MLT, or with both. IL-2 was injected i.p. twice a day at 8 and 16 h, whereas MLT was injected s.c. at 16 h only. The values represent the mean ± the standard deviation of three experiments with 5 mice/group.

(reviewed in Conti & Maestroni, 1995). Similar findings were obtained in other studies in which MLT was combined with IFN-γ in metastatic renal cell carcinoma (Neri et al., 1994, 1998). In addition, MLT in combination with low-dose IL-2 neutralized surgery-induced lymphocytopenia in cancer patients (Lissoni et al., 1995).

In another series of studies, we reported that MLT may rescue hematopoiesis in mice transplanted with Lewis lung carcinoma (LLC) and treated with cancer chemotherapeutic compounds (Table I, Maestroni et al., 1994). This effect apparently involved the endogenous release of granulocyte-macrophage colony-stimulating factor (GM-CSF) (Maestroni, Conti, & Lissoni, 1994; Maestroni, Covacci, et al., 1994). Interestingly, a recent report confirms the protective effect of MLT in rats treated with cytotoxic drugs (Anwar, Mahfouz, & Sayed, 1998). In contrast, a clinical-double blind study investigating the myeloprotective effect of MLT given in combination with carboplatin and etoposide to advanced lung cancer patients shows that MLT did not influence the chemotherapy-induced hematopoietic toxicity [Ghielmini, submitted].

To study the mechanisms underlying these surprising hematopoietic effects of MLT, we compared the ability of MLT to protect hematopoiesis in LLC-bearing mice and in tumor-free normal mice treated with the cytotoxic drug cyclophosphamide. This experiment was suggested by the fact that MLT added in GM-CFU cultures could directly enhance the number of GM-CFU but only in presence of a suboptimal concentration of GM-CSF, and bone marrow adherent cells. (Maestroni, Conti, et al., 1994; Maestroni, Covacci, et al., 1994) In addition,

TABLE I Effect of Melatonin and Cancer Chemotherapy Agents in LLC-Bearing Mice

Groups (n)	Leukocytes / μL	Platelets / μL (×10³)	GM-CFU / Femur	Primary tumor (cm²)	No. of metastases
Control (10)	10300±1070	253±69.5	8459±1674	—	—
PBS (64)	17128±3264***	300±79.6	10303±2907	4.09±0.87	16.8±6.7
ME (46)	12960±2667	287±74.4	9835±4067	3.97±0.73	12.8±5.2
CY160 (10)	5650±980	161±43.3	2471±490	0	0
CY160 + ME (12)	11083±2882*	316±59.7*	5927±1898**	0	0
CY40 (20)	8310±1343	209±45.7	6569±1791	2.8±0.88	3.95±1.47
CY40 + ME (20)	16875±2754*	344±51.9*	12644±2479**	2.9±1.48	4.3±4.4
ET40 (14)	8943±251	149±23.8	4089±1528	1.65±0.76	1.4±1.4
ET40 + ME (14)	10912±1352*	316±77*	6459±2826***	1.23±0.87	1±0.9
ET20 (22)	8673±1184	238±44.4	3916±1343	2.56±0.6	3.09±2.2
ET20 + ME (27)	13215±2845***	272±44.8	8052±3407***	2.44±1.25	2.8±2.5

Note: Cyclophosphamide (CY) and etoposide were injected at the doses indicated (mg/kg b.w.) in C57 BL/6 mice from Day 8 through Day 12 after LLC transplantation. Melatonin (ME) was injected from Day 8 throughout the experiments. The values represent the mean ± the standard deviation. Leukocytes and platelets were evaluated 16 days after tumor transplantation, whereas the remaining parameters were measured at the end of the experiments (Days 20–22). Control: normal healthy mice; PBS: phosphate saline. (From Maestroni et al., *Cancer Research*, 1994, 54: 2429–2432, with permission).

*: $p < 0.001$;

**: $p < 0.005$;

***: $p < 0.01$.

LLC is known to produce GM-CSF and exert myelopoietic activity in vivo (Young, Young, & Kim, 1988). MLT did not exert any hematopoietic protection in tumor-free mice but rather increased the bone marrow toxicity of cyclophosphamide (Maestroni, 1998). However, both in tumor-free and LLC-bearing mice, the effect of MLT was neutralized by naltrexone, which suggested the involvement of MIO. The MIO and/or the known κ-opioid agonist dynorphin A were found to be acting on a single κ1-opioid binding site present in adherent bone marrow cells. In fact, antisense oligodeoxynucleotide to κ-opioid receptor could neutralize the colony stimulating activity of dynorphin A (Figure 6). Activation of these opioid receptors possibly results in IL-1 release (Maestroni, Zammaretti, κ Pedrinis, 1999).

VII. CONCLUSION AND PERSPECTIVES

MLT binds to specific MLT receptors in Th cells and/or monocytes stimulating the production of IFN-γ, IL-2, MIO, IL-1, IL-6, and IL-12, which in turn up-regulate the immune response. Second messengers are not completely understood but include G-protein and inhibition of cAMP (Guerrero et al., 1996). The important immunotherapeutic effect of MLT against encephalitis viruses or bacterial infections (Ben-Nathan et al., 1995, 1997; Bonilla et al., 1997) might be explained by the increased production of IL-1, IL-12, IFN-γ and/or IL-2, as well as by an increased myelopoiesis due to the hematopoietic action of the MIO. A mechanism involving Th type 1 cytokines might also account for the capacity of MLT to restore immunodeficiency states secondary to aging (Caroleo et al., 1992; Pioli et al., 1993), trauma-hemorrhage (Wichmann, Zellweger, et al., 1996; Wichmann, Haisken, Ayala, & Chaudry, 1996), or to synergize with IL-2 in cancer patients (Conti & Maestroni 1995). In this regard, it is noteworthy to recall that MLT is most active on antigen or cytokine activated cells (Konakchieva et al., 1995; Maestroni et al., 1986, 1987). Consistently, IL-2 treatment in patients results in activation of the whole immune system and creates the most suitable biological background for MLT. The finding that MLT can stimulate IL-12 production from human monocytes only if incubated in the presence of IL-2 further supports this concept (Lissoni, Pittalis, et al., 1997). In fact, the plasma concentration of IL-12 was increased in patients who showed a partial response to the MLT/IL-2 (Lissoni, Rovelli, et al., 1997). This finding seems important because IL-12, which is mainly produced by monocytes/macrophages, plays a relevant role in cytokine-based cancer therapy (Banks, Patel, & Selby, 1995).

The ability of MLT to counteract the thymus involution and immunodepression caused by stress or corticosteroid treatment seems to be mediated by

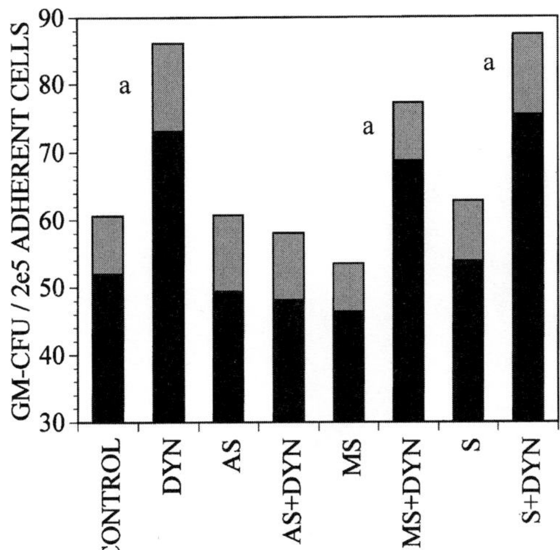

FIGURE 6 Effect of dynorphin A on adherent cells incubated with AS oligodeoxynucleotide to kappa-opioid receptors. Adherent cells were incubated overnight with AS, MS, and S oligodeoxynucleotides and then plated in a GM-CFU assay in presence of dynorphin A (DYN) 10^{-9} M. The values are relative to three experiments and represent the mean ± the standard deviation. a: $p < 0.01$.

the MIO. Whether the MIO action is exerted on peripheral immunocompetent cells and in the thymus or whether the hematopoietic effects of these putative novel opioid cytokines are also involved remains to be elucidated. However, it seems clear that the hematopoietic effects of MLT depend on a complex series of events involving the effects of the MIO on κ-opioid receptors expressed on bone marrow macrophages (Figure 6). This seems of considerable relevance for understanding the MLT effects and, in general, the physiology of hematopoiesis. MIO might belong to a new family of endogenous κ-opioid agonists which, in the case of hematopoietic protection, seem to synergize with GM-CSF on stromal cell κ-receptors and induce IL-1 (Maestroni et al., 1999). This would explain MIO rescue hematopoiesis against the toxic action of cancer chemotherapy in LLC-bearing mice. LLC is, in fact, known to release GM-CSF (Young et al., 1988). The fact that activated Th cells also may produce GM-CSF might account for the therapeutic and positive hematopoietic effects of MLT when administered together with IL-2 in cancer patients (Conti & Maestroni, 1995).

The cytokines involved in the immune-hematopoietic action of MLT may exert an influence on the production of MLT by the pineal gland. The pineal gland, in fact, is located outside the blood-brain barrier and some reports show that IFN-γ may directly affect the synthesis of MLT in the pineal gland (Withyachumnarnkul, Nonaka, Santana, Attia, & Reiter, 1990). Relevant to the hematopoietic link of MLT, it also has been reported that colony stimulating factors may enhance MLT synthesis (Zylinska, Komorowski, Robak, Mucha, & Stepien, 1995). A hypothetical pineal/MLT-immune-hematopoietic network, therefore, is taking shape (Figure 7). The proper functioning of such a network might be crucial in the adaptative response of the organism to environmental demands and, thus, in the maintenance of health. However, we are still far from a complete understanding of the mechanism underlying the immunological and hematopoietic action of MLT. In fact, MLT seems to exert both a pro- and antiinflammatory action. The latter, as evidenced by its effect on NO in LPS-treated mice, is related to inhibition of the nuclear trasncription factor NFκB. How this relates to the ability of MLT to enhance cytokine production remains to be studied. Perhaps the key point to understand in the MLT mechansim of action is the presence and the relative role of both membrane and nuclear receptors in immunocompetent cells Garcia-Mauriño et al., 1997, 1998; Garcia-Perganeda et al., 1997). Relevant to a possible role of nuclear receptors is the recent and intriguing finding that murine and human bone marrow cells contain MLT at a concentration that seems to be two or three orders of magnitude higher than that found in the circulation. Apparently, MLT is synthesized in these cells because MLT and the enzymatic machinery for its synthesis are present in cultures of immunocompetent and bone marrow cells (Conti et al., in press). In addition, it is not clear whether MLT acts on Th1 or Th2 cells or on both. Most evidences points to the involvement of Th1 cells; however, a recent report suggests that MLT acts by selectively activating Th2-type immune responses (Shaji, Kulkarni, & Agrewala, 1998) This seems a rather important question, as the Th1/Th2 balance and the resulting cytokine production are crucial for a successful immune response and may be relevant in immune-based pathologies (Del Prete, Maggi, & Romagnani, 1994). Another interesting issue relates to the possible direct action of MLT in the cell cycle of immunocompetent cells. This possibility is suggested by the reported ability of MLT to inhibit growth of tumor cells expressing MLT receptors (Blask, 1993).

Physiologically, it seems possible to distinguish two different MLT roles. The first one occurs under acute conditions during a viral or bacterial infection that produces a substantial activation of the immune system. In that condition, endogenous and/or exogenous MLT may optimize the immune response by sustaining Th cell and macrophage functions and production of cytokines, part of which (MIO, IL-1,

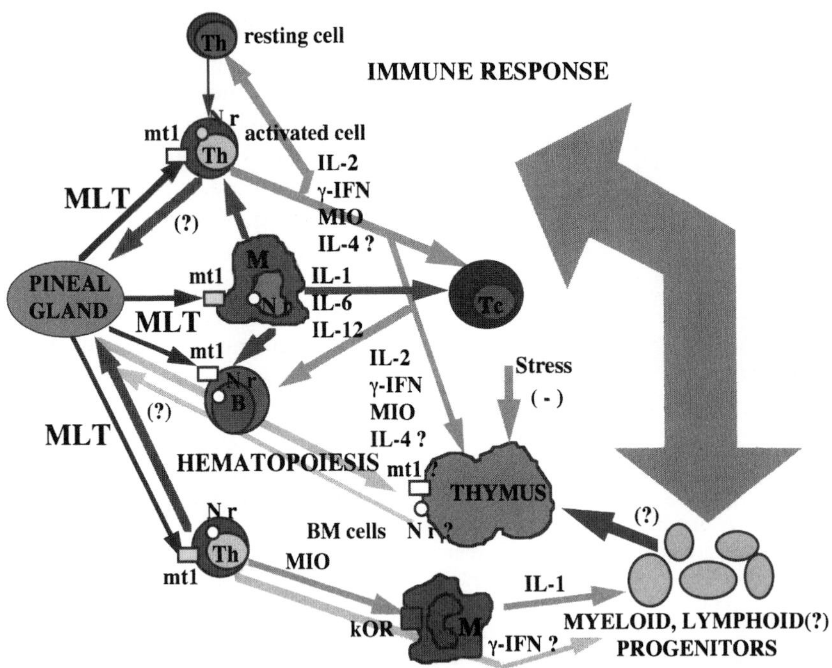

FIGURE 7 The pineal gland/MLT immune-hematopoietic network. MLT is secreted by the pineal gland during the dark phase of the photoperiod and binds to membrane (mt1) and/or nuclear receptors (Nr) in antigen or cytokine activated peripheral T helper (Th) cells, in peripheral macrophages (M), and in bone marrow Th cells. In contrast to peripheral Th cells, bone marrow Th cells seem to express constitutively MLT receptors. Activation of the receptors expressed antigen or cytokine activation of the immune system results in an increased production of cytokines and of MIO, which in turn act on immune effector cells such as B cell and T cytotoxic cells (Tc) and may counteract the depressive effect of stress (corticosteroids) on the thymus. This mechanism may account for the ability of MLT to counteract secondary immunodeficiencies, protect against viral and bacterial infections, and synergize with IL-2 or IFN-γ in mice and cancer patients. On the other hand, Th cells in the bone marrow seem to secrete MIO and, perhaps, IFN-γ which affect hematopoiesis. The MIO released by either activated peripheral Th cells or by bone marrow Th cells binds to kappa-opioid receptors (kOR) in bone marrow macrophages and stimulates IL-1 production, which in turn may synergize with GM-CSF released by activated immunocompetent cells and enhance myelopoiesis and, perhaps, lymphopoiesis. At lower concentrations of GM-CSF such as those sustaining physiological hematopoiesis, the effect of the MIO-induced IL-1 and IFN-γ might result in an inhibitory effect. The cytokines and MIO together with thymic hormones might act directly on the pineal gland and modulate MLT production to optimize the function of the pineal-immune-hematopoietic network.

IL-6) may also affect hematopoiesis. A second more general role may be exerted at the hematopoietic-immune level by a chronic circadian resetting of the immunological machinery to maintain the immune homeostasis. This is suggested by the observation that in healthy mice, i.e., in absence of any infection and immunological activation, only the Th cells that reside in the bone marrow are sensitive to MLT (Maestroni et al., 1996; Maestroni, 1993). Both the acute and chronic mechanisms might be exploited in the use of MLT as an immunotherapeutic agent to correct secondary immunodeficiency or to fight viral diseases. The use of MLT in combination with IL-2 in cancer neuroimmunotherapy might prolong survival and improve the patients' quality of life (Conti & Maestroni et al., 1995). These encouraging results therefore, deserve, to be expanded and challenged in other studies. In addition, MLT might be useful in enhancing the dendritic cell-induced T cell immune response against tumor antigens, a promising therapeutic strategy for cancer vaccines. With respect to the use of MLT in combination with cancer chemotherapeutic drugs, the clinical results obtained so far are disappointing. MLT administered alone seems to worsen the bone marrow toxicity of common cancer chemotherapeutic regimens or, at best, be ineffective. However, this result is similar to that obtained in tumor-free mice. A possible explanation of these negative results is that MLT stimulation, bone marrow Th cells might produce, together with MIO, inhibitory cytokines such as IFN-γ. This would result in an inhibition of hematopoiesis in the absence of a substantial amount of GM-CSF such as would be derived from a systemic immune activation would synergize with the MIO-induced IL-1. Once again, it appears that a state of systemic immune activation plays a permissive role in MLT action. Last but not least, I would like to emphasize the need for a large double-blind study in human immunodeficiency virus (HIV)-positive patients. In the presence of normal Th cell counts, the apparent ability of MLT to sustain Th cell functions and IL-2 and IFN-γ production might result in delayed development or occurrence of AIDS. Reduction of plasma viremia was associated with an increased IL-2 mRNA expression in lymph nodes of HIV-infected patients (Sei et al., 1996). IL-2 is the most potent cytokine capable of inducing the CD8+ T cell-mediated inhibition of HIV replication, which seems to override the ability of IL-2 to stimulate HIV expression (Kinter, Bende, Hardy, Jackson, & Fauci, 1995). If effective, MLT administration would be a relatively inexpensive and safe prevention of this devastating disease. Alternatively, MLT might be associated with low-dose IL-2, which seems to be beneficial in HIV-associated malignancies (Bernstein, et al. 1995) or with HIV protease inhibitors.

In conclusion, MLT seems to be an extremely interesting immunomodulatory hormone. Its mechanism of action and physiopathological relevance as well as its therapeutic potential need to be explored in well-controlled studies without forgetting that MLT also may exert adverse effects.

References

Angeli, A., Gatti, G., Sartori, M. L., Del Ponte, D., & Cerignola, R. (1988). Effect of exogenous melatonin on human natural killer (NK) cell activity. An approach to the immunomodulatory role of the pineal gland. In D. Gupta, A. Attanasio, & R. J. Reiter (Eds.), *The pineal gland and cancer* (pp. 145–157). Tübingen: Müller and Bass.

Anwar, M. M., Mahfouz, H. A., & Sayed, A. S. (1998). Potential protective effects of melatonin on bone marrow of rats exposed to cytotoxic drugs. *Comparative Biochemistry and Physiology, 119*, 493–591.

Banks, R. E., Patel, P. M., & Selby, P. J. (1995). Interleukin-12: A new player in cytokine therapy. *British Journal of Cancer, 71*, 655–659.

Barath, P., & Csaba, G. (1974). Histological changes in the lung, thymus and adrenal one and half year after pinealectomy. *Acta Biologica Academiae Scientiarum Hungaricae, 25*, 123–125.

Barjavel, M. J., Mamdouh, Z., Raghbate, N., & Bakouche, O. (1998). Differential expression of the melatonin receptor in human monocytes. *Journal of Immunology, 160*, 1191–1197.

Barron, R. L. (1993). Pathophysiology of septic shock and implications for therapy. *Clinical Pharmacology, 12*, 829–845.

Beasley, D., & Eldridge, M. (1994). Interleukin-1β and tumor necrosis factor-α synergistically induce NO synthase in rat vascular smooth muscle cells. *American Journal of Physiology, 266*, R1197–R1203.

Becker, J., Veit, G., Handgretinger, R., Attanasio, G., Bruchett, G., Trenner, I., Niethammer, D., & Gupta, D. (1988). Circadian variations in the immunomodulatory role of the pineal gland. *Neuroendocrinology Letters, 10*, 65–80.

Ben-Nathan, D., Maestroni, G. J. M., & Conti, A. (1995). Protective effect of melatonin in mice infected with encephalitis viruses. *Archives of Virology, 140*, 223–230.

Ben-Nathan, D., Maestroni, G. J. M., & Conti, A. (1997). Protective effect of melatonin in viral and bacterial infections. In G. J. M. Maestroni, A. Conti, & J. R. Reiter (Eds.), *Frontiers in Hormone Research* (pp. 72–81). Basel: Karger.

Blask, D. E. (1993). Melatonin in oncology. In H.-S. Yu, & R. J. Reiter (Eds.), *Melatonin. Biosynthesis, physiological effects, and clinical applications* (pp. 447–477). Boca Raton, FL: CRC Press.

Bonilla, E., Valerofuenmajor, N., Pons, H., & Chacin-Bonilla, L. (1997). Melatonin protects mice infected with Venezuelan equine encephalomyelitis virus. *Cellular and Molecular Life Sciences., 53*, 430–434.

Carlberg, C., & Wiesenberg, I. (1995). The orphan receptor family RZR/ROR, melatonin and 5-lipoxygenase: An unexpected relationship. *Journal of Pineal Research, 18*, 171–178.

Caroleo, M. C., Frasca, D., Nistico, G., & Doria, G. (1992). Melatonin as immunomodulator in immunodeficient mice. *Immunopharmacology, 23*, 81–89.

Champney, T. H., & McMurray, D. N. (1991). Spleen morphology and lymphoproliferative activity in short photoperiod exposed hamsters,. In F. Fraschini, & R. J. Reiter (Eds.), *Role of melatonin and pineal peptides in neuroimmunomodulation* (pp. 219–225). London: Plenum Publishing.

Colombo, L. L., Chen, G.-J., Lopez, M. C., & Watson, R. R. (1992). Melatonin induced increase in gamma-interferon production by murine splenocytes. *Immunology Letters, 33*, 123–126.

Conti, A., Haran-Ghera, N., & Maestroni, G. J. M. (1992). Role of pineal melatonin and melatonin-induced-immuno-opioids in murine leukemogenesis. *Medical Oncology and Tumor Pharmacotherapy, 9*, 87–92.

Conti, A., & Maestroni, G. J. M. (1995). The clinical neuroimmunotherapeutic role of melatonin in oncology. *Journal of Pineal Research, 19*, 103–110.

Conti, A., Conconi, S., Hertens, E., Skwarlo-Sonta, K., Markowska, M., & Maestroni, G. J. M. (in press). Melatonin synthesis in mouse and human bone marrow cells. *Journal of Pineal Research.*

Csaba, G., & Barath, P. (1975). Morphological changes of thymus and the thyroid gland after postnatal extirpation of pineal body. *Endocrinologia Experimentalis, 9*, 59–67.

Csaba, G., Bodocky, M., Fischer, J., & Acs, T. (1965). The effect of pinealectomy and thymectomy on the immune capacity of the rat. *Experientia, 22*, 168–175.

Cunha, F. Q., Assreuy, J., Moss, D. W., Rees, D., Leal, L. M. C., Moncada, S., Carrier, M., O'Donnel, C. A., & Liew, F. Y. (1994). Differential induction of nitric oxide synthase in various organs of the mouse during endotoxaemia: Role of TNF-α and IL-1-β. *Immunology, 81*, 211–215.

Del Gobbo, V., Libri, V., Villani, N., Caliò, R., & Nistico, G. (1989). Pinealectomy inhibits interleukin-2 production and natural killer activity in mice. *International Journal of Immunopharmacology, 11*, 567–577.

Del Prete, G., Maggi, E., & Romagnani, S. (1994). Human Th1 and Th2 cells: Functional properties, mechanisms of regulation and role in disease. *Laboratory Investigation, 70*, 299–307.

Evans, T., Carpenter, A., Silva, A., & Cohen, J. (1994). Inhibition of nitric oxide synthase in experimental gram-negative sepsis. *Journal of Infectious Diseases, 169*, 343–349.

Feychting, M., Osterlund, B., & Ahlbom, A. (1998). Reduced cancer incidence among the blind. *Epidemiology, 9,* 490–494.

Florquin, S., Amraoui, Z., Dubois, C., Decuyper, J., & Goldman, M. (1994). The protective role of endogenously synthesized nitric oxide in staphylococcal enterotoxin B-induced shock in mice. *Journal of Experimental Medicine, 180,* 1153–1158.

Garcia-Mauriño, S., Gonzales-Haba, M. G., Calvo, J. R., Goberna, R., & Guerrero, J.-M. (1998). Involvement of nuclear binding sites for melatonin in the regulation of IL-2 and IL-6 production in human blood mononuclear cells. *Journal of Neuroimmunology, 92,* 76–84.

Garcia-Mauriño, S., Gonzales-Haba, M. G., Calvo, J. R., Rafii-El-Idrissi, M., Sanchez-Margalet, V., Goberna, R., & Guerrero, J. M. (1997). Melatonin enhances IL-2, Il-6, and IFN- production by human circulating CD4+ cells. *Journal of Immunology, 159,* 574–581.

Garcia-Perganeda, A., Pozo, D., Guerrero, J. M., & Calvo, J. R. (1997). Signal transduction for melatonin in human lymphocytes. Involvement of a pertussis toxin-sensitive G protein. *Journal of Immunology, 159,* 3774–3781.

Gilad, E., Wong, H. R., Zingarelli, B., Virag, L., O'Connor, M., Salzman, A. L., & Szabo, C. (1998). Melatonin inhibits expression of the inducible isoform of nitric oxide synthase in murine macrophages: Role of inhibition of NFκB activation. *FASEB Journal, 12,* 685–693.

Giordano, M., & Palermo, M. S. (1991). Melatonin-induced enhancement of antibody dependent cellular cytotoxicity. *Journal of Pineal Research, 10,* 117–121.

Guerrero, J.-M., Garcia-Maurino, S., Gil-Haba, M., Rafii-El-Idrissi, M., Pozo, D., Garcia-Perganeda, A., & Calvo, J. R. (1996). Mechanisms of action on the human immune system: Membrane receptors versus nuclear receptors. In G. J. M. Maestroni, A. Conti, & R. J. Reiter (Eds.), *Therapeutic potential of the pineal hormone melatonin* (pp. 43–52). Basel: Karger.

Haldar, C., Haussler, D., & Gupta, D. (1992). Response of CFU-GM (colony forming units for granulocytes and macrophages) from intact and pinealectomized rat bone marrow to macrophage colony stimulating factor (rGM-CSF) and human recombinant erythropoietin (rEPO). *Progress in Brain Research, 91,* 323–325.

Hibbs, J. B. Jr., Taintor, R. R., Vavrin, Z., Granger, D. L., Drapier, J. C., Amber, I. J., & Lancaster, J. R. Jr. (1991). Synthesis of nitric oxide from a terminal guanidino atom of L-arginine: a molecular mechanism regulating cellular proliferation that targets intracellular iron. In S. Moncada, & E. A. Higgs (Eds.), *Nitric oxide from L-arginine: A bioregulatory system* (pp. 189–205.). Amsterdam: Excerpta Medica Elsevier.

Hofbauer, L. C., & Heufelder, A. E. (1996). Endocrinology meets immunology: T lymphocytes as novel targets for melatonin. *European Journal of Endocrinology, 134,* 424–425.

Kinter, A. L., Bende, S. M., Hardy, E. C., Jackson, R., & Fauci, A. S. (1995). Interleukin 2 induces CD8+ T cell-mediated suppression of human immunodeficiency virus replication in CD4+ T cells and this effect overrides its ability to stimulate virus expression. *Proceedings Natliobal Academy of Sciences USA, 92,* 19985–10989.

Konakchieva, R., Kyurkchiev, S., Kehayov, I., Taushanova, P., & Kanchev, L. (1995). Selective effect of methoxyndoles on the lymphocyte proliferation and melatonin binding to activated human lymphoid cells. *Journal of Neuroimmunology, 63,* 125–132.

Lerner, A. B., Case, J. D., Takahashi, Y., Lee, T. H., & Mori, W. (1958). Isolation of melatonin, the pineal gland factor that lightens melanocytes. *Journal of the American Chemical Society, 80,* 2587–2592.

Lewinsky, A., Zelazowsky, P., Sewerynek, E., Zerek-Melen, G., & Szudlinsky, M. (1989). Melatonin-induced immunosuppression of humal lymphocyte natural killer activity in vitro. *Journal of Pineal Research, 7,* 153–164.

Lissoni, P., Brivio, F., Brivio, O., Fumagalli, L., Gramazio, F., Rossi, M., Emanuelli, G., Alderi, G., & Lavorato, F. (1995). Immune effects of preoperative immunotherapy with high-dose subcutaneous interleukin-2 versus neuroimmunotherapy with lowdose interleukin-2 plus the neurohormone melatonin in gastrointestinal tract tumor patients. *Journal of Biological Regulatory Homeostatic Agents, 9,* 31–33.

Lissoni, P., Brivio, F., Tancini, G., Cattaneo, G., Archili, C., Conti, A., & Maestroni, G. J. M. (1990). Neuroimmunotherapy of human cancer with interleukin-2 and the neurohormone melatonin: Its efficacy in preventing hypotension. *Anticancer Research, 10,* 1759–1763.

Lissoni, P., Pittalis, S., Barni, S., Rovelli, F., Fumagalli, L., & Maestroni, G. J.-M. (1997). Regulation of interleukin-2/interleukin-12 interactions by the pineal gland. *International Journal of Thymology, 5,* 443–447.

Lissoni, P., Rovelli, F., Brivio, F., Pittalis, S., Maestroni, G. J. M., & Fumagalli, L. (1997). In vivo study of the modulatory effect of the pineal hormone melatonin on interleukin-12 secretion in response to interleukin-2. *International Journal of Thymology, 5,* 482–486.

Lissoni, P., Tisi, E., Barni, S., Ardizzoia, A., Rovelli, F., Rescaldani, R., Ballabio, D., Benenti, C., Angeli, M., Tancini, G., Conti, A., & Maestroni, G. J. M. (1992). Biological and clinical results of a neuroimmunotherapy with interleukin-2 and the pineal hormone melatonin as a first line treatment in advanced non-small cell lung cancer. *British Journal of Cancer, 66,* 155–158.

Maestroni, G., Hertens, E., Galli, P., Conti, A., & Pedrinis, E. (1996). Melatonin-induced T-helper cell hematopoietic cytokines resembling both interleukin-4 and dynorphin. *Journal of Pineal Research, 21,* 131–139.

Maestroni, G. J. M. (1993). The immunoneuroendocrine role of melatonin. *Journal of Pineal Research, 14,* 1–10.

Maestroni, G. J. M. (1995). T helper 2 lymphocytes as a peripheral target of melatonin. *Journal of Pineal Research, 18,* 84–89.

Maestroni, G. J. M. (1996). Melatonin as a therapeutic agent in experimental endotoxic shock. *Journal of Pineal Research, 20,* 84–89.

Maestroni, G. J. M. (1998). Kappa-opioid receptors in marrow stroma mediate the hematopoietic effects of melatonin-induced opioid cytokines. In M. S., J. M. Lipton, E. M. Sternberg, G. P. Chrousos, P. W. Gold, & C. C. Smith (Eds.), *Neuroimmunomodulation: Molecular aspects, integrative systems, and clinical advances* (pp. 411–420). New York: Academy of Science.

Maestroni, G. J. M., & Conti, A. (1989). Beta-endorphin and dynorphin mimic the circadian immunoenhancing and anti-stress effects of melatonin. *International Journal of Immunopharmacology,* 11, 333–340.

Maestroni, G. J. M., & Conti, A. (1990). The pineal neurohormone melatonin stimulates activated CD4+, Thy-1+ cells to release opioid agonist(s) with immunoenhancing and anti-stress properties. *Journal of Neuroimmunology, 28,* 167–176.

Maestroni, G. J. M., & Conti, A. (1991). Anti-stress role of the melatonin-immuno-opioid network. Evidence for a physiological mechanism involving T cell-derived, immunoreactive β-endorphin and met.enkephalin binding to thymic opioid receptors. *International Journal of Neurosciences, 61,* 289–298.

Maestroni, G. J. M., & Conti, A. (1993). Melatonin in relation to the immune system. In H.-S. Yu, & R. J. Reiter (Eds.), *Melatonin. Biosynthesis, physiological effects and clinical applications* (pp. 290–306). Boca Raton, FL: CRC Press.

Maestroni, G. J. M., Conti, A., & Lissoni, P. (1994). Colony-stimulating activity and hematopoietic rescue from cancer chemothereapy compounds are induced by melatonin via endogenous interleukin 4. *Cancer Research, 54*, 4740–4743.

Maestroni, G. J. M., Conti, A., & Pierpaoli, W. (1986). Role of the pineal gland in immunity. Circadian synthesis and release of melatonin modulates the antibody response and antagonize the imunosuppressive effect of corticosterone. *Journal of Neuroimmunology, 13*, 19–30.

Maestroni, G. J. M., Conti, A., & Pierpaoli, W. (1987). Role of the pineal gland in immunity: II. Melatonin enhances the antibody response via an opiatergic mechanism. *Clinical and Experimental Immunology, 68*, 384–391.

Maestroni, G. J. M., Covacci, V., & Conti, A. (1994). Hematopoietic rescue via T-cell-dependent, endogenous GM-CSF by the pineal neurohormone melatonin in tumor bearing mice. *Cancer Research, 54*, 2429–2432.

Maestroni, G. J. M., & Pierpaoli, W. (1981). Pharmacological control of the hormonally modulated immune response. In R. Ader (Ed.), *Psychoneuroimmunology* (pp. 405–425). New York: Academic Press.

Maestroni, G. J. M., Zammaretti, F., & Pedrinis, E. (1999). Hematopoietic effect of melatonin. Involvement of k1-opioid receptor on bone marrow macrophages and interleukin-1. *Journal of Pineal Research, 27*, 145–153.

Morrey, M. K., McLachlan, J. A., Serkin, C. D., & Bakouche, O. (1994). Activation of human monocytes by the pineal neurohormone melatonin. *Journal of Immunology, 153*, 2671–2680.

Natanson, C., Hoffman, W. D., Suffredini, A. F., Eichacker, P. Q., & Danner, R. L. (1994). Selected treatment strategies for septic shock based on proposed mechanisms of pathogenesis. *Annals of Internal Medicine, 120*, 771–783.

Neri, B., DeLeonardis, V., Gemelli, M. T., DiLoro, M., Mottola, A., Ponchietti, R., Raugei, A., & Cini, G. (1998). Melatonin as biological response modifier in cancer patients. *Anticancer Research, 18*, 1329–1332.

Neri, B., Fiorelli, C., Moroni, F., Nicita, G., Paoletti, M. C., Ponchietti, R., Raugei, A., Santoni, G., Trippitelli, A., & Grechi, G. (1994). Modulation of human lymphoblastoid interferon activity by melatonin in metastatic renal cell carcinoma. A phase II study. *Cancer, 73*, 3015–3019.

Palermo, M. S., Vermeulen, M., & Giordano, M. (1994). Modulation of antibody-dependent cellular cytotoxicity by pineal gland. In G. J. M. Maestroni, A. Conti, & R. J. Reiter (Eds.) *Advances in pineal research* (pp. 143–147). London: John Libbey.

Petrovsky, N., & Harrison, L. (1996). Diurnal rhythmicity of human cytokine production. A dynamic disequilibrium in T helper cell type 1/T helper cell type 2 balance. *Journal of Immunology, 158*, 5163–5168.

Pioli, C., Caroleo, M. C., Nistico, G., & Doria, G. (1993). Melatonin increases antigen presentation and amplifies specific and non specific signals for T-cell proliferation. *International Journal of Immunopharmacology, 15*, 463–469.

Poon, A. M., Liu, Z. M., Pang, C. S., Brown, G. M., & Pang, S. F. (1994). Evidence for a direct action of melatonin on the immune system. *Biological Signals, 3*, 107–117.

Pozo, D., Reiter, R. J., Calvo, J. R., & Guerrero, J. M. (1994). Physiological concentrations of melatonin inhibit nitric oxide synthase in rat cerebellum. *Pharmacology Letters, 55*, 455–460.

Rafii-El-Idrissi, M., Calvo, J. R., Harmouch, A., Garcia-Maurino, S., & Guerrero, J. M. (1998). Specific binding of melatonin by purified cell nuclei from spleen and thymus of the rat. *Journal of Neuroimmunology, 86*, 190–197.

Reppert, S. M., & Weaver, D. R. (1995). Melatonin madness. *Cell, 83*, 1059–1062.

Sei, S., Akiyoshi, H., Bernard, J., Venzon, D. J., Fox, C. H., Schwartzentruber, D. J., Anderson, B. D., Kopp, J. B., Mueller, B. U., & Pizzo, P. A. (1996). Dynamics of virus versus host interaction in children with human immunodeficiency virus type 1 infection. *Journal of Infectious Diseases, 173*, 1485–1490.

Shaji, A. V., Kulkarni, S. K., & Agrewala, J. N. (1998). Regulation of secretion of IL-4 and IgG1 isotype by melatonin-stimulated ovalbumin specific T cells. *Clinical and Experimental Immunology, 111*, 181–185.

Vanecek, J. (1998). Cellular mechanisms of melatonin action. *Physiological Reviews, 78*, 687–721.

Vaughan, M. K., & Reiter, R. J. (1971). Transient hypertrophy of the ventral prostate and coagulating glands and accelerated thymic involution following pinealectomy in the mouse. *Texas Reproduction Biology Medicine, 29*, 579–586.

Wichmann, M., Zellweger, R., DeMaso, A., Ayala, A., & Chaudry, I. (1996). Melatonin administration attenuates depressed immune functions trauma-hemorrhage. *Journal of Surgical Research, 63*, 256–262.

Wichmann, M. W., Haisken, J. M., Ayala, A., & Chaudry, I. H. (1996). Melatonin administration following hemorrhagic shock decreases mortality from subsequent septic challenge. *Journal of Surgical Research, 65*, 109–114.

Withyachumnarnkul, B., Nonaka, K. O., Santana, C., Attia, A. M., & Reiter, R. J. (1990). Interferon-gamma modulates melatonin production in rat pineal gland in organ culture. *Journal of Interferon Research, 10*, 403–411.

Young, M. R. I., Young, M. E., & Kim, K. (1988). Regulation of tumor-induced myelopoiesis and the associated immune suppressor cells in mice bearing metastatic Lewis lung carcinoma by prostaglandin E2. *Cancer Research, 48*, 6826–6831.

Yu, H.-S., & Reiter, R. J. (1993). *Melatonin. Biosynthesis, physiological effects, and clinical applications.* Boca Raton, FL: CRC Press.

Yu, H.-S., Tsin, A. T. C., & Reiter, R. J. (1993). Melatonin: History, biosynthesis, and assay methodology. In H.-S. Yu, & R. J. Reiter (Eds.), *Melatonin. Biosynthesis, physiological effects, and clinical applications* (pp. 1–17). Boca Raton, FL: CRC Press.

Zylinska, K., Komorowski, J., Robak, T., Mucha, S., & Stepien, H. (1995). Effect of granulocyte-macrophage colony stimulating factor and granulocyte colony stimulating factor on melatonin secretion in rats in vivo and in vitro studies. *Journal of Neuroimmunology, 56*, 187–190.

CHAPTER

17

Biological Rhythms and Immune Function

ROBERT B. SOTHERN, BEATRICE ROITMAN-JOHNSON

I. BIOLOGIC RHYTHMS

A. Introduction

Immunology has generally overlooked the fact that life is not only structured in space, but also in time. The many naturally occurring daily and other body rhythms have a regulating influence on the "normal" functioning of the body's many processes. In addition to responses to external stimuli, the metabolism of living organisms involves constantly changing processes that are not random, but undergo genetically anchored, built-in, periodic, and thus predictable variations. Therefore, in the organism itself, the process of homeostasis does not try to maintain a constant, fixed set point (reactive homeostasis), but rather tries to maintain a set point that itself is rhythmic (predictive homeostasis), having evolved due to the predictable changes in the environment such as light and darkness, temperature, food availability, and predator activity (Moore-Ede, 1986). In addition, it is also now clear that different variables and processes, although synchronized in time, are not all timed together, but have their own times of highs and lows. In some cases, a coordination or sequencing in time is apparent, such as has been shown in mitoses between organs in the mouse (Halberg & Howard, 1958) and for cell cycle functions (G1-phase [phospholipids, RNA], S-phase [DNA] and G2-phase [glycogen]) in the mouse liver (Barnum, Jardetzky, & Halberg, 1958; Halberg, Halberg, Barnum, & Bittner, 1959; Halberg, 1960). In humans, a larger proportion of bone marrow cells may be in the DNA S-phase at midday, whereas the actual number of mature red and white cells spilling into the bloodstream may reach highest numbers about 12 hours later near midnight. Some hormones, such as cortisol and testosterone, are highest in the morning when a person rises, whereas others, such as gastrin, insulin, and renin, are highest in the afternoon or early evening, and yet others, such as melatonin, prolactin, thyroid-stimulating hormone (TSH), and growth hormone, reach their peak levels while a person sleeps. At the physiologic level, body temperature, heart rate, and blood pressure are generally highest in the afternoon, yet hearing and sensitivity to pain are more acute in the evening. Circadian rhythms are thus a normal part of health, and although these body rhythms continue during illness, their alteration may be involved with or reveal troublesome health problems. Similarly, an individual's response to medications or other stimuli also shows a circadian rhythm, since the body does not respond the same at different times of the day. Thus, medicine taken at the right time may improve its effectiveness, while reducing any side effects.

Bioperiodicity has been shown to be a ubiquitous trait of any biological entity, with bioperiodic rhythmic networks interacting at different orders of complexity. The field of study encompassing this broad area of research into the time structure of living organisms is called "chronobiology" (Halberg, 1969). The frequencies of biological rhythms are divided into 3 categories. The narrowest region is the appoximately 24 h rhythm or *circadian* (from *circa* = about and *dies* = daily), a term introduced by Halberg and colleagues in 1959. The term *circadian* is broadly used when describing 24 h rhythms, regardless of the endogenous or exogenous causative mechanism (Moore-Ede, 1973). Frequencies shorter than circadian are called *ultradian* and longer are called *infradian* (Halberg, Carandente, Cornélissen, & Katinas, 1977). Much effort is also focused on understanding mechanisms underlying these 'biological clocks'. The genetic basis of endogenous rhythms is a topic of great interest to chronobiologists in many areas, from the molecular level of various clock genes (Barinaga, 1997; Schibler, 1998; Bjarnason, Jordan, Li, Sothern, & Ben-David, 1999; Takahashi & Hoffman, 1995), to cell cycle clock characteristics (Edmunds, 1984), and to the heritability of circadian characteristics in human twins (Barcal, Sova, Krizanovska, Levy, & Matousek, 1968; Hanson et al., 1984). Even along the infradian scale, a circannual rhythm in antibody formation by murine spleen against sheep red blood cells revealed a genetic-based difference in the season of highest values between two strains (Ratajczak, Thomas, Sothern, Vollmuth, & Heck, 1993).

All of this information suggests an endogenous, built-in, genetically determined foundation for the biological rhythmicity at multiple frequencies seen in all living organisms. It is now quite obvious that all life forms on earth, from single cell organisms to higher order species in each phylum, are traveling through time on waves of biological rhythms as their body functions wax and wane along a scale of interrelated periodicities that range from seconds to a year or more.

B. Circadian Rhythms of Life, Disease, and Death

Virtually every body function, whether physiologic or psychologic, has been shown to display a circadian rhythm in healthy individuals (Kanabrocki et al., 1983; Kanabrocki et al. 1990; Touitou & Haus, 1992), which persists well into old age (Haus, Nicolau, Lakatua, Sackett-Lundeen, & Petrescu, 1989) with remarkable precision and stability (Czeisler et al., 1999). These rhythms generally have known times of highest and lowest values in relation to each individual's sleep-wake schedule, which acts as a synchronizer for the body clock (Sothern, 1995).

On a population basis, epidemiological studies have shown that the time of day plays a role in when one is born and when one might die. Labor onset usually occurs at night and a peak in births is found in the early morning hours (Smolensky, Halberg, & Sargent, 1972). Morbidity and mortality from cardiovascular disease have repeatedly been shown to be more prevalent in the morning hours for the incidence of angina and ischemic episodes, myocardial infarction, sudden cardiac death, and cerebral infarction or hemorrhage (reviewed by Bogaty & Waters, 1989). Sudden death from pulmonary embolism was also reported to be circadian rhythmic with a peak in the morning (Manfredini et al., 1991).

Allergic conditions, such as asthma, hay fever, hives, and other allergies, display a circadian rhythm in symptoms, with itching, sneezing, wheezing, breaking out in rashes, and bronchial constriction more severe at night, during sleep and/or near awakening. Similarly, symptoms (pain, stiffness, dexterity) of rheumatoid- or osteoarthritis of the knee (Bellamy, Sothern, & Campbell, 1990) or hand (Bellamy, Sothern, Campbell, & Buchanan, 1991; Bellamy et al., 1997) are worse at night and improve during the day. Peptic ulcers are more likely to perforate and require hospitalization around noon if the site is duodenal or gastric, with a secondary peak around midnight in perforations requiring hospitalization if the site is gastric (Svanes, Sothern, & Sørbye, 1998).

C. Circannual Rhythms of Life, Disease, and Death

Through epidemiological and longitudinal data collection, it has become apparent that the time of year is also an important factor in influencing outcome, not only in quantitative characteristics of animals (Sothern, Farber, & Gruber, 1993), but in humans, as well (Haus, Nicolau, Lakatua, & Sackett-Lundeen, 1988; Reinberg, & Lagoguey, 1978). On a population basis, humans are more likely to be conceived in the late winter or spring than at other times (Smolensky et al., 1972), with the maximum occurring later in the year with increasing latitude (Roennenberg & Aschoff, 1990a, 1990b). In addition to the modifying effects of the natural photoperiod at different latitudes, the pattern of the circannual rhythm in human natality is undoubtedly reflective of modifying effects by society from religious practices and birth control. However, a possible mechanism underlying this phenomenon may be the influence of seasonal variations in human sperm quality and count, which have been reported to be greatest in the spring (Spira, 1984; Tjoa, Smolensky, Hsi, Steinberger, & Smith, 1982), which in turn may be affected by the circannual rhythm in testosterone, which has been shown to be highest in men in the winter (Dabbs, 1990).

Large seasonal variations in several immune defense mechanisms, including all white blood cell subtypes, have been reported in humans (Touitou & Haus, 1992). Circannual cycling in immunity may play a role in the seasonality of vulnerability to microorganisms (Hejl, 1977; Pöllman, 1982) and tumors (Cohen, Wax, & Modan, 1983; Hostmark, Laerum, & Farsund, 1984; Newell, Lyncy, Gibeau, & Skitz, 1985; Swerdlow, 1985). For example, childhood infectious diseases, such as chicken pox, mumps, rubella, and rubeola are more frequently diagnosed in the late winter and spring than at other times of the year (Smolensky, 1983) and a parallel circannual rhythm in rubella antibody titers has been shown (Rosenblatt, Shifrine, Hetherington, Paglieroni, & MacKenzie, 1982). With regard to cancer incidence, thyroid tumors are more frequently diagnosed in the late autumn and winter, with size and proliferation indicators (cells in S and G2M-phases) also showing highest values in autumn and winter, indicating that these tumors were growing faster at one time of the year than another (Akslen & Sothern, 1998).

Parameters of the coagulation system have also been reported to differ predictably throughout the year (Kanabrocki et al., 1995; Nicolau, Haus, Popescu, Sackett-Lundeen, & Petrescu, 1991). This may play a role in circannual rhythms reported in symptoms and/or deaths from coronary artery disease, including the incidence of myocardial infarction (Dunningan & Harland, 1970), sudden cardiac death (Beard, Fuster, & Elveback, 1982), and cerebral infarction or hemorrhage (Haberman, Capildeo, & Rose, 1981; Ramirez-Lassepas, Haus, Lakatua, Sackett, & Swoyer, 1980; Shinkawa, Veda, Hasuo, Kiyohara, & Fujishima, 1990). Peaks in these conditions are generally located in late winter or spring.

Respiratory morbidity and mortality have been reported to peak in the winter months in both hemispheres, with deaths greatest during February in the northern hemisphere and during July in the southern hemisphere (reviewed by Smolensky et al., 1972). There are more asthma attacks in late summer and fall than in the late winter, which may be associated not only with the amount of antigens (pollen, dust, etc.) in the air, but also with seasonal changes in the immune system. Depression and suicides have been reported to peak in the spring (Lester, 1971) and may be related to circannual changes in hormone levels, as well as light duration and quality. Sexually transmitted diseases also show a circannual rhythm in incidence, with more new cases diagnosed in late summer for gonorrhea and in early winter for syphilis (Smolensky, 1981). In addition, a seasonal incidence of cervical pathology (infections and neoplasia) has been reported (Rietveld, Rietveld, Boon, Sothern, & Hrushesky, 1988; Rietveld, Boon, & Meulman, 1997).

D. Rhythms Associated with the Menstrual Cycle

Many functions have been shown to vary predictably during the menstrual cycle, including hypothalamic, pituitary, and gonadal hormones, such as luteinizing hormone, follicle-stimulating hormone estradiol, progesterone, estrogen, estrone sulfate, growth hormone, and aldosterone (Dyrenfurth, Jewelewicz, Warren, Ferin, & Vande Wiele, 1974). Melatonin also shows menstrual cycle variations with the highest values near menstruation and the lowest values at ovulation (Wetterberg et al., 1976). In addition, many other circamensual rhythms have been described for a large number of neurological, cardiovascular, respiratory, hematologic, enzymatic, and hormonal biological activities, and for several aspects of cervical and endometrial physiology (Bisdee, Garlick, & James, 1989; Reinberg & Smolensky, 1974). Menstrual cycle coordination of cellular immunity was shown to play a role in outcome of breast cancer surgery. When resection of a mammary carcinoma was performed near the time of estrus (fertile stage) in mice there were 2.5 times as many cures compared with the infertile stages (Ratajczak, Sothern, & Hrushesky, 1988). Extending this finding to premenopausal women with breast cancer, the 10-year disease-free survival was more than four fold better when resection was performed near midcycle than near menstruation (Hrushesky, Bluming, Gruber, & Sothern, 1989). Others have confirmed this finding that timing of surgery within 7–10 days near or following ovulation favorably affects breast cancer outcome (Fentiman, Gregory, & Richards, 1994; Hagen & Hrushesky, 1998; Hrushesky, 1996).

Several disorders, both physiological and psychological, have been linked to the menstrual cycle (Brush & Goodsmit, 1988; Pirke, Wuttke, & Schweiger, 1989). The days preceding and during menstruation have been linked with an increase in psychopathologic behavior, including psychiatric hospitalizations, suicide attempts, sickness in industry, and accidents (O'Conner, Shelly, & Stern, 1974). A temporal relationship between the onset and duration of manic episodes and the first half of the menstrual cycle was reported for a woman who recorded her manic episodes, daily basal temperature on arising, and dates of menstruation over an 11-year span (Sothern, Slover, & Morris, 1993). These disorders may arise from alterations or a pronounced imbalance between the various sex and stress hormones that occurs at certain stages of the menstrual cycle.

In addition to the possibility that female subjects might get pregnant during a study, the plethora of information concerning changes associated with the menstrual cycle has led researchers to generally exclude ovulating women from research protocols. Instead, they choose men or postmenopausal or surgically altered women, assuming the fertility cycle as a source of variability is reduced, if not eliminated. However, these researchers often overlook the fact that variability to the same extent as occurs over the menstrual cycle can manifest itself as circadian variability in many of the same variables in each 24-h period. Although less is known about monthly cycles in men, there have been a few reports of infradian variations in human males, including testosterone excretion (Harkness, 1974), grip strength, body weight, and beard growth (Kühl et al., 1974; Levine, Halberg, Sothern, Bartter, & Delea, 1974; Sothern, 1974). In a 15-year series of 24-h urine collections by one man, several rhythmic components in urine volume and 17-ketosteroids were found, including 1, 7, 20, 30, and 365 days (Halberg, Engeli, Hamburger, & Hillman, 1965; Halberg & Hamburger, 1964). Such low frequency rhythms and their possible interaction with other components in the spectrum of rhythms in males constitute a potentially important, yet overlooked source of variability that needs to be studied further. For example, it is not known why low-frequency rhythms in males tend to be shorter than those found in females (about 20 days vs. about 30 days, respectively).

E. Circadian Time: Clock Hour vs. Stage of Rhythm

When comparing results from different synchronizing schedules, between species (such as mice vs. humans) or when suggesting sampling or treatment times, a certain amount of misconception and inaccuracy can arise whenever "time of day" (external, solar time) is used, rather than "stage of rhythm" (internal, biologic time) (Sothern, 1995). In preclinical studies, it is often mistakenly assumed that physiologic function is constant if the lighting regimen is fixed as continuous light or darkness. However, although circadian rhythms are anchored genetically (endogenously), they are synchronized by (entrained) and maintain certain phase relationships to external (exogenous) factors, especially the sleep portion of the light-dark (LD) schedule (Aschoff, 1960; Halberg, 1960). These rhythms will persist with a period different from 24 h when external time cues are suppressed or removed, such as during complete social isolation or in constant light or darkness (Aschoff, Hoffman, Pöhl, & Wever, 1975; Bruce, 1960; Halberg & Barnum, 1961). In addition, if the LD schedule is changed due to shifts in work or other social schedules, including a change to or from daylight savings time or transmeridian flights across one or more time zones, circadian rhythms do not shift immediately, but will begin to shift by about an hour a day so that peak/trough times will ultimately reset to the same phase relationship on the new sleep-wake schedule as the old one. On reviewing the synchronizing effect of LD, Aschoff and colleagues concluded that circadian rhythms are synchronized to a typical time relationship with respect to the environmental cycle and that sleep onset had immediate effects in determining a rhythm's timing. This is also the case in rodent studies, in which light onset (= sleep onset) is the dominant reference point of the LD regimen, when synchronization is complete and no other factors, such as feeding or treatment times, are present. Indeed, the coding of preclinical test- times in hours after lighting onset (HALO) facilitates comparison of results from studies with the same photofraction (i.e., LD 12:12) but with differing times of L-onset (Sothern, 1995). Use of circadian time, such as HALO, should also facilitate the often erroneous extrapolation of test times from nocturnally active rodents to diurnally active humans. For example, 8 AM means something completely opposite to a mouse and a human. Testing a mouse at 8 AM, which may be 2 h after light onset and thus during a mouse's usual time of sleeping, would be the physiologic equivalent to testing a human at midnight, 2 h after having gone to bed at 10 PM.

Different sleep-wake times will also result in apparent timing differences in humans when a peak in a variable is referred to an arbitrary external reference point (most commonly local midnight), whereas adjustment to an internal time reference, such as the beginning, middle or end of sleep, may reveal the same phase relationship between individuals on different sleep schedules. Thus, specification of a certain clock hour without regard to usual sleep-wake times may unintentionally result in sampling or treatment being assigned to an incorrect circadian stage. If a treatment is prescribed for 6 AM, it will be delivered 1 h after awakening for someone arising at 5 AM or 2 h before awakening for someone arising at 8 AM. In the case of a night worker, 6 AM will represent the end of the activity span, which may be an undesirable stage for treatment. Thus, it is the stage of rhythm (or circadian time) and not time of day that will ultimately result in a successful diagnosis or chronotherapy. Whenever possible, a physiologic variable that is generally known to display a prominent circadian rhythm, such as body temperature, total leukocytes, plasma cortisol, or urinary potassium can be measured as a marker rhythm to confirm an individual's synchrony and ensure and/or guide the correct timing of a prescribed treatment (Hermida, Halberg, & Langevin, 1986; Mormont, Claustrat, Waterhouse, Touitou, & Lévi, 1998; Smaaland, Sothern, et al., 1995). For economic and technical reasons, a reasonable alternative to repeated sampling of blood or urine for marker rhythms or use of machines to determine physiologic marker rhythms (activity, blood pressure, temperature, etc.), is to record the times a patient went to bed and got up for the past week and try to maintain this schedule throughout treatment. A treatment time based on an appropriate quadrant of the 24-h day, which has previously proved successful in the treatment of humans or rodents, is then selected according to circadian stage (hours after awakening or from midsleep) rather than arbitrary clock hours (time of day) (Sothern, 1995). A case in point is a recent study on the cardiovascular effects of aspirin that reported results from three dosing times in relation to time awakening or going to bed, which found that the time most effective in reducing blood pressure and its associated cardiovascular risk was when a low dose of aspirin was taken within 2 h of bedtime (Hermida, Fernández, Ayala, Mojón, & Iglesias, 1997).

II. STATISTICAL DETECTION AND DESCRIPTION OF RHYTHMS

The existence of biologic rhythms makes their detection and objective analysis very important in the health sciences. If individual values or time-point means appear to differ from each other or there is a recurring pattern that is obvious to the naked eye, it may appear that a circadian or other variation is present. However, until the time series is objectively evaluated by appropriate statistical procedures, one should refrain from using the word *rhythm* and may only describe the pattern as a variation.

To determine whether there is a systematic effect of time in a variable, it is necessary to collect data by making repeated measurements over several hours, days, weeks, months or years, to constitute a time series. When only two test times are being evaluated for time effect (e.g., sampling at only two times of the day), they are usually compared for significant differences by a t-test (for means) or by chi-square (for proportions). If these tests result in a probability level of 0.05 or less, it may be concluded that a statistically significant effect of time is present that may be a reflection of an underlying rhythm, but the complete characteristics of the rhythm itself cannot be described because only two times were measured.

When three or more test times are available, the time series may be tested for time effect by chi-square (if comparing proportions) or by an analysis of variance (ANOVA) for a comparison of means. With three or preferably more time-points available, the time series can also be tested for the presence of a rhythm, often by the fit of an appropriate model, such as a cosine. There are several methods in use to analyze times series, each with their advantages and disadvantages depending on the type and schedule of data collection. Periodogram and power spectra methods have been proposed by many authors (Enright, 1981; Martin, 1981; Martin & Brinkmann, 1976; van Cauter, 1974; Winfree, 1980). However, these classical methods generally require equally-spaced data over integral multiples of the period investigated. In addition, when using these analysis methods, there can be no missing values in a time series, which is often the case in a biologic time series. For analytical purposes, an interpolated value is used in place of a missing value, which may or may not be a reflection of the true value that might have been obtained had a measurement been taken at the missing time. In-depth reviews of the many procedures and other considerations in data acquisition and analysis are available (DePrins, Cornélissen, & Malbecq, 1986; Minors and Waterhouse, 1989; Morgan and Minors, 1995; Reinberg and Smolensky, 1983).

A. The Cosinor Technique

A common quantitative method used for analysis of periodic phenomena is the cosinor technique, involving the least-squares fit of a cosine to a time series (Halberg, Johnson, Nelson, Runge, & Sothern, 1972). The cosinor technique is very robust in that it can analyze a time series in which the data are not always equidistant or sampled over integral multiples of the period in question. It also can be useful in objectively quantifying individual rhythm characteristics, which can later be summarized for groups of individuals (Bingham, Arbogast, Cornélissen-Guillaume, Lee, & Halberg, 1982; Nelson, Tong, Lee, & Halberg, 1979).

The cosinor method analyzes a time series according to predefined criteria using a least-squares technique based on a cosine wave of variable period, phase, amplitude, and level. Detection of a statistically significant cosine fit with a given period implies a regular recurring, and therefore nonrandomness in a time series, with values oscillating at that frequency. Often the waveform of a time series can be more accurately approximated by the least squares fit of a multiple-component cosine model involving a concomitant fit of two or more components (i.e., 24 h plus 12 or 8 or 3 h, etc.) (Tong, Nelson, Sothern, & Halberg, 1977). Some cosinor programs are available for the personal computer (Bourden, Buguet, Cucherat, & Radomski, 1995; Mattes, Witte, Hohmann, & Lemmer, 1991; Monk & Fort, 1983; Sothern, Voegele, Mattson, & Hrushesky, 1989). A program called ChronoLab, written for the Macintosh computer (Mojón, Fernandez, & Hermida, 1992), is one of the easiest cosinor programs to use and is available free of charge over the Internet by contacting its authors at http://www.tsc.uvigo.es/BIO/References.html.

The detection of a significant rhythm will depend on several factors, including adequate sampling over an adequate number of cycles. It may be necessary to increase the sample size by collecting more data at more time-points over a longer timespan or from more individuals to detect a significant rhythm. Also, if it is not possible to quantify a rhythm mathematically, a waveform that is (1) reproducible from one day to the next or among several individuals or (2) that will change in a predictable way following manipulation of one or more synchronizers (lighting, feeding) may be evidence of a rhythm (Minors & Waterhouse, 1989).

B. Rhythm Parameters Estimated by Cosinor Analysis

Several parameters are derived from the best-fitting curve to describe the rhythm's characteristics (see Figure 1). These include the (1) period (duration of one complete cycle); (2) mesor (the midvalue of the cosine curve representing a rhythm-adjusted mean [from *meson* = middle of and *rhythm*]); (3) amplitude (the distance from the mesor to the peak or trough of the fitted cosine indicating the predictable rise and fall around the mesor); and (4) acrophase (the time of the peak of the fitted curve, representing the calculated average time of high values in the data). The time of

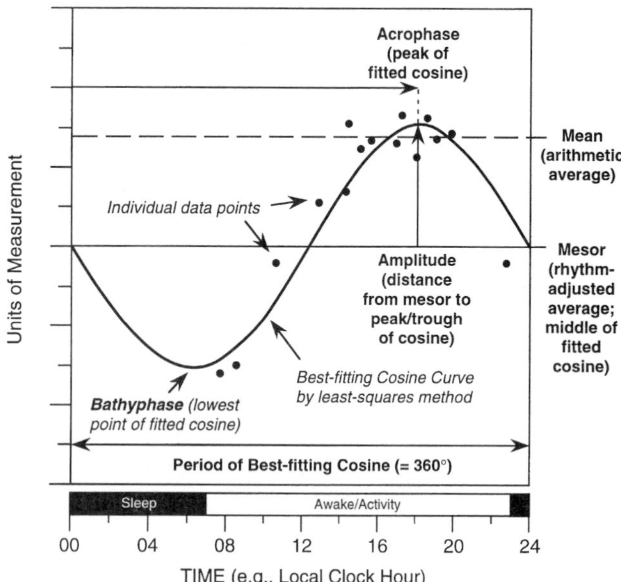

FIGURE 1 Use of the cosinor method in rhythm detection and description of characteristics of a rhythm. Due to unequidistant sampling, with more values in the afternoon and none during the night, the arithmetic mean is closer to the higher values and may not be representative of the actual overall 24-h mean. The fit of a 24-h cosine by the least-squares (cosinor) method reveals that the best-fitting curve follows, and therefore describes, the actual pattern in the data more closely than a flat line (the mean). Several rhythm parameters and their 95% confidence limits also can be computed. The midvalue of the fitted curve, the mesor, represents a rhythm-adjusted mean, not biased by dense sampling at some times and not at others (but equals the arithmetic mean when sampling is equidistant). Other characteristics of the rhythm include the calculated midtime of maximal values, the acrophase, (or low values, the bathyphase) and the extent of predictable variation above and below the mesor, the amplitude. Note that even with the lack of data at night, a rhythmic pattern appears obvious to the naked eye.

the lowest point of a rhythm is called the bathyphase (bathy = deep), whereas the peak of a multiple-component cosine is called the orthophase (ortho = right, correct). The objective statistically determined mesor, amplitude, and acrophase, as opposed to a subjective "eye-balled" evaluation, can be extremely useful in describing the characteristics of a rhythm and when comparing two or more rhythms in an individual, or between individuals or groups.

III. RHYTHMS OF THE IMMUNE SYSTEM

A. The Bone Marrow

It is well established that the different cellular elements of peripheral blood, such as granulocytes, lymphocytes, erythrocytes, and many other elements that constitute the immune system, undergo significant circadian variations when sampled over time (Haus, Lakatua, Swoyer, & Sackett-Lundeen, 1983). Since these cells arise from the bone marrow (BM) (Figure 2), it is surprising that only recently have more detailed data assessing time-dependent variations in cell kinetics in human BM become available (Laerum, Smaaland, & Sletvold, 1989). The patterns of proliferation of BM cells have been thought to be characterized by a steady-state cytokinetic rate equaling the rate at which cells in the peripheral blood are removed (Beck, 1991), which is accompanied by a rise and fall ("reactive" homeostasis) occurring under certain abnormal physiologic or pathologic conditions (Butcher, 1990). The production and migration of mature granulocytes into peripheral blood is both dependent on the actual needs of the body and on several hormonal and regulatory factors. For example, physical exercise and cortisone/cortisol are strong mobilizers of granulocytes, as are acute bacterial infections. Classic textbooks (Beck, 1991) teach that the cell division cycle is about 24 h in length, with phase M (the period of mitosis) lasting 0.5–1 h, phase G1 (the postmitotic/presynthetic gap) lasting 10 h, phase S (the period of DNA synthesis) lasting about 9 h, and phase G2 (the postsynthetic/premitotic gap) lasting about 4 h, while a resting cell is in phase G0. No mention is made, however, about a possible coordination in time, such that more cells might be in a certain cell cycle phase at one time of the day than another. It has been estimated that every second, up to 2 million red cells, 2 million platelets, and 700,000 granulocytes are produced in the bone marrow (Spivak, 1984) (Figure 2), resulting in an estimated production every 24 h of more than 170 billion each of red cells and platelets and more than 60 billion white cells. Granulocytes, with an average life-span of only 6–14 h need to be replaced every day, whereas other cells may live 1 or 2 weeks or longer before needing replacement (Nathan, 1987, 1988).

The continuous extremely high proliferative capacity of the bone marrow is rivaled only by the skin, intestinal mucosa and oral mucosa, each of which has been shown to exhibit circadian rhythms in humans (Bjarnason, Jordan, & Sothern, 1999; Buchi, Moore, Hrushesky, Sothern, & Rubin, 1991; Fisher, 1968; Scheving, 1959). New information related to proliferation in the BM has emerged, however, and it has become increasingly clear that hematopoiesis is not a temporally fixed phenomenon, but that there are strong endogenous rhythmic variations in the bone marrow's proliferative and mobilizing processes (Figure 2) as a part of an organism's "predictive" homeostasis. Circadian rhythms of proliferation in human and murine BM have recently been reviewed (Smaaland & Sothern, 1994). In addition, rhythmic activity of many normal organ functions, including the BM and adrenals, has been deduced from certain laboratory tests, all of which express a degree of circadian rhythmicity (Haus et al., 1983, 1984, 1988; Lévi et al., 1985; Lévi, Canon, Blum, Reinberg, & Mathé, 1983).

Killman, Cronkite, Fliedner, and Bond (1962) and Mauer (1965) first reported circadian variations in normal human BM proliferation with a mitotic peak around midnight. Two other reports indirectly confirmed a circadian rhythm in BM by finding a circadian variation in circulating human myeloid progenitor cells (CFU-GM), with highest colony number during the day in healthy men (Ross, Pollak, Akman, & Bachur, 1980; Verma et al., 1980). Smaaland and colleagues (1991) found a statistically significant circadian rhythm in DNA synthesis (percentage of cells in S-phase) in the total BM cell population in healthy men, with the lowest counts around midnight and the highest counts in the afternoon. A circadian rhythm in the number of colony-forming units of the myeloid progenitor cells (CFU-GM) in the same BM samples also was discovered (Smaaland et al., 1992). This 24-h rhythm was found to co-vary with the percentage of cells in DNA synthesis, with values 150% higher at midday than at midnight. In this group of healthy men, both DNA and CFU-GM in BM demonstrated a circannual rhythm, as well, with higher values observed in the late summer (Sothern, Smaaland, & Moore, 1995). In addition, similar significant circadian variations in BM erythropoietic and myeloid precursor cells have been demonstrated, with higher proliferation during the day as opposed to the night (Abrahamsen, Smaaland, Sothern, & Laerum, 1997). A recent circadian study on the proliferative activity and cell yield of the human BM stem cell progenitor population in 5 healthy men found that a lower yield of CD34+ cells occurred in each subject when BM was aspirated in the evening or during night, whereas an average six fold higher yield occurred during the daytime (Abrahamsen, Smaaland, Sothern, & Laerum, 1998). It has also been shown that cancer patients with a normal circadian cortisol rhythm and no metastases to the bone marrow also had the same circadian pattern, with highest BM S-phase fractions during the day (Smaaland, Abrahamsen, Svardal, Lote, & Ueland, 1992). It has thus become increasingly clear that hematopoiesis is not a temporally fixed phenomenon. Assuming an average hourly production of approximately 2.5 billion granulocytes per hour (see above), a circadian amplitude of 50% would indicate that the bone marrow might be actively producing

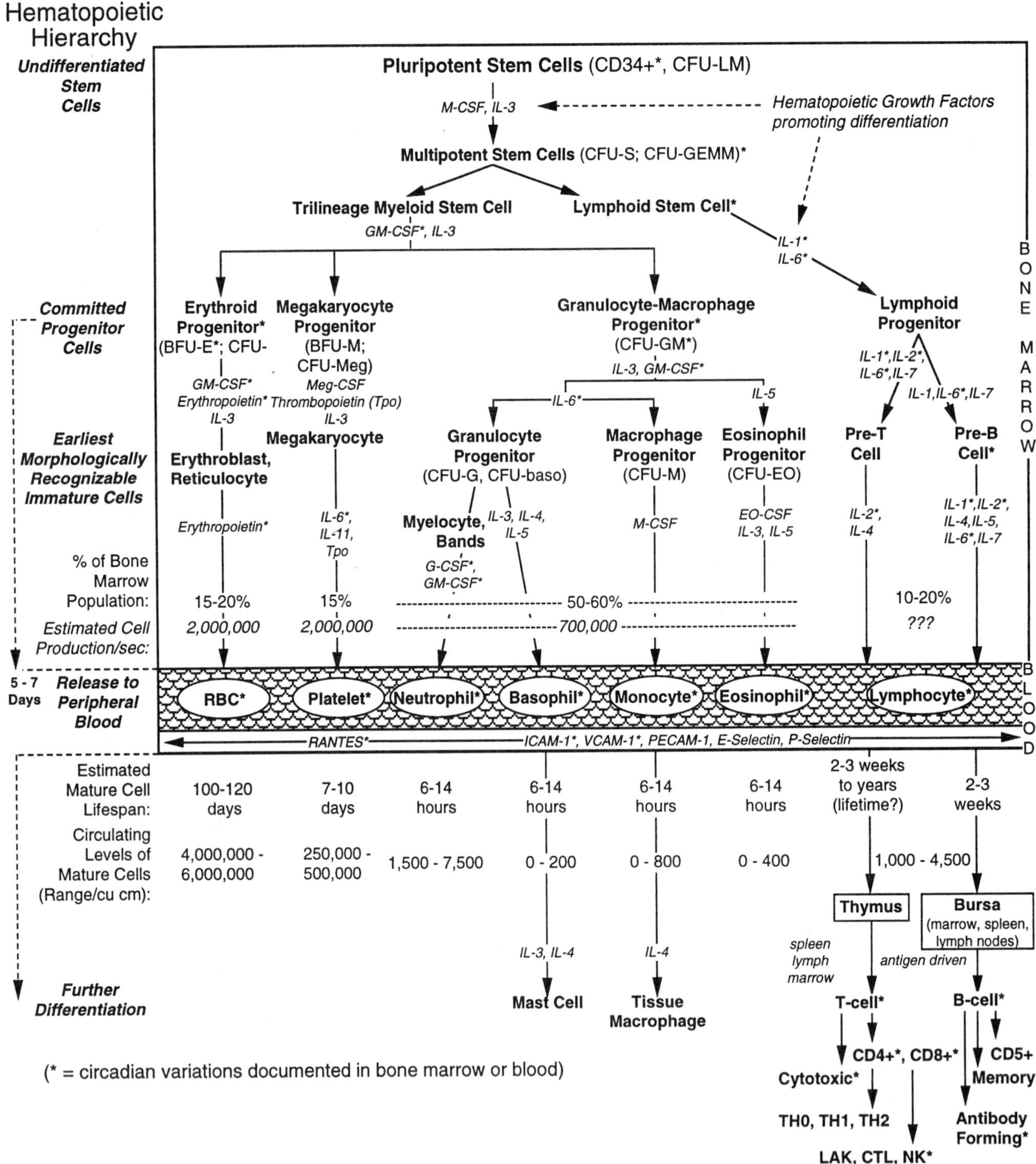

FIGURE 2 Scheme for hematopoiesis: the development of lymphoid, myeloid, and erythroid blood cells in the bone marrow. The maturation sequence from pluripotent stem cells to morphologically recognizable immature cells to mature cells that are released into the circulation is tightly controlled by both positive and negative growth factors and endogenous and exogenous needs. Many of the parameters and dynamics have now been shown to be circadian rhythmic in humans (designated by an asterisk).

50% more myeloid cells at midday (approximately 3.75 billion cells/h), and producing half the hourly average (1.25 billion/h) during the night. This can be taken advantage of in several ways, both in relation to diagnostics of the immune system and to primary diseases of the bone marrow, such as myelodysplastic conditions, and cytotoxic side effects of cancer and other therapies (see Section III).

B. Circadian Immune Functions

Virtually all immunological and related variables investigated to date in animals and humans have been shown to display circadian (and other) rhythms (Barnes, 1989; Levi Reinberg, & Canon, 1989; Smaaland & Sothern, 1994; Smolensky, 1983). A series of tables summarize circadian information about the timing of highest values for a wide range of variables of interest in the study of the immune network in humans. These include circulating cells (Table I); lymphocyte metabolism and transformability (Table II); circulating hormones and other substances that may exert various actions on different targets of the immune system (Table III); cytokines, receptors, and adhesion molecules (Table IV); cell cycle events in health and cancer (Table V); lung function (Table VI); reactions to antigen challenge (Table VII); and disease etiology and symptoms (Table VIII).

There may be disturbances or alterations in some of these circadian rhythms during the disease process and this in turn may sometimes prevent a rhythm from being described for an individual or for a group of patients (Bruguerolle et al., 1986; Focan, 1995). This was the case for serum neopterin, a marker of cellular immune system activation, which showed a significant circadian rhythm with a peak in the morning for a group of 7 clinically healthy individuals, but not for a group of 6 HIV-infected subjects (Table III) (Rhame et al., 1989), due to an alteration in the timing of peak values in 2 patients (subjects 22 and 26) (Figure 3). In other disease conditions, rhythms may persist that are comparably- timed with controls. This is the case for

TABLE I Circadian Immune Functions in Humans: Circulating Cells

Variable	Units, assay, or method	Time(s) or range of maxima	Author	Year
Total WBC	cells/cu mm	2156–2308	Haus, et al.	1988
Neutrophils, total	cells/cu mm	1820–2032	Haus, et al.	1988
Neutrophils, adult	cells/cu mm	1808–1948	Haus, et al.	1988
Neutrophils, bands	cells/cu mm	1736–0216	Haus, et al.	1988
Lymphocytes	cells/cu mm	0004–0108	Haus, et al.	1988
Monocytes	cells/cu mm	1816–2256	Haus, et al.	1988
Eosinophils	cells/cu mm	0056–0332	Haus, et al.	1988
Basophils	cells/cu mm	1840–0156	Kanabrocki, et al.	1990
CD34+	cell/cu mm	0000	Bjarnason, et al.	1996
T lymphocytes (OKT3+)	cells/cu mm	0000–0400	Lévi, Canon, Touitou, Sulon, et al.	1988
T-helper lymphocytes (OKT4+)	cells/cu mm	0000	Lévi, et al.	1985
T-suppressor-cytotoxic lymphocytes (OKT8+)	cells/cu mm	2030	Lévi, et al.	1983
T-helper/T-suppressor cytotoxic ratio	OKT4/OKT8	0030–0430	Lévi, Canon, Touitou, Sulon, et al.	1988
NK cells	CD3+/CD16+	1701–1915	Born, et al.	1997
Activated T-cells	HLA-DR+	2030–0306	Born, et al.	1997
Activated B-cells	OKIA	1150 & 2350	Lévi, Canon, Touitou, Sulon, et al.	1988
B lymphocytes (SIg+)	cells/cu mm	2000	Lévi, Canon, Touitou, Sulon, et al.	1988
Pre-B lymphocytes	CALLA	0150	Canon, et al.	1985
Light-chain-bearing B lymphocytes	anti-κ+	0900 & 2100	Lévi, et al.	1985
Light-chain-bearing B lymphocytes	anti-λ+	2040	Lévi, et al.	1985452

Notes: Results from healthy, diurnally active subjects unless otherwise noted. Time in local clock H:Min (range for highest values or 95% limits from cosinor analysis).

TABLE II Circadian Immune Functions in Humans: Lymphocyte Metabolism and Transformability

Variable	Units, assay, or method	Time(s) or range of maxima	Author	Year
DNA	synthesis	1000 & 2300	Carter, et al.	1975
RNA polymerase B	activity	0000	Heitbrock, et al.	1976
Total RNA	content	0600 & 1800	Sanchez, et al.	unpubl
Total RNA-cancer patients	content	0612–1140	Hrushesky, et al.	1980
Glucose-6-phosphate dehydrogenase	activity	1600	Ramot, et al.	1976
6-Phosphodehydrogenase	activity	2000	Ramot, et al.	1976
Lactate dehydrogenase	activity	1600	Ramot, et al.	1976
Hexokinase	activity	1200 & 2000	Ramot, et al.	1976
Glutamate-oxaloacetate transaminase	activity	2000	Ramot, et al.	1976
NK activity of mononuclear cells	51Cr-labeled K562 CML cells	1100	Williams, et al.	1980
NK activity of mononuclear cells	51Cr-labeled SRBC (ADCC)	1300	Abo, et al.	1981
NK activity of mononuclear cells	HNK1 monoclonal ab	1115	Ritchie, et al.	1983
NK activity of mononuclear cells	HNK1 monoclonal ab	1130	Lévi, Canon, Touitou, Reinberg, et al.	1988
PMN phagocytic activity	particles ingested/cell	2218–0332	Melchart, et al.	1992
Isolated lymphocyte transformability	PHA-induced	0800–1000	Tavidia, et al.	1972
Isolated lymphocyte transformability	spontaneous	1000 & 2200	Carter, et al.	1975
Whole blood lymphocyte transformability	PHA-induced	2000	Carter, et al.	1975
Isolated lymphocyte transformability	PHA-induced	1200	Eskola, et al.	1976
Whole blood lymphocyte transformability	spontaneous	0800 & 2000	Eskola, et al.	1976
Isolated lymphocyte transformability	ConA induced	2000	Haus, et al.	1983
Isolated lymphocyte transformability	PPD induced	0200	Haus, et al.	1983
Isolated lymphocyte transformability	PWM induced	1200	Haus, et al.	1983

Notes: Results from healthy, diurnally active subjects unless otherwise noted. Time in local clock H:Min (range for highest values or 95% limits from cosinor analysis). ADCC=antibody-dependent cell cytotoxicity; CML=chronic myelogenous leukemia; conA=convalin A; HNK1=human natural killer cells; PHA=phytohemagglutinin; PMN=polymorphonuclear; PPD=purified protein derivative; PWM=pokeweed mitogen; SRBC=sheep red blood cells.

prostate-specific antigen (PSA). As can be seen in Figure 4, reanalysis of normalized data from Maatman (1989) shows that men with prostatic cancer and elevated PSA levels had the identical circadian pattern in PSA as clinically healthy men (Mermall et al., 1995), with higher values in the late afternoon. Similarly, the circadian rhythm in the higher number of mitoses in tumor nodules in a woman with metastatic epidermoid carcinoma was shown to be comparably timed with the lower number of mitoses in normal skin, with an evening peak and a morning valley, indicating that the cell type of cancer origin may confer specific circadian cytokinetic time-keeping characteristics on the analogous cancer cell (Hrushesky, Lannin, & Haus, 1999).

Response to treatment may also involve the re-establishment of synchronized circadian rhythms. This was the case for carcinoembryonic antigen (CEA) in a group of 25 cancer patients (Touitou et al., 1988). Prior to treatment, a circadian rhythm as a group phenomenon was not significant due to several individuals having highest values near midnight rather than near midday, as is found in healthy subjects (Table III). A return to normal circadian rhythmicity was observed in all patients after 4 or 8 courses of timed treatments (Table III). Either circadian-specified tumor therapy or cancer control per se allowed for the normalization of the circadian rhythm in CEA. The normalization of circadian rhythms in cancer patients following treatment has also been observed for leukocyte differential counts (Blaauw et al., 1997) and for liver enzymes and lactate dehydrogenase (Karlsdottir et al., 1997).

Phase relationships between bone marrow cell proliferation and circulating leukocytes have been established in health (Abrahamsen et al., 1999; Smaaland, Sothern, et al., 1995). However, it is of interest to point out that although DNA synthesis in

TABLE III Circadian Immune Functions in Humans: Circulating Substances

Variable	Units, assay, or method	Time(s) or range of maxima	Author	Year
Adrenaline—health & asthma	nmol/L	1600	Barnes, et al.	1980
Cortisol—asthma	nmol/L	0700	Barnes, et al.	1980
Cyclic AMP	nmol/L	1600	Barnes, et al.	1980
Histamine	nmol/L	0400	Barnes, et al.	1980
Cortisol—saliva	μg/dL	0540–0820	Sothern, et al.	1994
Cortisol—serum	μg/dL	0626–0824	Sothern, et al.	1994
Cortisol—urine	μg/h	0646–0916	Sothern, et al.	1994
Melatonin—saliva	ng/dL	0216–0413	Sothern, et al.	1994
Melatonin—serum	ng/dL	0204–0347	Sothern, et al.	1994
Melatonin—urine	ng/h	0334–0506	Sothern, et al.	1994
Immunoglobulins				
IgA in health	mg/L	1210–1517	Reinberg, Schuller, et al.	1977
IgG in health	mg/L	1418–1600	Reinberg, Schuller, et al.	1977
IgM in health	mg/L	1428–1747	Reinberg, Schuller, et al.	1977
IgE in asthma	IU/L	0744–1550	Gaultier, et al.	1987
Complement, Protein				
Complement C3	mg/dL	1156–1932	Pallansch, et al.	1979
Total proteins	gm/L	1430–1803	Reinberg, Schuller, et al.	1977
C-reactive protein—rheumatoid arthritis	mg/L	2336	Herold & Günther	1992
Antigen, Immune Activity				
Carcinoembryonic antigen (CEA)—men	ng/mL	0628–0928	Touitou, et al.	1988
CEA—women	ng/mL	1448–2020	Touitou, et al.	1988
CEA—ovarian cancer	ng/mL	0828–1348	Touitou, et al.	1988
CEA—bladder cancer	ng/mL	0816–1514	Touitou, et al.	1988
Prostate—specific antigen (PSA)	ng/mL	1440–1924	Mermall, et al.	1995
PSA—prostate cancer	ng/mL	1424–1940	Maatman	1989
Neopterin—blood	ng/mL	0628–0928	Rhame, et al.	1989
Neopterin—urine	nmol/4h	0030–0830	Auzeby, et al.	1988

Notes: Results from healthy, diurnally active subjects unless otherwise noted. Time in local clock H:Min (range for highest values or 95% limits from cosinor analysis).

the bone marrow shows similarly timed circadian rhythms in health (Smaaland et al., 1991) and cancer (Smaaland, Abrahamsen, et al., 1992), with peak values near midday (Table V), the DNA synthesis rhythm in non-Hodgkin's lymphoma cells reached their peak around midnight (Smaaland, Lote, Sothern, & Laerum, 1993). Thus, normal and disease-state circadian phase relationships need to be established to optimize interventions and procedures (Mormont et al., 1998; Smaaland, Laerum, Abrahamsen, Sothern, & Lote, 1995).

C. Cytokines

The coordinated expression of cytokines and adhesion molecules is essential for the development of immune and inflammatory processes. Cytokine molecules are normally soluble, and their various effects are initiated by their binding to membrane-bound receptors on cells. Many receptors also have been identified as soluble in blood and urine. Following binding, signal transduction produces a cascade of intracellular signals and effects, wherein cells are instructed to alter their proliferation, differentiation phenotype, secretion, or rate of migration (Thompson, 1994).

More than 60 different cytokines have been identified and can be placed in distinct families such as interleukins and colony-stimulating factors (generally immunomodulatory and regulating factors for hematopoiesis), interferons (antiviral and immunomodulatory functions), chemokines (chemoattractant

TABLE IV Circadian Immune Functions in Humans: Cytokines, Receptors, Adhesion Molecules

Variable	Units, assay, or method	Time(s) or range of maxima	Author	Year
		Cytokines		
IL-1α	ng/mL	2030	Bourin, et al.	1990
IL-1α	ng/mL	2100	Petrovsky, et al.	1998
IL-1β	pg/mL	2120–0008	Hohagen, et al.	1993
IL-1β	U/mL	0225	Entzian, et al.	1996
IL-1β (sleep apnea)	U/mL	0104	Entzian, et al.	1996
IL-2	pg/mL	1330–1630	Young, et al.	1995
IL-2	pg/mL	0100	Lissoni, et al.	1998
IL-6 (rheumatoid arthritis)	pg/mL	0730	Arvidson, et al.	1994
IL-6	pg/mL	0200	Sothern, et al.	1995
IL-6	ng/mL	0211	Entzian, et al.	1996
IL-6 (sleep apnea)	ng/mL	2047	Entzian, et al.	1996
IL-6 (urine)	pg/h	1800	Sothern, et al.	1995a
IL-10	pg/mL	0730 & 1930	Young, et al.	1995
IL-12	pg/mL	2300	Petrovsky, et al.	1998
GM-CSF	pg/mL	1330 & 1930	Young, et al.	1995
GM-CSF	pg/mL	0657	Akbulut, et al.	1999
IFN-γ	pg/mL	2352–0148	Hohagen, et al.	1993
IFN-γ	U/mL	2202	Entzian, et al.	1996
IFN-γ (sleep apnea)	U/mL	1720	Entzian, et al.	1996
IFN-γ	pg/mL	0000	Petrovsky, et al.	1998
TNF-α	pg/mL	0730 & 1330	Young, et al.	1995
TNF-α	ng/mL	0232	Entzian, et al.	1996
TNF-α	ng/mL	2130	Petrovsky, et al.	1998
TNF-α (colorectal cancer)	pg/mL	0040	Muc-Wierzgon, et al.	1998
		Receptors		
IL-2sR	U/mL	1229	Lemmer, et al.	1992
IL-2sR - rheumatoid arthritis	U/mL	1608	Herold & Günther	1992
Transferrin receptor (sTfR)	ng/mL	1616–1948	Sothern, et al.	1995
IL-6sR	ng/mL	1619	Roitman-Johnson, et al.	1996
TNF-R55	ng/mL	0557–0945	Liebmann, et al.	1998
		Adhesion Molecules		
VCAM-1	ng/mL	1505	Sothern, et al.	1997
ICAM-1	ng/mL	0730–1330	Roitman-Johnson, et al.	1998

Notes: Results from healthy, diurnally active subjects unless otherwise noted. Time in local clock H:Min (range for highest values or 95% limits from cosinor analysis).

and growth regulating functions), growth factors (connective tissue functions), and tumor necrosis/nerve growth factors (immunomodulatory and growth regulators) (Callard & Gearing, 1994). Adhesion molecules are cell surface structures that primarily determine the migration route of cells, but they also affect other cell functions, such as cytotoxicity and antigen presentation (Harlan & Liu, 1992). The main adhesion molecule families include selectin adhesins (initial phases of cell adhesion to capture leukocytes from the circulation onto the vascular endothelium); immunoglobulin adhesins (establishes firm adhesion of leukocytes), and integrins (emigration into tissues and activation and cytolytic function of lymphocytes).

Both cytokine and adhesion molecule systems are therefore important components of inflammation and immunity and their interdependent network will be

TABLE V Circadian Immune Functions in Humans: Cell Cycle Events

Variable	Units, assay, or method	Time(s) or range of maxima	Author	Year
		Bone marrow		
Total cells	DNA S-phase (%)	1052–1440	Smaaland, et al.	1991
Total cells	CFU-GM (colonies)	1100–1608	Smaaland, Laerum, et al.	1992
Total cells (cancer)	DNA S-phase (%)	1100	Smaaland, Abrahamsen, et al.	1992
Erythroid precursors	DNA S-phase (%)	0800–1600	Abrahamsen, et al.	1997
Myeloid precursors	DNA S-phase (%)	0800–2000	Abrahamsen, et al.	1997
Pluripotent precursors (CD34+ cells)	DNA S-phase (%)	1024–1448	Abrahamsen, et al.	1998
		Rectal mucosa		
Total cells	DNA S-phase (DPM/μg DNA)	0320–1128	Buchi, et al.	1991
		Oral mucosa		
Late G1-phase	p53	0800–1400	Bjarnason, et al.	1999
G1, early S-phase	Cyclin-E	1400–1600	Bjarnason, et al.	1999
G2-phase	Cyclin-A	1400–1800	Bjarnason, et al.	1999
M-phase	Cyclin-B1	1800–0000	Bjarnason, et al.	1999
Proliferating cells	Ki67	0000–0500	Bjarnason, et al.	1999
		Cancer		
Mammary	mitotic index	1300–1500	Voutilainen	1953
Skin	mitotic index	2200	Tahti	1956
Skin	DNA synthesis	0600–1200	Focan & Pierard	1976
Ovarian	DNA synthesis	1100–1500	Klevecz, et al.	1987
Non-Hodgkins lymphoma	DNA S-phase	2220–0348	Smaaland, et al.	1993
Head & neck	DNA synthesis	1000	Focan	1995
Lung	DNA synthesis	0000–0600	Focan	1995
Lung	mitotic index	1800–2400	Focan	1995
Uterine/cervix	DNA synthesis	1200	Focan	1995
Uterine/cervix	mitotic index	0000	Focan	1995

Notes: Results from healthy, diurnally active subjects unless otherwise noted. Time in local clock H:Min (range for highest values or 95% limits from cosinor analysis).

TABLE VI Circadian Immune Functions in Humans: Lung Function

Variable	Units, assay, or method	Time(s) or range of maxima	Author	Year
FEV1	L/sec	1600	Guberan, et al.	1969
Specific airway conductance	plethysmograph	1200	Kerr	1973
PEF	L/min	1128–1624	Smolensky & Halberg	1977
Lung secretions	mucociliary clearance	1200–1800	Bateman, et al.	1978
PEF—asthma	L/min	1600	Barnes, et al.	1980
PEF—health & asthma	L/min	1600	Hetzel & Clark	1980
FEV1—extrinsic asthma	L/sec	1119-1706	Todisco, et al.	1995
FEV1—intrinsic asthma	L/sec	0938-1743	Todisco, et al.	1995

Notes: Results from healthy, diurnally active subjects unless otherwise noted. Time in local clock H:Min (range for highest values or 95% limits from cosinor analysis).

TABLE VII Circadian Immune Functions in Humans: Reactions

Variable	Units, assay, or method	Time(s) or range of maxima	Author	Year
	Challenge			
Histamine—induced Itching	pruritus	0000	Cormia	1952
Histamine—inhalation	bronchial reactivity	0000–0400	DeVries, et al.	1962
Grass pollen—skin testing	skin reactivity	1900–2300	Reinberg, et al.	1965
Histamine—skin testing	skin reactivity	2144–0048	Reinberg, et al.	1969
House dust—skin testing	skin reactivity	1632–0108	Reinberg at el	1969
Penicillen—skin testing	skin reactivity	1848–0400	Reinberg, et al.	1969
Acetycholine—inhalation	bronchial reactivity (FEV1)	2300	Reinberg at el	1971
House dust—inhalation—asthmatics	bronchial reactivity (FEV1, PEF)	2300	Gervais, et al.	1977
Tuberculin challenge	response	0700	Cove-Smith, et al.	1978
Allergen exposure—single daytime	dyspnea	night	Taylor, et al.	1979
	Antigen stimulation			
IFN-γ Response to purified protein derivative	U/mL	2230–0130	Petrovsky, et al.	1994
IFN-γ Response to tetanus toxoid	U/mL	2300–0200	Petrovsky, et al.	1994
	Vaccination			
Venezuelian equine encephelomyelitis virus	antibody levels	0800	Feigin	1970
A/Philippines & A/Chili viruses	antibody levels	1200	Langlois, et al.	1986
Hepatitis B	antibody levels	1300–1500	Pöllman et al.	1988

Notes: Results from healthy, diurnally active subjects unless otherwise noted. Time in local clock H:Min (range for highest values or 95% limits from cosinor analysis).

crucial in fully understanding their roles in health and disease, including selecting appropriate times for diagnostic sampling and therapies. For example, lymphoid cell responsiveness to IL-2 was shown to be dependent on the circadian time of exposure, suggesting that optimal delivery of immunotherapy to cancer patients might be guided by considering immunological rhythms (Lévi, Canon, Dipalma, Florentin, & Misset, 1991).

Reports on circadian rhythms in these molecules in healthy subjects indicate that there may be different times of the day for highest circulating levels that are unique for each molecule (Table IV).

D. Temporal and/or Functional Relationships

Relationships between circulating levels of biological parameters, like cytokines with cortisol and leukocytes, are often studied to determine functional relationships between variables in health or disease. However, rarely are samples collected around the clock, such as was done for cytokines and cortisol in 4 healthy humans (Hohagen et al., 1993), or is the time of day of sampling even mentioned. Since circadian variation is a fact of life, correlations of rhythmic variables may produce spurious results due to inadequate sampling. This can be illustrated for serum IL-6 when compared with cortisol and leukocytes in a group of men who were studied for 24 h in 1993 as part of the ongoing Medical Chronobiology Aging Project (Kanabrocki et al., 1990). When 11 men, 46–72 years of age, were sampled every 3 h for 24 h, a statistically significant circadian rhythm was found for each variable, and a specific temporal relationship was observed (Sothern, Roitman-Johnson, Kanabrocki, Yager, Fuerstenberg, et al., 1995b). The sequence of calculated peaks occurred at 02:03 for IL-6, 07:47 for cortisol, 16:27 for neutrophils, 19:54 for total WBC, 22:27 for monocytes, 23:17 for basophils, 23:54 for lymphocytes and 01:35 for eosinophils (see Figure 5 & Table IX). Thus, the peak in IL-6 was about 5–6 h before that in cortisol and from 1 to 10 h after peaks in leukocytes. To test for any functional relationships between circulating IL-6 levels and the other parameters, simple linear correlations were performed using only the values at 07:00, only values at 10:00, all 3-hourly values or the overall 24 h means (07:00 and 10:00 were selected since they are often standard times for scheduling clinical sampling). Significant correlations were observed depending on which time-points were used (Table X). For example,

TABLE VIII Circadian Immune Functions in Humans: Disease, Pain

Variable	Units, assay, or method	Time(s) or range of maxima	Author	Year
		Etiology		
Fever—bacterial	onset	0500–1200	Hejl	1977
Fever—viral	onset	1500–2200	Hejl	1977
Renal allograft	rejection	0600	Knapp, et al.	1979
Ulcer—duodenal	perforation	1620–1908	Svanes, et al.	1998
Ulcer—gastric	perforation	1200 & 0000	Svanes, et al.	1998
		Symptoms		
Asthma	attacks	night	Reinberg, et al.	1963
Atopic dermatitis	pruritus	1900–2300 & 0700	Borelli, et al.	1966
Hay fever	all symptoms	morning	Nicholson & Bogie	1973
Asthma	dyspnea rating	0400	Reinberg, Guillet, et al.	1977
Rheumatoid arthritis (hand)	joint circumference	0604–0848	Kowanko, et al.	1982
Rheumatoid arthritis (hand)	stiffness rating	0752–1012	Kowanko, et al.	1982
Asthma—untreated	wheeze & cough	night	Turner-Warwick	1984
Asthma—treated	wheeze & cough, dyspnea	night	Turner-Warwick	1988
		Pain		
Headache—migraine	onset	0400–1200	Ostfeld	1963
Headache—cluster	onset	2300–0600	Ekbom	1970
Headache—muscle	onset	0800–1200	Waters & O'Connor	1971
Intractable pain	self-rating	2200	Folkard	1976
Toothache	onset	0300-0800	Pöllman & Harris	1978
Osteoarthritis—knee	pain rating	1640-0132	Bellamy, et al.	1990
Rheumatoid arthritis—hand	pain rating	0216-0652	Bellamy, et al.	1991
Fibromyalgia	aches, pain, stiffness	early morning	Yunus, et al.	1981
Osteoarthritis—hand	pain rating	0028-0712	Bellamy, et al.	1997

Notes: Results from diurnally active patients unless otherwise noted. Time in local clock H:Min (range for highest values or 95% limits from cosinor analysis).

a significant correlation was found between IL-6 and cortisol values measured only at 10:00, but not when using all time-points, the 24 h mean or values from 07:00. Significant correlations between IL-6 and all leukocyte subtypes may simply have arisen since the circadian pattern in each variable was similarly timed, whereas the significant correlation between the overall 24-h means for IL-6 and monocytes and eosinophils may truly imply an overall functional relationship, at least as much as it can be ascertained in these clinically symptom-free subjects.

In this same group of 11 clinically healthy men, temporal and/or functional circadian relationships have been established between a number of other variables including serum PSA and testosterone (Mermall et al., 1995); atrial natiuretic peptides (ANF) and blood pressure (Sothern, Vesely, et al., 1995); serum IL6 and its soluble receptor (IL6sR) (Roitman-Johnson et al., 1996); circulating ANF, serum sodium, and chloride (Sothern et al., 1996); ANF, serum calcium, and phosphate (Vesely et al., 1996); and plasma fibrinogen, blood platelets, and serum IL6 (Kanabrocki et al., 1999).

Thus, around-the-clock studies can provide important clues to the overall functional relationships between biologic parameters, including cytokines and other variables hypothesized to be involved with their regulation and function, since each exhibits a significant circadian rhythm. A temporal coordination may be biologically significant between two or more parameters even though one or more of the amplitudes may be small enough to seem statistically insignificant, such as between testosterone, peaking at 08:38 h, with an average circadian range of change of 202 ng/mL, and PSA, peaking at 17:02 h, with a average circadian range of change of 0.4 ng/mL (Mermall et al., 1995). Although the small range of change in PSA makes a single, time-unqualified

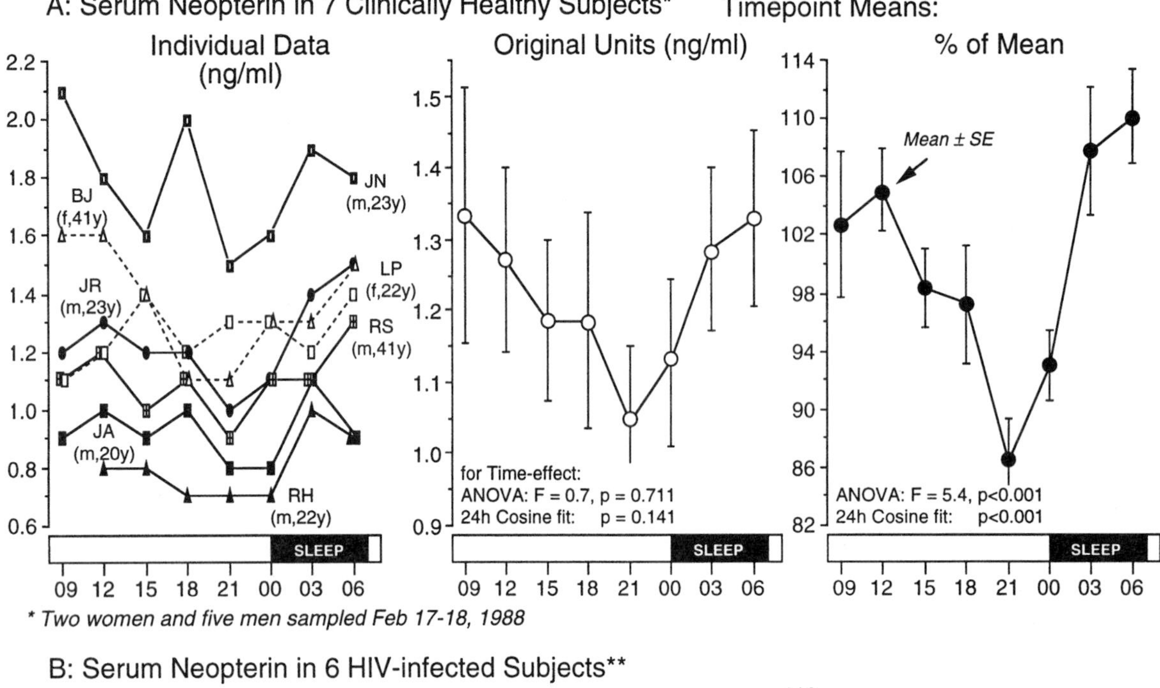

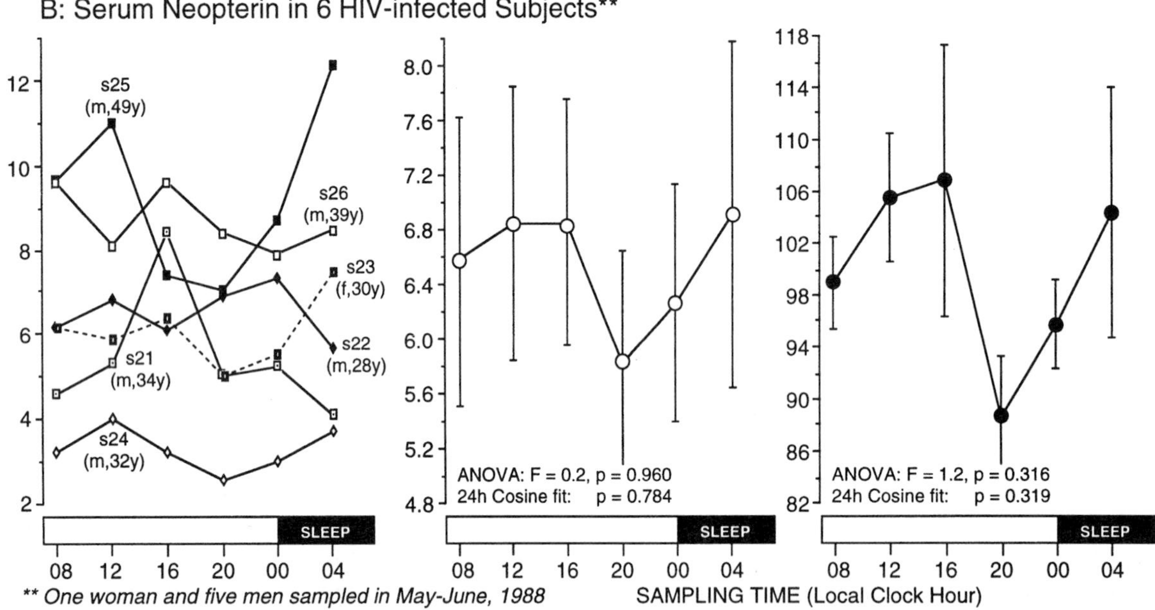

FIGURE 3 Circadian variations in serum neopterin, a measure of immune system activation (especially T lymphocytes), in clinically- healthy individuals (A) and patients with HIV infection (B). In health, neopterin levels are highest during sleep and showed lowest levels in the evening. Some HIV patients had higher levels during the day than at night (Subjects 22 and 26), indicating a possible disease-induced alteration of the circadian rhythm in this variable, and thereby preventing detection of a significant circadian rhythm for the patients as a group.

sample diagnosis reliable, relationships among a cytokine such as IL-6 and other variables determined at only a single time-point may be misleading due to differences in timing of circadian highs and lows. That the times of circadian maxima, as well as the range of change from lowest to highest values over 24 h, vary widely among variables can be compared in Table IX for a number of cytokines and related immunologic variables measured in the same group of 11 clinically healthy men cited above. It should be noted that several other cytokines and biologicals (IL-1-beta, IL-8, IL-4sR, RANTES, FGF-basic) usually showed large circadian variations, but a significant group rhythm could not be detected, possibly due to low levels in healthy individuals (Sothern, unpublished). When comparing individuals, the highest

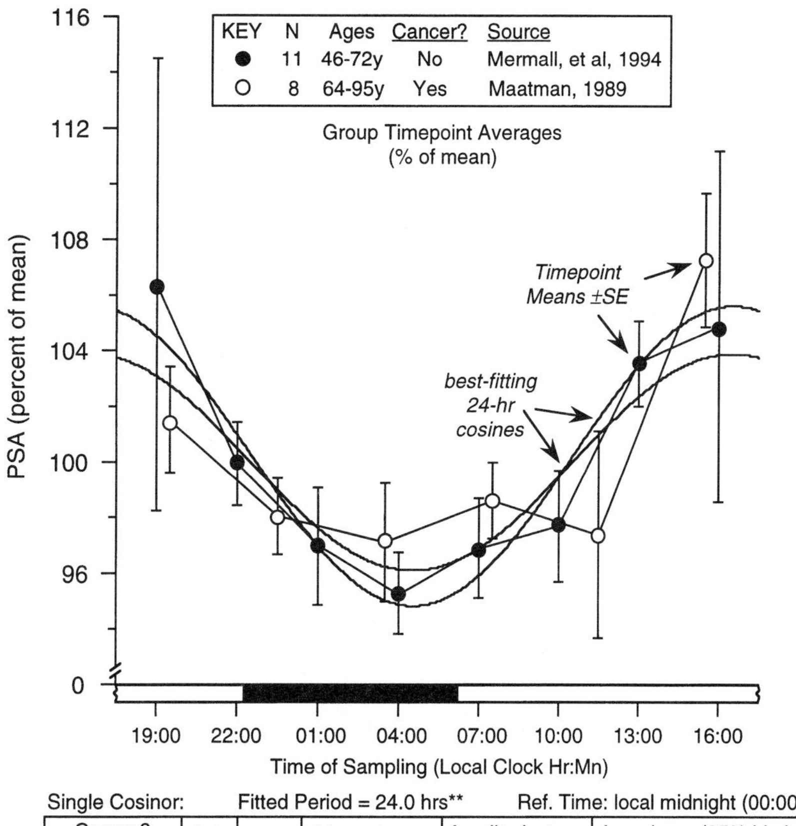

Single Cosinor: Fitted Period = 24.0 hrs** Ref. Time: local midnight (00:00 h)

Cancer?	#pts	p	Mesor ± s.e.		Amplitude ± s.e.		Acrophase (95% Limits)
No	85	0.011	100%	1.2	5.4%	1.8	17:02 h (14:40 ,19:24 h)
Yes	48	0.024	100%	1.0	3.9%	1.4	17:00 h (14:24 ,19:40 h)

FIGURE 4 Circadian rhythm in serum prostate specific antigen (PSA) in men without and with prostate cancer. In spite of increased levels of PSA in the cancer patients, expression of individual data as percentage of mean reveals a circadian pattern nearly identical to that found in health. For both groups, the amplitude was about 4 to 5% and highest values were in the mid-to late afternoon between 2 and 7 P.M. This suggests that the mechanism for PSA production remains intact in the disease state. Data were analyzed by the least-squares fit of a 24-h cosine, resulting in a (1) p-value from zero-amplitude (no rhythm) test, (2) mesor = rhythm-adjusted average; (3) amplitude = half peak-trough difference of cosine; and (4) acrophase = peak of fitted cosine in H: Min from local midnight (see Figure 1).

24-h mean was usually at least twice that of the lowest 24-h mean. Thus, 24-h measurements or an optimally timed measurement at only a single time-point might increase diagnostic accuracy, as well as guide in the selection of time(s) to optimize responses to a pharmacologic agent. As a minimum, time of day of measurements and/or procedures should be recorded and reported for future reference.

IV. DIAGNOSIS AND MEDICAL TREATMENTS

A. Chronodiagnosis

Since nearly every variable measured in mice and humans has been found to be more or less circadian rhythmic, it follows that the body is in a constant state of flux throughout the day and night. Circadian rhythms, as well as ultradian and infradian rhythms, are thus likely to influence the outcome of procedures. In the circadian domain, certain values and functions may be predictably higher at one time of the day and lower 12 h later and vice versa. White blood cells (WBCs), as representative of the immune system, are a case in point. Lower values in the morning and higher values in the evening reflect the normal circadian rhythm in WBCs (Table I). WBCs in blood sampled at 10 AM may be 4,500 cell/cu mm, whereas 12 h later at 10 PM WBCs in a new blood sample may be twice as high (9,000 cells/cu mm) in the same individual. This range of change is a completely normal daily event due to the circadian rhythm in hematopoiesis mentioned earlier. Such a large,

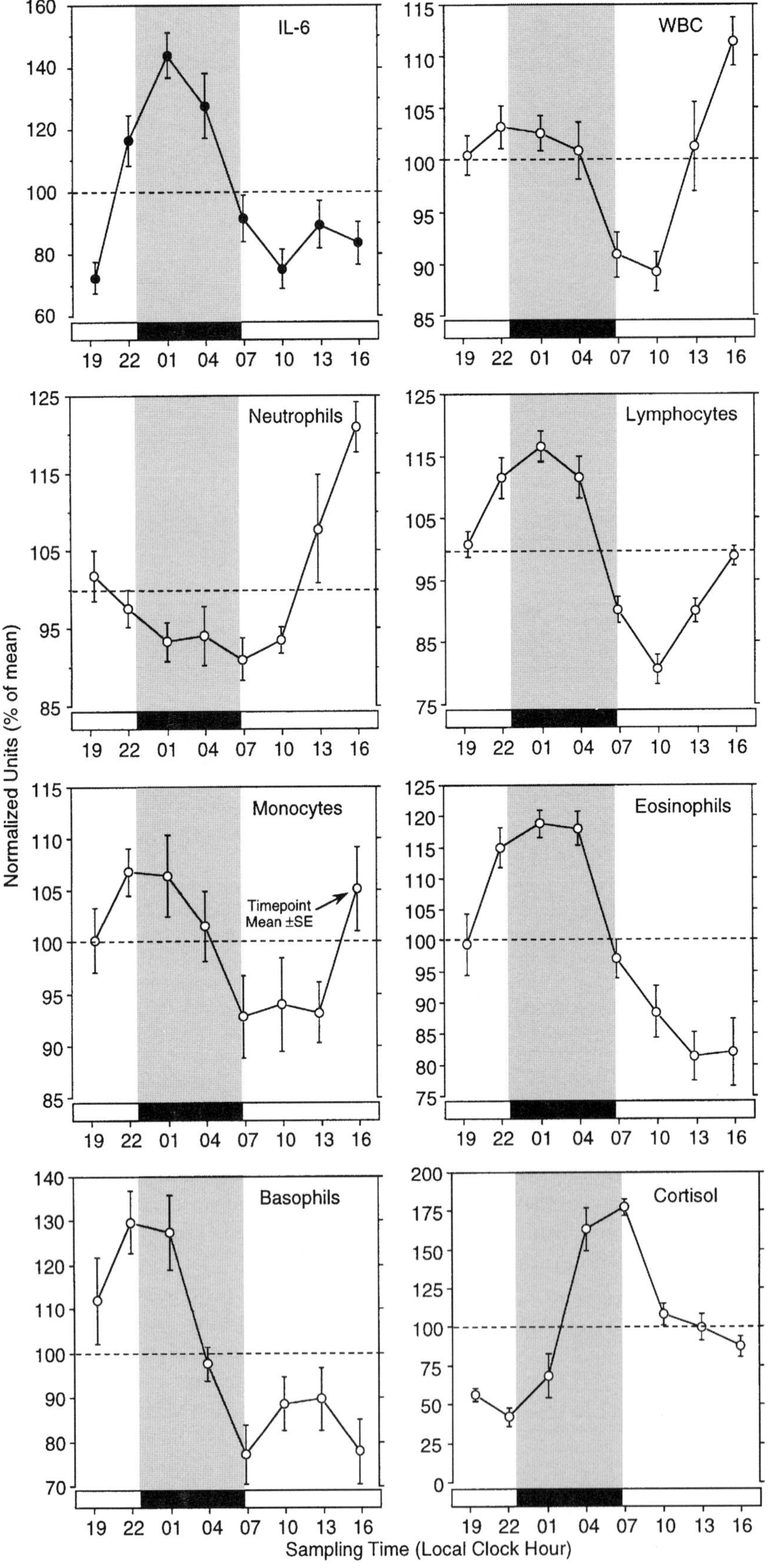
IL-6
WBC
Neutrophils
Lymphocytes
Monocytes
Eosinophils
Basophils
Cortisol
Timepoint Mean ±SE
Normalized Units (% of mean)
Sampling Time (Local Clock Hour)
19 22 01 04 07 10 13 16

TABLE IX Circadian Averages, Range of Variation, and Sequence of Timing over 24 h for Cytokines & Related Variables in the Blood of 11 Clinically Healthy Men

Variable	24 h Units	Average		Range of change (%)		Time of peak values
		Mean	(lowest, highest)	Mean (%)	(Low, high)	
Cortisol	μg/dL	10.3	(8.2, 13.7)	502	(242, 795)	07:47 h
IL-10	pg/mL	71.9	(8, 266.4)	989	(23, 6925)	08:28 h
Fibrinogen	mg/dL	253	(182, 375)	34	(13, 188)	09:47 h
ICAM-1	ng/mL	210	(162, 310)	22	(8, 48)	11:09 h
IL-2	pg/mL	2708	(1226, 12658)	476	(31, 1367)	12:48 h
TNF-alpha	pg/mL	69	(53.9, 109)	62	(16, 131)	14:00 h
VCAM-1	ng/mL	644	(379, 1096)	28	(12, 57)	15:05 h
IL-6sR	ng/mL	40	(50, 52)	16	(8, 37)	16:19 h
Neutrophils	cells/cu mm	4602	(2010, 7067)	53	(23, 118)	16:27 h
Platelets	thous/cu mm	240	(167, 306)	19	(6, 34)	16:57 h
sTfR	ng/mL	2196	(1499, 3012)	26	(13, 42)	18:02 h
GM-CSF	pg/mL	62	(16, 147)	1664	(32, 12684)	19:28 h
Total WBC	thous/cu mm	8.0	(5.0, 12.0)	36	(24, 63)	19:54 h
Monocytes	cells/cu mm	533	(336, 775)	48	(25, 74)	22:27 h
Basophils	cells/cu mm	82	(40, 206)	168	(29, 734)	23:17 h
Lymphocytes	cells/cu mm	2332	(1634, 3459)	56	(33, 84)	23:54 h
Eosinophils	cells/cu mm	299	(83, 582)	80	(57, 296)	01:35 h
IL-6	pg/mL	3.4	(1.7, 6.5)	167	(49, 297)	02:03 h
Melatonin	ng/dL	12.3	(2.5, 30.0)	>241,000	(3167, 868900)	02:55 h
FGF basic	pg/mL	1.36	(0.68, 3.68)	291	(62, 517)	n.s.
IL-1-beta	pg/mL	n.d.		n.d.		n.s.
IL-4sR	pg/mL	28.6	(22.4, 42.3)	28	(15, 39)	n.s.
IL-8	pg/mL	26.5	(22.1, 30.7)	83	(35, 191)	n.s.
RANTES	pg/mL	14276	(6164, 25426)	89	(38, 158)	n.s.

Notes: Men, median age 50 years (range: 46–72 years), sampled every 3 h for 24 h (sleep: 23: 15–06:45 h). Circadian average = mean of 8 samples/subject. n.d. = not detectable. Circadian variation is indicated as the range of change from lowest to highest value within 24 h (in percentages). The clock times of the average highest values are listed if a circadian rhythm was detected at $p \leq 0.05$ from the least-squares fit of a 24 h cosine to all data from the group of subjects or not shown (n.s. = not significant) if $p > 0.05$. IL = interleukin; FGF = fibroblast growth factor; sTfR = serum transferrin receptor; GM-CSF = granulocyte-macrophage colony-stimulating factor; TNF = tumor necrosis factor; ICAM = intercellular adhesion molecule; VCAM = vascular cell adhesion molecule; RANTES = regulated on activation normal T-cell expressed and presumably secreted.

predictable change over the course of a day in WBCs has been shown to occur with comparable timing in groups of diurnally active, clinically healthy individuals studied in several locations around the world (Halberg, Sothern, et al., 1977). Even when absolute levels may differ between individuals, the circadian patterns are nevertheless similar, as has been documented in a man and a woman who each provided 20 circadian profiles for analysis (Figure 6).

Similarly, adrenal corticosteroids in humans have been shown to be at their peak in the morning hours and lower at night (Bartter, Delea, & Halberg, 1962). In a clinical setting, adrenal gland abnormality may be diagnosed with a single sample of cortisol at

FIGURE 5 Circadian patterns in circulating interleukin-6 (IL-6), cortisol, and leukocytes in 11 clinically healthy men, ages 46–72 years, sampled every 3 h for 24 h beginning at 19:00. Since each variable shows a prominent circadian rhythm, correlations of variables at only one time and not others may show spurious relationships that may or may not be present if all times or the overall 24-h mean are compared. Dark bar/shaded area = sleep and/or rest.

TABLE X Correlations between Values for Interleukin-6 (IL-6) and Other Variables in Blood Measured Every 3 h for 24 h in Clinically Healthy Men

IL-6 vs.	7 AM values			10 AM values			24 h means			All 3-hourly values		
	N	r	*p*	N	r	*p*	N	r	*p*	N	r	*p*
Cortisol	11	0.20	0.563	11	0.71	*0.015*	11	0.31	0.346	88	0.02	0.850
WBC	"	0.42	0.204	"	0.06	0.855	"	0.42	0.199	"	0.36	*<0.001*
Neutrophils	"	0.37	0.267	"	0.01	0.985	"	0.36	0.280	"	0.23	*0.032*
Lymphocytes	"	0.22	0.511	"	−0.01	0.975	"	0.26	0.435	"	0.33	*0.002*
Monocytes	"	0.70	*0.016*	"	0.08	0.826	"	0.63	*0.039*	"	0.54	*<0.001*
Eosinophils	"	0.71	*0.015*	"	0.70	*0.018*	"	0.72	*0.013*	"	0.63	*<0.001*
Basophils	"	0.03	0.923	"	0.10	0.761	"	0.39	0.236	"	0.33	*0.002*

Notes: Eleven men, ages 46–72 years, sampled every 3 h around the clock beginning at 19:00 h on May 14, 1993.

the right time. A very low level in the morning may be used to diagnose adrenal hypofunction (Addison's disease), since such a patient has low cortisol levels over the 24 h, whereas a very high level of cortisol at night may indicate adrenal hyperfunction (Cushing's syndrome), since these patients have high levels of cortisol throughout the 24 h (Bartter, 1974).

Circadian rhythms are a fundamental feature of health and their alteration can indicate some abnormality. For example, symptoms of asthma, perhaps the most rhythmic of all diseases (Smolensky, Scott, Barnes, & Jonkman, 1986), are usually worse at night. Although lung capacity in general is reduced, the 24-h amplitude for peak expiratory flow (PEF) is much greater than in healthy subjects. When values for PEF fall more than 10% during sleep from their daytime levels, persons are identified as "night dippers" and may require medical treatment. On the other hand, in patients with suspected high blood pressure, the circadian amplitude may increase prior to the clinical diagnosis of hypertension, with blood pressure being above acceptable limits only at certain times of the day (so-called amplitude-hypertension) (Halberg, Drayer, Cornélissen, & Weber, 1984). Too much blood pressure variability over 24 h has recently been shown to be a diagnostically significant risk factor for vascular disease (Cornelissen et al., 1999) and has been labeled CHAT for "circadian hyperamplitude tension."

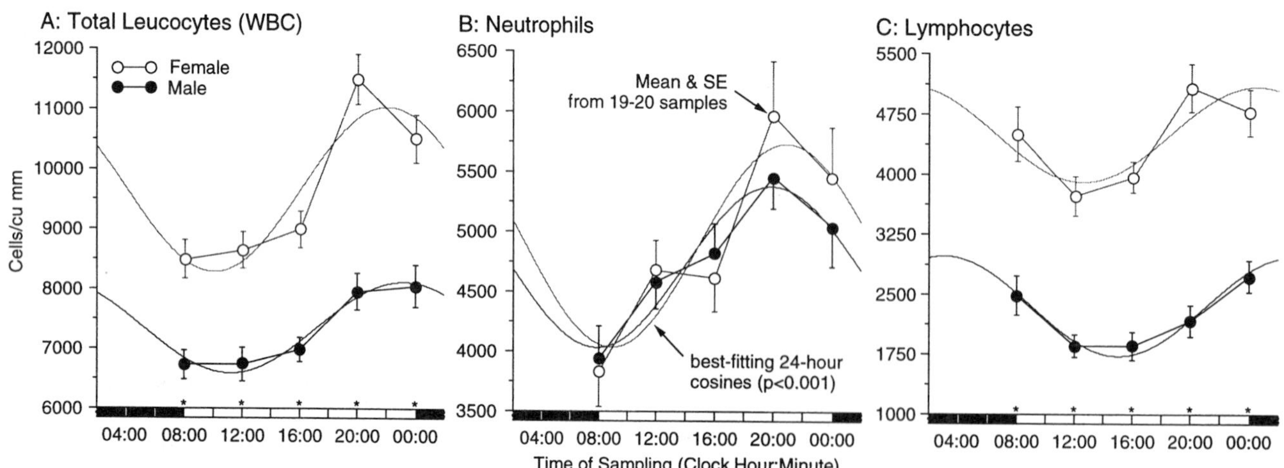

FIGURE 6 Circadian rhythm in fingertip blood sampled every 4 h on 20 separate days over the course of 10 months (May 25–Mar 19, $n = 98$ samples) in a clinically healthy, nonatopic man (RBS) and woman (BRJ), both 27–28 years of age. Similar circadian patterns with highest values in the evening, all significant at $p < 0.001$ for fit of 24-h cosine, were present in each variable in spite of significant differences in absolute counts between the 2 subjects in some variables (from *t*-test, denoted by an asterisk).

A high body temperature early in the day or late at night may be indicative of an illness of bacterial or viral origin, respectively (Hejl, 1977), whereas changes in the sleep-wake cycle may accompany clinical depression or seasonal affective disorder (SAD). Changes in the circadian temperature patterns of a breast, not only by elevated levels but more ultradian oscillations, may indicate the presence of a small tumor (Simpson, 1987).

The timing of circadian rhythms in the immune system (as gauged by T and B lymphocytes) is apparently altered with advancing stages of HIV infection, with a loss of rhythm or more erratic times of highs and lows characterizing infected individuals even if the total numbers of cells is within the normal range (Bourin et al., 1989; Martini et al., 1988; Swoyer et al., 1990). Unusual acrophases (high values at night) were also noted in the oral temperature of some HIV-infected individuals, indicating altered phase relations among variables in this viral infection (Sothern et al., 1990). However, the timing for the cortisol rhythm has been reported to remain unaltered with advancing stages of HIV-infection (Bourin et al., 1989).

B. Chronotoxicity

In the reactive homeostatic view, a stimulus is thought to provoke similar positive and/or negative effects regardless of when it is applied or more or less the same value of some bodily variable will be obtained at all times of the day (Figure 7, top left). However, in the chronobiologic (predictive homeostatic) view, a periodic system will respond differently to the same stimulus if applied at different times of the day, or bodily values will vary predictably (Figure 7, top right). Many experiments have been performed that overwhelmingly confirm the latter.

As early as 1955, chronotoxicity was shown when an unequal number of audiogenic-induced convulsions and deaths in mice resulted after exposure to identical auditory stimulation (e.g., a ringing bell) at different times of the day (Halberg, Bittner, Gully, Albrecht, & Brackney, 1955). Nearly 50% of the mice convulsed and died following exposure to loud sound early in the daily dark/activity span, whereas only 10% convulsed and 2% died if exposed to the same loud sound during the middle of the daily light/resting span. Similar large differences in survival, though with a difference in the best and worst times compared with the previous example, were observed following exposure of mice to *E. coli* endotoxin (Halberg, Johnson, Brown, & Bittner, 1960; Halberg & Stephens, 1958). Fewer than 10% of the mice died following exposure in the middle of the daily dark/activity span, whereas more than 80% mortality occurred following the same exposure late in the daily light/resting span. A susceptibility rhythm of mice to a toxic dose of ethanol was also shown decades ago (Haus & Halberg, 1959), with more mice succumbing following exposure at the beginning of the daily dark/activity span.

In a dramatic display of host chronotoxicity, experiments done in 1957–58 documented virtually an all or none phenomenon in deaths from whole body X-irradiation (Haus, Halberg, Loken, & Kim, 1974). When different groups of male C-mice (16/timepoint) were irradiated with the same dose of radiation (550r) at one of six circadian stages 4 h apart, a circadian rhythm in radiosensitivity was observed. Eight days after exposure, all 16 mice irradiated in the middle of the daily dark/activity span were dead, whereas all 16 mice exposed late in the light/resting span were alive. A similarly timed rhythm was also demonstrated in susceptibility of bone marrow cells to whole body irradiation in Balb/c mice, leading the authors to suggest that a higher number of hematopoietic stem cells surviving at some times and not others may be the underlying cause for differences in the mortality of mice irradiated at different circadian times (Haus, Halberg, & Loken, 1974).

Since the late 1950s and early 1960s there has been a multitude of reports on chronotoxicity observed for a wide range of agents and species, including mortality of mice from insulin, amphetamine, strychnine, nicotine, and phenobarbital (reviewed by Scheving, Tsai, & Pauly, 1986). This has led to the concept of "hours of diminished resistance" (Halberg, 1960) and "hours of changing responsiveness or susceptibility" (Reinberg, 1967). As to any underlying mechanism(s), circadian rhythms in the rates of absorption, metabolism, and excretion may all contribute toward the overall variation in the responsiveness to a drug, whether it be the drug's effectiveness or toxicity (Moore-Ede, 1973).

It can now be generalized that administration of certain treatments without regard to physiologic rhythms will result in the varying positive or negative effects as displayed in Figure 7, top right. Reduction in dose at all times to reduce toxicity also may reduce efficacy (Figure 7, bottom left), whereas adjusting the dose according to the stage of the susceptibility rhythm may reach the desired effect while minimizing the risk from toxicity (Figure 7, bottom right). This has far-reaching implications, not only for the timing of anticancer procedures and medications, but, also for screening procedures, immunotherapy, allergy shots, and many other treatments. For example, the

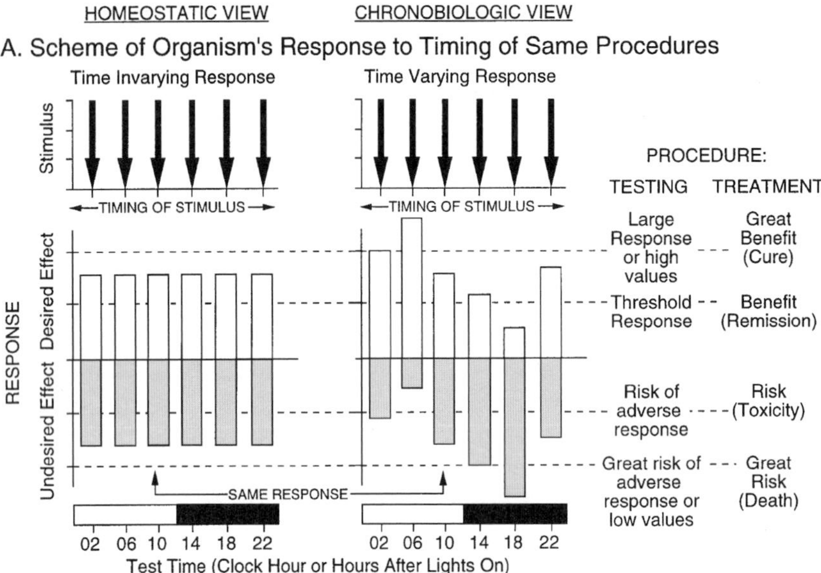

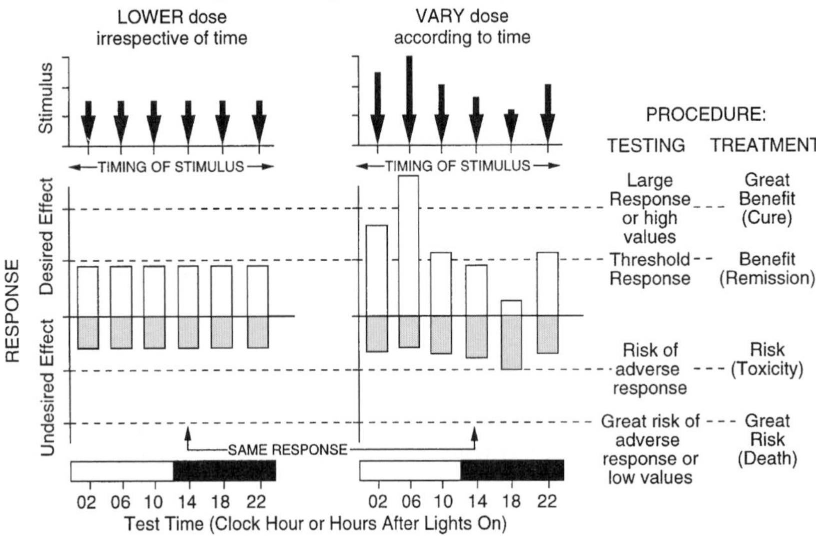

FIGURE 7 An organism's response to a stimulus, such as skin testing or drug treatment, or the value of on a variable, such as lymphocyte count or cortisol levels, depends on when the procedure is performed. Whereas it is usually assumed that the same result will be obtained from an identical procedure regardless of time of day (upper left panel), it is usually the case that the observed results vary in a circadian rhythmic pattern (upper right panel). As a consequence, a procedure may not have the desired effect or the effect may be unexpectedly negative because it is administered at the wrong time. The response may be to lower the doses at all times (lower left panel) or to either treat with a higher dose at the best time or to vary the doses according to time of day to achieve a greater response with lowered toxicity (lower right panel).

size of the erythema resulting from skin testing with a standard dose of histamine can vary more than 100% in the same individual depending on the time of day with the same challenge (Table VII; Figure 8), yet skin testing for allergies is generally not scheduled with this in mind. Likewise, the recovery from a standardized exercise, as gauged by blood glucose levels, has been shown to occur faster in the morning than in the late afternoon, which not only has implications for conditioned athletes, but also for patients with diabetes mellitus (Weydahl & Sothern, 1997).

C. Chronotherapy—The Timing of Treatment

The application of biological rhythms endeavors to find ways to use rhythms to ensure positive and cost-effective outcomes of various events, such as blood

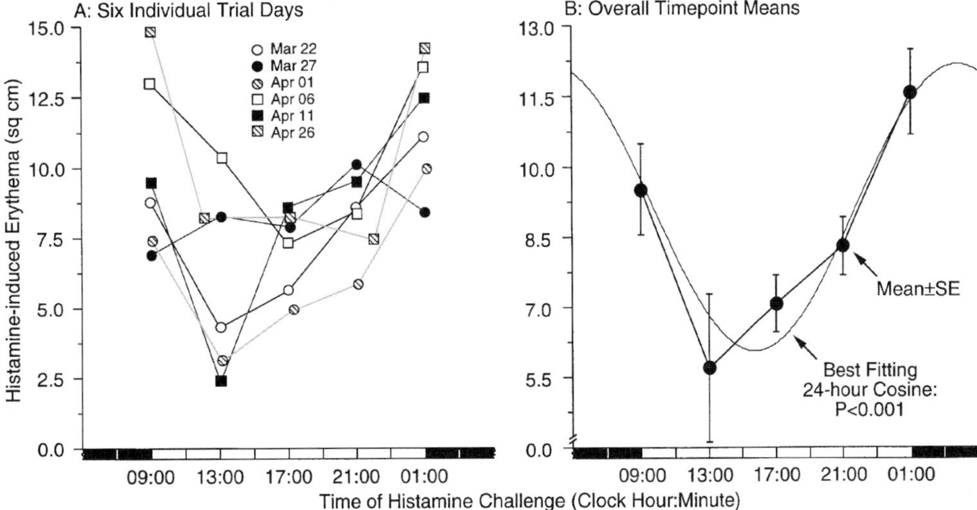

FIGURE 8 Circadian rhythm in cutaneous response to histamine challenge in a nonatopic man (RBS, 28 years of age). On six different days, subject self-injected 0.5 cc of a histamine solution (1/5000,000) subcutaneously into a forearm every 4 h during waking. Erythema was traced after 15 min and area computed. Responses were reproducibly larger when histamine was introduced near awakening or just before bedtime.

sampling, drug treatment, medical and surgical procedures, performance and exercise scheduling, natural family planning, and dieting, among others. For centuries, traditional Chinese medicine has intuitively developed the concept of timing when administering treatment for a wide variety of diseases or ailments (Wu, 1982). Thus, the site of a treatment (e.g., for acupuncture or moxibustion) or a dose (e.g., of herbs and other medications) will differ depending on the natural cycles of the patient, which may involve the time of day, day of the week or menstrual cycle, phase of the moon, or the season. In Western medicine, therapies routinely employed in the treatment of diseases are, for the most part, not administered with regard to biological rhythms, but usually at the convenience of the health care-givers or on a schedule that assures patient compliance, i.e., three times a day with meals. This was once called the "stupidity of a three times a day" drug administration approach (translation from the original German text of Jores, 1935a, 1935b), which can now be restated as "the imprudence of equal dosing at equal intervals throughout the day."

Many therapies, especially powerful anticancer agents, are accompanied by undesired and even life-threatening toxicities, since cytostatic (cell killing) and other effects are exerted in all tissues, diseased or not. Thus, healthy tissue undergoing rapid proliferation, such as the bone marrow, hair, oral mucosa, and gut, is often damaged by chemotherapy and leads to dose reductions and/or delays in treatment. Therefore, doses of chemotherapy represent an inherent compromise between toxicity in the cancer (the desired target) and the host (the undesired target) while an attempt is made to deliver the maximal dose possible (Figure 7, top). Many anticancer drugs have been shown to work better at some times of the day than others, thereby resulting in less toxicity, increased dosage, better disease control, and more cures. Some areas in which proper timing (chronotherapy) of medications or other procedures has been implicated in improved diagnosis and/or efficacy are listed in Table XI.

Due to the rhythmic time structure of the host, we now know that constant dosing does not result in

TABLE XI Medical Areas in Which Symptoms and Treatments Have Been Studied Rhythmically

Arthritis	HIV Infection
Asthma, pulmonary diesease	Irradiation
Adrenal response	Jet-lag shiftwork
Anesthesiology	Menstrual cycle
Alcohol	Psychiatric disorders
Blood disorders	Pain
Cancer	SAD, Light-dark effects
Diet, meal-timing, nutrition	Sexual dysfunction
Epilepsy	Transplants
Hypertension, other cardiovascular morbidity	Ulcer, gastric disorders

constant blood levels. For example, constant dosing of the anticancer drug 5-Fluorouracil (5-FU) at a flat rate over 5 days resulted in a nearly 100% difference in plasma and urine levels of this anticancer drug between peak (at 01:00) and trough (at 10:00) (Lévi, Adam, et al., 1988). Similarly, a circadian rhythm in the anticoagulant effect of heparin infused at a constant rate was demonstrated in 6 patients with venous thromboembolism (Decousus et al., 1985). Variations between night and day ranged from 40–60% in standard anticoagulation parameters (APTT, TT), with maxima occurring at night. Circadian variations were noted in serum and urine trough levels of zidovudine (AZT) in 3 HIV-infected individuals receiving 4-hourly constant dosing (Sothern et al., 1990). Highest concentrations of AZT were seen following the evening doses, with a range of change from lowest to highest concentrations of nearly 400% in serum and urine in 1 patient. Just as with cancer chronotherapy, proper timing of AZT (or other newly developed medications) by varying the number of tablets taken throughout the day (e.g., 3, 2, 1 at 8-h intervals) rather than constant dosing (equal numbers of tablets at equal intervals) has the potential of improving the toxicity:efficacy ratio of this and other drugs being used by an ever-increasing number of HIV-infected individuals worldwide.

The time factor may be even more relevant to the effective use of biological response modifiers. The circadian stage (time of day) when interleukins, interferons, and growth factors are given will ultimately determine how effective these factors will be (Wood, 1995). Therefore, it is important to define the time structure of the pharmacodynamic effects of biological agents. A potentially important consequence of the circadian pattern and phasing of bone marrow DNA synthesis, as well as CFU-GM, is the possibility of increasing the effect of biological response modifiers such as GM-CSF, G-CSF, and regulatory peptides (Ohdo et al., 1998; Paukovits et al., 1990) by administering the optimal dose at the time of greatest responsiveness of the bone marrow. This may increase the usefulness and efficacy of these biological substances, and also possibly reduce side effects. Indeed, a study administering G-CSF to healthy volunteers at six different times around the clock has shown that dosing near midday resulted in a greater increase in the 24-h overall production of CD34+ cells by the bone marrow (Bjarnason et al., 1996). However, the circadian rhythm in circulating CD34+ cells was maintained in the presence of vastly elevated levels, indicating that harvesting of these cells for greatest yield should still be at midnight, near their circadian peak in the circulation.

1. *Asthma*

Circadian differences have been found in the effectiveness of selected inhaled or injected bronchodilaters, including terbutaline, corticosteroids, and theophylline, among others (Smolensky, D'Alonzo, & Reinberg, 1990; Smolensky et al., 1986). It was concluded that proper evaluation of any antiasthmatic drug should include at least three different drug administration times throughout the 24 h, since a drug that might exhibit only minimal potency when given in the morning may prove more efficacious when administered in the evening. Studies to date, even of sustained-release preparations, have usually shown that evening, as opposed to morning, treatments have been more effective in controlling the symptoms of asthma (D'Alonzo, Smolensky, Gianotti, Emerson, Staudinger, & Steinijans, 1990; Migrom, Barnhart, Gaddy, Bush, & Busse, 1990; Smolensky & D'Alonzo, 1988; Steinijans, Trautmann, Sauter, & Staudinger, 1990). It was also shown that while on a 12-h constant dose regime of theophylline, 70% of the use of a steroid inhaler occurred between 8 PM and 8 AM, indicating that an equal-interval, equal-dose medication schedule was not effective in controlling the nocturnal symptoms of asthma (Brown, Smolensky, & D'Alonzo, 1990). Prescribed dosing with corticoids only in the morning has been shown to be effective in the control of asthma and resulted in the fewest side effects (Reinberg, Touitou, Botbol, & Gervais, 1990). In an attempt to prolong the action of administered steroids, recent studies have shown that corticosteroid dosing in the morning and midafternoon also effectively controls airway inflammation without the undue side effects when steroids are taken at night (Pincus, Humeston, & Martin, 1997). It has also been suggested that small, late evening or 2 AM doses of short-acting glucocorticoids may alleviate early morning inflammatory symptoms and minimize side effects for immunoinflammatory disorders such as asthma (Petrovsky, McNair, & Harrison, 1998) and rheumatoid arthritis (Arvidson, Gudbjornsson, Larsson, & Hallgren, 1997).

2. *Cancer—Murine Models*

There is an overwhelming body of experimental evidence in murine systems unequivocally demonstrating that lethal and organ-specific nonlethal chemotherapeutic toxicity, as well as cancer cure, each depend to some extent on the circadian timing of drug administration. Chronotoxicity of more than 30 anticancer agents has been reviewed (Bjarnason & Hrushesky, 1994; Lévi, Boughattas, & Blazsek, 1988; Mormont, Boughattas, & Lévi, 1989).

The earliest demonstration of chronotoxicity from an anticancer drug was shown following the administration of cytosine arabinosyl (ara-C) at different times of the day (Cardoso, Scheving, & Halberg, 1970). The mortality of healthy mice from a single dose of ara-C given at one of six different circadian stages was greatest following injection in the daily dark/activity span for mice housed in LD12:12, a time, we now know, of maximal bone marrow DNA S-phase synthesis (Smaaland & Sothern, 1994). This finding was later confirmed in experiments on mice that received repeated injections of ara-C over 5 to 6 days, always at the same time of day (Scheving, Cardoso, Pauly, Halberg, & Haus, 1974). In an attempt to further reduce the hematologic chronotoxicity to mice caused by ara-C, Li, Souland, Filipski, Deschamps de Paillatte, and Lévi (1998) have recently shown that continuous infusion of a negative regulator of hematopoiesis (AcSDKP) and/or rhG-CSF given at 09 HALO further improved the tolerability of the bone marrow to ara-C beyond that already achieved with optimal circadian timing.

When tumor-bearing animals were treated with eight equal doses of ara-C or with eight doses varying in a sinusoidal manner such that the peak dose was in the middle of the daily light/resting span (see Figure 7), an increased tolerance to ara-C was demonstrated in leukemic mice treated on the schedule adjusted to their circadian system (Haus et al., 1972). The survival rate was more than double that of the conventionally treated animals even though the same total 24-h dose was used for each treatment schedule. In an extension of this work, the location of the peak dose was moved around the clock to occur at each of the eight injection times (Haus, Halberg, Kühl, & Lakatua, 1974). A circadian rhythm gauged by both survival and cures was found, with maximal responses located in the second half of the daily light/resting span. Thus, the timing of the highest and lowest doses, and not the pattern of dosing, was the critical factor in survival. When compared with the homeostatic reference treatment schedule of equal doses, survival of non-leukemic mice was nearly tripled (from 25 to 58–70%) when the peak sinusoidal dose was given during the daily light span and was at least equal or slightly increased when placed in the daily dark/activity span. Cures of leukemic mice were either doubled (from 10 to 20%) when peak dose was placed in the light/resting span (the "right time"), or halved (to less than 5%) when peak doses were placed in the second half of the daily dark/activity span (the "wrong time"). Thus, improperly timed chronotherapy was actually less effective than the homeostatic reference schedule in the attempt to cure leukemic mice. These experiments involving several thousand mice showed that the same number of injections (eight) and total 24-h dose increased tolerance and efficacy with properly timed "sinusoidal" chronotherapy when compared with eight equal-dose "homeostatic" injections. Similarly, greatest tumor response, more remissions, and longer survival were reported (Sothern, Lévi, Haus, Halberg, & Hrushesky, 1989) for rats bearing an immunocytoma when treated with two drugs, each at its best time: doxorubicin near the end of the daily light (resting) span (Sothern, Nelson, & Halberg, 1977) and cisplatin in the middle or latter part of the daily activity (dark) span (Lévi et al., 1982).

3. *Cancer—Human Trials*

The preclinical results in the previous section served as the basis for the first chronotherapeutic schedules with these drugs in clinical trials in humans (Hrushesky, 1985). In this crossover study, cumulative bone marrow toxicity was reported to be less, platinum clearance was greater, and there were fewer episodes of nausea when the drugs were delivered at circadian stages comparable to the best times (circadian stages) found in the rats (Schedule A: early morning for doxorubicin, late afternoon for cisplatin) when compared with an opposite schedule (Schedule B: early morning for cisplatin, late afternoon for doxorubicin). In further studies using a fixed schedule of doxorubicin and cisplatin (Schedule A or B), there were half as many reductions in dose, one fourth as many delays in treatment, half as many complications (transfusions, infections, bleeding) and greater survival for patients receiving Schedule A when compared with patients treated on Schedule B, in spite of the fact that Schedule B patients had many more delays in treatments and dose reductions. Schedule B-treated patients, however, still performed better than randomly treated, time-unspecified controls. These preclinical and clinical findings on chronotherapy with doxorubicin and cisplatin have been summarized by Hrushesky, Roemeling, and Sothern, (1989a, 1989b).

Many other clinical trials have reported that proper timing of chemotherapy can improve clinical outcome (Bjarnason, 1995; Wood and Hrushesky, 1996). For example, Focan (1979) reported on patients with solid tumors who received the same combination of drugs (methotrexate, 5-FU, vinblastine, cyclophosphamide) at equal doses, but on two differently timed schedules. Significant differences in tumor responses were found (58 vs. 23% partial response rate). A 5-year disease-free survival of children with acute lymphoblastic leukemia was better depending on the timing of their maintenance chemotherapy (6-mercaptopurine and methotrexate): 80% with evening treatment vs. 40% morning treatment (Rivard, Infante-Rivard, Hoyeux, & Champagne, 1985). Lévi and colleagues (1990) showed that THP-Adriamycin, like Adriamycin (doxorubicin), was better tolerated by patients with ovarian cancer when given in the morning at 06:00. They also studied 124 cases with lung cancer who received cisplatin at 18:00 and etoposide daily either at 06:00 or 18:00 and found less hematological toxicity with etoposide at 06:00 (Lévi & Reinberg, 1990). In treating patients with metastatic adenocarcinoma, Bjarnason, Kerr, Doyle, MacDonald, & Sone (1993) reported an increase in dose intensity and a reduction in toxicity when 5-FU and leucovorin were delivered around 21:00-22:00 on a sinusoidal schedule via a programmable drug pump. Similarly, Lévi and colleagues (1994) reported less toxicity and higher dose intensities when treating patients with colorectal cancer on a chronomodulated schedule of oxaliplatin, 5-FU, and leucovorin vs. a fixed (flat) infusion rate. A similar chronotherapy has been tested with success in phase II trials of non small cell lung and esophagus cancers (Focan, Denis, Kruetz, Focan-Henrard, & Lévi, 1995; Focan, Kreutz, Denis, Focan-Henrard, & Moeneclay, 1997). Due to these studies showing the importance of timing of anticancer medications, ongoing clinical cancer trials in Europe since 1998 have been designed to include a chronotherapy arm for each treatment (Dogliatti, Tampellini, & Lévi, 1998).

V. SUMMARY

Biologic processes in living organisms have both a physical and a temporal organization as the result of a genetically controlled predictive, rather than a reactive, homeostasis (Moore-Ede, 1986). "Normal" values change throughout the 24-h day, such that the same value may be too high at one time, too low at another, or considered acceptable at other times. Although arising endogenously from within, biologic rhythms are synchronized by external factors, such as the sleep-wake schedule, which ultimately determine the phase-relationships for high and low values. Thus, for diagnostic purposes, time of day, or more correctly, stage of rhythm, needs to be taken into account. This is also the case for stage of the menstrual cycle and time of the year. Findings to date suggest that when something is done should become as critical as what and how much for interpretation and treatment of many conditions and illnesses, thereby adding a fourth dimension (time) to our understanding of biology, physiology, and especially medicine.

Acknowledgments

We wish to acknowledge the cooperation of Dr. Eugene L. Kanabrocki, director of the Medical Chronobiology Aging Project at the Hines V.A. Hospital in Hines, IL, and thank Robert M. Stupar for useful editorial comments and suggestions. This chapter is dedicated to the memory of Professor Lawrence E. Sdeving

References

Abo, T., Kawate, K., Itoh, K., & Kumagia, K. (1981). Studies in the bioperiodicity of the immune response. I. Circadian rhythms of human T, B and K cell traffic in the peripheral blood. *Journal of Immunology, 126*, 1360–1363.

Abrahamsen, J. F., Sothern, R. B., Sandberg, S., Aakvaag, A., Laerum, O. D., & Smaaland, R. (1999). Circadian variations in human peripheral blood on days with and without bone marrow sampling and relation to bone marrow cell proliferation. *Biological Rhythm Research, 30*(1), 29–53.

Abrahamsen, J. F., Smaaland, R., Sothern, R. B., & Laerum, O. D. (1997). Circadian cell cycle variations of erythro- and myelopoiesis in humans. *European Journal of Haematology, 58*, 333–345.

Abrahamsen, J. F., Smaaland, R., Sothern, R. B., & Laerum, O. D. (1998). Variation in cell yield and proliferative activity of positive selected human CD34+ bone marrow cells along the circadian time scale. *European Journal of Haematology, 60*, 7–15.

Akslen, L., & Sothern, R. B. (1998). Seasonal variations in the presentation and growth of thyroid cancer. *British Journal of Cancer, 77*, 1174–1179.

Akbulut, H., Icli, F., Büyükcelik, A., Akbulut, K. G., & Demirci, S. (1999). The role of granulocyte-macrophage-colony stimulating factor, cortisol, and melatonin in the regulation of the circadian rhythms of peripheral blood cells in healthy volunteers and patients with breast cancer. *Journal of Pineal Research, 26*(1), 1–8.

Arvidson, N. G., Gudbjornsson, B., Elfman, L., Rydén, A.-C., Tötterman, T. H., & Hallgren, R. (1994). Circadian rhythm of serum interleukin-6 in rheumatoid arthritis. *Annals of the Rheumatic Diseases, 53*, 521–524.

Arvidson, N. G., Gudbjornsson, B., Larsson, A., & Hallgren, R. (1997). The timing of glucocorticoid administration in rheumatoid arthritis. *Annals of the Rheumatic Diseases, 56*(1): 27–31.

Aschoff, J. (1960). Exogenous and endogenous components in circadian rhythms. In *Biological clocks. Cold Spring Harbor Symposia on Quantitative Biology* (vol. 25, pp. 11–28). New York: Biological Laboratory.

Aschoff, J., Hoffman, K., Pöhl, H., & Wever, R. (1975). Re-entrainment of circadian rhythms after phase-shifts of the Zeitgeber. *Chronobiologia, 2*, 23–78.

Auzéby, A., Bogdan, A., Krozi, Z., & Touitou, Y. (1988). Time-dependence of urinary neopterin, a marker of cellular immune activity. *Clinical Chemistry, 34*, 1866–1867.

Barcal, R., Sova, J., Krizanovska, M., Levy, J., & Matousek, J. (1968). Genetic background of circadian rhythms. *Nature, 220*, 1128–1131.

Barinaga, M. (1997). New clues found to circadian clocks — including mammals. *Science, 276*, 1030–1031.

Barnes, P., Fitzgerald, G., Brown, M., & Dollery, C. (1980). Nocturnal asthma and changes in circulating epinephrine, histamine and cortisol. *New England Journal of Medicine, 303*, 263–267.

Barnes, P. J. (1989). Circadian rhythms in the respiratory system. In J. Arendt, D. S. Minors, & J. M. Waterhouse, (Eds.), *Biological rhythms in clinical practice* (pp. 71–82). London: Wright.

Barnum, C. P., Jardetzky, C. D., & Halberg, F. (1958). Time relations among metabolic and morphologic 24h changes in mouse liver. *American Journal of Physiology, 195*, 301–310.

Bartter, F. C. (1974). Periodicity and medicine. In L.E. Scheving, F. Halberg, & J. E., Pauly, (Eds.), *Chronobiology* (pp. 6–13). Tokyo: Igaku Shoin Ltd.

Bartter, F. C., Delea, C. S., & Halberg, F. (1962). A map of blood and urinary changes related to circadian variations in adrenal cortical function in normal subjects. *Annals of the New York Academy of Sciences, 98*, 969–983.

Bateman, J. R. M., Pavia, D., & Clarke, S. W. (1978). The retention of lung secretions during the night in normal subjects. *Clinical Science, 55*, 523–527.

Beard, C. M., Fuster, V., & Elveback, L. R. (1982). Daily and seasonal variation in sudden cardiac death, Rochester, Minnesota, 1950–1975. *Mayo Clinic Proceedings, 57*, 704–761.

Beck, W. S. (1991). Hematopoiesis. In W. S. Beck (Ed.), *Hematology* (5th ed., pp. 1–21), Cambridge, MA: MIT Press.

Bellamy, N., Campbell, J., Sothern, R., Soucy, E., Flynn, J., & Buchanan, W. W. (1997). Circadian rhythm in pain, stiffness and manual dexterity in osteoarthritis (OA) of the hand: A study of the relationship between discomfort and disability (Abstract). *Chronobiology International, 14*(suppl. 1), 16.

Bellamy, N., Sothern, R. B., & Campbell, J. (1990). Rhythmic variations in pain perception in osteoarthritis of the knee. *Journal of Rheumatology, 17*, 364–372.

Bellamy, N., Sothern, R. B., Campbell, J., & Buchanan, W. W. (1991). Circadian rhythm in pain, stiffness, and manual dexterity in rheumatoid arthritis: relation between discomfort and disability. *Annals of Rheumatic Disease, 50*, 243–248.

Bingham, C., Arbogast, B., Cornélissen-Guillaume, G., Lee, J. K., & Halberg, F. (1982). Inferential statistical methods for estimating and comparing cosinor parameters. *Chronobiologia, 9*, 397–439.

Bisdee, J. T., Garlick, P. J., & James, W. P. T. (1989). Metabolic changes during the menstrual cycle. *British Journal of Nutrition, 61*, 641–650.

Bjarnason, G. A. (1995). Clinical cancer chronotherapy: a review. *Journal of Infusional Chemotherapy, 5*, 31–37.

Bjarnason, G. A., & Hrushesky, W. J. M. (1994). Cancer Chronotherapy. In W. J. M. Hrushesky (Ed.), *Circadian cancer therapy* (pp. 241–263). Boca Raton: CRC Press.

Bjarnason, G. A., Jordan, R., & Sothern, R. B. (1999). Circadian variation in the expression of cell-cycle proteins in human oral epithelium. *American Journal of Pathology, 154*, 613–622.

Bjarnason, G. A., Jordan, R., Li, Q., Sothern, R. B., & Ben-David, Y. (1999). Circadian rhythm in proliferation and expression of clock genes in human epithelium over 24 hours: clinical implications (Abstract). *Chronobiology International, 16*(suppl. 1), 14.

Bjarnason, G. A., Kerr, I. G., Doyle, N., MacDonald, M., & Sone, M. (1993). Phase I study of 5-fluorouracil and leucovorin by a 14 day circadian infusion in patients with metastatic adenocarcinoma. *Cancer Chemotherapy and Pharmacology, 33*(3), 221–228.

Bjarnason, G. A., Reis, M., Robinson, J. B., Sothern, R. B., Crump, M., Brown, G., DeBoer, G., & Perkins, N. (1996). Circadian variation in CD34+ count and response to G-CSF in healthy volunteers: Implications for harvesting efficacy (Abstract). *Blood, 88*(suppl. 1), 395a.

Blaauw, A., Karlsdottir, A., Brydøy, M., Schem, B. C., Ekanger, R., Dalene, R., Sandberg, S., Sothern, R. B., & Smaaland, R. (1997). Altered circadian variations in leucocyte differential counts may be normalized during chemotherapy in cancer patients (Abstract). *Chronobiology International, 14*(suppl. 1), 18.

Bogaty, P., & Waters, D. D. (1989). Possible mechanisms accounting for the temporal distribution of anginal attacks. In B. Lemmer, (Ed.), *Chronopharmacology. Cellular and biochemical interactions* (pp. 509–524). New York: Marcel-Dekker.

Borelli, S., Chlebarov, S., & Flach, E. (1966). Atopic neurodermatitis, and the problem of its 24h rhythm and its dependence on weather and climate. *Munchener Medizinische Wochenschrift, 108*, 474–480.

Born, J., Lange, T., Hansen, K., Mölle, M., & Fehm, H.-L. (1997). Effects of sleep and circadian rhythm on human circulating immune cells. *Journal of Immunology, 158*, 4454–4464.

Bourdon, L., Buguet, A., Cucherat, M., & Radomski, M. W. (1995). Use of a spreadsheet program for circadian analysis of biological/physiological data. *Aviation, Space and Environmental Medicine, 66*, 787–791.

Bourin, P., Mansour, I., Lévi, F., Villette, J.-M., Roué, R., Fiet, J., Rouger, P., & Doinel, C. (1989). [Early disturbance of the circadian rhythm of T and B lymphocytes in human immunodeficiency virus infection]. [French] *Comptes Rendus de l'Academie des Sciences — Serie III, Sciences de la Vie, 308*, 431–436,

Brown, A. C., Smolensky, M. H., & D'Alonzo, G. E. (1990). Day-night pattern of isoproterenol (ISO) use for relief of acute asthma symptoms. In A. Reinberg, M. Smolensky, & G. Labrecque, (Eds.), *Annual review of chronopharmacology* (vol. 6, pp. 317). Oxford: Pergamon Press.

Bruce, V. G. (1960). Environmental entrainment of circadian rhythms. In *Biological clocks. Cold Spring Harbor Symposia on Quantitative Biology* (vol. 25, pp. 29–48). New York: Biological Laboratory.

Bruguerolle, B., Lévi, F., Arnaud, C., Bouvenot, G., Mechkouri, N., Vannetzel, J., & Touitou, Y. (1986). Alteration of physiologic circadian time structure of six plasma proteins in patients with advanced cancer. In A. Reinberg, M. Smolensky, & G. Labrecque, (Eds.), *Annual review of chronopharmacology*, (vol. 3, pp. 207–210.). Oxford: Pergamon Press.

Brush, M. G., & Goodsmit, E. M., (Eds.), (1988). *Functional disorders of the menstrual cycle.* Chichester: John Wiley & Sons.

Buchi, K. N., Moore, J. G., Hrushesky, W. J. M., Sothern, R. B., & Rubin, N. H. (1991). Circadian rhythm of cellular proliferation in the human rectal mucosa. *Gastroenterology, 101*, 410–415.

Butcher, E. C. (1990). Cellular and molecular mechanisms that direct leukocyte traffic. *American Journal of Pathology, 136*, 3–11.

Callard, R. E., & Gearing, A. J. H. (1994). *The cytokine facts book.* San Diego: Academic Press.

Canon, C., Lévi, F., Reinberg, A., & Mathé, G. (1985). Circulating CALLA positive lymphocytes (L) exhibit a circadian rhythm in man. *Leukemia Research, 9*, 1539–1546.

Cardoso, S. S., Scheving, L. E., & Halberg, F. (1970). Mortality of mice as influenced by the hour of the day of drug (ara-C) administration (Abstract). *Pharmacologist, 12*, 302.

Carter, J. B., Barr, G. D., Levin, A. S., Byers, V. S., Ponce, B., & Fudenberg, H. (1975). Standardization of tissue culture conditions for spontaneous thymidine-2 ^{14}C incorporation by unstimulated normal peripheral lymphocytes: Circadian rhythm of DNA synthesis. *Journal of Allergy and Clinical Immunology, 56*, 191–205.

Cohen, P., Wax, Y., & Modan, B. (1983). Seasonality in the occurrence of breast cancer. *Cancer Research, 43*, 892–896.

Cormia, F. E. (1952). Experimental histamine pruritis. I. Influence of physical and psychological factors on threshold reactivity. *Journal of Investigative Dermatology, 19*, 21–34.

Cornelissen, G., Halberg, F., Schwartzkopff, O., Delmore, P., Katinas, G., Hunter, D., Tarquini, B., Tarquini, R., Perfetto, F., Watanabe, Y., & Otsuka, K. (1999). Chronomes, time structures, for chronobioengineering for a "full life." *Biomedical Instrumentation & Technology, 33*(2), 152–187.

Cove-Smith, M. S., Kabler, P. A., Pownall, R., & Knapp, M. S. (1978). Circadian variation in an immune response in man. *British Journal of Medicine, ii*, 253.

Czeisler, C. A., Duffy, J. F., Shanahan, T. L., Brown, E. N., Mitchell, J. F., Rimmer, D. W., Ronda, J. M., Silva, E. J., Allan, J. S., Emens, J. S., Dijk, D.-J., & Kronauer, R. E. (1999). Stability, precision, and near-24-hour period of the human circadian pacemaker. *Science, 284*, 2177–2181.

Dabbs, J. M. Jr. (1990). Age and seasonal variation in serum testosterone concentration among men. *Chronobiology International, 7*(3), 245–249.

D'Alonzo, G. E., Smolensky, M. H., Gianotti, L., Emerson, M., Staudinger, H., & Steinijans, V. (1990). Chronotherapeutically optimized theophylline therapy. In A. Reinberg, M. Smolensky, and G. Labrecque, (Eds.), *Annual review of chronopharmacology* (vol. 6, pp. 319–322). New York: Pergamon Press.

Decousus, H. A., Croze, M., Lévi, F. A., Jaubert, J. C., Perpoint, B. M., Bonadona, J. F. D., Reinberg, A., & Queneau, P. M. (1985). Circadian changes in anticoagulant effect of heparin infused at a constant rate. *British Medical Journal, 290*, 341–344.

DePrins, J., Cornélissen, G., & Malbecq, W. (1986). Statistical procedures in chronobiology and chronopharmacology. In A. Reinberg, M. Smolensky, & G. Labrecque, (Eds.), *Annual review of chronopharmacology* (vol. 2, pp. 27–141). New York: Pergamon Press.

DeVries, K., Goei, J. T., Booy-Noord, H., & Orie, N. G. (1962). Changes during 24 hours in the lung function and histamine hyperreactivity of the bronchial tree in asthmatic and bronchitis patients. *International Archives of Allergy, 20*, 93–101.

Dogliatti, L., Tampellini, M., & Lévi, F. (1998). Chronochemotherapy of colorectal cancer. From Villejuif to Europe. In Y. Touitou, (Ed.), *Biological clocks. Mechanisms and applications* (pp. 475–481). Amsterdam: Elsevier.

Dunningan, M. G., & Harland, W. A. (1970). Seasonal incidence and mortality of ischemic heart disease. *Lancet, i*, 793–797.

Dyrenfurth, I., Jewelewicz, R., Warren, M., Ferin, M., & Vande Wiele, R. L. (1974). Temporal relationships of hormonal variables in the menstrual cycle. In M. Ferin, F. Halberg, R. M. Richart, & R. L. Vande Wiele, (Eds.), *Biorhythms and human reproduction* (pp. 171–201). New York: John Wiley & Sons.

Edmunds, L. (Ed). (1984). *Cell cycle clocks*. New York: Marcel-Dekker.

Ekbom, K. A. (1970). Patterns of cluster headache with a note on the relations to angina pectoris and peptic ulcer. *Acta Neurologica Scandinavica, 46*, 225–237.

Enright, J. T. E. (1981). Data analysis. In J. Aschoff (Ed.), *Biological rhythms. Handbook of behavioral neurobiology* (vol. 4, pp. 21–39). New York: Plenum Press.

Entzian, P., Linnemann, K., Schlaak, M., & Zabel, P. (1996). Obstructive sleep apnea syndrome and circadian rhythms of hormones and cytokines. *American Journal of Respiratory & Critical Care Medicine, 153*, 1080–1086.

Eskola, J., Frey, H., Molnar, G., & Soppi, E. (1976). Biological rhythm of cell-mediated immunity in man. *Clinical and Experimental Immunology 26*, 253–257.

Feigin, R. (1970). Metabolic changes in infectious diseases. *Clinical Pediatrics, 9*, 84–93.

Fentiman, I., Gregory, W., & Richards, M. (1994). Effects of menstrual phase on surgical treatment of breast cancer. *Lancet, 344*, 402.

Fisher, L. B. (1968). The diurnal mitotic rhythm in the human epidermis, *British Journal of Dermatology, 60*, 75–80.

Focan, C. (1995). Marker rhythms for cancer chronotherapy. From laboratory animals to human beings. *in vivo, 9*, 283–298.

Focan, C. (1979). Sequential chemotherapy and circadian rhythm in human solid tumors. *Cancer Chemotherapy and Pharmacology, 3*, 197–202.

Focan, C., Denis, B., Kreutz, F., Focan-Henrard, D., & Lévi, F. (1995). Ambulatory chronotherapy with 5-fluorouracil, folinic acid and carboplatin for advanced non-small cell lung cancer. A phase II feasibility trial. *Journal of Infusional Chemotherapy, 5*, 148–152.

Focan, C., Kreutz, F., Denis, D., Focan-Henrard, D., & Moeneclay, N. (1997). Ambulatory chronotherapy with 5-fluorouracil (5FU), folinic acid (FOL) and carboplatin (CB) for advanced non-small cell lung (NSCLC) and esophagus cancer (C). An interesting therapeutic index [Abstract]. *Proceedings of the American Society of Clinical Oncology, 16*, 468a.

Focan, G., & Pierard, G. (1976). Variations circadiennes de la prolifération cellulaire dans des tumeurs épidermiques. *Bulletin de la Societe Francaise de Dermatologie et Syphiligraphie, 83*, 331–334.

Folkard, S. (1976). Diurnal variation and individual differences in the perception of intractable pain. *Journal of Psychosomatic Research, 20*, 289–301.

Gaultier, C., De Montis, G., Reinberg, A., & Motohashi, Y. (1987). Circadian rhythm of serum total immunoglobulin E (IgE) in asthmatic children. *Biomedicine and Pharmacotherapy, 41*, 186–188.

Gervais, P., Reinberg, A., Gervais, C., Smolensky, M. H., & DeFrance, O. (1977). Twenty-four hour rhythm in the bronchial hyperreactivity to house dust in asthmatics. *Journal of Allergy and Clinical Immunology*, 59, 207-213.

Guberan, E., Williams, M. K., Walford, J., & Smith, M. M. (1969). Circadian variation in FEV1 in shift workers. *British Journal of Industrial Medicine, 26*, 121–125.

Haberman, S., Capildeo, R., & Rose, F. C. (1981). The seasonal variation in mortality from cerebrovascular disease. *Journal of Neurological Sciences, 52*, 25–36.

Hagen, A. A., & Hrushesky, W. J. M. (1998). Menstrual timing of breast cancer surgery. *The American Journal of Surgery, 104*, 245–261.

Halberg, F. (1969). Chronobiology. *Annual Review of Physiology, 31*, 675–725.

Halberg, F. (1960). Temporal coordination of physiologic function. In *Biological clocks. Cold Spring Harbor Symposia on Quantitative Biology* (vol. 25, pp. 289–310). New York: Biological Laboratory.

Halberg, F., & Barnum, C. F. (1961). Continuous light or darkness and circadian periodic mitosis and metabolism in C and D8 mice. *American Journal of Physiology, 201*, 227–230.

Halberg, F., Bittner, J. J., Gully, R. J., Albrecht, P. G., & Brackney, E. L. (1955). 24h periodicity and audiogenic convulsions in I mice of various ages. *Proceedings of the Society of Experimental Biology and Medicine, 88*, 169–173.

Halberg, F., Carandente F., Cornélissen G., & Katinas G. S. (1977). Glossary of chronobiology, *Chronobiologia, 4*(suppl. 1), 1–189.

Halberg, F., Drayer, J. I. M., Cornélissen, G., & Weber, M. A. (1984). Cardiovascular reference data for recognizing circadian mesor- and amplitude-hypertension in apparently healthy men. *Chronobiologia, 11*, 275–298.

Halberg, F., Engeli, M., Hamburger, C., & Hillman, D. (1965). Spectral resolution of low-frequency, small amplitude rhythms in excreted 17-ketosteroid; probable androgen-induced circaseptan desynchronization. *Acta Endocrinologica (Kbh), 103*(suppl.), 5–54.

Halberg, F., Halberg, E., Barnum, C. P., & Bittner, J. J. (1959). Physiologic 24 h periodicity in human beings and mice, the lighting regimen and daily routine. In R. B. Withrow (Ed.), *Photoperiodism and related phenomena in plants and animals* (Ed Publication No. 55, pp. 803–878). Washington, DC: American Association for the Advancement of Science.

Halberg, F., & Howard, R. B. 24 h periodicity and experimental medicine. (1958). Examples and interpretations. *Postgraduate Medicine, 24*, 349–358.

Halberg, F., Johnson, E., Brown, B. W., & Bittner, J. J. (1960). Susceptibility rhythm to *E. coli* endotoxin and bioassay. *Proceedings of the Society of Experimental Biology, 103*, 142–144.

Halberg, F., Johnson, E. A., Nelson, W., Runge, W., & Sothern, R. B. (1972). Autorhythmometry—procedures for physiologic self-measurement and their analysis. *Physiology Teacher, 1*, 1–11.

Halberg, F., Sothern, R. B., Roitman, B., Halberg, E., Halberg, Francine, Mayersbach, H. v., Haus, E., Scheving, L. E., Kanabrocki, E. L., Bartter, F. C., Delea, C., Simpson, H. W., Tavadia, H. B., Fleming, K. A., Hume, P. , & Wilson, C. (1977). Agreement of circadian characteristics for total leucocyte counts in different geographic locations. In *Proceedings of the XII International Conference of the International Society for Chronobiology, Washington, DC, Aug 10–13, 1975* (pp. 3–17). Milan: Il Ponte.

Halberg, F., & Stephens, A. N. (1958). 24 h periodicity in mortality of C mice from E. coli lipopolysaccharide [Abstract]. *Federation Proceedings, 17*, 439.

Hanson, B. R., Halberg, F., Tuna, N., Bouchard, T. J. Jr., Lykken, D. T., Cornelissen, G., Heston, L. L. (1984). Rhythmicity reveals heritability of circadian characteristics of heart rate of human twins reared apart. *Cardiologia, 29*, 267–282.

Harkness, R. A. (1974). Variations in testosterone excretion in man. In M. Ferin, F. Halberg, R. M. Richart, & R. L. Vande Wiele, (Eds.), *Biorhythms and human reproduction* (pp. 469–478). New York: John Wiley & Sons.

Harlan, J. M., & Liu, D. Y. (1992). *Adhesion: Its role in inflammatory disease.* New York: W. H. Freeman.

Haus, E., & Halberg, F. (1959). 24 h rhythm in susceptibility of C-mice to a toxic dose of ethanol. *Journal of Applied Physiology, 14*, 878–880.

Haus, E., Halberg, F., Kühl, J. F. W., & Lakatua, D. J. (1974). Chronopharmacology in animals. In J. Aschoff, F. Ceresa, & F. Halberg, (Eds.), *Chronobiological aspects of endocrinology* (pp. 122–156). Stuttgart: F. K. Schattauer-Verlag.

Haus, E., Halberg, F., & Loken, M. K. (1974). Circadian susceptibility-resistance cycle of bone marrow cells to whole body x-irradiation in Balb/c mice. In L. E. Scheving, F. Halberg, & J. E. Pauly, (Eds.), *Chronobiology* (pp. 435–474). Tokyo: Igaku-Shoin Ltd.

Haus, E., Halberg, F., Loken, M. K., & Kim, Y. S. (1974). Circadian rhythmometry of mammalian radiosensitivity. In C. A. Tobias & P. Todd, (Eds.), *Space radiation biology* (pp. 435–474). New York: Academic Press.

Haus, E., Halberg, F., Scheving, L. E., Pauly, J. E., Cardoso S.S., Kühl, J. F. W., Sothern, R. B., Shiotsuka, R. N., & Hwang, D. S. (1972). Increased tolerance of leukemic mice to arabinosyl cytosine with schedule adjusted to circadian system. *Science, 177*, 80–82.

Haus, E., Lakatua, D. J., Swoyer, J., & Sackett-Lundeen, L. (1983). Chronobiology in hematology and immunology. *American Journal of Anatomy, 168*, 467–517.

Haus, E., Lakatua, D. J., Swoyer, J., and Sackett-Lundeen, L. (1984). Chronobiology in laboratory medicine. In W. T. Rietveld, (Ed.), *Clinical aspects of chronobiology* (pp. 13–82). Baarn, The Netherlands: Bakker Publishing.

Haus, E., Nicolau, G. Y., Lakatua, D., & Sackett-Lundeen, L. (1988). Reference values for chronopharmacology. In A. Reinberg, M. Smolensky, & G. Labrecque, (Eds.), *Annual review of chronopharmacology* (vol. 4, pp. 333–424). Oxford: Pergamon Press.

Haus, E., Nicolau, G., Lakatua, D. J., Sackett-Lundeen, L., & Petrescu, E. (1989). Circadian rhythm parameters of endocrine functions in elderly subjects during the seventh to the ninth decade of life. *Chronobiologia, 16*, 331–352.

Heitbrock, H. W., Mertelsmann, R., & Garbrecht, M. (1976). Circadian rhythm of RNA polymerase B activity in human peripheral blood lymphocytes. *International Journal of Chronobiology, 3*, 255–261.

Hejl, Z. (1977). Daily, lunar, yearly and menstrual cycles and bacterial or viral infections in man. *Journal of Interdisciplinary Cycle Research, 8*, 250–253.

Hermida, R. C., Fernández, J. R., Ayala, D. E., Mojón, A., & Iglesias, M. (1997). Influence of aspirin usage on blood pressure: Dose and administration-time dependencies. *Chronobiology International, 14*, 619–637.

Hermida, R. C., Halberg, F., & Langevin, T. R. (1986). Serial white blood cell counts and chronochemotherapy according to highest values (macrophases) or by model characteristics (acrophases). In F. Halberg, L. Reale, & B. Tarquini, (Eds.), *Proceedings of the 2nd International Conference on Medico-Social Aspects of Chronobiology* (pp. 327–343). Rome: Instituto Italiano di Medicina Sociale.

Herold, M., & Günther, R. (1992). Circadian rhythm of erythrocyte sedimentation rate, C-reactive protein and soluble interleukin-2 receptor in patients with active rheumatoid arthritis. *Journal of Interdisciplinary Cycle Research, 22*, 129–130.

Hetzel, M. R., & Clark, T. J. H. (1980). Comparison of normal and asthmatic circadian rhythms in peak expiratory flow. *Thorax, 35*, 732–738.

Hohagen, F., Timmer, J., Weyerbrock, A., Fritsch-Montero, R., Ganter, U., Krieger, S., Berger, M., & Bauer, J. (1993). Cytokine production during sleep and wakefulness and its relationship to cortisol in healthy humans. *Neuropsychobiology, 28*, 9–16.

Hostmark, J., Laerum, O. D., & Farsund, T. (1984). Seasonal variations of symptoms and occurrence of human bladder carcinomas. *Scandinavian Journal of Urology and Nephrology, 18*, 107–111.

Hrushesky, W. J. M. (1996). Breast cancer, timing of surgery, and the menstrual cycle: Call for prospective trial. *Journal of Women's Health, 5*, 555–566.

Hrushesky, W. J. M. (1985). Circadian timing of cancer chemotherapy. *Science, 228*, 73–75.

Hrushesky, W. J. M., Bluming, A. Z., Gruber, S. A., & Sothern, R. B. (1989). Menstrual influence on surgical cure of breast cancer. *Lancet, 8669*, 949–952.

Hrushesky, W. J. M., Lannin, D., & Haus, E. (1999). Evidence for an ontogenetic basis for circadian coordination of cancer cell proliferation. *Journal of the National Cancer Institute, 90*, 1480–1484.

Hrushesky, W. J. M., Levi, F., Halberg, F., Haus, E., Scheving, L., Sanchez, S., Medini, E., Brown, H., & Kennedy, B. J. (1980). Clinical chrono-oncology. In L. E. Scheving, & F. Halberg, (Eds.), *Chronobiology: Principles and applications to shifts in schedules* (pp. 513–533). Alphen aan den Rijn, The Netherlands: Sijthhoff and Noordhoff.

Hrushesky, W. J. M., Roemeling, R. v., & Sothern, R. B. (1989b). Circadian chronotherapy: From animal experiments to human cancer chemotherapy. In B. Lemmer, (Ed.), *Chronopharmacology: Cellular and biochemical interactions* (pp. 439–473). New York: Marcel Dekker.

Hrushesky, W. J. M., Roemeling, R. v., & Sothern, R. B. (1989a). Preclinical and clinical cancer chemotherapy. In J. Arendt, D. S. Minors, & J. M. Waterhouse, (Eds.), *Biological rhythms in clinical practice* (pp. 225–252). London: Butterworth & Co.

Jores, A. (1935b). Das problem der tagesperiodik in der biologie. *Medizinische Klinik, 31*, 1139–1142.

Jores, A. (1935a). Physiologie und pathologie der 24-stundenrhythmik des menschen. *Ergebnisse der Inneren Medizin und Kinderheilkunde, 48*, 574–629.

Kanabrocki, E. L., Scheving, L. E., Olwin, J. H., Marks, J. S., McCormick, J. B., Halberg, F., Pauly, J. E., Greco, J., DeBartolo, M., Nemchausky, B. A., Kaplan, E., & Sothern, R. (1983). Circadian variations in the urinary excretion of electrolytes and trace elements in man. *American Journal of Anatomy, 166*, 121–148.

Kanabrocki, E. L., Sothern, R. B., Bremner, W. F., Demakis, J. G., Bean, J. T., Ringelstein, J. G., Riley, C., Fabbrini, N., Crosby, T. J., Mermall, H., Third, J. L. H. C., Shirazi, P., & Olwin, J. H. (1995). Weekly and yearly rhythms in plasma fibrinogen in hospitalized male military veterans. *American Journal of Cardiology, 76*, 628–631.

Kanabrocki, E. L., Sothern, R. B., Messmore, H. L., Roitman-Johnson, B., McCormick, J. B., Dawson, S., Bremner, W. F., Third, J. L. H. C., Nemchausky, B. A., Shirazi, P., & Scheving, L. E. (1999). Circadian inter-relationships among levels of plasma fibrinogen, blood platelets, and serum interleukin-6. *Clinical Applications in Thrombosis and Hemostasis, 5*(1), 37–42.

Kanabrocki, E. L., Sothern, R. B., Scheving, L. E., Vesely, D. L., Tsai, T. H., Shelstad, J., Cournoyer, C., Greco, J., Mermall, H., Nemchausky, B. M., Bushnell, D. L., Kaplan, E., Kahn, S., Augustine, G., Holmes, E., Rumbyrt, J., Sturtevant, R. P., Sturtevant, F., Bremner, F., Third, J. L. H. C., McCormick, J. B., Mudd, C. A., Dawson, S., Sackett-Lundeen, L., Haus, E., Halberg, F., Pauly, J. E., & Olwin, J. H. (1990). Reference values for circadian rhythms of 98 variables in clinically healthy men in fifth decade of life. *Chronobiology International, 7*, 445–461.

Karlsdottir, A., Brydøy, M., Blaauw, A., Schem, B. C., Ekanger, R., Dalene, D., Sandberg, S., Sothern, R. B., & Smaaland, R. (1997). Circadian rhythms in liver enzymes and lactate dehydrogenase (LDH) before and during cytotoxic chemotherapy courses in cancer patients [Abstract]. *Chronobiology International, 14*(suppl. 1), 80.

Katschinski, D. M., Wiedemann, G. J., Mentzel, M., Mulkerin, D. L., Touhidi, R., & Robins, H. I. (1997). Influence of circadian rhythm on 41.8°C whole body hyperthermia induction of haematopoietic growth factors. *International Journal of Hyperthermia, 13*, 571–576.

Kerr, H. D. (1973). Diurnal variation of respiratory function independent of air quality. *Archives of Environmental Health, 26*, 144–152.

Killman, S. A., Cronkite, E. P., Fliedner, T. M., & Bond, V. T. (1962). Mitotic indices of human bone marrow cells. I. Number and cytologic distribution of mitoses. *Blood, 19*, 743–750.

Klevecz, R. B., Shymko, R. M., Blumenfeld, D., & Braly, P. S. (1987). Circadian gating of S phase in human ovarian cancer. *Cancer Research, 47*, 6267–6271.

Knapp, M. S., Cove-Smith, M. S., Dugdale, R., MacKenzie, N., & Pownall, R. (1979). Possible effect of time on renal allograft rejection. *British Medical Journal, i (6155)*, 75–77.

Kowanko, I. C., Knapp, M. S., Pownall, R., & Swannell, A. J. (1982). Domiciliary self-measurement in rheumatoid arthritis and the demonstration of circadian rhythmicity. *Annals of Rheumatic Disease, 41*, 453–455.

Kühl, J. F. W., Lee, J. K., Halberg, F., Haus, E., Günther, R., & Knapp, E. (1974). Circadian and lower frequency rhythms in male grip strength and body weight. In M. Ferin, F. Halberg, R. M. Richart, & R. L., Vande Wiele, (Eds.), *Biorhythms and human reproduction* (pp. 529–548). New York: John Wiley & Sons.

Laerum, O. D., Smaaland, R., & Sletvold, O. (1989). Rhythms in blood and bone marrow: Potential therapeutic implications. In B. Lemmer, (Ed.), *Chronopharmacology: Cellular and biochemical interactions* (pp. 371–393). New York: Marcel Dekker.

Langlois, P. H., White, R. F., & Glezen, W. P. (1986). Diurnal variation in human response to influenza vaccination? A pilot study of 125 volunteers. In A. Reinberg, M. Smolensky, & G. Labrecque, (Eds.), *Annual review of chronopharmacology* (vol. 3, p. 123). Oxford: Pergamon Press.

Lemmer, B., Schwulera, U., Thrun, A., & Lissner, A. (1992). Circadian rhythm of soluble interleukin-2 receptor in healthy individuals. *European Cytokine Network, 3*, 335–336.

Lester, D. (1971). Seasonal variation in suicidal deaths. *British Journal of Psychiatry, 118*, 627–628.

Lévi, F., Adam, R., Soussan, A., Caussanel, J. P., Benavides, M., Misset, J. L., Burki, F., Reinberg, A., Smolensky, M., Bismuth, H., & Mathé, G. (1988). Ambulatory 5-day chronotherapy of colorectal cancer with continuous venous infusion of 5-fluorouracil (5-FU) at circadian-modulated rate. Preliminary results. In A. Reinberg, M. Smolensky, & G. Labrecque, (Eds.), *Annual review of chronopharmacology* (vol 5, pp. 419–422). New York: Pergamon Press.

Lévi, F., Benavides, M., Chevelle, C., Le Saunier, F., Bailleul, F., Misset, J.-L., Regensberg, C., Vannetzel, J.-M., Reinberg, A., & Mathé, G. (1990). Chemotherapy of advanced ovarian cancer with 4′-O-tetrahyropyranyl doxorubicin and cisplatin a randomized phase II trial with an evaluation of circadian timing and dose-intensity. *Journal of Clinical Oncology, 8*, 705–714.

Lévi, F., Boughattas, N. A., & Blazsek, I. (1988). Comparative murine chronotoxicity of anti-cancer agents and related mechanisms. In A. Reinberg, M. Smolensky, & G. Labrecque, (Eds.), *Annual review of chronopharmacology* (vol. 4, pp. 283–331). New York: Pergamon Press.

Lévi, F. A., Canon, C., Blum, J. P., Mechkouri, M., Reinberg, A., & Mathé, G. (1985). Circadian and/or circahemidian rhythms in nine lymphocyte-related variables from peripheral blood of healthy subjects. *Journal of Immunology, 134*, 217–220.

Lévi, F., Canon, C., Blum, J. P., Reinberg A., & Mathé, G. (1983). Large-amplitude circadian rhythm in helper:suppressor ratio of peripheral blood lymphocytes. *Lancet, 2*, 462–463.

Lévi, F. A., Canon, C., Dipalma, M., Florentin, I., & Misset, J. L. (1991). When should the immune clock be rest? From circadian pharmacodynamics to temporally optimized drug delivery. *Annals of the New York Academy Sciences, 618*, 312–329.

Lévi, F., Canon, C., Touitou, Y., Reinberg, A., & Mathé, G. (1988). Seasonal modulation of the circadian time structure of circulating T and natural killer lymphocyte subsets from healthy subjects. *Journal of Clinical Investigation, 81*, 407–413.

Lévi, F. A., Canon, C., Touitou, Y., Sulon, J., Mechkouri, M., Demey-Ponsard, R., Touboul, J. P., Vannetzel, J. M., Mowrowicz, I., Reinberg, A., & Mathé, G. (1988). Circadian rhythms in circulating T lymphocyte subtypes, and plasma testosterone, total and free cortisol and in five healthy men. *Clinical and Experimental Immunology, 71*, 329–335.

Lévi, F., Hrushesky, W. J. M., Halberg, F., Langevin, T. R., Haus, E., & Kennedy, B. J. (1982). Lethal nephrotoxicity and hematologic toxicity to cis-diamminedichloroplatinum ameliorated by optimal circadian timing and hydration. *European Journal of Cancer and Clinical Oncology, 18*, 471–477.

Lévi, F., & Reinberg, A. (1990). Meeting report. Chronobiology and chronotherapy of cancer. *Chronobiology International, 5/6*, 471–474.

Lévi, F. A., Reinberg, A., & Canon, C. (1989). Clinical immunology and allergy. In J. Arendt, D. S. Minors, & J. M. Waterhouse, (Eds.), *Biological rhythms in clinical practice* (pp. 99–135). Wright: London.

Lévi, F. A., Zidani, R., Vannetzel, J. M., Perpoint, B., Focan, C., Faggiuolo, R., Chollet, P., Garufi, C., Itzhaki, M., Dogliatti, L., Iacobelli, S., Adam, R., Kumstlinger, F., Gastiaburu, J., Bismuth, H., Jasmin, C., & Misset, J.-L. (1994). Chronomodulated versus fixed-infusion-rate delivery of ambulatory chemotherapy with oxaliplatin, fluorouracil, and folinic acid (Leucovorin) in patients with colorectal cancer metastases: A randomized multi-institutional trial. *Journal of the National Cancer Institute, 86*, 1608–1617.

Levine, H., Halberg, F., Sothern, R. B., Bartter, W. J., & Delea, C. (1974). Circadian phase-shifting with and without geographic displacement. In M. Ferin, F. Halberg, R. M. Richart, & R. L. Vande Wiele, (Eds.), *Biorhythms and human reproduction* (pp. 557–574). New York: John Wiley & Sons.

Li, X.-M., Soulard, C., Filipski, E., Deschamps de Paillatte, E., & Lévi, F. (1998). Circadian-based effects of AcSDKP, with or without rhG-CSF on hematologic toxicity of chemotherapy in mice. *European Journal of Haematology, 60*(3), 181–188.

Liebmann, P. M., Reibnegger, G., Lehofer, M., Moser, M., Pürstner, P., Mangge, H., & Schauenstein, K. (1998). Circadian rhythm of the soluble p75 tumor necrosis factor (sTNF-R75) receptor in humans—a possible explanation for the circadian kinetics of TNF-α effects. *International Immunology, 10*, 1393–1396.

Lissoni, P., Rovelli, F., Brivio, F., Brivio, O., & Fumagalli, L. (1998). Circadian secretions of IL-2, IL-12, IL-6 and IL-10 in relation to the light/dark rhythm of the pineal hormone melatonin in healthy humans. *Natural Immunity, 16*(1), 1–5.

Maatman, T. J. (1989). The role of prostate specific antigen as a tumor marker in men with advanced adenocarcinoma of the prostate. *Journal of Urology, 141*, 1378–1380.

Manfredini, R., Gallerani, M., Ricci, L., Lalo, G., Pareschi, P. L., & Fersini, C. (1991). Circadian rhythm of sudden death from pulmonary embolism [Abstract]. *Journal of Interdisciplinary Cycle Research, 22*, 151.

Martin, W. (1981). Estimation of parameters of circadian rhythms, if measurements cannot be performed around the clock. The case of a band limited signal plus noise. In A. Reinberg, N. Vieux, & P. Andlauer, (Eds.), *Night and shiftwork: Biological and social aspects* (pp. 37–44). Oxford: Pergamon Press.

Martin, W., & Brinkmann, K. (1976). A computer program system for the analysis of equispaced time series. *Journal of Interdisciplinary Cycle Research, 7*(3), 251–258,

Martini, E., Muller, J.-Y., Doinel, C., Gastal, C., Roquin, H., Douay, L., & Salmon, C. (1988). Disappearance of CD4-lymphocyte circadian cycles in HIV-infected patients: Early event during asymptomatic infection. Short communication. *AIDS, 2*, 133–134.

Mattes, A., Witte, K., Hohmann, W., & Lemmer, B. (1991). Pharmfit—a nonlinear fitting program for pharmacology. *Chronobiology International, 8*, 460–476.

Mauer, A. M. (1965). Diurnal variation of proliferative activity in the human bone marrow. *Blood, 26*, 1–7.

Melchart, D., Martin, P., Hallek, M., Holzmann, M., Jurcic, X., & Wagner, H. (1992). Circadian variation of the phagocytic activity of polymorphonuclear leukocytes and of various other parameters in 13 healthy male adults. *Chronobiology International, 9*, 35–45.

Mermall, H., Sothern, R. B., Kanabrocki, E. L., Quadri, S. F., Bremner, F. W., Nemchausky, B. M., & Scheving, L. E. (1995). Temporal (circadian) and functional relationship between prostate-specific antigen and testosterone in healthy men. *Urology, 46*(1), 45–53.

Migrom, H., Barnhart, A., Gaddy, J., Bush, R., & Busse, W. (1990). The effect of chronotherapy with a 24 h sustained release theophylline preparation (Uniphyl) on A. M. and P. M. differences in airway patency and responsiveness. In A., Reinberg, M. Smolensky, & G. Labrecque, (Eds.), *Annual review of chronopharmacology* (vol. 6, pp. 301–304). Oxford: Pergamon Press.

Minors, D. S., & Waterhouse, J. M. (1989). Analysis of biological time series. In J. Arendt, D. S. Minors, & J. M. Waterhouse, (Eds.), *Biological rhythms in clinical practice* (pp. 272–293). London: Wright.

Mojón, A., Fernandez, J. R., & Hermida, R. C. (1992). ChronoLab: An interactive software package for chronobiologic time series analysis written for the Macintosh computer. *Chronobiology International, 9*, 403–412.

Monk, T. H., & Fort, A. (1983). "Cosina": A cosine curve fitting program suitable for small computer. *International Journal of Chronobiology, 8*, 193–224.

Moore-Ede, M. (1973). Circadian rhythms of drug effectiveness and toxicity. *Clinical Pharmacology & Therapeutics, 14*, 925–935.

Moore-Ede, M. (1986). Physiology of the circadian timing system: Predictive versus reactive homeostasis. *American Journal of Physiology, 19*, R735–752.

Morgan, E., & Minors, D. D., (Eds.). Methods in biological time-series analysis. (1995). *Biological Rhythm Research, 26*, 124–252.

Mormont, C., Boughattas, N. A., & Lévi, F. (1989). Mechanisms of circadian rhythms in the toxicity and efficacy of anticancer drugs: relevance for the development of new analogues. In B. Lemmer, (Ed.), *Chronopharmacology. cellular and biochemical interactions* (pp. 395–437). New York: Marcel Dekker.

Mormont, M. C., Claustrat, B., Waterhouse, J., Touitou, Y., & Lévi, F. (1998). Clinical relevance of circadian rhythm assessment in cancer patients. In Y. Touitou, (Ed.), *Biological Clocks—mechanisms and applications* (pp. 497–505). Amsterdam: Elsevier.

Muc-Wierzgon, M., Madej, K., Baranowski, M., & Wierzgon, J. (1998). Circadian rhythmometry of serum endogenous tumor necrosis factor-alpha in patients with colorectal cancer metastases. *European Cytokine Network, 9*(2), 193–196.

Nathan, D. G. (1988). Hematologic diseases, In J. B. Wyngaardan, & L. H. Smith, (Eds.), *Textbook of medicine* (pp. 873–878). Philadelphia: W. B. Saunders.

Nathan, D. G. (1987). Stem cells and hematopoiesis, In D. J. Weatherall, J. G. G. Ledingham, & D. A. Warrell, (Eds.), *Oxford textbook of medicine* (2nd ed.) (vol. II, pp. 19.7–19.12). Oxford: Oxford University Press.

Nelson, W., Tong, Y. L., Lee, J. K., & Halberg, F. (1979). Methods for cosinor rhythmometry. *Chronobiologia, 6*, 305–323.

Newell, G. R., Lyncy, H. K., Gibeau, J. M., & Skitz, M. R. (1985). Seasonal diagnosis of Hodgkin's disease among young adults. *Journal of the National Cancer Institute, 74*, 53–56.

Nicholson, P. A., & Bogie, W. (1973). Diurnal variation in the symptoms of hay fever: Implications for pharmaceutical development. *Current Medical Research and Opinion, 1*, 395–400.

Nicolau, G. Y., Haus, E., Popescu, M., Sackett-Lundeen, L., & Petrescu, E. (1991). Circadian, weekly, and seasonal variations in cardiac mortality, blood pressure, and catecholamine excretion. *Chronobiology International, 8*, 149–159.

O'Conner, J. F., Shelley, E. M., & Stern, L. O. (1974). Behavioral rhythms related to the menstrual cycle. In M. Ferin, F. Halberg, R. M. Richart, & R. L. Vande Wiele, (Eds.), *Biorhythms and human reproduction* (pp. 309–324). New York: John Wiley & Sons.

Ohdo, S., Arata, N., Furukubo, T., Yukawa, E., Higuchi, S., Nakano, S., & Ogawa, N. (1998). Chronopharmacology of granulocyte colony-stimulating factor in mice. *Journal of Pharmacology and Experimental Therapeutics, 285*(1), 242–246.

Ostfeld, A. M. (1963). The natural history and epidemiology of migraine and muscle contraction headache. *Neurology, 13*, 11–15.

Paukovits, W. R., Guigon, M., Binder, K. A., Hergl, A., Laerum, O. D., & Schulte-Hermann, R. (1990). Prevention of hematotoxic side effects of cytostatic drugs in mice by a synthetic hemoregulatory peptide, *Cancer Research, 50*, 328–332.

Pallansch, M., Kim, Y., Halberg, E., Halberg Francine, Rowe, N., Carandente, F., Tarquini, B., Neri, B., Reissmann, G., Halberg, F., & Cagnoni, M. (1979). Circadian rhythm in several components of the complement cascade in healthy women [Abstract]. *Chronobiologia, 6*, 139–140.

Petrovsky, N., McNair, P., & Harrison, L. C. (1994). Circadian rhythmicity of interferon-gamma production in antigen-stimulated whole blood. *Chronobiologia, 21*, 293–300.

Petrovsky, N., McNair, P., & Harrison, L. C. (1998). Diurnal rhythms in pro-inflammatory cytokines: Regulation by plasma cortisol and therapeutic implications. *Cytokine, 10*(4), 307–312.

Pincus, D. J., Humeston, T. R., & Martin, R. J. (1997). Further studies on the chronotherapy of asthma with inhaled steroids: The effect of dosage timing on drug efficacy. *Journal of Allergy and Clinical Immunology, 100*, 771–774.

Pirke, K. M., Wuttke, W., & Schweiger, U., (Eds.). (1989). *The menstrual cycle and its disorders*. Berlin: Springer-Verlag.

Pöllman, L. (1982). Circannual variations in the frequency of some diseases of the oral mucosa. *Journal of Interdisciplinary Cycle Research, 13*, 249–256.

Pöllman, L., & Harris, P. H. P. (1978). Rhythmic changes in pain sensitivity in teeth. *International Journal of Chronobiology, 5*, 459–464.

Pöllman, L., & Pöllman, B. (1988) Circadian variations of the efficiency of hepatitis B vaccination. In A. Reinberg, M. Smolensky, & G. Labrecque, (Eds.), *Annual review of chronopharmacology* (vol. 5, pp. 45–48). Oxford: Pergamon Press.

Ramirez-Lassepas, M., Haus, E., Lakatua, D. J., Sackett, L., & Swoyer, J. (1980). Seasonal (circannual) periodicity of spontaneous intracerebral hemorrhage in Minnesota. *Annals of Neurology, 8*, 539–541.

Ramot, B., Brok-Simoni, F., Chiveidman, E., & Ashkenazi, Y. E. (1976). Blood leucocyte enzymes. III. Diurnal rhythm of activity in isolated lymphocytes of normal subjects and chronic lymphatic leukemia patients. *British Journal of Haematology, 34*, 79–85.

Ratajczak, H. V., Sothern, R. B., & Hrushesky, W. J. M. (1988). Estrous influence on surgical cure of a mouse breast cancer. *Journal of Experimental Medicine, 168*, 73–83.

Ratajczak, H. V., Thomas, P. T., Sothern, R. B., Vollmuth, T., & Heck, J. D. (1993). Evidence for genetic basis of seasonal differences in antibody formation between two mouse strains. *Chronobiology International, 10*, 383–394.

Reinberg, A. (1967). The hours of changing responsiveness or susceptibility. *Perspectives in Biology and Medicine, 11*, 111–128.

Reinberg, A., Gervais, P., Morin, M., & Abulker, C. (1971). Rythme circadien humain du seuil de la réponse bronchique a l'acétylcholine. *Comptes Rendus de l'Academie des Sciences—Serie III, Sciences de la Vie, 272*, 1879–1881.

Reinberg, A., Ghata, J., & Sidi, E. (1963). Nocturnal asthma attacks: Their relationship to the circadian adrenal cycle. *Journal of Allergy and Clinical Immunology, 34*, 323–330.

Reinberg, A., Guillet, P., Gervais, P., Ghata, J., Vignaud, D., & Abulker, C. (1977). One month chronocorticotherapy (Dutimelan, 8-15 mite). Control of the asthmatic condition without adrenal suppression and circadian rhythm alteration. *Chronobiologia, 4*, 295–312.

Reinberg, A., & Lagoguey, M. (1978). Annual endocrine rhythms in healthy young adult men: Their implication in human biology and medicine. In I. Assenmacher, & D. S. Farner, (Eds.), *Environmental endocrinology* (pp. 113–121). Berlin: Springer-Verlag.

Reinberg, A., Schuller, E., Delasnerie, N., Clench, J., & Helary, M. (1977). Rythmes circadiens et circannuels des leucocytes, protéines totales, immunoglobulines A, G et M, etude chez 9 adultes jeunes et sains. *Nouvelle Presse Médicale, 6*, 3819–3823.

Reinberg, A., Sidi, E., & Ghata, J. (1965). Circadian rhythms of human skin to histamine or allergen and the adrenal cycle. *Journal of Allergy and Clinical Immunology, 36*, 279–283.

Reinberg, A., & Smolensky, M. H. (1974). Circatrigintan secondary rhythms related to the hormonal changes in the menstrual cycle: General considerations. In M. Ferin, F. Halberg, R. M. Richart, & R. L. Vande Wiele, (Eds.), *Biorhythms and human reproduction* (pp. 241–258). New York: John Wiley & Sons.

Reinberg, A., & Smolensky, M. H. (1983). Investigative methodology for chronobiology. In A. Reinberg, & M. H. Smolensky, (Eds.), *Biological rhythms and medicine. Cellular, metabolic, physiopathologic, and pharmacologic aspects* (pp. 23–46). New York: Springer-Verlag.

Reinberg, A., Touitou, Y., Botbol, M., & Gervais, P. (1990). Preservation of the adrenal function with oral morning dosing of corticoids in long term (3 to 11 years) treated corticodependent asthmatics. In A. Reinberg, M. Smolensky, & G. Labrecque, (Eds.), *Annual review of chronopharmacology* (vol. 6, pp. 327–330). Oxford: Pergamon Press.

Reinberg, A., Zagulla-Mally, Z., Ghata, J., Halberg, F. (1969). Circadian reacitivity rhythms of human skin to house dust, penicillin and histamine. *Journal of Allergy, 44*, 292–306.

Rhame, F., Sothern, R. B., Sackett-Lundeen, L., Suarez, C., Hrushesky, W. J. M., & Haus, E. (1989). Aberrant circadian physiologic, immune and endocrine rhythms in HIV-infected individuals [Abstract]. *Proceedings of the V International Conference on AIDS*, Montreal, June 4–9.

Rietveld, W. J., Boon, M. E., & Meulman, J. J. (1997). Seasonal fluctuations in the cervical smear detection rates for (pre)malignant changes and for infections. *Diagnostic Cytopathology, 17*, 452–455.

Rietveld, P. E. M., Rietveld, W. J., Boon, M. E., Sothern, R. B., & Hrushesky, W. J. M. (1988). The incidence of cervical pathology in Dutch women. Seasonal rhythms in infections and neoplasia [Abstract]. *Journal of Interdisciplinary Cycle Research, 19*, 206.

Ritchie, W. S., Oswald, I., Micklem, H. S., Boyd, J. E., Elton, R. A., Jazwinska, E., & James, K. (1983). Circadian variation of lymphocyte subpopulations: A study with monoclonal antibodies. *British Journal of Medicine, 286*, 1773–1775.

Rivard, G., Infante-Rivard, C., Hoyeux, C., & Champagne, J. (1985). Maintenance chemotherapy for childhood acute lymphoblastic leukemia: Better in the evening. *Lancet, 2*, 1264–1266.

Roennenberg, T., & Aschoff, J. (1990a). Annual rhythm of human reproduction. I. Biology, sociology or both? *Journal of Biologic Rhythms, 5*, 195–216.

Roennenberg, T., & Aschoff, J. (1990b). Annual rhythm of human reproduction. II. Environmental correlations. *Journal of Biologic Rhythms, 5*, 217–239.

Roitman-Johnson, B., Sothern, R. B., Kanabrocki, E. L., Nemchausky, B. M., & Scheving, L. E. (1998). Circadian rhythm in human serum intercellular adhesion molecule (ICAM-1) [Abstract]. *Journal of Allergy and Clinical Immunology, 101*, S18.

Roitman-Johnson, B., Sothern, R. B., Kanabrocki, E. L., Yager, J. G., Corcoran, K., Fuerstenberg, R. K., Weatherbee, J. A., Nemchausky, B. M., & Scheving, L. E. (1996). Circadian rhythm in serum interleukin-6 soluble receptor (IL6sR): Temporal and functional relationship to IL6 (Abstract). *Journal of Allergy and Clinical Immunology, 97*(1, part 3), 413.

Rosenblatt, L. S., Shifrine, M., Hetherington, N. W., Paglieroni, T., & MacKenzie, M. R. (1982). A circannual rhythm in rubella antibody titers. *Journal of Interdisciplinary Cycle Research, 13*, 81–88.

Ross, D. D., Pollak, A., Akman, S. A., & Bachur, N. R. (1980). Diurnal variation of circulating human myeloid progenitor cells. *Experimental Hematology, 8*, 954–960.

Scheving, L. E. (1959). Mitotic activity in the human epidermis. *Anatomical Record, 135*, 7–19.

Scheving, L. E., Cardoso, S. S., Pauly, J. E., Halberg, F., & Haus, E. (1974). Variation in susceptibility of mice to the carcinostatic agent arabinosyl cytosine. In L. E. Scheving, F. Halberg, & J. E. Pauly, (Eds.), *Chronobiology* (pp. 213–217). Tokyo: Igaku Shoin Ltd.

Scheving, L. E., Tsai, T. H., & Pauly, J. E. (1986). Chronotoxicology and chronopharmacology with emphasis on carcinostatic agents. In A. Reinberg, M. Smolensky, & G. Labrecque, (Eds.), *Annual review of chronopharmacology* (vol. 2, pp. 177–197). New York: Pergamon Press.

Schibler, U. (1998). New cogwheels in the clockworks. *Nature 393*, 620–621.

Shinkawa, A., Veda, K., Hasuo, Y., Kiyohara, Y., & Fujishima, M. (1990). Seasonal variation in stroke incidence in Hisayama, Japan. *Stroke, 21*, 1262–1267.

Simpson, H. W. (1987). Human thermometry in health and disease: The chronobiologist's perspective. In L. E. Scheving, F. Halberg, & C. F. Ehret, (Eds.), *Chronobiotechnology and chronobiological engineering (NATO ASI Series)* (pp. 141–188). Dordrecht: Martinus Mijhoff.

Smaaland, R., Abrahamsen, J. F., Svardal, A. M., Lote, K., & Ueland, P. M. (1992). DNA cell cycle distribution and glutathione (GSH) content according to circadian stage in bone marrow of cancer patients. *British Journal of Cancer, 66*, 39–45.

Smaaland, R., Laerum, O. D., Abrahamsen, J. F., Sothern, R. B., & Lote, K. (1995). Cytokinetic circadian patterns in human host and tumor. *Journal of Infusional Chemotherapy, 5*, 11–14.

Smaaland, R., Laerum, O. D., Lote, K., Sletvold, O., Sothern, R. B., & Bjerknes, R. (1991). DNA synthesis in human bone marrow is circadian stage dependent. *Blood, 77*, 2603–2611.

Smaaland, R., Laerum, O. D., Sothern, R. B., Lote, K., Sletvold, O., & Bjerknes, R. (1992). CFU-GM and DNA synthesis of human bone marrow are circadian stage dependent and show covariation. *Blood, 79*, 2281–2287.

Smaaland, R., Lote, K., Sothern, R. B., & Laerum, O. D. (1993). DNA synthesis and ploidy in non-Hodgkin's lymphomas demonstrate intrapatient variation depending on circadian stage of cell sampling. *Cancer Research, 53*, 3129–3138.

Smaaland, R., & Sothern, R. B. (1994). Cytokinetic basis for circadian pharmacodynamics: Circadian cytokinetics of murine and human bone marrow and human cancer. In W. J. M. Hrushesky (Ed.), *Circadian cancer therapy* (pp. 119–163). Boca Raton: CRC Press.

Smaaland, R., Sothern, R. B., Lote, K., Sandberg, S., Aakvaag, A., & Laerum, O. D. (1995). Circadian phase relationships between peripheral blood variables and bone marrow proliferative activity in clinical health. *in vivo, 9*, 379–389.

Smolensky, M. H. (1983). Aspects of human chronopathology. In A. Reinberg, & M. H. Smolensky, (Eds.), *Biological rhythms and medicine. Cellular, metabolic, physiopathologic, and pharmacologic aspects* (pp. 131–209). Springer-Verlag: New York.

Smolensky, M. H. (1981). Chronobiologic factors related to the epidemiology of human reproduction. In J. Cortéz-Prieto, A. Campos da Paz, & M. Nevese-Castro, (Eds.), *Research on fertility and sterility* (pp. 157–181). Lancaster: MTP Press.

Smolensky, M. H., & D'Alonzo, G. E. (1988). Biologic rhythms and medicine. *American Journal of Medicine, 85*, 34–46.

Smolensky, M. H., D'Alonzo, G. E., & Reinberg, A. (1990). Current developments in the chronotherapy of nocturnal asthma. In A. Reinberg, M. Smolensky, & G. Labrecque, (Eds.), *Annual review of chronopharmacology* (vol. 6, pp. 81–112). Oxford: Pergamon Press.

Smolensky, M. H., & Halberg, F. (1977). Circadian rhythms in airway patency and lung volumes. In J. P McGovern, M. H. Smolensky, & A. Reinberg, (Eds.), *Chronobiology in allergy and immunology* (pp. 117–138). Springfield, IL: C. C. Thomas.

Smolensky, M., Halberg, F., & Sargent, F. (1972). Chronobiology of the life sequence. In S. Ito, K. Ogata, & H. Yohimura, (Eds.), *Advances in climatic physiology* (pp. 281–318). Tokyo: Igaku Shoin Ltd.

Smolensky, M. H., Scott, P. H., Barnes, P. J., & Jonkman, J. H. G. (1986). The chronopharmacology and chronotherapy of asthma. In A. Reinberg, M. Smolensky, & G. Labrecque, (Eds.), *Annual review of chronopharmacology* (vol. 2, pp. 229–273). Oxford: Pergamon Press.

Sothern, R. B. (1974). Low frequency rhythms in the beard growth of a man. In L. E. Scheving, F. Halberg, & J. E. Pauly, (Eds.), *Chronobiology* (pp. 241–244). Tokyo: Igaku Shoin Ltd.

Sothern, R. B. (1995). Time of day versus internal circadian timing references. *Journal of Infusional Chemotherapy, 5*, 24–30.

Sothern, R. B., Farber, M. S., & Gruber, S. A. (1993). Circannual variations in baseline blood values of dogs. *Chronobiology International, 10*, 364–382.

Sothern, R. B., Kanabrocki, E. L., Boles, M. A., Nemchausky, B. M., Olwin, J. H., & Scheving, L. E. (1994). Marker rhythmometry: Comparison of simultaneous circadian variations for cortisol & melatonin in 3 biological fluids of adult men [Abstract]. In *Biological rhythms and medications. Proceedings of the 6th International Conference of Chronopharmacology & Chronotherapeutics.*

Sothern, R. B., Lévi, F., Haus, E., Halberg, F., & Hrushesky, W. J. M. (1989). Control of a murine plasmacytoma with doxorubicin–cisplatin Dependence on circadian stage of treatment. *Journal of the National Cancer Institute, 81*, 135–145.

Sothern, R. B., Nelson, W. L., & Halberg, F. (1977). A circadian rhythm in susceptibility of mice to the anti-tumor drug, adriamycin. In *Proceedings of the XII International Conference of the International Society for Chronobiology* (pp. 433–438). Milan: Il Ponte.

Sothern, R. B., Rhame, F., Suarez, C., Fletcher, C., Sackett-Lundeen, L., Haus, E., & Hrushesky, W. J. M. (1990). Oral temperature rhythmometry and substantial within-day variation in zidovudine levels following steady state dosing in human immunodeficiency virus (HIV) infection. In D. K. Hayes, J. E. Pauly, & R. J. Reiter, (Eds.), *Chronobiology: Its role in clinical medicine, general biology and agriculture, part A* (pp. 67–76). New York: Wiley-Liss Inc.

Sothern, R. B., Roitman-Johnson, B., Kanabrocki, E. L., Nemchausky, B. M., & Scheving, L. E. (1995). Circadian rhythm in serum transferrin receptor in healthy men [Abstract 221]. *Biological Rhythm Research*, 26, 444–445.

Sothern, R. B., Roitman-Johnson, B., Kanabrocki, E. L., Nemchausky, B. M., Scheving, L. E., & Olwin, J. H. (1997). Circadian rhythm in serum vascular cell adhesion molecule-1 in men. [Abstract]. *Chronobiology International, 14*(suppl. 1), 160.

Sothern, R. B., Roitman-Johnson, B., Kanabrocki, E. L., Yager, J. G., Fuerstenberg, R. K., Weatherbee, J. A., Young, M. R. I., Nemchausky, B. M., & Scheving, L. E. (1995a). Circadian characteristics of interleukin-6 in blood and urine of clinically-healthy men. *in vivo, 9*, 331–339.

Sothern, R. B., Roitman-Johnson, B., Kanabrocki, E. L., Yager, J. G., Fuerstenberg, R. K., Weatherbee, J. A., Young, M. R. I., Nemchausky, B. M., & Scheving, L. E. (1995b). Temporal and functional relationship between interleukin-6, leukocytes and serum cortisol in men [Abstract]. *Journal of Allergy and Clinical Immunology*, *95*(1, part 2), 37.

Sothern, R. B., Roitman-Johnson, B., Kanabrocki, E. L., Yager, J. G., Roodell, M. M., Weatherbee, J. A., Young, M. R. I. , Nemchausky, B. M., & Scheving, L. E. (1995). Circadian characteristics of circulating interleukin-6 in adult men. *Journal of Allergy and Clinical Immunology*, *95*, 1029–1035.

Sothern, R. B., Smaaland, R., & Moore, J. M. (1995). Circannual rhythm in DNA Synthesis (S-Phase) in healthy human bone marrow and rectal mucosa. *FASEB Journal*, *9*, 397–403.

Sothern, R. B., Slover, G. P. T., & Morris, R. W. (1993). Circannual and menstrual rhythm characteristics in manic episodes and body temperature. *Biological Psychiatry*, *33*, 194–203.

Sothern, R. B., Vesely, D. L., Kanabrocki, E. L., Bremner, F. W., Third, J. L. H. C., McCormick, J. B., Dawson, S., Ryan, M., Greco, J., Bean, J. T., Nemchausky, B. M., Shirazi, P., & Scheving, L. E. (1996). Circadian relationships between circulating atrial natriuretic peptides and serum sodium and chloride in healthy humans. *American Journal of Nephrology*, *16*, 462–470.

Sothern, R. B., Vesely, D. L., Kanabrocki, E. L., Hermida, R. C., Bremner, F. W., Third, J. L. H. C., Boles, M. A., Nemchausky, B. M., Olwin, J. H., & Scheving, L. E. (1995). Temporal (circadian) and functional relationship between atrial natriuretic peptides and blood pressure. *Chronobiology International*, *12*(2), 106–120.

Sothern, R. B., Voegele, M. , Mattson, O., & Hrushesky, W. J. M. (1989). A chronobiological statistical package for personal computer [Abstract]. *Chronobiologia*, *16*, 184.

Spira, A. (1984). Seasonal variations in sperm characteristics. *Archives of Andrology*, *12*, 23–28.

Spivak, J. L. (1984). Normal hematopoiesis, In A. M. Harvey, R. J. Johns, V. A. McKusick, A. H. Owens, & R. S. Ross, (Eds.), *The principles and practice of medicine*, 21st ed. (pp. 461–466). Norwalk, CT: Appleton-Century-Crofts.

Steinijans, V. W., Trautmann, H., Sauter, R., & Staudinger, H. (1990). Theophylline therapeutic drug monitoring in the case of a new sustained-release pellet formulation for once-daily evening administration. In A. Reinberg, M. Smolensky, & G. Labrecque, (Eds.), *Annual review of chronopharmacology* (vol. 6, pp. 323–326). Oxford: Pergamon Press.

Svanes, C., Sothern, R. B., & Sørbye, H. (1998). Rhythmic patterns in incidence of peptic ulcer perforation over 5.5 decades in Norway. *Chronobiology International*, *15*(3), 241–264

Swerdlow, A. J. (1985). Seasonality of presentation of cutaneous melanoma, squamous cell cancer and basal cell cancer in the Oxford region. *British Journal of Cancer*, *52*, 893–900.

Swoyer, J., Rhame, F., Hrushesky, W., Sackett-Lundeen, L., Sothern, R., Gale, H., & Haus, E. (1990). Circadian rhythm alterations in HIV infected subjects. In D. K. Hayes, J. E. Pauly, & R. J. Reiter, (Eds.), *Chronobiology: Its role in clinical medicine, general biology and agriculture, part A*, (pp. 437–449). New York: Wiley-Liss, Inc.

Tahti, E. (1956). Studies of the effect of X-irradiation on 24 hour variations in the mitotic activity in human malignant tumours. *Acta Pathologica et Microbiologica Scandinavica*, *117*(suppl.), 1–166.

Takahashi, J. S., & Hoffman, M. (1995). Molecular biological clocks. *American Scientist*, *83*, 158–165.

Tavidia, H. B., Fleming, K. A., Hume, P. D., & Simpson, H. W. (1972). Circadian rhythmicity of plasma cortisol and PHA-induced lymphocyte transformation. *Clinical and Experimental Immunology*, *22*, 190–193.

Taylor, A. J., Davies, R. J., Hendrick, D. J., & Pepys, J. (1979). Recurrent nocturnal asthmatic reactions to bronchial provocation tests. *Clinical Allergy*, *9*, 213–219.

Tjoa, W. S., Smolensky, M. H., Hsi, B., Steinberger, E., & Smith, K. D. (1982). Circannual rhythm in human sperm count revealed by serially independent sampling. *Fertility and Sterility*, *38*, 454–459.

Thompson, A. W. (1994). *The cytokine handbook*, 2nd ed. San Diego: Academic Press.

Todisco, T., Eslami, A., Baglioni, S., Dottorini, M., Bruni, L., & Grassi, Y. (1995). Circadian behavior of extrinsic and intrinsic asthma [Abstract]. *Biological Rhythm Research*, *26*, 450–451.

Tong, Y. L., Nelson, W. L., Sothern, R. B., & Halberg, F. (1977). Estimation of the orthophase—timing of the high values on a non-sinusoidal rhythm—illustrated by the best timing for experimental cancer chronotherapy. In *Proceedings of the XII International Conference of the International Society for Chronobiology* (pp. 765–769). Milan: Il Ponte.

Touitou, Y., & Haus, E., (Eds.) (1992). *Biological rhythms in clinical and laboratory medicine*. Berlin: Springer-Verlag.

Touitou, Y., Sothern, R. B., Lévi, F., Focan, C., Bogdan, A., Auzéby, A., Franchimont, P., Roemeling, R. v., & Hrushesky, W. J. M. (1988). Sources of predictable tumor marker variation within the so-called normal range: Circadian and circannual aspects of plasma carcinoembryonic antigen (CEA) in health and cancer. *Journal of Tumor Marker Oncology*, *3*, 351–359.

Turner-Warwick, M. (1984). Definition and recognition of nocturnal asthma. In P. J. Barnes, & J. Levy, (Eds.), *Nocturnal asthma* (pp. 3–5). Oxford: Oxford University Press.

Turner-Warwick, M. (1988). Management of chronic asthma. In P. J. Barnes, N. C. Thomson, & I. Rodger, (Eds.), *Asthma: Basic mechanisms and clinical management* (pp. 731–742). San Diego: Academic Press.

van Cauter, E. (1974). Methods for the analysis of multifrequency biological time series. *Journal of Interdisciplinary Cycle Research*, *5*, 131–148.

Verma, D. S., Fisher, R., Spitzer, G., Zander, A. R., McCredie, K. B., & Dick, K. A. (1980). Diurnal changes in circulating myeloid progenitor cells in man. *American Journal of Hematology*, *9*, 185–192.

Vesely, D. L., Sothern, R. B., Scheving, L. E., Bremner, F. W., Third, J. L. H. C., McCormick, J. B., Dawson, S., Kahn, S., Augustine, G., Ryan, M., Greco, J., Nemchausky, B. M., Shirazi, P., & Kanabrocki, E. L. (1996). Circadian relationships between circulating atrial natriuretic peptides and serum calcium and phosphate in healthy humans. *Metabolism*, *45*, 1021–1028.

Voutilainen, A. (1953). Uber die 24 stunden rhythmik der mitosen frequenz on malignen tumoren. *Acta Pathologica et Microbiologica Scandinavica*, *99*(suppl.), 1–104.

Waters, W. E., & O'Connor, P. J. (1971). Epidemiology of headache and migraine in women. *Journal of Neurology, Neurosurgery and Psychiatry*, *34*, 148–153.

Wetterberg, L., Arendt, J., Paunier, L., Sizonenko, P. C., Donselaar, W. van., & Heyden, T. (1976). Human serum melatonin changes during the menstrual cycle. *Journal of Clinical Endocrinology and Metabolism*, *42*, 185–188.

Weydahl, A., & Sothern, R. B. (1997). Seasonal variation in glycemic response to exercise in the subarctic. *Biological Rhythm Research*, *28*, 42–55.

Williams, R., Kraus, L. J., Dubey, D. P., Yunis, E. J., & Halberg, F. (1980). Circadian bioperiodicity in natural killer cell activity in human blood. *Chronobiologia*, *6*, 172.

Winfree, A. T. (1980). *The geometry of biological time. Biomathematics*, vol. 8. New York: Springer-Verlag.

Wood, P. (1995). Chronotherapy of growth factors. *Journal of Infusional Chemotherapy*, *5*, 20–23.

Wood, P., & Hrushesky, W. J. M. (1996). Circadian rhythms and cancer chemotherapy. *Critical Reviews in Eukaryotic Gene Expression, 6*(4), 299–343.

Wu, J. (1982). Neijing chronobiologic medical theories. *Chinese Medical Journal, 95*, 569–578.

Young, M. R. I., Matthews, J. P., Kanabrocki, E. L., Sothern, R. B., Roitman-Johnson, B., & Scheving, L. E. (1995). Circadian rhythmometry of serum interleukin-2, interleukin-10, tumor necrosis factor-α, and granulocyte-macrophage colony-stimulating factor in men. *Chronobiology International, 12*, 19–27.

Yunus, M., Masi, A. T., Calabro, J. J., Miller, K. A., & Feigenbaum, S. L. (1981). Primary fibromyalgia (fibrositis): Clinical study of 50 patients with matched normal controls. *Seminars in Arthritis and Rheumatism, 11*, 151–171.

PART

III

IMMUNE SYSTEM EFFECTS ON THE NERVOUS SYSTEM

C H A P T E R

18

Cytokines, CVOs, and the Blood-Brain Barrier

WILLIAM A. BANKS

I. INTRODUCTION

Circulating cytokines communicate with the central nervous system (CNS) to inform, protect, and destroy the tissues behind the blood-brain barrier (BBB). How blood-borne cytokines influence CNS events is a topic of great importance and any mechanism invoked must deal with the fact that large molecular weight cytokines in the blood are separated from neuronal tissues by the BBB. In theory, the mechanisms available to the cytokines for influencing the CNS are many and include actions on afferent nerves, alterations in cerebral blood flow, alteration of the blood levels of other circulants that affect the CNS, alterations of the functioning and integrity of the BBB, entry at the circumventricular organs (CVOs), or passage across the BBB. Evidence for each of these mechanisms exists, at least under certain conditions, and it is likely that one or the other predominates under specific pathophysiologic states. We review here the evidence for those mechanisms in which cytokines make direct contact with brain tissues by (1) interacting at the CVOs, or (2) crossing the BBB.

II. CONSIDERATIONS OF THE BBB

A. History of the BBB

The evidence for a separation between the circulation and the CNS first arose from experiments with dyes by Erlich and others in late 19th century Germany (Davson, 1967). These dyes could stain most tissues except for the brain and spinal cord after their peripheral administration. At first, explanations such as the inability of CNS tissue to be stained by these particular dyes or the presence of a very small interstitial fluid space within the CNS were offered. As these explanations were discounted, it became increasingly clear that a hematoencephalic barrier existed. Elegant experiments in 1940s and 1950s by Davson and others characterized many of the physiological aspects of this barrier (Davson, 1967), and in the late 1960s the ultrastructure was studied by Brightman and Reese (Reese & Brightman, 1968). These studies showed that the BBB greatly restricted the blood-to-brain leakage of serum proteins because the endothelial cells comprising the capillaries and lining the venules and arterioles were cemented together by tight junctions. This effectively eliminates the plasma ultrafiltrate produced by the Starlings forces and nearly excludes large serum proteins. For example, the cerebrospinal fluid (CSF)-to-serum ratio for albumin is 1:200.

In the 1970s, Oldendorf introduced the brain uptake index (BUI) that allowed a new level of quantifying BBB permeability (Oldendorf, 1971). Use of this method and others by several investigators showed that the degree to which many substances crossed the BBB could be predicted based on their physicochemical characteristics, in particular being related directly to lipid solubility and indirectly to the square root of molecular weight. Some compounds crossed the BBB to an extent greater than that predicted by their physicochemical characteristics because saturable systems transported them into the brain, and other compounds crossed less than predicted because of efflux (brain to blood) transporters or other factors such as protein binding.

The BUI is an excellent method for substances with about a 5% extraction from blood with a single pass through the brain, such as glucose, large neutral amino acids, heroine, ethanol, and nicotine (Cornford, Braun, Oldendorf, & Hill, 1982; Oldendorf, 1973, 1974). However, this method is too insensitive for substances with lower extraction rates such as morphine, most peptides, and cytokines. Extremely sensitive methods introduced in the early 1980s included an in vivo graphical method (Blasberg, Fenstermacher, & Patlak, 1983; Patlak, Blasberg, & Fenstermacher, 1983), later termed multiple-time regression analysis, and in situ methods (Barrera, Kastin, Fasold, & Banks, 1991; Takasato, Rapoport, & Smith, 1984; Zlokovic, Begley, Djuricic, & Mitrovic, 1986). In addition, some of the in vitro methods are sensitive enough to study some peptides (Raeissi & Audus, 1989). The introduction of these very sensitive methods coupled with techniques such as high performance liquid chromatography, capillary depletion, and radioactive labeling made it possible to study the permeability of the BBB to peptides and regulatory proteins.

B. Concepts of the BBB

The mammalian BBB largely defines the internal fluid milieu of the CNS by regulating the movement of substances between the blood and the fluid spaces of the CNS (CSF and interstitial fluid). The BBB is often divided into the vascular, or endothelial, barrier and the epithelial barrier at the choroid plexus. The endothelial cells that comprise the capillaries and line the arterioles and venules constitute the BBB of the spinal cord (Rapoport, 1976). The endothelial cells are modified .in that circumferential belts of tight junctions between contiguous nonfenestrated endothelial cells of the CNS preclude the leakage found in the capillary beds of peripheral tissues. Likewise, intracellular tight junctions comparable to those of the BBB endothelium exist between contiguous ependymal cells at the choroid plexus (Johanson, 1988) and between arachnoid mater cells (Balin, Broadwell, Salcman, & el-Kalliny, 1986). The endothelia of the BBB have other modifications as well. They engage in endocytosis of blood-borne macromolecules and a recycling of the luminal plasmalemma but to a lesser degree than peripheral endothelia (Broadwell & Banks, 1993). Secondary lysosomes hydrolyze many but not all macromolecules undergoing endocytosis within the BBB endothelia (Broadwell & Salcman, 1981; Broadwell et al., 1993). These modifications of the endothelia effectively eliminate the plasma ultrafiltrate characteristic of capillary beds in peripheral tissues and serve to define the restrictive permeability of the BBB.

Between the CSF and the interstitial fluid of the CNS, no anatomical barrier exists in the adult mammal. However, diffusion of molecules from the cerebral ventricles into the brain parenchyma is time-dependent, and distinct concentration gradients for biologically active molecules can occur within the periventricular stratum (Maness, Kastin, Banks, & Zadina, 1991; van der Ploeg et al., 1991). For example, the concentration of the tetrapeptide Tyr-MIF-1 (Tyr-Pro-Leu-Gly-NH_2) after intraventricular (icv) injection was found to decrease by half per 0.29 mm distance from the midline (Maness, Banks, Zadina, & Kastin, 1996). Diffusion within the brain parenchyma is also very limited (Cserr, 1984). The concentration of model compounds is reported to decrease to 10% at a distance of 1–3 mm from their site of introduction (de Lange, Bouw, Danhof, De Boer, & Breimer, 1993). These gradients are likely to be especially sharp for peptides and proteins with a high suseptibility to enzymatic degradation, which serves to limit the time available for diffusion. In addition, CNS-to-blood efflux by saturable transport systems or with the reabsorption of CSF (bulk flow) into the blood also limits residence time within the CNS. These considerations suggest that for enzymatically degradable molecules, such as the cytokines, sites of action within the CNS cannot be far removed from sites of injection or release.

The CVOs include the pineal gland, the subfornical organ, the median eminence, the neural lobe of the pituitary, the area postrema, the subcommissural organ, and the organum vasculosum of the lamina terminalis (Weindl, 1973). The total mass of these tissues is small, accounting for less than 1% of total brain weight. Most functions associated with CVOs relate to neuroendocrine secretions or to events requiring rapid or stereotypical responses, such as emesis in response to toxic materials or drinking and cardiovascular reactions in response to volume contraction (Ferguson & Marcus, 1988; Gross & Weindl, 1987; Johnson & Gross, 1993). The CVOs are not a uniform group of tissues, but each has unique neuroanatomical characteristics (Gross & Weindl, 1987). In most regions of a typical CVO, the majority of capillaries are not engaged in the formation of a BBB. This allows blood-borne substances a ready access to a small area of the CNS. Neural connections between the CVOs and areas of the CNS with a BBB provide a way that blood-borne substances can affect deep brain function (Johnson & Gross, 1993). However, CVOs are not homogenous, but consist of distinct regions, some of which can have a BBB (Johnson & Gross, 1993; Gross & Weindl, 1987). The ependymal cells that define the interface between the CVOs and the CSF are typically sealed together by tight junctions so that leakage out of the CVOs and into the CSF is limited. The interface between the interstitial fluids of the CVOs and the adjacent brain tissues has been studied extensively and most authorities agree that they are separated by a barrier that limits the exchange (Krisch, 1986; Krisch & Leonhardt, 1989). However, the extent to which that barrier is defined by the constraints of diffusion vs. a cellular barrier is in some dispute (Krisch, 1986; Krisch & Leonhardt, 1989; Ross, Broadwell, Poston, & Lawhorn, 1994). If a cellular barrier does exist between the CVOs and the adjacent brain interstitial fluid, the possibility exists that transport systems and the physicochemical characteristics of a compound govern exchange at this interface just as they do in other regions of BBB function. In general, CVOs are a likely route through which signals from the periphery are transmitted into the CNS by neural relay or translocation of substances (Ferguson & Marcus, 1988; Gross & Weindl, 1987; Johnson & Gross, 1993).

C. Mechanisms of Passage across the BBB

A clear understanding of the basic fundamentals underlying BBB permeability is critical to understanding how cytokines and the BBB interact. This section gives a brief overview of those fundamentals. This overview clearly demonstrates that the BBB is not a simple rigid or inert barrier. Instead, the endothelial and epithelial monolayers that constitute the BBB are dynamic, biologically active interfaces between the CNS and the blood. The BBB restricts but also regulates the exchange of substances between the blood and the CNS and, as will be demonstrated in other sections below, is engaged in the pathophysiology of the neuroimmune axis.

Blood-borne substances use a limited number of well-defined pathways to enter the CNS: residual leakiness, membrane diffusion, saturable transport systems, and diapedesis. Major pathways for efflux are CSF reabsorption at the arachnoid villi, membrane diffusion, transport, and drainage by way of the brain's primitive lymphatics.

The restrictive function of the BBB is formidable, but not absolute. The patent, extracellular pathways found at the pial surface/subarachnoid space and elsewhere allows passage between the blood and the CNS interstitial fluid/CSF (Broadwell & Banks, 1993; Broadwell & Sofroniew, 1993). These extracellular pathways may underlie the establishment of a quasi-equilibrium between blood and the fluids of the CNS for serum proteins such as albumin (Broadwell et al., 1993). The concentrations in CSF of serum proteins entering the CNS by this pathway are low; for example, the concentration of albumin in the CSF is about 1/200th of that in the serum. The CSF/serum ratios are influenced not only by the low rates of infux but also by enzymatic stability within the CNS and rates of efflux. The unidirectional influx constant (Ki) for albumin is 10^{-5} to 10^{-6} mL/g-min. This means that the amount of albumin found in 0.01 to 0.001 microliter of serum enters each gram of brain every minute.

Many endogenous molecules and drugs diffuse through the cell membranes that comprise the BBB. Lipid solubility/hydrogen bonding correlates directly and the square root of the molecular weight inversely with the rate of passage across the BBB (Chikhale, Ng, Burton, & Borchardt, 1994; Cornford et al., 1982; Oldendorf, 1974; Rapoport, 1976). However, even water soluble molecules, as exemplified by morphine and some peptides, can cross to some degree by this mechanism to induce CNS effects (Banks & Kastin, 1985a, 1994a; Begley, 1994; Oldendorf, 1974).

Other substances are transported across the BBB by saturable carrier systems (Davson, Welch, & Segal, 1987a). A transport system tends to be highly specialized for molecules with closely related structures, such as hexoses (Oldendorf, 1971), or large neutral amino acids (Oldendorf, 1971, 1973), organic acids (Barany, 1972; Kannan, Kuhlenkamp, Ookhtens, & Kaplowitz, 1992), or small peptides with N-terminal tyrosines (Banks, Kastin, Fischman, Coy, & Strauss, 1986). Transporters can be unidirectional, with movement of substances only into or out of the CNS, or bidirectional, with net movement of substances from the side of higher to the side of lower concentration.

Diapedesis is the process by which cells cross the intact walls of blood vessels (Lossinsky et al., 1991). Mature immune cells are able to cross such walls, including the high endothelium (Chin, Sackstein, & Cai, 1991; Tavassoli & Minguell, 1991) of the bone marrow and the endothelial BBB. Diapedesis involves a coordination between invagination of the endothelial cell and podocytosis of the immune cell. This results in the immune cell tunneling through the endothelial cell or, apparently less typically, crossing between cells at the tight junctions. Cytokines may modulate both the immune cell and the barrier cell actions in diapedesis (Chin et al., 1991; Tavassoli et al., 1991). Cytokines are likely involved at both the high epithelium of the bone marrow and the endothelium of the BBB, modulating both the immune and endothelial cells (Male, 1995; Persidsky et al., 1997; Sharief, Noori, Ciardi, Cirelli, & Thompson, 1993). Release of response to other secreted substances by both the endothelial and immune cell result in an intimate communication which underlies diapedesis.

Efflux of a substance from the CNS to the blood can be due to CSF reabsorption at the arachnoid villi, membrane diffusion, transport, and drainage by way of the brain's primitive lymphatics. For some substances, their efflux mechanisms are so robust that their levels in the blood are nearly identical after injecting them either icv or infusing them iv (Davson & Segal, 1996a). Any substance present in the CSF will enter the blood together with the usual reabsorption of CSF from the CNS at the arachnoid villi (Passaro, Debas, Oldendorf, & Yamada, 1982). Lipid solubility can be an important determinant in the rate at which a substance exits the CNS (de Lange et al., 1993). Such passage is not saturable. Similarly, drainage by way of the brain's lymphatic system is not saturable (Davson et al., 1996a). The mechanisms that dictate which substances are drained by the lymphatics, which provides a direct pathway to the cervical lymph nodes, are unclear but can have important consequences for immune responses (Knopf, Cserr, Nolan, Wu, & Harling-Berg, 1995; Yamada, DePasquale, Patlak, & Cserr, 1991).

Saturable efflux systems are responsible for the CNS-to-blood transport of many key substances including electrolytes, free fatty acids, peptides, amino acids, metabolic degradation products, and toxins (Banks, Kastin, & Rapoport, 1997; Begley, 1992; Chen, Castro, Chow, & Reichlin, 1997; Daniel, Love, & Pratt, 1978; Davson et al., 1996a; Martins, Banks, & Kastin, 1997a; Tsuji et al., 1992). Efflux systems can play important roles in establshing and maintaining the nutritive and homeostatic environment of the CNS (Davson et al., 1996a), can be affected by disease states (Plotkin, Banks, Waguespack, & Kastin, 1997), and participate in the neuroimmune axis (Cserr & Knopf, 1992; Martins, Banks, & Kastin, 1997b).

Insults to the BBB, in addition to altering any of the normal mechanisms of BBB permeability outlined above, may alter unique or quiescent pathways. Adsorptive endocytosis (AE) is one such pathway that can be induced by lectins, such as wheatgerm agglutinin, binding to the oligosaccharides on the luminal surface of BBB endothelial cells (Broadwell, 1989). The resulting endocytosis can overwhelm the process for clearing internalized membrane, and the vesicular traffic is then diverted to the Golgi complex. Subsequent vesicles originating from the Golgi complex may be routed to the abluminal surface of the BBB endothelium, thereby completing the process of adsorptive transcytosis, that is, blood-to-brain transfer (Banks & Broadwell, 1994; Broadwell, Balin, & Salcman, 1988; Villegas & Broadwell, 1993). Such transfer effectively defines a disruption of the BBB. AE differs from other vesicular processes of the normal brain endothelial cell such as diapedesis, receptor-mediated endocytosis, and fluid phase endocytosis (Villegas et al., 1993; Broadwell, 1989) and is probably induced by a wide range of insults to the BBB and CNS (Dux, Doczi, Joo, Szerdahelyi, & Siklos, 1988; Hardebo & Kahrstrom, 1985; Lossinsky, Vorbrodt, & Wisniewski, 1983; Vorbrodt, 1994).

Cytokines have the potential to interact with the BBB in many different ways. These interactions can be globally divided into at least two major categories. The first is a determination of whether cytokines can cross the BBB by any of the previously listed mechanisms or interact at the CVOs. The second major category is whether cytokines alter BBB function. This is a broader, less well-studied category and includes such questions as whether cytokines disrupt the BBB or alter AE, diapedesis, membrane diffusion, CSF reabsorption, or transporters.

III. INTERACTIONS OF CYTOKINES AT THE CVOS

A. Background

When the consideration of how blood-borne cytokines could affect the CNS first arose in the mid 1980s, the consensus was that they should be virtually excluded by the BBB because of their large size but might enter the brain at the organum vasculosum laminae terminalis, a CVO (Blatteis, 1992; Breder,

Dinarello, & Saper, 1988; Katsuura, Arimura, Koves, & Gottschall, 1990; Komaki, Arimura, & Koves, 1992; Sirko, Bishai, & Coceani, 1989; Stitt, 1990). As already discussed, the CVOs represent a diverse group of tissues that, in general, have capillaries that are not modified so as to produce a BBB. The hypothesis that blood-borne cytokines could enter the CVOs was, therefore, reasonable.

Once within the CVO, a substance has a number of possible mechanisms through which to exert effects on the CNS (Davson & Segal, 1996c; Gross et al., 1987; Johnson et al., 1993; Weindl, 1973). Many of these mechanisms have been investigated for cytokines. In general, the substance can interact with neurons or nerve terminals to relay information to other areas of the CNS or it can interact with cells within the CVO to release substances that diffuse to other cells within or adjacent to the CVO. In particular, several laboratories have postulated that prostaglandins (Blatteis, 1992; Breder et al., 1988; Komaki et al., 1992; Sirko et al., 1989; Stitt, 1990) could be released from CVOs to diffuse into deeper regions of the brain to stimulate nearby cells to release brain-derived cytokines or other substances. Because the diffusion distances required are small and prostaglandins cross barrier membranes well, these pathways have a great deal of appeal.

Some hypothesized that once within the CVOs, cytokines could diffuse throughout the brain. This aspect of the hypothesis was at variance with generally accepted views of the roles played by the CVOs because, as reviewed in a previous section, influx from CVOs to adjacent brain tissues and CSF is limited by diffusion rates within the CNS and epithelial barrier function. Influx at the CVOs and other extracellular pathways (Broadwell & Banks, 1993; Broadwell & Sofroniew, 1993; Campbell & Erwin, 1993; Richards, 1978; Ross et al., 1994) is well defined, and substances using these pathways imitate albumin. Therefore, these pathways could not account for CSF/serum ratios much different from 0.5%, the ratio for albumin. Significant movement of cytokines from CVOs to deep brain tissue would likely require transport at the CVO/brain tissue interface.

B. Cytokine Uptake from Blood

Despite the large number of hypotheses incorporating CVOs in cytokine blood-to-brain communication and an extensive number of papers on this topic, no data showing that cytokines actually entered the CVOs or quantifying such entry existed. Therefore, we compared the uptake of radioactively labeled interleukin (IL)-1α by a number of CVOs to that of brain uptake. These studies used radioactively labeled albumin as a measure of nonspecific diffusion (Plotkin, Banks, & Kastin, 1996). The pineal, median eminence, and area postrema took up 20–160 times more albumin and IL-1α than the non-CVO regions of the brain (e.g., cerebellum, cortex) and contained about 5% of the total IL-1α taken up by the brain. The pineal was over 4 times more permeable to IL-1α than was the median eminence. However, the CVOs contained 6-10 times more IL-1α than albumin, and the uptake of radioactively labeled IL-1α could be decreased significantly with unlabeled IL-1α. Therefore, the vasculature of the CVO also contains the transporter for IL-1α.

C. The CVO-Brain Interface

The interface between a CVO (subfornical organ; SFO) and the rest of the brain has also been investigated with regard to IL-1α permeability in the CVO to brain direction (Maness, Kastin, & Banks, 1998). That study found that IL-1α does not have free passage across the interface, but is retarded by the row of CVO cells that abut next to the adjacent brain. The zone 30 μm on either side of the CVO/non-CVO interface formed a sharp demarcation that totally separated the concentrations of the two regions.

The permeability of IL-1α in the CSF to CVO direction also has been assessed by studying the distribution of radioactively labeled albumin and IL-1α after icv injection (Plotkin et al., 1996). The uptake of both IL-1α and albumin by CVOs was greater than regions of the brain with a BBB, even when analysis was restricted to periventricular non-CVO regions. The IL-1α/albumin ratio was about one for most regions, indicating that diffusion was the major mechanism for distribution. Only the median eminence had an IL-1α/albumin ratio that was significantly greater than the other regions, which suggests selective uptake. However, the ratio was not decreased with unlabeled IL-1α.

In conclusion, the CVOs represent a likely area for interactions of blood-borne cytokines and brain tissue. Several mechanisms are available by which CVOs could respond to cytokines, including neuronal relay and the release of substances that could diffuse within the CVO or into areas of the brain that are immediately adjacent to the CVO. The vasculature of the CVO does not form a BBB, and therefore allows cytokines to leak into its tissue area. In addition, the CVO vasculature transports IL-1α into the CVO, increasing the concentration of IL-1α 6–10 times higher than it would be otherwise. The CVO/non-CVO brain tissue interface forms a barrier to diffusion of IL-1α in the CVO-to-deep-brain tissue direction but is less robust in the opposite direction. CVOs differ in their permeabilities to IL-1α, with the median eminence being the least permeable (when compared with the area postrema and the pineal) in the blood-to-CVO-direction and the most permeable when movement into the CVO after icv injection is measured. Therefore, if other cytokines behave like IL-1α, blood-borne cytokines enter the CVOs readily by leakage and transport, but are unable to use CVOs as a pathway into areas behind the BBB (unless they are transported at the CVO/brain interface barrier), whereas cytokines injected icv are likely to enter the CVO in substantial amounts.

IV. TRANSPORT OF BLOOD-BORNE CYTOKINES ACROSS THE BBB

A. Early Perceptions

Studies throughout the 1980s established that cytokines given by peripheral routes had widespread effects on the CNS. Papers that considered what mechanism might explain these effects usually rejected the possibility that cytokines might cross the BBB, due to their size. These rejections were seldom referenced and, indeed, were often made for cytokines that had yet to be examined for BBB permeability. Meanwhile, in other fields, common proteins as large as transferrin (MW 90,000) were being found to be transported across the BBB by saturable systems (Banks, Kastin, Fasold, Barrera, & Augereau, 1988; Fishman, Rubin, Handrahan, Connor, & Fine, 1987; Hill, Ruff, Weber, & Pert, 1985; Raub & Newton, 1991). Although consideration of the low lipid solubility and large molecular weight of cytokines did reassure that they were unlikely to cross the BBB by virtue of their physicochemical characteristics, such consideration gave no insight into the possibilities of transport by saturable systems (Table I).

TABLE I Transport of Cytokines and Related Substances across the Murine BBB

Saturable transport	No saturable transport
Murine IL-1α	IL-2
Human IL-1α	IL-1 soluble receptors
Murine IL-1β	TNF-α soluble receptors
IL-1 receptor antagonist	MIP-1α (aggregated and nonaggregated)
GM-CSF	MIP-1β (aggregated and nonaggregated)
Murine IL-6	IFNα
Human IL-6	Human TNF-α
Murine TNF-α	
IFN gamma	

Note: The table lists substances that have been studied for BBB permeability and been categorized with regard to the presence or absence of saturable transport in mice.

B. The IL-1s

1. *IL-1α*

IL-1α was one of the first cytokines to be studied regarding BBB permeability and is currently the most studied cytokine in this regard. IL-1α has offered many advantages for BBB studies. For example, it is easily labeled with radioactive iodine, after which it retains 100% of its biological activity (Dower et al., 1986). Both human and murine IL-1α cross the mouse BBB but immunoassays are available that distinguish between the two species; thus, the studies described under Chronic Infusions were possible.

The ability of human or murine IL-1α to cross the mouse BBB has been studied by several methods including multiple-time regression analysis, brain-washout of the vascular space, capillary depletion, and CSF sampling (Banks & Kastin, 1991; Banks, Kastin, & Durham, 1989; Banks, Kastin, & Gutierrez, 1993; Banks, Ortiz, Plotkin, & Kastin, 1991) and all of these have shown that it crosses the BBB by a specific, saturable transport system. Binding sites for Il-1α or message for IL-1 receptors are found on brain vasculature and the choroid plexus (Ban, Milon, Prudhomme, Fillion, & Haour, 1991; Cunningham & De Souza, 1993; Cunningham, et al., 1991, 1992; Ericsson, Liu, Kasckow, Hart, & Sawchenko, 1993; Hashimoto et al., 1991; Wong & Licinio, 1994); these binding sites likely represent a combination of receptors for intracellular signalling and transporters. More recently, passage of radioactively labeled IL-1α across brain vasculature has been visualized by autoradiography (Maness, Kastin, & Banks, 1998). The Ki for IL-1α is about 10–40 times greater than the Ki for albumin (Table II), and about 0.05 to 0.08% of an intravenously injected dose of Il-1α enters a gram of brain. In comparison, about one third this amount of morphine and about one thirtieth this amount of the shellfish neurotoxin domoic acid enter the brain (Advokat & Gulati, 1991; Banks & Kastin 1991, 1994a; Banks et al., 1989, 1991; Preston & Hynie, 1991). Therefore, although the amount of IL-1α entering the brain is modest, it is likely to be sufficient to affect some aspects of brain function. For example, a correlation exists between food intake and CSF levels of IL-1α (Opara, Laviano, Meguid, & Yang, 1995).

TABLE II Unidirectional Influx Constants in Mice for Cytokines and Related Substances

	Ki (μL/g-min)	Citation
Substance transported		
Murine IL-1α	1.35	Banks et al., 1991
Human IL-1α	0.427	Banks et al., 1989
Murine IL-1β	0.473	Banks et al., 1991
IL-1 receptor antagonist	0.519	Gutierrez et al., 1994
Murine IL-6	0.305	Banks et al., 1994
Human IL-6	0.454	Banks et al., 1994
Murine TNF-α (adults)	0.225	Gutierrez et al., 1993
Murine TNF-α (neonates)	0.812	Gutierrez et al., 1993
IFN gamma	0.736	Pan et al., 1997b
Murine GM-CSF	0.29	McLay et al., 1997
Selected reference substances		
Human albumin	0.00972	Banks et al., 1989
Morphine	0.251	Banks et al., 1994a
Glucose	19.1[a]	Davson & Segal, 1996b
Arachidonate	10.3[a]	Washizaki, Purdon, DeGeorge, Robinson, Rapoport, & Smith, 1991

[a]Approximated from PS or K_{out} values.

Aluminum (Al), a neurotoxin with complex interactions on the BBB (Banks & Kastin, 1983, 1985a, 1985b, 1989, 1994b), inhibits the transport of IL-1α across the BBB (Banks et al., 1989). Al has been found to selectively inhibit other BBB transport systems (Banks, Kastin, & Fasold, 1988; Banks et al., 1989; Banks & Kastin, 1994b) and exerts many of its other biological effects by displacing ions such as calcium and iron (Arispe, Rojas, & Pollard, 1993; Cannata et al., 1991; Kinraide & Parker, 1987; Oteiza, Fraga, & Keen, 1993; Shortle & Smith, 1988; Zatta, Bordin, & Favarato, 1993). Since Al does not inhibit some forms of vesicular transport (Banks et al., 1989), the ability of Al to inhibit the blood-to-brain uptake of IL-1α is consistent with an ion dependent, nonvesicular saturable transport system. In comparison, dexamethosone, α-MSH, indomethacin, and morphine, agents shown to modify IL-1α activity, had no effect on BBB transport (Banks et al., 1991).

Antibodies directed at either the IL-1α molecule or its receptor have shown that the site of the IL-1α molecule that binds to the BBB transporter is very similar or identical to the site that binds to the murine T lymphocyte type I receptor. In comparison, the binding site of the BBB transporter is distinct from the type I receptor (Banks et al., 1991). The type I soluble receptor does not cross the BBB (Banks, Plotkin, & Kastin, 1995). Binding of IL-1α to its soluble receptor, which does not cross the BBB (Banks et al., 1995), retards IL-1α entry into the CNS. However, entry is not completely inhibited, suggesting that the BBB transporter can strip IL-1α from the soluble receptor or transport the free fraction.

Studies demonstrating that IL-1α is transported into the spinal cord by a saturable transport system similar to the one in brain (Banks, Kastin, & Ehrensing, 1994) have demonstrated that the BBB transporter must be located on brain endothelium since the spinal cord does not contain CVOs or choroid plexus tissue (Davson, Welch, & Segal, 1987b). The rate at which IL-1α is transported is the same for cervical, thoracic, and lumbar spinal cord but is only about 80% of the transport rate for brain. Almost none of the blood-borne IL-1α entering the spinal cord is due to diffusion of IL-1α from the cranial CSF (Banks et al., 1994). The ability of blood-borne IL-1α to cross the BBB of the spinal cord and the brain raises the possibility that some of the effects of peripherally administered IL-1α, such as analgesia (Nakamura, Nakanishi, Kita, & Kadokawa, 1988), might be directly mediated through entry at the spinal cord, whereas other effects, such as sleep and temperature (Imeri, Opp, & Krueger, 1993; Opp & Krueger, 1991), are mediated through entry at the brain. It should be noted that although these studies clearly demonstrate that IL-1α is transported across the endothelial barrier, the studies do not address the possibility that IL-1α is also transported at the choroid plexus.

2. *IL-1β and the Receptor Antagonist*

An early study examined the ability of a crude preparation of human IL-1β given intravenously to cross the BBB in the cat (Coceani, Lees, & Dinarello, 1987). Blood levels were not measured, but enough IL-1β (about 1 μg/cat) was given to produce fever. No increase in CSF IL-1β levels was seen. Later studies with radioactively labeled murine recombinant IL-1β showed that it crossed the BBB by a self-inhibitable system that it shares to some extent with IL-1α (Banks et al., 1991) and with the IL receptor antagonist (Gutierrez, Banks, & Kastin, 1994) (IL-1ra). Cross-inhibition studies among these three species of IL-1, however, do show that there is probably a family of closely related transporters with some of the subtypes showing a preference for one or the other of the IL-1s. Such a mix of transporter specificity may result in a differential inhibition of blood-to-brain entry among the three IL-1s as serum levels of the three cytokines rise or fall during pathophysiological events, thereby altering their relative proportions in the CNS

(Gutierrez et al., 1994). These two studies (Coceani et al., 1987; Gutierrez et al., 1994) can be reconciled by the greater senstivity in detecting transport with radioactively labeled materials as well as the probability that human IL-1β does not cross the BBB of the cat, whereas murine IL-1β studied in the mouse has no species differences to consider.

The unidirectional influx constant for IL-1ra is similar to that of the other IL-1s at about 0.519 μL/g-min (Gutierrez et al., 1994). However, there were other differences in comparison to the other IL-1s. First, the amount of unlabeled IL-1ra needed to self-inhibit was 59.4 μg/kg (Gutierrez et al., 1994). This compares with 29.7 μg/kg for human IL-1α, 0.0637 μg/kg for murine IL-1α, and 0.0438 μg/kg for murine IL-1β self-inhibition (Banks et al., 1991). This indicates a higher capacity transport for IL-1ra. IL-1ra was very effective at inhibition of IL-1α but less so for IL-1β (Gutierrez et al., 1994). The percentage of an intravenously injected dose entering the brain was also the highest for any cytokine yet determined: 0.33% for IL-1ra labeled with radioactive iodide and 0.65% for IL-1ra labeled with ^{35}S (Gutierrez et al., 1994). The value for I-IL-1α is about 0.05–0.08% (Banks et al., 1991).

Autoradiography has shown that blood-borne IL-1α, IL-1β, and IL-1ra are taken up by the cerebral vasculature and sequestered at the choroid plexus (Maness, Banks, Zadina, & Kastin, 1995). IL-1α is intensely concentrated by the posterior division of the septum (PDS), an area that does not concentrate IL-1β or IL-1ra. IL-1α uptake at the PDS can be blocked by an excess of unlabeled IL-1α but not by unlabeled IL-1β or IL-1ra. The PDS, therefore, represents an area of selective transport into the CNS for IL-1α. The PDS consists of the triangular septal nucleus and the septofimbrial nucleus (Loo, 1931; Ramon y Cajal, 1901) both of which receive projections from the hippocampus and the subiculum (Raisman, 1966; Swanson & Cowan, 1979). The PDS, in turn, projects to the ipsilateral medial and possibly the contralateral medial and lateral habenular nuclei; the habenular nuclei project to the interpeduncular nuclei (Herkenham & Nauta, 1977; Morley, 1986; Swanson & Cowan, 1979). Therefore, this neural network provides a pathway through which IL-1α input at the PDS could modulate input from the hippocampal region into the limbic and midbrain regions.

In summary, the IL-1s are transported across the BBB by one or more saturable systems located at the endothelium and probably at the choroid plexus. Transport shows regional variation, with entry at the PDS providing a way for blood-borne IL-1α to influence limbic and midbrain functions.

C. IL-2

In a study by Saris et al. (1988) 37 patients with cancer but no evidence of CNS metastasis received recombinant IL-2 intravenously and CSF was sampled from the lumbar region for up to 26 h later. IL-2 was recovered from the CSF and the CSF/serum ratio was 0.5. A later study with radioactively labeled IL-2 in mice showed that it does not cross the BBB by a saturable transport system (Waguespack, Banks, & Kastin, 1994). An influx rate can be measured for IL-2 that exceeds that of albumin, and is presumably due to the ability of IL-2 to enter at sites of residual leakage. Autoradiography that compared IL-2 with the IL-1s and to tumor necrosis factor (TNF) has shown that IL-2 is not taken up by the cerebral vasculature, the choroid plexus, or the PDS in the mouse (Maness et al., 1995). Sabo, Ni, Nadeau, Liberato, and Loh (1992) used ^{14}C-labeled IL-2 to demonstrate entry into many tissues, including brain. Uptake by brain was small but measurable and exceeded levels in testis and abdominal fat by 2 h. However, no effort was made to determine whether the radioactivity taken up by these tissues represented intact IL-2.

D. IL 6

The transport of IL-6 across the BBB has been studied in two separate laboratories. Both have concluded that IL-6 crosses the BBB (Banks, Kastin, & Gutierrez, 1994; Luheshi, Gay, & Rothwell, 1994). Both human and murine IL-6 cross the murine BBB (Banks et al., 1994). The transporter is distinct from those for the IL-1α, IL-6, and TNF-α; and IL-6 is recoverable from the brain interstitial fluid and from the CSF (Banks et al., 1994).

E. TNF-α

TNF-α has been studied extensively with regard to its ability to cross the BBB. It does so by a transport system that is distinct from those described for other cytokines (Gutierrez, Banks, & Kastin, 1993). Blood-borne radioactively labeled TNF-α enters both brain interstitial fluid and the CSF as an intact molecule. It also has been shown to enter various regions of the spinal cord (Pan, Banks, & Kastin, 1997a). Autoradiographic studies have shown TNF-α to be taken up by the vasculature and choroid plexus but not by the PDS (Maness et al., 1995). The TNF-α transporter, unlike the transporter for IL-1α, is not affected by Al. Treatment with desferoxamine also does not affect the transport of TNF-α, which further supports the idea that ions such as iron are not involved in the transport of TNF-α even though iron is involved in other functions of TNF-α (Helyar & Sherman, 1987; Tanaka, Araki, Nitta, & Tateno, 1987). The soluble p75 receptor for TNF-α does not cross the BBB (Banks et al., 1995) and, unlike the results for IL-1α and its soluble receptor, the BBB transport system for TNF-α appears unable to strip TNF-α from its soluble receptor.

F. Other Cytokines and Related Substances

Macrophage inflammatory protein (MIP)-1α and -1β have been studied for their abilities to cross the BBB (Banks & Kastin, 1996). These substances do not cross the BBB either in their monomeric or polymeric forms. These compounds did interact with the endothelial cells comprising the BBB in a unique manner not noted for other cytokines. Blood-borne MIP-1s immediately associated to a high degree with the luminal side of the BBB vasculature in a reversible, nonsaturable manner. This association could underlie a mechanism by which blood-borne MIP-1s could alter the functioning of the BBB.

Interferon (IFN)-α and IFN-γ have been characterized for their entry into the CNS (Pan, Banks, & Kastin, 1997b). Although a low entry rate for IFN-α could be measured, no saturable component could be measured. By contrast, IFN-γ entered by a saturable mechanism at a rate about three times faster than that of TNF-α and about nine times faster than that of IFN-α. IFN-γ also entered throughout the spinal cord, but in contrast to studies with IL-1α, entry into the spinal cord was higher than for the brain. Human interferon has also been found to cross the blood-CSF barrier of the monkey (Habif, Lipton, & Cantell, 1975).

Murine granulocyte-macrophage colony-stimulating factor (GM-CSF) crosses the murine BBB to enter the brain and spinal cord by saturable transport (McLay, Kimura, Banks, & Kastin, 1997). The rate of uptake by spinal cord is about half the rate of uptake by brain. GM-CSF is transported across the BBB at the same rate in male and female mice. Murine GM-CSF is also transported across the rat BBB.

V. TRANSPORT OF BLOOD-BORNE CYTOKINES ACROSS THE BBB: CHRONIC INFUSIONS

Most studies that have investigated the question of cytokine transport across the BBB have relied on single injections of radioactive materials. This approach is ideal for determining influx constants and other acute aspects of brain-blood interactions. However, cytokine levels in the blood are often sustained, raising the question of the contribution of blood to the CNS at steady state. This question was addressed by chronically infusing (48 h) human IL-1α to the mouse (Banks & Kastin, 1997). Both murine and human IL-1α cross the murine BBB but immunoassay kits exist that can distinguish the two moieties. Therefore, two questions could be addressed by this method: (1) how much of brain IL-1α is derived from blood and (2) does blood-borne IL-1α stimulate the release of IL-1α from the brain?

No murine IL-1α was present in blood or brain before or during the 48 h infusion of human IL-1α. The lack of murine IL-1α in blood or brain with infusion means that blood-borne IL-1α does not stimulate its own release in either the blood or brain. However, human IL-1α did appear in the brain tissue of mice, demonstrating blood-to-brain transport of IL-1α. The brain/serum ratio for human IL-1α was relatively high at 0.126 mL/g.

These studies show that with a chronic elevation in blood levels, blood-borne human IL-1α does not stimulate the production or release of IL-1α in deep brain structures, as has been postulated to occur in CVOs. Furthermore, the studies show that the brain/serum ratio for IL-1α is relatively high in comparison to other, even smaller, regulatory substances.

VI. CNS TO BLOOD TRANSPORT OF CYTOKINES

The CNS to blood passage, or efflux, of cytokines was first considered for IL-1α in 1989 (Banks et al.). Efflux was found to be somewhat faster than could be accounted for by CSF reabsorption. Pretreatment with aluminum decreased efflux, suggesting an inhibitable component. However, subsequent studies were not able to demonstrate self-inhibition (Banks et al., 1991). Therefore, the passage of IL-1α across the BBB is bidirectional with only the blood-to-brain component being due to a saturable transport system. The nature of the efflux mechanism is not totally resolved, but likely to be due in large part to reabsorption with the CSF (bulk flow).

Other cytokines also have been examined for their abilities to cross the BBB in the brain-to-blood direction. IL-1β (Banks et al., 1991) and IL-2 (Waguespack et al., 1994), like IL-1α, have efflux rates faster than can be typically accounted for by reabsorption of CSF but are not self-inhibited. The rate of efflux of IL-6 is indistinguishable from that attributable to reabsorption of CSF (Banks et al., 1994; Chen et al., 1997; Romero, Ildiko, Lechan, & Reichlin, 1996).

TNF-α has the distinction of having been studied by three separate laboratories and having been found to have an efflux rate faster, slower, and equal to that explicable by bulk flow (Bodnar et al., 1989; Chen & Reichlin, 1998; Gutierrez et al., 1993). Some of this contradiction is no doubt due to species differences in the cytokine and animal used. Human TNF-α injected into the brain of the rat yielded blood levels similar to those produced by iv injection (Bodnar et al., 1989; Chen et al., 1997). In comparison, murine TNF-α injected into the mouse brain exited from the brain more slowly than expected based on reabsorption of CSF (Gutierrez et al., 1993), suggesting that TNF-α is sequestered by periventricular tissues from the CSF.

At this time, no cytokine has been demonstrated by self-inhibition to possess a saturable component to its efflux system. Nevertheless, it has now been clearly demonstrated that even the slower efflux of bulk flow is a pathway by which CNS cytokines can make substantial contributions to blood levels (Chen et al., 1997; Chen & Reichlin, 1998; Romero et al., 1996). The combination of a slow efflux from brain and favorable pharmacokinetics in the blood (small volume of distribution and long half-life) result in high blood levels. These principles have since been shown to be active for leptin (Maness, Kastin, Farrell, & Banks, 1998), another compound with similar characteristics. Such efflux is likely to be significant in two major conditions: (1) cytokines produced in high amounts in the CNS are likely to produce high levels of cytokines in the blood; (2) cytokines experimentally injected into the CNS in high doses are likely to produce high levels in the blood, raising the possibility that some of the effects seen are due to activation of peripheral, not CNS, receptors.

VII. ALTERATIONS IN BBB TRANSPORT IN PATHOPHYSIOLOGICAL CONDITIONS

Alterations in the function of BBB transporters for substances other than cytokines has long been appreciated and often has been correlated with altered metabolic demands of the CNS in healthy maturation (Duffy & Pardridge, 1987; Johanson, 1989), aging (Banks & Kastin, 1986; Daniel et al., 1978; Kannan et al., 1992; Mooradian, Morin, Cipp, & Haspel, 1991; Shah & Mooradian, 1997), and disease (Banks, Jaspan, & Kastin, 1997; Fugisawa, Sasaki, & Akiyama, 1991; Greenwood & Pratt, 1983; Harik & Kalaria, 1991; Lorenzi, 1990; Mooradian, 1987; Pan, Banks, Kennedy, Gutierrez, & Kastin, 1996; Plotkin et al., 1997). Such alterations in BBB function can result from, as well as cause, disease. (Bodnar et al., 1989; Caro et al., 1996; De Vivo et al., 1991; Fazakerley & Webb, 1985; Greenwood et al., 1983; Hill, Mervis, Avidor, Moody, & Brenneman, 1993; Moses & Nelson, 1994; Schinkel et al., 1994; Schwartz, Figlewicz, Baskin, Woods, & Porte, Jr., 1994; Schwartz, Peskind, Raskind, Boyko, & Porte, 1996; van Heek et al., 1997; Zlokovic et al., 1993). Several examples currently exist for altered transport rates of cytokines in healthy and disease states.

A diurnal variation in the uptake of IL-1α by the brain, spinal cord, testis, and muscle was found in the mouse. Peak uptake rates occurred for these tissues between 0800 and 1200 and nadirs between 2400 and 0400 for all compounds. For muscle, the highest and lowest uptake rates differed less than 2-fold, but the difference was almost 10-fold for spinal cord. No changes were seen in the tissue uptakes of human TNF-α, which does not cross the BBB of the ICR (CD-1) mouse (Banks, Kastin, & Ehrensing, 1998).

Some of the most dramatic variations in transport rates have been noted for TNF-α and are consistent with its proposed roles in brain development and neuroimmunomodulation. TNF-α is transported about three times faster in neonates than in adults, suggesting a role for blood-borne TNF-α in brain maturation (Gutierrez et al., 1993). In addition, transport of TNF-α is enhanced in experimental allergic encephalomyelitis, an animal model of multiple sclerosis. The enhanced transport mirrors disease activity anatomically and temporally (Pan et al., 1996). In spinal cord transection, TNF-α transport is enhanced about 2 h after injury and is especially robust proximal to the site of injury. These correlations between TNF-α transport and immunologic and traumatic CNS injury suggests that blood-borne TNF-α could play a role in the progression of injury by being transported into the CNS.

Efflux of cytokines also may be altered by pathophysiological events, as suggested by the finding that clearance of TNF-α from the CNS is enhanced by lipopolysaccharide (Chen et al., 1998). It is currently unclear whether this is due to the induction of a saturable component to efflux, enhancement of the rate of reabsorption of CSF, shuttling of TNF to the cervical lymphatics, or another mechanism.

VIII. SUMMARY AND NEW DIRECTIONS

Cytokines enter the CVOs from the blood and, as exemplified by IL-1α, such entry is a combination of leakage and saturable transport. Saturable transport increases the concentration of IL-1α in CVOs between 6–10 times. CVOs are not equally permeable to either serum proteins or cytokines, with the median eminence being the least permeable of the CVOs surveyed. However, not all CVOs have been examined. The movement of IL-1α out of the CVO into the adjacent brain tissue is highly restricted by the layer of CVO cells at the brain-CVO interface. Other cytokines need to be investigated to determine whether the findings for IL-1α extend to them.

Several blood-borne cytokines are transported across the BBB to reach areas deep within the brain. Some of these areas, such as the PDS, may provide mechanisms by which cytokines originating from the blood may affect many CNS activities and regions through neural relays. Cytokines, as exemplified by IL-1α, cross the vascular BBB in the brain and spinal cord and probably can also cross at the choroid plexus. Alteration of the transport of cytokines in the diseased or injured CNS likely contributes to the deranged neuroimmune axis. The role of altered BBB function in disease states deserves increased attention.

The reabsorption of CSF provides a pathway by which significant amounts of cytokine originating within the CNS can enter the circulation. No self-inhibitable transport system has yet been described for a cytokine in the CNS-to-blood direction, although several exit the CNS at a rate faster than CSF reabsorption can explain. CNS to CVO movement of cytokines also occurs, usually at rates explained by diffusion within the CNS. The median eminence had an uptake rate from the adjacent CNS that exceeded that explicable by diffusion. The role of movement of cytokines from CNS to blood and CNS to CVO in those disease states with high brain levels of cytokines needs further study. In addition, experimenters who rely on injection of cytokines into the CSF to study the CNS should realize that some of their cytokines reach the CVOs and peripheral tissues as well.

Mechanisms exist by which cytokines administered or secreted on one side of the BBB can affect events on the other. These mechanisms include pathways by which some cytokines themselves are transferred across the BBB in modest amounts. Which cytokine affects which behavior by which mechanism under which pathophysiological circumstance remains largely unresolved.

References

Advokat, C., & Gulati, A. (1991). Spinal transection reduces both spinal antinociception and CNS concentration of systemically administered morphine in rats. *Brain Research, 555*, 251–258.

Arispe, N., Rojas, E., & Pollard, H. B. (1993). Alzheimer disease amyloid β protein forms calcium channels in bilayer membranes: Blockade by tromethamine and aluminum. *Proceedings of the National Academy of Sciences USA, 90*, 567–571.

Balin, B. J., Broadwell, R. D., Salcman, M., & el-Kalliny, M. (1986). Avenues for entry of peripherally administered protein to the central nervous system in mouse, rat, and squirrel monkey. *Journal of Comparative Neurology, 251*, 260–280.

Ban, E., Milon, G., Prudhomme, N., Fillion, G., & Haour, F. (1991). Receptors for interleukin-1 (α and β) in mouse brain: Mapping and neuronal localization in hippocampus. *Neuroscience, 43*, 21–30.

Banks, W. A., & Broadwell, R. D. (1994). Blood to brain and brain to blood passage of native horseradish peroxidase, wheat germ agglutinin and albumin: Pharmacokinetic and morphological assessments. *Journal of Neurochemistry, 62*, 2404–2419.

Banks, W. A., Jaspan, J. B., & Kastin, A. J. (1997). Effect of diabetes mellitus on the permeability of the blood-brain barrier to insulin. *Peptides, 18*, 1577–1584.

Banks, W. A., & Kastin, A. J. (1986). Aging, peptides, and the blood-brain barrier: Implications and speculations. In T. Crook, R. Bartus, S. Ferris, & S. Gershon (Eds.), *Treatment development strategies for Alzheimer's disease* (pp. 245–265). Madison, CT: Mark Powley Associates.

Banks, W. A., & Kastin, A. J. (1985b). Aluminum alters the permeability of the blood-brain barrier to some non-peptides. *Neuropharmacology, 24*, 407–412.

Banks, W. A., & Kastin, A. J. (1985a). Peptides and the blood-brain barrier: Lipophilicity as a predictor of permeability. *Brain Research Bulletin, 15*, 287–292.

Banks, W. A., & Kastin, A. J. (1983). Aluminium increases permeability of the blood-brain barrier to labelled DSIP and β-endorphin: Possible implications for senile and dialysis dementia. *Lancet, ii*, 1227–1229.

Banks, W. A., & Kastin, A. J. (1989). Aluminum-induced neurotoxicity: Alterations in membrane function at the blood-brain barrier. *Neuroscience and Biobehavioral Reviews, 13*, 47–53.

Banks, W. A., & Kastin, A. J. (1991). Blood to brain transport of interleukin links the immune and central nervous systems. *Life Sciences, 48*, PL117–PL121.

Banks, W. A., & Kastin, A. J. (1994b). Effects of aluminum on blood-brain barrier structure and function. *Life Chemistry Reports, 11*, 141–149.

Banks, W. A., & Kastin, A. J. (1994a). Opposite direction of transport across the blood-brain barrier for Tyr-MIF-1 and MIF-1: Comparison with morphine. *Peptides, 15*, 23–29.

Banks, W. A., & Kastin, A. J. (1997). Relative contributions of peripheral and central sources to levels of IL-1α in the cerebral cortex of mice: assessment with species-specific enzyme immunoassays. *Journal of Neuroimmunology, 79*, 22–28.

Banks, W. A., & Kastin, A. J. (1996). Reversible association of the cytokines MIP-1α and MIP-1β with the endothelia of the blood-brain barrier. *Neuroscience Letters, 205*, 202–206.

Banks, W. A., Kastin, A. J., & Durham, D. A. (1989). Bidirectional transport of interleukin-1 alpha across the blood-brain barrier. *Brain Research Bulletin, 23*, 433–437.

Banks, W. A., Kastin, A. J., & Ehrensing, C. A. (1998). Diurnal uptake of circulating interleukin-1α by brain, spinal cord, testis and muscle. *Neuroimmunomodulation, 5*, 36–41.

Banks, W. A., Kastin, A. J., & Ehrensing, C. A. (1994). Transport of blood-borne interleukin-1α across the endothelial blood-spinal cord barrier of mice. *Journal of Physiology (London), 479*, 257–264.

Banks, W. A., Kastin, A. J., & Fasold, M. B. (1988). Differential effect of aluminum on the blood-brain barrier transport of peptides, technetium and albumin. *Journal of Pharmacology and Experimental Therapeutics, 244*, 579–585.

Banks, W. A., Kastin, A. J., Fasold, M. B., Barrera, C. M., & Augereau, G. (1988). Studies of the slow bidirectional transport of iron and transferrin across the blood-brain barrier. *Brain Research Bulletin, 21*, 881–885.

Banks, W. A., Kastin, A. J., Fischman, A. J., Coy, D. H., & Strauss, S. L. (1986). Carrier-mediated transport of enkephalins and N-Tyr-MIF-1 across blood-brain barrier. *American Journal of Physiology, 251*, E477–E482.

Banks, W. A., Kastin, A. J., & Gutierrez, E. G. (1993). Interleukin-1α in blood has direct access to cortical brain cells. *Neuroscience Letters, 163*, 41–44.

Banks, W. A., Kastin, A. J., & Gutierrez, E. G. (1994). Penetration of interleukin-6 across the blood-brain barrier. *Neuroscience Letters, 179*, 53–56.

Banks, W. A., Kastin, A. J., & Rapoport, S. I. (1997). Permeability of the blood-brain barrier to circulating free fatty acids. In S. Yehuda & D. I. Mostofsky (Eds.), *Handbook of essential fatty acid biology: Biochemistry, physiology, and behavioral neurobiology* (pp. 3–14). Totowa, NJ: Human Press.

Banks, W. A., Ortiz, L., Plotkin, S. R., & Kastin, A. J. (1991). Human interleukin (IL) 1α, murine IL-1α and murine IL-1β are transported from blood to brain in the mouse by a shared saturable mechanism. *Journal of Pharmacology and Experimental Therapeutics, 259*, 988–996.

Banks, W. A., Plotkin, S. R., & Kastin, A. J. (1995). Permeability of the blood-brain barrier to soluble cytokine receptors. *Neuroimmunomodulation, 2*, 161–165.

Barany, E. H. (1972). Inhibition by hippurate and probenecid of in vitro uptake of iodipamide and O-iodohippurate. A composite uptake system for iodipamide in choroid plexus, kidney cortex and anterior uvea of several species. *Acta Physiologica Scandinavica, 86*, 12–27.

Barrera, C. M., Kastin, A. J., Fasold, M. B., & Banks, W. A. (1991). Bidirectional saturable transport of LHRH across the blood-brain barrier. *American Journal of Physiology, 261*, E312–E318.

Begley, D. J. (1992). The interaction of some centrally active drugs with the blood-brain barrier and circumventricular organs. *Progress in Brain Research, 91*, 163–169.

Begley, D. J. (1994). Strategies for delivery of peptide drugs to the central nervous system: Exploiting molecular structure. *J.Control.Release, 29*, 293–306.

Blasberg, R. G., Fenstermacher, J. D., & Patlak, C. S. (1983). Transport of α-aminoisobutyric acid across brain capillary and cellular membranes. *Journal of Cerebral Blood Flow and Metabolism, 3*, 8–32.

Blatteis, C. M. (1992). Role of the OVLT in the febrile response to circulating pyrogens. In A. Ermisch, R. Landgraf, & H.-J. Ruhle (Eds.), *Circumventricular organs and brain fluid environment* (pp. 409–412). Amsterdam: Elsevier.

Bodnar, R. J., Pasternak, G. W., Mann, P. E., Paul, D., Warren, R., & Donner, D. B. (1989). Mediation of anorexia by human recombinant tumor necrosis factor through a peripheral action in the rat. *Cancer Research, 15*, 6280–6284.

Breder, C. D., Dinarello, C. A., & Saper, C. B. (1988). Interleukin-1 immunoreactive innervation of the human hypothalamus. *Science, 240*, 321–324.

Broadwell, R. D. (1989). Transcytosis of macromolecules through the blood-brain barrier: A cell biological perspective and critical appraisal. *ACTA Neuropathologica (Berlin), 79*, 117–128.

Broadwell, R. D., Balin, B. J., & Salcman, M. (1988). Transcytotic pathway for blood-borne protein through the blood-brain barrier. *Proceedings of the National Academy of Sciences USA, 85*, 632–636.

Broadwell, R. D., & Banks, W. A. (1993). Cell biological perspective for the transcytosis of peptides and proteins through the mammalian blood-brain fluid barriers. In W. M. Pardridge (Ed.), *The blood-brain barrier* (pp. 165–199). New York: Raven Press.

Broadwell, R. D., & Salcman, M. (1981). Expanding the definition of the blood-brain barrier to protein. *Proceedings of the National Academy of Sciences USA, 78*, 7820–7824.

Broadwell, R. D., & Sofroniew, M. V. (1993). Serum proteins bypass the blood-brain barrier for extracellular entry to the central nervous system. *Experimental Neurology, 120*, 245–263.

Campbell, A. D., & Erwin, V. G. (1993). Chronic ethanol administration downregulates neurotensin receptors in long- and short-sleep mice. *Pharmacology Biochemistry and Behavior, 45*, 95–106.

Cannata, J. B., Fernandez-Soto, I., Fernandez-Menendez, M. J., Fernandez-Martin, J. L., McGregor, S. J., Brock, J. H., & Halls, D. (1991). Role of iron metabolism in absorption and cellular uptake of aluminum. *Kidney International, 39*, 799–803.

Caro, J. F., Kolaczynski, J. W., Nyce, M. R., Ohannesian, J. P., Opentanova, I., Goldman, W. H., Lynn, R. B., Zhang, P. -L., Sinha, M. D., & Considine, R. V. (1996). Decreased cerebrospinal-fluid/serum leptin ratio in obesity: A possible mechanism for leptin resistance. *Lancet, 348*, 159–161.

Chen, G., Castro, W. L., Chow, H.-H., & Reichlin, S. (1997). Clearance of ^{125}I-labelled interleukin-6 from brain into blood following intracerebroventricular injection in rats. *Endocrinology, 138*, 4830–4836.

Chen, G., & Reichlin, S. (1998). Clearance of [^{125}I]-tumor necrosis factor-α from the brain into the blood after intracerebroventricular injection into rats. *Neuroimmunomodulation, 5*, 261–269.

Chikhale, E. G., Ng, K. Y., Burton, P. S., & Borchardt, R. T. (1994). Hydrogen bonding potential as a determinant of the in vitro and in situ blood-brain barrier permeability of peptides. *Pharmaceutical Research, 11*, 412–419.

Chin, Y.-H., Sackstein, R., & Cai, J.-P. (1991). Lymphocyte-homing receptors and preferential migration pathways. *Proceedings of the Society for Experimental Biology and Medicine, 196*, 374–380.

Coceani, F., Lees, J., & Dinarello, C. A. (1987). Occurence of interlukin-1 in cerebralspinal fluid of the conscious cat. *Brain Research, 446*, 245–250.

Cornford, E. M., Braun, L. D., Oldendorf, W. H., & Hill, M. A. (1982). Comparison of lipid-mediated blood-brain-barrier penetrability in neonates and adults. *American Journal of Physiology, 243*, C161–C168.

Cserr, H. F. (1984). Convection of brain interstitial fluid. In K. Shapiro, A. Marmarou, & H. Portnoy (Eds.), *Hydrocephalus* (pp. 59–68). New York: Raven Press.

Cserr, H. F., & Knopf, P. M. (1992). Cervical lymphatics, the blood-brain barrier and the immunoreactivity of the brain: A new view. *Immunology Today, 13*, 507–512.

Cunningham, E. T., Jr., & De Souza, E. B. (1993). Interleukin 1 receptors in the brain and endocrine tissues. *Immunology Today, 14*, 171–176.

Cunningham, E. T. Jr., Wada, E., Carter, D. B., Tracey, D. E., Battey, J. F., & De Souza, E. B. (1991). Localization of interleukin-1 receptor messenger RNA in murine hippocampus. *Endocrinology, 128*, 2666–2668.

Cunningham, E. T. Jr., Wada, E., Carter, D. B., Tracey, D. E., Battey, J. F., & De Souza, E. B. (1992). In situ histochemical localization of type I interleukin-1 receptor messenger RNA in the central nervous system, pituitary, and adrenal gland of the mouse. *Journal of Neuroscience, 12*, 1101–1114.

Daniel, P. M., Love, E. R., & Pratt, O. E. (1978). The effect of age upon the influx of glucose into the brain. *Journal of Physiology (London), 274*, 141–148.

Davson, H. (1967). The blood-brain barrier. In *Physiology of the cerebrospinal fluid.* (pp. 82–103). London: J. and A. Churchill.

Davson, H., & Segal, M. B. (1996c). Morphological aspects of the barriers. In *Physiology of the CSF and blood-brain barriers* (pp. 93–192). Boca Raton, FL: CRC Press.

Davson, H., & Segal, M. B. (1996b). Special aspects of the blood-brain barrier. In *Physiology of the CSF and blood-brain barriers* (pp. 303–485). Boca Raton: CRC Press.

Davson, H., & Segal, M. B. (1996a). The return of the cerebrospinal fluid to the blood: The drainage mechanism. In *Physiology of the CSF and blood-brain barriers* (pp. 489–523). Boca Raton: CRC Press.

Davson, H., Welch, K., & Segal, M. B. (1987a). Some special aspects of the blood-brain barrier. In *Physiology and pathophysiology of the cerebrospinal fluid* (pp. 247–374). Edinburgh: Churchill Livingstone.

Davson, H., Welch, K., & Segal, M. B. (1987b). *The physiology and pathophysiology of the cerebrospinal fluid*. Edinburgh: Churchill Livingstone.

de Lange, E. C. M., Bouw, M. R., Danhof, M., De Boer, A. G., & Breimer, D. D. (1993). Application of intracerebral microdialysis to study regional distribution kinetics of atenolol and acetaminophen in rat brain. In *The use of intracerebral microdialysis to study the blood-brain barrier transport characteristics of drugs (thesis, Leiden/Amsterdam Center for Drug Research)* (pp. 93–106). Leiden: Sinteur.

De Vivo, D. C., Trifiletti, R. R., Jacobson, R. I., Ronen, G. M., Behmand, R. A., & Harik, S. I. (1991). Defective glucose transport across the blood-brain barrier as a cause of persistent hypoglycorrhachia, seizures, and developmental delay. *New England Journal of Medicine, 325*, 703–709.

Dower, S. K., Kronheim, S. R., Hopp, T. P., Cantrel, M., Deely, M., Gillis, S., Henney, C. S., & Urdal, D. L. (1986). The cell surface receptors for interleukin-1α and interleukin-1β are identical. *Nature, 324*, 266–268.

Duffy, K. R., & Pardridge, W. M. (1987). Blood-brain barrier transcytosis of insulin in developing rabbits. *Brain Research, 420*, 32–38.

Dux, E., Doczi, T., Joo, F., Szerdahelyi, P., & Siklos, L. (1988). Reverse pinocytosis induced in cerebral endothelial cells by injection of histamine into the cerebral ventricle. *ACTA Neuropathologica (Berlin), 76*, 484–488.

Ericsson, A., Liu, C., Kasckow, J., Hart, B. P., & Sawchenko, P. E. (1993). Distribution of the type 1 interleukin-1 receptor mRNA in the central nervous system of the rat [Abstract]. *Society for Neuroscience Abstracts, 19*, 95.

Fazakerley, J. K., & Webb, H. E. (1985). Cyclosporin, blood-brain barrier, and multiple sclerosis. *Lancet, 2*, 889–890.

Ferguson, A. V., & Marcus, P. (1988). Area postrema stimulation induced cardiovascular changes in the rat. *American Journal of Physiology, 255*, R855–R860.

Fishman, J. B., Rubin, J. B., Handrahan, J. V., Connor, J. R., & Fine, R. E. (1987). Receptor-mediated transcytosis of transferrin across the blood-brain barrier. *Journal of Neuroscience Research, 18*, 299–304.

Fugisawa, Y., Sasaki, K., & Akiyama, K. (1991). Increased insulin levels after OGTT load in peripheral blood and cerebrospinal fluid of patients with dementia of the Alzheimer type. *Biological Psychiatry, 30*, 1219–1228.

Greenwood, J., & Pratt, O. E. (1983). The effect of ethanol upon thiamine transport across the blood-brain barrier in the rat. *Journal of Physiology (London), 348*, 61P.

Gross, P. M., & Weindl, A. (1987). Peering through the windows of the brain. *Journal of Cerebral Blood Flow and Metabolism, 7*, 663–672.

Gutierrez, E. G., Banks, W. A., & Kastin, A. J. (1994). Blood-borne interleukin-1 receptor antagonist crosses the blood-brain barrier. *Journal of Neuroimmunology, 55*, 153–160.

Gutierrez, E. G., Banks, W. A., & Kastin, A. J. (1993). Murine tumor necrosis factor alpha is transported from blood to brain in the mouse. *Journal of Neuroimmunology, 47*, 169–176.

Habif, D. V., Lipton, R., & Cantell, K. (1975). Interferon crosses the blood-cerebrospinal fluid barrier in monkeys. *Proceedings of the Society for Experimental Biology and Medicine, 149*, 287–289.

Hardebo, J. E., & Kahrstrom, J. (1985). Endothelial negative surface charge areas and blood-brain barrier function. *Acta Physiologica Scandinavica, 125*, 495–499.

Harik, S. I., & Kalaria, R. N. (1991). Blood-brain barrier abnormalities in Alzheimer's disease. *Annals of the New York Academy of Sciences, 640*, 47–52.

Hashimoto, M., Ishikawa, Y., Yokota, S., Goto, F., Bando, T., Sakakibara, Y., & Iriki, M. (1991). Action site of circulating interleukin-1 on the rabbit brain. *Brain Research, 540*, 217–223.

Helyar, I., & Sherman, A. R. (1987). Iron deficiency and interleukin 1 production by rat leukocytes. *American Journal of Clinical Nutrition, 46*, 346–352.

Herkenham, M., & Nauta, W. J. (1977). Afferent connections of the habenular nuclei in the rat. A horseradish peroxidase study, with a note on the fiber-of-passage problem. *J.Comp.Neurol., 173*, 123–146.

Hill, J. M., Mervis, R. F., Avidor, R., Moody, T. W., & Brenneman, D. E. (1993). HIV envelope protein-induced neuronal damage and retardation of behavioral development in rat neonates. *Brain Research, 603*, 222–233.

Hill, J. M., Ruff, M. R., Weber, R. J., & Pert, C. B. (1985). Transferrin receptors in rat brain: Neuropeptide-like pattern and relationship to iron distribution. *Proceedings of the National Academy of Sciences USA, 82*, 4553–4557.

Imeri, L., Opp, M. R., & Krueger, J. M. (1993). An IL-1 receptor and an IL-1 receptor antagonist attenuate muramyl dipeptide- and IL-1-induced sleep and fever. *American Journal of Physiology, 265*, R907–R913.

Johanson, C. E. (1988). The choroid plexus-arachnoid membrane-cerebrospinal fluid system. In A. A. Boulton, G. B. Baker, & W. Walz (Eds.), *Neuromethods; the neuronal microenvironment* (pp. 33–104). Clifton, NJ: Humana Press.

Johanson, C. E. (1989). Ontogeny and phylogeny of the blood-brain barrier. In E. A. Neuwelt (Ed.), *Implications of the blood-brain barrier and its manipulation* (vol. 1, pp. 157–198). New York: Plenum Publishing.

Johnson, A. K., & Gross, P. M. (1993). Sensory circumventricular organs and brain homeostatic pathways. *FASEB, 7*, 678–686.

Kannan, R., Kuhlenkamp, J. F., Ookhtens, M., & Kaplowitz, N. (1992). Transport of glutathione at blood-brain barrier of the rat: Inhibition by glutathione analogs and age-dependence. *Journal of Pharmacology and Experimental Therapeutics, 263*, 964–970.

Katsuura, G., Arimura, A., Koves, K., & Gottschall, P. E. (1990). Involvement of organum vasculosum of lamina terminalis and preoptic area in interleukin 1β-induced ACTH release. *American Journal of Physiology, 258*, E163–E171.

Kinraide, T. B., & Parker, D. R. (1987). Cation amelioration of aluminum toxicity in wheat. *Plant Physiology, 83*, 546–551.

Knopf, P. M., Cserr, H. F., Nolan, S. C., Wu, T.-Y., & Harling-Berg, C. J. (1995). Physiology and immunology of lymphatic drainage of interstitial and cerebrospinal fluid from the brain. *Neuropathology and Applied Neurobiology, 21*, 175–180.

Komaki, G., Arimura, A., & Koves, K. (1992). Effect of intravenous injection of IL-1β on PGE_2 levels in several brain areas as determined by microdialysis. *American Journal of Physiology, 262,* E246–E251.

Krisch, B. (1986). The functional and structural borders between the CSF- and blood-dominated milieus in the choroid plexuses and the area postrema of the rat. *Cell and Tissue Research, 245,* 101–115.

Krisch, B., & Leonhardt, H. (1989). Relations between leptomeningeal compartments and the neurohemal regions of circumventricular organs. *Biomedical Research, 10 (suppl 3),* 155–168.

Loo, Y. T. (1931). The forebrain of the opossum, *Didelphis virginiana. Journal of Comparative Neurology, 52,* 1–148.

Lorenzi, M. (1990). The blood-brain barrier in diabetes mellitus. In J. C. Porter & D. Jezova (Eds.), *Circulating regulatory factors and neuroendocrine function* (pp. 381–390). New York: Plenum Press.

Lossinsky, A. S., Pluta, R., Song, M. J., Badmajew, V., Moretz, R. C., & Wisniewski, H. M. (1991). Mechanisms of inflammatory cell attachment in chronic relapsing experimental allergic encephalomyelitis: A scanning and high-voltage electron microscopic study of the injured mouse blood-brain barrier. *Microvascular Research, 41,* 299–310.

Lossinsky, A. S., Vorbrodt, A. W., & Wisniewski, H. M. (1983). Ultracytochemical studies of vesicular and canalicular transport structures in the injured mammalian blood-brain barrier. *ACTA Neuropathologica (Berlin), 61,* 239–245.

Luheshi, G. N., Gay, J., & Rothwell, N. J. (1994). Circulating IL-6 is transported into the brain via a saturable transport mechanism in the rat [Abstract]. *British Journal of Pharmacology, 112,* 637P.

Male, D. (1995). The blood-brain barrier—no barrier to a determined lymphocyte. In J. Greenwood, D. J. Begley, & M. B. Segal (Eds.), *New concepts of a blood-brain barrier* (pp. 311–314). New York: Plenum Press.

Maness, L. M., Banks, W. A., Zadina, J. E., & Kastin, A. J. (1996). Periventricular penetration and disappearance of icv Tyr-MIF-1, DAMGO, tyrosine, and albumin. *Peptides, 17,* 247–250.

Maness, L. M., Banks, W. A., Zadina, J. E., & Kastin, A. J. (1995). Selective transport of blood-borne interleukin-1α into the posterior division of the septum of the mouse brain. *Brain Research, 700,* 83–88.

Maness, L. M., Kastin, A. J., & Banks, W. A. (1998). Relative contributions of a CVO and the microvascular bed to delivery of blood-borne IL-1α to the brain. *American Journal of Physiology, 275,* E207–E212.

Maness, L. M., Kastin, A. J., Banks, W. A., & Zadina, J. E. (1991). In vivo translocation and selective removal of ^{125}I-Tyr-MIF-1 from the rat brain after icv injection. *Society for Neuroscience Abstracts, 17,* 240–240.

Maness, L. M., Kastin, A. J., Farrell, C. L., & Banks, W. A. (1998). Fate of leptin after intracerebroventricular injection into the mouse brain. *Endocrinology, 139,* 4556–4562.

Martins, J. M., Banks, W. A., & Kastin, A. J. (1997a). Acute modulation of the active carrier-mediated brain to blood transport of corticotropin-releasing hormone. *American Journal of Physiology, 272,* E312–E319.

Martins, J. M., Banks, W. A., & Kastin, A. J. (1997b). Transport of CRH from mouse brain directly affects peripheral produciton of β-endorphin by the spleen. *American Journal of Physiology, 273,* E1083–E1089.

McLay, R. N., Kimura, M., Banks, W. A., & Kastin, A. J. (1997). Granulocyte-macrophage colony-stimulating factor crosses the blood-brain and blood-spinal cord barriers. *Brain, 120,* 2083–2091.

Mooradian, A. D. (1987). Blood-brain barrier choline transport is reduced in diabetic rats. *Diabetes, 36,* 1094–1097.

Mooradian, A. D., Morin, A. M., Cipp, L. J., & Haspel, H. C. (1991). Glucose transport is reduced in the blood-brain barrier of aged rats. *Brain Research, 551,* 145–149.

Morley, B. J. (1986). The interpeduncular nucleus. *International Review of Neurobiology, 28,* 157–182.

Moses, A. V., & Nelson, J. A. (1994). HIV infection of human brain capillary endothelial cells-Implications for AIDS dementia. *Advances in Neuroimmunology, 4,* 239–247.

Nakamura, H., Nakanishi, K., Kita, A., & Kadokawa, T. (1988). Interleukin-1 induces analgesia in mice by a central action. *European Journal of Pharmacology, 149,* 49–54.

Oldendorf, W. H. (1971). Brain uptake of radio-labelled amino acids, amines and hexoses after arterial injection. *American Journal of Physiology, 221,* 1629–1639.

Oldendorf, W. H. (1974). Lipid solubility and drug penetration of the blood-brain barrier. *Proceedings of the Society for Experimental Biology and Medicine, 147,* 813–816.

Oldendorf, W. H. (1973). Stereo-specificity of blood-brain barrier permeability to amino acids. *American Journal of Physiology, 224,* 967–969.

Opara, E. I., Laviano, A., Meguid, M. M., & Yang, Z.-J. (1995). Correlation between food intake and CSF IL-1α in anorectic tumor bearing rats. *Neuroreport, 6,* 750–752.

Opp, M. R., & Krueger, J. M. (1991). Interleukin 1-receptor antagonist blocks interleukin 1-induced sleep and fever. *American Journal of Physiology, 260,* R453–R457.

Oteiza, P. I., Fraga, C. G., & Keen, C. L. (1993). Aluminum has both oxidant and antioxidant effects in mouse brain membranes. *Archives of Biochemistry and Biophysics, 300,* 517–521.

Pan, W., Banks, W. A., & Kastin, A. J. (1997a). BBB permeability to ebiratide and TNF in acute spinal cord injury. *Experimental Neurology, 146,* 367–373.

Pan, W., Banks, W. A., & Kastin, A. J. (1997b). Permeability of the blood-brain barrier and blood-spinal cord barriers to interferons. *Journal of Neuroimmunology, 76,* 105–111.

Pan, W., Banks, W. A., Kennedy, M. K., Gutierrez, E. G., & Kastin, A. J. (1996). Differential permeability of the BBB in acute EAE: Enhanced transport of TNF-α. *American Journal of Physiology, 271,* E636–E642.

Passaro, E. Jr., Debas, H., Oldendorf, W., & Yamada, T. (1982). Rapid appearance of intraventricularly administered neuropeptides in the peripheral circulation. *Brain Research, 241,* 338–340.

Patlak, C. S., Blasberg, R. G., & Fenstermacher, J. D. (1983). Graphical evaluation of blood-to-brain transfer constants from multiple-time uptake data. *Journal of Cerebral Blood Flow and Metabolism, 3,* 1–7.

Persidsky, Y., Stins, M., Way, D., Witte, M. H., Weinand, M., Kim, K. S., Bock, P., Gendelman, H. E., & Fiala, M. (1997). A model for monocyte migration through the blood-brain barrier during HIV-1 encephalitis. *Journal of Immunology, 158,* 3499–3510.

Plotkin, S. R., Banks, W. A., & Kastin, A. J. (1996). Comparison of saturable transport and extracellular pathways in the passage of interleukin-1α across the blood-brain barrier. *Journal of Neuroimmunology, 67,* 41–47.

Plotkin, S. R., Banks, W. A., Waguespack, P. J., & Kastin, A. J. (1997). Ethanol alters the concentration of met-enkephalin in brain by affecting peptide transport system-1 independent of preproenkephalin mRNA. *Journal of Neuroscience Research, 48,* 273–280.

Preston, E., & Hynie, I. (1991). Transfer constants for blood-brain barrier permeation of the neuroexcitatory shellfish toxin, domoic acid. *Le Journal Canadien des Sciences Neurologiques, 18,* 39–44.

Raeissi, S., & Audus, K. L. (1989). In-vitro characterization of blood-brain barrier permeability to delta sleep-inducing peptide. *Annals of the New York Academy of Sciences, 41,* 848–852.

Raisman, G. (1966). The connexions of the septum. *Brain, 89,* 317–348.

Ramon y Cajal, S. (1901). Estructura del septum lucidum. *Trab.Lab.Invest.Biol.Univ.Madrid, 1,* 159–188.

Rapoport, S. I. (1976). *Blood brain barrier in physiology and medicine.* New York: Raven Press.

Rapoport, S. I., Ohata, M., & London, E. D. (1981). Cerebral blood flow and glucose utilization following opening of the blood-brain barrier and during maturation of the rat brain. *Federation Proceedings, 40,* 2322–2325.

Raub, T. J., & Newton, C. R. (1991). Recycling kinetics and transcytosis of transferrin in primary cultures of bovine brain microvessel endothelial cells. *Journal of Cellular Physiology, 149,* 141–151.

Reese, T. S., & Brightman, M. W. (1968). Similarity instructure and permeability to peroxidase of epithelia overlying fenestrated cerebral capillaries [Abstract]. *Anatomical Record, 160,* 414.

Richards, J. G. (1978). Permeability of intercellular junctions in brain epithelia and endothelia to exogenous amine: Cytochemical localization of extracellular 5-hydroxydopamine. *Journal of Neurocytology, 7,* 61–70.

Romero, L. I., Ildiko, K., Lechan, R. M., & Reichlin, S. (1996). Interleukin-6 (IL-6) is secreted from the brain after intracerebroventricular injection of IL-1β in rats. *American Journal of Physiology, 270,* R518–R524.

Ross, J. F., Broadwell, R. D., Poston, M. R., & Lawhorn, G. T. (1994). Highest brain bismuth levels and neuropathology are adjacent to fenestrated blood vessels in mouse brain after intraperitoneal dosing of bismuth subnitrate. *Toxicology and Applied Pharmacology, 124,* 191–200.

Sabo, J., Ni, G., Nadeau, D. J., Liberato, D. J., & Loh, A. (1992). Comparative tissue distribution of ^{125}I- and U-^{14}C-labeled recombinant human interleukin-2 in the rat. *Lymphokine and Cytokine Research, 11,* 229–233.

Saris, S. C., Rosenberg, S. A., Friedman, R. B., Rubin, J. T., Barba, D., & Oldfield, E. H. (1988). Penetration of recombinant interleukin-2 across the blood-cerebrospinal fluid barrier. *Journal of Neurosurgery, 69,* 29–34.

Schinkel, A. H., Smit, J. J. M., van Tellingen, O., Beijnen, J. H., Wagenaar, E., van Deemter, L., Mol, C. A. A. M., van der Valk, M. A., Robanus-Maandag, E. C., te Riele, H. P. J., Berns, A. J. M., & Borst, P. (1994). Disruption of the mouse mdr1a p-glycoprotein gene leads to a deficiency in the blood-brain barrier and to increased sensitivity to drugs. *Cell, 77,* 491–502.

Schwartz, M. W., Figlewicz, D. P., Baskin, D. G., Woods, S. C., & Porte, D. Jr. (1994). Insulin and the central regulation of energy balance: Update 1994. *Endocrine Reviews, 2,* 109–113.

Schwartz, M. W., Peskind, E., Raskind, M., Boyko, E. J., & Porte, D., Jr. (1996). Cerebrospinal fluid leptin levels: Relationship to plasma levels and adiposity in humans. *Nature Medicine, 2,* 589–593.

Shah, G. N., & Mooradian, A. D. (1997). Age-relatedhanges in the blood-brrain barrier. *Experimental Gerontology, 32,* 501–519.

Sharief, M. K., Noori, M. A., Ciardi, M., Cirelli, A., & Thompson, E. J. (1993). Increased levels of circulating ICAM-1 in serum and cerebrospinal fluid of patients with active multiple sclerosis. Correlation with TNF-α and blood-brain barrier damage. *Journal of Neuroimmunology, 43,* 15–22.

Shortle, W. C., & Smith, K. T. (1988). Aluminum-induced calcium deficiency syndrome in declining red spruce. *Science, 240,* 1017–1018.

Sirko, S., Bishai, I., & Coceani, F. (1989). Prostaglandin formation in the hypothalamus in vivo: effect of pyrogens. *American Journal of Physiology, 256,* R616–R624.

Stitt, J. T. (1990). Passage of immunomodulators across the blood-brain barrier. *Yale Journal of Biology and Medicine, 63,* 121–131.

Swanson, L. W., & Cowan, W. M. (1979). The connections of the septal region of the rat. *Journal of Comparative Neurology., 186,* 621–656.

Takasato, Y., Rapoport, S. I., & Smith, Q. R. (1984). An in situ brain perfusion technique to study cerebrovascular transport in the rat. *American Journal of Physiology, 247,* H484–H493.

Tanaka, T., Araki, E., Nitta, K., & Tateno, M. (1987). Recombinant human tumor necrosis factor depresses serum iron in mice. *Journal of Biological Response Modifiers, 6,* 484–488.

Tavassoli, M., & Minguell, J. J. (1991). Homing of hemopoietic progenitor cells to the marrow. *Proceedings of the Society for Experimental Biology and Medicine, 196,* 367–373.

Tsuji, A., Terasaki, T., Takabatake, Y., Tenda, Y., Tamai, I., Yamashima, T., Moritani, S., Tsuruo, T., & Yamashita, J. (1992). P-glycoprotein as the drug efflux pump in primary cultured bovine brain capillary endothelial cells. *Life Sciences, 51,* 1427–1437.

van der Ploeg, I., Cintra, A., Altiok, N., Askelöf, P., Fuxe, K., & Fredholm, B. B. (1991). Limited distribution of pertussis toxin in rat brain after injection into the lateral cerebral ventricles. *Neuroscience, 44,* 205–214.

van Heek, M., Compton, D. S., France, C. F., Tedesco, R. P., Fawzi, A. B., Graziano, M. P., Sybertz, E. J., Strader, C. D., & Davis, H. R. Jr. (1997). Diet-induced obese mice develop peripheral, but not central, resistance to leptin. *Journal of Clinical Investigation, 99,* 385–390.

Villegas, J. C., & Broadwell, R. D. (1993). Transcytosis of protein through the mammalian cerebral epithelium and endothelium: II. Adsorptive transcytosis of WGA-HRP and the blood-brain and brain-blood barriers. *Journal of Neurocytology, 22,* 67–80.

Vorbrodt, A. W. (1994). Glycoconjugates and anionic sites in the blood–brain barrier. In M. Nicolini & P. F. Zatta (Eds.), *Glycobiology and the brain* (pp. 37–62). Oxford: Pergamon Press.

Waguespack, P. J., Banks, W. A., & Kastin, A. J. (1994). Interleukin-2 does not cross the blood-brain barrier by a saturable transport system. *Brain Research Bulletin, 34,* 103–109.

Washizaki, K., Purdon, D., DeGeorge, J., Robinson, P. J., Rapoport, S. I., & Smith, Q. R. (1991). Fatty acid uptake and esterification by the in situ perfused rat brain [Abstract]. *Society for Neuroscience Abstracts, 17,* 864.

Weindl, A. (1973). Neuroendocrine aspects of circumventricular organs. In W. F. Ganong & L. Martini (Eds.), *Frontiers in neuroendocrinology* (pp. 3–32). New York: Oxford University Press.

Wong, M.-L., & Licinio, J. (1994). Localization of interleukin 1 type 1 receptor mRNA in rat brain. *Neuroimmunomodulation, 1,* 110–115.

Yamada, S., DePasquale, M., Patlak, C. S., & Cserr, H. F. (1991). Albumin outflow into deep cervical lymph from different regions of rabbit brain. *American Journal of Physiology, 261,* H1197–H1204.

Zatta, P., Bordin, C., & Favarato, M. (1993). The inhibition of trypsin and alpha-chymotrypsin proteolytic activity by aluminum (III). *Archives of Biochemistry and Biophysics, 303,* 407–411.

Zlokovic, B. V., Begley, D. J., Djuricic, B. M., & Mitrovic, D. M. (1986). Measurement of solute transport across the blood-brain barrier in the perfused guinea pig brain: Method and application to N-methyl-α-aminoisobutyric acid. *Journal of Neurochemistry, 46,* 1444–1451.

Zlokovic, B. V., Ghiso, J., Mackic, J. B., McComb, J. G., Weiss, M. H., & Frangione, B. (1993). Blood-brain barrier transport of circulating Alzheimer's amyloid β. *Biochemical and Biophysical Research Communications, 197,* 1034–1040.

CHAPTER

19

Secretion of Immunomodulatory Mediators from the Brain: An Alternative Pathway of Neuroimmunomodulation

SEYMOUR REICHLIN

I. INTRODUCTION

Many different mechanisms by which the brain can influence immune function have been identified or suggested (Ader, Felten, & Cohen, 1991; MacLean & Reichlin, 1981; Reichlin, 1998, 1999a) (Table I). Best established is control by the sympathetic nervous system, acting through noradrenergic innervation of lymphatic tissue, and by the action of catecholamines on circulating and fixed immunocompetent and natural killer cells (Irwin, 1994; Madden, Sanders, & Felten, 1995; Sundar, Sierpial, Kilts, Ritchie, & Weiss, 1990; Vredevoe, Moser, Gan, & Bonavida, 1995). Neural control can also be mediated by anterior pituitary hormones, whose secretion is regulated by the hypothalamus. Anterior pituitary hormones influence directly, or through target gland secretions, many different aspects of immune function (Ader et al., 1991, Reichlin, 1995). Most important of the pituitary hormones is corticotropin, which regulates the secretion of glucocorticoids, which in turn exert a profound influence on immunocompetent cells and appear to serve as a homeostatic feedback signal to modulate overexuberant (potentially harmful) inflammatory responses (Chrousos, 1995; Sternberg, 1997). Growth hormone and prolactin generally stimulate lymphocyte function, as do the gonadotropins acting mainly by way of sex steroids. Other postulated mechanisms include the secretion of neuropeptides such as Substance P, vasoactive intestinal peptide, and somatostatin from nerve endings (Goetzl et al., 1998), and vasomotor regulation of gut immunocompetent cells and cell trafficking (Ottaway & Husband, 1994). Undernutrition, which can be a consequence of psychological disturbance, can profoundly inhibit immune function. These topics are dealt with in detail in other chapters of this book.

TABLE I Established Pathways by Which the CNS Can Influence Immunity

Eating behavior and nutritional state
Psychogenic anorexia
Vagal-afferent mediated ("sickness behavior," other)
Hypothalamic-pituitary axis
Glucocorticoids
Prolactin
Growth hormone
Sex steroids
Sympathetic nervous system
Noradrenergic innervation of lymphatic tissue
Circulating epinephrine
Control of regional blood supply
Sensory afferent fibers
Axone reflexes [tachykinins substance P, K], somatostatin, CGRP, CRH)
Vasomotor changes in gut
Regulation of lymphocyte trafficking in gut lymphatic system
Regulation of salivary gland secretion

The purpose of this review is to summarize the evidence that the brain itself can serve as a secretory source of immunomodulatory cytokines and other immuneregulators and thereby play a role in neuroimmunomodulation.

II. MECHANISMS BY WHICH MACROMOLECULES ENTER THE BLOOD FROM THE BRAIN

The brain traditionally has been considered to be immunologically privileged. Tight junctions between the endothelial cells that line brain capillaries almost completely prevent entry to the brain parenchyma and cerebrospinal fluid of antigens and of other macromolecules from the circulation (Rapaport, 1976). Even relatively small molecules such as glucose, amino acids, and electrolytes enter the brain from the blood by way of specific endothelial membrane transporters (Pardridge, 1983). In a few highly specialized areas that surround the third and fourth ventricle (the periventricular organs) endothelia are fenestrated so that blood constituents can come into direct contact with nerve cell bodies and endings (McKinley, McAllen, & Mendelsohn, 1990). But even in these structures, which include the median eminence of the hypothalamus, OVLT (organum vasculosum of the lamina terminalis), and the area postrema of the fourth ventricle, uptake into the brain is localized and they do not provide a route of entry of blood constituents into the bulk of the brain.

Other reasons for considering the brain to be "immune-privileged" are that intracerebral implants of foreign tissues are not rejected as readily as those implanted in peripheral tissues, and antigen recognizing cells are not present in normal brain under basal conditions (Hickey, 1990).

Considered in this frame of reference, it would seem most reasonable to assume that the brain would influence systemic immune processes mainly through its efferent neural and neuroendocrine pathways—the autonomic nervous system, the hypothalamic-pituitary axis, and possibly through other peripheral nerve-mediated actions.

A. Transfer of Macromolecules from Brain to Venous Circulation

Contrary to this view of an immunologically isolated brain is the finding that macromolecules such as immunoregulatory cytokines arising autochthonously in the brain can readily enter the blood. Unlike peripheral tissues, the brain does not have a lymphatic system that can drain intercellular spaces. Instead, all types of cells of the brain, neurons, and supporting cells are in communication with the cerebrospinal fluid by way of channels that surround the cells, and which drain into the cerebrospinal fluid (CSF) (Rapaport 1976). Classical studies of Dandy (1929) and Weed (1914) indicated that most cerebrospinal fluid was resorbed into the blood from the subarachnoid space by way of the arachnoidal villi that project into the lumen of the superior sagittal sinus (SSS), the principal pathway of venous drainage from the brain. As Greitz (1993) quotes McComb, "for more than a generation now, standard texts and teaching have limited CSF drainage solely to the arachnoid."

B. Transfer from CSF to Regional Lymphatics by Bulk Flow

The Weed hypothesis of arachnoidal villus transfer has been modified significantly by studies of clearance of particulate substances from the subarachnoid space. Early work in this area was summarized and expanded by Field and Brierley (1948) who showed that india ink introduced into the subarachnoid space of the rabbit appears mainly in lymph nodes located in deep cervical nodes in the neck and in the retroperitoneal space. India ink, a suspension of carbon particles, exits the brain by way of perineuronal

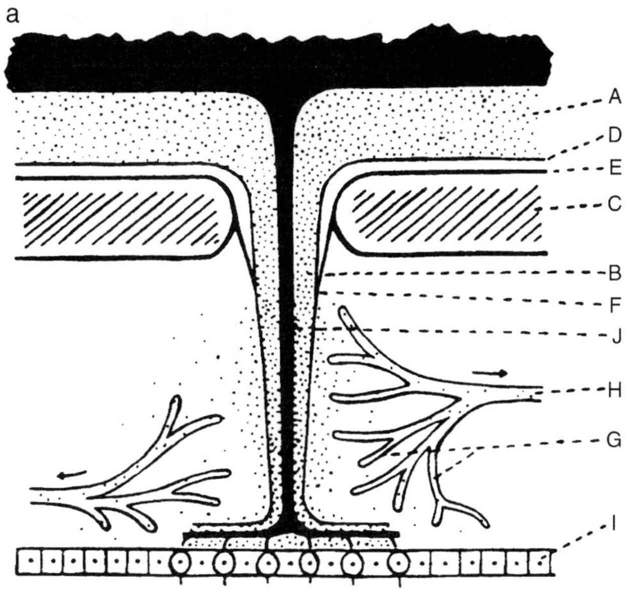

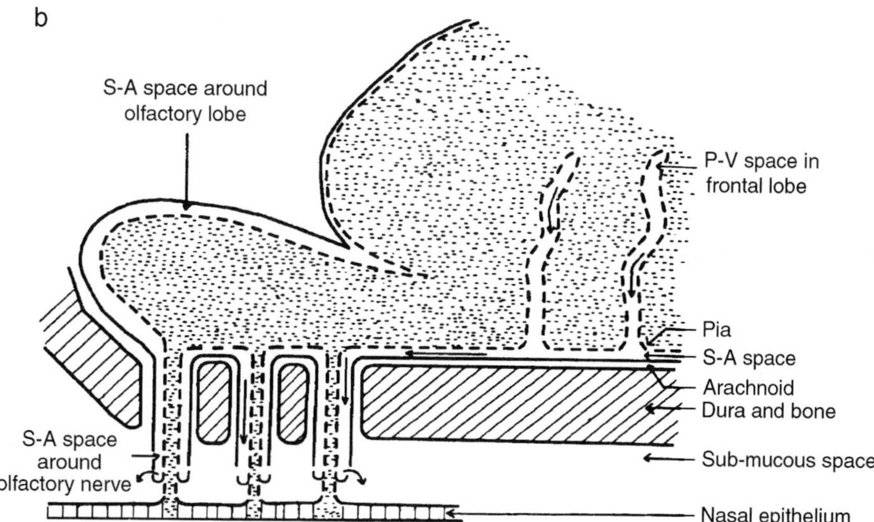

FIGURE 1 (a) Schematic diagram of route for the bulk flow of CSF including dissolved macromolecules from the brain into the submucous space of the nasopharynx. The black dots represent india ink particles, which move in the subarachnoid space to sleeve-like extensions, which exit the CNS around the olfactory neurons as they pass through the cribriform plate. The arachnoid extensions terminate in the submucosal space of the nasal mucosa. Larger molecules (over 5000 Kd) are taken up into lymphatic capillaries thence drain into the deep cervical lymph node chain. Smaller molecules are taken up by capillaries and enter the general circulation. A, subarachnoid space containing india ink oldi splace; C, cribriform plate; D, arachnoid; E, dura; F, fusion of dura and arachnoid with epineurium; G, lymphatic capillaries; H, lymphatic collecting trunk; I, mucous membrane of nose; J, olfactory nerve bundle. From Field & Brierly (1948). (b) Diagram of hypothesized route for movement of injected protein from the subarachnoid space into the submucous space of the nose. After leaving the perivascular spaces in the brain, CSF moves into the subarachnoid space of the olfactory lobe. From Cserr & Knopf (1992).

extensions of the subarachnoid space that surround all nerves that enter and leave the neuroaxis (Figure 1). From the brain, the principal route of exit is by way of the channels that surround the olfactory neuronal fibers as they pass through the cribriform plate of the sphenoid sinus (Bradbury, Cserr, & Westrop, 1981; Kida, Patazis, & Weller, 1993; Zhang, Richards, Kida, & Weller, 1992). These channels terminate in the nasal submucosa. Macromolecules (and particles) in excess of 5000 Da in size are taken up by lymphatic capillaries, which then drain into the deep cervical lymph nodes and cervical lymph channels and ultimately into the systemic circulation. Anatomical channels of this size oppose no molecular size barrier; this form of exit, termed "bulk transport" Rapaport (1976) does not depend on energetic reactions and is nonselective. Imaging methods in humans demonstrate that the pulsatile expansion of the brain (in the fixed cranial cavity) during cardiac systole is the major factor forcing flow of tracers out of the brain, into the CSF, and into the blood (Greitz, 1993).

The magnitude of bulk flow drainage from the brain was first determined in experimental animals by measurements of the rate with which inert labeled tracers such as albumin, dextrans, or polyethylene glycols were diluted in CSF after they had been introduced into the lateral cerebral ventricle. Given a steady state of CSF volume, the rate of dilution is the rate at which tracer leaves the brain. Efflux rate is equal to the rate of formation and of secretion of cerebrospinal fluid (Bradbury and Cserr, 1985; Bradbury et al., 1981; Cserr, Harling-Berg, & Knopf, 1992). Over a wide range of molecular sizes, the rates with which macromolecules leave the brain are equal.

The relative proportion of brain derived macromolecules that enter the lymphatic system (as compared with sagittal sinus drainage) has been measured in several species by collecting lymphatic fluid draining the head. In rabbits, for example, that proportion appears to be in the range of 40% (Bradbury & Cserr, 1985; Bradbury et al., 1981).

That proinflammatory cytokines introduced into the CSF also leave the brain was first documented by Bodnar and colleagues (1989) who showed that radioiodinated hTNF-α appeared in peripheral blood after icv injection in rats. They suggested that some of the central actions attributed to tumor necrosis factor on the basis of effects induced by central administration could be due to its peripheral actions. In the light of recent observations that have implicated cytokine receptors on abdominal vagal afferents in the pathogenisis of cytokine-induced anorexia in rats (Maier, Goehler, Fleshner, & Watkins, 1998), their suggestion may indeed be correct. In mice, Banks and colleagues (Banks, Kastin, & Broadwell, 1995; Banks, Kastin, & Durham, 1989; Banks, Kastin, & Gutierrez, 1994) also showed that interleukin (IL)-6 and IL-1 left the brain of the mouse after intracerebral injection. Since the rate of efflux was approximately the same as that of albumin, these workers concluded that transport out was by bulk flow.

Our group has carried out pharmacokinetic studies of the efflux of radioiodinated tracer hIL-6 (Chen, Castro, Chow, & Reichlin, 1997), hTNF-α (Chen & Reichlin, 1998) (Figure 2), and hIL-1β (Chen & Reichlin, 1999) and LPS (Chen, McCuskey, & Reichlin, 2000) after icv injection in the rat (Figure 3) (Table II). The four substances, of molecular weight in excess of 17 kDa were all cleared from brain to blood by first order kinetics compatible with a two compartment (brain-to-blood) system. Rates of clearance from brain to blood for IL-6, TNF-α, and LPS are virtually identical despite the fact that the rate of peripheral clearance of each is quite different. The rate of clearance of IL-1β is approximately double that of the other tracers, a difference attributable to the fact that IL-1 is transferred from brain to blood by an active transport system as well as by bulk flow. Over the first 4 h, 31.6 and 41.8% of the injected dose of IL-6 and TNF-α had appeared in peripheral blood (as determined by measurements of the area under the curve (AUC) compared with iv injection). In the case of IL-1β, which has a very large volume of peripheral distribution as compared with the other two cytokines, the AUC after icv injection over the first 2 h was 89.9% of that after iv injection, and blood levels of IL-1β after icv injection were significantly higher than those after iv injection at one hour and thereafter. Di Santo, Benignia, Angnelloa, Sipeb, & Ghezzi, (1999) also report that blood levels of hIL-1β after icv injection are higher than after iv injection (in the mouse). They attribute the difference to the brain pool acting as a reservoir from which the injected cytokine is gradually cleared.

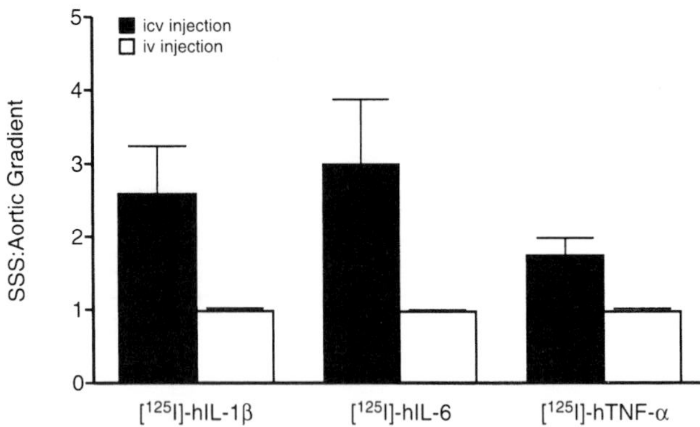

FIGURE 2 Sagittal sinus concentration of radioiodinated IL-1, IL-6, and TNF- is higher than blood levels following icv injection of tracer-labeled cytokine. This is evidence of passage of cytokine from brain to peripheral blood. Classical work of Weed (1914) and Dandy (1929) indicates that this flow is by way of arachnoid villi in the superior sagittal sinus, which have fenestrated endothelia.

All of the studies cited above are based on pharmacokinetic analysis after a single icv bolus injection. Measurements of brain-to-blood clearance of hIL-1 receptor antagonist (IL-1RA) under presumably steady-state conditions have been made by Kakuscka, Qi, Clark, & Lechan (1993) who adminis-

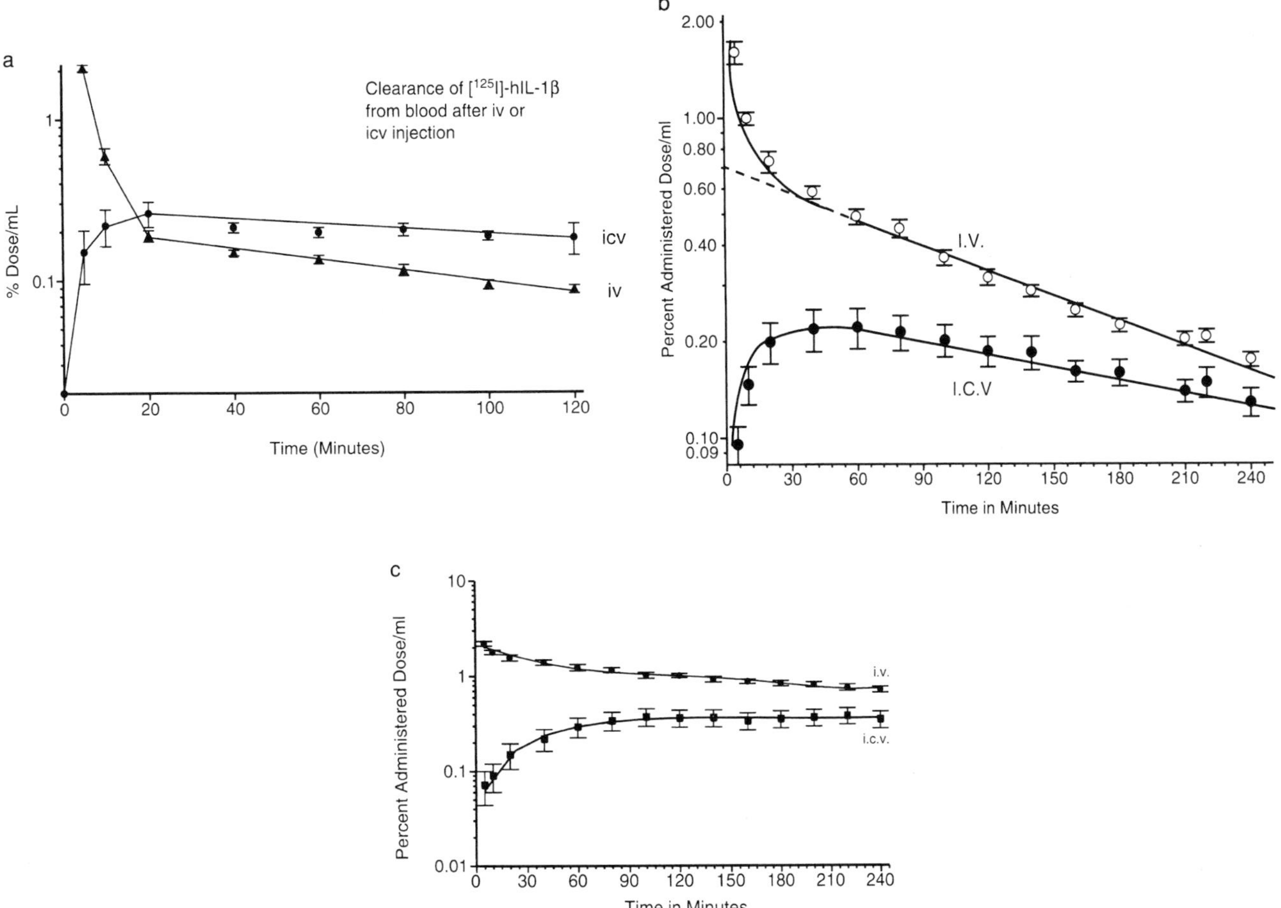

FIGURE 3 Clearance from brain to blood of radioiodide-labeled hIL-1β (a), IL-6 (b), and TNF-α (c) after icv injection as compared with clearance after iv injection. Values are expressed as percentage of injected dose per milliliter of blood. Note that the blood level of IL-1 after icv injection reaches that after iv injection at approximately 20 min after injection, and significantly exceeds iv concentration for the rest of the time followed (up to 120 min). Blood levels of IL-6 after icv injection peak at 60 min, but do not reach the levels seen after iv injection. Blood levels of TNF-α approach the levels observed at 120 min after icv injection, but both levels remain elevated over the next 240 min. The brain-to-blood clearance for each substance is virtually the same (see Table II); differences in blood levels reflect differences in the volume of distribution and rate of peripheral clearance of the respective cytokine in the blood. Higher values late after injection reflect the continued release of labeled cytokine from the brain depot.

tered human IL-1 receptor antagonist (IL-1RA) icv or iv to rats for 9 h by means of an Alzet minipump after an initial priming dose (Figure 4). The icv dose was three times higher than the iv dose. Blood levels of IL-1RA after icv injection were not significantly different from values after iv administration, indicating that approximately one third of the icv administered cytokine had left the brain, a value reasonably close to those obtained after bolus injection. They also observed incidently that blood levels of hIL-1RA after icv injection were higher when the animals had been treated with lipopolysaccharide (LPS).

Bacterial endotoxin also exits the brain by the mechanism of bulk flow (Chen, McCuskey, & Reichlin, 2000). Approximately 70% of an administered dose enters the blood within 4 h of icv injection (Figure 5). These high values, as compared with clearance of labeled cytokines, are probably due to differences in metabolic degradation; there is substantial "first-pass" degradation of labeled cytokines, but no degradation of LPS. Faggioni et al. (1995b) documented the appearance of LPS in peripheral blood after icv injection (in mice).

Values for brain-to-blood clearance of various inert markers, obtained by measuring the rate at which the concentration of tracer in CSF declines after icv injection in rats, are reasonably close to those measured in rats by pharmacokinetic analysis of blood secretion patterns. Some representative values (Percentage of brain content cleared to blood per

TABLE II Pharmacokinetic Analysis of Brain-to-Blood Clearance of Radioiodinated hIL-1β, hIL-6, hTNF-α, and *E. coli* Endotoxin (lipopolysaccharide, LPS) and Percentage of Injected Dose that Enters the Blood Following icv Injection in Rats

	Brain-to-blood clearance (%min)		Area under the curve (% of iv AUC)
IL-1	2.00 ± 0.01		89.9
IL-6	1.16	0.22	41.8
TNF-α	1.12	0.30	31.6
LPS	1.00	0.21	70.0

Clearance is expressed as percentage of total brain content entering the blood per minute. Percentage of injected dose that enters the blood is expressed by comparing the area under the curve (AUC) after icv injection with the value after iv injection. (Data from Chen & Reichlin, 1997, 1998, 1999; Chen, McCuskey & Reichlin, 2000). Clearance data on IL-1 based on 2 h observation. The others were observed over a 4 h period.

minute) are: 0.75, (Bass & Lundborg, 1973) 0.88, (Cserr, DePasquale, Harling-Berg, Park, & Knopf, 1965) 1.1, (Kawakami, Yamamoto, Sawada, & Iga, 1994) 1.60.

These data taken together indicate clearly that a substantial proportion of macromolecules arising in the brain can rather quickly enter the blood, and, as in the case of IL-1β, blood levels after icv injection can persist much longer than after iv injection.

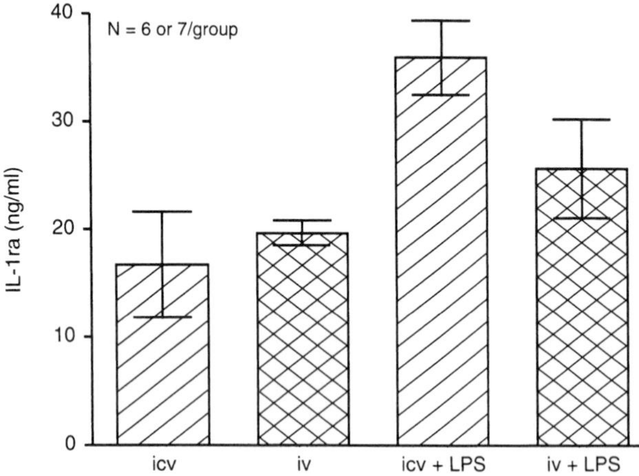

FIGURE 4 Steady-state blood levels of human IL-1 receptor antagonist (hIL-1RA) in rats after a priming pulse and 8 h of icv perfusion. Concentrations were determined by immunoassay. The amount of material injected icv was three times that of the iv injection, yet the achieved blood levels were indistinguishable. This finding is interpreted to indicate that under steady-state conditions, approximately one third of the cytokine introduced into the brain appeared in peripheral blood. In this study, a significantly higher blood level was achieved if the rats also had been given peripheral injection of LPS.

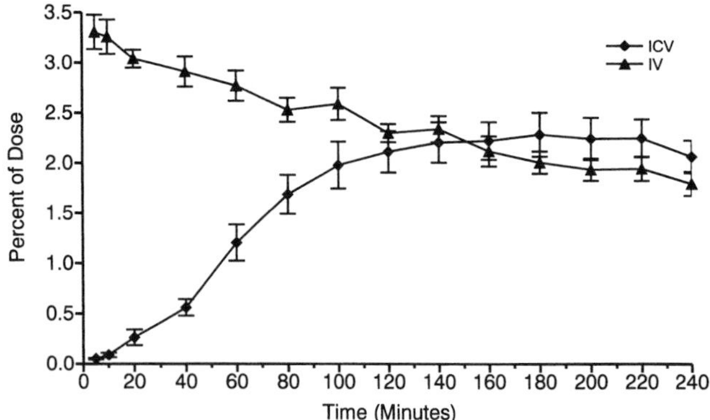

FIGURE 5 Brain-to-blood clearance of radioiodinated LPS after icv injection in rats. Blood levels of LPS reach those after iv injection at approximately 120 min, and both remain elevated for the remainder of the observation period.

The ease with which a relatively large fraction of macromolecules introduced into the cerebral ventricles rapidly appears in peripheral blood contrasts dramatically with the extreme difficulty with which macromolecules in peripheral blood gain entry to the brain through the blood-brain barrier (Banks et al., 1995). Inward transport is slow and specific, whereas outward flow is relatively rapid and nonspecific.

To the historically minded neuroendocrinologist, the idea that substances in the CSF can drain through the cribriform plate into the nasal submucosa bears an uncanny, though superficial, resemblance to the 2nd century views of Galen, modified by Vesalius in the 16th century. Quoting Vesalius' 1543 paper, Toni & Lechan (1993) wrote,

> it is now required to list each part needed for mucous excretion [from the brain]. There are two ducts in the brain substance, then a thin portion of membrane shaped as the infundibulum, then the gland that receives the tip of this infundibulum and the ducts that drive the mucus [*pituita*] from this gland to the palate and nares. . . . and I said that one [duct] . . . from the middle of the common cavity[third ventricle] descends . . . into the brain substance, and the end of this duct is . . . the sinus of the gland where the brain mucus is collected.

Consideration of the bulk flow of water and macromolecules via perineuronal channels should not obscure the fact that macromolecules also exit the brain by way of the fenestrated arachnoidal villi that drain into the superior sagittal sinus. With specific reference to brain efflux of cytokines, the concentration of IL-6 in superior sagittal sinus blood is higher than its concentration in aortic blood entering the brain, whether the IL-6 has been induced within the brain by icv injection of IL-1β (Romero, Kakucska, Lechan, & Reichlin, 1996) (see below) or LPS (Gottschall, Komaki, & Arimura, 1992; Chen,

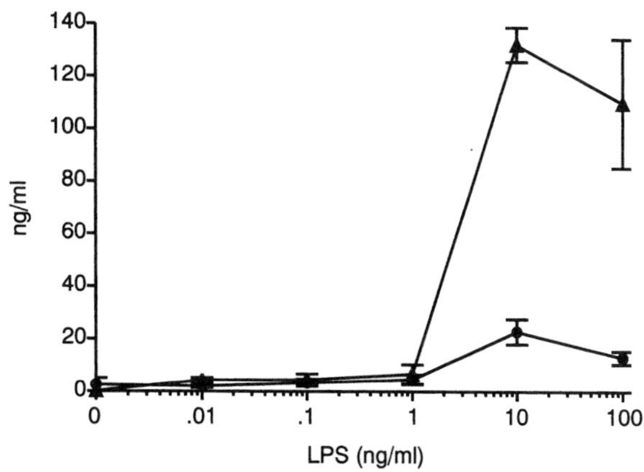

FIGURE 6 Effect of LPS on IL-6 secretion by human choroid plexus dispersed cell culture. The culture consists of epithelial, endothelial, and interstitial cells. (Reichlin, 1999)

McCuskey, & Reichlin, 2000), or if an IL-6 tracer has been introduced into the brain by icv injection (Chen et al., 1997). (Figure 5). Similarly, there is a positive SSS:aortic gradient for bioactive TNF-α after icv injection of LPS (Chen, McCuskey, & Reichlin, 2000), and of labeled TNF-α after icv injection of tracer (Chen & Reichlin, 1998) (Figure 5). A positive SSS:aortic gradient after icv injection of radioiodinated hIL-1β was observed (Figure 6), but not of radioiodinated LPS (Chen, McCuskey, & Reichlin, 2000). Failure to document a SSS: aortic gradient after icv injection of labeled LPS may be attributed to the extremely low rate of peripheral clearance, which leads to a relatively high rate of recirculation of labeled tracer into the brain arterial supply.

The fact that IL-1β, IL-6, TFN-α, and LPS, all molecules larger than 17 KDa, enter the peripheral blood from the cerebral ventricle by bulk transport, and that other macromolecules are similarly transported makes it likely that virtually any cytokine or product of injured or dying cells or bacterial toxin that arises in the brain could enter the peripheral circulation, and depending on its concentration, materially influence both peripheral metabolic and immunological activity.

Release of other classes of biologically significant brain-derived molecules into peripheral blood have been reported. These include estradiol in male songbirds (Schlinger & Arnold, 1991), brain-derived neurotrophic factor (BDNF) after subarachnoid hemorrhage in humans (Berendes et al., 1997), and catecholamine metabolites in several species (Esler et al., 1990). Leptin concentration in jugular vein blood was reported to be higher than arterial blood concentration in men, a finding interpreted to mean that the brain is a site of leptin secretion (Esler et al., 1998), but in studies carried out in this laboratory (Reichlin, Chen, & Nicolson, 2000) SSS leptin levels were slightly but significantly less than aortic levels, a finding interpreted to mean that cerebral cortex extracted leptin from the blood.

That substances arising in the brain or introduced by injection enter peripheral blood has practical implications for the interpretation of experiments in which antibodies and other antagonists have been injected into the brain to block particular brain functions. Turnbull and Rivier (1998a, 1998c) have shown that antibodies injected icv in rats can enter the circulation in sufficient concentration to block peripheral functions. The same reservations may apply to their own studies on icv injection of IL-1β, which appears to be a more potent inhibitor of testicular responses to chorionic gonadotropin than when administered iv (Turnbull & Rivier, 1997).

III. SOURCES OF CYTOKINES ARISING IN THE BRAIN AND THEIR REGULATION

A relatively large number of cytokines have been shown to arise in the brain from cellular components of brain parenchyma, brain vasculature, meninges, and choroid plexus, which are candidate peripheral immunoregulators (Table III). (Andersson, Perry, & Gordon, 1992; Benveniste, 1994; Faggioni et al., 1995;

TABLE III Immunomodulatory Cytokines Known to Arise in Brain Which Are Candidate Peripheral Immunoregulators

Stimulatory
Interleukins-1 (,), -2, -3, -5, -6, -8, -11, -12 ,-15
TNF-α
Interferon-γ
Monocyte chemotactic and activating factor
Granulocyte-macrophage-colony simulating factor
Leukemia inhibitory factor
Erythropoietin
Hepatocyte growth factor
Inhibitory
IL-1 receptor antagonist
Transforming growth factor-β
Interleukin-10
TNF-α receptor

(List of brain cytokines compiled from Steinberg, 1997; Reichlin, 1999a).

Gatti & Bartfai, 1993; Griffin, 1997; Licinio & Wong, 1997; Plata-Salaman, 1991; Schöbitz, Holsboer, & deKloet, 1994; Sternberg, 1997; Hopkins & Rothwell, 1995). In general, proinflammatory cytokines are not expressed in these tissues under basal conditions but appear after inflammatory challenges, or in the case of IL-1β and IL-6 after physical or emotional stress.

Known cellular sites of synthesis of cytokines in the brain are neurons (IL-1, IL-6, TNF-α) (Breder, Tsujimoto, Terano, Scott, & Saper, 1993; Hopkins & Rothwell, 1995; Ringheim, Burgher, & Heroux, 1995), choroid plexus (Tarlow et al., 1993), endothelia (Licinio & Wong, 1997; Van Dam et al., 1996), astrocytes, (Lee, Kiu, Dickson, Brosnan, & Berman, 1993), and microglia (Benveniste, 1994; Chao, Hu, Sheng, & Peterson, 1995). In response to inflammatory stimuli, the most intense and best characterized response is that of resident microglia and circulating activated monocytes/lymphocytes/macrophages that enter the brain under the stimulation of locally induced chemokines (Hickey, 1991). LPS and proinflammatory cytokines that circulate in blood can induce the appearance of cytokines and other inflammatory products such as prostaglandins and nitric oxide within the brain.

LPS-induced inflammation is a highly conserved response developed over billions of years by the evolution of eukaryotes in a hostile bacterial environment (see Reichlin, 1999a for review). LPS, a constitutent of the cell wall of all gram-negative bacteria coupled to the LPS binding protein, binds to the LPS-LPSbp-CD14 receptor (in the case of LPS) (Ulevitch & Elias, 1994) and to cytokine receptors on brain endothelia (Figure 5). The LPS receptor is homologous to the IL-1 receptor (Yang et al., 1998). Genes encoding IL-1, IL-6, IL-1 receptor antagonists and type 1 IL-1 receptors are expressed by brain microvessel endothelia (Fabry et al., 1993; Licinio & Wong, 1997; Van Dam et al., 1996). Also expressed is caspase 1, a regulatory enzyme that converts pro-IL-1 into its active form (Licinio & Wong, 1997).

LPS and proinflammatory cytokines acting on brain endothelia thus can induce complementary inflammatory changes inside the blood-brain barrier by cellular transduction (Licinio & Wong, 1997). Presumably, the same activation pathways could stimulate cytokine production for export from the brain. The well-characterized sympathetic innervation of cerebral blood vessels (Palmer, 1986) is a potential neural pathway of control of their proinflammatory response.

Supportive elements in the brain (meninges, blood vessels, and choroid) are activated early following inflamatory signals; intraparenchymal changes (including glial responses) occur relatively late (Andersson et al., 1992). It is likely that after central inflammatory stimulation with LPS or IL-1, venous and CSF drainage from the brain contains components secreted by circumventricular structures (including ependyma), endothelia, vascular smooth muscle, and various elements of the choroid plexus (which drain directly into the superior sagittal sinus). Later in the course of central inflammation, cytokines arising from brain parenchymal elements such as glia and neurons could enter the brain interstitial space (which is in continuity with the CSF and enter the blood via the superior sagittal sinus and by perineuronal cranial nerve channels (Bradbury et al., 1981; Weller, Kida, & Zhang, 1992; Yamada, Depasquale, Patlak, & Cserr, 1991). Indeed, it is likely that all of these mechanisms are operative to varying degrees depending on the cause of the central nervous system damage and the time course of the illness.

A. Choroid Plexus as a Source of Central Cytokines

The choroid plexus is a potentially important source of immunoregulatory factors from the brain. It is a highly vascular structure that closely contacts both CSF and peripheral blood and is situated at the blood-brain interface where it could influence bidirectional transport of neuroregulators and cytokines as well as antigens (Nathanson & Chun, 1989). Whole rat choroid, whole human choroid, and mixed endothelial-epithelial cultures of human choroidal epithelia cells all secrete IL-6 following exposure to either IL-1β or LPS (Figure 6). Whole choroid also secretes TNF-α when exposed to LPS (Figure 6), but not in response to IL-1β. All three components of the choroid, epithelium, matrix (containing macrophages, antigen presenting cells, and fibroblasts), and endothelia have receptors for IL-1 and IL-6 (Wong & Licinio, 1997). When exposed to LPS, choroidal epithelia express TNF-α (Tarlow et al., 1993). It is likely that choroid plexus-derived cytokines contribute to the rise in CSF cytokines after icv injection of IL-1 or LPS. The idea that the choroid plexus is a site of antigen-recognizing cells and can serve as a transfer point of brain-derived antigens to the peripheral blood was proposed by Nathanson and Chun (1989).

The choroid plexus is a candidate neuroregulatory structure. It displays a large repertoire of neurotransmitter, neuropeptide, and hormone receptors (Nilsson, Lindvall-Axelsson, & Owman, 1992; Reichlin, 1998) (Table IV) and is innervated by nerve fibers arising in the hypothalamus and the sympathetic nervous system.

TABLE IV Neuroendocrine Receptors Expressed on Choroid Plexus (Modified from Nilsson et al., 1992; Reichlin, 1998)

Noradrenergic $\beta 1$, $\beta 2$
Dopamine (D1)
Histamine (H2)
Melatonin
Muscarinic
Serotonin
Atriopeptin
Vasopressin (1)
Angiotensin-II
IGF-1
Insulin
Growth Hormone
Prolactin
GABA
Benzodiazepine
tryptamine (2), IL-1, TNF-α, Leptin

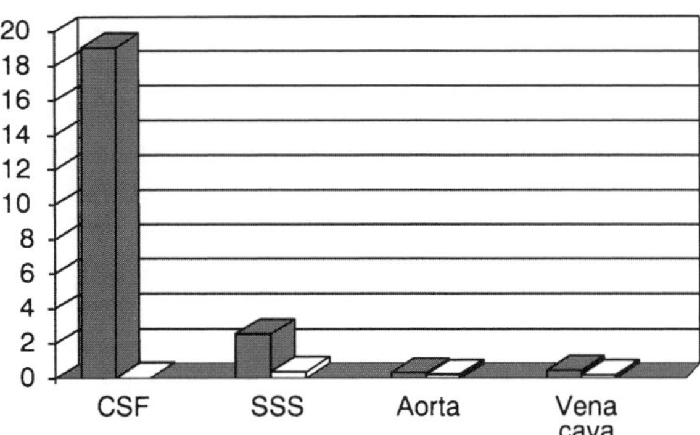

FIGURE 7 IL-6 in cerebrospinal fluid, SSS, aorta, and vena cava in a rat with a subarachnoid hemorrhage induced by passage of nylon thread into the middle cerebral artery. As compared with contral levels (shown in white), concentration in CSF was dramatically elevated, the concentration in superior sagittal sinus was higher than control, and higher than in aortic and vena cava blood. Peripheral blood levels also were elevated as compared with control. (Ritter, Funk, Chen, & Reichlin, 1998, unpublished.)

IV. FUNCTIONAL IMPLICATIONS OF BRAIN-TO-BLOOD TRANSFER OF CYTOKINES AND OTHER MACROMOLECULES

Brain-to-blood passage may be the mechanism by which closed head injury (Goodman, Robertson, Grossman, & Narayan, 1990; Ott, McLain, Gillespie, & Young, 1994; McClain, Cohen, Phillips, Ott, & Young, 1991; Robertson et al., 1991, 1992; Young, Ott, Beard, Dempsey, Tibbs, & McClain, 1988), ischemic stroke (Beamer, Coull, Clark, Hazel, & Silberger, 1995; Feuerstein, Liu, & Barone, 1994; Feuerstein, Wang, & Barone, 1996, 1998), meningitis (Sharief, Ciardi, & Thompson, 1992) and brain death (Amado et al., 1995) can induce the circulating inflammatory cytokines and metabolic changes that are characteristic of the acute phase response (fever, muscle wasting, catabolic state, hypercoaguability). After ischemic stroke in humans persistence of the acute phase response (as marked by elevated blood levels of fibrinogen) increases the risk of later stroke (Beamer et al., 1998). Brain-to-blood transfer of cytokines has been demonstrated after subarachnoid hemorrhage in an animal model of stroke. In a series of rats in which the middle cerebral artery was deliberately occluded by passing a fine nylon filament into the internal carotid artery (Ritter, Funk, Reichlin, unpublished) one particular animal had an unusually high peripheral blood level of IL-6 and a markedly elevated superior sagittal sinus-to-aortic IL-6 concentration gradient (Figure 7). At autopsy 24 h later the animal was found to have a large amount of blood in the subarachnoid space, undoubtedly due to inadvertent puncture of the artery. Dramatic increase in CSF IL-6 was also noted.

Brain-to-blood clearance may be the mechanism by which brain natriuretic factor (BNF) appears in peripheral blood of patients with subarachnoid hemorrhage (Berendes et al., 1997) accounting for the hyponatremia and "salt wasting" in these patients.

Cytokine products derived from brain tumors may circulate in blood and produce immunological and other peripheral reponses. For example, the anergic state that commonly occurs in patients with neuroblastoma has been attributed to secretion by the tumor of transforming growth factor-β (TGF-β) (Bodmer, Huber, Heid, & Fontana, 1991). Brain-to-blood transfer of TNF-α also has been shown in rats bearing intracranial tumors (Tracey et al., 1990). In addition to passage by way of the CSF, tumors may develop direct vascular connections with the general circulation.

Since toxins introduced into the brain enter the blood from the brain it is likely that bacterial toxins generated within the brain by infections such as meningitis and brain abscess could induce peripheral inflammation by their peripheral effects.

A. Regulation of Brain Cytokines by Noninflammatory Stimuli

In contrast to the rich literature on inflammation and ischemia-induced brain cytokines little is known about purely neural factors that could regulate central cytokine secretion. Open field stress (LeMay, Vander, & Kluger, 1990), forced immobilization (Nukina et al., 1998), and adrenaline administration (DeRijk, Boelen, Tilders, & Berkenbosch, 1994; Van Gool, van Vugt, Helle, & Aarden, 1990) increase peripheral IL-6 levels. Immobilization stress also has been reported to increase brain IL-1 concentration (Minami et al., 1991), a response that is partially suppressed by the feedback effects of stress-induced pituitary–adrenal activation (Nguyen et al., 1998).

As determined in cerebral cell culture systems, a number of neuropeptides have been shown to increase IL-6 production including vasoactive intestinal peptide (VIP) (Gottschall, Komaki, & Arimura, 1994; Schettini et al., 1994) and pituitary adenylate cyclase activating polypeptide (PACAP) (Gottschall et al., 1994). It is likely that these peptides act through the cAMP response element on the IL-6 gene since cAMP will also stimulate IL-6 secretion (Schettini et al., 1994). Adenosine can also activate IL-6 secretion in vitro (Fiebich et al., 1996). It is conceivable that changes in central neuropeptide milieu could influence brain secretion of Il-6 and perhaps of other cytokines as well.

That inflammatory and ischemic changes in brain can modify peripheral cytokine levels is well established. There is also evidence that certain neurotransmitters can influence the secretion of brain cytokines. On the other hand, there is as yet no hard evidence to support the hypothesis that changes in brain function, such as those seen in emotional stress, can exert immunomodulatory control by modulating the pattern of flow of cytokines from the brain into peripheral blood.

V. BRAIN REGULATION OF PERIPHERAL CYTOKINE PRODUCTION: NEURAL VS. HUMORAL CONTROL

In the search for mechanisms of neuroimmunomodulation, Di Simoni and colleagues (Di Simoni, De Luigi, et al., 1993; Di Simoni, Sironi, De Luigi, Manfridi, & Ghezzi, 1993) were the first to show that intracerebral injection of hIL-1β in rats induced higher blood levels of IL-6 than the same amount of IL-1β administered by intravenous route (Figure 8). Subsequently, these workers (De Simoni, Del Bo, De Luigi, Simard, & Forloni, 1995) and others (Gottschall et al., 1992) showed that icv injection of LPS also induced peripheral blood levels of IL-6. Peripheral levels of IL-1 were also increased by central administration of LPS (Gottschall et al., 1992) as was the

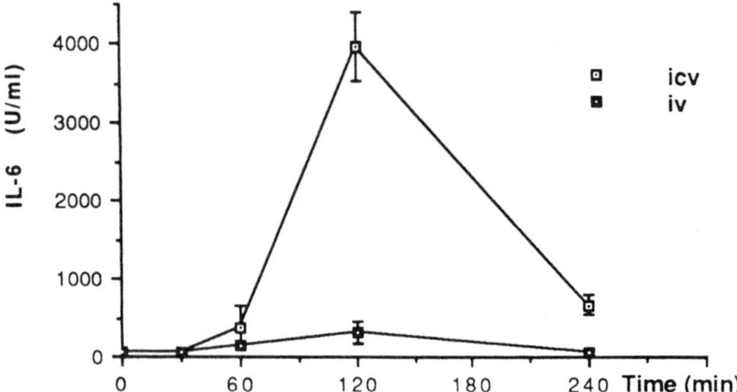

FIGURE 8 Icv injection of IL-1β in rats is followed by the appearance in peripheral blood of IL-6. Concentration of IL-6 in blood is much higher than that observed after iv injection. (From De Simoni et al., 1990.)

expression of IL-1 mRNA in several peripheral tissues (De Simoni et al., 1995). In contrast to the greater effect of icv than iv injection on peripheral IL-6 after IL-1β injection, peripheral and centrally induced effects of LPS on IL-6 were virtually the same (Gottschall et al., 1992).

A number of hypotheses have been considered in attempts to explain the effect of centrally administered IL-1 or LPS on peripheral cytokines. One possibility is that the central inflammatory state induced a massive sympathetic discharge. Increased catecholamine secretion after central injection of IL-1β has been well documented (Kannan et al., 1996; Petit et al., 1994; Sundar et al., 1990) and a number of studies support the view that peripheral catecholamines can modify acute immunity. There are several reasons to consider that the sympathetic nervous system might mediate peripheral response to centrally administered IL-1. Emotional stress (LeMay et al., 1990; Soszynski, Kozak, Conn, Rudolph, & Kluger, 1996; Takaki, Huang, Somogyvári-Vigh, & Arimura, 1994; Zhou, Kusnecov, Shurin, DePaoli, & Rabin, 1993) and catecholamine administration (DeRijk et al., 1994; Van Gool et al., 1990) induce increased peripheral IL-6 levels; icv administration of IL-1β leads to increased sympathetic nervous system activity (Kannan et al., 1996; Petit et al., 1994; Sundar et al., 1990); destruction of the peripheral sympathetic system with 6-hydroxy dopamine reduces the peripheral IL-6 response to restraint stress (Takaki et al., 1994); and adrenergic blocking agents reduce the peripheral IL-6 response to emotional stress (Soszynski et al., 1996). A hepatic origin of IL-6 release controlled by the sympathetic nervous system is suggested by the finding that infused catecholamines stimulate the release of IL-6 from rat liver perfused in vitro (Liao, Keiser, Scales, Kunkel, &

Kluger, 1995) and that the induction of hepatic glycogenolysis induced by central administration of IL-1 is blocked by several adrenolytic agents (Petit et al., 1994). Immobilization stress brings about increased expression of IL-6 mRNA in hepatic parenchymal cells Kitamsura et al. (1997) and Finck, Dantzer, Kelley, Woods, & Johnson (1997) reported that the peripheral TNF-α response to icv injection of LPS is blocked by pretreatment with phenotolamine, a nonselective α-adrenergic blocker.

On the other hand, other experimental findings suggest that peripheral catecholamine rise does not mediate the release of IL-6 into peripheral blood following central administration of IL-1. Chlorisondamine, a quaternary amine that blocks presynaptic transmission at preganglionic synapses, was shown to have no effect on peripheral IL-6 elevation induced by icv IL-1 (Romero et al., 1996). Moreover, icv injections of CRF in doses known to activate the sympathetic nervous system did not induce elevation of peripheral IL-6 levels (Romero et al., 1996). Chemical sympathectomy by peripheral injections of 6-hydroxy dopamine did not block the early appearance of IL-6 in the blood after icv injection of LPS (De Luigi, Terreni, Sironi, & De Simoni, 1998); indeed, sympathetic nerve denervation appeared to enhance the LPS-induced response. Several classes of adrenergic receptor blockers failed to block centrally induced peripheral IL-6 responses in studies carried out by Chen and Reichlin (1999). These included propanalol, a nonselective β-adrenergic blocker; butoxamine, a selective β2-blocker; and phentolamine, a nonselective α-blocker.

Thus, the data attempting to link the peripheral IL-6 response to centrally administered IL-1β (LPS) to sympathetic activation is contradictory. Other than the liver response cited above, catecholamines and the sympathetic nervous system appear to inhibit IL-6 responses to inflammatory stimuli (Felsner, Hofer, Rinner, Porta, Korsatko, & Schauenstein, 1995; Madden et al., 1995; Sundar et al., 1990; Van der Poll, Jansen, Endert, Sauerwein, & van Deventer, 1994).

An alternative hypothesis proposed by our group was that centrally administered IL-1β induced IL-6 secretion within the brain, which was then transferred to blood (Reichlin, 1998; Romero et al., 1996).

To test this hypothesis, measurements were made of the IL-6 concentration in cerebrospinal fluid and the gradient between blood draining the brain via the superior sagittal sinus and aortic blood entering the brain in rats in which IL-1β had been injected into the lateral cerebral ventricle. In confirmation of the earlier work of De Simoni and co-workers

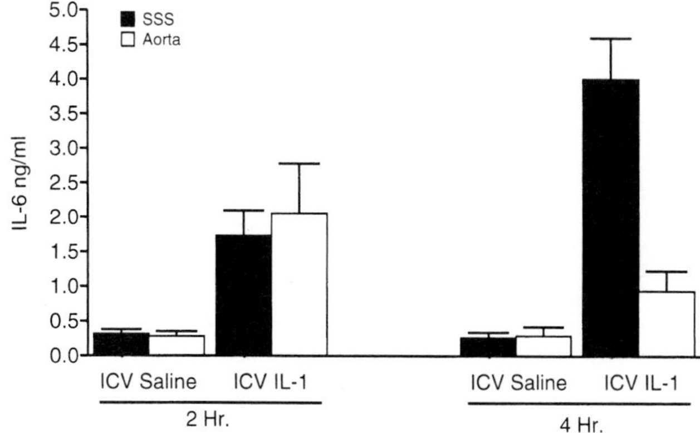

FIGURE 9 Concentration of IL-6 in superior sagittal sinus (SSS) compared with that in aorta at 2 and 4 h after icv injection of 100 ng of hIL-1 in rats. Note that aortic blood levels are elevated at both time intervals. At 2 h, SSS, and aortic blood levels are equal, but by 4 h, there is a marked SSS:Aorta gradient, indicating that the induced cytokine entered the peripheral blood, at least in part by secretion from brain (Romero et al., 1996).

(De Simoni, De Luigi, et al., 1993, De Simoni, Sironi, et al., 1993) peripheral blood levels of IL-6 were found to be elevated after icv injection (Reichlin, 1998). A significant SSS:aortic gradient was not evident at 2 h, but appeared in samples taken at 4 h (Figure 9) (Romero et al., 1996). On the basis of these findings, the conclusion was drawn that at 4 h release of IL-6 from the brain contributed to the elevated IL-6 levels. However, the reports of De Simoni, De Luigi, et al. (1993) and De Simoni, Sironi, et al. (1993) and our own observations show that peripheral blood IL-6 was higher at 2 than at 4 h. Since peripheral elevation of IL-6 preceeds the onset of CNS IL-6 activation (as indicated by comparison of peripheral and CSF levels of IL-6) and peripheral blood levels have returned to normal while the central response is reaching its maximum, it seems unlikely that release of IL-6 from CNS to blood could account for the early response. Similarly, the pattern of activation of IL-6 mRNA in brain and spleen observed by Di Simone et al. (1995) indicates that the peripheral preceeds the central response. It seems unlikly therefore that passage of induced brain IL-6 could explain the time course of peripheral IL-6 response to central administration of IL-1β. Similar findings have been observed after icv injection of LPS (Figure 10).

A third hypothesis to explain the elevation of peripheral blood IL-6 after icv injection of IL-1β is that the peripheral response is due to the early entry into the blood of the inciting cytokine. As noted above, radioiodinated IL-1β (as is also true for IL-6, TNF-α, IL-1β, and LPS) appears in peripheral blood within 5 min after icv injection and reaches peak levels

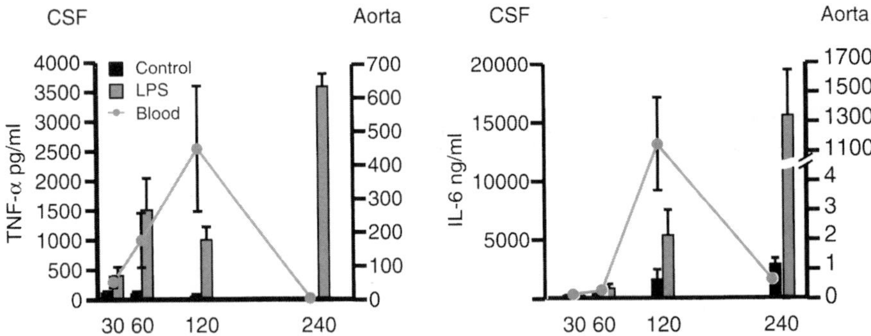

FIGURE 10 Effect of acute icv injection of 1 mcg LPS on CSF and aortic blood levels of IL-6 and TNF-α. IL-6 in CSF was not significantly increased at 60 min but was significantly increased at 60 min, continued to rise up to 240 min, the longest time observed. Blood levels of IL-6 were not detectably elevated until 120 min, and had fallen almost to baseline by 240 min. TNF-α appeared earlier in CSF and peripheral blood-CSF levels continued to rise at 240 min, whereas blood levels had falled to normal at that time. These results indicate that the changes in central cytokine secretion were not responsible for the peripheral changes.

between 60 and 120 min. Fully 89% of the injected dose has appeared in peripheral blood within the first 2 h after injection (Figure 3), and blood values after icv injection are higher than those after iv injection after the first hour of injection. Further, the time course of peripheral IL-6 response to centrally administered IL-1β is similar to that induced by iv administration. In mice, the blood level of hIL-1β achieved after icv injection is much higher than that after iv injection (Di Santo et al., 1999). Di Santo et al., postulated that the intracerebral space served as a reservoir that released IL-1β slowly into the blood.

The most reasonable explanation, to this reviewer, is that the early peripheral IL-6 response is mainly due to bulk flow of IL-1β from the brain into the blood with activation of peripheral reactive tissues, to which is added a limited contribution of locally induced IL-6 from the brain (Chen & Reichlin, 1999). Intravenous IL-1β, in contrast to icv IL-1β, has only minimal effects on central IL-6 responses and hence does not mobilize brain response as does the icv route of administration. Faggioni, Benigni, & Ghezzi (1995) also emphasized the possible role of brain-to-blood transfer to icv injected LPS in determining peripheral responses and Gottschall et al. (1992) reported that blood IL-6 levels after icv injection of LPS was not higher than levels after iv injection. Recently we have shown that the peripheral IL-6 response to icv LPS is much less than would be induced by the amount of LPS reaching the blood. From our finding that icv injection of LPS reduces the peripheral IL-6 response to LPS we attribute the blunted response after icv injection to the mobilization of brain-directed peripheral immune suppressing factors such as the pituitary-adrenal axis (Chen, McCuskey, & Reichlin, 2000).

VI. THE BRAIN AS A SELECTIVE ROUTE OF SYSTEMIC IMMUNIZATION: BRAIN-TO-BLOOD TRANSPORT AS A DETERMINANT OF IMMUNE RESPONSE

As noted above, the brain traditionally has been considered to be an immune-privileged site (c.f. Hickey et al., 1991; Weller et al., 1996). Antigens presented systemically are largely excluded from the brain by the blood-brain barrier, and the brain tolerates foreign grafts much more readily than it does transplantation under the skin or in parenchymal organs. Nevertheless, the nonselectivity of exit into peripheral blood of macromolecules arising from (or introduced into) the brain led Cserr and co-workers to determine whether antigens introduced into the brain were capable of inducing a peripheral specific immune response (Cserr et al., 1992, 1995; Cserr & Knopf, 1992; Gordon, Knopf, & Cserr, 1992; Knopf, Cserr, Nolan, Wu, & Harling-Berg, 1995). In confirmation of earlier studies (Panda, Dale, Loan, & Davis, 1965; Santos & Valdimarsson, 1982) they showed that ovalbumin or human serum albumin introduced into the CSF induced higher concentrations of IgG than when administered iv.

Their observations have been confirmed and extended in our own laboratory (Figure 11). Crystalline ovalbumin injected into the lateral cerebral ventricle induced a much greater increase in antiovalbumin IgG and IgA than by other routes, which included iv, sc, and intranasal administration. Furthermore, the response to icv injection occurred with a shorter latent period than did the response to other routes. IgM responses were the same after all routes of immunization.

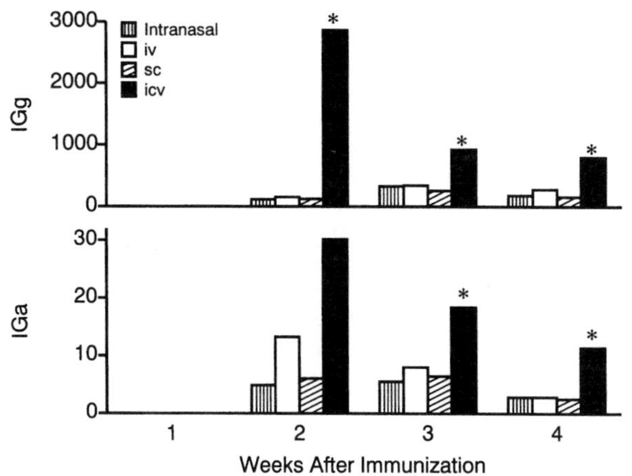

FIGURE 11 Ovalbumin, 90 mcg, administered by way of the lateral cerebral ventricle induces a more immediate and significantly greater antibody (IgG, and IgA) response in peripheral blood than when given by iv, sc, or intranasal routes.

The mechanisms by which intracerebral presentation of antigen induce higher immune responses than peripheral presentation are at this time not known. That excision of deep cervical lymph nodes prevented the rise in peripheral antibody production in response to ovalbumin (Harling-Berg, Knopf, Merriam, & Cserr, 1989) indicates that antigen drainage into this specific set of nodes is an essential component of the response. Excision of cervical lymph nodes also reduces the severity of experimental autoimmune disease of the brain in rats (Phillips, Needham, & Weller, 1997).

A number of other hypotheses to explain the selectivity of CNS presentation can be suggested. In light of our finding that cytokines leave the brain by bulk flow via the same pathways as the antigens it is possible that deep cervical nodes are exposed not only to the injected foreign antigen, but simultaneously to immune potentiating cytokines including IL-1β, IL-6, and IL-2.

It is also possible that the highly restricted drainage from brain to deep cervical lymph nodes through its funnel-like drainage pattern provides a critically high concentration of antigen that is sustained for a longer time than the same total amount present in low concentrations and for a shorter time of exposure when distributed throughout the body.

The icv antigen presentation system of the brain is similar to the general mucosal immune system (Brandtzaeg, 1995, 1996; Kramer, Sutherland, Bao, Husband, 1995; Neutra, Pringault, & Kraehenbuhl, 1996) in its capacity to induce tolerance to ingested antigens. The process, termed "tolerization" is mediated by a shift in the pattern of T cell activation from a so-called T1 to T2 pattern (Weiner, 1997). Autoimmune encephalomyelitis induced in rats by systemic injection of myelin basic protein and immune adjuvants is inhibited by icv injection of myelin basic protein (Harling-Berg, Knopf, & Cserr, 1991).

It is also possible that the immune privileged brain behaves like the immune privileged eye in expressing what is termed "anterior chamber-associated immune deviation" (ACAID) (Li, D'Orazio, & Niederkorn, 1996; Niederkorn & Mayhew, 1995; Streilin, Ksander, & Taylor, 1997). "ACAID" is defined as the suppression of delayed-type hypersensitivity with simultaneous induction of antibody production.

On the basis of detailed studies in mice it appears that foreign antigens presented to the anterior chamber of the eye are processed by local antigen recognition cells, which then leave the eye, enter the general circulation, localize to the spleen, and then induce immune globulin production at many sites thoughout the body as well as suppressing systemic delayed hypersensitivity. This selective pattern is mediated by a selective Th2 response, which suppresses Th1 reactions.

Immune deviation of the eye is a possible mechanism of neuroimmunomodulation as shown by studies of the neuropeptidic mediation of external lighting induced patterns of sensitization. (Ferguson, Fletcher, Herndon, & Griffith, 1995). VIP in the eye appears to increase susceptibility to ACAID whereas substance P decreases susceptibility. This conclusion is based on studies showing that ACAID can be induced in mice exposed to normal diurnal lighting, but not if they are exposed to constant light. VIP and substance P concentrations in the iris and ciliary body are also modulated by light. VIP disapears from the eyes of mice reared in the dark whereas substance P concentrations increase. In mice reared with normal diurnal lighting VIP receptor antagonist blocked ACAID in diurnal mice whereas SP receptor antagonist restored ACAID in dark-adapted mice. This mechanism is a potential pathway of neuroimmunomodulation. Whether neuropeptide regulation of immune response applies to antigens presented by the CNS route has not been determined.

VII. SUMMARY

In contrast to the highly selective control of entry of substances from blood to brain through the blood-brain barrier, exit of substances from the brain is nonselective and relatively rapid. Brain-to-blood transfer of macromolecules occurs through the arachnoid villi in the superior sagittal sinus and by way of perineuronal channels that are continuous with the subarachnoid space. These channels accompany spinal and cranial nerves as they leave the neuroaxis. In the head, the major exit route is by way of perineuronal cuffs around the olfactory nerves as they pass through the cribriform plate to terminate in the nasal submucosa. From this site, brain-derived macromolecules such as cytokines and antigens can enter the lymphatic drainage to the deep cervical lymph chain and ultimately into the systemic circulation. Between 30 and 70% of IL-1, IL-6, TNF-α, and *E. coli* endotoxin injected into the lateral cerebral ventricle leave the brain by bulk flow and have appeared in peripheral blood within 4 h. Antigen presented by way of the cerebral ventricles also induces an earlier and more intense humoral antibody response than by peripheral administration. Direct brain-to-blood secretion of cytokines and antigens present a potential route of neuroimmunomodulation, but it is still not known whether this pathway can be influenced by strictly neural and psychological factors.

Acknowledgments

Thanks are due to my collaborators, Drs. GuanJie Chen, Luz I. Romero, Janet Funk, Ronald M. Lechan, Sherry Hsiao-Chow, Robert S. McCuskey, Charles A. Dinarello, and W. Lester Castro. Ms. Jodie Field and Ms. Teresa Sherman have given invaluable technical support. I wish to thank Dr. William A. Banks and Christina J. Harling-Berg for valuable suggestions. Dr. Roberto Toni, Istituto di Anatomia Umana Normale, University of Bologna guided me to the original publication of Vesalius on the anatomy of the hypothalamus. Research supported by U.S. Public Health Service grant 16684.

References

Ader, R., Felten, D. L., & Cohen, N. (Eds.). (1991). *Psychoneuroimmunology, 2nd ed.* New York: Academic Press.

Amado, J. A., Lopez-Espadas, F., Vazquez-Barquero, A., Alas, E., Riancho, J. A., Lopez-Cordovilla, J. J., & Garcia-Unzueta, M. T. (1995). Blood levels of cytokines in brain dead patients. Relationship with circulating hormones and acute phase reactants. *Metabolism, 44*, 812–816.

Andersson, P. B., Perry, V. H., & Gordon, S. (1992). Intracerebral injection of proinflammatory cytokines or leukocyte chemotaxins induces minimal myelomonocytic cell recruitment to the parenchyma of the central nervous system. *Journal of Experimental Medicine, 176*, 255–259.

Banks, W. A., Kastin, A. J., & Broadwell, R. D. (1995). Passage of cytokines across the blood-brain barrier. *Neuroimmunomodulation, 2*, 241–248.

Banks, W. A., Kastin, A. J., & Durham, D. A. (1989). Bidirectional transport of interleukin-1 alpha across the blood-brain barrier. *Brain Research Bulletin, 23*, 433–437.

Banks. W. A., Kastin, A. J., & Gutierrez, E. G. (1994). Penetration of interleukin-6 across the murine blood-brain barrier. *Neuroscience Letters, 179*, 53–56.

Barrera, C. M., Kastin, A. J., Fasold, M. B., & Banks, W. A. (1991). Bidirectional saturable transport of LHRH across the blood-brain barrier. *American Journal of Physiology, 261*, E312–318.

Bass, N. H., & Lundborg, P. (1973). Postnatal development of bulk flow in the cerebrospinal fluid system of the albino rat: Clearance of carboxyl-[14C] Inulin *after* intrathecal injection. *Brain Research, 52*, 323–332.

Beamer, N. B., Coull, B. M, Clark, W. M., Hazel, J. M., & Silberger, J. R. (1995). Persistent inflammatory response in stroke survivors. *Neurology, 50*, 1722–1728.

Benveniste, E. N. (1994). Cytokine circuits in the brain. Implications for AIDS dementia complex. *Research Publications Association for Research in Nervous and Mental Disease, 72*, 71–88.

Berendes, E., Walter, M., Cullen, P., Praien, T., Van Aken, H., Horsthemke, J., Schulte, M., von Wild, K., & Scherer, R. (1997). Secretion of brain natriuretic peptide in patients with aneurysmal subarachnoid hemorrhage. *Lancet, 349*, 245–249.

Blatteis, C. M. (1992). Role of the OVLT in the febrile response to circulating pyrogens. *Progress in Brain Research, 91*, 409–412.

Bodmer, S., Huber, D., Heid, I., & Fontana, A. (1991). Human glioblastoma cell derived transforming growth factor-beta 2: Evidence for secretion of both high and low molecular weight biologically active forms. *Journal of Neuroimmunology, 34*, 33–42.

Bodnar, R. J., Pasternak, G. W., Mann, D., Paul, R., Warren, R., & Donner, D. B. (1989). Mediation of anorexia by human recombinant tumor necrosis factor through a peripheral action in the rat. *Cancer Research, 15*, 6280–6284.

Bradbury, M. W. B., & Cole, D. F. (1980). The role of the lymphatic system in drainage of cerebrospinal fluid and aqueous humour. *Journal of Physiology, London, 299*, 353–365.

Bradbury, M. W. B., & Cserr, H. F. (1985). Drainage of cerebral interstitial fluid and of cerebrospinal fluid into lymphatics. In M. G. Johnson (Ed.), *Experimental biology of the lymphatic circulation* (pp. 355–394). Amsterdam: Elsevier.

Bradbury, M. W. B., Cserr, H. F., & Westrop, R. J. (1981). Drainage of cerebral interstitial fluid into deep cervical lymph of the rabbit. *American Journal of Physiology, 240*, F329–F336.

Brandtzaeg, P. (1995). Molecular and cellular aspects of the secretory immunoglobulin system. *APMIS: Acta Pathologica, Microbiologica, et Immunologica Scandinavica., 103*(Suppl.), 1–19.

Brandtzaeg, P. (1996). The human intestinal immune system basic cellular and humoral mechanisms. *Bailliere's Clinical Rhematology, 10*, 1–24.

Breder, C. D., Tsujimoto, M. Terano, Y., Scott, D. W., & Saper, C. B. (1993). Distribution and characterization of tumor necrosis factor—like immunoreactivity in the murine central nervous system. *Journal of Comparative Neurology, 337*, 543–567.

Chao, C. C., Hu, S., Sheng, W. S., & Peterson, P. K. (1995). Tumor necrosis factor-alpha production by human fetal microglial cells: Regulation by other cytokines. *Developmental Neuroscience, 17*, 97–105.

Chen, G., & Reichlin, S. (1998). Clearance of 125I-TNF-β from the brain into the blood following intracerebroventricular injection in rats. *Neuroimmunomodulation, 5*, 221–276.

Chen G., & Reichlin, S. (1999). Mechanisms by which blood levels of IL-6 are elevated after intracerebroventricular (ICV) injectin of IL-1β in the rat: Neural vs. humoral control. *Endocrinology, 140*, 5549–5555.

Chen, G., Castro, W. L., Chow, H.-H., & Reichlin, S. (1997). Clearance of 125I-labeled interleukin-6 from brain into blood following intracerebroventricular injection in rats. *Endocrinology, 138*, 4830–4836.

Chen. G., McCuskey, R. S., & Reichlin, S. (2000). Blood interleukin-6 (IL-6) and tumor necrosis factor-α (TNF-α) elevation after intracerebroventricular injection of E. coli endotoxin (LPS) in the rat is determined by two opposing factors: Peripheral induction by LPS transferred from brain-to-blood and inhibition of peripheral response by a brain-mediated mechanism. *Neuroimmunomodulation* (in press).

Chrousos, G. P. (1995). The hypothalamic-pituitary-adrenal axis and immune-mediated inflammation. *New England Journal of Medicine, 332,* 1351–1362.

Cserr, H. F., DePasquale, M., Harling-Berg, C. J., Park, J. T., & Knopf, P. M. (1995). Afferent and efferent arms of the humoral immune response to CSF-administered albumins in a rat model with normal blood-brain permeability. *Journal of Neuroimmunology, 41,* 195–202.

Cserr, H. F., Harling-Berg, C. J., & Knopf, P. M. (1992). Drainage of brain extracellular fluid into blood and deep cervical lymph and its immunological significance. *Brain Pathology, 2,* 269–276.

Cserr, H. F., & Knopf, P. M. (1992). Cervical lymphatics, the blood-brain barrier and the immunoreactivity of the brain: A new view. *Immunology Today, 13,* 507–512.

Dandy, W. E. (1929). Where is cerebrospinal fluid absorbed? *Journal of the American Medical Association, 92,* 2012–2014.

DeRijk, R. H., Boelen, A., Tilders, F. J., & Berkenbosch, F. (1994). duction of plasma interleukin-6 by circulating adrenaline in the rat. *Psychoneuroendocrinology, 19,* 155–163.

De Luigi, A., Terreni, L., Sironi, M., & De Simoni, M. G. (1998) The sympathetic nervous system tonically inhibits peripheral interleukin-1β and interleukin-6 induction by central lipopolysaccharide. *Neuroscience, 83,* 1245–1250.

De Simoni, M. G., De Luigi, A., Gemma, L., Sironi, M., Manfridi, A., & Ghezzi, P. (1993). Modulation of systemic interleukin-6 induction by central interleukin-1. *American Journal of Physiology, 265,* R739–R742.

De Simoni, M. G., Sironi, M., De Luigi, A., Manfridi, A., & Ghezzi, P. (1993). Intracerebroventricular injection of interleukin-1 induces high circulating levels of interleukin-6. *Journal of Experimental Medicine, 171,* 1773–1778, 1990.

De Simoni, M. G., Del Bo, R., De Luigi, A., Simard, S., & Forloni, G. (1995). Central endotoxin induces different patterns of interleukin (IL)-1 beta and IL-6 messenger ribonucleic acid expression and IL-6 secretion in the brain and periphery. *Endocrinology, 136,* 897–902.

Di Santo, E., Benignia, F., Agnelloa, D., Sipeb, J. D., & Ghezzi, P. (1999). Peripheral effects of centrally-administered Interleukin-1β in relation to its clearance from the brain into the blood and tissue distribution. *Neuroimmunomodulation, 6,* 360–364

Erlich, S. S., McComb, J. G., Hyman, S., & Weiss, M. H. (1986). Ultrastructural morphology of the olfactory pathway for cerebrospinal fluid drainage in the rabbit. *Journal of Neurosurgery, 64,* 466–473.

Esler, M., Jennings, G., Lambert, G., Meredith, I., Horne, M., & Eisenhofer, G. (1990). Overflow of catecholamine neurotransmitters to the circulation: Source, fate and functions. *Physiological Reviews, 70,* 963–985.

Esler, M., Vaz, M., Collier, G., Nestel, P., Jennings, G., Kaye, D., Seals, D., & Lambert, G. (1998). Leptin in human plasma is derived in part from the brain, and cleared by the kidneys. *Lancet, 351,* 879.

Fabry, Z., Fitzsimmons, K. M., Herlaein, J. A., Moninger, T. O., Dobbs, M. B., & Hart, M. N. (1993). Production of the cytokines interleukin 1 and 6 by murine brain microvellel endothelium and smooth muscle pericytes. *Journal Neuroimmunology, 47,* 23–34.

Faggioni, R. F., Benigni, P., & Ghezzi, P. (1995). Proinflammatory cytokines as pathogenetic mediators in the central nervous system:brain-periphery connections. *Neuroimmunomodulation, 2,* 2–15.

Faggioni, R., Fantuzzi, G., Villa, P., Buurman, W., van Tits, L. J. H., & Ghezzi P. (1995). Independent down-regulation of central and peripheral tumor necrosis factor production as a result of lipopolysaccharide tolerance in mice. *Infection and Immunity,* 1473–1477.

Felten, D. L., Cohen, N., Ader, R., Felten, S. Y., Carlson, S. L., & Roszman, T. L. Central neural circuits involved in neural-immune interactions. (1991). In R. Ader, D. L. Felten, & N. Cohen, (Eds.), *Psychoneuroimmunology,* (2nd ed., pp. 3–26). San Diego: Academic Press.

Felsner, P., Hofer, D., Rinner, I., Porta, S., Korsatko, W., & Schauenstein, K. (1995). Adrenergic suppression of peripheral blood T cell reactivity in the rat is due to activation of peripheral alpha 2-receptors. *Journal of Neuroimmunology, 57,* 27–34.

Ferguson, T. A., Fletcher, S., Herndon, J., & Griffith, T. S. (1995). Neuropeptides modulate immune deviation induced via the anterior chamber of the eye. *Journal of Immunology,* 1746–1756.

Feuerstein, G. Z., Liu, T., & Barone, F. C. (1994). Cytokines, inflammation, and brain injury: Role of tumor necrosis factor. *Cerebrovascular and Brain Metabolism Reviews 6,* 341–360.

Feuerstein, G. Z., Wang, X., & Barone, F. C. (1997). Inflammatory gene expression in cerebral ischemia and trauma. Potential new therapeutic targets. *Annals of the New York Academy of Science, 825,* 179–193.

Feuerstein, G. Z., Wang, X., & Barone, F. C. (1998). Inflammatory mediators and brain injury: The role of cytokines and chemokines in stroke CNS Disease. In M. D. Ginsberg & J. Bogousslavsky (Eds.), *Cerebrovascular disease: Pathophysiology, diagnosis and management VI* (pp. 507–531). Malden MA: Blackwell Science.

Fiebich, B. L., Biber, K., Gyufko, K., Berger, M., Bauer, J., & van Calker, D. (1996). Adenosine A2b receptors mediate an increase in interleukin (IL)-6 mRNA and IL-6 protein synthesis in human astroglioma cells. *Journal of Neurochemistry, 66,* 1426–1431.

Field, E. J., & Brierley, J. B. (1948). The lymphatic connexions of the subarachnoid space. *British Medical Journal,* 1167–1171.

Finck, B. N., Dantzer, R., Kelley, K. W., Woods, J. A., & Johnson, R. W. (1997). Central lipopolysaccharide elevates plasma IL-6 concentration by an -adrenoreceptor-mediated mechanism. *American Journal of Physiology,* 272, R1880–R1887.

Földi, M. (1996a). The brain and the lymphatic system (I). *Lymphology, 29,* 1–9.

Földi, M. (1996b). The brain and the lymphatic system (II). *Lymphology,* 29, 10–14.

Gatti, S., & Bartfai, T. (1993). Induction of tumor necrosis factor-alpha mRNA in the brain after peripheral endotoxin treatment: Comparison with interleukin-1 family and interleukin-6. *Brain Research, 624,* 291–294.

Goetzl, E. J., Pankhaniya R. R., Gaufo, G. O., Mu, Y., Xia, M., & Sreedharan, S.P. (1998). Selectivity of effects of vasoactive intestinal peptide on macrophages and lymphocytes in compartmental immune responses. *Annals of the New York Academy of Sciences, 840,* 540–550.

Goodman, J. C., Robertson, C. S., Grossman, R. G., & Narayan, R. K. (1990). Elevation of tumor necrosis factor in head injury. *Journal of Neuroimmunology, 30,* 213–217.

Gordon, L. B., Knopf, P. M., & Cserr, H. F. (1992). Ovalbumin is more immunogenic when introduced into brain or cerebrospinal fluid than into extracerebral sites. *Journal of Neuroimmunology, 40,* 81–88.

Gottschall, P. E., Komaki, G., & Arimura, A. (1992). Increased circulating interleukin-1 and interleukin-6 after intracerebroventricular injection of lipopolysaccharide. *Neuroendocrinology, 56*, 935–938.

Gottschall, P. E., Tatsuno, I., & Arimura, A. (1994). Regulation of interleukin-6 (IL-6) secretion in primary cultured astrocytes: Synergism of interleukin-1 (IL-1) and pituitary adenylate cyclase activating polypeptide (PACAP). *Brain Research, 637*, 197–203.

Griffin, D. E. (1997). Cytokines in the brain during viral infections: Clues to HIV-associated dementia. *Journal of Clinical Investigation, 100*, 2948–2951.

Griffith, T. S., Herndon, J. M., Lima, J., Kahn, M., & Ferguson, T. A. (1995). The immune response and the eye. TCR-chain related molecules regulate the systemic immunity to antigen presented in the eye. *International Immunology, 7*, 1617–1625.

Greitz, D. (1993). Cerebrospinal fluid circulation and associated intracranial dynamics. *Acta Radiologica Supplementum, 386*, 1–23.

Harling-Berg, C., Knopf, P. M., Merriam, J., & Cserr, H. F. (1989). Role of cervical lymph nodes in the systemic humoral immune response to human serum albumin microinfused into rat cerebrospinal fluid. *Journal of Neuroimmunology, 25*, 185–193.

Harling-Berg, C. J., Knopf, P. M., & Cserr, H. F. (1991). Myelin basic protein infused into cerebrospinal fluid suppresses experimental autoimmune encephalitis. *Journal of Neuroimmunology, 35*, 45–51.

Hickey, W. F. (1991). T-lymphocyte entry and antigen recognition in the central nervous system. In R. Ader, D. L. Felten, & N. Cohen (Eds.), *Psychoneuroimmunology*, (2nd ed., pp. 149–175). San Diego: Academic.

Hopkins, S. J., & Rothwell, N. J. (1995). Cytokines and the nervous system I: Expression and recognition. *Trends in Neuroscience, 18*, 83–88.

Irwin, M. (1994). Stress-induced immune suppression: Role of brain corticotropin releasing hormone and autonomic nervous system mechanisms. *Advances in Neuroimmunology, 4*, 29–47.

Irwin, M., Hauger, R. L., & Brown, M., Britton, K. T. (1988). CRF activates autonomic nervous system and reduced natural killer cytotoxicity. *American Journal of Physiology, 255*, R744–R747.

Jackson, R. T., Tigges, J., & Arnold, W. (1979). Subarachnoid space of the CNS, nasal mucosa, and lymphatic system. *Archives of Otolaryngology, 105*, 180–184.

Jin, L., Burguera, B. G., Couce, M. E., Scheithauer, B. W., Lamsan, J., Eberhardt, N. L., Kulig, E., Lloyd, R. V. (1999). Leptin and leptin receptor expression in normal and neoplastic human pituitary: Evidence of a regulatory role for leptin on pituitary cell proliferation. *Journal of Clinical Endocrinology and Metabolism, 84*, 2903–2911.

Kakucska, I., Qi, Y., Clark, B. D., & Lechan, R. M. (1993). Endotoxin-induced corticotropin-releasing hormone gene expression in the hypothalamic paraventricular nucleus is mediated centrally by interleukin-1. *Endocrinology, 133*, 815–821.

Kannan, H., Tanaka, Y., Kunitake, T., Ueta, Y., Hayashida, Y., & Yamashita, H. (1996). Activation of sympathetic outflow by recombinant human interleukin-1β in conscious rats. *American Journal of Physiology, 39*, r479–r485.

Kawakami, J., Yamamoto, K., Sawada, Y., & Iga, T. (1994). Prediction of brain delivery of oflaxacin, a new quinolone, in the human from animal data. *Journal of Pharmacokinetics and Biopharmaceutics, 22*, 207–227.

Kida, S., Patazis, A., & Weller, R. O. (1993). CSF drains directly from the subarachnoid space into nasal lymphatics in the rat. Anatomy, histology and immunological significance. *Neuropathology and Applied Neurobiology, 19*, 480–488.

Kitamsura, H., Konno, A., Morimatsu, M., Jung, B. D., Kimura, K., & Saito, M. (1997). Immobilization stress increases hepatic IL-6 expression in mice. *Biochemical and Biophysical Research Communications, 238*, 707–711.

Kossmann, T., Hans, V. H., Imhof, H. G., Stocker, R., Grob, P., Trentz, O., & Morganti-Kossman, C. (1995). Intrathecal and serum interleukin-6 and the acute-phase response in patients with severe traumatic brain injuries. *Shock, 4*, 311–317.

Knopf, P. M., Cserr, H. F., Nolan, S. C., Wu, T. Y., & Harling-Berg, C. J. (1995). Physiology and immunology of lymphatic drainage of interstitial and cerebrospinal fluids from the brain. *Neuropathology and Applied Neurobiology, 21*, 175–180.

Kramer, D. R., Sutherland, R. M., Bao, S., & Husband, A. J. (1995). Cytokine mediated effects in mucosal immunity. *Immunol Cell Biol, 73*, 389–396.

Lee, S. C., Liu, W., Dickson, D. W., Brosnan, C. F., & Berman, J. W. (1993). Cytokine production by human fetal microglia and astrocytes. Differential induction by lipopolysaccharide and IL-1 beta. *Journal of Immunology, 150*, 2659–2667.

LeMay, L. G., Vander A. J., & Kluger, M. J. (1990). The effects of psychological stress on plasma interleukin-6 activity in rats. *Physiological Behavior*, 957–961.

Li, X.-Y., D'Orazio, T., & Niederkorn, J. Y. (1996). Role of Th1 and Th2 cells in anterior chamber-associated immune deviation. *Immunology, 89*, 34–40.

Liao, J., Keiser, J. A., Scales, W. E., Kunkel, S. L., & Kluger, M. J. (1995). Role of epinephrine in TNF and IL-6 production from isolated perfused rat liver. *American Journal of Physiology, 268*, R896–R901.

Licinio, J., & Wong, M.-L. (1997). Pathways and mechanisms for cytokine signaling of the central nervous system. *Journal of Clinical Investigation, 100*, 2941–2947.

MacLean, D., & Reichlin, S. (1981). Neuroendocrinology and the immune process. In R. Ader (Ed.), *Psychoneuroimmunology* (pp. 475–520). San Diego: Academic.

Madden, K. S., Sanders, V. M., & Felten, D. L. (1995). Catecholamine influences and sympathetic neural modulation of immune responsiveness. *Annual Review of Pharmacology and Toxicology, 35*, 417–448.

Maier, S. E., Goehler, L. E., Fleshner M., & Watkins, L. R. (1998). The role of the vagus nerve in cytokine-to-brain communication. *Annals of the New York Academy of Sciences, 840*, 289–300.

McClain, C., Cohen, D., Phillips, R., Ott, L., & Young, B. (1991). Increased plasma and ventricular fluid interleukin-6 fluid levels in patients with head injury. *Journal of Laboratory and Clinical Medicine, 118*, 225–231.

McComb, J. G. (1983). Recent research into the nature of the cerebrospinal fluid formation and absorption. *Journal of Neurosurgery, 59*, 369–383.

McGeer, P. L., & McGeer, E. G. (1995). The inflammatory response system of brain: Implications for therapy of Alzheimer and other neurodegenerative diseases. *Brain Research Reviews, 21*, 195–218.

McKinley, M. J., McAllen, R. M., Mendelsohn, F. A. O. et al. (1990). Circumventricular organs: Neuroendocrine interfaces between the brain and the hemal milieu. *Frontiers in Neuroendocrinology, 11*, 219–233.

Minami, M., Kuraishi, Y., Yamaguchi, T., Nakai, S., Hirai, Y., & Satoh, M. (1991). Immobilization stress induces interleukin-1 beta messenger RNA in rat brain. *Neuroscience Letters, 123*, 254–256.

Morash, B., Li, A., Murphy, P. R., Wilkinson, M., & Ur, E. (1999). Leptin gene expression in the brain and pituitary gland. *Endocrinology, 140*, 5995–5998.

Nakamori, T., Morimoto, A., Yamaguchi, K., Watanabe, T., Long, N. C., & Murakami, N. (1993). Organum vasculosum lamina terminalis (OVLT) is a brain site to produce interleukin-1β during fever. *Brain Research, 618*, 155–159.

Nathanson, J. A., & Chun, L. L. (1989). Immunological function of the blood-cerebrospinal fluid barrier. *Proceedings of the National Academy of Science USA, 86*, 1684–1688.

Neutra, M. R., Pringault, E., & Kraehenbuhl, J.-P. (1996). Antigen sampling across epithelial barriers and induction of mucosal immune responses. *Annual Review of Immunology, 14*, 275–300.

Nguyen, K. T., Deak, T., Owens, S. M., Kohno, P. T., Fleshner, T., Watkins, L. R., & Maier, S. F. (1998). Exposure to acute stress induces brain interleukin-1β protein in the rat. *Journal of Neuroscience, 18*, 2239–2240.

Niederkorn, J. Y., & Mayhew, E. (1995). Role of splenic B cells in the immune privilege of the anterior chamber of the eye. *European Journal of Immunology, 25*, 2783–2787.

Nilsson, C., Lindvall-Axelsson, M., & Owman, C. (1992). Neuroendocrine regulatory mechanisms in the choroid plexus-cerebrospinal fluid system. *Brain Research-Brain Research Reviews, 17*, 109–138.

Nukina, H., Sudo, N., Komaki, G., Yu, X.-N., Mine, K., & Kubo, C. (1998). The restraint stress-induced elevation in plasma interleukin-6 negatively regulates the plasma TNF- level. *Neuroimmunomodulation, 5*, 318–323.

Ott, L., McLain, C. J., Gillespie, M., & Young, B. (1994). Cytokines and metabolic dysfunction after severe head injury. *Journal of Neurotrauma, 11*, 447–472.

Ottaway, C. A., & Husband, A. J. (1994). The influence of neuroendocrine pathways on lymphocyte migration. *Immunology Today, 15*, 511–517.

Palmer, G. C. (1986). Neurochemical coupled actions of transmitters in the microvasculature of the brain. *Neuroscience & Biobehavioral Reviews, 10*, 79–101.

Panda, J. N., Dale, H. E., Loan, R. W., & Davis, L. E. (1965). Immunologic response to subarachnoid and intracerebral injection of antigens. *Journal of Immunology, 94*, 760–764.

Pardridge, W. M. (1983). Brain metabolism: A perspective from the blood-brain barrier. *Physiological Reviews, 63*, 1481–1535.

Petit, F., Jarrous, A., Dickenson, R. D., Molina, P. E., Abumrad, M. N., & Lang, C. H. (1994). Contribution of central and pertipheral adrenergic stimulation to the IL-1 alpha-mediated glucoregulation. *American Journal of Physiology, 267*, E49–56 1994.

Phillips, M. J., Needham, M., & Weller, R. O. (1997). Role of cervical lymph nodes in autoimmune encephalomyelitis in the Lewis rat. *Journal of Pathology, 182*, 457–464.

Plata-Salaman, C. R. (1991). Immunoregulators in the nervous system. *Neuroscience and Biobehavioural Reviews*, 185–215.

Rapaport, S. I. (1976). *Blood-brain barrier in physiology and medicine.* New York: Raven Press.

Reichlin, S. (1995). Endocrine-immune interaction. In L. J. DeGroot, (Ed.), *Endocrinology* (pp. 2964–3012). Philadelphia: W. B. Saunders.

Reichlin, S. (1999b). Editorial: Is leptin a secretion of the brain? *Journal of Clinical Endocrinology and Metabolism 84*, 2267–2269.

Reichlin, S. (1998). Alternative pathways of neural control of the immune process. *Annals of the New York Academy of Sciences, 840*, 301–316.

Reichlin, S. (1999a) Neuroendocrinology of infection and the innate immune system. *Recent Progress in Hormone Research, 54*, 133–183.

Reichlin, S., Chen, G., & Nicolson, M. (2000). Blood to brain transfer of leptin in normal and IL-1β treated male rats. *Endocrinology*, in press.

Ringheim, G. E., Burgher, K. L., & Heroux, J. A. (1995). Interleukin-6 mRNA expression by cortical neurons in culture: Evidence for neuronal sources of interleukin-6 production in the brain. *Journal of Neuroimmunology, 63*, 113–123.

Robertson, C. S. Inflammatory cells and the hyhpermetabolism of head injury. *Journal of Laboratory and Clinical Medicine, 118*, 205.

Romero, L. I., Kakucska, I., Lechan, R. M., & Reichlin, S. (1996). Interleukin-6 (IL-6) is secreted from the brain after intracerebroventricular injection of IL-1β in rats. *American Journal of Physiology, 270*, R518–524.

Santos, T. Q., & Valdimarsson, H. (1982). T-dependent antigens are more immunogenic in the subarachnoid space than in other sites *Journal of Neuroimmunology, 2*, 215–222.

Schettini, G., Grimaldi, M., Navarra, P., Pozzoli, G., Reichlin, S., & Preziosi, O. (1994). Regulation of interleukin-6 production by cAMP-protein kinase-A pathway in rat cortical astrocytes. *Pharmacological Research, 30*, 13–24.

Schlinger, B. A., & Arnold, A. P. (1991). Brain is the major site of estrogen synthesis in a male songbird. *Proceedings of the National Academy of Sciences USA, 88*, 4191–4194.

Schöbitz, B., Holsboer, F., & deKloet, E. R. (1994). Cytokines in the healthy and diseased brain. *News in Physiological Science, 9*, 138–142.

Sharief, M. K., Ciardi, M., & Thompson, E. J. (1992). Blood-brain barrier damage in patients with bacterial meningitis: Association with tumor necrosis factor-alpha but not interleukin-1 beta. *Journal of Infectious Disease, 166*, 350–358.

Sternberg, E. M. (1997). Neural-immune interactions in health and disease. *Journal of Clinical Investigation, 100*, 2641–2647.

Streilin, J. W., Ksander, B. R., & Taylor, A. W. (1997). Immune deviation in relation to ocular immune privilege. *Journal of Immunology, 158*, 3557–3560.

Sundar, S. K., Cierpial, M. A., Kilts, C., Ritchie, J. C., & Weiss, J. M. (1990). Brain IL-1 induced immunosuppression occurs through activation of both pituitary-adrenal axis and sympathetic nervous system by corticotropin releasing factor. *Journal of Neuroscience, 10*, 3701–3706.

Soszynski, D., Kozak, W., Conn, C. A., Rudolph, K., & Kluger, M. J. (1996). Beta-adrenoceptor antagonists suppress elevation in body temperature and increase in plasma IL-6 in rats exposed to open field. *Neuroendocrinology, 63*, 459–467.

Takaki, A., Huang, Q.-H., Somogyvári-Vigh, A., & Arimura, A. (1994). Immobilization stress may increase plasma interleukin-6 via central and peripheral catecholamines. *Neuroimmunomodulation, 1*, 335–342.

Tarkowski, E., Rosengren, L., Blomstrand, C., Wikkelso, C., Jensen, Ekholm, S., & Tarkowski, A. (1995). Early intrathecal production of interleukin-6 predicts the size of brain lesions in stroke. *Stroke, 26*, 1393–1398.

Tarlow, M. J., Jenkins, R., Comis, S. D., Osborne, M. P., Stephens, S., Stanley, P., & Crocker, J. (1993). Ependymal cells of the choroid plexus express tumour necrosis factor-. *Neuropathology and Appled Neurobiology, 19*, 324–328.

Turnbull, A., & Rivier, C. (1998a). Inhibition of gonadotropin-induced testosterone secretion by the intracerebroventricular injection of interleukin-1 beta in the male rat. *Endocrinology, 138*, 1008–1013.

Turnbull, A. V., & Rivier, C. (1998b). Intraventricular passive immunization I. The effect of intracerebroventricular administration of an antiserum to tumor necrosis factor- on the plasma adrenocorticotrophin response to lipopolysaccharide in rats. *Endocrinology, 139*, 119–127.

Turnbull, A. V., & Rivier, C. L. (1998c). Intracerebral passive immunization II. Intracerebroventricular infusion of neuropeptides antisera can inhibit neuropeptide signalling in peripheral tissues. *Endocrinology, 139*, 128–136.

Ulevitch, R. J., & Elias, P. S. (1994). Receptor-dependent mechanisms of cell stimulation by bacterial endotoxin. *Annual Review of Immunology, 13,* 437–457.

Van Dam, A. M., De Vries, H. E., Kuiper, J., Ziljlstra, F. J., De Boer, A. G., Tilders, F. J., & Berkenbosch, F. (1996). Interleukin-1 receptors on rat brain endothelial cells: A role in neuroimmune interaction? *FASEB Journal, 10,* 351–356.

Van Gool, J., van Vugt, H., Helle, M., & Aarden, L. A. (1990) The relation among stress, adrenaline, interleukin 6 and acute phase proteins in the rat. *Clinical Immunology and Immunopathology, 57,* 200–210

Van der Poll, T., Jansen, J., Endert, E., Sauerwein, H. P., & van Deventer, S. J. (1994) Noradrenaline inhibits lipopolysaccharide-induced tumor necrosis factor and interleukin 6 production in human whole blood. *Infection & Immunity, 62,* 2046–2050.

Vredevoe, D. L., Moser, D. K., Gan, X.-H., & Bonavida, B. (1995). Natural killer cell anergy to cytokine stimulants in a subgroup of patients with heart failure: Relationship to norepinephrine. *Neuroimmunomodulation, 2,* 16–24.

Weed, L. H. (1914). Studies on the cerebrospinal fluid III. The pathways of escape from the subarachnoid spaces with particular reference to the arachnoid villi. *Journal of Medical Research, 26,* 51–54.

Weiner, H. L. (1997). Oral tolerance for the treatment of autoimmune diseases. *Annual Review of Medicine, 48,* 341–351.

Wiesner, G., Vaz, M., Collier, G., Seals, D., Kaye, D., Jennings, G., Lambert, G., Wilkinson, D., & Esler, M. (1999). Leptin is released from the human brain: Influence of adiposity and gender. *Journal of Clinical Endocrinology and Metabolism, 84,* 2270–2274.

Weiss, J. M., Quan, N., & Sundar, S. K. (1994). Widespread activation and consequences of interleukin-1 in the brain. *Annals of the New York Academy of Sciences, 741,* 338–357.

Weller, R. O., Kida, S., & Zhang, E.-T. (1992). Pathways of fluid drainage from the brain-morphological aspects and immunological significance in rat and man. *Brain Pathology, 2,* 277–284.

Wilkinson, M., Morash, B., & Ur, E. (1999) The brain is a source of leptin. *In Neuroendocrinology of leptin* (pp. 106–125). Basel: Karger.

Yamada, S., DePasquale, M., Patlak, C. S., & Cserr H. (1991). Albumin outflow into deep cervical lymph from different regions of rabbit brain. *American Journal of Physiology, 261,* H1197–H1204.

Yang, R.-B., Mark, M. R., Gray, A., Huang, A., Xle, H. H., Zhang, M., Goddard, A., Wood, W. I., Gurney, A. L., & Godowski, P. J. (1998). Toll-like receptor-2 mediates lipopolysaccharide-induced cellular signalling. *Nature, 395,* 284–288.

Young, A. B., Ott, L. G., Beard, D., Dempsey, R. J., Tibbs, P. A., & McClain, C. J. (1988). The acute-phase response of the brain-injured patient. *Journal of Neurosurgery, 69,* 375–380.

Zhang, E. T., Richards, H. K., Kida, S., & Weller, R. O. (1992). Directional and compartmentalised drainage of interstitial fluid and cerebrospinal fluid from the rat brain. *Acta Neuropathologica, 83,* 233–239.

Zhou, D., Kusnecov, A. W., Shurin, M. R., DePaoli, M., & Rabin, B. S. (1993). Exposure to physical and psychological stsressors elevates plasma interleukin 6: Relationship to the activation of hypothalamic-pituitary-adrenal axis. *Endocrinology, 133,* 2523–2530.

CHAPTER

20

Central Cytokines: Effects on Peripheral Immunity, Inflammation, and Nociception

TETSURO HORI, TOSHIHIKO KATAFUCHI, TAKAKAZU OKA

I. INTRODUCTION

Cytokines play unique roles as signal molecules in the bidirectional communication between the central nervous system (CNS) and the biodefense system. Proinflammatory cytokines derived from the peripheral biodefense system signal the brain, thereby producing a variety of acute phase responses, such as fever, anorexia, sleep, modulation of the sympathetic nervous activity, various endocrine responses and the induction of cytokines in the brain (see review, Rothwell & Hopkins, 1995). It has progressively become clear that these CNS-mediated responses, in turn, may influence the biodefense system, and some responses are considered to have adaptive values for the infected host. For instance, fever has detrimental effects on invaded microorganisms and enhancing effects mainly on T cell-mediated immunity, thereby increasing the survival rate of infected hosts (Hori, Kaizuka, & Katafuchi, 1996; Kluger, Kozak, Conn, Leon, & Soszynski 1997; Roberts, 1991). The activation of the hypothalamus-pituitary-adrenocortical (HPA) system raises plasma levels of glucocorticoid, which, inhibits broad spectrum of immunological and inflammatory responses to limit overaction of the biodefense system, forming a negative feedback.

Emerging evidence has revealed that circulating cytokines transmit information to the brain through multiple mechanisms: (1) the cytokines-specific transport through the blood-brain barrier of cytokines (Banks, Kastin, & Broadwell, 1995); (2) the generation of secondary signal molecules (e.g., prostaglandins) at endothelial cells of the cerebral microvessels (Matsumura et al., 1998); (3) the transduction of immune signals to brain neural signals at the circumventricular organs where the blood-brain barrier is leaky (Blatteis & Sehic, 1997; Ota, Katafuchi, Takaki, & Hori, 1997); and (4) the detection of inflammatory signals by peripheral afferent nerves particularly by vagal afferents (Watkins, Maier, & Geohler, 1995). These mechanisms do not seem to be mutually exclusive and they may contribute, more or less, to the manifestation of acute phase responses with different time courses.

Besides their peripheral origins, many cytokines are also synthesized in the brain by astrocytes, microglia, vascular endothelial cells, meningeal cells, and probably also by neurons (see review, Liu, Takao, Hashimoto, & De Souza 1996; Wong, Al-Shehlee, Gold, & Licinio, 1996; Wong, Bongiorno, Rettori, McCann & Licinio 1997). The production of cytokines in the brain has been demonstrated as the increase in their gene expression, proteins, and biological activities after systemic administration of lipopolysaccharide (LPS) (Breder et al., 1994; Coceani, Lees, Mancilla, Berlizario, & Dinarello, 1993; van Dam, Brouns, Louisse, & Berkenbosch, 1992), during immobilization stress (Minami et al., 1991), and during various kinds of brain insults (meningitis, cerebral ischemia, some degenerative diseases) (Rothwell, 1996; Wong et al., 1996). Cytokines receptors also have been identified widely in the brain (see review, Faggioni, Benigni, & Ghezzi, 1995; Liu et al., 1996; Wong et al., 1996). Brain-derived cytokines also may produce acute phase responses that are almost identical with those caused by peripheral cytokines. Due to the well-known pleiotropic activities of cytokines and their ability to induce other cytokines to form a cytokine network, it is difficult to attribute any acute phase responses to particular cytokines.

Brain-derived proinflammatory cytokines may modulate the activities of the sympathetic nervous system and the HPA axis, that is two major communication channels from the brain to the biodefense system (Hori, Katafuchi, Take, Shimizu, & Niijima, 1995; Sundar, Cierpial, Kilts, Ritchie, & Weiss, 1990; Take, Mori, Katafuchi, & Hori, 1993). Therefore, it is expected that the brain may have some roles in the control of peripheral immune/inflammatory responses, which accompany the induction of cytokines in the CNS as well as in the local inflamed tissues. Proinflammatory cytokines such as interleukin-1 (IL-1), tumor necrosis factor-α (TNF-α) and interleukin-6 (IL-6) are released in the inflammatory tissues and sensitize nociceptors, thereby inducing local hyperalgesia (see review, Perkins & Davis, 1996). On the other hand, small quantities of these cytokines, when administered centrally, may modulate nociceptive behaviors, suggesting the involvement of brain cytokines in the central processing of nociceptive information (Hori, Oka, Hosoi, & Aou, 1998; Oka, Aou, & Hori, 1993). This chapter focuses on effects of central cytokines and their related substances on the peripheral immune responses, inflammation, and nociception.

II. INDUCTION OF CYTOKINES IN THE BRAIN DURING INFLAMMATORY AND NONINFLAMMATORY STRESSES

Although there is evidence that blood cytokines cross the blood-brain barrier by cytokines-specific transport systems (Banks et al., 1995), they may not be the major source of brain cytokines in terms of their absolute amount. It has been believed that the cytokines within the brain are those synthesized by brain cells such as microglia, astrocytes, and neurons. The induction of cytokines in the brain is substantiated by detection of protein and gene transcripts. Such cytokines include IL-1α, IL-1β IL-1 receptor antagonist (IL-1ra), IL-3, IL-6, IL-10, TNF-α, TNF-β, interferon α (IFN-α), and transforming growth factor β (TGF-β). Some cytokines are expressed constitutively in the brain. The production of central cytokines increases during peripheral inflammation as well as various brain insults including the cerebral ischemia and meningitis. The distribution of cytokines and their receptors in the brain has been extensively reviewed (Liu et al., 1996; Wong et al., 1996, 1997).

A. IL-1

Systemic administration of LPS (commonly used as an experimental model of systemic inflammation) has been reported to induce the expression of IL-1β at the gene and protein levels in various brain regions and the pituitary glands in rats, mice, and rabbits (Ban, Haour, & Lenstra, 1992; Hillhouse & Mosley, 1993; Laye, Parnet, Goujon, & Dantzer, 1994; Nakamori, Morimoto, Yamaguchi, Watanabe, & Murakami, 1994; Quan, Sundar, & Weiss, 1994; Van Dam et al., 1992) with less pronounced gene expression of IL-1ra and IL-10 (Wong et al., 1997). Subcutaneous injection of formalin into the hind paws (a model of persistent pain/inflammation) in rats provokes pronounced expression of IL-1β mRNA in glial cells of the hypothalamus (Yabuuchi, Maruta, Minami, & Satoh, 1996a). Noninflammatory stress such as immobilization also induces IL-1β mRNA in the rat hypothalamus (Minami et al., 1991).

B. TNF-α

TNF-α-like immunohistochemistry (Breder, Tsujimoto, Terano, Scott, & Saper, 1993) and in situ hybridization of TNF-α mRNA (Breder et al., 1994) have revealed detailed localization of this cytokine in the neurons in various brain regions including hypothalamic nuclei, pons, and medulla of mice in the baseline condition. Systemic injection of LPS increases

TNF-α levels in the cerebrospinal fluid in cats and rats (Coceani et al., 1993; Klir, Roth, Szelenyi, McClellan, & Kluger, 1993) and its mRNA particularly in the hypothalamic arcuate nucleus and circumventricular organs such as organum vasculosum laminae terminalis, median eminence, and area postrema in mice (Breder et al., 1994). Receptors for TNF-α are found in the mouse brain (Kinouchi, Brown, Pasternak, & Donner, 1991). TNF receptor types I and II have been expressed in microglia, astrocytes, and oligodendroglia and neurons.

C. IL-6 and Leukemia Inhibitory Factor

High levels of IL-6 have been found in the cerebrospinal fluid of cats and rats during LPS-induced fever (Coceani et al., 1993; Klir et al., 1993) and of patients with acute brain infection (Houssiau, Bukasa, & Sindic, 1988). IL-6 mRNA and IL-6 receptor mRNA are found in the hypothalamus and the limbic system including the dentate gyrus and piriform cortex in the rat (Gadient & Otten, 1995; Schöbitz, de Kloet, Sutanto, & Holsboer, 1993).

Leukemia inhibitory factor (LIF), a member of cytokines that share gp130 as a receptor subunit (IL-6, IL-11, ciliary neurotrophic factor, etc.), and LIF receptors are constitutively expressed in the murine hypothalamus and pituitary as assessed by reverse transcriptase-polymerase chain reaction (Z. Wang, Ren, & Melmed, 1996). Intraperitoneal injection of LPS increases the expression of LIF and LIF receptors in the hypothalamus and the pituitary gland, in association with increased release of adrenocorticotropic hormone (ACTH).

D. IFN-α

The brain produces high levels of IFN-α during infection (Ho-Yen & Carrington, 1987; Lloyd, Hickie, Brockman, Dwyer, & Wakefield, 1991; von Sydow, Sonnenborg, Gaines, & Strannegard, 1991). Recent studies have indicated the constitutive expression of IFN-α in human brain (Brandt et al., 1993; Ho-Yen & Carrington, 1987; Lloyd et al., 1991; von Sydow et al., 1991). Neurons and microglia in human brain of nonneurological and neurological cases are stained with an anti-IFN-α antibody (Akiyama, Ikeda, Katoh, McGeer, & McGeer, 1994; Yamada, Horisberger, Kawaguchi, Moroo, & Toyoda, 1994). Astrocytes of rats and mice in vitro produce IFN-α when stimulated with neurotropic viruses and endotoxin (Lieberman, Pitha, Shin, & Shin, 1989; Tedeschi, Barrett, & Keane, 1986). The binding sites for human IFN-α have been demonstrated in the rat brain, particularly in the hypothalamus (Janicki, 1992). Human microglia expresses IFN-α receptors constitutively (Yamada & Yamanaka, 1995). Astrocytes are suggested to have receptors for IFN-α/β because IFNs induce class 1 major histocompatibility complex (MHC) antigens on an astrocyte subpopulation and thus render them susceptible to the lytic actions of cytotoxic T cells (Borgeson, Tallent, & Keane, 1989).

Like other cytokines (IL-1, IL-6, and TNF-α), IFN-α, when injected centrally, produces a similar type of CNS-mediated acute phase responses including fever, sleep, anorexia, analgesia, altered activities of central neurons and sympathetic nerves, and decreased natural killer (NK) cytotoxicity in the spleen (see review, Hori, Katafuchi, Take, & Shimizu, 1998). However, IFN-α, unlike other proinflammatory cytokines, inhibits the HPA system (Saphier et al., 1994). Another unique characteristics of IFN-α is that its acute central effects are mediated, at least partially, by opioid receptor mechanisms, because the CNS responses so far examined are blocked by opioid antagonists. Such responses include analgesia (Blalock & Smith, 1981), fever (Nakashima et al., 1995), suppression of NK cytotoxicity (Take et al., 1993), the enhanced activity of splenic sympathetic nerve (Katafuchi, Take, & Hori, 1993), and altered activity of hypothalamic neurons (Kuriyama, Hori, Mori, & Nakashima, 1990; Nakashima, Hori, Kuriyama, & Matsuda, 1988). In fact, it has been demonstrated that IFN-α binds to opioid receptors in mice brain homogenates and rats brain nerve membranes competitively with dihydromorphine (Blalock & Smith, 1981) and naloxone (Menzies, Patel, Hall, O'Grady, & Rier, 1992), respectively.

E. IL-10

IL-10, which was initially found as a cytokine synthesis inhibitory factor (Fiorentino, Bond, & Mosmann, 1989), has been demonstrated to protect animals from lethal endotoxemia probably by its ability to inhibit the production of proinflammatory cytokines (Gerard et al; 1993; Howard, Muchamel, Andrade, & Menon, 1993; Moore, O'Garra, De Waal Malefyt, Vieira, & Mosmann, 1993; Sironi et al., 1993). IL-10 and its mRNA have been found in the astrocytes and microglia of human and animal brains of infectious, traumatic, neoplastic, and neurodegenerative diseases in the CNS (Diab et al., 1997; Tarkowski et al., 1997; Williams, Dooley, Ulvestad, Becher, & Antel, 1996). Systemic injection of LPS induces modest increases in IL-10 mRNA expression in the CNS of rats, although to a lesser degree than IL-1β gene expression (Wong et al., 1997).

III. EFFECTS OF CENTRAL CYTOKINES AND THE RELATED SUBSTANCES ON PERIPHERAL IMMUNITY

Several proinflammatory cytokines, neuropeptides, and the related substances in the brain have been demonstrated to alter various parameters of immunity in the periphery. Such actions of brain cytokines appear to constitute a negative feedback to prevent overactions of the peripheral cellular immunity.

A. IL-1

Intracerebroventricular (i.c.v.) injection of low doses (50 pg–5 ng) of IL-1β in rats has been shown to suppress various immune responses such as NK cell activity, mitogenic response to phytohemagglutinin (PHA), and IL-2 production of blood and splenic lymphocytes ((Sundar et al., 1989, 1990), specific antibody production (Irwin, 1993), and secretion of IL-1 from splenic macrophages (Brown et al., 1991). The reduction of immune responses is suppressed by i.c.v. pretreatment with α-melanocyte stimulating hormone (α-MSH), which is known to inhibit many actions of IL-1 (Catania & Lipton, 1994). Furthermore, the central IL-1β-induced immunosuppression is prevented by i.c.v. pretreatment with anticorticotropin releasing factor (CRF) antibody (Sundar et al., 1990) and mimicked by i.c.v. injection of CRF (Irwin, 1993; Irwin, Hauger, Brown, & Britton, 1988). An i.c.v. injection of IL-1β (100 ng) markedly induces c-fos protein expression in the paraventricular nucleus (PVN) and the arcuate nucleus of rat hypothalamus together with ACTH release (Rivest, Torres, & Rivier, 1992). The c-fos protein positive cells in the PVN contain CRF. These findings suggest the mediation of IL-1-induced immunosuppression by activation of CRF neurons in the brain.

An i.c.v. injection of LPS, a potent inducer of proinflammatory cytokines (Quan et al., 1994), also results in the suppression of the peripheral cellular immunity, which is likewise attenuated by simultaneous i.c.v. infusion of α-MSH (Sundar et al., 1989). Furthermore, i.c.v., but not intravenous (i.v.), administration of gp120, the envelope protein of human immunodeficiency virus (HIV), reduces the peripheral cellular immunity of blood and splenic lymphocytes (Concanavalin A [Con A] mitogenic response and NK activity) in rats (Sundar et al., 1991). This immunosuppression is considered to be mediated by central induction of IL-1β, because IL-1 activity is detected in the brain after gp120 infusion (Quan et al., 1996) and thymocyte stimulation, which is produced by active fractions of gp120-infused brains, is inhibited by anti-IL-1 receptors antibody (Sundar et al., 1991). Simultaneous i.c.v. administration of gp120 with α-MSH abolishes the reduced NK activity and glucocorticoid response. Although the site(s) of actions of gp120 in the brain to induce IL-1 is not known, its injection into the hippocampus stimulated IL-1 production more readily than i.c.v. administration. These findings implicate that IL-1 production in the brain occurs after HIV infection and central IL-1 may be responsible, at least in part, for certain pathological changes in the CNS.

The brain IL-1β-induced immunosuppression is considered to be brought about by activation of both the HPA axis and the sympathetic nervous system. Either adrenalectomy, sympathectomy, or sympathetic ganglion blockade alone only partially inhibits the immunosuppression (Brown et al., 1991; Sundar et al., 1989, 1990). The activation of the splenic sympathetic nerve following i.c.v. injection of IL-1β (1–5 ng) has been confirmed by recording its firing activity in anesthetized rats (Ichijo, Katafuchi, & Hori, 1994). The IL-1β-induced increase in the splenic sympathetic activity is blocked by i.c.v. pretreatment with α-MSH as well as IL-1ra. The enhancement of the splenic sympathetic activity plays a critical role, at least partially, in the central IL-1β-induced immunosuppression. In fact, electrical stimulation of the splenic sympathetic nerve in rats has been shown to suppress the splenic NK activity through β-adrenergic receptor mechanisms (Figure 1) (Katafuchi, Take, et al., 1993). Furthermore, activation of the sympathetic nervous system by a ganglionic stimulant suppresses NK activity, mitogen-induced proliferation, and production of IL-2 and IFN-γ in rat splenic lymphocytes (Fecho, Maslonek, Dykstra, & Lysle, 1993).

B. IFN-α

An i.c.v. injection of IFN-α, like that of IL-1β, also suppresses the NK activity of blood and splenic lymphocytes for a period of 30–120 min in mice and rats (Take, Mori, Katafuchi, Kaizuka, & Hori, 1992; Take et al., 1993). A brain microinjection study has revealed that the most sensitive site to microinjected IFN-α for reducing the splenic NK activity is located in the medial preoptic area (MPO) in the hypothalamus. The microinjection of IFN-α into the lateral preoptic area (LPO), the lateral hypothalamus (LHA), the ventromedial hypothalamus (VMH), and the PVN caused no changes in NK activity (Figure 2) (Take, Uchimura, Kanemitsu, Katafuchi, & Hori, 1995).

The suppression of NK activity after i.c.v. or intra-MPO injection of IFN-α is abolished by naltrexone (i.c.v.), an opioid antagonist (Take et al., 1993, 1995),

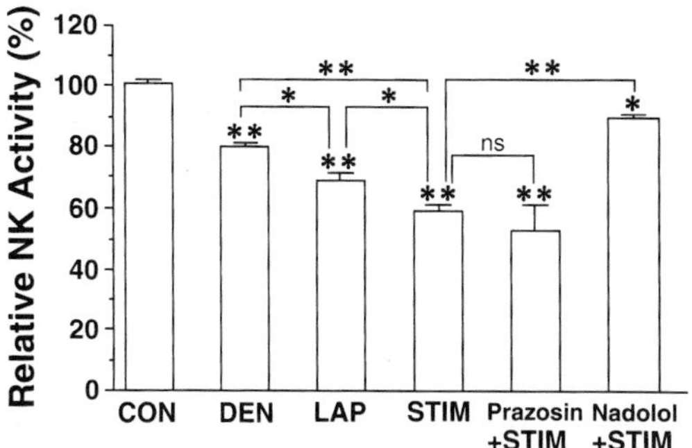

FIGURE 1 Effects of splenic sympathetic nerve stimulation on the splenic NK cell activity. Relative NK cell activity at an effector:target cells ratio of 100:1 were expressed as percentage of mean values of the nontreated controls (CON, $n = 11$). The splenic NK cell activity after laparotomy for 20 min with sham-denervation (LAP) was reduced to $69.3 \pm 3.0\%$ ($n = 5$) of the CON. The splenic denervation performed immediately after the laparotomy resulted in an increase in the NK cell activity compared with LAP (DEN, $80.3 \pm 1.3\%$). An electrical stimulation of the peripheral cut end of the splenic nerve (20 Hz for 20 min) lowered the NK activity to $59.2 \pm 2.4\%$ (STIM, $n = 5$). The stimulation-induced suppression of NK activity was almost completely blocked by an intravenous injection of a peripheral acting β-adrenergic receptor antagonist, nadolol (2 mg/kg) (nadolol + STIM, $n = 3$), but not by that of an α-adrenergic antagonist, prazosin (3 mg/kg) (prazosin + STIM, $n = 3$). $^{*}P < 0.05$, $^{**}P < 0.01$, and n.s., not significant. From Katafuchi, et al., 1993b.

suggesting the involvement of opioid receptors mechanisms (see section II-D). Electrophysiologi-cally, a majority of MPO neurons in rats is known to decrease the firing rate to direct application of IFN-α in a naloxone preventable way (Nakashima et al., 1988). Furthermore, the IFN-α-induced suppression of NK activity is abolished by pretreatment with α-helical CRF_{9-41}, a CRF antagonist, indicating the mediation through activation of CRF neurons (Take et al., 1993). Since the reduced NK activity caused by i.c.v. injection of CRF is not affected by naltrexone, the opioid-dependent alteration of MPO neurons by IFN-α occurs before the process involving the activation of CRF neurons.

The IFN-α-induced reduction of NK activity is completely blocked by surgical interruption of the splenic nerve, whereas adrenalectomy failed to alter the immunosuppressive responses to central IFN-α. Centrally (i.c.v. and MPO) administered IFN-α inhibits the activity of the HPA axis in rats (Saphier et al., 1994) and augments the electrical activity of the splenic sympathetic nerve in anesthetized rats (Katafuchi, Take et al., 1993; Katafuchi, Ichijo, Take, & Hori, 1993). Therefore, the reduced NK activity by central IFN-α, unlike that by IL-1β, seems to depend solely on the intact splenic innervation.

C. Other Cytokines

An i.c.v. infusion of IL-2 (20 ng), IL-6 (20 ng), or TNF-α (40 ng) had no effect on Con A-induced splenic lymphocyte proliferation and the activity of the HPA axis in rats assessed 45 min after infusion, although the equimolar IL-1β (i.c.v.) was able to reduce the lymphocyte mitogenic response and activate hormonal responses (Connor, Song, Leonard, Merali, & Anisman, 1998).

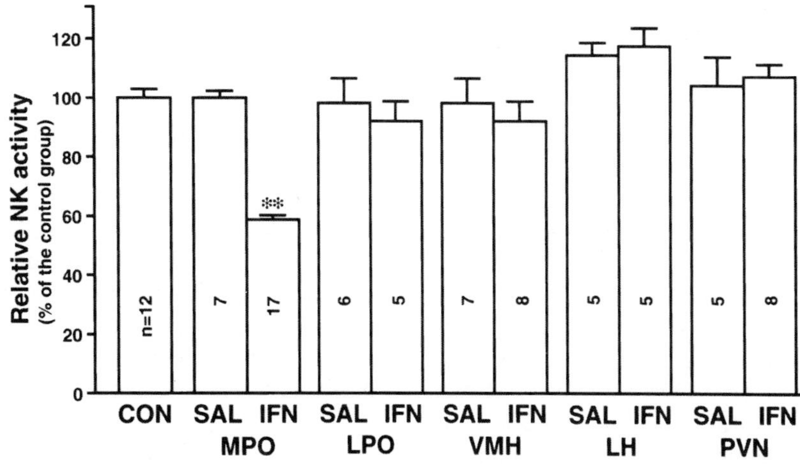

FIGURE 2 Effects of microinjection of IFN-α into hypothalamic areas on splenic NK cell activity. Relative NK cell activity at an effector:target cells ratio of 100:1 was expressed as percentage of mean value of noncannulated and nontreated control group (CON). IFN-α at 200U or saline (SAL) was microinjected into the medial preoptic area (MPO), the lateral preoptic hypothalamus (LPO), the ventromedial hypothalamic nucleus (VMH), the lateral hypothalamic area (LHA), and the paraventricular nucleus (PVN). $^{**}P < 0.01$. From Take et al., 1995, with permission.

D. Opioids

Opioid peptides inhibit various parameters of cellular immunity (lymphocyte proliferation, NK activity, and IFN-γ production) by their actions within the CNS (see review, Hall, Suo, & Weber, 1998). The immunosuppression by endogenous opioids in the brain was for the first time found by a study showing that a form of footshock stress causing opioid-dependent, but not opioid-independent, analgesia produced the suppression of NK cell cytotoxicity in rats in a naloxone reversible way (Shavit, Lewis, Terman, Gale, & Liebeskind, 1984). Subsequently, it became clear that stimulation of opioid receptors in the brain, but not in the periphery, resulted in the reduced NK activity, as an i.c.v. injection of morphine, but not peripheral administration of N-methylmorphine, which does not cross the blood-brain barrier, provoked the immunosuppression (Shavit et al., 1986). In addition, the reduced NK activity after i.c.v. injection of IFN-α, which was known to stimulate brain opioid receptors, was found to be abolished by i.c.v. pretreatment with naltrexone (Take et al., 1993). Furthermore, endogenous opioid activity in the CNS is involved in conditioned stimulus-induced alterations of immune functions (Lysle, Luecken, & Maslonek, 1992). After establishing a conditioning of suppression of cellular immunity in rats (Con A-induced proliferation of splenic lymphocytes and NK activity) by presentation of an innocuous stimulus (a conditioned stimulus) paired with footshock stimulus (an aversive unconditioned stimulus), subcutaneous injection of naltrexone just before reexposure to the conditioned stimulus resulted in the attenuation of the conditioned stimulus-induced immunosuppression. But administration of N-methylnaltrexone, which does not cross the blood-brain barrier, failed to affect it, indicating the involvement of endogenous opioids in the brain.

The brain site(s) of actions of opioid peptides have not been examined systematically. At present, microinjection of β-endorphin or morphine into the MPO, the anterior hypothalamus, and the periaqueductal gray matter is known to suppress splenic NK cell activity and blood lymphocyte proliferation in rats (Hernandez, Flores, & Bayer, 1993; Hori et al., 1991; Weber & Pert, 1989). Although microinjection of morphine in the periaqueductal gray matter increases plasma levels of ACTH and glucocorticoid temporarily in association with suppression of NK activity and lymphocyte proliferation in rats, pretreatment with a glucocorticoid receptor antagonist (RU486) does not prevent the immunosuppression (Hall et al., 1998). This suggests that the central morphine induces immunosuppression predominantly through a glucocorticoid-independent mechanism. It appears that the sympathetic nervous system is closely involved in the central morphine-induced immunosuppression (Hall et al., 1998), because stimulation of hypothalamic opioid receptors by IFN-α reduces splenic NK activity through an activation of the splenic sympathetic nerve (Take et al., 1993).

Concerning the opioid receptor subtypes responsible for the central morphine-induced immunosuppression, studies using selective μ, δ, and κ agonists and antagonists showed that μ receptors were the most potent in inducing the reduction of blood lymphocyte proliferative responses to Con A (Mellon & Bayer, 1998) and splenic NK cell activity (Band et al., 1992).

E. Corticotropin-Releasing Factor

It has been demonstrated that both central IL-1β- and IFN-α-induced immunosuppression is completely blocked by pretreatment with anti-CRF antibody or a CRF antagonist (α-helical CRF_{9-41}) (Sundar et al., 1990; Take et al., 1993). In addition, the enhancement of the splenic sympathetic activity induced by i.c.v. IL-1β was also blocked by α-helical CRF_{9-41} (Ichijo et al., 1994). An i.c.v. injection of CRF decreased the splenic and blood NK cell activity (Irwin et al., 1988; Take et al., 1993) and a specific in vivo antibody production in rats (Irwin, 1993). An i.c.v. pretreatment with a sympathetic ganglionic blocker completely blocked the CRF-induced reduction in NK cell activity and increase in plasma noradrenaline, whereas the same dose of this blocker did not affect the increase in plasma levels of ACTH and corticosterone (Irwin et al., 1988). Therefore, it is suggested that the sympathetic nervous system, but not the HPA axis, plays a significant role in the CRF-induced immunosuppression. The splenic sympathetic nerve activity increases in a dose-dependent manner following i.c.v. infusion of CRF in rats (Katafuchi, Ichijo, & Hori, 1997). Consistent with this finding, an in vivo microdialysis study in rats has shown that noradrenaline release from the sympathetic nerve terminals in the spleen is enhanced by i.c.v. injection of CRF (Shimizu, Hori, & Nakane, 1994).

F. Prostaglandin E_2

Prostaglandin E_2 (PGE_2, 0.5–2 μg, i.c.v.), a principal mediator of many proinflammatory cytokines, decreases proliferative responses of splenic lymphocytes by its action within the brain in rats (Rassnick, Zhou,

& Rabin, 1995). Since this response is accompanied by increased plasma concentrations of ACTH and corticosterone, the activation of HPA axis is likely to mediate the altered immune reactivity. However, electrical activity of the splenic sympathetic nerve also increases after i.c.v. infusion of PGE_2 at 1 ng (Katafuchi et al., 1997) through its action on EP1 receptor subtype for PGE_2 (Ando, Ichijo, Katafuchi, & Hori, 1995). Furthermore, an increase in noradrenaline turnover in the spleen has been observed after i.c.v. injection of PGE_2 but not that of PGD_2 or $PGF_{2\alpha}$ (Terao, Kitamura, Asano, Kobayashi, & Saito, 1995). These data indicate that the sympathetic nervous system is involved also in the PGE_2-induced immunosuppression.

Brain IL-1β-induced acute phase responses such as ACTH release (Katsuura, Arimura, Koves, & Gottschall, 1990), fever (Stitt, 1986), hyperalgesia (Oka et al., 1993) and altered activity of hypothalamic neurons (Kuriyama et al., 1990) are abolished by inhibition of a key enzyme of prostanoids syntheses (cyclooxygenase, COX), and such acute phase responses may be mimicked by central injection of PGE_2. It has not been examined whether the central administration of COX inhibitors blocks the central IL-1β-induced immunosuppression. However, the enhancement of the splenic sympathetic activity (Ichijo, et al., 1994) and the noradrenaline turnover in the spleen by central IL-1β (Terao et al., 1995) are blocked by inhibition of COX activity. Therefore, the synthesis of prostanoids is likely to be involved in the IL-1β-induced reduction of cellular immunity.

The i.c.v. IL-1β-induced enhancement of the splenic sympathetic activity was blocked by a CRF antagonist, α-helical CRF_{9-41} (Ichijo et al., 1994). An increase in the splenic nerve activity induced by i.c.v. PGE_2 was blocked by i.c.v. pretreatment with α-helical CRF_{9-41}, whereas the CRF-induced enhancement of the nerve activity was not affected by sodium salicylate at a dose 100 times more than that required for suppressing the IL-1β-induced activation of the nerve (Katafuchi et al., 1997). Therefore, it is likely that an activation of prostanoids (most probably PGE_2)-dependent process is followed by that of CRF system in the brain, resulting in the enhanced splenic nerve activity. A similar sequential relationship between the prostanoids-dependent process and CRF mechanisms has been suggested in the IL-1-induced activation of the HPA axis (Watanabe, Morimoto, Sakata, & Murakami, 1990). In fact, it has been shown that PGE_2 but not $PGF_{2\alpha}$ stimulates the release of CRF from rat hypothalamic explants (Pozzoli et al., 1994).

G. Involvement of Brain Cytokines in the Noninflammatory Stress-Induced Immunomodulation

Irwin, Vale, and Rivier (1990) demonstrated that footshock stress-induced reduction of splenic NK cell activity was mediated by brain CRF independently of the HPA activation. Related to this, it has been reported that the splenic sympathetic nerve may be a significant mediator of immunosuppression by noninflammatory stresses, for example footshock-induced suppression of lymphocyte proliferative responses and IgM plaque-forming cell responses (Wan et al., 1993) and immobilization-induced reduction of splenic NK cell activity (Shimizu, Kaizuka, Hori, & Nakane, 1996). As described already, both IL-1β and IFN-α in the brain can induce suppression of the peripheral immunity, which is dependent on central CRF and is mediated, at least in part, by activation of the sympathetic nervous system. These cytokines are known to be produced in the brain during noninflammatory stresses such as immobilization (see section II). These findings raise a possibility that such brain cytokines are involved in the stress-induced immunosuppression. Supporting this hypothesis, reduction of lymphocyte proliferation responses and NK cell activity following footshock and immobilization stress was attenuated by i.c.v. pretreatment with anti-IL-1 antibody and α-MSH, respectively (Saperstein et al., 1992; Katafuchi, Kondo, Take, & Hori, 1998).

At least two hypothalamic nuclei (MPO and PVN) play roles in the immunomodulation by hypothalamic IL-1β and IFN-α. Although chemical or electrical stimulation of MPO neurons decreases the splenic sympathetic activity, electrolytic lesioning of the MPO increases it in association with reduced NK activity (Katafuchi, Ichijo, et al., 1993). A majority of MPO neurons decreases the firing rate to direct applications of IL-1 and IFN-α (Hori et al., 1988; Nakashima et al., 1988), intra-MPO or i.c.v. injection of which augments the splenic sympathetic activity (Ichijo et al., 1994; Katafuchi, Take, et al., 1993). By contrast, the excitation of PVN neurons, putative CRF containing neurons, enhances the splenic sympathetic activity. There is a direct neural connection from the MPO to the PVN (Swanson, 1976) and this projection is thought to be inhibitory, that is the electrical stimulation of the MPO inhibits the multiple unit activity of the PVN in conscious rats (Saphier & Feldman, 1986). These findings, taken together, suggest a following mechanism of immunosuppression (Figure 3). IL-1 and IFN-α in the brain inhibit the activity of MPO neurons. The decreased firing rate of MPO neurons

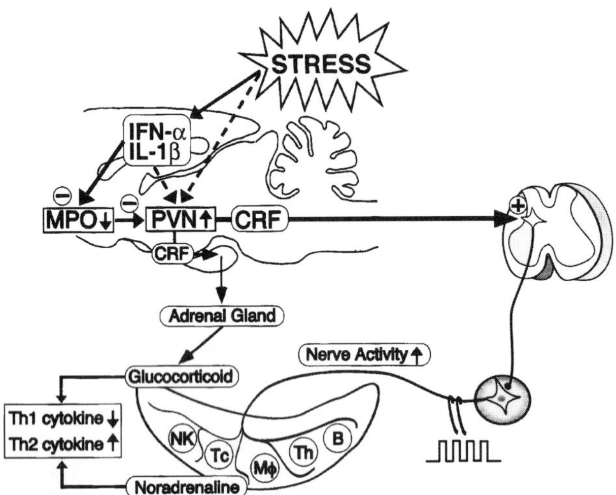

FIGURE 3 Involvement of hypothalamic cytokines in stress-induced immunomodulation.

elicits a disinhibition of PVN neurons, putative CRF neurons, and the resultant enhancement of the activity of CRF neurons stimulates the sympathetic nervous system and the HPA axis, thereby reducing the cellular immunity. In addition, activation of CRF neurons is suggested to occur in response to direct actions of cytokines and neurosensory signals from the lower brain stem and limbic brain.

The HPA axis and the sympathetic nervous system are two major communication channels that convey stress messages from the brain to the immune system. It has long been believed that actions of glucocorticoids and catecholamines are, in general, immunosuppressive. However, recent studies have revealed that these stress mediators alter differentially the production of cytokines controlling T helper 1 (Th1) cells and Th2 cells (see review, Webster, Torpy, Elenkov, & Chrousos, 1998). Catecholamines inhibit the production of Th1-type cytokines (IL-2, IFN-γ, TNF-α, and IL-12) by their actions on β_2 receptors of mononuclear phagocytes and Th1 cells, but they increase or do not affect the synthesis of Th2-type cytokines (IL-4, IL-10, IL-13). It has been found that Th1 cells have high density of β_2-adrenergic receptors, whereas Th2 cells do not (Ramer-Quinn, Baker, & Sanders, 1997). This may provide, at least in part, a basis for differential influences of catecholamines on Th1- and Th2-type of immunity. Corticosteroids also exert similar differential actions by inhibiting IL-12 production from monocytes (Blotta, DeKruyff, & Umetsu, 1997). These effects elicit the immune system toward Th2 dominance (Figure 3).

H. Other Neuropeptides

Little is known about effects of central administration of neuropeptides on peripheral immunity. Since the enhancement of the sympathetic nervous system by central CRF alters peripheral immune functions, the other central neuropeptides that stimulate the sympathetic nerve are expected to modulate immunity. Chronic i.c.v. infusion of angiotensin II and substance P in rats for a period of 28 days and 14 days, respectively, both of which have been known to facilitate the sympathetic nervous system, result in an increase in the percentage of total T cells measured by flow cytometry. The percentage of B-cell population decreased by infusion of angiotensin II but not by that of substance P (Fannon & Phillips, 1991). These effects are most likely due in part to the increased activity of the sympathetic nervous system. It remains to be elucidated whether the above effects of central angiotensin II are mediated by an increase in vasopressin release.

Nerve growth factor (NGF) is known as a retrograde trophic messenger in the brain as well as in the peripheral nervous system. It has been shown that NGF might be involved in the modulation of stress-induced responses. For instance, intermale aggressive behavior in mice leads to a massive release of biologically active NGF from the submaxillary salivary gland into the bloodstream (Aloe, Alleva, Boehm, & Levi-Montalcini, 1986) and a profound increase in NGF mRNA and protein in the hypothalamus with no changes in other sites in the brain (Spillantini et al., 1989). In addition, NGF is involved in the modulation of inflammatory/immune reactions locally. IL-1 stimulates NGF release in the brain (Strijbos & Rothwell, 1995) and NGF induces IL-1 expression in PC12 cells (Alheim et al., 1991). An i.c.v. administration of NGF, the amount of which was comparable to those released in mice hypothalamus during aggressive behavior, enhanced PHA-induced splenocyte proliferation but suppressed splenic NK cell activity in rats (Sacerdote, Manfredi, Aloe, Micera & Panerai, 1996). Intravenous injection of NGF augmented lymphocyte proliferation only at very high doses compared with i.c.v. injection and did not affect NK cell activity. The effects of i.c.v. NGF disappeared by i.c.v. pretreatment with an anti-NGF antibody, but not by i.v. injection of the antibody, indicating the central action of NGF. These altered immune responses were not mediated by the HPA axis since i.c.v. NGF did not modify the concentration of plasma corticosterone. Since NGF is shown to modulate release of growth hormone and prolactin (Patterson & Childs, 1994), the immunomodulatory effects of central NGF might be mediated by these pituitary hormones (Sacerdote et al., 1996). The involvement of autonomic nervous system remains to be determined. The NGF-induced increase in lymphocyte proliferation may be interpreted as a mechanism of counterbalance with the immunosuppression by other central modulators including proinflammatory cytokines (Sacerdote et al., 1996).

IV. EFFECTS OF CENTRAL CYTOKINES AND THE RELATED SUBSTANCES ON PERIPHERAL INFLAMMATION

A. Central Modulation of Peripheral Inflammation

Although inflammation in the peripheral tissues primarily is regulated by local factors, there is much evidence that signals originating within the CNS influence the peripheral inflammation. For instance, earlier studies reported that carrageenan-induced acute edema in the paw of rats was attenuated by central injection of $PGF_{2\alpha}$ (Bhattacharya & Das, 1984b), noradrenaline (Bhattacharya & Das, 1986), serotonin (Bhattacharya & Das, 1985a), histamine (Bhattacharya & Das, 1985b), γ-aminobutyric acid, and glycine (Bhattacharya & Sarkar, 1986). On the other hand, the enhancement of the paw edema was observed after central injection of PGE_2 (Bhattacharya & Das, 1984b), PGD_2 (Bhattacharya, Mohan Rao, & Das Gupta, 1989), acetylcholine (Das & Bhattacharya, 1985), bradykinin (Bhattacharya, Mohan Rao, Das, & Das Gupta, 1988), and glutamate (Bhattacharya & Sarkar, 1986). Furthermore, the turnover rate of noradrenaline and serotonin, but not of dopamine, in the hypothalamus increased during the course of carrageenan-induced acute paw edema, possibly in an attempt to limit the inflammation by activating these aminergic system (Bhattacharya, Das, & Mohan Rao, 1988). A neuropeptide α-MSH in the hypothalamus is also known to be released by actions of some proinflammatory cytokines, thereby inhibiting peripheral inflammation in which cytokines are involved (Lipton, 1989). These findings suggest that there are bidirectional interactions between the CNS and the peripheral inflamed tissues.

The CNS may influence the peripheral inflammation by glucocorticoids through activation of HPA axis. The presence of peripheral inflammation modulates the activity of HPA axis by neural (nociceptive afferents) and humoral (cytokines) signals arising from inflamed tissues. An on-going inflammation at one site (Freund's adjuvant injection on the hindpaw) in rats has been demonstrated to produce a negative feedback inhibition on bradykinin-induced plasma extravasation at another site (knee joint) (Green, Miao, Janig, & Levine, 1995). The studies involving capsaicin treatment, spinal cord transection, hypophysectomy, inhibition of corticosterone synthesis, and adrenalectomy have revealed a negative feedback inhibition of an inflammatory process. The information is conveyed neurally (C-fiber afferents) from inflamed tissue to the hypothalamus and the CNS exerts antiinflammatory actions through activation of the HPA axis. An acute local inflammation caused by intramuscular injection of a small volume of turpentine has been shown to produce an activation of HPA axis, which is mediated by synergistic actions of CRF and vasopressin with both stimulatory (prostanoids) and inhibitory (nitric oxide) intermediates (Turnbull & Rivier, 1996). Although Green et al. (1995) showed that the feedback inhibition stated above was not mediated via activation of sympathetic efferents, the centripetal neural pathways that involve β_2 receptors also may be suggested in the modulation of peripheral inflammation by centrally administered α-MSH (Macaluso et al., 1994).

B. Modulation of Peripheral Inflammation by Central Cytokines

A number of cytokines synthesized at inflamed tissues have been reported to modulate the processes of inflammation by their local actions, that is positively by IL-1β, TNF-α, IL-6, and IL-8 and negatively by IL-4, IL-10, IL-13, IFN-γ, and TGF-β (Marie, Pitton, Fitting, & Cavaillon, 1996; Moore et al., 1993; Pober & Cotran, 1990). However, much attention had not been directed to the possible influence of brain-derived cytokines on the peripheral inflammation. It was demonstrated that an i.c.v. injection of leukocyte pyrogen, produced by rabbit leucocytes incubated with LPS, enhanced picryl-chloride-induced edema in the mouse pinna (Dulaney et al., 1992). Since leukocyte pyrogen is considered to contain proinflammatory cytokines such as TNF and IL-1, this finding suggests that central proinflammatory cytokines might likewise promote inflammation in the periphery. As described in section II, cytokines and their gene transcripts are expressed widely in the brain during peripheral inflammation (Quan et al., 1994; Wong et al., 1997; Yabuuchi, Maruta, et al., 1996). These findings, together, suggest that the brain produces cytokines on messages from the inflammatory tissues and, in turn, sends modulatory signals back to the peripheral tissues. Proinflammatory cytokines thus induced centrally may promote the peripheral inflammation (Dulaney et al., 1992), forming a positive feedback. This is in contrast to the inhibitory actions of centrally administered IL-1β and IFN-α on the peripheral cellular immunity (Sundar et al., 1990; Take et al., 1993). The biological significance of opposite types of actions of central proinflammatory cytokines on the two host defense responses (peripheral inflammation and cellular immunity) remains to be determined.

IL-10, an antiinflammatory cytokine, is also synthesized in the brain during cerebral diseases (see II-E). IL-10 mRNA is expressed in the rat brain after systemic injection of LPS (Wong et al., 1997). An i.c.v. injection of IL-10 has been shown to inhibit LPS-induced production of TNF and IL-1β in the brain without affecting the HPA axis (DiSanto et al., 1995). Central IL-10, in addition to peripheral one, might inhibit the peripheral inflammation by its ability to inhibit the production of proinflammatory cytokines in the brain.

A neurocytokine ciliary neurotrophic factor (CNTF), like other cytokines that share gp130 as a receptor subunit (IL-6, IL-11, LIF, cardiotropin-1, and oncostatin M), inhibits the production of peripheral and central TNF, induces serum amyloid A protein, and potentiates the IL-1-induced HPA axis activation (Benigni et al., 1995, 1996). Carrageenan-induced inflammation in mice was markedly inhibited by an i.c.v. injection of CNTF, but not by its i.v. or local injection (Meazza et al., 1997). This antiinflammatory action was associated with high serum levels of corticosterone and disappeared by adrenalectomy, suggesting that an intact HPA axis is required for it. Furthermore, a CNTF receptor antagonist (i.c.v.) enhanced inflammation, indicating endogenous CNTF in the brain might be a negative regulator of peripheral inflammation (Meazza et al., 1997). At present, it is unknown whether peripheral inflammatory stimuli induces CNTF in the brain, although CNTF is detected in the blood of septic patients (Guillet, Fourcin, Chevalier, Pouplard, & Gascan, 1995). LIF, another gp130 utilizing cytokine, is expressed in mouse hypothalamus and pituitary by systemic challenge of LPS (Wang, Z. et al., 1996). Further studies are required to determine whether other gp-130 family of cytokines in the brain has antiinflammatory actions.

C. Modulation of Peripheral Inflammation by Central Prostaglandins

Prostaglandins, principal mediators of many proinflammatory cytokines, in the CNS as well as in the periphery play important roles in the mediation and modulation of peripheral inflammation. The levels of PGE_2 and $PGF_{2\alpha}$ in the rat brain have been reported to increase during carrageenan-induced inflammation in the rat paw (Bhattacharya & Das, 1984a). The carrageenan-induced paw inflammation in rats is enhanced by i.c.v. injection of PGE_2 and PGD_2, whereas the inflammation is attenuated by i.c.v. injection of $PGF_{2\alpha}$, a phospholipase inhibitor (hydrocortisone) and COX inhibitors (paracetamol and mefenamic acid) (Bhattacharya & Das, 1984b; Bhattacharya et al., 1989). Similarly, the other COX inhibitors (lysine acetylsalicylate and sodium salicylate), when injected into the lateral cerebroventricle but not systemically, attenuate the picryl chloride-induced edema in the mouse pinna (Catania, Arnold, Macaluso, Hiltz, & Lipton, 1991). However, this antiinflammatory effect of COX inhibition is not observed after central administration of indomethacin, another COX inhibitor, in doses that inhibit the peripheral inflammation when given intraperitoneally (Catania et al., 1991). Furthermore, i.c.v. injection of dexamethasone (a phospholipase inhibitor) and PGE_2 (0.25–1µg) do not affect the inflammatory edema in mouse pinna (Catania et al., 1991). Although the authors have concluded that salicylates work in the brain to inhibit acute peripheral inflammation, their data have suggested that PGs are not important for central modulation of this inflammatory model in mice.

D. Modulation of Peripheral Inflammation by Central CRF

Brain CRF, a key mediator for manifestation of stress responses, is induced by IL-1β (Sapolosky, Rivier, Yamamoto, Plotsky, & Vale, 1987; Tsagarakis, Gillies, Rees, Besser, & Grossman, 1989; Watanobe & Takebe, 1994) as well as by neurotransmitters during inflammatory and noninflammatory stresses. Systemic administration of LPS stimulates CRF gene expression in the PVN by a mechanism that involves the central actions of IL-1, because the LPS-induced CRF mRNA response is completely abolished by central, but not peripheral, treatment with IL-1ra (Kakcuscka, Qi, Clark, & Lechan, 1993). This peptide modulates immune/inflammatory reactions through activation of the HPA axis and the sympathetic nervous system. The final signal molecules, glucocorticoid and noradrenaline, profoundly suppress various inflammatory/immune functions such as leukocyte migration, release of inflammatory mediators, production of cytokines, NK activity and mitogen-induced proliferation of T cells (see review, Madden & Felten, 1995).

Although the expression of CRF in the PVN is enhanced after acute injection of LPS and IL-1β (Kakcuscka et al., 1993; Sapolsky et al., 1987), it has been reported that CRF mRNA in the PVN and CRF levels in the hypophysial portal vein are reduced as a chronic inflammation (adjuvant-induced arthritis) progresses, despite the signs of chronic activation of the HPA axis (an increase in proopiomelanocortine (POMC) mRNA in the anterior pituitary and elevated circulating corticosterone levels) (Harbuz et al., 1992). This paradoxical decrease in PVN CRF mRNA is accompanied by increased arginine vasopressin (AVP) mRNA in the PVN, increased AVP contents in the portal blood, and elevated AVP receptor concentration in the anterior pituitary (Harbuz et al., 1992; Chowdrey et al., 1995). These data suggest that the regulation of the HPA axis by CRF in the PVN may be transferred to AVP which is colocalized with CRF in the PVN neurons during the chronic inflammation (Chowdrey et al., 1995; Shanks et al., 1998).

Lewis rats, which have a genetically determined CRF deficiency and hyporesponsiveness to CRF, exhibit an increased susceptibility to inflammation (Sternberg et al., 1989), whereas Fischer rats, which show CRF hyperresponsiveness, are less susceptible to infection (Sternberg, Wilder, Gold & Chrousos, 1990; Zelazowski et al., 1992). Quite recently, it was demonstrated that i.c.v. transplantation of fetal hypothalamic tissue from inflammatory resistant Fischer (F344/N) rats into inflammatory susceptible Lewis (LEW/N) rats resulted in the reduction of subcutaneous carrageenan inflammation (>85% compared with those of naive or sham-operated LEW/N rats or LEW/N rats transplanted with F344/N spinal cord) (Misiewicz et al., 1997). LEW/N rats transplanted with LEW/N hypothalamic tissues also showed >50% decrease in the peripheral inflammation. These LEW/N rats transplanted with F344/N or LEW/N hypothalamic tissues expressed greater hypothalamic CRF mRNA within the host PVN, but not in the graft, than naive LEW/N rats. Furthermore, higher increases in corticosterone levels to LPS challenge were observed in LEW/N rats transplanted with F344/N hypothalamus. It thus appears that these effects of transplantation on peripheral inflammation may be mediated, at least in part, through the improvement of HPA axis, which otherwise is deficient, secondary to defect in biosynthesis of CRF (Sternberg et al., 1989) in naive LEW/N rats. However, there is no consistent correlation between the changes in CRF mRNA and the changes in peripheral inflammation in both strains of rats transplanted with neuronal tissues from different sources (Misiewicz et al., 1997). This implicates that other factors in addition to CRF may contribute to modulation of peripheral inflammation. In contrast, the transplantation of hypothalamic tissues did not alter the higher percentage of circulating naive versus memory T helper cells in LEW/N rats, suggesting that the hypothalamus has a greater role in the innate inflammatory responses than in the acquired immune processes. These findings suggest the contribution of specific neural tissues and central signal molecules to modulation of peripheral inflammation and to susceptibility to inflammatory diseases (Misiewicz et al., 1997).

Recent studies have revealed that CRF and its receptors are expressed outside the brain. CRF is produced in immune cells and peripheral nerves (sensory nerves and postganglionic sympathetic nerves) particularly under inflammatory conditions, and regulates the inflammation in an autocrine/paracrine fashion. The functional significance of peripheral CRF in the immune/inflammatory responses and nociception was recently reviewed (Schafer, Mousa, & Stein, 1997; Webster et al., 1998).

E. Modulation of Peripheral Inflammation by Central α-MSH

The POMC derivative α-MSH, which occurs widely in the brain, pituitary organs, and peripheral tissues, is a potent inhibitor of acute phase responses including fever, sleep, lymphocyte proliferation, and inflammation (Cannon, Tatro, Reichlin, & Dinarello, 1986; Catania & Lipton, 1994; Hiltz & Lipton, 1989; Lipton, 1989). This peptide may inhibit all the acute phase responses, so far examined, to proinflammatory cytokines such as IL-1, IL-6, and TNF. However, α-MSH cannot antagonize IFN-α-induced firing rate responses of thermosensitive neurons and glucose-responsive neurons in the hypothalamus, although the IL-1β-induced responses of same neurons are abolished by this peptide (Kuriyama et al., 1990; Hori et al., 1991). Similarly, α-MSH suppresses IL-1-induced augmentation of thymocyte proliferation, but not the IL-2-induced proliferation of lymphocytes (Cannon et al., 1986).

α-MSH(1-13) and α-MSH(11-13), when administered systemically (i.v. or i.p.), inhibit an increase in rabbit skin vascular permeability evoked by histamine or leukocyte pyrogen (Lipton, 1988) and edema caused by picryl chloride in the mouse ear (Hiltz & Lipton, 1989). These antiinflammatory effects are considered to be due, at least partially, to actions of α-MSH in the periphery, perhaps directly on inflamed tissues. α-MSH inhibits inflammation by acting on host cells (neutrophils, macrophages) in the periphery through multiple mechanisms, that is the inhibition of production of proinflammatory cytokines and chemokines (IFN-γ, TNF-α, IL-8, monocyte chemotactic protein 1) (Chiao, Foster, Thomas, Lipton, & Star, 1996; Taylor, Streilein, & Cousins, 1992), nitric oxide

(Star et al., 1995) and PGE (Cannon et al., 1986), and the augmentation of production of an antiinflammatory cytokine IL-10 (Bhardwaj et al., 1996).

Furthermore, α-MSH acts centrally to inhibit peripheral inflammation. α-MSH and α-MSH(11-13), when given i.c.v., inhibit peripheral inflammation in mice caused by challenge with several stimuli such as picryl chloride, IL-1β, IL-8, leukotriene B4, and platelet-activating factor (Ceriani, Macaluso, Catania, & Lipton, 1994; Lipton, Macaluso, Hiltz, & Catania, 1991). α-MSH is produced in the POMC-containing neurons in the arcuate nucleus of hypothalamus. Binding sites for the peptide are widely distributed in the brain and several subtypes of melanocortin receptors have been identified within the septal region, hypothalamus, thalamus, and midbrain (Tatro, 1996). α-MSH is released in the brain and the periphery by actions of IL-1 and leukocyte pyrogen (Bell & Lipton, 1987; Martin and Lipton, 1990). It is therefore suggested that proinflammatory cytokines cause various forms of acute phase responses on one hand and evoke central and peripheral release of α-MSH on the other, and this peptide in turn acts centrally and peripherally to prevent overactions of proinflammatory cytokines (Lipton, 1989).

The antiinflammatory messages of central α-MSH seem to be conveyed by descending neural pathway(s), because spinal cord transection completely eliminates the antiinflammatory action of centrally administered α-MSH in mice (Macaluso et al., 1994), and there is no increase in plasma levels of corticosterone after central injection of α-MSH (Lipton et al., 1991).

The perfusion of the medial preoptic hypothalamus with α-MSH in rats, but not that of the ventromedial nucleus, stimulates serotonin activity and inhibits dopamine release locally, as assessed by microdialysis (Gonzalez, Kalia, Hole, & Wilson, 1997). These monoaminergic responses are suggested to mediate the stimulation of aggressive behavior and the inhibition of release of luteinizing hormone caused by α-MSH. The α-MSH-induced increase in serotonin in the medial preoptic area is suggested to be responsible, at least in part, for antiinflammatory activity of α-MSH, because central administration of serotonin, but not dopamine, is shown to attenuate acute peripheral inflammation (Bhattacharya & Das, 1985a).

A pharmacological study of receptors blockade has revealed that β_2-adrenergic receptors in the periphery, but not in the brain, are involved in the suppression of peripheral inflammation by central injection of α-MSH (Macaluso et al., 1994). Blocking of α- and β_1-adrenergic receptors and cholinergic receptors has no effect on the antiinflammatory actions of central α-MSH. Thus, the antiinflammatory action of brain α-MSH is mediated by neural pathways that involve peripheral β_2-adrenergic receptors. In fact, β-adrenergic agonists have been shown to exhibit antiinflammatory actions locally, for example, the inhibition of bradykinin-induced macromolecular leakage from postcapillary venules by β_2-agonist (Svensjo, Persson, & Rutili, 1977) and inhibitory effects of β-adrenergic stimulants on increased vascular permeability caused by allergic mediators (Inagaki, Miura, Daikoku, Nagai, & Koda, 1989).

F. Modulation of the Peripheral Inflammation by Noradrenaline and Serotonin

Proinflammatory cytokines have been shown to modulate the turnover of classical neurotransmitters such as noradrenaline, dopamine, or serotonin. IL-1β increases the turnover of noradrenaline and serotonin in the brain after its i.c.v., intrahypothalamic, or intrafrontal cortical injection in rats and mice (Gemma, Ghezzi, & De Simoni, 1991; Kamikawa, Hori, Nakane, Aou & Tashiro, 1998; Mohankumar, Thyagarajan & Quadri, 1993; Shintani et al., 1993) as well as after its systemic injection (Clement et al., 1997; Dunn, 1988, 1992; Mohankumar & Quadri, 1993; Zalcman et al., 1994). Intrahypothalamic, but not i.p., injection of IL-1β also increases dopamine release in the brain (Dunn, 1992; Shintani et al., 1993). I.c.v. administration of IL-2 increases the concentration of noradrenaline and serotonin in the olfactory bulbectomized rat, an animal model of depression (Song & Leonard, 1995). I.p. injection of IL-2 increased turnover of noradrenaline and dopamine, whereas that of IL-6 increased serotonin and dopamine turnover in the mouse brain (Zalcman et al., 1994). Conversely, neurotransmitters modulate cytokines synthesis and secretion in the brain. Serotonin increases the expression of mRNA of IL-6, TNF-α and TGF-β in rat hippocampal astrocytes (Pousset et al., 1996). Noradrenaline and vasoactive intestinal peptide induce IL-6 secretion by rat astrocytes through cAMP formation (Maimone et al., 1993).

It has long been known that i.c.v. injection of noradrenaline attenuates carrageenan-induced acute edema (Bhattacharya & Das, 1986). The antiinflammatory action of central noradrenaline is substantiated by a finding that depletion of noradrenaline in the PVN by direct injection of 6-hydroxydopamine results in an increase in the severity of adjuvant arthritis, a T-cell-mediated chronic inflammation (Harbuz, Chover-Gonzalez, Biswas, Lightman, &

Chowdrey, 1994). Moreover, the presence of adjuvant arthritis or carrageenan-induced acute edema has been found to increase the noradrenaline turnover in the hypothalamic PVN (Bhattacharya, Das, et al., 1988; Harbuz et al., 1994). It thus appears that the peripheral inflamed tissues signal the brain to activate the central noradrenergic system and the noradrenaline-induced stimulation of the PVN neurons leads to inhibition of inflammatory processes probably via the HPA axis and the sympathetic nervous system. It is possible to suggest that IL-1 plays a role in this feedback loop.

As for the modulatory actions of central serotonin, the results of studies are contradictory. Central administration of serotonin diminishes the carrageenan-induced edema (Bhattacharya & Das, 1985). On the other hand, total body depletion of serotonin (Harbuz et al., 1996), as well as lesions of central serotonergic neurons (Harbuz, Conde, Marti, Lightman, and Jessop, 1997), reduces the severity of the adjuvant arthritis, suggesting a proinflammatory role for central serotonin in this chronic inflammation.

V. EFFECTS OF CENTRAL CYTOKINES AND THE RELATED SUBSTANCES ON NOCICEPTION

There is cumulative evidence that several cytokines and cytokine-induced substances such as prostaglandins, CRF, and noradrenaline in the brain, modulate nociception. Many studies have revealed that an i.c.v. administration of proinflammatory cytokines may alter nociceptive threshold in rats and mice, as assessed by hot-plate test, tail-flick test, and writhing test. However, some of the findings are contradictory. Hyperalgesia was reported after i.c.v. injection of IL-1β, IL-6, and TNF-α, whereas analgesia was observed after that of IL-1α, IL-1β, IL-2, IFN-α, and TNF-α (Table I).

A. Modulation of Nociception by Central Cytokines

1. IL-1β

Among the cytokines produced in the brain, the most intensive studies have focused on the pain

TABLE I Effects of i.c.v. Injection of Cytokines on Nociception

Cytokine	Effect	Dose	Duration	Animal	Method	Possible involvement	Other effects	References[a]
IL-1β	Hyperalgesia	3 pg–0.3 ng	5–60	rat	Hot-plate test	IL-1 receptor, PGs	3–300 ng: no effect	[a]
	Hyperalgesia	3 pg–0.3 ng	5–60	rat	Recording of WDR neuron	IL-1 receptor, PGs	3–300 ng: no effect	[a]
	Hyperalgesia	10 pg	15–30	rat	Hot-plate test	100 ng: no effect		[c]
	Hyperalgesia	5–50 ng	15–55	rat	Tail-flick test			[d]
	No effect	125–2000 (=0.25–4 ng)		rat	Cold-water tail-flick test Hot-plate test		Fever	[e]
	Biphasic							
	Hyperalgesia	10–100 pg	60–180	rat	Paw-pressure test	IL-1 receptor, PGs, CRF		[f]
	Analgesia	1–10 ng	120–180		IL-1 receptor, CRF		Fever	
IL-1α	Analgesia	48 ng/kg[b]	5–20	mouse	Writhing test			[g]
		1 ng		mouse	Writhing test	Peripheral CRF		[h]
	Analgesia	2.5–15 ng	3–5	rat	Hot-plate test			[i]
		5 ng	3	rat	Hot-plate test	central CRF and NA		[j]
	No effect	250–1000 U (=2.5–10 ng)		rat	Cold-water tail-flick test Hot-plate test		Fever	[e]
IL-2	Analgesia			rat	Tail flick test	Opioid receptor		[k]
IL-6	Hyperalgesia	0.3–300 ng	15–30	rat	Hot-plate test	PGs		[l]
TNF-α	Analgesia	1–3.5 ng	3–5	rat	Hot-plate test	IL-1	Decreased locomotion	[i]
	Hyperalgesia	10 pg–1 ng	60	rat	Plantar test	IL-1, PGs		[m]
IFN-α	Analgesia	250–500 U[d]	5	mouse	Hot-plate test	Opioid receptor		[n]
	Analgesia	15000 U		rat	Cold-water tail-flick test			[d]

[a] *a*, Oka et al., 1993; *b*, Oka et al., 1994a; *c*, Tonosaki & Sugimura, 1998; *d*, Wiertelak et al., 1994b; *e*, Adams et al., 1993; *f*, Yabuuchi et al., 1996b; *g*, Nakamura et al., 1988; *h*, Kita et al., 1993; *i*, Bianchi et al., 1992; *j*, Bianchi & Panerai, 1995; *k*, Jiang et al., 1994; *l*, Oka, Oka, Hosoi, & Hori, 1995; *m*, Oka, Wakugawa, et al.,1996; *n*, Blalock & Smith, 1981.

[b] Fifty percent inhibition in 20 g mice.

[c] Time of the maximal effect.

modulatory action of IL-1β, but the findings are conflicting. For example, behavioral studies have suggested that i.c.v. injection of IL-1β induces analgesia (Yabuuchi, Nishiyori, Minami, & Satoh, 1996), hyperalgesia (Oka et al., 1993; Tonosaki & Sugiura, 1998; Watkins, Wiertelak, Goehler, Smith, et al. 1994b; Yabuuchi, Nishiyori, et al., 1996), or has no effect on nociception (Adams, Bussiere, Geller, & Adler, 1993) in rats (Table I). These different results may be attributed partly to the difference of doses of IL-1β administered. The studies on the effect of IL-1β (i.c.v.) at wide dose ranges have revealed that the dose-response relationship is U-shaped (Oka et al., 1993) or biphasic (Yabuuchi, Nishiyori, et al., 1996). Namely, i.c.v. injections of IL-1β at picogram order induce hyperalgesia and those at nanogram order produce either analgesic or no effect (Figure 4A, 4B). In fact, i.c.v. injection of IL-1β at the intermediate doses failed to affect nociceptive behaviors (Adams et al., 1993).

An electrophysiological study in anesthetized rats has shown that i.c.v. injection of IL-1β enhanced responses of wide dynamic range (WDR) neurons in the trigeminal nucleus caudalis to noxious stimuli, (Oka, Aou, & Hori, 1994a) (Figure 4C). The WDR neurons are members of nociceptive neurons and relay somatosensory signals from the nociceptors to the thalamic nuclei. The enhancement of nociceptive neuronal responses is in accordance with the behavioral hyperalgesia in terms of the effective doses

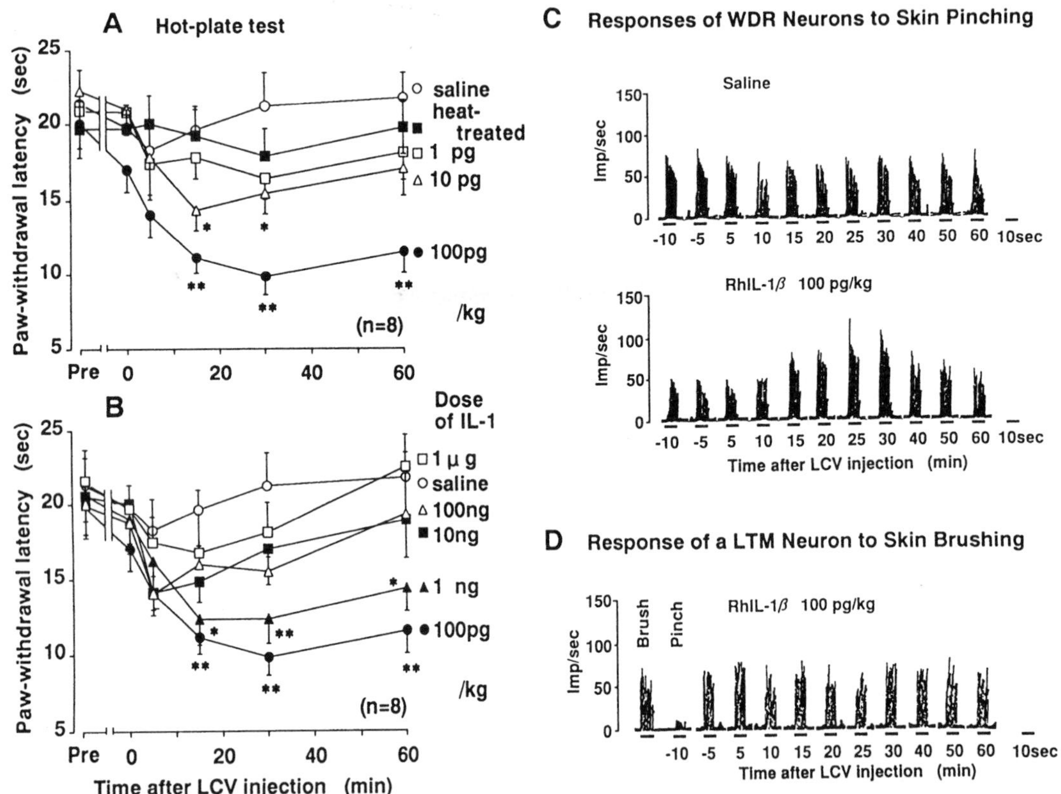

FIGURE 4 Hyperalgesic effects of lateral cerebroventricular (LCV) injection of recombinant human IL-1β (rhIL-1β) on nociception as assessed by a hot-plate test (A and B) and by changes in responses of WDR neurons to noxious pinching (C). In A and B, rats weighing 300–350 g were injected with rhIL-1β at 1 pg/kg (open square, A), 10 pg/kg (open triangle, A), 100 pg/kg (closed circle), 1 ng/kg (closed triangle), 10 ng/kg (closed square, B), 100 ng/kg (open triangle, B) 1 μg/kg (open square, B) or heat-inactivated rhIL-1β at 100 pg/kg (closed square, A), or saline (open circle). Each point represents mean ± SEM. Symbols adjacent to points represent the level of significance when compared with saline-injected controls. $^{*}P < 0.05$;$^{**}P < 0.01$. C: Changes in the responses of WDR neurons to noxious pinching after LCV injection at time 0 of saline and rhIL-1β at 100 pg/kg. Pinching stimuli were applied to the receptive field of the rat's face for a period of 10 sec at the scheduled times. D: The effect of LCV injection of rhIL-1β at 100 pg/kg on the response of a LTM neuron to brushing. Noxious pinching and brushing was applied during the underlined 10-s periods. From Oka et al., Intracerebroventricular injection of interleukin-1β induces hyperalgesia in rats. *Brain Res 624* (1993) 61–68 and Intracerebroventricular injection of interleukin-1β enhances nociceptive neuronal responses of the trigeminal nucleus caudalis in rats. *656* (1994) 236–244 with permission of Elsevier Science, Amsterdam.

(3–300 pg) and the duration of responses (5–60 min). On the other hand, IL-1β did not affect the response of the low threshold mechanoreceptive neurons, which relay the information of innocuous tactile stimuli (Figure 4D). This indicates that the modulatory action of IL-1β on the responsiveness of somatosensory neurons is modality specific.

Furthermore, microinjection studies have demonstrated that the modulatory effects of IL-1β on nociception differ also depending on the injected sites in the brain in rats (Oka, Oka, Hosoi, Aou, & Hori, 1995; Sellami & de Beaurepaire, 1995). Oka, Oka, Hosoi, Aou, et al. (1995) found that the microinjection of IL-1β (1.5–15 pg) into the MPO induced thermal hyperalgesia 15–60 min after injection, showing a maximal response at a dose of 6 pg (Figure 5A, 5B). Since the intraMPO injection of IL-1β at 6 pg did not affect the body temperature, the changes in the nociceptive behavior were not caused secondarily by the altered body temperature (Figure 5C). A similar hyperalgesia was observed after injection of IL-1β at 6 pg into the LPO, the median preoptic nucleus

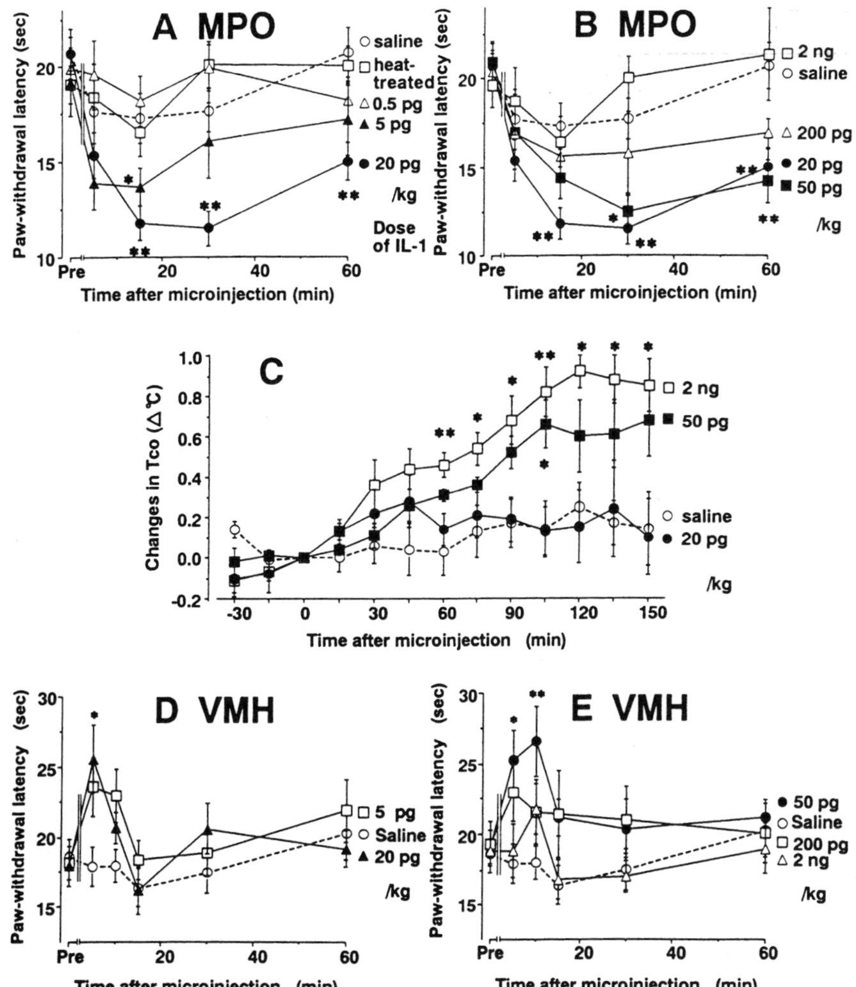

FIGURE 5 The opposing effects of rhIL-1β microinjected into the medial part of the preoptic area (MPO; A, B) and the ventromedial hypothalamus (VMH; D and E) on nociception as assessed by a hot-plate test. C: The effect of intra MPO microinjection of rhIL-1β on body temperature. In A-C, rats weighing 320–350 g were injected with rhIL-1β at 0.5 pg/kg (open triangle, A), 5 pg/kg (closed triangle), 20 pg/kg (closed circle), 50 pg/kg (closed square), 200 pg/kg (open triangle, B) or 2 ng/kg (open square, B and C), or heat inactivated rhIL-1β at 20 pg/kg (open square, A), saline (open circle). In D and E, rats were injected with rhIL-1β at 5 pg/kg (open square, D), 20 pg/kg (closed triangle), 50 pg/kg (closed circle), 200 pg/kg (open square, E) 2 ng/kg (open triangle), saline (open circle), $n = 8$–14. Each point represents mean ± SEM. Symbols adjacent to points represent the level of significance when compared with saline-injected controls. $^{*}P < 0.05$; $^{**}P < 0.01$. From Oka et al., The opposing effects of interleukin-1β microinjected into the preoptic hypothalamus and the ventromedial hypothalamus on nociceptive behavior in rats. *Brain Res 700* (1995) 271–278 with permission of Elsevier Science, Amsterdam.

(MnPO), and the diagonal band of Broca (DBB). However, the microinjection of IL-1β (6–15 pg) into the ventromedial hypothalamus (VMH) produced analgesia with rapid onset and short duration (5–10 min after injection) (Figure 5D, 5E). Another study (Sellami & de Beaurepaire, 1995) demonstrated that IL-1β induces hyperalgesia in the PVN of the hypothalamus and analgesia in the centromedial and gelatinous nuclei of the thalamus. These site-specific effects of IL-1β on nociception might be another explanation for the conflicting reports on altered nociceptive behaviors after i.c.v. injection of IL-1β. It should be noted that both the IL-1β-induced hyperalgesia in the MPO and the analgesia in the VMH are inhibited by pretreatment with either IL-1ra or sodium salicylate and, therefore, hypothalamic IL-1β is suggested to modulate pain through its receptor-mediated and prostanoids-dependent actions (Oka, Oka, Hosoi, Aou, et al., 1995).

Changes in nociception, which are induced by systemic injection of LPS (van Dam et al., 1992), subcutaneous injection of formalin (Yabuuchi, Maruta, et al., 1996), and exposure to repeated cold stress (Tagoh et al., 1995), are known to be associated with expression of IL-1β mRNA in the brain including the nuclei where the microinjection of IL-1β alters nociception. For example, subcutaneous injection of formalin into the rat hindpaws, which is considered to be a model of persistent pain, induced IL-1β mRNA exclusively in the PVN and the dorsomedial hypothalamic nucleus (DMH) (Yabuuchi, Maruta, et al., 1996). An i.c.v. injection of isoproterenol, a β-adrenoceptor agonist, produced a long-lasting analgesia with two peaks (60 and 180 min) and IL-1β mRNA expression in the hypothalamus including the MPO, the PVN and the VMH, the hippocampus, the paraventricular thalamic nucleus, and the central gray matter (Yabuuchi et al., 1997). The second peak of analgesia was antagonized by coadministration of IL-1ra. These findings provide further evidence that IL-1β synthesized in the brain modulates nociception.

2. *IL-1α*

The analgesic responses have been reported after the i.c.v. injection of IL-1α at pyrogenic doses in mice (Kita, Imano, & Nakamura, 1993; Nakamura, Nakanishi, Kita, & Kadokawa, 1988) and that of IL-1α at 2.5–15 ng in rats (Bianchi, Sacerdote, Ricciardi-Castagnoli, Mantegazza, & Panerai, 1992). But it remains to be investigated whether i.c.v. injection of IL-1α at picogram order, like that of IL-1β (Oka et al., 1993; Yabuuchi, Nishiyori, et al., 1996), produces hyperalgesia. The short time course (3–5 min) of the IL-1α-induced analgesia in rats (Bianchi et al., 1992) may be compared with those of the analgesia observed after intra-VMH administration of IL-1β (Oka, Oka, Hosoi, Aou, et al., 1995) and after i.c.v. injection of a high pyrogenic dose of PGE_2 (Oka, Aou, & Hori, 1994b). As to the mechanism of IL-1α-induced analgesia, one report suggested the mediation by central CRF and noradrenaline (Bianchi and Panerai, 1995), whereas another study indicated the involvement of peripheral, but not central, CRF (Kita et al., 1993).

3. *IL-6*

I.c.v. injection of recombinant human IL-6 at doses between 300 pg and 300 ng produced hyperalgesia without febrile responses or, if any, during the period before the development of fever in rats (Oka, Oka, Hosoi, & Hori, 1995). This hyperalgesia was abolished by simultaneous i.c.v. injection of sodium salicylate, suggesting the involvement of prostanoid synthesis. Although it was shown that IL-6 in the peripheral tissues caused hyperalgesia by its ability to produce IL-1 locally (Cunha, Poole, Lorenzetti, & Ferreira, 1992), such a mechanism of IL-1 mediation of the IL-6-induced hyperalgesia is unlikely to operate in the brain because IL-1ra (i.c.v.) did not affect the IL-6-induced hyperalgesia (Oka, Oka, Hosoi, & Hori 1995).

4. *TNF-α*

TNF-α, like IL-1β, produces hyperalgesia at low doses (Oka, Wakugawa, Hosoi, Oka, & Hori, 1996) and analgesia at high doses (Bianchi et al., 1992). I.c.v. injection of TNF-α (10 pg–1 ng) induced a slow and long-lasting (30–90 min) hyperalgesia without affecting the body temperature in rats (Oka, Wakugawa, et al., 1996). This hyperalgesia was blocked by IL-1ra and diclofenac, suggesting the mediation by TNF-α-induced IL-1 production and subsequent synthesis of prostanoids. On the other hand, another study (Bianchi et al., 1992) demonstrated that i.c.v. injection of TNF-α (1–3.5 ng) induced a rapid brief (3–5 min after injection) analgesia. This analgesia was antagonized by anti-IL-1 antibodies. However, it was not blocked by neither indomethacin (a COX inhibitor), naloxone (an opioid receptor antagonist), nor antisera against β-endorphin, met-enkephalin, and dynorphin. This indicates that the TNF-α-induced analgesia is also mediated by IL-1 but not by prostanoids or opioid peptides.

5. *IFNα*

Central administration of IFN-α has been demonstrated to induce analgesia in mice and rats (Adams et al., 1993; Blalock & Smith, 1981). Since this analgesia

(Bianchi et al., 1995). This noradrenaline-induced analgesia is compatible with antiinflammatory action of central noradrenaline. On the other hand, analgesia induced by the activation of central noradrenergic system is suggested to be mediated in part by induction of IL-1β in the brain (Yabuuchi et al., 1997). The involvement of central serotonin in the pain modulatory actions of cytokines is not known at present. Although the catecholaminergic and serotonergic systems are involved in the descending pain inhibitory system in the lower brainstem, little is known about their involvement in the cytokine-induced alteration of nociception. More detailed studies are required to elucidate the complicated mechanisms of pain modulatory actions of central noradrenaline and serotonin.

F. Biological Significance of Pain Modulatory Actions of Central Cytokines

The hyperalgesia induced by central cytokines and PGE_2 in small, nonpyrogenic amounts might explain systemic hyperalgesia clinically observed in the early phase of infectious diseases. It would serve as a warning signal of infection before the development of typical sickness symptoms including fever, sleepiness, anorexia, activation of the HPA axis and the sympathetic nervous system, and hypoalgesia. The switching of nociception from hyperalgesia to hypoalgesia that is accompanied by other sickness symptoms may be understood to reflect the changes of the strategy of the host for fighting microbial invasion with the progress of diseases.

Acknowledgments

This work was supported by grants-in-aid for scientific research (No.10307001 and No. 09557006 to T. Hori and No. 10557008 and No. 08457021 to T. Katafuchi) from the Ministry of Education, Science, and Culture, Japan.

References

Adams, J. U., Bussiere, J. L., Geller, E. B., & Adler, M. W. (1993). Pyrogenic doses of intracerebroventricular interleukin-1 did not induce analgesia in the rat hot-plate or cold-water tail flick tests. *Life Sciences, 53*, 1401–1409.

Ahmed, M. S., Llanos-Q, J., Dinarello, C. A., & Blatteis, C. M. (1985). Interleukin 1 reduces opioid binding in guinea pig brain. *Peptides, 6*, 1149–1154.

Akiyama, H., Ikeda, K., Katoh, M., McGeer, E. G., & McGeer, P. L. (1994). Expression of MRP14, 27E10, interferon-α and leukocyte common antigen by reactive microglia in postmortem human brain tissue. *Journal of Neuroimmunology, 50*, 195–201.

Alheim, K., Andersson, C., Tingsborg, S., Ziolkowska, M., Shulzberg, M., & Bartfai, T. (1991). Interleukin-1 expression is inducible by nerve growth factor in PC12 pheochromocytoma cells. *Proceedings of the National Academy of Sciences of the United States of America, 88*, 9302–9306.

Aloe, L., Alleva, E., Bohm, A., & Levi-Montalcini, R. (1986). Aggressive behavior induces release of nerve growth factor from mouse salivary gland into the bloodstream. *Proceedings of the National Academy of Sciences of the United States of America, 83*, 6184–6187.

Ando, T., Ichijo, T., Katafuchi, T., & Hori, T. (1995). Intracerebroventricular injection of prostaglandin E_2 increases splenic sympathetic nerve activity in rats. *American Journal of Physiology, 269*(3 Pt2), R662–R668.

Ban, E., Haour, F., & Lenstra, R. (1992). Brain interleukin-1 gene expression induced by peripheral lipopolysaccharide administration. *Cytokine, 4*, 48–54.

Band, L. C., Pert, A., Williams, W., de Costa, B. R., Rice, K. C. & Weber R. J. (1992). Central μ-opioid receptors mediate suppression of natural killer activity in vivo. *Progress in Neuroendocrinimmunology, 5*, 95–101.

Banks, W. A., Kastin, A. J., & Broadwell, R. D. (1995). Passage of cytokines across the blood-brain barrier. *Neuroimmunomodulation, 2*, 241–248.

Bell, R. C., & Lipton, J. M. (1987). Pulsatile release of antipyretic neuropeptide α-MSH from septum of rabbit during fever. *American Journal of Physiology, 252*(6 Pt2), R1152–R1157.

Benigni, F., Fantuzzi, G., Sironi, M., Sacco, S., Pozzi, P., Dinarello, C. A., Sipe, J. D., Poli, V., Cappelletti, M., Paonessa, G., Panayotatos, N., Pennica, D., & Ghezzi, P. (1996). Six different cytokines that share gp130 as a receptor subunit, induce serum amyloid A and potentiate the induction of interleukin-6 and the activation of the hypothalamus-pituitary-adrenal axis by interleukin-1. *Blood, 87*, 1851–1854.

Benigni, F., Villa, P., Demitri, M. T., Sacco, S., Sipe, J. D., Lagunowich, L., Panayotatos, N., & Ghezzi, P. (1995). Ciliary neurotrophic factor (CNTF) inhibits brain and peripheral TNF production and, in association with its soluble receptor, protects mice against LPS toxicity. *Molecular Medicine, 1*, 568–575.

Besedovsky, H. O., Del Rey, A., Klusman, I., Furukawa, H., Monge Arditi, G., & Kabiersch, A. (1991). Cytokines as modulators of the hypothalamus-pituitary-adrenal axis. *Journal of Steroid Biochemistry and Molecular Biology, 40*, 613–618.

Bester, H., Menendez, L., Besson, J. M., & Bernard, J. F. (1995). Spino (trigemino) parabrachiohypothalamic pathway: Electrophysiological evidence for an involvement in pain processes. *Journal of Neurophysiology, 73*, 568–585.

Bhardwaj, R. S., Schwarz, A., Becher, E., Mahnke, K., Aragane, Y., Schwarz, T, & Luger, T. A. (1996). Proopiomelanocortin-derived peptides induce IL-10 production in human monocytes. *Journal of Immunology, 156*, 2517–2521.

Bhattacharya, S. K. (1986). The antinociceptive effect of intracerebroventricularly administered prostaglandin D_2 in the rat. *Psychopharmacology, 89*, 121–124.

Bhattacharya, S. K., & Das, N. (1984a). Effect of carrageenan-induced pedal oedema on rat brain prostaglandins. *Neurochemical Pathology, 2*, 163–169.

Bhattacharya, S. K., & Das, N. (1984b). Effect of central prostaglandins on carrageenan-induced pedal oedema in rats. *Journal of Pharmacy and Pharmacology, 36*, 768–769.

Bhattacharya, S. K., & Das, N. (1985a). Central serotonergic modulation of carrageenan-induced pedal inflammation in rats. *Pharmaceutical Research, 6*, 315–318.

Bhattacharya, S. K., & Das, N. (1985b). Anti-inflammatory effect of intracerebroventricular administrated histamine in rats. *Agents Actions, 17*, 150–152.

Bhattacharya, S. K., & Das, N. (1986). Central catecholaminergic modulation of carrageenan-induced pedal oedema in rats. *Research in Experimental Medicine, 186*, 365–374.

Bhattacharya, S. K., Das, N., & Mohan Rao, P. J. (1988). Brain monoamines during carrageenan-induced acute paw inflammation in rats. *Journal of Pharmacy and Pharmacology, 40*, 518–520.

Bhattacharya, S. K., Mohan Rao, P. J., Das, N., & Das Gupta, G. (1988). Intracerebroventricularly administered bradykinin augments carrageenan-induced paw oedema in rats. *Journal of Pharmacy and Pharmacology, 40*, 367–369.

Bhattacharya, S. K., Mohan Rao, P. J., & Das Gupta, G. (1989). Effect of centrally administered prostaglandin D2 and some prostaglandin synthesis inhibitors on carrageenan-induced paw oedema in rats. *Journal of Pharmacy and Pharmacology, 41*, 569–571.

Bhattacharya, S. K., & Sarkar, M. K. (1986). Effect of some centrally administered putative amino acid neurotransmitters on carrageenan-induced paw oedema in rats. *Journal of Pharmacy and Pharmacology, 38*, 144–146.

Bianchi, M., & Panerai, A. (1995). CRH and the noradrenergic system mediate the antinociceptive effect of central interleukin-1α in the rat. *Brain Research Bulletin, 36*, 113–117.

Bianchi, M., Sacerdote, P., Ricciardi-Castagnoli, P., Mantegazza, P., & Panerai, A. E. (1992). Central effects of tumor necrosis factor-α and interleukin-1α on nociceptive thresholds and spontaneous locomotor activity. *Neuroscience Letters, 148*, 76–80.

Bjorkman, R. L., Hedner, T., Hallman, K. M., Henning, M., & Hedner, J. (1992). Localization of the central antinociceptive effects of diclofenac in the rat. *Brain Research, 590*, 66–73.

Blalock, J. E., & Smith, E. M. (1980). Human leukocyte interferon: structural and biological relatedness to adrenocorticotropic hormone and endorphins. *Proceedings of the National Academy of Sciences of the United States of America, 77*, 5972–5974.

Blalock, J. E., & Smith, E. M. (1981). Human leukocytic interferon (HuIFN-α): Potent endorphin-like opioid activity. *Biochemical and Biophysical Research Communications, 101*, 472–478.

Blatteis, C. M., & Sehic, E. (1997). Prostaglandin E2: A putative fever mediator. In P. A. Mackowiak (Ed.), *Fever: Basic mechanisms and management* (pp. 117–145), Philadelphia: Lippincott-Raven.

Blotta, M. H., DeKruyff, R. H., & Umetsu, D. T. (1997). Corticosteroids inhibit IL-12 production in human monocytes and enhance their capacity to induce IL-4 synthesis in CD4+ lymphocytes. *Journal of Immunology, 158*, 5589–5595.

Borgeson, M., Tallent, M. W., & Keane, R. W. (1989). Astrocyte modulation of central nervous system immune responses. In E. J. Goetzl and N. H. Spector (Ed.), *Neuroimmune networks: Physiology and diseases*, (pp. 51–55), New York: Alan R. Liss.

Brandt, E. R., Mackay, I. R., Hertzog, P. J., Cheetham, B. A., Sherritt, M., & Bernard, C. C. (1993). Molecular detection of interferon-α expression in multiple sclerosis brain. *Journal of Neuroimmunology, 44*, 1–5.

Breder, C. D., Hazuka, C., Ghayur, T., Klug, C., Huginin, M., Yasuda, K., Teng, M., & Saper, C. B. (1994). Regional induction of tumor necrosis factor α expression in the mouse brain after systemic lipopolysaccharide administration. *Proceedings of the National Academy of Sciences of the United States of America, 91*, 11393–11397.

Breder, C. D., Tsujimoto, M., Terano, Y., Scott, D. W., & Saper, C. B. (1993). Distribution and characterization of tumor necrosis factor-α-like immunoreactivity in the murine central nervous system. *Journal of Comparative Neurology, 337*, 543–567.

Brown, R., Li, Z., Vriend, C. Y., Nirula, R., Janz, L., Falk, J., Nance, D. M., Dyck, D. G. & Greenberg, A. H. (1991). Suppression of splenic macrophage interleukin-1 secretion following intracerebroventricular injection of interleukin-1β: Evidence for pituitary-adrenal and sympathetic control. *Cellular Immunology, 132*, 84–93.

Burstein, R., Dado, R. J., Cliffer, K. D., & Giesler, G. J. Jr. (1991). Physiological characterization of spinohypothalamic tract neurons in the lumbar enlargement of rats. *Journal of Neurophysiology, 66*, 261–284.

Cannon, J. G., Tatro, J. B., Reichlin, S., & Dinarello, C. A. (1986). Alpha melanocyte stimulating hormone inhibits immunostimulatory and inflammatory actions of interleukin 1. *Journal of Immunology, 137*, 2232–2236.

Carstens, E., MacKinnon, J. D., & Guinan, M. J. (1982). Inhibition of spinal dorsal horn neuronal responses to noxious skin heating by medial preoptic and septal stimulation in the cat. *Journal of Neurophysiology, 48*, 981–991.

Catania, A., Arnold, J., Macaluso, A., Hiltz, M. E., & Lipton, J. M. (1991). Inhibition of acute inflammation in the periphery by central action of salicylates. *Proceedings of the National Academy of Sciences of the United States of America, 88*, 8544–8547.

Catania, A., & Lipton, J. M. (1994). The neuropeptide alpha-melanocyte-stimulating hormone: a key component of neuroimmunomodulation. Neuroimmunomodulation, *1*, 93–99.

Ceriani, G., Macaluso, A., Catania, A., & Lipton, J. M. (1994). Central neurogenic antiinfllammatory action of α-MSH: Modulation of peripheral inflammation induced by cytokines and other mediators of inflammation. *Neuroendocrinology, 59*, 138–143.

Chiao, H., Foster, S., Thomas, R., Lipton, J. M., & Star, R. A. (1996). Alpha-melanocyte-stimulating hormone reduces endotoxin-induced liver inflammation. *Journal of Clinical Investigation, 97*, 2038–2044.

Chowdrey, H. S., Larsen, P. J., Harbuz, M. S., Jessop, D. S., Aguilera, G., Eckland, D. J., & Lightman, S. L. (1995). Evidence for arginine vasopressin as the primary activator of the HPA axis during adjuvant-induced arthritis. *British Journal of Pharmacology, 116*, 2417–2424.

Clement, H. W., Buschmann, J., Rex, S., Grote, C., Opper, C., Gemsa, D., & Wesemann, W. (1997). Effects of interferon-γ, interleukin-1β, and tumor necrosis factor-α on the serotonin metabolism in the nucleus raphe dorsalis of the rat. *Journal of Neural Transmission, 104*, 981–991.

Coceani, F., Lees, J., Mancilla, J., Berlizario, J., & Dinarello, C. A. (1993). Interleukin-6 and tumor necrosis factor in cerebrospinal fluid: Changes during pyrogen fever. *Brain Research, 612*, 165–171.

Coleman, R. A., Smith, W. L., & Narumiya, S. (1994). VIII. International Union of Pharmacology classification of Prostanoid receptors: properties, distribution and structure of the receptors and their subtypes. *Pharmacological Reviews, 46*, 205–229.

Connor, T. J., Song, C., Leonard, B. E., Merali, Z. & Anisman, H. (1998). An assessment of the effects of central interleukin-1b, -2, -6, and tumor necrosis factor-a administration on some behavioural, neurochemical, endocrine and immune parameters in the rat. *Neuroscience, 84*, 923–933.

Cunha, F. Q., Poole, S., Lorenzetti, B. B., & Ferreira, S. H. (1992). The pivotal role of tumor necrosis factor α in the development of inflammatory hyperalgesia. *British Journal of Pharmacology, 107*, 660–664.

Das, N., & Bhattacharya, S. K. (1985). Central cholinergic modulation of carrageenan-induced pedal inflammation in rats. *Pharmaceutical Research, 3*, 137–139.

DeLeo, J. A., Colburn, R. W., Nichols, M., & Malhotra, A. (1996). Interleukin-6-mediated hyperalgesia/allodynia and increased spinal IL-6 expression in a rat mononeuropathy model. *Journal of Interferon and Cytokine Research, 16*, 695–700.

Diab, A., Zhu, J., Lindquist, L., Wretlind, B., Link, H., & Bakhiet, M. (1997). Cytokine mRNA profiles during the course of experimental Haemphilius influenzae bacterial meningitis. *Clinical Immunology and Immunopathology, 85*, 236–245.

DiSanto, E., Sironi, M., Pozzi, P., Gnocchi, P., Isseta, A. M., Delvaux, A., Goldman, M., Marchant, A., & Ghezzi, P. (1995). Interleukin-10 inhibits lipopolysaccharide-induced tumor necrosis factor and interleukin-1β production in the brain without affecting the activation of the hypothalamus-pituitary-adrenal axis. *Neuroimmunomodulation, 2*, 149–154.

Dulaney, R., Macaluso, A., Woerner, J., Hiltz, M. A., Catania, A., & Lipton, J. M. (1992). Changes in peripheral inflammation induced by the central actions of an α-MSH analog and of endogenous pyrogen. *Progress in Neuroendocrinimmunology, 5*, 179–186.

Dunn, A. J. (1988). Systemic interleukin-1 administration stimulates hypothalamic norepinephrine metabolism paralleling the increased plasma corticosterone. *Life Sciences, 43*, 429–435.

Dunn, A. J. (1992). Endotoxin-induced activation of cerebral catecholamine and serotonin metabolism: comparison with interleukin-1. *Journal of Pharmacology and Experimental Therapeutics, 261*, 964–969.

Faggioni, R., Benigni, F., & Ghezzi, P. (1995). Proinflammatory cytokines as pathogenetic mediators in central nervous system: Brain-periphery connection. *Neuroimmunomodulation, 2*, 2–15.

Fannon, L. D., & Phillips, M. I. (1991). Chronic ICV infusion of neuropeptides alters lymphocyte populations in experimental rodents. *Regulatory Peptides, 34*, 189–195.

Fecho, K., Maslonek, K. A., Dykstra, L. A., & Lysle, D. T. (1993). Alterations of immune status induced by the sympathetic nervous system: immunomodulatory effects of DMPP alone and in conjunction with morphine. *Brain, Behavior, and Immunity, 7*, 253–270.

Fiorentino, D. F., Bond, M. W., & Mosmann, T. R. (1989). Two types of mouse T helper cell. IV. TH2 clones secrete a factor that inhibits cytokine production by TH1 clones. *Journal of Experimental Medicine, 170*, 2081–2095.

Follenfant, R. L., Nakamura-Craig, M., Henderson, B., & Higgs, G. A. (1989). Inhibition by neuropeptides of interleukin-1β-induced, prostaglandin-independent hyperalgesia. *British Journal of Pharmacology, 98*, 41–43.

Gadient, R. A., & Otten, U. (1995). Interleukin-6 and interleukin-6 receptor mRNA expression in rat central nervous system. *Annals of the New York Academy of Sciences, 762*, 403–406.

Gemma, C., Ghezzi, P., & De Simoni, M. G. (1991). Activation of the hypothalamic serotoninergic system by central interleukin-1. *European Journal of Pharmacology, 209*, 139–140.

Gerard, C., Bruyns, C., Marchant, A., Abramowicz, D., Vandenabeele, P., Delvaux, A., Fiers, W., Goldman, M., & Velu, Y. (1993). Interleukin 10 reduces the release of tumor necrosis factor and prevents lethalty in experimental endotoxemia. *Journal of Experimental Medicine, 177*, 547–550.

Green, P. G., Miao, F. J. P., Janig, W., & Levine, J. D. (1995). Negative feedback neuroendocrine control of the inflammatory response in rats. *Journal of Neuroscience, 15*, 4678–4686.

Gonzalez, M. I., Kalia, V., Hole, D. R., & Wilson, C. A. (1997). α-melanocyte-stimulating hormone (α-MSH) and melanin-concentrating hormone (MCH) modify monoaminergic levels in the preoptic area of the rat. *Peptides, 18*, 387–392.

Guillet, C., Fourcin, M., Chevalier, S., Pouplard, A., & Gascan, H. (1995). ELISA detection of circulating levels of LIF, OSM, and CNTF in septic shock. *Annals of the New York Academy of Sciences, 762*, 407–409.

Hall, D. M., Suo, J.-L., & Weber, R. J. (1998). Opioid mediated effects on the immune system: sympathetic nervous system involvement. *Journal of Neuroimmunology, 83*, 29–35.

Hansen, M. K., Taishi, P., Chen, Z., & Krueger, J. M. (1998). Vagotomy blocks the induction of interleukin-1β (IL-1β) mRNA in the brain of rats in response to systemic IL-1β. *The Journal of Neuroscience, 18*, 2247–2253.

Harbuz, M. S., Chover-Gonzalez, A. J., Biswas, S., Lightman, S. L., & Chowdrey, H. S. (1994). Role of central catecholamines in the modulation of corticotrophin-releasing factor mRNA during adjuvant-induced arthritis in the rat. *British Journal of Rheumatology, 33*, 205–209.

Harbuz, M. S., Conde, G. L., Marti, O., Lightman, S. L., & Jessop, D. S. (1997). The hypothalamic-pituitary-adrenal axis in autoimmunity. *Annals of the New York Academy of Sciences, 823*, 214–224.

Harbuz, M. S., Perveen-Gill, Z., Lalies, M. D., Jessop, D. S., Lightman, S. L., & Chowdrey, H. S. (1996). The role of endogenous serotonin in adjuvant-induced arthritis in the rat. *British Journal of Rheumatology, 35*, 112–116.

Harbuz, M. S., Rees, R. G., Eckland, D., Jessop, D. S., Brewerton, D., & Lightman, S. L. (1992). Paradoxical responses of hypothalamic corticotropin-releasing factor (CRF) messenger ribonucleic acid (mRNA) and CRF-41 peptide and adenohypophysial proopiomelanocortin mRNA during chronic inflammatory stress. *Endocrinology, 130*, 1394–1400.

Hargreaves, K. M., Dubner, R., & Costello, A. H. (1989). Corticotropin releasing factor (CRF) has a peripheral site of action for antinociception. *European Journal of Pharmacology, 170*, 275–279.

Hargreaves, K. M., Flores, C. M., Dionne, R. A., & Mueller, G. P. (1990). The role of pituitary β-endorphin in mediating corticotropin-releasing factor-induced antinociception. *American Journal of Physiology, 258* (2 Pt1), E235–E242.

Hernandez, M. C., Flores, L. R., & Bayer, B. M. (1993). Immunosuppression by morphine is mediated by central pathways. *Journal of Pharmacology and Experimental Therapeutics, 267*, 1336–1341.

Hillhouse, E. W., & Mosley, K. (1993). Peripheral endotoxin induces hypothalamic immunoreactive interleukin-1β in the rat. *British Journal of Pharmacology, 109*, 289–290.

Hiltz, M. E., & Lipton, J. M. (1989). Antiinflammatory activity of a COOH-terminal fragment of the neuropeptide α-MSH. *FASEB Journal, 3*, 2282–2284.

Hori, T., Kaizuka, Y., & Katafuchi, T. (1996). Thermoregulation and immunity: the brain-immune interaction mechanisms. In K. Shiraki, K., S. Sagawa & M. K. Yousef (Ed.), *Physiological basis of occupational health: stressful environments*, (pp. 31–40). Amsterdam: SPB Academic Publishing bv.

Hori, T., Katafuchi, T., Take, S., and Shimizu, N. (1998). Neuroimmunomodulatory actions of hypothalamic interferon-α. *Neuroimmunomodulation, 5*, 172–177.

Hori, T., Katafuchi, T., Take, S., Shimizu, N., & Niijima, A. (1995). The autonomic nervous system as a communication channel between the brain and the immune system. *Neuroimmunomodulation, 2*, 203–215.

Hori, T., Nakashima, T., Take, S., Kaizuka, Y., Mori, T., & Katafuchi, T. (1991). Immune cytokines and regulation of body temperature, food intake and cellular immunity. *Brain Research Bulletin, 27*, 309–313.

Hori, T., Oka, T., Hosoi, M., & Aou, S. (1998). Pain modulatory actions of cytokines and prostaglandin E2 in the brain. *Annals of the New York Academy of Sciences, 840*, 269–281.

Hori, T., Shibata, M., Nakashima, T., Yamasaki, M., Asami, A., Asami, T., & Koga, H. (1988). Effects of interleukin-1 and arachidonate on the preoptic and anterior hypothalamic neurons. *Brain Research Bulletin, 20*, 75–82.

Hosoi, M., Oka, T., & Hori, T. (1997). Prostaglandin E receptor EP_3 subtype is involved in thermal hyperalgesia through its actions in the preoptic hypothalamus and the diagonal band of Broca in rats. *Pain, 71*, 303–311.

Houssiau, F. A., Bukasa, K., & Sindic, C. J. M. (1988). Elevated levels of the 26K human hybridoma growth factor (interleukin 6) in cerebrospinal fluid of patients with acute infection of the central nervous system. *Clinical and Experimental Immunology, 71*, 320–323.

Howard, M., Muchamel, T., Andrade, S., & Menon, S. (1993). Interleukin 10 protects mice from lethal endotoxemia. *Journal of Experimental Medicine, 177*, 1205–1208.

Ho-Yen, D. O., & Carrington, D. (1987). Alpha-interferon responses in cerebrospinal fluid of patients with suspected meningitis. *Journal of Clinical Pathology, 40*, 83–86.

Ichijo, T., Katafuchi, T., & Hori, T. (1994). Central administration of interleukin-1β enhances splenic sympathetic nerve activity in rats. *Brain Research Bulletin, 34*, 547–553.

Inagaki, N., Miura, T., Daikoku, M., Nagai, H., & Koda, A. (1989). Inhibitory effects of β-adrenergic stimulants on increased vascular permeability caused by passive cutaneous anaphylaxis, allergic mediators, and mediator releasers in rats. *Pharmacology, 39*, 19–27.

Irwin, M. (1993). Brain corticotropin-releasing hormone- and interleukin-1 β-induced suppression of specific antibody production. *Endocrinology, 133*, 1352–1360.

Irwin, M., Hauger, R., Brown, M. & Britton, K. T. (1988). CRF activates autonomic nervous system and reduces natural killer cytotoxicity. *American Journal of Physiology, 255*(5 Pt2), R744–R747.

Irwin, M., Vale, W., & Rivier, C. (1990). Central corticotropin-releasing factor mediates the suppressive effect of stress on natural killer cytotoxicity. *Endocrinology, 126*, 2837–2844.

Janicki, P. K. (1992). Binding of human alpha-interferon in the brain tissue membranes of the rat. *Research Communication of Chemistry, Pathology and Pharmacology, 75*, 117–120.

Jiang, C., Xu, D., Zheng, Z., Fan, P., Liu, X., You, Z., Song, C., Wang, C., & Lu, C. (1994). The central analgesic effect of IL-2. *Chinese Journal of Applied Physiology, 10*, 322–324.

Kakucska, I., Qi, Y., Clark, B. D., & Lechan, R. M. (1993). Endotoxin-induced corticotropin-releasing hormone gene expression in the hypothalamic paraventricular nucleus is mediated centrally by interleukin-1. *Endocrinology, 133*, 815–821.

Kamikawa, H., Hori, T., Nakane, H., Aou, S., & Tashiro, N. (1998). IL-1β increases norepinephrine level in rat frontal cortex: Involvement of prostanoids, NO, and glutamate. *American Journal of Physiology, 275*(3 Pt2), R803–R810.

Katafuchi, T., Ichijo, T., & Hori, T. (1997). Sequential relationship between actions of CRF and PGE_2 in the brain on splenic sympathetic nerve activity in rats. *Journal of the Autonomic Nervous System, 67*, 200–206.

Katafuchi, T., Ichijo, T., Take, S., & Hori, T. (1993). Hypothalamic modulation of natural killer cell activity in rats. *Journal of Physiology (Lond.), 471*, 209–221.

Katafuchi, T., Kondo, T., Take, S., & Hori, T. (1998). Hypothalamic modulation of delayed-type hypersensitivity and splenic natural killer cell activity. In Y. Oomura & T. Hori (Eds.), *Brain and biodefence*, (pp. 3–11). Tokyo: Japan Scientific Societies Press & Basel: S. Karger AG.

Katafuchi, T., Take, S., & Hori, T. (1993). Roles of sympathetic nervous system in the suppression of cytotoxicity of splenic natural killer cells in the rat. *Journal of Physiology (Lond.), 465*, 343–357.

Katsuura, G., Arimura, A., Koves, K., & Gottschall, P. E. (1990). Involvement of organum vasculosum lamina terminalis and preoptic area in interleukin-1β-induced ACTH release. *American Journal of Physiology, 258*(1 Pt1), E163–E171.

Kinouchi, K., Brown, G., Pasternak, G., & Donner, D. B. (1991). Identification and characterization of receptors for tumor necrosis factor–alpha in the brain. *Biochemistry, Biophysics Research Communication, 181*, 1532–1538.

Kita, A., Imano, K., & Nakamura, H. (1993). Involvement of corticotropin-releasing factor in the antinociception produced by interleukin-1 in mice. *European Journal of Pharmacology, 237*, 317–322.

Klir, J. J., Roth, J., Szelenyi, Z., McClellan, J. L., & Kluger, M. J. (1993). Role of hypothalamic interleukin-6 and tumor necrosis factor-α in LPS fever in rat. *American Journal of Physiology, 265*(3 Pt2), R512–R517.

Kluger, M. J., Kozak, W., Conn, C. A., Leon, L. R., & Soszynski, D. (1997). The adaptive value of fever. In P. A. Mackowiak (Ed.), *Fever: Basic mechanisms and management*, (pp. 255–266), Philadelphia: Lippincott-Raven.

Komaki, G., Arimura, A., & Koves, K. (1992). Effect of intravenous injection of IL-1β on PGE_2 levels in several brain areas as determined by microdialysis. *American Journal of Physiology, 262*(2 Pt1), E246–E251.

Kuriyama, K., Hori, T., Mori, T., & Nakashima, T. (1990). Actions of interferon-α and interleukin-1β on glucose-responsive neurons in the ventromedial hypothalamus. *Brain Research Bulletin, 24*, 803–810.

Lacroix, S., & Rivest, S. (1998). Effect of acute systemic inflammatory response and cytokines on the transcription of the genes encoding cyclooxygenase enzymes (COX-1 and COX-2) in the rat brain. *Journal of Neurochemistry, 70*, 452–466.

Laye, S., Bluthe, R. M., Kent, S., Combe, C., Medina, C., Parnet, P., Kelley, K., & Dantzer, R. (1995). Subdiaphragmatic vagotomy blocks induction of IL-1β mRNA in mice brain in response to peripheral LPS. *American Journal of Physiology, 268*(5 Pt2), R1327–R1331.

Laye, S., Parnet, P., Goujon, E., and Dantzer, R. (1994). Peripheral administration of lipopolysaccharide induces the expression of cytokines transcripts in the brain and pituitary of mice. *Molecular Brain Research, 27*(1), 157–162.

Lieberman, A. P., Pitha, P. M., Shin, H. S., & Shin, M. L. (1989). Production of tumor necrosis factor and other cytokines by astrocytes stimulated with lipopolysaccharide or a neurotropic virus. *Proceedings of the National Academy of Sciences of the United States of America, 86*, 6348–6352.

Lipton, J. M. (1988). α-MSH in CNS control of fever and its influence on inflammation/immune responses. In M. E. Hadley (Ed.), *The melanotropic peptides*, (pp. 97–113), Boca Raton, FL: CRC Press.

Lipton, J. M. (1989). Neuropeptide α-melanocyte-stimulating hormone in control of fever, the acute phase response, and inflammation. In E. J. Goetzl & N. H. Spector (Eds.) *Neuroimmune networks: Physiology and diseases*, (pp. 243–250). New York: Alan R. Liss.

Lipton, J. M., Macaluso, A., Hiltz, M. E., & Catania, A. (1991). Central administration of the peptide α-MSH inhibits inflammation in the skin. *Peptides, 12*, 795–798.

Liu, C. H., Takao, T., Hashimoto, K., & De Souza, E. B. (1996). Interleukin-1 receptors in the nervous system. In N. J. Rothwell (Ed.) *Cytokines and the nervous system* (pp. 21–40), Austin, TX: R. G. Landes.

Lloyd, A., Hickie, I., Brockman, A., Dwyer, J., & Wakefield, D. (1991). Cytokine levels in serum and cerebrospinal fluid in patients with chronic fatigue syndrome and control subjects. *Journal of Infectious Diseases, 164*, 1023–1024.

Low, K. G., Allen, R. G., & Melner, M. H. (1992). Differential regulation of proenkephalin expression in astrocytes by cytokines. *Endocrinology, 131*, 1908–1914.

Lysle, D. T., Leucken, L. J., & Masloned, K. A. (1992). Modulation of immune status by a conditioned aversive stimulus: Evidence for the involvement of endogenous opioids. *Brain, Behavior, and Immunity, 6*, 179–188.

Macaluso, A., McCoy, D., Watanabe, T., Biltz, J., Catania, A., & Lipton, J. M. (1994), Antiinflammatory influence of α-MSH molecules: Central neurogenic and peripheral actions. *Journal of Neuroscience, 14*, 2377–2382.

Madden, K. S., & Felten, D. L. (1995). Experimental basis for neural-immune interactions. *Physiological Reviews, 75*, 77–106.

Maimone, D., Cioni, C., Rosa, S., Macchia, G., Aloisi, F., & Annunziata, P. (1993). Norepinephrine and vasoactive intestinal peptide induce IL-6 secretion by astrocytes: Synergism with IL-1β and TNFα. *Journal of Neuroimmunology, 47*, 73–82.

Marie, C., Pitton, C., Fitting, C., & Cavaillon, J. M. (1996). IL-10 and IL-4 synergize with TNF-α to induce IL-1ra production by human neutrophils. *Cytokine, 8*, 147–151.

Martin, L. W., & Lipton, J. M. (1990). Acute phase response to endotoxin; rise in plasma α-MSH and effects of α-MSH injection. . *American Journal of Physiology, 259*(4 Pt2), R768–R772.

Matsuda, T., Hori, T., & Nakashima, T. (1992). Thermal and PGE_2 sensitivity of the organum vasculosum lamina terminalis region and preoptic area in rat brain slices. *Journal of Physiology, 454*, 197–212.

Matsumura, K., Cao, K., Ozaki, M., Morii, H., Nakadate, K., & Watanabe, Y. (1998). Brain endothelial cells express cyclooxygenase-2 during lipopolysaccharide-induced fever: Light and electron microscopic immunocytochemical studies. *Journal of Neuroscience, 18*, 6279–6289.

Matsumura, K., Watanabe, Y., Imai-Matsumura, K., Connoly, M., Koyama, Y., Onoe, H., & Watanabe, Y. (1992). Mapping of prostaglandin E_2 binding sites in rat brain using quantitative autoradiography. *Brain Research, 581*, 292–298.

Meazza, C., DiMarco, A., Fruscella, P., Gloaguen, I., Laufer, R., Sironi, M., Sipe, J. D., Villa, P., Romano, M., & Ghezzi, P. (1997). Centrally mediated inhibition of local inflammation by ciliary neurotrophic factor. *Neuroimmunomodulation, 4*, 271–276.

Meller, S. T., Dykstra, C., Grzybycki, D., Murphy, S., & Gebhart, G. F. (1994). The possible role of glia in nociceptive processing and hyperalgesia in the spinal cord of the rat. *Neuropharmacology, 33*, 1471–1478.

Mellon, R. D., & Bayer, B. M. (1998). Role of central opioid receptor subtypes in morphine-induced alterations in peripheral lymphocyte activity. *Brain Research, 789*, 56–67.

Menzies, R. A., Patel, R., Hall, N. R. S., O'Grady, M. P., & Rier, S. E. (1992). Human recombinant interferon alpha inhibits naloxone binding to rat brain membranes. *Life Sciences, 50*, PL227–232.

Minami, M., Kuraishi, Y., Yamaguchi, T., Nakai, S., Hirai, Y., & Satoh, M. (1991). Immobilization stress induces interleukin-1β mRNA in the rat hypothalamus. *Neuroscience Letters, 123*, 254–256.

Misiewicz, B., Poltorak, M., Raybourne, R. B., Gomez, M., Listwak, S., & Sternberg, E. M. (1997). Intracerebroventricular transplantation of embryonic neuronal tissue from inflammatory resistant into inflammatory susceptible rats suppresses specific components of inflammation. *Experimental Neurology, 146*, 305–314.

Mohankumar, P. S., & Quadri, S. K. (1993). Systemic administration of interleukin-1 stimulates norepinephrine release in the paraventricular nucleus. *Life Sciences, 52*, 1961–1967.

Mohankumar, P. S., Thyagarajan, S., & Quadri, S. K. (1993). Interleukin-1β increases 5-hydroxyindoleacetic acid release in the hypothalamus in vivo. *Brain Research Bulletin, 31*, 745–748.

Mokha, S. S., Goldsmith, G. E., Hellon, R. F., & Puri, R. (1987). Hypothalamic control of nocireceptive and other neurones in the marginal layer of the dorsal horn of the medulla (trigeminal nucleus caudalis) in the rat. *Experimental Brain Research, 65*, 427–436.

Moore, K. W., O'Garra, A., De Waal Malefyt, R., Vieira, P., & Mosmann, T. R. (1993). Interleukin-10. *Annual Review of Immunology, 11*, 165–190.

Mousa, S. A., Schaefer, M., Mitchell, W. M., Hassan, A. H., & Stein, C. (1996). Local upregulation of corticotropin-releasing hormone and interleukin-1 receptors in rats with painful hindlimb inflammation. *European Journal of Pharmacology, 311*, 221–231.

Nakamori, T., Morimoto, A., Yamaguchi, K., Watanabe, T., & Murakami, N. (1994). Interleukin-1β production in the rabbit brain during endotoxin-induced fever. *Journal of Physiology (Lond.), 476*, 177–186.

Nakamura, H., Nakanishi, K., Kita, A., & Kadokawa, T. (1988). Interleukin-1 induces analgesia in mice by a central action. *European Journal of Pharmacology, 149*, 49–54.

Nakashima, T., Hori, T., Kuriyama, K., & Matsuda, T. (1988). Effects of interferon-α on the activity of preoptic thermosensitive neurons in tissue slices. *Brain Research, 454*, 361–367.

Nakashima, T., Hori, T., Mori, T., Kuriyama, K., & Mizuno, K. (1989). Recombinant human interleukin-1β alters the activity of preoptic thermosensitive neurons in vitro. *Brain Research Bulletin, 23* 209–213.

Nakashima, T., Murakami, T., Murai, Y., Hori, T., Miyata, S., & Kiyohara, T. (1995). Naloxone suppresses the rising phase of fever induced by interferon-α. *Brain Research Bulletin, 37*, 61–66.

Navarra, P., Pozzoli, G., Brunetti, L., Ragazzoni, E., Besser, M., & Grossman, A. (1992). Interleukin-1β and interleukin-6 specifically increase the release of prostaglandin E_2 from rat hypothalamic explants in vitro. *Neuroendocrinology, 56*, 61–68.

Negro, A., Tavella, A., Facci, L., Callegaro, L., & Skaper, S. D. (1992). Interleukin-1β regulates proenkephalin gene expression in astrocytes cultured from rat cortex. *Glia, 6*(3), 206–212.

Ohkubo, T., Shibata, M., Takahashi, H., & Inoki, R. (1983). Effect of prostaglandin D_2 on pain and inflammation. *Japanese Journal of Pharmacology, 33*, 264–266.

Ohkubo, T., Shibata, M., Takahashi, H., & Naruse, S. (1985). Naloxone prevents the analgesic action of α-MSH in mice. *Experientia, 41*, 627–628.

Oka, T., Abe, M., Oka, K., Hori, T., & Takahashi, S. (1998). The preoptic hypothalamus mediates hyperalgesia induced by intravenous administration of lipopolysaccharide in rats. *Society for Neuroscience Abstracts, 24*, 882.

Oka, T., Aou, S., & Hori, T. (1993). Intracerebroventricular injection of interleukin-1β induces hyperalgesia in rats. *Brain Research, 624*, 61–68.

Oka, T., Aou, S., & Hori, T. (1994a). Intracerebroventricular injection of interleukin-1β enhances nociceptive neuronal responses of the trigeminal nucleus caudalis in rats. *Brain Research, 656*, 236–244.

Oka, T., Aou, S., & Hori, T. (1994b). Intracerebroventricular injection of prostaglandin E_2 induces thermal hyperalgesia in rats: the possible involvement of EP_3 receptors. *Brain Research, 663*, 287–292.

Oka, T., Hori, T., Hosoi, M., Oka, K., Abe, M., & Kubo, C. (1997). Biphasic modulation in the trigeminal nociceptive neuronal responses by the intracerebroventricular prostaglandin E_2 may be mediated through different EP receptors subtypes in rats. *Brain Research, 771*, 278–284.

Oka, T., Hosoi, M., Oka, K., & Hori, T. (1997). Biphasic alteration in the trigeminal nociceptive neuronal responses after intracerebroventricular injection of prostaglandin E_2 in rats. *Brain Research, 749*, 354–357.

Oka, T., Oka, K., Hosoi, M., Aou, S., & Hori, T. (1995). The opposing effects of interleukin-1β microinjected into the preoptic hypothalamus and the ventromedial hypothalamus on nociceptive behavior in rats. *Brain Research, 700*, 271–278.

Oka, T., Oka, K., Hosoi, M., & Hori, T. (1995). Intracerebroventricular injection of interleukin-6 induces thermal hyperalgesia in rats. *Brain Research, 692*, 123–128.

Oka, T., Oka, K., Hosoi, M., & Hori, T. (1996). Inhibition of peripheral interleukin-1β-induced hyperalgesia by the intracerebroventricular administration of diclofenac and α-melanocyte-stimulating hormone. *Brain Research, 736*, 237–242.

Oka, T., Wakugawa, Y., Hosoi, M., Oka, K., & Hori, T. (1996). Intracerebroventricular injection of tumor necrosis factor-α induces thermal hyperalgesia in rats. *Neuroimmunomodulation, 3*, 135–140.

Ota, K., Katafuchi, T., Takaki, A., & Hori, T. (1997). AV3V neurons that send axons to hypothalamic nuclei respond to the systemic injection of IL-1β. *American Journal of Physiology, 272*(6 Pt2), R532–R540.

Patterson, J. C., & Childs, G. V. (1994). Nerve growth factor in the anterior pituitary: Regulation of secretion. *Endocrinology, 135*, 1689–1696.

Perkins, M. N., & Davis, A. J. (1996). Cytokines and nociception. In N. J. Rothwell (Ed.), *Cytokines and the nervous system* (pp. 179–202). Austin, TX: R. G. Landes.

Perlstein, R. S., Whitnall, M. H., Abrams, J. S., Mougey, E. H., & Neta, R. (1993). Synergistic roles of interleukin-6, interleukin-1, and tumor necrosis factor in the adrenocorticotropin response to bacterial lipopolysaccharide in vivo. *Endocrinology, 132*, 946–952.

Pober, J. S., & Cotran, R. S. (1990). Cytokines and endothelial cell biology. *Physiological Reviews, 70*, 427–451.

Poddubiuk, Z. M. (1976). A comparison of the central actions of prostaglandins A_1, E_1, E_2, $F_{1\alpha}$ and $F_{2\alpha}$ in the rat, I. behavioral, antinociceptive and anticonvulsant actions of intraventricular prostaglandins in the rat. *Psychopharmacology, 50*, 89–94.

Poole, S., Bristow, A. F., Lorenzetti, B. B., Das, R. E., Smith, T. W., & Ferreira, S. H. (1992). Peripheral analgesic activities of peptides related to α-melanocyte stimulating hormone and interleukin-$1\beta^{193-195}$. *British Journal of Pharmacology, 106*, 489–492.

Poree, L. R., Dickenson, A. H., & Wei, E. T. (1989). Corticotropin-releasing factor inhibits the response of trigeminal neurons to noxious heat. *Brain Research, 502*, 349–355.

Pousset, F., Fournier, J., Legoux, P., Keane, P., Shire, D., & Soubrie, P. (1996). Effect of serotonin on cytokine mRNA expression in rat hippocampal astrocytes. *Molecular Brain Research, 38*, 54–62.

Pozzoli, G., Costa, A., Grimaldi, M., Schettini, G., Preziosi, P., Grossman, A., & Navarra, P. (1994). Lipopolysaccharide modulation of eicosanoid and corticotrophin-releasing hormone release from rat hypothalamic explants and astrocyte cultures in vitro: Evidence for the involvement of prostaglandin E_2 but no prostaglandin F_{2a} and lack of effect of nerve growth factor. *Journal of Endocrinology, 140*, 103–109.

Quan, N., Sundar, S. K., & Weiss, J. M. (1994). Induction of interleukin-1 in various brain regions after peripheral and central injections of lipopolysaccharide. *Journal of Neuroimmunology, 49*, 125–134.

Quan, N., Zhang, Z., Emery, M., Lai, E., Bonnsall, R., Katyanaraman, V. S., & Weiss, J. M. (1996). In vivo induction of interleukin-1 bioactivity in brain tissue after intracerebral infusion of native gp 120 and gp 160. *Neuroimmunomodulation, 3*, 56–61.

Ramer-Quinn, D. S., Baker, R. A., and Sanders, V. M. (1997). Activated T helper 1 and T helper 2 cells differentially express the beta-2-adrenergic receptor: a mechanism for selective modulation of T helper 1 cell cytokine production. *Journal of Immunology, 159*, 4857–4867.

Rassnick, S., Zhou, D., & Rabin, B. S. (1995). Central administration of prostaglandin E_2 suppresses in vitro cellular immune responses. *American Journal of Physiology, 269*(1 Pt2), R92–R97.

Rhodes, D. L., & Liebeskind, J. C. (1978). Analgesia from rostral brain stem stimulation in the rat. *Brain Research, 143*, 521–532.

Rivest, S., Torres, G., & Rivier, C. (1992). Differential effects of central and peripheral injection of interleukin-1β on brain c-fos expression and neuroendocrine functions. *Brain Research, 587*, 13–23.

Rizvi, T. A., Ennis, M., & Shipley, M. T. (1992). Reciprocal connections between the medial preoptic area and the midbrain periaqueductal gray in rat: A WGA-HRP and PHA-L study. *Journal of Comparative Neurology, 315*, 1–15.

Roberts, N. J. Jr. (1991). Impact of temperature elevation on immunologic defenses. *Reviews of Infectious Diseases, 13*, 462–472.

Robertson, B., Xu, X. J., Hao, J. X., Wiesenfeld-Hallin, Z., Mhlanga, J., Grant, G., & Kristensson, K. (1997). Interferon-γ receptors in nociceptive pathways: Role in neuropathic pain-related behaviour. *NeuroReport, 8*, 1311–1316.

Rothwell, N. J. (1996). The role of cytokines in neurodegeneration. In N. J. Rothwell (Ed.), *Cytokines and the nervous system*, (pp. 145–162), Austin, TX: R. G. Landes.

Rothwell, N. J., & Hopkins, S. J. (1995). Cytokines and the nervous system. II: Actions and mechanisms of actions. *Trends in Neurosciences, 18*, 130–136.

Ruzicka, B. B., Thompson, R. C., Watson, S. J., & Akil, H. (1996). Interleukin-1β-mediated regulation of μ-opioid receptor mRNA in primary astrocyte-enriched cultures. *Journal of Neurochemistry, 66*, 425–428.

Saperstein, A., Brand, H., Audhya, T., Nabriski, D., Hutchinson, B., Rosenzweig, S., & Hollander, C. S. (1992). Interleukin 1β mediates stress-induced immunosuppression via corticotropin-releasing factor. *Endocrinology, 130*, 152–158.

Sacerdote, P., Manfredi, B., Aloe, L., Micera, A., & Panerai, A. E. (1996). Centrally injected nerve growth factor modulates peripheral immune responses in the rat. *Neuroendocrinology, 64*, 274–279.

Saphier, D., & Feldman, S. (1986). Effects of stimulation of the preoptic area on hypothalamic paraventricular nucleus unit activity and corticosterone secretion in freely moving rats. *Neuroendocrinology, 42*, 167–173.

Saphier, D., Roerig, S. C., Ito, C., Vlasak, W. R., Farrar, G. E., Broyles, J. E., & Welch, J. E. (1994). Inhibition of neural and neuroendocrine activity by α-interferon: Neuroendocrine, electrophysiological, and biochemical studies in the rat. *Brain, Behavior, and Immunity, 8*, 37–56.

Sapolsky, R., Rivier, C., Yamamoto, G., Plotsky, P., & Vale, W. (1987). Interleukin-1 stimulates the secretion of hypothalamic corticotropin-releasing factor. *Science, 238*, 522–524.

Schaefer, M., Carter, L., & Stein, C. (1994). Interleukin-1β and corticotropin-releasing factor inhibit pain by releasing opioids from immune cells in inflamed tissue. *Proceedings of the National Academy of Sciences of the United States of America, 91*, 4219–4223.

Schafer, M., Mousa, S. A., & Stein, C. (1997). Corticotropin-releasing factor in antinociception and inflammation. *European Journal of Pharmacology, 323*, 1–10.

Schöbitz, B., de Kloet, E. R., Sutanto, W., & Holsboer, F. (1993). Cellular localization of interleukin 6 mRNA and interleukin 6 receptor mRNA in rat brain. *European Journal of Neuroscience, 5*, 1426–1435.

Sehic, E., Szekely, M., Ungar, A. L., Oladehin, A., & Blatteis, C. M. (1996). Hypothalamic prostaglandin E_2 during lipopolysaccharide-induced fever in guinea pigs. *Brain Research Bulletin, 39*, 391–399.

Sellami, S., & de Beaurepaire, R. (1995). Hypothalamic and thalamic sites of action of interleukin-1β on food intake, body temperature and pain sensitivity in the rat. *Brain Research, 694*, 69–77.

Shanks, N., Harbuz, M. S., Jessop, D. S., Perks, P., Moore, P. M., & Lightman, S. L. (1998) Inflammatory disease as chronic stress. *Annals of the New York Academy of Sciences, 840*, 599–607.

Shavit, Y., Depaulis, A., Martin, F. C., Terman, G. W., Pechnick, R. N., Zane, C. J., Gale, R. P., & Liebeskind, J. C. (1986). Involvement of brain opiate receptors in the immune-suppressive effect of morphine. *Proceedings of the National Academy of Sciences of the United States of America, 83*, 7114–7117.

Shavit, Y., Lewis, J. W., Terman, G. W., Gale, R. P., & Liebeskind, J. C. (1984). Opioid peptides mediate the suppressive effect of stress on natural killer cell cytotoxicity. *Science, 223*, 188–190.

Sherman, J. E., & Kalin, N. H. (1986). ICV-CRH potently affects behavior without altering antinociceptive responding. *Life Sciences, 39*, 433–441.

Shimizu, N., Hori, T., & Nakane, H. (1994). An interleukin-1β-induced noradrenaline release in the spleen is mediated by brain corticotropin-releasing factor: An in vivo microdialysis study in conscious rats. *Brain, Behavior and Immunity, 7*, 14–23.

Shimizu, N., Kaizuka, Y., Hori, T., & Nakane, H. (1996). Immobilization increases norepinephrine release and reduces NK cytotoxicity in spleen of conscious rat. *American Journal of Physiology, 271*(3 Pt2), R537–R544.

Shintani, F., Kanba, S., Nakaki, T., Nibuya, M., Kinoshita, N., Suzuki, E., Yagi, G., Kato, R., & Asai, M. (1993). Interleukin-1β augments release of norepinephrine, dopamine, and serotonin in the rat anterior hypothalamus. *Journal of Neuroscience, 13*, 3574–3581.

Shyu, K. W., & Lin, M. T. (1985). Hypothalamic monoaminergic mechanisms of aspirin-induced analgesia in monkeys. *Journal of Neural Transmission, 62*, 285–293.

Sironi, M., Munoz, C., Pollicino, T., Sibioni, A., Sciacca, FlL., Bernasconi, S., Vecchi, A., Colotta, F., & Mantovani, A. (1993), Divergent effects of interleukin-10 on cytokine production by mononuclear phagocytes and endothelial cells. *European Journal of Immunology, 23*, 2692–2695.

Song, C., & Leonard, B. E. (1995). Interleukin-2-induced changes in behavioural, neurotransmitter, and immunological parameters in the olfactory bulbectomized rat. *Neuroimmunomodulation, 2*, 263–273.

Song, Z. H., & Takemori, A. E. (1990). Involvement of spinal kappa opioid receptors in the antinociception produced by intrathecally administered corticotropin-releasing factor in mice. *Journal of Pharmacology and Experimental Therapeutics, 254*, 363–368.

Spillantini, M. G., Aloe, L., Alleva, E., Desimone, R., Goedert, M., & Levi-Montalcini, R. (1989). Nerve growth factor mRNA and protein increase in hypothalamus in a mouse model of aggression. *Proceedings of the National Academy of Sciences of the United States of America, 86*, 8555–8559.

Star, R. A., Rajora, N., Huang, J., Stock, R. C., Catania, A., & Lipton, J. M. (1995). Evidence of autocrine modulation of macrophage nitric oxide synthase by alpha-melanocyte-stimulating hormone. *Proceedings of the National Academy of Sciences of the United States of America, 92*, 8016–8020.

Sternberg, E. M., Wilder, R. L., Gold, P. W., & Chrousos, G. P. (1990). A defect in the central component of the immune system-hypothalamic-pituitary-adrenal axis feedback loop is associated with susceptibility in experimental arthritis and other inflammatory diseases. *Annals of the New York Academy of Sciences, 594*, 289–292.

Sternberg, E. M., Young, W. B., Bernardini, R., Calogero, A. E., Chrousos, G. P., Gold, P. W., & Wilder, R. L. (1989). A central nervous system defect in biosynthesis of corticotropin-releasing hormone is associated with susceptibility to streptococcal cell wall-induced arthritis in Lewis rat. *Proceedings of the National Academy of Sciences of the United States of America, 86*, 4771–4775.

Stitt, J. T. (1986). Prostaglandin E as the neural mediator of the febrile response. *Yale Journal of Biology and Medicine, 59*, 137–149.

Strijbos, P. J., & Rothwell, N. J. (1995). Interleukin-1-beta attenuates excitatory amino-acid-induced neurodegeneration in vitro: Involvement of nerve growth factor. *Journal of Neuroscience, 15*(5 Pt1), 3468–3474.

Sugimoto, Y., Shigemoto, R., Namba, T., Negishi, M., Mizuno, N., Narumiya, S., & Ichikawa, A. (1994). Distribution of the messenger RNA for the prostaglandin E receptor subtype EP_3 in the mouse nervous system. *Neuroscience, 62*, 919–928.

Sundar, S. K., Becker, K. J., Cierpial, M. A., Carpenter, M. D., Rankin, L. A., Fleener, S. L., Ritchie, J. C., Simson, P. E., & Weiss, J. M. (1989). Intracerebroventricular infusion of interleukin 1 rapidly decreases peripheral cellular immune responses. *Proceedings of the National Academy of Sciences of the United States of America, 86*, 6398–6402.

Sundar, S. K., Cierpial, M. A., Kamaraju, L. S., Long, S., Hsieh, S., Lorenz, C., Aaron, M., Ritchie, J. C., & Weiss, J. M. (1991). Human immunodeficiency virus glycoprotein (gp120) infused into rat brain induces interleukin 1 to elevate pituitary-adrenal activity and decrease peripheral cellular immune responses. *Proceedings of the National Academy of Sciences of the United States of America, 88*, 11246–11250.

Sundar, S. K., Cierpial, M. A., Kilts, C., Ritchie, J. C., & Weiss, J. M. (1990). Brain IL-1-induced immunosuppression occurs through activation of both pituitary-adrenal axis and sympathetic nervous system by corticotropin-releasing factor. *Journal of Neuroscience, 10*, 3701–3706.

Svensjo, E., Persson, C. G. A., & Rutili, G. (1977). Inhibition of bradykinin-induced macromolecular leakage from post-capillary venules by a β-adrenoreceptor stimulant, terbutaline. *Acta Physiologica Scandinavica, 101*, 514–516.

Swanson, L. W. (1976). An autoradiographic study of the efferent connections of the preoptic region in the rat. *Journal of Comparative Neurplogy, 167*, 227–256.

Tagoh, H., Nishijo, H., Uwano, T., Kishi, H., Ono, T., & Muraguchi, A. (1995). Reciprocal IL-1β gene expression in medial and lateral hypothalamic areas in SART-stressed mice. *Neuroscience Letters, 184*, 17–20.

Take, S., Mori, T., Katafuchi, T., & Hori, T. (1993). Central interferon-α inhibits natural killer cytotoxicity through sympathetic innervation. *American Journal of Physiology, 265*(2 Pt2), R453–R459.

Take, S., Mori, T., Katafuchi, t., Kaizuka, Y., & Hori, T. (1992). Central interferon-α suppresses the cytotoxic activity of natural killer cells in the mouse spleen. *Annals of the New York Academy of Sciences, 650*, 46–50.

Take, S., Uchimura, D., Kanemitsu, Y., Katafuchi, T., & Hori, T. (1995). Interferon-α acts at the preoptic hypothalamus to reduce natural killer cytotoxicity in rats. *American Journal of Physiology, 268*(6 Pt2), R1406–R1410.

Takeshige, C., Sato, T., Mera, T., Hisamitsu, T., & Fang, J. (1992). Descending pain inhibitory system involved in acupuncture analgesia. *Brain Research Bulletin, 29*, 617–634.

Tarkowski, E., Rosengren, L., Blomstrand, C., Wikkelso, C., Jensen, C., Ekholm, S., & Tarkowski, A. (1997). Intrathecal release of pro- and anti-inflammatory cytokines during stroke. *Clinical and Experimental Immunology, 110*, 492–499.

Tatro, J. B. (1996). Receptor biology of the melanocortins, a family of neuroimmunomodulatory peptides. *Neuroimmunomodulation, 3*, 259–284.

Taylor, A. W., Streilein, J. W., & Cousins, S. W. (1992). Identification of alpha-melanocyte-stimulating hormone as a potential immunosuppressive factor in aqueous humor. *Current Eye Research, 11*, 1199–1209.

Tedeschi, B., Barrett, J. N., & Keane, R. W. (1986). Astrocytes produce interferon that enhances the expression of H-2 antigens on a subpopulation of brain cells. *Journal of Cell Biology, 102*, 2244–2253.

Terao, A., Kitamura, H., Asano, A., Kobayashi, M., & Saito, M. (1995). Roles of prostaglandins D_2 and E_2 in interleukin-1-induced activation of norepinephrine turnover in the brain and peripheral organs of rats. *Journal of Neurochemistry, 65*, 2742–2747.

Tonosaki, Y., & Sugiura, Y. (1998). α-MSH modulates Fos expression in the paraventricular nucleus and hyperalgesia induced by intracerebroventricular administration of interleukin-1β in rats. *Annals of the New York Academy of Sciences, 840*, 615–618.

Tsagarakis, S., Gillies, G., Rees, L. H., Besser, M., & Grossman, A. (1989). Interleukin-1 directly stimulates the release of corticotrophin releasing factor from rat hypothalamus. *Neuroendocrinology, 49*, 98–101.

Turnbull, A. V., & Rivier, C (1996). Corticotropin-releasing factor, vasopressin, and prostaglandins mediate, and nitric oxide restraints, the hypothalamic-pituitary-adrenal response to acute local inflammation in the rat. *Endocrinology, 137*, 455–463.

van Dam, A. M., Brouns, M., Louisse, S., & Berkenbosch, F. (1992). Appearance of interleukin-1 in macrophages and in ramified microglia in the brain of endotoxin-treated rats: A pathway for the induction of non-specific symptoms of sickness? *Brain Research, 588*, 291–296.

von Sydow, M., Sonnenborg, A., Gaines, H., & Strannegard, O. (1991). Interferon-alpha and tumor necrosis factor-alpha in serum of patients in various stages of HIV-1 infection. *AIDS Research Human Retroviruses, 7*, 375–380.

Walker, J. M., Akil, H., & Watson, S. J. (1980). Evidence for homologous actions of pro-opiomelanocortin products. *Science, 210*, 1247–1249.

Walker, K., Dray, A., & Perkins, M. (1996). Hyperalgesia in rats following intracerebroventricular administration of endotoxin: Effect of bradykinin B_1 and B_2 receptor antagonist treatment. *Pain, 65*, 211–219.

Wan, W., Vriend, C. Y., Wetmore, L., Gartner, J. G., Greenberg, A. H., & Nance, D. M. (1993). The effects of stress on splenic immune function are mediated by the splenic nerve. *Brain Research Bulletin, 30*, 101–105.

Wang, Y., Li, L., Liu, J., Wang, Z., Jiang, C., & Liu, X. (1997). The analgesic domain of IL-2. *Biochemical and Biophysical Research Communications, 230*, 542–545.

Wang, Y., Pei, G., Cai, Y. C., Zhao, Z. Q., Wang, J. B., Jiang, C. L., Zheng, Z. C., & Liu, X. Y. (1996). Human interleukin-2 could bind to opioid receptor and induce corresponding signal transduction. *NeuroReport, 8*, 11–14.

Wang, Z., Ren, S. G., & Melmed, S. (1996). Hypothalamic and pituitary leukemia inhibitory factor gene expression in vivo: A novel endotoxin-inducible neuro-endocrine interface. *Endocrinology, 137*, 2947–2953.

Watanabe, T., Morimoto, A., Sakata, Y., & Murakami, N. (1990). ACTH response induced by interleukin-1 is mediated by CRF secretion stimulated by hypothalamic PGE. *Experientia, 46*, 481–484.

Watanabe, Y., Watanabe, Y., & Hayaishi, O. (1988). Quantitative autoradiographic localization of prostaglandin E_2 binding sites in monkey diencephalon. *Journal of Neuroscience, 8*, 2003–2010.

Watanobe, H., & Takebe, K. (1994). Effects of intravenous administration of interleukin-1-β on the release of prostaglandin E_2, corticotropin-releasing factor, and arginine vasopressin in several hypothalamic areas of freely moving rats: estimation by push-pull perfusion. *Neuroendocrinology, 60*, 8–15.

Watkins, L. R., Maier, S. F., & Geohler, L. E. (1995). Cytokine-to-brain communication: a review and analysis of alternative mechanisms. *Life Science, 57*, 1011–1026.

Watkins, L. R., Martin, D., Ulrich, P., Tracey, K. J., & Maier, S. F. (1997). Evidence for the involvement of spinal cord glia in subcutaneous formalin induced hyperalgesia in the rat. *Pain, 71*, 225–235.

Watkins, L. R., Wiertelak, E. P., Goehler, L. E., Mooney-Heiberger, K., Martinez, J., Furness, L., Smith, K. P., & Maier, S. F. (1994). Neurocircuitry of illness-induced hyperalgesia. *Brain Research, 639*, 283–299.

Watkins, L. R., Wiertelak, E. P., Goehler, L. E., Smith, K. P., Martin, D., & Maier, S. F. (1994). Characterization of cytokine-induced hyperalgesia. *Brain Research, 654*, 15–26.

Weber, R. J., & Pert, A. (1989). The periaqueductal gray matter mediates opiate-induced immunosuppression. *Science, 245*, 188–190.

Webster, E. L., Torpy, D. J., Elenkov, I. J., & Chrousos, G. P. (1998). Corticotropin-releasing hormone and inflammation. *Annals of the New York Academy of Sciences, 840*, 21–32.

Weidenfeld, J., Crumeyrolle-Arias, M., & Haour, F. (1995). Effect of bacterial endotoxin and interleukin-1 on prostaglandin biosynthesis by the hippocampus of mouse brain: role of interleukin-1 receptors and glucocorticoids. *Neuroendocrinology, 62*, 39–46.

Williams, D. W. Jr., Lipton, J. M., & Giesecke, A. H. Jr. (1986). Influence of centrally administered peptides on ear withdrawal from heat in the rabbit. *Peptides, 7*, 1095–1100.

Williams, K., Dooley, N., Ulvestad, E., Becher, B., & Antel, J. P. (1996). IL-10 production by adult human derived microglial cells. *Neurochemistry International, 29*, 55–64.

Wong, M. L., Al-Shehlee, A., Gold, P. W., & Licinio, J. (1996). Cytokines in the brain. In N. J. Rothwell (Ed.), *Cytokines and the nervous system* (pp. 3–20). Austin, TX: R. G. Landes

Wong, M. L., Bongiorno, P. B., Rettori, V., McCann, S. M., & Licinio, J. (1997). Interleukin (IL)-1β, IL-1 receptor antagonist, IL-10, and IL-13 gene expression in the central nervous system and anterior pituitary during systemic inflammation: Pathophysiological implications. *Proceedings of the National Academy of Sciences of the United States of America, 94*, 227–232.

Xin, L., & Blatteis, C. M. (1992). Blockade by interleukin-1 receptor antagonist of IL-1β-induced neuronal activity in guinea pig preoptic area slices. *Brain Research, 569*, 348–352.

Xu, X. J., Hao, J. X., Olsson, T., Kristensson, K., van der Meide, P. H., & Wiesenfeld-Hallin, Z. (1994). Intrathecal interferon-γ facilitates the spinal nociceptive flexor reflex in the rat. *Neuroscience Letters, 182*, 263–266.

Yabuuchi, K., Maruta, E., Minami, M., & Satoh, M. (1996). Induction of interleukin-1β mRNA in the hypothalamus following subcutaneous injections of formalin into the rat hind paws. *Neuroscience Letters, 207*, 109–112.

Yabuuchi, K., Maruta, E., Yamamoto, J., Nishiyori, A., Takami, S., Minami, M., & Satoh, M. (1997). Intracerebroventricular injection of isoproterenol produces its analgesic effect through interleukin-1β production. *European Journal of Pharmacology, 334*, 133–140.

Yabuuchi, K., Nishiyori, A., Minami, M., & Satoh, M. (1996). Biphasic effects of intracerebroventricular interleukin-1β on mechanical nociception in the rat. *European Journal of Pharmacology, 300*, 59–65.

Yamada, T., Horisberger, M. A., Kawaguchi, N., Moroo, I., & Toyoda, T. (1994). Immunohistochemistry using antibodies to α-interferon and its induced protein, MxA, in Alzheimer's and Parkinson's disease brain tissues. *Neuroscience Letters, 181*, 61–64.

Yamada, T., & Yamanaka, I. (1995). Microglial localization of α-interferon receptor in human brain tissues. *Neuroscience Letters, 189*, 73–76.

Zalcman, S., Green-Johnson, J. M., Murray, L., Nance, D. M., Dyck, D., Anisman, H., & Greenberg, A. H. (1994). Cytokine-specific central monoamine alterations induced by interleukin-1, -2 and -6. *Brain Research, 643*, 40–49.

Zelazowski, P., Smith, M. A., Gold, P. W., Chrousos, G. P., Wilder, R. L., & Sternberg, E. M. (1992) In vitro regulation of pituitary ACTH secretion in inflammatory disease susceptible Lewis (LEW/N) and inflammatory disease resistant Fischer (F344/N) rats. *Neuroendocrinology, 56*, 474–482.

CHAPTER

21

Production and Influence of Inflammatory Cytokines in Diseases of the Adult Central Nervous System

JEAN E. MERRILL

I. INTRODUCTION

This chapter focuses on two diseases of the adult human nervous system involving inflammation in which cytokines and free radicals have been implicated. One disease is an autoimmune disease and the other is a neurodegenerative disease. Both illustrate the role of cytokines in inflammation and are of interest for comparison in that the cytokines are induced by quite different pathological events in the two diseases, they are present in different areas of the central nervous system (CNS), and their presence yields different outcomes in terms of the cells that are the targets of the pathology. Interesting similarities between the two pathologies include the activation of endogenous microglia and presence of free radicals. Therefore, there is some instructive advantage in analyzing cytokines in the context of such different human diseases.

A. Multiple Sclerosis

1. *Role of Cytokines in Disease*

Multiple sclerosis (MS) is considered an inflammatory, autoimmune, demyelinating disease of the CNS in which myelin and the cells that produce myelin (oligodendrocytes), are damaged and destroyed. Myelin, the multilamellar membrane required for efficient nerve conduction, as well as the axons sheathed by myelin, may be targets in the disease process leading to plaque formation. When myelin is disrupted, conduction slows and clinical signs become evident. In the plaque itself oligodendrocytes die; the form of death is necrotic. Evidence of necrosis is supported by findings of hypertrophied cell bodies and disrupted plasma and mitochondrial membranes. The presence of activated phagocytic cells in the plaques has implicated microglia and blood-borne macrophages as mediators of myelin and oligodendrocyte damage. Their presence infers that, among other toxins, free radicals of oxygen and nitrogen are at work in this pathology.

Interferon gamma (IFN-γ), interleukin 1 beta (IL-1β), and tumor necrosis factor alpha (TNF-α) can activate macrophages and glia to produce free radicals of oxygen and nitrogen in the rodent. This is also true for activation by ligand-crosslinking of the

Fc receptor (FcR) and complement receptor (C3biR) (Murphy, Grzybicki, & Simmons, 1995). Although nitric oxide (NO) cannot be directly induced by proinflammatory cytokines in adult human macrophages and glia, cytokines probably amplify NO production incurred by additional membrane perturbations or the crosslinking of cell surface molecules other than cytokine receptors (Bukrinsky et al., 1995; DeMaria et al., 1994; Vouldoukis et al., 1995). Thus, proinflammatory cytokines could play a role in NO production in the peripheral immune system as well as in the CNS. Proinflammatory cytokines have been examined both at the protein and/or mRNA levels in MS patients' blood plasma, cerebrospinal fluid (CSF), brain tissue, and cultured blood leukocytes. There is evidence that among other proinflammatory cytokines, IFN-γ, IL-1β, IL-6, transforming growth factor beta (TGF-β), and TNF-α are elevated (Hofman et al., 1986; Hofman, Hinton, Johnson, & Merrill, 1989; Merrill, Strom, Ellison, & Myers, 1989; Hauser, Doolittle, Lincoln, Brown, & Dinarello, 1990; Link, Soderstrom, Olsson, Hojeberg, Ljungdahl, & Link, 1994; Merrill & Benveniste, 1996).

Elevations in TNF-α and IFN-γ appear to predict relapses in MS. Additionally, the number of circulating IFN-γ-positive blood cells correlates with moderate to severe disability (Beck, Rondot, Catinot, Falcoff, Kirchner, & Wietzerbin, 1988; Link et al., 1994). In clinical trials, treatment of MS patients with IFN-γ exacerbated the disease (IFNγ MS Study Group, 1993), whereas treatment with (IFN-β) improved patients' clinical scores. Therefore it is believed that IFN-β may benefit MS patients by inhibiting IFN-γ-inducible genes such as the major histocompatibility antigen class II (MHCII) genes (Ransohoff, Devajyothi, Estes, Babcock, & Rudick, 1991). IL-1 is constitutively produced by MS patients' freshly isolated lymphocytes in vitro in the absence of stimulation, suggesting in vivo activation (Merrill et al., 1989). IL-6 has been shown to be associated with disease onset and to inhibit demyelination in the animal model of MS, experimental allergic encephalomyelitis (EAE) (Gijbels, Brocke, Abrams, & Steinman, 1995; Rodriguez, Pavelko, McKinney, & Leibowitz, 1994) IL-6 may function to down-regulate IL-1β and TNF-α. In that regard, IL-6 is desirable in MS lesions. Nevertheless, IL-6 contributes to the expansion and differentiation of B cells, and it is known that antimyelin antibodies exacerbate EAE (Genain et al., 1996). Furthermore, IL-6 knock-out mice fail to be susceptible to EAE (Fontana, Eugster, Frei, Lassmann, Malipiero, & Sahrbacher, 1998). Anti-IL6, while decreasing the disease course in EAE animals, leads to a 20-fold increase in IL-6 levels in these animals (Gijbels et al., 1995). These two observations suggest that IL-6 may be proinflammatory leading to autoantibodies and, therefore, IL-6 would be undesirable in MS. Interestingly, the mRNAs for TGF-β and IL-4, cytokines, which can be both pro- and antiinflammatory, are also elevated in MS patients' blood cells as determined by in situ hybridization (Link et al., 1994). Such biological oxymorons exist in autoimmune states and warn us to be cautious in treating the disease with modulators of cytokines (Merrill & Benveniste, 1996).

2. *NO in MS: Regulation of and by Cytokines*

NO is a small, biologically active molecule involved in neuronal signaling, gene regulation, and toxic events in certain intracellular biochemical pathways. NO has been shown to be capable of modulating the induction of the immune response, the permeability of the blood–brain barrier (BBB), trafficking of cells to the CNS, and local responses in the inflammatory milieu. Therefore, it might be predicted that NO could be both beneficial and harmful in an autoimmune disease such as MS.

Within the demyelinated lesions in MS brain, activation of both astrocytes and microglia in the form of gliosis and NO production has been reported (reviewed in Merrill & Murphy, 1996). Evidence to support this includes the presence of astrocyte-associated NADPH diaphorase staining in chronic and acute MS brain lesions. Type II or inducible NO synthase (iNOS) mRNA has been detected in these plaques by reverse transcriptase-polymerase chain reaction (RT-PCR) (Bö et al., 1995); iNOS protein, nitrotyrosine staining, and in situ RT-PCR for iNOS colocalizes with *Ricinus communis* agglutinin-1 staining, a marker for macrophages/microglia. iNOS and NO were found in MS but not control brain tissue (Bagasra, et al., 1995). Recently, DeGroot, Ruuls, Theeuwes, Dijkstra, and Van der Walk (1997) also found strong iNOS positivity in cells in MS lesions; the cells were identified as parenchymal and perivascular macrophgages and were only iNOS positive in active demyelinating areas. In our laboratory, studies suggest that astrocytes, microglia, inflammatory macrophages, and even endothelial cells make iNOS in MS tissue (manuscript in preparation). Increased NO production probably occurs in MS given that there are elevated levels of nitrite and nitrate levels in the CSF of patients (Johnson et al., 1995). In the same study, increased levels of neopterin, a precursor of the iNOS enzyme cofactor tetrahydrobiopterin, was also reported in CSF from MS patients. The reaction of NO with superoxide anion (O2-) forms peroxynitrite

($ONOO^-$), a strong trans-nitrosating agent capable of nitrosating susceptible protein thiols, such as cysteine. This chemical reaction may result in formation of nitroso-amino acids, such as nitrosocysteine, potentially making them immunogenic. Thus, it is of interest that MS patients have elevated circulating antibodies to conjugated S-nitrosocysteine epitopes, suggesting nitrosation of proteins in vivo (Boullerne, Petry, Meynard, & Geffard, 1995). We have identified the nitration of tyrosines by nitrotyrosine-specific antibody staining in MS tissue suggesting that the identified iNOS staining is characterizing a functional enzyme; in other words, that NO is being produced in vivo in MS brain (manuscript in preparation; Merrill, De Rosa, & Franklin, 1998).

Much of the regulation of NO production in macrophages and glia has been studied in the rodent. In humans, such cells are clearly turned on to produce iNOS and NO when certain cell surface receptors are crosslinked; these include CD4, a non-CD4 binding site for HIV-1; CD23; and CD69 (Bukrinsky et al., 1995; DeMaria et al., 1994; Koka et al., 1995; Nicholson et al.,1996; Reiling et al., 1994; Vodovotz et al., 1996; Vouldoukis et al., 1995). The role of cytokines in augmenting NO induction in human glia and macrophages in vitro may be very different from that in rodent cells in vitro and even different from effects in vivo in human disease. IFN-γ is a strong inducer of iNOS and NO in rat glia and macrophages and this production is synergistically increased in the presence of TNF-α or lipopolysaccharide (LPS) (Dileepan, Page, Li, & Stechschulte, 1995; Merrill, Ignarro, Sherman, Melinek, & Lane, 1993; Murphy et al., 1995; Reiling et al., 1994). IFN-γ and IL-1β, but not LPS, are inducers of iNOS and NO in human glial cells derived from fetal brain tissue (Ding et al., 1997; Koka et al., 1995; Lee, Dickson, Liu, & Brosnan, 1993), but not from neonatal or adult brain-derived glial cells (Murphy et al., 1995; this laboratory's unpublished observations). Stevenson, Tam, Wolf, and Sher (1995) have shown that IL-12, probably through the induction of TNF-α and IL-1β induces NO. IL-2 in mice and humans in vivo induces NO (Yim et al., 1995). IL6 has no effect on NO induction (Rockett, Awburn, Aggarwal, Cowden, & Clark, 1992; Tanaka et al., 1995).

There is interest in the presence of elevated IL-4 in MS and its potential link to NO production in the CNS of these patients. In the rodent, the capacity of IL-4 and IL-10 to inhibit iNOS and NO appears to depend on pretreatment of the cells being stimulated with IFN-γ; activated mouse cells are barely inhibited by IL-4 and IL-10 (Bogdan, Vodovitz, Paik, Xie, & Nathan, 1994; Gazzinelli, Oswald, James, & Sher, 1992; Schneemann, Schoedon, Frei, & Schaffner, 1993). Multiple mechanisms for this inhibition have been suggested: (1) through the reduction of TNF-α (Fiorintino, Zlotnik, Mosmann, Howard, & O'Garra, 1991; Gazzinelli et al., 1992) (2) inhibition of the activation of protein kinase Cε (Sands, Bulut, Severn, Xu, & Liew, 1993); or (3) induction of arginase (Corraliza, Soler, Eichmann, & Modolell, 1995). These cytokines may synergize with each other or with TGF-β (Alleva, Burger, & Elgert, 1994). Still other studies have found modest or no inhibition of NO (Murphy et al., 1995; Strassmann, Patil-Koota, Finkelman, Fong, & Kambayashi, 1994) or an increase in NO by IL-10 (Chesrown, Monnier, Visner, & Nick, 1994). As with the rodent, depending on the state of activation of human monocytes/macrophages, IL-4 may up- or down-regulate NO. Nevertheless, IL-4 regulation of NO in the human works in an apparently opposite fashion from that in the rodent. IL-4 can directly induce iNOS and NO production in resting monocytes from normal healthy human donors (reviewed in Merrill & Benveniste, 1996). This activation can be amplified by pretreatment with IFN-γ (Pierre-Kolb et al., 1994). In spontaneously high NO producer monocytes, especially those from allergy patients, IL-4 abrogates NO (Mautino et al., 1994). Nevertheless, in one study IL-4 also has been shown to induce NO in murine splenocytes (Tian & Lawrence, 1995). The production of elevated NO in allergy patients and the ability of IL-4 to induce NO indirectly in peripheral blood mononuclear cells is probably related to the fact that crosslinking of the molecule CD23, the low affinity IgE Fc receptor [FcεRII], by IgE or anti-FcεR antibody leads to NO (Becherel et al., 1994; Vouldoukis et al., 1995). IL-4 induces IgE production as well as an increase in soluble CD23. Interestingly, high levels of IL-4 and NO could feed back negatively, possibly through the elevation of cAMP, on both IgE production and NO (Becherel et al., 1994), which may explain the IL-4 inhibition of "spontaneously" produced NO from allergy patients (Mautino et al., 1994).

In studies in our own laboratory, IL-4 inhibited human glial cell production of TNF-α at nanogram per milliliter and NO production at milligram per milliliter concentrations. Although it inhibited rat TNF-α at nanogram per milliliter concentrations, IL-4 had no effect on rat NO production. The induction of the iNOS gene in rodents and humans is different, suggesting that the regulation of the gene may also be species-specific. In our studies, rat microglia are in an activated state in vivo at birth; therefore they may have been refractory to inhibition by IL-4 and IL-10 in our in vitro studies (St. Pierre, Wong, & Merrill, 1997).

In our hands, IL-13 inhibited NO in rodent glia and human glial cell cultures. The inhibition of TNF-α and microglial cell cytotoxicity by IL-13 may be unrelated events: IL-13 down-regulation of IL-1 may account for the depression in TNF-α production, whereas cytotoxicity may be inhibited partially because of the NO inhibition (Cash et al., 1994; Doyle et al., 1994). St. Pierre et al. (1997) have shown that IFN-γ/LPS induction of rat microglial cell TNF-α was strongly inhibited by IFN-β whereas NO was only weakly inhibited. This suggests that there are even differences in NO regulation by cytokines between mice and rats. Furthermore, the significant inhibition of human glial cells' NO and TNF-α point out the complex mechanisms of actions and species-specific differences in IFN-γ regulatory pathways.

In some autoimmune diseases, including MS, a pernicious proinflammatory cycle may account for the clinical and histopathological chronicity. In this regard, it is quite noteworthy that NO and/or $ONOO^-$ directly up-regulate production of IL-1β, TNF-α, IL-8, and IL-12,) and hydrogen peroxide (H_2O_2) in macrophages. Exposure of a mouse macrophage cell line to S-nitroso-N-acetylpenicillamine (SNAP) induces IL-12 p40 mRNA (Rothe, Hartmann, Geerlings, & Kolb, 1996). Nitrogen radicals also indirectly enhance cytokine induction of TNF-α (Eigler, Sinha, Endres, 1993; Fülle et al., 1991; Lander, Ogiste, Teng, & Novogrodsky, 1995; Magrinat, Mason, Shami, & Weinberg, 1992; Rothe et al., 1996). This induction is mediated at the transcriptional level possibly through the induction of NFκB (Lander et al., 1995). Lander suggests that NO, through enhancement of GTPase activity and G-protein-mediated events, stimulates the translocation of NFκB to the nucleus. Nevertheless, in some cases, NO inhibits LPS-induced IL-1β and TNF-α in macrophages (Eigler et al., 1993; Fülle et al., 1991). In endothelial cells, NO inhibits NFκB translocation by stabilizing the NFκB:IκB complex by preventing IκB degradation (DeCaterina et al., 1995; Peng, Rajavashidsth, Libby, Liao., 1995). These cases illustrate the complexity of the effects of free radicals in signal transducing events in the macrophage at different stages of activation and point to the danger in generalizing NO effects on NFκB in all cells.

3. *NO and Antiinflammatory Effects on the Immune System*

Although it is clearly a proinflammatory molecule locally at sites of tissue damage, NO also may protect against autoimmune disease when acting early and systemically. Mutant mice, in which the *iNOS* gene is defective, as well as IFN-γ receptor knock-out mice (with impaired NO production), have a significantly stronger anti-CD3 response and the T helper cell type 1 (Th1) response to infectious agents than wild type mice (Matthys et al., 1995). This suggests that NO may inhibit T-cell responses leading to delayed type hypersensitivity by inhibiting T-cell proliferation (Matthys et al., 1995), either through suppression of IFN-γ or induction of prostaglandin E2 (PGE2) (Blanco, Geng, & Lotz, 1995). NO also has been shown to inhibit leukocyte adhesion and migration by its interference with CD11/CD18 (leukocyte functional antigen-1, [LFA-1]) expression (Kubes, Suzuki, & Granger, 1991). NO also down-regulates MHCII expression in macrophages, thereby inhibiting antigen presentation (Sicher Vazquez, & Lu, 1994). In other words, early in the disease process in MS or EAE, NO might actually protect against autoimmune events initiated in the peripheral blood.

B. Alzheimer's Disease

1. *Involvement of Cytokines*

Alzheimer's disease (AD) is a neurodegenerative process involving pathological changes in neurons and glia; microglia and astrocytes are activated in the brains of AD patients, while oligodendrocytes and myelin are normal and intact. Unlike MS, AD does not involve infiltration of blood-borne T and B cells or macrophages. Nevertheless, nonsteroidal antiinflammatory drugs have been claimed to be protective in individuals with AD, raising the interesting hypothesis that immune-like activities of microglia and cytokine production in the CNS contribute to inflammation and ultimately to neuronal loss (Dickson et al., 1996). The classes of neurons lost include pyramidal neurons in the hippocampus and neocortex and cholinergic neurons in the basal forebrain (reviewed in Merrill & Murphy, 1997). Although neither IL-1 nor IL-6 are increased in AD patients' peripheral blood, analysis by enzyme-linked immuno sorbent assay and immunohistochemical staining of AD brain tissue shows that there are elevations of both cytokines, especially in parenchymal microglia. There is increased TNF-α in AD sera, and this is associated with increased CNS disease; TNF-α is also elevated in AD brain tissue (Dickson et al., 1996). The actual role of cytokines in AD must be inferred since there are no animal models close enough to the human disease to dissect the interrelations between pathology and immune-like activities in AD CNS.

Hallmarks of the cytopathology of AD include neurofibrillary tangles and senile plaques. There are no real links between immune-like activities in the CNS and the production of hyperphosphorylated tau protein within paired helical filaments (PHF) comprising the tangles. However, more research is needed to identify the putative effects of cytokines on signal transduction pathways in neurons as they might interface with cytoskeletal changes leading to PHF.

In contrast, there may be an immune-like component in the origin of amyloid plaques that consist of beta amyloid protein (Aβ) cleaved from the larger amyloid precursor protein (APP). Immunocytochemical studies have identified that Aβ in AD patients differs from that in the normal aging brains in a number of ways. A more highly fibrillogenic form of Aβ (Aβ1-42) is present in AD brain parenchyma and blood vessels, and it is present to a greater extent in AD than aging brain. In AD, the amyloid is denser in appearance and the core is associated with molecules not seen in aging brain. These acute phase reactants include serum amyloid P protein, complement proteins, α2 macroglobulin, α1-antichymotrypsin, heparin sulfate proteoglycans, and apolipoprotein-E (Dickson et al., 1996; Selkoe, 1991). Astrocytes and microglia are the cellular source of these proteins. The role of these molecules in stabilization or "nucleation" of the plaque core is a topic of wide interest. Because of its role in stimulating the induction of these entities elsewhere in the body and in other inflammatory milieus, IL-6 is the suspected inducer of these proteins in AD tissue.

There is no appropriate animal model for AD, thus hindering our ability to adequately test hypotheses for treatments and cures for this disease. Since it is believed that overexpression of mediators of inflammation within the CNS might mimic the disease, a variety of surrogate animals models have been examined for the nature of the pathology in vivo. Chronic infusion of LPS into the fourth ventricle over an extended period of time in the young rat brain produces components of the neuropathology of AD. These include reactive microglia and astrogliosis in the hippocampal area, induction of IL-1β and APP mRNA in the basal forbrain and hippocampus, and degeneration of CA3 pyramidal neurons, and spatial memory impairment. Transgenic mice genetically engineered to overexpress IL-6 behind the neuron-specific enolase produce greater amounts of IL-1β, IL-6, and TNF-α in response to peripherally injected LPS than wild type mice but suffer no neuronal injury (Di Santo et al., 1996; Fattori et al., 1995). In contrast, animals in which IL-6 is produced under the regulatory control of glial fibrillary acidic protein develop neurologic disease correlating with the level of expression of the transgene. High IL-6 expressors demonstrate astrogliosis, neuronal loss, and induction of acute phaase reactant proteins all AD features. Cognitive decline in these transgenics is age-dependent. Long-term potentiation in the dentate gyrus and abnormal hippocampal paroxysmal discharge are also seen (Campbell et al., 1993, 1997).

IL-1, IL-2, IL-3, IL-6, TGF-β, and granulocyte-macrophage colony stimulating factor up-regulate APP mRNA expression in rodent primary and human tumor cell cultures (Dickson et al., 1996; Ringheim et al., 1998). The exact mechanism of induction in human primary cells is less well understood, especially since most human cultures are derived from embryonic and not adult tissue. Furthermore, TGF-β induces Aβ deposition in cerebral blood vessels and meninges of aged transgenic mice overexpressing this cytokine from astrocytes (Wyss-Coray, Masliah et al., 1997). Interestingly, Aβ activates microglia in vitro to produce O2-, NO, IL-1β, and TNF-α (McDonald, Brunden, & Landreth, 1997; Meda, et al., 1995). These findings suggest that cytokines can induce APP production and Aβ deposition, which then induces more cytokines leading to a chronic stimulation of plaque formation and microglial activation.

2. *NO's Role in Pathology*

Aβ interacts with the cell surface receptor for advanced glycation end products on neurons and microglia as well as to an unrelated class A scavenger receptor on microglia, inducing oxidative stress in microglia (Yan et al., 1996). Aβ induces NO production in neurons by activation of type I NOS (nNOS) (Hu & el-Fakahany, 1993). A recent report also suggested that iNOS could be seen in neurons in AD brain (Vodovotz et al., 1996). Since the consequence of O_2^- and NO production is the formation of $ONOO^-$, the ensuing lipid peroxidation would disrupt cell membranes, alter ion homeostasis, and trigger a cascade of events leading to neuronal death.

II. CYTOKINES, RECEPTORS, AND SIGNALING PATHWAYS

A. IL-1β and TNF-α

1. *Receptors*

Although there are several members of the IL-1 receptor family, IL-1 signals only through the type I receptor (IL-1RI). The type II receptor (IL-1RII) has a short nonsignaling cytoplasmic tail, and the soluble type I receptor (solIL1RI) completely lacks a cytoplasmic tail. IL-1 signaling, which can lead to activation or modulation of many significant pathways in the CNS in addition to inflammation—including social investigation, fever, sleep, appetite, neurotransmitter, and neuroendocrine balance, and permeability of the BBB—can be inhibited by the solIL1RI and the IL-1R antagonist (IL1Ra) (reviewed in Otero & Merrill, 1994; Rothwell, Busbridge, Humphray, & Hissey, 1990; Rothwell & Hopkins, 1995). Functional IL-1 receptors are found on astrocytes, microglia, oligodendrocytes, and most neurons.

The TNF cytokine receptor family, with at least 12 members sharing structural homology in the extracellular domain, binds ligands that also belong to a family of related proteins. The two TNF receptors are named p55 type I and p75 type II receptors. Signaling is mediated through the type I receptor predominantly, as a consequence of trimerization of the receptor and the binding of trimers of TNF-α or TNF-β (more commonly called lymphotoxin). Other members of the receptor family include the low-affinity nerve growth factor receptor, Fas, and CD40. Distinguishing features of the receptor family include the shared, homologous, cysteine-rich extracellular domains, and the shared cytoplasmic "death domain" seen in Fas and the type I receptor (Otero & Merrill, 1994; St. Pierre, Merrill, & Dopp, 1996). Most CNS cell types express both type I and II receptors, although one type usually predominates. In our in vitro studies we determined that microglia express both type I and II TNF-α receptors, whereas rat oligodendrocytes and astrocytes express almost exclusively type I (Dopp, Mackenzie-Graham, Otero, & Merrill, 1996). The type I receptor is increased by IFN-γ and TNF-α in most cell types.

2. *Signaling by IL-1β and TNF-α*

Both cytokines, IL-1β and TNF-α activate several signaling pathways. In ceramide signaling, ligand binding initiates the conversion of sphingomyelin to ceramide by virtue of the action of neutral or acidic sphingomyelinase (nSMase or aSMase). The nSMase triggers p38 kinase (mitogen activated protein kinase 2 [MAP2]) and at lower concentrations triggers extracellular signal-regulated kinases (ERK1/2 MAP kinases). The aSMase activates NFκB translocation to the nucleus (Hamilton, Tannenbaum, & Tebo, 1996). IL-1 receptor associated kinase autophosphorylates and is activated to phosphorylate further downstream kinases such as those in the family of TNF receptor associated factor (TRAF) kinases. TRAF2 activates TNF-α-induced NFκB whereas TRAF6 is the IL-1 specific family member. Another signaling pathway proceeding from IL-1 or TNF-α receptor binding is via the activation of phospholipase C to phosphatidylcholine and diacerglycerol and activation of an AP-1 site via PKC zeta. Yet another transcription factor implicated in IL-1 and TNF-α signaling is NF-IL-6. The signaling will be different in different cell types and generate a diverse array of patterns of gene expression depending on the biological context (Hamilton, et al., 1996).

3. *Response to IL-1β and TNF-α*

Although neurons and astrocytes produce IL-1β and TNF-α at least in vitro, microglia produce significantly more of these cytokines. IL-1β causes microgliosis and microglial nodule formation, as well as contributing to multinucleated giant cell formation in microglia and astrogliosis and proliferation of astrocytes, all hallmarks of activation and inflammatory perturbation in these glial cells (Merrill & Benveniste, 1996; St. Pierre et al. 1996). IL-1β activates microglial adhesion molecules: very late antigen-4, intercellular adhesion molecule-1 (ICAM-1), and lymphocyte function associated antigen-1 as well as Fc and complement receptors on microglia, all of which contribute to the ability of microglia to mediate cytotoxicity of neurons, oligodendrocytes, or virally infected and tumor cells. IL-1β induces free radical formation in microglia and NO production in rodent microglia and astrocytes. In addition to inducing TNF-α, which produces many of the same changes as IL-1, IL-1β can lead to substantial changes in the BBB, otoxicity of neurons, oligodendrocytes, or virally infected and tumor cells (Merrill & Benveniste, 1996).

TNF-α has a greater effect on the induction of colony stimulating factors that modulate the proliferation of microglia and on the expression of MHCII molecules on glial cell membranes than does IL-1α (Merrill & Benveniste, 1996). TNF-α and lymphotoxin (LT) also have also been implicated in toxicity as well as protection of neurons and oligodendrocytes. Both IL-1β and TNF-α have been shown to induce the production of other cytokines and growth factors, some of which are beneficial to the health of cells in the CNS. These include TGF-β, IL-6, nerve growth factor, leukemia inhibitory factor (LIF), and basic fibroblast growth factor (Gadient & Otten, 1997; Strijbos & Rothwell, 1995). Thus, IL-1β and TNF-α could contribute to substantial damage or protection within the CNS, to be determined, once again, by the context in which these events occur. (Hamilton et al., 1996; Merrill & Benveniste, 1996). Careful considerations must be given to modulating these cytokines in AD and MS.

B. IL-6

1. *IL-6 Receptor*

IL-6 binds to a specific receptor (IL6R) on the surface of neurons and glia, giving rise to the additional binding to ligand and association of two molecules of the signal transducing protein gp130; gp130 dimerization leads to two different kinase-mediated signaling pathways in IL-6-stimulated cells (Gadient & Otten, 1997). Although gp130 is ubiquitously expressed and utilized by other members of the IL-6 cytokine family (LIF, ciliary neurotrophic factor [CNTF]), the IL6R is specific for IL-6 binding but structurally related to receptors for IL-2, -3, -4, -5, -7, -9, LIF, CNTF, and colony stimulating factors (Gruol & Nelson, 1997).

In addition to the membrane-bound form of the IL-6 receptor, proteolysis releases a soluble form of the receptor, which when complexed with ligand can trigger gp130 on the surface of cells. This rather unique trans-signaling pathway is not common in other cytokine families and endows CNTF and IL-6 responsiveness in cells otherwise lacking the specific receptor (Gadient & Otten, 1997).

2. *Signaling*

IL-6 binds to IL6R, causing dimerization of gp130 and activation of intracellular kinases of the Janus kinase family (JAK1, Jak2, TYK2). Transphosphorylation of JAKs, kinase activation, and tyrosine phosphorylation on gp130 allows for the interaction of signal transducers and activators of transcription (STAT1, STAT3) to interact with JAKs and the gp130 chain. STAT proteins are then activated themselves by tyrosine phosphorylation, after which they dimerize and translocate to the nucleus, binding to IL-6 response elements and transducing the signal to IL-6-specific genes (Gadient & Otten, 1997; Merrill & Benveniste, 1996; St. Pierre et al., 1996).

Alternatively, a second pathway may be induced involving the G protein Ras binding Raf, leading to downstream activation of MEK, MAPK, and the phosphorylation of a different set of transcription factors at threonine residues (Gadient & Otten, 1997).

3. *Responses to IL-6*

IL-6 is produced by and there are IL6R on microglia, macroglia, and neurons, suggesting autocrine and paracrine functions for this cytokine. Areas of the CNS expressing high levels of both receptors and ligand include hippocampus, hypothalamus, neocortex, and cerebellum (Cornfield & Sills, 1991). IL-6 can be induced by IL-1β and TNF-α. In astrocytes, IL-6 production is stimulated by neurotransmitters such as noradrenaline, histamine, vasoactive intestinal peptide, and substance P (Gadient & Otten, 1997).

IL-6 is a centrally acting endogenous pyrogen and may interfere with pain via induction of prostaglandins (Gadient & Otten, 1997; Rothwell, Busbridge, Lefeuvre, & Hardwick, 1991). IL-6 may be proinflammatory in that it contributes to astrogliosis, but there is a growing list of anti-inflammatory events that IL-6 modulates including the down-regulation of adhesion molecules, MHCII, and TNF-α in astrocytes (Benveniste, Tang, & Law, 1995; Merrill & Benveniste, 1996; Tilg, Dinarello, & Mier, 1997). IL-6 inhibits the differentiation of monocytes into macrophages (Tilg et al., 1997). IL-6 induces IL1Ra and enhances tissue metalloproteinases, thereby significantly inhibiting IL-1 responses, most importantly IL-1-mediated degradation of tissues. IL-6 inhibits ICAM-1 expression at the protein and mRNA levels in both astrocytes and microglia. IL-6 induces acute phase proteins, some of which are protective in vivo, such as α2-macroglobulin in EAE (Tilg et al., 1997). Acute phase proteins induce IL1Ra and soluble TNF receptors, both of which blunt the effects of their cognate ligands.

IL-6 promotes survival and differentiation of oligodendrocytes and neurons (Gadient & Otten, 1997; Merrill & Benveniste, 1996). In neurons, the protective effect of IL-6 has been postulated to be due to its capacity to modulate calcium transport. IL-6 protects neurons against other forms of insult such as MPP+ toxicity, ischemia, and free radicals and can postulated to do so by induction of the antiapoptotic protein Bcl-xL (Schwartze & Hawley, 1995; Fujio, Kunisada, Hirato, Yamauchi-Takihara, & Kishimoto, 1997). Nevertheless, this hypothesis needs to be formally tested in neuronal models. IL-6 induces neurite outgrowth in both PC12 cells and primary hippocampal neurons. Neuronal differentiation of PC12 cells by IL-6 seems to involve STAT3 signaling and an active ras-GTP complex (Gadient & Otten, 1997). Thus, in the context of both MS and AD, it would appear that IL-6 might have more beneficial features than detrimental ones and that one might not necessarily want to interfere with its production or function.

C. TGF-β

1. *Receptor Complex*

The three cloned and sequenced isoforms of mammalian TGF-β (TGF-β1, TGF-β2, TGF-β3) in their mature biologically active form are 25kDa homodimeric, nonglycosylated polypeptides with shared homologies and overlapping but distinct functional capabilities. TGF-βs regulate cell cycle progression, differentiation, adhesion, migration, and extracellular matrix production and are, therefore, functionally related to other family members that include bone morphogenic factors, activins, and inhibins (Kriegelstein, Rufer, Suter-Crazzolara, & Unsicker, 1995). Mature TGF-β is bound by a heterodimeric or trimeric receptor complex, and signal transduction proceeds as a result of serine-threonine kinase phosphorylations by the two receptor molecules (Wrana et al., 1992).

The three different receptor molecules compromising the signaling complex have been cloned and sequenced and are designated TGF-β receptors I and II and betaglycan (Ebner et al., 1993; Lin, Wang, Ng-Eaton, Weinberg, & Lodish, 1992) The constitutively active kinase type II receptor binds TGF-β, allowing the ligand to be recognized and bound by receptor I, which then is phosphorylated by receptor II (Wrana, Attisano, Wieser, Venture, Massague, 1994). Phosphorylation allows the type I receptor to propagate downstream signaling (Wrana et al., 1994). Betaglycan is a transmembrane proteoglycan with a cytoplasmic tail that is too short for signaling. Rather, betaglycan acts as a docking site for TGF-β and is required for high-affinity binding to the TGF-β type II receptor (St. Pierre et al., 1996).

2. *TGF-β Signaling*

The mechanisms of signal transduction from serine/threonine kinase receptors to the nucleus have been unraveled through studies in lower species. *C. elegans Sma* genes were identified to be homologous to TGF-β-activatable *Drosophila Mad* genes. Vertebrate homologues of *Sma* and *Mad* have been called SMAD; these are proteins that become phosphorylated by specific type I serine/threonine kinase receptors (Heldin, Miyazowa, & ten Dijke, 1997). TGF-β binding leads to activation of pathway-restricted Smad2 and Smad3 phosphorylation, following which heterotrimerization with Smad4 occurs. Smad4 is a common mediator SMAD. This hetero-oligomeric complex is translocated to the nucleus, where it binds directly or in complex with other proteins to DNA and affects transcription of specific genes (Heldin et al., 1997). Inhibitory Smads (6 and 7) bind to receptors and block the signaling of the pathway-restricted SMADs; whether they must be in multimers to function in this fashion is unknown. Other parallel signal transduction pathways may also exist. In certain cell types, TGF-β also activates TAK-1, a serine/threonine kinase of the MAPKKK family, Ras-Rac families of GTP-binding proteins, and MAPKs ERK-1/2 and stress-activated protein kinase/Jun-N-terminal kinase (SAPK/JNK) (Heldin et al., 1997). It remains to be determined which pathways are activated and under what circumstances in neurons and glia.

3. *Anti- and Proinflammatory Effects of TGF-β*

Transgenic animals in which TGF-β1 has been disrupted show no gross developmental abnormalities at birth. However, soon thereafter these animals succumb to a wasting syndrome, having acquired a multifocal inflammatory cell response that causes tissue necrosis and organ failure. These data suggest that TGF-β is necessary for homeostatic maintenance of a quiescent immune response (Shull et al., 1992). TGF-β has been thought to be antiinflammatory due to its ability to inhibit many inflammatory activities of astrocytes and microglia (Merrill & Benveniste, 1996). TGF-β blocks the ability of T-cell lines to adoptively transfer EAE by preventing their antigen-specific activation. In fact, myelin basic protein (MBP)-tolerized T cells secrete TGF-β. TGF-β ameliorates, whereas anti-TGF-β antibodies exacerbate EAE when injected in vivo (St. Pierre et al., 1996).

TGF-β has been shown to enhance or inhibit (Lindholm, Castren, Kiefer, Zafra, & Thoenen, 1992; Merrill & Benveniste, 1996; Toru-Delbauffe et al., 1989) astrogliosis and astrocyte proliferation. TGF-β inhibits C3 complement component, intercellular adhesion molecule (ICAM-1), and neural cell adhesion molecule (NCAM-1) but up-regulates L1 in astrocytes (Barnum & Jones, 1994; Saad et al., 1991; Shrikant, Lee, Kalvakolanu, Ransohoff, & Benveniste, 1996; Xiao, Zhang, Ma, & Link, 1996). TGF-β inhibits transcription of MHCII and B7 molecules and thus antigen presentation; it also inhibits transcription and translation of NOS, thereby inhibiting NO production in vitro in rat astrocytes and microglia (Merrill & Benveniste, 1996; Panek & Benveniste, 1995; Schluesener, 1990). The ability of TGF-β to inhibit both reactive nitrogen and oxygen species by glia and macrophages means that the cytotoxicity of neurons and oligodendrocytes by these effectors can be prevented (Chao et al., 1994; Merrill & Benveniste, 1996). In this context, TGF-β might be considered antiinflammatory and of benefit in an autoimmune disease like MS or neurodegenerative processes in AD. Nevertheless, overproduction of TGF-β within the nervous system can lead to hyperimmune responses, notably through the induction of infiltration of macrophages and neutrophils (Wahl et al., 1987; Wyss-Coray, Barrow, Brooker, & Mucke, 1997); this is postulated to be because TGF-β induces alpha and beta chemokine production, thereby activating these cells that are known contributors to pathology in the CNS (Wahl et al., 1987; Wyss-Coray et al., 1997).

In contrast to the effects on immune-like functions of glia, TGF-βs are potently protective of neurons in the CNS and can directly or indirectly (by induction of other trophic factors and/or by inhibiting proliferation) drive neurons and oligodendrocyte precursors to differentiate (Kriegelstein et al., 1995; Merrill & Benveniste, 1996). TGF-βs are therefore important developmentally. Interestingly, TGF-β2 is structurally similar to NGF (Swindells, 1992). TGF-β induces the production of neuroprotective factors from astrocytes such as IL-6 (Benveniste et al., 1994) and NGF (Lindholm, Hengerer, Zafra, & Thoenen, 1990; Saad et al., 1991); TGF-β's induction of IL-6 may account for its ability to regulate Ca++ levels and induce bcl-2 increases in neurons, thereby aiding in their survival (Kriegelstein et al., 1995).

III. ADHESION MOLECULES, CHEMOKINES, AND FREE RADICALS

Cell migration from blood to brain and within the CNS plays a critical role in the pathology of the autoimmune disease MS. Although inflammatory cell migration does not seem to occur in AD, migration of microglia within the CNS parenchyma may be critical in plaque formation. Adhesion molecules and chemokines are probably involved. Production of these molecules is modulated transcriptionally, posttranscriptionally, and posttranslationally by free radicals present in the inflammatory milieu. The interactions of these entities is thus an important topic for exploration.

A. Extravasation of Cells across the BBB

Activation and adherence of blood-borne leukocytes to cerebrovascular endothelial cells (EC) involves ICAM-1 on EC and its integrin receptor on leukocytes, LFA-1. Crosslinking of ICAM-1 activates T cells and macrophages, resulting in the production of the proinflammatory molecules IFN-γ, IL-1, and NO (reviewed in Merrill & Murphy, 1997). Induction of NO and cytokines alters the permeability of the BBB, increases ICAM-1 and LFA-1, and induces another adhesion molecule called vascular cell adhesion molecule-1 (VCAM-1) on EC and glia. VCAM-1 is a ligand for a constitutively expressed integrin found on leukocytes, VLA-4. It is the expression of VLA-4 and its interaction with VCAM-1 that is crucial for the preferential entry of CD4+ T cells into the CNS. Leukocyte transendothelial extravasation involves homophilic interactions between leukocyte and EC CD31 (PECAM-1) (Merrill & Benveniste, 1996; Ransohoff, Glabinski, & Tani, 1996). Once cells have crossed the BBB, they are directed to migrate toward gradients created by chemoattractant cytokines called chemokines, which can be quite specific in determining the immigration patterns of lymphocytes and macrophages to certain inflammatory regions. Chemokines are also capable of enhancing activation by integrins through redistribution of adhesion molecules, thereby modulating leukocyte-EC interactions (Merrill & Benveniste, 1996; Ransohoff et al., 1996).

B. Chemokines

Chemokines are small cytokines produced by many different cell types in response to various stimuli. In the CNS, macrophages/microglia, astrocytes, EC, and other cells associated with the cerebral vasculature produce a wide but signatory array of chemokines. These are divided into two families. The α family, including IL-8, KC, and IFN-γ inducible protein (IP-10) is specific for neutrophils. The β family, whose members include monocyte chemoattractant peptide-1 (MCP-1), regulated on activation, normal T cell expressed and secreted (RANTES), and macrophage inflammatory protein-1 (MIP-1), acts on monocytes and T cells. The receptors for these chemokines are classic seven-transmembrane, G protein-coupled proteins. These receptors are designated as CXCR-1 thru-4 for the α family and CCR-1 thru-5 for the β family of ligands (Merrill & Murphy, 1997).

Induction of or an increase in chemokine expression is commonplace in neuropathologies. Chemokine expression is invariably associated with inflammation at the onset of acute EAE and selectively elevated during relapses. Antibodies to MIP-1α preclude development of EAE (Karpus et al., 1995). The β chemokines RANTES, MCP-1, and MIP-1α (but not IP-10) are elevated following trauma. Microglia produce MCP-1 in response to Aβ, suggesting a role in aging and AD (Meda et al., 1996). This is augmented by the presence of IFN-γ and in large part mediated by TNF-α.

C. Regulation of Molecules Influencing Cell Trafficking at the BBB

1. *Free Radicals and Chemokines*

The biological interactions between NO and chemokines are significant. NO inhibits expression of the chemokines IL-8 and MCP-1 in EC but upregulates IL-8 transcription in leukocytes and melanoma cells. Still other studies have shown that reactive oxygen species (ROS) H_2O_2 and hydroxyl radical (OH-) as well as paraquat up-regulate IL-8 in stimulated cells. Antioxidants such as DMSO, mannitol, ethanol, and thiourea inhibit this induction (Merrill & Murphy, 1996, 1997). This suggests that ECs use a different pathway of IL-8 induction than inflammatory and other cells, and that there may exist a protection mechanism in vasculature to prevent the recruitment of leukocytes and extravasation into the nervous system in the absence of other signals indicating the initiation of and/or requirement for an immune response.

2. *Free Radicals and Cytokines*

NFκB influences the inflammatory response, and not insignificantly it affects those cytokines and chemokines influencing BBB permeability and cell trafficking into the CNS: IL-1β, IL-6, TNF-α, IFN-γ, CSFs, IL-8, MCP-1, HLA-DR, VCAM-1, and ICAM-1 (Dröge et al., 1994; Raes, Renard, & Remacle, 1995). As previously discussed, IL-1β, TNF-α, IL-6, and NO are all elevated in EAE and MS (Merrill & Benveniste, 1996). IL-1β and TNF-α induce IL-6 and NO. With some exceptions, NO and ROS increase TNF-α, IL-6, and IL-1β gene expression in vitro and in vivo. The Th1 response is driven by IL-12, which has been shown to be critical in unmasking latent EAE in resistant mouse strains (Segal & Shevach, 1996). NO induces the transcription of the p40 chain of the IL-12 heterodimer (Rothe et al., 1996). Blocking ROS or NO production with mitochondrial inhibitors or antioxidants abrogates transcription of and subsequent production of these proinflammatory cytokines, supporting the hypothesis that free radicals can regulate gene transcription and subsequent events at the BBB (Merrill & Benveniste, 1996).

3. *Free Radicals and Adhesion Molecules*

MHC II, induced by IFN-γ or LPS in murine macrophages and rat astrocytes, is inhibited by NO donors or stimulants that induce NO. In vascular smooth muscle cells and EC, NO inhibits ICAM-1 and VCAM-1. In murine brain microvascular EC, inhibition of Na+/K+ ATPase by ouabain activates NF-κB, leading to the expression of VCAM-1 and iNOS. In a variety of cell types, AP-1 dependent transcriptional activation can be induced both by pro- and antioxidant conditions. Interestingly, the ICAM-1 promoter also contains a functional AP-1 site. Pyrolidone dithiocarbamate (PDTC) induces ICAM-1 via the stimulation of c-*fos* and c-*jun* binding to the AP-1 consensus site (Muñoz et al., 1996), suggesting that ICAM-1 and VCAM-1 are up-regulated by prooxidants through NF-κB. These adhesion molecules are usually inhibited by scavengers like NO and PDTC (DeCaterina et al., 1995; Marui et al., 1993), though ICAM-1 can be up-regulated by antioxidants through the AP-1 site. ROS can also regulate the amplification of cells and their migration across the BBB. Oxygen intermediates induce, whereas NO inhibits, macrophage colony-stimulating factor (M-CS) (Merrill & Benveniste, 1996; Merrill & Murphy, 1997). Since the thiol compound diethyldithiocarbamate (DDTC) increases M-CS factors in other cells, there is the suggestion that NO may be acting as an oxygen radical scavenger preventing M-CS factor gene transcriptional activation (East, Abboud, & Borch, 1992).

D. Redox Sensitive Transcription Factors in CNS Inflammation

The transcription factors AP-1 and NF-κB are involved in the regulation of expression of a very large number of genes that have been implicated in AD and MS. These include iNOS, cyclooxygenase 2 (COX-2), neuronal and oligodendrocyte trophic factors, cytokines, chemokines, and adhesion molecules, all of which are capable of being modified by ROS and NO. Critical steps in signaling pathways can be influenced by ROS and NO and thus these radicals have the potential to regulate the expression or activation of transcription factors. Because NO reacts with metals and thiols, which may be located at strategic allosteric or active sites, signaling components containing transition metals or thiols will be susceptible to nitrosative attack (Stamler, 1994).

1. *NF-κB*

Nuclear factor (NF)-κB is present constitutively in cells as a protein dimer p50/065. It remains in an inactive state in the cytoplasm while bound to IκB. Phosphorylation and degradation of IκB release NF-κB to move to the nucleus and bind to DNA. This event is induced by a variety of different stimuli and, depending on the cell type, NO and ROS are implicated both as activators and inhibitors of this translocation (reviewed in Merrill & Murphy, 1997). NF-κB is activated by alternative pathways, so it is not universally true that oxidants activate and antioxidants block this transcription factor.

NO influences NF-κB activation in astrocytes in that exogenous NO donors appear to cause translocation of NF-κB to the nucleus (Park, Lin, & Murphy, 1994). Specific DNA binding of NF-κB is inhibited by oxidants and stimulated by reducing agents, and these effects appear to be mediated by the p50 DNA-binding subunit. Serine substitution of a cysteine residue at the N-terminal binding region reduces binding and renders the protein insensitive to reducing agents. NO donors also block NF-κB binding to DNA in a reversible manner, possibly through nitrosylation of the same cysteine residue (Park, Lin, & Murphy, 1997). However, in human vascular endothelial cells, NO donors stabilize IκB and activate its transcription, thus inhibiting NF-κB translocation (Peng, Libby, & Liao, 1995).

2. *AP-1*

AP-1 is a dimeric complex of Jun-Jun or Jun-Fos proteins. Cysteine residues within the leucine zipper and basic domains of Fos and Jun are important for their dimerization. Increased binding of AP-1 to DNA occurs following O_2^- up-regulation of Fos and Jun; indeed, ROS facilitate AP-1 activity stimulated by TNF-α and bFGF (Merrill & Murphy, 1997). It appears that, in general, oxidative conditions increase expression, phosphorylation, and binding of Jun to DNA in many cell types. NO also leads to increased expression of Fos and Jun in neurons; the mechanisms have been variously described as being cGMP/PKG dependent, cGMP independent, and cAMP/CREB dependent. Again, as with ROS, paradoxically, NO donors decrease AP-1 binding (Tabuchi, Sano, Tsuchiya, & Tada, 1994).

Certain factors that are trophic and survival factors for both glia and neurons are dependent on c-fos and are induced in cells by H_2O_2. These include bFGF, epidermal growth factor (EGF), platelet derived growth factor (PDGF), and NGF. Early gene expression in striatal neurons, neurite outgrowth, dendritic remodeling, and synaptic function of hippocampal granule cells are all increased both in vitro and in vivo by generators of NO and $ONOO^-$.

3. *Other CNS Genes*

NO and nitroso-containing molecules could potentially destabilize zinc finger motifs in transcription factors and eject metal groups from biochemically important proteins within cells, thus rendering them nonfunctional. Therefore, it might be speculated that nitrogen radicals could affect type IIII NOS (ecNOS) in vascular endothelial cells, the neurofilament gene in neurons, and myelin genes in oligodendrocytes, all of which are regulated by zinc finger-containing transcription factors (Elder, Liang, Li, & Lazzarini, 1992). NO appears to downregulate the myelin genes: myelin basic protein, myelin associated glycoprotein, and proteolipid protein (Mackenzie-Graham, Mitrovic, Smoll, & Merrill, 1994). The implications of this in vitro finding, if upheld in vivo, are that in the presence of activated microglia producing NO, remyelination might not occur in MS lesions.

IV. CONCLUSIONS

The importance of the effects of cytokines, chemokines, adhesion molecules, and free radicals in diseases of the adult human nervous system such as AD and MS can only be evaluated in the pathological context of their presence, both temporally and spatially. The proposed role of radicals and cytokines in the causation of particular neuropathologies is mostly conjecture inspite of the highly suggestive data from animal studies. Continued research in designing and engineering better models to assess these hypotheses is necessary. Awareness of the subtle fundamental effects of cytokines and free radicals on gene expression will be especially relevant to the clinical applications made in treating disease.

References

Alleva, D. G., Burger, C. J., & Elgert, K. D. (1994). Tumor-induced regulation of suppressor macrophage nitric oxide and TNFα production. Role of tumor-derived IL-10, TGFβ, and prostaglandin E2. *Journal of Immunology, 153*, 1674–1686.

Bagasra, O., Michaels, F. H., Zheng, Y. M., Bobroski, L. E., Spitsin, S. V., Fu, Z. F., Tawadros, R., & Koprowski, H. (1995). Activation of the inducible form of nitric oxide synthase in the brains of patients with multiple sclerosis. *Proceedings of the National Academy of Sciences, 92*, 12041–12045.

Barnum, S. R., & Jones, J. L. (1994). Transforming growth factor—β1 inhibits inflammatory cytokine-induced C3 gene expression in astrocytes. *Journal of Immunology, 152*, 765–773.

Becherel, P. A., Mossalayi, M. D., Le-Goff, L., Ouaaz, F., Dugas, B., Guillosson, J. J., Debre, P., & Arock, M. (1994). IgE-dependent activation of FcεRII/CD23+ normal human keratinocytes: The role of cAMP and nitric oxide. *Cellular and Molecular Biology, 40*, 283–290.

Beck, J., Rondot, P., Catinot, L., Falcoff, E., Kirchner, H., & Wietzerbin, J. (1988). Increased production of interferon gamma and tumor necrosis factor precedes clinical manifestation in multiple sclerosis: Do cytokines trigger off exacerbations? *Acta Neurologica Scandanavica, 78*, 318–326.

Benveniste, E. N., Kwon, J., Chung, W. J., Sampson, J., Pandya, K., & Tang, L. P. (1994). Differential modulation of astrocyte cytokine gene expression by TGF-β. *Journal of Immunology, 153*, 5210–5221.

Benveniste, E. N., Tang, L., & Law, R. M. (1995). Differential regulation of astrocyte TNF-α expression by the cytokines TGF-β, IL-6 and IL-10. *International Journal of Developmental Neuroscience, 13*, 341–349.

Blanco, F. J., Geng, Y., & Lotz, M. (1995). Differentiation-dependent effects of IL-1 and TGFβ on human articular chondrocyte proliferation are related to inducible nitric oxide synthase expression. *Journal of Immunology, 154*, 4018–4026.

Bö, L., Dawson, T. M., Wesselingh, S., Mork, S., Choi, S., Kong, P. A., Hanley, D., & Trapp, B. D. (1995). Induction of nitric oxide synthase in demyelinating regions of multiple sclerosis brains. *Annals of Neurology, 36*, 778–786.

Bogdan, C., Vodovotz, Y., Paik, J., Xie, Q.-W., & Nathan, C. (1994). Mechanisms of suppression of nitric oxide synthase expression by interleukin-4 in primary mouse macrophages. *Journal of Leukocyte Biology, 55*, 227–233.

Boullerne, A. I., Petry, K. G., Meynard, M., & Geffard, M. (1995). Indirect evidence for nitric oxide involvement in multiple sclerosis by characterization of circulating antibodies directed against conjugated S-nitrosocysteine. *Journal of Neuroimmunology, 60*, 117–124.

Bukrinsky, M. I., Nottet, H. S. L. M., Schmidtmayerova, H., Dubrovsky, L., Flanagan, C. R., Mullins, M. E., Lipton, S. A., & Gendelman, H. E. (1995). Regulation of nitric oxide synthase activity in human immunodeficiency virus type 1 (HIV-1)-infected monocytes: Implications for HIV-associated neurological disease. *Journal of Experimental Medicine, 181*, 735–745.

Campbell, I. L., Abraham, C. A., Masliah, E., Kemper, P., Inglis, J. D., Oldstone, M.B.A., & Mucke, L. (1993). Neurologic disease induced in transgenic mice by cerebral overexpression of interleukin 6. *Proceedings of the National Academy of Sciences, 90*, 10061–10065.

Campbell, I. L., Stalder, A. K., Chiang, C.-S., Bellinger, R., Heysey, C. J., Steffensen S., Masliah, E., Powell, H. C., Gold L. H., Henriksen, S. J., & Siggins, G. R. (1997). Cytokines in the brain: Transgenic models to access the pathogenic acrtions of cytokines in the central nervous system. *Molecular Psychiatry, 2*, 125–129.

Cash, E., Minty, A., Ferrara, P., Caput, D., Fradelizi, D., & Rott, O. (1994). Macrophage-inactivating IL-13 suppresses experimental autoimmune encephalomyelitis in rats. *Journal of Immunology, 153*, 4258–4267.

Chao, C. C., Hu, S., Kravitz, F. H., Tsang, M., Anderson, W. R., & Peterson, P. K. (1994). Transforming growth factor-β protects human neurons against β-amyloid-induced injury. *Molecular and Cellular Neuropathology, 23*, 150–161.

Chao, C. C., Hu, S., Molitor, T. W., Shaskan, E. G., & Peterson, P. K. (1992). Activated microglia mediate neuronal cell injury via a nitric oxide mechanism. *Journal of Immunology, 149*, 2736–2741.

Chesrown, S. E., Monnier, J., Visner, G., & Nick, H. S. (1994). Regulation of inducible nitric oxide synthase mRNA levels by LPS, IFN-γ, TGF-β, and IL-10 in murine macrophage cell lines and rat peritoneal macrophages. *Biochemical and Biophysical Research Communication, 200*, 126–134.

Cornfield, L. J., & Sills, M. A. (1991). High affinity interleukin-6 binding sites in bovine hypothalamus. *European Journal of Pharmacology, 220*, 113–115.

Corraliza, I. M., Soler, G., Eichmann, K., & Modolell, M. (1995). Arginase induction by suppressors of nitric oxide synthesis (IL-4, IL-10, and PGE2) in murine bone-marrow-derived macrophages. *Biochemical and Biophysical Research Communication, 206*, 667–673.

De Caterina, R., Libby, P., Peng, H.-B., Thannickal, V. J., Rajavshisth, T. B., Gimbrone, M. A. Jr., Shin, W. S., & Liao, J. K. (1995). Nitric oxide decreases cytokine-induced endothelial activation. *Journal of Clinical Investigations, 96*, 60-68.

De Groot, C. J. A., Ruuls, S. R., Theeuwes, J. W. M., Dijkstra, C. D., & Van der Walk, P. (1997). Immunocytochemical characterization of the expression of inducible and constitutive isoforms of nitric oxide synthase in demyelinating multiple sclerosis lesions. *Journal of Neuropathology and Experimental Neurology, 56*, 10–20.

De Maria, R., Cifone, M. G., Trotta, R., Rippo, M. R., Festuccia, C., Santoni, A., & Testi, R. (1994). Triggering of human monocyte activation through CD69, a member of the natural killer cell gene complex family of signal transducing receptors. *Journal of Experimental Medicine, 180*, 1999–2004.

Dickson, D. W., Lee, S. C., Brosnan C. F., Sinicropi, S., Vlassara, H., & Yen, S.-H. C. (1996). Neuroimmunology of aging and Alzheimer's disease with emphasis on cytokines. In R. M. Ransohoff & E. N. Benveniste (Eds.), *Cytokines and the CNS*, (pp. 239–268). Baton Rouge: CRC Press.

Dileepan, K. N., Page, J. C., Li, Y., & Stechschulte, D. J. (1995). Direct activation of murine peritoneal macrophages for nitric oxide production and tumor cell killing by interferon-γ. *Journal of Interferon and Cytokine Research, 15*, 387–394.

Ding, M., St. Pierre, B. A., Parkinson, J. F., Medberry, P., Wong, J. L., Rogers, N. E., Ignarro, I. J., & Merrill, J. E. (1997). Inducible nitric oxide synthase and nitric oxide production in human fetal astrocytes and microglia: A kinetic analysis, *Journal of Biological Chemistry, 272*, 11327–11335.

Di Santo, E., Alonzi, T., Fattori, E., Poli, V., Ciliberto, G., Sironi, M., Gnocchi, P., Ricciardi-Castagnoli, P., & Ghezzi, P. (1996). Overexpression of the interleukin-6 in the central nervous system of transgenic mice increases central but not systemic proinflammatory cytokine production. *Brain Research, 740*, 239–244.

Dopp, J. M., Mackenzie-Graham, A., Otero, G. C., & Merrill, J. E. (1996). Differential expression, cytokine modulation, and specific functions of type-1 and type-2 tumor necrosis factor receptors in rat glia. *Journal of Neuroimmunology, 75*, 104–112.

Doyle, A G., Herbein, G., Montener, L. J., Minty, A. J., Caput, D., Ferrara, P., & Gordon, S. (1994). Interleukin-13 alters the activation state of murine macrophages in vitro: Comparison with interleukin-4 and interferon-γ. *European Journal of Immunology, 24*, 1441–1445.

Dröge, W., Schulze-Osthoff, K., Mihm, S., Galter, D., Schenk, H., Eck, H.-P., Roth, S., & Gmünder, H. (1994). Functions of glutathione and glutathione disulfide in immunology and immunopathology. *FASEB Journal, 8*, 1131–1138.

East, C. J., Abboud, C. N., & Borch, R. F. (1992). Diethyldithiocarbamate induction of cytokine release in human long-term bone marrow cultures. *Blood 80*, 1172–1177.

Ebner, R., Chen, R.-H., Shum, L., Lawler, S., Zioncheck, T. F., Lee, A., Lopez, A. R., & Derynck, C. (1993). Cloning of the type I TGF-β receptor and its effect on TGF-β binding to the type II receptor. *Science, 260*, 1344–1348.

Eigler, A., Sinha, B., & Endres, S. (1993). Nitric oxide-releasing agents enhance cytokine-induced tumor necrosis factor synthesis in human mononuclear cells. *Biochemical, Biophysical and Research Communication, 196*, 494–501.

Elder, G. A., Liang, Z., Li, C., & Lazzarini, R. A. (1992). Targeting of Sp1 to a non-SP1 site in the human neurofilament (H) promoter via an intermediary DNA-binding protein. *Nucleic Acids Research, 23*, 6281–6285.

Fattori, E., Lazzaro, D., Musiani, P., Modesti, A., Alonzi, T., & Ciliberti, G. (1995). IL-6 expression in neurons of transgenic mice causes reactive astrogliosis and increase ramified mciroglial cells but no neuronal damage. *European Journal of Neuroscience, 7*, 2441–2449.

Fiorentino, D. F., Zlotnik, A., Mosmann, T. R., Howard, M., & O'Garra, A. (1991). IL-10 inhibits cytokine production by activated macrophages. *Journal of Immunology, 147*, 3815–3822.

Fontana, A., Eugster, H.-P., Frei, K., Lassmann, H., Malipiero, U., & Sahrbacher, U. (1998). Experimental autoimmune encephalomyelitis in cytokine gene knockout [Abstract]. *Journal of Neuroimmunology, 90*, 4.

Fujio, Y., Kunisada, K., Hirota, H., Yamauchi-Takihara, K., & Kishimoto, T. (1997). Signals through gp130 upregulate *bcl-x* gene expression via STAT1-binding cis-element in cardiac myocytes. *Journal of Clinical Investigation, 99*, 2898–2905.

Fülle, H.-J., Enders, S., Sinha, B., Stoll, D., Weber, P. C., & Gerzer, R. (1991). Effects of SIN-1 on cytokine synthesis in human mononuclear cells. *Journal of Cardiovascular Pharmacology, 17*, S113–S116.

Gadient, R. A., & Otten U. H. (1997). Interleukin-6—a molecule with both beneficial and destructive potentials. *Progress in Neurobiology, 52*, 379–390.

Gazzinelli, R. T., Oswald, I. P., James, S. L., & Sher, A. (1992). IL-10 inhibits parasite killing and nitrogen oxide production by IFN-γ-activated macrophages. *Journal of Immunology, 148*, 1792–1796.

Genain, C. P., Abel, K., Belmar, N., Villinger, F., Rosenberg, D. P., Linington, C., Raine, C. S., & Hauser, S. L. (1996). Late complications of immune deviation therapy in a nonhuman primate. *Science, 274*, 2054–2057.

Gijbels, K., Brocke, S., Abrams, J. S., & Steinman, L. (1995). Administration of neutralizing antibodies to interleukin-6 (IL-6) reduces experimental autoimmune encephalomyelitis and is associated with elevated levels of IL-6 bioactivity in central nervous system circulation. *Molecular Medicine, 1*, 795–805.

Gruol, D. L., & Nelson T. E. (1997). Physiological and pathological roles of interleukin-6 in the central nervous system. *Molecular Neurobiology, 15*, 307–339.

Hamilton, T. A., Tannenbaum, C. S., & Tebo, J. M. (1996). Cytokine-initiated intracellular signaling pathways. In R. M. Ransahoff & E. N. Benveniste (Eds.), *Cytokines and the CNS*. (pp. 25–46). Baton Rouge: CRC Press.

Hauser, S. L., Doolittle, D. H., Lincoln, R., Brown, R. H., & Dinarello, C. A. (1990). Cytokine accumulations in CSF of multiple sclerosis patients: Frequent detection of interleukin-1 and tumor necrosis factor but not interleukin-6. *Neurology, 40*, 1735–1739.

Heldin, C.-H., Miyazono, K., & ten Dijke, P. (1997). TGF-β signalling from cell membrane to nucleus through SMAD proteins. *Nature, 390*, 465–471.

Hofman, F. M., Hinton, D. R., Johnson, K., & Merrill, J. E. (1989). Tumor necrosis factor identified in multiple sclerosis brain. *Journal of Experimental Medicine, 170*, 607–612.

Hofman, F. M., von Hanwehr, R. I., Dinarello, C. A., Mizel, S. B., Hinton, D., & Merrill, J. E. (1986). Immunoregulatory molecules and IL2 receptors identified in multiple sclerosis brain. *Journal of Immunology, 136*, 3239–3245.

Hu, J., & el-Fakahany E. E. (1993). β amyloid 25-35 activates nitric oxide synthase in a neuronal clone. *Neuroreport, 4*, 760–762.

IFN-beta Multiple Sclerosis Study Group. (1993). Interferon beta-1 is effective in relapsing-remitting multiple sclerosis. I. Clinical results of a multicenter, randomized, double-blind, placebo-controlled trial. *Neurology, 43*, 655–661.

Johnson, A. W., Land, J. M., Thompson, E. J., Bolanos, J. P., Clark, J. B., & Heales, S. J. (1995). Evidence for increased nitric oxide production in multiple sclerosis. *Journal of Neurology, Neurosurgery, and Psychiatry, 58*, 107–116.

Karpus, W. J., Lukacs, N. W., McRae, B. L. Strieter, R. M., Kunkel, S. L., & Miller, S. D. (1995). An important role for the chemokine macrophage inflammatory protein-1a in the pathogenesis of the T cell-mediated autoimmune disease, experimental autoimmune encephalomyelitis. *Journal of Immunology, 155*, 5003–5010.

Koka, P., He, K., Zack, J. A., Kitchen, S., Peacock, W., Fried, I., Tran, T., Yashar. S. S., & Merrill, J. E. (1995). Human immunodeficiency virus 1 envelope proteins induce interleukin 1, tumor necrosis factor α and nitric oxide in glial cultures from fetal, neonatal, and adult human brain. *Journal of Experimental Medicine, 182*, 941–952.

Kriegelstein, K., Rufer, M., Suter-Crazzolara, C., & Unsicker, K. (1995). Neural functions of the transforming growth factors β. *International Journal of Developmental Neuroscience, 13*, 301–315.

Kubes, P., Suzuki, M., & Granger, D. N. (1991). Nitric oxide: an endogenous modulator of leukocyte adhesion. *Proceedings of the National Academy of Sciences, 88*, 4651–4654.

Lander, H. M., Ogiste, J. S., Teng, K. K., & Novogrodsky, A. (1995). p21ras as a common signaling target of reactive free radicals and cellular redox stress. *Journal of Biological Chemistry, 270*, 21195–21198.

Lee, S. C., Dickson, D. W., Liu. W., & Brosnan, C. F. (1993). Induction of nitric oxide synthase activity in human astrocytes by interleukin-1β and interferon-γ. *Journal of Neuroimmunology, 46*, 19–24.

Lin, H. Y., Wang, X.-F., Ng-Eaton, E., Weinberg, R. A., & Lodish, H. A. (1992). Expression cloning of the TGF-β type II receptor, a functional transmembrane serine/threonine kinase. *Cell, 68*, 775–785.

Lindholm, D., Castren, E., Kiefer, R., Zafra, F., & Thoenen, H. (1992). Transforming growth factor-β1 in the rat brain: Increase after injury and inhibition of astrocyte proliferation. *Journal of Cell Biology, 117*, 395–400.

Lindholm, D., Hengerere, B., Zafra, F., & Thoenen, H. (1990). Transforming growth factor-β1 stimulates expression of nerve growth factor in the rat CNS. *Neuroreport, 1*, 9–12.

Link, J., Soderstrom, M., Olsson, T., Hojeberg, B., Ljungdahl, A., & Link, H. (1994). Increased transforming growth factor-β, interleukin-4, and interferon-γ in multiple sclerosis. *Annals of Neurology, 36*, 379–386.

MacKenzie-Graham, A. J., Mitrovic, B., Smoll, A., & Merrill, J. E. (1994). Differential sensitivity to nitric oxide in immortalized cloned murine oligodendrocyte cell lines. *Developmental Neuroscience 16*, 162–171.

Magrinat, G., Mason, S. N., Shami, P. J., & Weinberg, J. B. (1992). Nitric oxide modulation of human leukemia cell differentiation and gene expression. *Blood, 80*, 1880–1884.

Marui, N., Offermann, M. K., Swerlick, R., Kunsch, C., Rosen, C. A., Ahmad, M., Alexander, R. W., & Medford, R. M. (1993). Vascular cell adhesion molecule-1 (VCAM-1) gene transcription and expression are regulated through an antioxidant-sensitive mechanism in human vascular endothelial cells. *Journal of Clinical Investigation, 92*, 1866–1874.

Matthys, P. Froyen, G., Verdot, L., Huang, S., Sobis, H., Van Damme, J., Vray, B., Aguet, M., & Billiau, A. (1995). IFN-γ receptor deficient mice are hypersensitive to the anti-CD3-induced cytokine release syndrome and thymocyte apoptosis. *Journal of Immunology, 155*, 3823–3829.

Mautino, G., Paul-Eugene, N., Chanez, P., Vignola, A. M., Kolb, J. P., Bousquet, J., & Dugas, B. (1994). Heterogeneous spontaneous and interleukin-4-induced nitric oxide production by human monocytes. *Journal of Leukocyte Biology, 56*, 15–20.

McDonald, D., Brunden, K., & Landreth, G. (1997). Amyloid fibrils activate tyrosine kinase-dependent signaling and superoxide production in microglia. *Journal of Neuroscience, 17*, 2284–2294.

Meda, L., Bernasconi, S., Bonaiuto, C., Sozzani, S., Zhou, D., Otvos, L., Mantovani, A., Rossi, F., & Cassatella, M. A. (1996). β amyloid (25-35) peptide and IFNγ synergistically induce the production of the chemotactic cytokine MCP-1/JE in monocytes and microglial cells. *Journal of Immunology, 157*, 1213–1218.

Meda, L., Cassatella, M. A., Szendrei, G. I., Otvos, L., Baron, P., Villalba, M., Ferrari, D., & Rossi, F. (1995). Activation of microglial cells by β-amyloid protein and interferon γ. *Nature, 374*, 647–650.

Merrill, J. E., & Benveniste, E. N. (1996). Cytokines in inflammatory brain lesions: Helpful and harmful. *TINS, 19*, 331–338.

Merrill, J. E., De Rosa, M., & Franklin, R. J. M. (1998). New concepts in nitric oxide in demyelination and remyelination [Abstract]. *Journal of Neuroimmunology, 90*, 50.

Merrill, J. E., Ignarro, L. J., Sherman, M. P., Melinek, J., & Lane, T. E., (1993). Microglial cell cytotoxicity of oligodendrocytes is mediated through nitric oxide. *Journal of Immunology, 151*, 2132–2141.

Merrill, J. E., & Murphy, S. (1996). Nitric oxide. In M. Aschner & H. K. Kimelberg (Eds.), *The role of glia in neurotoxicity* (pp. 263–281). New York: CRC Press.

Merrill, J. E., & Murphy, S. P. (1997). Regulation of gene expression in the nervous system by reactive oxygen and nitrogen species. *Metabolic Brain Disease, 12*, 97–112.

Merrill, J. E., Strom, S.R., Ellison, G. W., & Myers, L. W. (1989). In vitro study of mediators of inflammation in multiple sclerosis. *Journal of Clinical Immunology, 9*, 84–96.

Muñoz, C., Castellanos, M. C., Alfranca, A., Vara, A., Esteban, M. A., Redondo, J. M., & de Landázuri, M. O. (1996). Transcriptional up-regulation of intercellular adhesion molecule-1 in human endothelial cells by the antioxidant pyrrolidine dithiocarbamate involves the activation of activating protein-1. *Journal of Immunology, 157*, 3587–3597.

Murphy, S., Grzybicki, D. M., & Simmons, M. L. (1995). Glial Cells as nitric oxide sources and targets. In S. Vincent (Ed.), *Nitric oxide in the nervous system* (pp. 164–190). San Diego: Academic Press.

Nicholson, S., da Gloria Bonecini-Almeida, M., Lapa da Silva, J. R., Nathan, C., Xie, Q.-W., Mumford, R., Weidner, J. R., Calaycay, J., Geng, J., Boechat, N., Linhares, C., Rom, W., & Ho., J. L. (1996). Indicible nitric oxide synthase in pulmonary alveolar macrophages from patients with tuberculosis. *Journal of Experimental Medicine, 183*, 2293–2302.

Otero G. C. & Merrill, J. E. (1994). Cytokine receptors on glial cells. *GLIA, 11*, 117–128.

Panek, R. B., & Benveniste, E. N. (1995) Class II MHC gene expression in microglia. *Journal of Immunology, 154*, 2846–2854.

Park, S. K., Lin, H. L., & Murphy, S. (1994). Nitric oxide limits transcriptional induction of nitric oxide synthase in CNS glial cells. *Biochemical and Biophysical Research Communication, 201*, 762–768.

Park, S. K., Lin, H. L., & Murphy, S. (1997). Nitric oxide regulates nitric oxide synthase-2 gene expression by inhibiting NF-κB binding to DNA. *Biochemical Journal, 322*, 609–613.

Peng, H., Libby, P., & Liao, J. K. (1995). Induction and stabilization of IkBa by nitric oxide mediates inhibition of NF-κB. *Journal of Biological Chemistry, 270*, 14214–14219.

Peng, H.-B., Rajavashidsth, T. B., Libby, P., & Liao, J. K. (1995). Nitric oxide inhibits macrophage-colony stimulating factor gene transcription in vascular endothelial cells. *Journal of Biological Chemistry, 270*, 17050–17055.

Pierre Kolb, J., Paul-Eugene, N., Damais, C., Yamaoka, K., Drapier, J. C., & Dugas, B. (1994). Interleukin-4 stimulates cGMP production by IFN-γ-activated human monocytes. *Journal of Biological Chemistry, 269*, 9811–9816.

Raes, M., Renard, P., & Remacle, J. (1995) Free radicals as second messengers. *Critical Reviews Social Biology, 189*, 355–366.

Ransohoff, R. M., Devajyothi, C., Estes, M. L., Babcock, G., & Rudick, R. A. (1991). Interferon-β specifically inhibits interferon γ-induced class II major histocompatibility complex gene transcription in a human astrocytoma cell line. *Journal of Neuroimmunology, 33*, 103–112.

Ransohoff, R. M., Glabinski, A., & Tani, M. (1996). Chemokines in immune-mediated inflammation of the central nervous system. *Cytokine and Growth Factor Review, 7*, 35–46.

Reiling, N., Ulmer, A. J., Duchrow, M., Ernst, M., Flad, H.-D., & Hauschildt, S. (1994). Nitric oxide synthase: mRNA expression of different isoforms in human monocytes/macrophages. *European Journal of Immunology, 24*, 1941–1944

Ringheim, G. E., Szczepanik, A. M., Petko, W., Burgher, K. L., Zhu, S. Z., & Chao, C. C. (1998). Enhancement of beta-amyloid precursor protein transcription and expression by the soluble interleukin-6 receptor/interleukin-6 complex. *Molecular Brain Research, 55*, 35–44.

Rockett, K. A., Awburn, B. M. M., Aggarwal, B. B., Cowden,W. B., & Clark, I. A. (1992). In vivo induction of nitrite and nitrate by tumor necrosis factor, lymphotoxin, and interleukin-1: Possible roles in malaria. *Infection and Immunity, 60*, 3725–3730.

Rodriguez, M., Pavelko, K. D., McKinney, C. W., & Leibowitz, J. L. (1994). Recombinant human IL-6 suppresses demyelination in a viral model of multiple sclerosis. *Journal of Immunology, 153*, 3811–3821.

Rothe, H., Hartmann, B., Geerlings, P., & Kolb, H. (1996). Interleukin-12 gene expression of macrophages is regulated by nitric oxide. *Biochemical and Biophysical Research Communication, 224*, 159–163.

Rothwell, N. J., Busbridge N. J., Humphray, H., & Hissey, P. (1990). Central actions of interleukin-1β on fever and thermogenesis. In C. A. Dinarello (Ed.), *Proceedings of 2nd international workshop on cytokines*. Philadelphia: W.B. Saunders.

Rothwell, N. J., Busbridge, N. J., Lefeuvre, R. A., & Hardwick, A. J. (1991). Interleukin-6 is a centrally acting endogenous pyrogen in the rat. *Canadaian Journal of Physiology and Pharmacology, 69*, 1465–1469.

Rothwell, N. J., & Hopkins, S. J. (1995) Cytokines and the nervous system II: Actions and mechanisms of action. *TINS, 18*, 130–136.

Saad, R., Constam, D. B., Ortmann, R., Moos, M., Fontana, A., & Schachner, M. (1991). Astrocyte-derived TGF-β2 and NGF differentially regulate neural recognition molecule expression by cultured astrocytes. *Journal of Cell Biology, 115*, 473–484.

Sands, W. A., Bulut, V., Severn, A., Xu, D., & Liew, F. Y. (1994). Inhibition of nitric oxide synthase by interleukin-4 may involve inhibiting the activation of protein kinase Cε. *European Journal of Immunology, 24*, 2345–2350.

Schluesener, H. J. (1990). Transforming growth factors type β1 and β2 suppress rat astrocyte autoantigen presentation and antagonize hyperinduction of class II major histocompatibility complex antigen expression by interferon-γ and tumor necrosis factor-α. *Journal of Neuroimmunology, 27*, 41–47.

Schneemann, M., Schoedon, G., Frei, K., & Schaffner, A. (1993). Immunovascular communication: Activation and deactivation of murine endothelial cell nitric oxide synthase by cytokines. *Immunology Letters, 35*, 159–162.

Schwarze, M. M. K., & Hawley, R. G. (1995). Prevention of myeloma cell apoptosis by ectopic *bcl-2* expression or interleukin 6-mediated up-regulation of *bcl-xL*. *Cancer Research, 55*, 2362–2265.

Segal, B. M., & Shevach, E. M. (1996). IL-12 unmasks latent autoimmune disease in resistant mice. *Journal of Experimental Medicine, 184*, 771–775.

Selkoe, D. J. (1991). The molecular pathology of Alzheimer's disease. *Neuron, 6*, 487–498.

Shrikant, P., Lee, S. J., Kalvakolanu, I., Ransohoff, R. M., & Benveniste, E. N. (1996). Stimulus-specific inhibition of intercellular adhesion molecule-1 gene expression by TGF-β. *Journal of Immunology, 157*, 892–900.

Shull, M. M., Ormsby, I., Kier, A. B., Pawlowski, S., Diebold, R. J., Yin, M., Allen, R., Sidman, C., Proetzel, G., Calvin, D., Annunziata, N., & Doetschman, T. (1992). Targeted disruption of the mouse transforming growth factor-β1 gene results in multifocal inflammatory disease. *Nature, 359*, 693–699.

Sicher, S. C., Vazquez, M. A., & Lu, C. Y. (1994). Inhibition of macrophage Ia expression by nitric oxide. *Journal of Immunology, 153*, 1293–1300.

Stamler, J. S. (1994). Redox-signalling. *Cell, 78*, 931–936.

Stevenson, M. M., Tam, M. F., Wolf, S. F., & Sher, A. (1995). IL-12 induced protection against blood-stage *Plasmodium chabaudi* AS requires IFN-γ and TNF-α and occurs via a nitric oxide-dependent mechanism. *Journal of Immunology, 155*, 2545–2556.

St. Pierre, B., Wong, J. L., & Merrill, J. E. (1997). Inhibition of human and rat glial cell function by antiinflammatory cytokines, antioxidants, and elevators of cAMP. In R. M. Devon, R. Doucette, B. H. J. Juurlink, A. J. Nazarali, D. J. Schreyer, & V. M. K. Verge (Eds.), *Cell biology and pathology of myelin: Evolving biological concepts and therapeutic approaches* (pp., 265–276), New York: Plenum Publishing.

St. Pierre, B. A., Merrill J. E., & Dopp, J. M. (1996). Effects of cytokines on CNS cells: Glia. In R. M. Ransohoff & E. N. Benveniste (Eds.), *Cytokines and the CNS* (pp. 152–168). Baton Rouge, LA: CRC Press.

Strassmann, G., Patil-Koota, V., Finkelman, F., Fong, M., & Kambayashi, T. (1994). Evidence for the involvement of interleukin 10 in the differential deactivation of murine peritoneal macrophages by prostaglandin E2. *Journal of Experimental Medicine, 180*, 2365–2370.

Strijbos, P. J. L. M., & Rothwell, N. J. (1995). Interleukin-1β attenuates excitatory amino acid-induced neurodegeneration in vitro: Involvement of nerve growth factor. *Journal of Neuroscience, 15*, 3468–3474.

Swindells, M. B. (1992). Structural similarity between transforming growth factor-β2 and nerve growth factor. *Science, 258*, 1160–1161.

Tanaka, T., Akira, S., Yoshida, K., Umemoto, M., Yoneda, Y., Shirafuji, N., Fujiwara, H., Suematsu, S., Yoshida, N., & Kishimoto, T. (1995). Targeted disruption of the NF-IL6 gene discloses its essential role in bacteria killing and tumor cytotoxicity by macrophages. *Cell, 80*, 353–361.

Tian, L., & Lawrence, D. A. (1995). Lead induces nitric oxide production in vitro by murine spenic macrophages. *Toxicology and Applied Pharmacology, 132*, 156–163.

Tilg, H., Dinarello, C. A. S., & Mier, J. W. (1997). IL-6 and APPs: Anti-inflammatory and immunosuppressive mediators. *Immunology Today, 18*, 428–432.

Toru-Delbauffe, D., Baghdassarian-Chalaye, D., Gavaret, J. M., Courtin, F., Pomerance, M., & Pierre, M. (1990). Effects of transforming growth factor β1 on astroglial cells in culture. *Journal of Neurochemistry, 54*, 1056–1061.

Vodovotz, Y., Lucia, M. S., Flanders, K. C. Chesler, L., Xie, Q.-W., Smith T. W., Weidner, J., Mumford, R., Webber, R., Nathan, C., Roberts, A. B., Lippa, C.F., & Sporn, M. B. (1996). Inducible nitric oxide synthase in tangle-bearing neurons of patients with Alzheimer's Disease. *Journal of Experimental Medicine, 184*, 1425–1433.

Vouldoukis, I., Riveros-Moreno, V., Dugas, B., Ouaz, F., Becherel, P., Debre, P., Moncada, S., & Djavad Mossalayi, M. (1995). The killing of *Leishmania major* by human macrophages is mediated by nitric oxide induced after ligation of the FceRII/CD23 surface antigen. *Proceedings of the National Academy of Sciences, 92*, 7804–7808.

Wahl, S. M., Hunt, D. A., Wakefield, L. M., McCartney-Francis, N., Wahl, L. M., Roberts, A. B., & Sporn, M. B. (1987). Transforming growth factor type β induces monocyte chemotaxis and growth factor production. *Proceedings of the National Academy of Sciences, 84*, 5788–5792.

Wrana, J. L., Attisano, L., Carcamo, J., Zentella, A., Doody, J., Laiho, M., Wang, X.-F., & Massague, J. (1992). TGFβ signals through a heteromeric protein kinase receptor complex. *Cell, 72*, 1003–1014.

Wrana, J. L., Attisano, L., Wieser, R., Venture, F., & Massague, J. (1994). Mechanism of activation of the TGF-β receptor. *Nature, 370*, 341–347.

Wyss-Coray, T., Barrow, P., Brooker, M. J., & Mucke, L. (1997). Astroglial overproduction of TGF-β1 enhances inflammatory central nervous system disease in transgenic mice. *Journal of Neuroimmunology, 77*, 45–50.

Wyss-Coray, T., Masliah, E., Mallory, M., McConlogue, L., Johnson-Wood, K., Lin, C., & Mucke, L. (1997). Amyloidogenic role of cytokine TGF-β1 in transgenic mice and in Alzheimer's disease. *Nature, 389*, 603–606.

Xiao, B. G., Zhang, G.-X., Ma, C.-G., and Link, H. (1996). Transforming growth factor-beta 1 (TGF-β1)-mediated inhibition of glial cell proliferation and down-regulation of intercellular adhesion molecule-1 (ICAM-1) are interrupted by gamma interferon (IFN-γ). *Clinical and Experimental Immunology, 103*, 475–481.

Yan, S. D., Chen, X., Fu, J., Chen, M., Zhu, H., & Roher, A. (1996). RAGE and amyloid-β peptide neurotoxicity in Alzheimer's disease. *Nature, 382*, 685–691.

Yim, C.-Y., McGregor, J. R., Kwon, O.-D., Bastian, N. R., Rees, M., Mori, M., Hibbs, J. B. Jr., & Samlowski, W. E. (1995). Nitric oxide synthesis contributes to IL-2-induced antitumor responses against intraperitoneal meth A tumor. *Journal of Immunology, 155*, 4382–4390.

CHAPTER

22

Multiple Routes of Action of Interleukin-1 on the Nervous System

STEVEN F. MAIER, LINDA R. WATKINS, DWIGHT M. NANCE

I. INTRODUCTION

It is well accepted that the central nervous system (CNS) can modulate many aspects of immune function via its regulation of autonomic and neuroendocrine outflow pathways that contact organs and cells of the immune system. In recent years it has also become clear that products of immune cells can communicate to the CNS, potently altering neural activity and the products of neural activity such as behavior, hormone release, and autonomic function (Besedovsky & Del Rey, 1996; Dantzer, Bluthi, Kent, & Goodall, 1993; Maier & Watkins, 1998; Turnbull & Rivier, 1999). In this capacity the immune cells function as a diffuse sense organ, informing the CNS about events in the periphery relating to infection and injury (Blalock, Smith, & Meyer, 1985). Thus, the brain and immune system form a bidirectional communication network, with immune products signaling the brain, and the brain regulating immune function and coordinating host defense.

Studies of immune signaling to the brain have largely focused on the cytokine interleukin-1β (IL-1β). This is at least in part because the original interest in this area focused on fever. It was known as early as 1960 (Atkins, 1960) that fever was mediated by phagocytic cells that released endogenous pyrogens into the blood in response to infectious agents. It was also known that fever was mediated by cells in the preoptic region of the hypothalamus (Cooper, Cranston, & Honour, 1967), and so something in endogenous pyrogen (EP) had to be able to communicate to the brain. A variety of experiments indicated that IL-1β was the critical constituent of EP (see Kluger, 1991, for a description of the history of this work), and so IL-1β became a focus. IL-1β is a 17.5 kDa protein synthesized and secreted by a variety of cell types in the periphery including monocytes and macrophages (Dinarello, 1991), and by glial cells and neurons in the CNS (Buttini & Boddeke, 1995; Lechan et al., 1990; Tringali et al, 1996; Van Dam, Brouns, Louisse, & Berken-Bosch, 1992). IL-1β is well known for its role in T-cell activation in which it induces IL-2 production and the expression of IL-2 receptors by T-cells. However, peripheral IL-1 also is a key participant in the communication to the CNS that follows infection or injury, and brain IL-1 is an important component of the neural link in the bidirectional immune–brain loop. The purpose of this chapter is to summarize what is known concerning these IL-1β actions on brain.

II. IL-1β AND IMMUNE-TO-BRAIN COMMUNICATION

The best known role of IL-1β in immune-to-brain communication is as an element of the innate or nonspecific immune response. This type of immunity is called innate because the cells involved are germline coded and exist before infection by a microbial invader or injury. In contrast, in acquired immunity the responding cells are not germline coded but are determined by a random rearrangement of genes that code for the T cell or B cell receptor and are developed by clonal expansion after infection. Innate immunity is also called nonspecific immunity because it does not involve pathogen-specific receptors, but rather relies on detection of general patterns that characterize microbial products (see Medzhitov & Janeway, 1998).

The fact that the responding cells and processes in nonspecific immunity already exist when a challenge occurs and do not require a clonal expansion of cells suggests that this form of immunity is temporally the first line of host defense. Indeed, the effectors of specific immunity (cytotoxic T cells, antibody, etc.) do not appear until several days after infection. Some aspects of innate immunity are structural and passive. For example, the skin keeps many microorganisms outside the body and a large number of microorganisms cannot survive the low pH of the stomach. However, other innate immune processes are more active and can be engaged rapidly after infection. Phagocytic cells such as monocytes/macrophages are key cellular elements in many of these processes. Cells such as macrophages are capable of distinguishing self from nonself, but here this is accomplished by receptors on the phagocyte that recognize molecular structures that are shared by large groups of pathogens (see Medzhitov & Janeway, 1997, for review). For example, the general structure of lipopolysaccharide (LPS, endotoxin) is shared by all gram-negative bacteria, and macrophages have a membrane receptor (CD14) that recognizes LPS and therefore can respond to diverse gram-negative bacteria via a single receptor molecule.

Phagocytic cells not only recognize microbes, but can also engulf them and kill them via lysosomal enzymes. In addition, activated phagocytic cells such as macrophages release a variety of products, such as nitric oxide, that can interfere with pathogen growth. Activated macrophages sequentially release the proinflammatory cytokines tumor necrosis factor-α (TNF-α), IL-1α and β, and IL-6. These secreted peptides are called cytokines because they play a key role in communicating between immune cells and orchestrating and coordinating immune defenses. These particular cytokines are called proinflammatory because one of their major functions is to initiate and coordinate the inflammatory response at the site of infection, a response that limits the spread of the infectious agent from a wound site or other points of entry.

These cytokines are also critical in initiating a complex host defense response called the acute phase response (APR) (Baumann & Gauldie, 1994). This response has numerous components. Liver metabolism is shifted away from normal liver products such as carrier proteins to the production of acute phase proteins including C-reactive protein, haptoglobin, etc. There are alterations in plasma zinc, copper, and iron, increased numbers of circulating white blood cells, and so on. These changes have diverse functions, but many operate to limit pathogen growth. For example, iron is needed for many microbes to proliferate, and so the reduction in plasma iron serves to limit pathogen growth.

Many aspects of the APR are mediated at the periphery, with IL-6 being a key signal to the liver to initiate the APR. However, the early response to microbial infection or injury also involves a number of CNS mediated responses. The best known is fever. Fever is a pervasive reaction to infection or injury that occurs within a short period of time of the initiating event. Fever is not a pathological reaction, but is an adaptive mechanism of host defense. Many microbes replicate best at the normal core body temperature of the host, and a number of enzymatic processes involved in phagocytosis as well as the speed of replication of white blood cells are augmented by increases in core body temperature (see Hart, 1988, and Kluger, Kozek, Conn, Leon, & Soszynski, 1996, for reviews). Indeed, inhibition of fever has been shown to be detrimental to survival under a variety of circumstances (Kluger, 1966). A regulated increase in core body temperature during infection is mediated via neurons in the anterior hypothalamus. There are concurrent autonomic and behavioral adjustments (shivering, vascular changes, etc.) that sustain and regulate the pyrogenic response. The point is that this complex, but integrated, set of changes is mediated in the brain, not just in the periphery.

In addition to fever, there are a number of other physiological sequelae of infection and macrophage activation that are mediated by the CNS. For example, sleep is increased, particularly slow wave sleep (Krueger & Majde, 1994). In addition, there is both hypothalamo-pituitary-adrenal (HPA) and sympathetic nervous system (MacNeil, Jansen, Greenberg, & Nance 1996) activation 20–30 min after infection or activation of macrophages with substances such as LPS (Turnbull & Rivier, 1999 for review). There are also numerous behavioral adjustments that occur following infection, and behavior is, of course, regulated by the CNS. Food and water intake, exploration, social interaction, sexual behavior, and maternal behavior are all reduced, and pain sensitivity/reactivity is enhanced (see Kent et al., 1992, Maier & Watkins, 1999, and Yirmiya, 1997, for reviews).

This pattern has been called "sickness behavior" (Kent et al., 1992) and has been argued to be an adaptive response to infection and injury, rather than a pathological set of changes resulting from debilitation (Hart, 1988). The adaptive nature of these changes can be rationalized within the context of the high energy costs of fever (in mammals, each 1°C rise in core body temperature requires an estimated extra 10–13% of energy) and the cellular proliferation that occurs during host defense (Kluger, 1979). Many of the behavioral changes reduce the energetic cost of behavior, and the end products of HPA and sympathetic activation both function to liberate energy from bodily stores (e.g., they convert glycogen to glucose). In addition, these behavioral changes may reduce the risk of exposure to predation during a time of weakness. Only the CNS would appear to be capable of orchestrating such a widespread pattern of changes.

For these reasons the immune system must be able to signal the CNS, informing the brain that infection or injury has occurred. Indeed, both the electrical and chemical activity of the brain changes soon after infection with a virus or bacterial product (Dunn, 1995, for review). A substantial body of evidence supports the concept that IL-1β is a key signal that is released at the periphery to signal the brain that infection has occurred, and thereby to initiate the sickness syndrome. First, the peripheral administration of IL-1β produces the full pattern of sickness behavior. Fever (Dinarello et al., 1986), increased sleep (Opp, Obal, & Krueger, 1991), anorexia and adipsia (Bluthé, Beaudu, Kelley, & Dantzer, 1995), decreased locomotion and exploration (Dantzer et al., 1993), decreased social interaction (Dantzer et al., 1993), decreased sexual behavior (Yirmiya et al., 1995), hyperalgesia (Watkins, Maier, & Goehler, 1995), and HPA activation (Besedovsky, del Ray, Sorkin, & Dinarello, 1986) all result. Furthermore, the peripheral administration of IL-1β produces alterations in brain monoamines that are similar to those produced by LPS or viral infection (Dunn, 1995). Second, the peripheral immunoneutralization of IL-1β and the blockade of peripheral IL-1 receptors with the IL-1 receptor antagonist (IL-1ra) block or reduce many of the consequences of peripheral infection and immune activation. Fever (Long, Otterness, Kunkel, Vander, & Kluger, 1990), anorexia and adipsia (Bluthé, Dantzer, & Kelley, 1992), locomotor reductions (Dantzer et al., 1993), decreased social interaction (Bluthe et al., 1995), hyperalgesia (Watkins et al., 1995), and HPA activation (Rivier, Chizzonite, & Vale, 1989) produced by LPS are all reduced by blocking IL-1β action in the periphery. In addition, monoaminergic and other alterations in brain that normally follow infection are reduced (Dunn, 1995).

However, it should be noted that IL-1ra and the immunoneutralization of IL-1β rarely produce a complete blockade of the effects of LPS and viral infection. This suggests that IL-1β is not a solitary messenger between the immune system and the brain. In addition, it is likely that the communication mechanisms between the immune system and the brain may vary depending on the immune activating agents as well as the region of the body exposed to the immune stimulus. For example, the effects of IL-1β, LPS, and influenza virus on food intake are differently affected by IL-1ra and cyclooxygenase inhibitors (Dunn & Swiergiel, 1998; Swiergiel, Smagin, & Dunn, 1997). Also, the fever induced by LPS, bacterial infection induced by cecal ligation and puncture, and macrophage inflammatory protein-1 is mediated by different mechanisms (Gourine, Rudolph, Tesfaigzi, & Kluger, 1998; Minanao et al., 1990). Despite these complexities, IL-1β continues to be a primary candidate for one of the key messengers between the immune system and brain involved in the initiation of the sickness syndrome.

III. MECHANISMS BY WHICH IL-1β COMMUNICATES TO THE BRAIN

Although it is clear that IL-1β is a messenger between the immune system and the CNS, the manner in which the message is delivered remains a topic of controversy. A number of facts lead very naturally to the suggestion that the communication pathway is direct, with IL-1β accumulating in the bloodstream, traveling to the brain via the blood, and entering the brain to exert its actions. These facts are that (a) the brain expresses receptors for IL-1β on neurons and glial cells (Cunningham et al., 1992); (b) administering IL-1b directly into the brain produces many of the same responses as does peripheral injection of IL-1 or immune activating agents (e.g., Plata-Salaman, Oomura, & Kai, 1988); and (c) blocking brain IL-1 receptors with IL-1 receptor antagonist or immunoneutralizing IL-1 in brain blocks some of the sickness responses produced by peripheral IL-1β or immune activation (see review by Rothwell & Hopkins, 1995).

The difficulty with the simple idea that IL-1β signals the brain by diffusing into the brain parenchyma from the bloodstream is that IL-1β and other cytokines are relatively large proteins (IL-β is roughly 17.5 kDa) and are quite lipophobic. Thus, it is very unlikely that IL-1β could enter the brain by passive diffusion across the blood-brain barrier.

A. Blood-Borne Mechanisms

However, the idea that IL-1 accumulates in blood and signals the brain via transport to the brain in blood is still appealing, partly because this is a frequently used pathway by which peripheral products such as hormones signal the CNS. However, specialized mechanisms are then required to allow blood-borne IL-1 to deliver its message to the brain, and a number have been proposed.

1. *Active Transport*

The brain requires many substances from the periphery that are unable to cross the blood-brain barrier by passive diffusion. Some neuroactive peptides can enter via a noncompetitive, nonsaturable mechanism determined by physiochemical characteristics of the substances. However, cytokines such as IL-1β do not have the requisite characteristics (Banks & Kastin, 1987). In addition, a variety of substances are actively transported by protein complexes that can bind the substance and move it across the barrier. Examples are amino acids, fatty acids, thyroid hormones, organic acids, hexoses, and transferrin. Such carrier-mediated transport is saturable, and may be able to transport proteins against a gradient (Banks & Kastin, 1987).

Banks and his colleagues have clearly demonstrated that IL-1β and other cytokines can be transported into brain parencyhma by a saturable process that has the characteristics of being carrier mediated (see Chapter 18). These studies involve assessing the presence of radiolabled cytokines in brain that have been injected peripherally, typically intravenously (iv). Careful multiple-time regression analyses revealed a greater presence of radiolabled cytokines in brain than could be accounted for by passive diffusion, and studies involving the addition of competing unlabeled cytokines indicated that the process is saturable (Banks, Ortiz, Plotkin, & Kastin, 1991). Furthermore, analyses of neurons separated from brain capillaries indicated that the cytokines did cross into the brain parenchyma, rather than simply being sequestered in blood vessels (Guttierez, Banks, & Kastin, 1993).

Thus, there is little doubt that IL-1β and other cytokines can be actively transported into brain. However, the amounts that are transported are quite small. For example, only 0.07% of iv injected IL-1β enters the brain (Banks et al., 1991), and since entry by active transport is regionally nonselective, much of the entry that does occur is in regions that do not have a documented function in mediating sickness behaviors. For example, cerebral cortices and cerebellum accounted for 60% of uptake of IL-1β (Banks, Kastin, & Durham, 1989). This may not be a major problem when dealing with large iv, injections of IL-1β, but it may be a very significant problem when considering the small levels of IL-1β that circulate under physiological conditions during a peripheral infection. Although active transport of IL-1β into brain clearly exists, the physiological role of this process remains to be elucidated.

2. *Entry at Circumventricular Organs*

The blood-brain barrier prevents passage of substances into the brain because of the low rate of pinocytosis in endothelial cells and the existence of tight junctions joining adjacent endothelial cells. There are a number of specialized regions in the brain that have fenestrated capillaries, thereby allowing plasma passage to occur. These are called circumventricular organs (CVOs), with the area postrema and organum vasculosum of the lamina terminalis (OVLT) being examples. Cytokines such as IL-1β could readily cross into these organs. IL-1β would have to bind to IL-1 receptors at these sites and exert its actions locally in the CVOs since IL-1β and other cytokines would be unlikely to be able to diffuse to other brain sites from the CVOs. This is because tight junctions between ependymal cells form a barrier between the CVOs and the rest of the brain. The most popular argument has been that binding of IL-1β to its receptors in CVOs such as the OVLT leads to prostaglandin (PG) synthesis (Saper & Breder, 1994). PGs are small molecules and are lipophilic, and would therefore be able to penetrate the tight junctions separating the OVLT from the brain. PGs are excitatory, and thus could activate adjacent neurons by diffusion, thereby initiating the neural cascade of events that follow peripheral immune stimulation (Ericsson, Arias, & Sawchenko, 1997). For example, it has been proposed that PGs activate neurons in the medial preoptic area that borders on the OVLT (Saper & Breder, 1994), which then project to a variety of endocrine and autonomic control regions that mediate a pyrogenic response.

Recent attention has also been focused on the area postrema, particularly with regard to its role in mediating the HPA response to iv IL-1β. Removal of the area postrema with an aspiration lesion substantially reduced the increase in plasma adinocorticotropic hormone (ACTH) produced by iv administration of IL-1β (Lee, Whiteside, & Herkenham, 1998). Furthermore, the lesion altered the usual pattern of neural activation produced by iv IL-1β as measured by c-fos mRNA. Of particular interest for HPA activation, the lesion abolished IL-1β-induced increases in c-fos mRNA in the paraventricular nucleus. Area postrema lesions also have been reported to reduce release of norepinephrine in the hypothalamus produced by peripheral IL-1β (Ishizuka et al., 1997).

However, there are ambiguities concerning the role of the area postrema. The area postrema lesions in the Lee et al. (1998) experiment produced significant damage to the neighboring nucleus tractus solitarius (NTS), particularly the region of the NTS containing the sites of termination of vagal nerve afferent fibers (see below). A further study employed smaller area postrema lesions that did not destroy parts of the NTS, but the effects of this lesion on the ACTH response to IL-1β and c-fos mRNA in the paraventricular nucleus were modest (Lee et al., 1998). Furthermore, even the large area postrema lesions left c-fos mRNA increases to iv IL-1β in a number of brain areas undiminished, and so the more general role of the area postrema in mediating immune-to-brain communication beyond the HPA axis response is unclear. Moreover, Ericsson and colleagues (1997) failed to find any effect of area postrema lesions on c-fos immunoreactivity in the paraventricular nucleus. However, Ericsson et al. (1997) used a much higher dose of iv IL-1β than did Lee et al. (1998) (1.87 versus 0.5 μg/kg), an issue to which we will return.

3. *Binding to Sites on the Cerebral Vasculature*

The cerebral vasculature has a number of associated cell types such as endothelial cells and microglia that express IL-1 receptors (Ericsson, Liu, Hart, & Sawchenko, 1995; Wong & Licinio, 1994; Yabuuci, Minami, Katsumata, & Satoh, 1994). It has been argued that circulating IL-1β binds to these receptors and thereby induces these cells to synthesize and secrete other products whose chemical and physical nature allows them to cross into the brain parenchyma from these perivascular cells. These substances, in turn, then activate neurons in the region at which they cross into the brain (Ericsson et al., 1997; Scammell, Elmquist, Griffin, & Saper, 1996). Cells associated with the cerebral vasculature also express CD14, and so LPS can bind directly to these cells, thereby potentially inducing a signal that can cross into brain parenchyma (Lacroix & Rivest, 1998).

PGs have most often been argued to be the critical mediator that is produced in response to IL-1β by perivascular cells, and that then diffuses into brain tissue to excite neurons. As noted previously, PGs are small lipophilic molecules and so they can diffuse into brain quite readily. PGs are produced from their precursor arachidonic acid via the activity of the enzyme cyclooxygenase (COX). This enzyme exists in several isoforms, one of which (COX-2) is inducible and is induced in cerebral blood vessel cells by IL-1β (Cao, Matsumura, Yamagata, & Watanabe, 1996) or by peripheral injection of LPS (Breder & Saper, 1996). Indeed, COX-2 mRNA and protein increase in both microglial (Elmquist et al., 1997) and endothelial (Matsumura et al., 1998) cells in the cerebral vasculature after LPS. As would be expected, prostaglandin E2 (PGE2) immunoreactivity has been found to be increased in the cerebral vasculature after peripheral injection of LPS (Van Dam, Brouns, Man-A-Hing, & Berkenbosch, 1993). Furthermore, IL-1β mRNA expression in barrier cells associated with the meninges, choroid plexus, and CVOs is stimulated by peripheral injection of LPS (Quan et al., 1999), with the IL-1β formed in these cells inducing COX-2 and PGs.

In addition to detection in perivascular cells after peripheral injections of LPS or IL-1β, PGE2 can also be detected in brain (Sehic, Székely, Ungar, Oladehin, & Blatteis, 1996). Furthermore, a number of different PG receptor subtypes have been localized in brain (Matsumura et al., 1992) and PGs are known to be able to excite neurons via a number of different mechanisms. A potential difficulty for the idea that neurally mediated aspects of sickness responses are mediated by perivascular PGs is that PGs would be expected to be produced throughout the cerebral vasculature, but peripheral immune activation produces a very discrete pattern of activation of brain regions (Brady, Lynn, Herkenham, & Gottesfeld, 1994; Ericsson, Kovacs, & Sawchenko, 1994; Wan et al., 1993; Wan , Wetmore, Sorensen, Greenberg, & Nance 1994) and a selective set of sickness responses. However, Ericsson and colleagues (1997) argued that the density of PG receptors, particularly the EP3 receptor, is especially high in regions of the brain that are involved in mediating responses such as HPA activation and fever. Thus, the selective distribution of PG receptors in brain might allow regional selectivity of response to PGs that are widely produced. Finally, it can be noted that inhibition of PG synthesis by COX inhibitors, such as indomethacin, blunts or blocks most of the endocrine, autonomic, and sickness responses produced by peripheral IL-1 or LPS (e.g., Katsuura, Gottschall, Dahl, & Arimura, 1988; MacNeil et al., 1994; Wan et al., 1994). There can be no question that central PGs play an important role in mediating the neural effects of peripheral immune stimulation.

B. Neural Communication: The Vagus Nerve

Communication between the immune system and the CNS in which IL-1 or some other molecule travels to the brain in the blood is of obvious adaptive value when infections become systemic. Of course, experiments in which IL-1β or LPS are injected iv in large amounts capitalize on such a potential situation. However, brain-mediated sickness responses such as fever can occur when LPS or cytokines are injected at doses and routes of administration such that neither IL-1, other cytokines, nor even LPS itself is detectable in the blood (Kluger, 1991). Moreover, this is not a problem of assay sensitivity since the iv doses of cytokines required to produce sickness responses such as fever are orders of magnitude above the detection limits of the assays.

An obvious alternative to blood-borne communication is that immune-derived signals such as IL-1 act locally at their site of synthesis and release to activate afferent sensory neural fibers. Under such a scenario increases in blood levels of cytokines would not be needed, only a local increase in tissue levels. In addition, neural signaling would be in keeping with the idea that the immune system, in addition to its other functions, operates as a diffuse sense organ scattered throughout the body to inform the brain about events in the body relating to infection and injury (Blalock, Smith, & Meyer, 1985). After all, sense organs communicate to the brain via peripheral sensory nerves.

The vagus nerve is a prime candidate to function as such a nerve. The vagus innervates points of pathogen entry such as the lung, and parts of organs that screen for pathogens and toxins such as the liver, as well as many other visceral organs. Importantly, over half of the vagal fibers are afferents conveying sensory input to the brain. Vagal signaling to the brain of peripheral immune activation would be consistent with the general afferent function of the vagus of providing the CNS with a variety of information relating to homeostasis in internal tissues. Furthermore, afferent vagal fibers terminate in the NTS and the associated area postrema in the brain stem. This is of note because the NTS and area postrema are the first regions of the brain to become activated after peripheral administration of IL-1β or LPS, and do so at the lowest doses (Brady et al., 1994; Ericsson et al., 1994). In addition, catecholaminergic pathways that ascend from the NTS and ventrolateral medulla are required for the central activational effects of peripheral immune activation (Ericsson et al., 1994; Nance, Greenberg, & Jackson et al., 1995; Sehic & Blatteis, 1996).

The idea that IL-1β conveys its signal to the brain by activating afferent vagal fibers requires that peripheral inflammatory stimuli and IL-1β activate sensory vagal fibers and that this vagal communication to the brain is important in producing sickness responses that are mediated by the brain. Nijima (1998) was the first to suggest that peripheral IL-1β activates vagal fibers, and demonstrated increased hepatic vagal electrical activity after hepatoportal injection of IL-1β. Vagal activation is not restricted to hepatic events, and both iv and intraperitoneal (ip) injection of LPS (Gaykema et al., 1998) and IL-1β (Goehler et al., 1998a) induce Fos protein in the nodose ganglia, the site of afferent vagal cell bodies. Subdiaphragmatic vagotomy blocked the appearance of Fos in the nodose ganglia following ip injection, demonstrating that c-fos activation was a result of the stimulation of vagal sensory fibers below the cut (Gaykema et al., 1998).

1. *Subdiaphragmatic Vagotomy*

The fact that IL-1β and LPS activate the vagus does not, by itself, indicate that the vagus carries a signal to the brain that is critical for the mediation of brain-mediated sickness responses. In addition, vagal signaling between the immune system and brain requires that severing the vagus reduces or abolishes sickness responses mediated by the CNS. The ideal experiment would involve bilaterally severing the vagus at a cervical level just before it enters the brain. However, animals do not survive bilateral cervical vagotomy. Vagotomy procedures generally involve cutting the vagal trunk just below the diaphragm, in combination with dissection of individual fibers that innervate visceral organs such as the liver but that are not contained in the vagal trunk at the level of the cut. This procedure is not ideal since it leaves intact the vagus above the diaphragm and its connection to the brain. The vagus innervates organs above the cut such as the lungs, and iv injected substances would have rapid and direct access to intact vagal fibers above the cut. Substances injected iv pass directly through the heart and then to the lungs, an area heavily innervated by the vagus.

For this reason most of the experiments that have examined the impact of subdiaphragmatic vagotomy on sickness responses have employed ip injection of LPS, IL-1β, or other substances, since subdiaphragmatic vagotomy denervates only the gut and associated organs. There are now a substantial number of such experiments and those that found subdiaphragmatic vagotomy to block or reduce sickness responses to ip administered substances are summarized in Table I. As can be seen, a wide array of behavioral, physiological, and neural responses to LPS and IL-1β are blocked or reduced.

TABLE I Outcomes Blocked or Attenuated by Subdiaphragmatic Vagotomy

Behavioral/physiological		
Fever	IL-1	Watkins et al., 1995
Fever	IL-1	Bluthe et al., 1996
Fever	LPS	Sehic & Blatties, 1996
Fever	LPS	Goldbach et al., 1997
Fever	IL-1	Hansen & Krueger, 1997
Fever	LPS	Romanovsky et al., 1997
Food motivated behavior	IL-1	Bret-Dibat et al., 1995
Food motivated behavior	LPS	Bret-Dibat et al., 1995
Hyperalgesia	LPS	Watkins et al., 1994
Hyperalgesia	IL-1	Watkins et al., 1991
Immobility	LPS	Laye et al., 1995
Sleep	IL-1	Hansen & Krueger, 1997
Sleep	IL-1	Opp & toth, 1997
Sleep	LPS	Kapas et al., 98
Social interaction	LPS	Bluthe et al., 1995
Social interaction	IL-1	Bluthe et al., 1996
Taste aversion learning	IL-1	Goehler et al., 1995
Brain		
c-fos in PVN, SON	LPS	Wan et al., 1994
c-fos in PVN CRH neurons	LPS	Gaykema et al., 1995
Hypothalamic NE depletion	IL-1	Fleshner et al, 1995
IL-1 mRNA	LPS	Laye et al., 1995
PGE2 in preoptic area	LPS	Sehic & Blatties, 1996
Hypothalamic NE release	IL-1	Ishizuka et al., 1997
NO release in PVN	IL-1	Ishizuka et al., 1998
IL-1 mRNA	IL-1	Hansen et al., 1998
HPA		
Plasma ACTH	LPS	Gaykema et al., 1995
Plasma ACTH	IL-1	Kapcala et al., 1996
Plasma ACTH	IL-1	Fleshner et al., 1995
Plasma CORT	TNF	Fleshner et al., 1998

2. *Controversial Aspects of Vagotomy*

The vagotomy experiments have been controversial and have stimulated much discussion. One issue has concerned the effects of vagotomy on sickness responses elicited by iv administration of LPS and IL-1β. Some experiments have found subdiaphragmatic vagotomy to reduce responses to iv LPS or IL-1β (e.g., Fleshner et al., 1995; Romanovksy, Kulchitsky, Simons, Sugimoto, & Szekeley, 1997b; Sehic & Blatties, 1996), whereas others have found no effect (e.g., Arias et al., 1997; Wan et al., 1994). As noted above, iv injected substances have direct and rapid access to intact vagal fibers, as well as eventually circulating to denervated areas, and so variable effects would be expected even if the vagus was the sole route of communication. Indeed, iv administration of IL-1β and LPS does activate afferent vagal fibers as indicated by Fos in the nodose and electrical multi-unit activity of nodose neurons (Ek, Kurosawa, Lundeberg, & Ericsson, 1998). Furthermore, subdiaphragmatic vagotomy reduces, but does not eliminate Fos induction in the nodose following iv administration of LPS (Gaykema et al., 1998). This suggests that iv injected substances circulate to regions innervated by the abdominal vagus, and that iv injected substances are able to activate the vagus at sites above and below the region of a subdiaphragmatic cut. Similarly, Goldbach et al. (1997) compared the effects of subdiaphragmatic vagotomy on fever following ip and intramuscular (im) injection of LPS. Vagotomy blocked the fever following ip administration, but had no effect on the fever produced by im LPS. Whether the fever produced by im administration was mediated by cutaneous nerves, vagal fibers above the cut, or blood-borne routes is unknown.

A second issue concerns not whether vagotomy is or is not effective in reducing sickness responses following peripheral immune activation, but rather the interpretation of the effects of vagotomy. The preceding discussion assumes that vagotomy has blocked behavioral, physiological, and neural responses to LPS and IL-1β because it interrupts communication between the immune system and the CNS. However, an alternative is that vagotomy interferes with the ability of the organism to respond. The vagus contains efferent parasympathetic fibers, and sympathetic fibers are also intermingled with the vagus. It is possible that an interruption of this efferent signaling to the periphery interferes with the ability of an organism to mount a fever, show an HPA response, etc. In addition, vagotomy might interfere with peripheral immune processes so that macrophages no longer function properly, cytokines do not become systemic in normal quantities, and so on.

This issue has been most extensively addressed with regard to fever and temperature regulation. One strategy is to determine whether vagotomized animals display normal fever to thermogenic stimuli that do not require immune-to-brain communication. If normal fever results, then vagotomy does not disrupt the ability of organism to mount a fever. This approach was used by Milligan et al. (1998) who administered PGE2 directly into the brain. PGE2 is thermogenic when administered into the brain, and produced a completely normal fever in vagotomized animals. Using a somewhat different approach, Romanovasky, Kulchitsky, Somons, Sugimoto, and Szekeley (1997a) investigated the thermoregulatory capability of rats that had received subdiaphragmatic vagotomy. Tail vasoconstriction in response to cold, brown adipose tissue thermogenesis, and fever in response to the sympathomimetic ephedrine (which does not produce fever via IL-1 or other cytokines) were all normal. Sickness responses other than fever have not been extensively investigated in this regard, but it can be noted that we (Fleshner, Gaykema, Goehler, Watkins, & Maier, unpublished observations) have found a normal HPA response to a tail-shock stressor in vagotomized subjects. Similarly, Wan et al. (1994) showed that footshock-induced c-fos in the brain was unaffected by subdiaphragmatic vagotomy. Finally, Bluthé et al. (1994) has reported normal levels of dehydrogenase activity of peritoneal macrophages in vagotomized subjects.

Another form of the argument that vagotomy is effective for reasons other than interruption of afferent signaling is that vagotomy interferes with the tendency for ip injected LPS or cytokines to become systemic. The experiments described above do not address this issue, since by this hypothesis the ability to mount a fever, etc., is still intact, it is just that ip injected substances in vagotomized animals do not become blood-borne and so are unable to participate in normal blood-borne signaling. This possibility is made plausible by a recent report by Lenczowski, Van Dam, Poole, Larrick, and Tilders (1997). These investigators injected LPS ip and measured LPS, IL-1β, and IL-6 in blood and peritoneum at various times later. The interesting result was that LPS, IL-1β, and IL-6 only became systemic in a proportion of the subjects. For some subjects, LPS remained in the peritoneal cavity, as did IL-1β and IL-6. Clearly, if vagotomy altered the kinetics of LPS or cytokine exit from the peritoneum it could alter sickness responses for this reason, rather than because afferent signals to the brain were interrupted. To examine this possibility, Hansen et al. injected 10, 50, or 100 μg/kg LPS ip and measured LPS, IL-1β, and IL-6 in blood at various times thereafter (Hansen, Nguyen, Fleshner, Goehler, & Gaykema, 1999). Vagotomy had little, if any, effect on plasma values. LPS, IL-1, and IL-6 increased in blood in a time and dose dependent manner, and vagotomy had no effect at all on the pattern observed following the 10 and 50 μg/kg doses, and produced only a very small reduction following 100 μg/kg LPS.

A third issue has involved the health of vagotomized subjects (Opp & Toth, 1997). This is an issue because subdiaphragmatic vagotomy generally denervates the stomach and intestine, and vagotomized subjects will eat poorly and may be malnourished unless special precautions are taken. It has been speculated that perhaps vagotomy blocks various effects because the subjects are in poor condition or because complications from vagotomy lead to bacterial translocation across the gut, resulting in LPS tolerance (Scammel, Griffin, Elmquist, & Saper, 1998). However, special care procedures such as postoperative feeding of highly palatable diets yield vagotomized animals that eat and gain weight normally. This issue has been extensively studied by Romanovsky et al. (1997b), who concluded that vagotomized animals that had been given a variety of special care procedures and who gained weight and thermoregulated normally still failed to develop fever to ip LPS.

Another approach to this question has been to conduct selective vagotomies. The gastric and celiac (innervates the intestines) branches are by far the most important with respect to eating, nutrition, and the health of the subject. However, the hepatic branch is likely to be important for immune-to-brain communication since ip substances such as LPS are initially processed in the liver, and the liver contains a specialized population of macrophages (Kupffer cells) that respond rapidly to LPS. The hepatic branch of the vagus is quite small and mostly afferent, and contributes only very minimally to the innervation of the gut. Significantly, selective hepatic vagotomy, which leaves the innervation of the gut undisturbed, blocks both the hyperalgesia (Watkins et al., 1994) and the fever (Simons et al., 1998) that results from LPS.

3. *Vagal Signal Transduction*

It is reasonable to conclude from the above discussion that at least under some circumstances the vagus carries a signal to the brain from peripheral immune activity that is necessary for the occurrence of sickness behaviors. This leaves the question of how immune signals such as those provided by IL-1β are transduced into vagal activity. The simplest possibility would be that there are IL-1 or other cytokine receptors expressed on vagal nerve fibers. Goehler et al. (1997) examined the binding of biotinylated IL-1 receptor antagonist (IL-1ra) to the vagus and associated structures and failed to observe specific binding to vagal fibers. However, there was intense binding to cells in paraganglia that surround vagal fibers. These are clusters of chemosensory glomus cells that are in close proximity to vagal nerve fibers, and provide afferent innervation of vagal fibers involving catecholamine and indoleamine transmitters. Thus, it is possible that IL-1β released near vagal fibers binds to sites on paraganglia, which then in turn release transmitters onto adjacent vagal fibers, thereby activating these neurons. In addition, Ek et al. (1998) recently reported detecting mRNA for IL-1 receptor type 1 in the cell bodies of afferent vagal fibers in the nodose ganglion, and so vagal fibers themselves may also express IL-1 receptor. Only a very small number of IL-1 receptors (approximately 10) are required on a cell to produce signaling (see below), and the binding technique used by Goehler et al. (1997) was likely not sensitive enough to detect receptors on the vagus itself.

This leaves the issue of the source of IL-1β. If vagal signaling plays a special role under circumstances in which there are not appreciable levels of circulating cytokines, then what is the source of IL-1 or other cytokines? CNS-mediated responses to infection occur fairly rapidly, with fever and other responses occurring in less than an hour following ip administration of LPS. Consistent with this timecourse, glutamate is released within the NTS at the site of vagal sensory nerve termination within 60 min of ip LPS injection (Mascarucci, Perego, Terrazzino, & De Simoni, 1998). How does LPS, or other infective or inflammatory agents, lead to a cytokine signal that could reach vagal terminals within the necessary timeframe without cytokines appearing in the circulation?

One possibility is provided by a series of experiments reported by Goehler et al. (1999). These investigators sacrificed subjects 30, 45, or 60 min after ip injection of either LPS or vehicle. The ventral abdominal vagus nerve, a section of the cervical vagus nerve distal to the carotid bifurcation, and a section of the proximal sciatic nerve distal to the pelvis and proximal to the knee were dissected out and removed for study. The nerves of separate groups were examined either immunohistochemically or by enzyme-linked immunosorbent assay (ELISA). The ventral abdominal vagus, and especially the hepatic branch, contained abundant connective tissue around and between vagal fibers, which constitutively contained large aggregates of lymphoid/myeloid-like cells that we called "NALC" (nerve-associated lymphoid cells). In contrast, connective tissue associated with the cervical vagus and the sciatic nerve was much more limited. The NALC associated with the abdominal vagus contained large numbers of dendritic cells (OX-6 positive cells with the morphological characteristics of dendritic cells) and macrophages (ED1 positive cells). OX-6 and ED1 positive lymphoid cells were also present on and between vagal fibers, as well as in the NALC. IL-1β immunoreactivity (IL-1β-IR) was not detectable in any of the nerves plus associated lymphoid tissue for animals that had received only saline, or in any nerve 30 min after ip LPS. However, IL-1β-IR was evident 45 min after LPS, but only in the abdominal vagus nerve plus associated connective tissue. By 60 min after LPS the increase in IL-1β-IR was quite prominent, but occurred only in the abdominal vagus nerve. IL-1β-IR was not detectable in either cervical vagus plus connective tissue or sciatic nerve plus connective tissue. Interestingly, the IL-β-IR occurred in cells that were either OX-6 or ED1 positive, as revealed by double-label immunofluorescence. Extracts for nerves plus associated connective tissue were also assayed for IL-1β protein content by ELISA. IL-1β protein was essentially undetectable in any nerve plus connective tissue under vehicle conditions. However, IL-1β protein content of the abdominal vagus increased by 45 min after LPS, and was even greater 60 min after ip LPS. IL-1β protein was not increased by ip LPS in any of the other nerves. Immuohistochemical analyses suggested that the IL-1β was in the connective tissue around the vagus, and in lymphoid tissue between vagal fibers.

In summary, immune cells capable of expressing IL-1 are resident in connective tissue associated with the abdominal vagus, as well as between and on vagal fibers. These cells rapidly express IL-1β following ip administration of LPS, a process detectable even at the protein level. Does this mean that these cells synthesize IL-1β in response to LPS in this rapid timeframe? There is evidence that there is constitutive expression of pro-IL-1β (the precursor of IL-1β) (Tringali et al., 1997), and LPS rapidly increases the activity of the enzyme (ICE) that cleaves pro-IL-1β (Yao & Johnson, 1997). Thus, it is possible that these specialized cells associated with the abdominal vagus store a constitutive pool of pro-IL-1β, and LPS leads to the rapid cleavage of pro-IL-1β, yielding the biologically active IL-1β. The data obtained by Goehler et al.

(1999) are consistent with this possibility because the antibodies directed at IL-1β used for both the immunohistochemical and ELISA studies have high affinity for mature IL-1β, but very poor affinity for pro-IL-1β. Thus, neither immunohistochemistry nor ELISA would detect constitutive pro-IL-1β. Of course, it is always possible that IL-1β is synthesized rapidly.

The final step would be release of mature IL-1β from the dendritic cells and macrophages resident in the NALC around the vagus, with the IL-1β then binding to receptors on paraganglia to activate catecholamine and indoleamine input to the vagus, as well as binding to receptors on the vagus itself, thereby initiating vagal activation. Thus, IL-1β would be able to signal the vagus by a paracrine action, rather than requiring entry into blood and transport to the vagus. This allows a rapid action, and an action without measurable blood levels. Indeed, plasma IL-1β was measured in the studies reported by Goehler et al. (1999), and IL-1β-IR and IL-1β protein increases following ip LPS appeared in vagal nerve before increases in plasma IL-1β were detectable. This type of data may also help to explain why sickness responses following ip injection sometimes do not correlate with blood or peritoneal lavage levels of cytokines (Lenzkowski et al., 1997). It should also be noted that IL-1β by itself need not be the only product involved in the activation of vagal fibers. IL-1β and LPS can induce a variety of neuroactive substances, any of which could have independent actions on vagal fibers. For example, IL-1β induces PG synthesis and release, and Ek et al. (1998) have demonstrated mRNA for the EP3 subtype of the PG receptor in afferent vagal cells. Furthermore, the PG inhibitor indomethacin reduced both c-fos mRNA in nodose ganglia neurons after the administration of IL-1β, as well as vagal afferent electrical activity.

4. *Other Peripheral Nerves*

Although neural communication of immune signals to the brain has focused on the vagus nerve, there is no a priori reason why the vagus should be unique. Immune signals are generated at many sites of inflammation such as the skin, which are not innervated by the vagus. A number of recent studies have explored sickness responses such as fever and HPA activation following injection of turpentine under the skin. The sickness responses that follow are mediated by IL-1β and TNF-α released locally at the site of inflammation because blocking these cytokines peripherally blocks the sickness responses, yet neither cytokine increases in the circulation (Luheshi et al., 1997; Turnbull et al., 1997). The only cytokine that increases in the circulation is IL-6 (Luheshi et al., 1997), but iv injected IL-6 does not induce COX-2 in brain barrier cells (Lacroix & Rivest, 1998), nor does it potently produce brain-mediated sickness responses (Wang, Ando, & Dunn, 1997). It may well be that either IL-1β or TNF-α activates cutaneous nerves, thereby signaling the brain. Interestingly, TNF-α is known to rapidly activate the sciatic nerve, possibly because it inserts itself into the lipid bilayer, thereby forming sodium channels (Myers, Wagner, & Sorkin, 1999). IL-1β has not been studied in this regard.

5. *Summary and Analysis*

The first issue is whether either the blood-borne or neural route hypothesis is capable of explaining all of the data by itself. Most of the recent work on blood-borne routes has focused on cytokine and PG induction in CVOs and cells of the cerebral vasculature. It is clear that PG inhibitors can block most or all sickness responses. However, it would be difficult for these mechanisms to explain all of immune-to-brain communication because brain-mediated responses such as fever can be observed as quickly as 15 min following iv LPS (e.g., Blatties, 1974), yet COX-2 and IL-1β increases in CVOs and barrier cells do not generally occur until 1.5 to 2 h after iv LPS or IL-1β (e.g., Matsumura et al., 1998), although an increase in COX-2 mRNA as rapidly as 45 min has been reported (Breder & Saper, 1996). Actual PG production, of course, would be delayed yet further. This creates somewhat of a paradox, however, since COX-2 inhibitors block even the early phase of fever and other sickness responses that appear before COX-2 is induced in barrier cells (Cao, Matsumura, Yamagata, & Watankbe, 1997). Perhaps the key to this riddle is provided by the observation that PG in the brain, measured by in vivo microdialysis, shows a rapid increase that accompanies the onset of fever (Sehic et al., 1996). This might lead to the conclusion that the constitutive form of COX, COX-1, is responsible for early fever. However, the effects of immune activation on fever are generally ascribed to COX-2 (e.g., Mastumura et al., 1998), and LPS does not increase COX-1 mRNA (Lacroix & Rivest, 1998). Potential resolution is provided by the finding that some neurons (but not glial cells, endothelial cells, etc.) express a constitutive form of COX-2 (Breder, Smith, Roz, & Kasferrer, 1992). This has led Blatties and colleagues (Li et al., 1999) to suggest that the early PG response is derived from neurons in response to noradrenergic input coming from the NTS after vagal activation by LPS and cytokines, whereas a later induction of COX-2 in barrier cells is produced by blood-borne cytokines acting at microglial or endothelial cells.

The blood-borne hypotheses as sole mechanisms also have difficulty with the fact that following ip administration of LPS or cytokines vagotomy reduces or blocks sickness responses, yet the effector mechanisms to produce fever, HPA increases, etc., are fully intact, and circulating LPS and cytokine levels are not reduced. If immune-to-brain communication is a simple matter of LPS or cytokines binding to receptors on barrier cells, then vagotomy should have no effect, given that it does not alter the kinetics of LPS and cytokine entry into the vasculature.

The vagal hypothesis also has difficulties as a sole communication route. The blockade of sickness responses by vagotomy is rarely complete, although this can always be attributed to activation of vagal fibers above the cut. Furthermore, vagotomy has no effect on sickness responses produced by im or sc administration of LPS, and has variable effects following iv administration, perhaps being effective only at very low doses (Romanovsky et al., 1997b). It is always possible to appeal to communication via the intact portion of the vagus, but Gaykema et al. (1998) did find that subdiaphragmatic vagotomy substantially reduces fos in the nodose ganglia following iv LPS. Thus, it is likely that iv LPS can act via nonvagal routes. Furthermore, cytokines and COX-2 are induced in barrier cells, and this should serve a function and sometimes correlates with sickness behavior (Cao et al., 1997).

Thus, it would appear that there are ample data to support both neural and blood-borne communication routes. Perhaps the existence of multiple routes for so important a function as immune-to-brain communication is not surprising. The current data are consistent with the argument that neural routes are important during the earliest phase of the response to inflammatory or infective agents before significant blood levels of cytokines develop. Neural routes may continue to be key if infection remains at levels below which significant blood levels of cytokines accumulate. Later during infection or at higher doses of inflammatory agents, blood-borne communication may play the predominant role. However, even here neural input may continue to operate because agents administered iv do activate afferent vagal fibers. Thus, the relative contributions of different signaling pathways may vary in complex ways with dose, time, and route of administration. A final point is that signaling also may vary with the agent. LPS has been suggested to exert some of its effects by inducing products other than IL-1β, TNF-α, and IL-6. Blocking all three cytokines does not entirely eliminate the effects of LPS (Dunn & Swiergiel, 1998). Since vagotomy effects are far more robust when cytokines are administered than when LPS is administered, the vagus may transduce cytokine signals, and so non-cytokine-mediated effects of LPS might still be intact (e.g., direct binding of LPS to CD14 sites in barrier cells). Perhaps the key question concerns how signaling occurs during an actual infection rather than after a bolus injection of LPS or cytokine. This issue is largely unexplored.

IV. BRAIN IL-1β

If IL-1β and other cytokines communicate to the brain by activating peripheral nerves, binding to receptors on cells of the cerebral vasculature and inducing other messengers such as PGs that then cross into the brain, and entering at CVOs such as the OVLT, why then are there IL-1 receptors on neurons and glia, particularly in areas distant from CVOs such as the hippocampus (Cunningham et al., 1992)? In addition, why does intracerebroventricular (icv) and regional microinjections into discrete brain nuclei of IL-1β produce sickness responses such as fever, HPA activation, reduced social behavior, and the like (Kent, Rodriguez, Kelley, & Dantzer, 1994; Plata-Salaman et al., 1988), and why does blocking IL-1 receptors in the brain block or reduce some sickness responses produced by peripheral injection of IL-1β, other cytokines, or LPS (see below)?

One answer to these questions is that neural and/or blood-borne signals induce IL-1β production by cells within the central nervous system. Glial cells and neurons are both capable of producing IL-1, and perhaps it is IL-1β produced within the brain that binds to IL-1 receptors in the brain, not IL-1β that is produced in the periphery.

A. Constitutive and Immune-Induced Brain IL-1β

There is little question that IL-1β is produced in brain following pathological conditions such as cerebral injury, ischemia, and inflammation (Rothwell & Hopkins, 1995). However, whether IL-1β is expressed in the "normal" brain, and whether IL-1β is increased by peripheral immune activation remain controversial issues. These issues are controversial because results using different procedures to measure IL-1β have sometimes yielded different outcomes. Assays measure IL-1β mRNA expression, protein level, or bioactivity. With regard to mRNA, in situ hybridization has generally failed to detect mRNA for IL-1β under normal basal conditions (e.g., Buttini & Boddeke, 1995), whereas reverse transcriptase-polymerase chain reaction (RT-PCR) has detected IL-1β mRNA (Hansen et al., 1998). In considering this issue, it is important to keep in mind that the mRNA for IL-1β is not an abundant mRNA, and in addition is unstable (Herzyk Allen, Marsh, & Wewers, 1992). Furthermore, only very small quantities of IL-1β are necessary for biological activity. The icv administration of only picograms to femtograms is neurally active (Sundar et al., 1989), possibly because only as few as 10 IL-1 receptors have to be occupied to produce signal transduction (Dinarello, 1999). Indeed, IL-1β is among the most potent neuroactive substances yet discovered, and so only small quantities are to be expected. Indeed, IL-1β is also among the most tightly regulated substances in the brain. At least five endogenous mechanisms oppose IL-1β action in brain (see Watkins et al., 1999, for a review of these processes).(a) There is an endogenous antagonist for IL-1 (IL-1ra), and production of IL-1ra increases under some conditions, thereby reducing IL-1 biological action. (b) There is a "decoy" receptor (IL-1 type II receptor) that does not lead to signaling following IL-1 binding. Thus, any IL-1 that binds to this receptor is essentially inactivated, and increases in Type II receptor production is a regulatable process. (c) There are soluble forms of the IL-1 receptor that inactivate IL-1 that is not bound to membrane receptors. (d) Mature IL-1β is formed by cleavage from a precursor molecule (pro-IL-1β) by IL-1 converting enzyme (ICE). Thus, alterations in ICE activity modulate the production of IL-1β. (e) A number of peptides such as alpha-melanocyte stimulating hormone (α-MSH) oppose the actions of IL-1β. This almost unprecedented level of regulation of IL-1β is consistent with its extreme potency and the idea that only low levels are needed for biological action. The remaining point that needs to be made is that RT-PCR is a more sensitive technique for detecting mRNA than is in situ hybridization. This is because a large amount of amplification is inherent in the RT-PCR technique. With in situ hybridization, the hybridization of a probe to a 10–20 μm slice of tissue on a slide is examined. If only a small proportion of cells express IL-1β mRNA, very few cells on the slide will contain IL-1β mRNA and the signal will be small and perhaps not reliably detectable above background staining. RT-PCR can detect as little as one molecule of cytokine mRNA per 10 cells (Pitossi, Del Ray, Kabiersch, & Besedovsky et al., 1997). Of course, the difficulty with a technique having this sensitivity is that it may detect levels of IL-1β mRNA that are not biologically meaningful.

Protein measurement utilizes antibodies directed against the protein to be measured. The antibodies can be used to conduct either immunocytochemistry or ELISAs. Again, there appear to be discrepant findings between these two methods for assessing IL-1β protein levels under basal conditions. In general, immunocytochemistry has failed to detect IL-1β protein in the "resting" brain (Van Dam et al., 1992), whereas ELISA has found measurable levels of protein (Nguyen et al., 1998). However, ELISA is conducted on extracts from large number of neurons such as the entire hippocampus. Not only is the product of a large numbers of neurons concentrated for assay, but also the brain samples are sonicated before extraction. Immunocytochemistry, on the other hand, examines the binding of the antibody to a 10–20 μm brain slice on a slide. Immunocytochemistry has the advantage that the location of IL-1β immunoreactivity can be examined, but it is likely to be less sensitive than is ELISA.

Finally, IL-1β activity in a bioassay has also been reported under basal conditions (Quan, Zhang, Emery, Bosnall, & Weiss, 1996). Specificity is always an issue with bioassays, but Quan et al. (1996) demonstrated that the bioactivity was blocked by IL-1ra, supporting the argument that it was IL-1β that was detected by the assay performed on homogenates from brain under basal conditions. Again, the homogenates were created from large samples of neural tissue, allowing many neurons to be concentrated. The conclusion is that IL-1β mRNA, protein, and bioactivity in brain under basal conditions has been detected by some techniques. Detection by other techniques has not met with success, but a reasonable argument can be made that the issue is one of sensitivity. An additional argument that the detected IL-1β is "physiological" is that both IL-1β mRNA (Krueger & Majde, 1994) and protein (Nguyen et al., 1998) have a circadian rhythm, being highest during the sleep part of the cycle, consistent with the proposed role of brain IL-1 in sleep (see Chapter 26). There is less controversy over whether peripheral administration of IL-1β or LPS induces IL-1β increases in brain. IL-1β mRNA has been reported to be increased following LPS even using in situ hybridization (e.g., Buttini & Bodekke, 1995; Quan, Whiteside, & Herkenham, 1998), and IL-1β protein also increases, even as assessed by immunocytochemistry (Van Dam et al., 1992), these effects being most prominent in microglial cells.

Data recently obtained by K. T. Nguyen and M. K. Hansen in the laboratory of S. F. Maier and L. R.

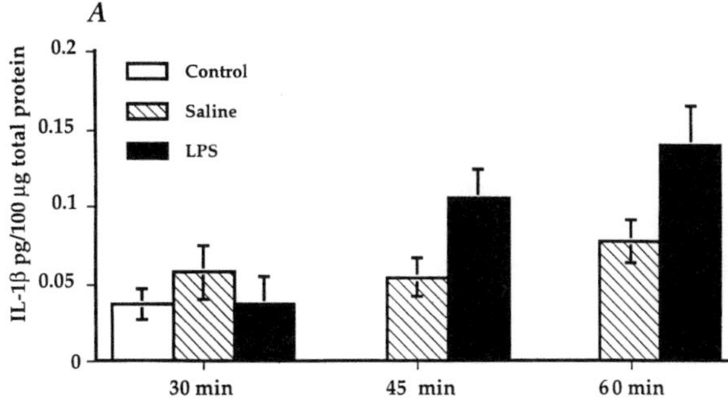

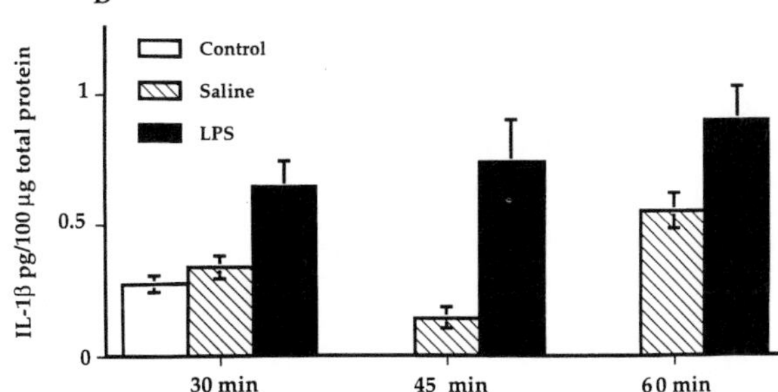

FIGURE 1 Mean level of IL-1β protein 30, 45, and 60 min after ip injection of LPS or saline. The IL-1β levels of home cage controls are shown at the 30 min point on the graphs for convenience. (A) Depicts levels for the hippocampus; (B) Depicts levels for the hypothalamus.

Watkins may be especially instructive. IL-1β protein was measured in discrete regions of the brain and spinal cord at various times following an ip injection of 100 µg/kg LPS. The unusual finding was that IL-1β protein was increased in as little as 30 min following LPS in some areas (e.g., hypothalamus), and by 45 min in other regions (e.g., hippocampus). These data are shown in Figure 1. Parenthetically, IL-1β increases in blood were not detectable until 60 min after ip LPS, again suggesting that there is an early non-blood-borne signal to the CNS.

These data are unusual because this IL-1β protein increase precedes the time at which increases in IL-1β mRNA in brain parenchyma are detected (e.g., Quan, Stern, Whiteside, & Herkenham, 1999; Quan et al., 1998). In any event, new protein in brain is not likely to be able to be transcribed and translated within 30 min, particularly in view of the fact that the injection was ip and so time is required to transduce a signal and transmit it to the brain. However, it is possible that the IL-1β that was observed reflects posttranslational processing of preformed IL-1β precursor. As noted above, IL-1β is synthesized as a 33 kDa precursor (pro-IL-1β) that is biologically inactive, with mature IL-1β being formed from pro-IL-1β by proteolytic cleavage by ICE (see Watkins et al., 1999, for a review of IL-1 processing). The active forms of ICE also result from proteolytic cleavage from an ICE precursor, and stimulation by LPS produces the rapid processing of ICE (Yao & Johnson, 1997), leading to the production of mature IL-1β. This process can indeed be quite rapid. For example, adenosine triphosphate (ATP) induces an increase in ICE activity that leads to the production of mature IL-1β from pro-IL-1β and IL-1β release within 7.5 min (Griffiths, Stam, Downs, & Otterness et al., 1995). LPS may well increase ATP levels, as stressors are known to do so (Minor & Saade, 1997), and neurons that utilize ATP as a transmitter project from the A1 cell group via the ventral noradrenergic bundle to the hypothalamus (Sperlagh, Sershen, Lojtha, & Vizi, 1998). Furthermore, there is some evidence that the brain may store pro-IL-1β in constitutive fashion, particularly in the hypothalamus. Tringali et al. (1996) found a rapid release of IL-1β, as measured by radioimmunoassay, from hypothalamic explants. Interestingly, this rapidly released IL-1β immunoreactivity was not decreased by inhibitors of IL-1β gene expression such as dexamethasone, IL-4, and IL-10. This can be explained by either a preexisting pool of readily releasable IL-β or pro-IL-1β that is rapidly cleaved. The rapid increase in overall protein levels found in the Nguyen et al. studies cannot be explained by a pool of releasable IL-1β, because the samples were sonicated and so the assay measures intracellular as well as extracellular IL-1β. If the IL-1β family member that is preformed is pro-IL-1β rather than IL-1β, then it might be readily understandable why "IL-1β" can be detected by the sensitive ELISA procedure, but not by immunocytochemistry. Most antibodies directed against IL-1β also bind to pro-IL-1β, but with much reduced affinity (Dinarello, 1992).

B. IL-1β Action in Brain

The remaining issue concerns whether IL-1β in the CNS plays a role in mediating the physiological and behavioral sickness responses produced by peripheral immune activation. The fact that icv and regional administration of small quantities of IL-1β produces many of the same sickness responses that follow peripheral immune activation is suggestive, but does not prove that IL-1β synthesized and released in the brain in response to peripheral cytokines, LPS, or other immune-activating agents is involved in the mediation of sickness. A physiological role for IL-1β can only be concluded if the blockade of IL-1β synthesis in brain, or the administration of IL-1 antisera or IL-1ra into the brain blocks or reduces sickness responses. There are a number of such studies. The icv administration of IL-1ra or IL-1β antiserum has been shown to block or reduce (a) fever produced by ip LPS (Luheshi et al., 1996), LPS injected into a subcutaneous airpouch (Miller, Hopkins, & Luheshi, 1997), turpentine injected im (Luheshi et al., 1997), and cecal ligation and puncture (Gourine et al., 1998); (b) the growth hormone reduction produced by iv LPS and by cecal ligation and puncture (Lang, Fan, Wojnar, Varg, & Cooney, 1998); (c) the increase in plasma glucose concentration and glucose production produced by iv LPS (Lang, Cooney, & Vary, 1996); (d) the reduction in plasma gonadotropin level produced by LPS (Ebisui et al., 1992); (e) the plasma catecholamine increase following iv LPS (Lang et al., 1996); (f) the increase in corticotropin releasing hormone (CRH) mRNA in the paraventricular nucleus (PVN) following ip LPS (Kakucksa, Qi, Clark, & Lechan, 1993); (g) the increase in extracellular levels of serotonin in hippocampus that follows ip LPS (Linthorst, Flachskamm, Muller-Prenss, Holsboer, & Real, 1995); (h) the increased nonrapid eye movement sleep produced by iv muramyl dipeptide and IL-1β (Imeri, Opp, & Krueger, 1993); (i) the reduction in social exploration produced by ip IL-1β (Kent et al., 1992); (j) the reduction in food intake produced by ip IL-1β (Kent et al., 1992); (k) the reduction in female sexual behavior produced by ip IL-1β (Avitsur, Pollak, & Yirmiya, 1997); (l) the gastrointestinal hypomotility produced by iv LPS (Plaza, Fioramonti, & Bueno, 1997); and (m) the intrathecal administration of IL-1ra blocks the hyperalgesia produced by ip LPS (Maier, Wiertelak, Martin, & Watkins, 1993).

An interpretive issue concerning icv administration of an agent is whether the effects obtained could be mediated by leakage to the periphery. The most common control for this possibility is to inject the same dose as was used icv either iv or ip, and this was determined in a number of the studies previously cited (e.g., Lang et al., 1996). In addition, the icv studies all utilized doses of IL-1ra in the microgram range, whereas milligram dosages are necessary to obtain effects on the measures cited above after peripheral administration (e.g., Luheshi et al., 1997). It should also be noted that not all sickness responses are reduced by icv IL-1ra. For example, the reduction in food intake (Kent, Kelley, & Dantzer, 1992), social exploration (Bluthé et al., 1992), and female sexual behavior (Avitsur et al., 1997) produced by LPS were unaffected. Interestingly, all three outcomes were blocked when induced by IL-1β (see above), again pointing to the fact that LPS can act independently of IL-1β. In addition, exactly how brain IL-1 is involved in the HPA response to LPS and cytokines is unclear. As noted, icv IL-1ra can completely block the increase in CRH mRNA in the PVN following LPS (Kakucksa et al., 1993), but has been reported to have little effect on plasma ACTH (Habu, Watanobe, Yasujima, & Suda, 1998). Whether this is an issue of dose and time of administration, or a more fundamental inconsistency is unknown. In sum, it can be concluded that brain IL-1β does play a role in the neural circuitry that produces at least some of the consequences of peripheral immune stimulation. This does not mean that IL-1β is the proximate mediator of any of these sickness behaviors. IL-1β has been shown to induce production and release of a number of neurotransmitters and neuromodulators—prostaglandins, nitric oxide, glutamate, serotonin, and norepinephrine are but examples. What the results do suggest is that IL-1β is critically involved somewhere in the central circuits that mediate many of the sickness responses.

C. Stress

The potential role of brain IL-1β in mediating neural, endocrine, physiological, and behavioral consequences of exposure to stressors deserves special comment. A similarity between the neurochemical, endocrine, physiological, and behavioral sequelae of peripheral immune activation and exposure to stressors has often been noted (Dunn, 1995; Maier & Watkins, 1998). Stressors and immune activation produce many of the same brain, endocrine, physiological, and behavioral changes (see Maier & Watkins, 1998, for review), as well as similar peripheral alterations. For example, the stressor inescapable tailshock increases plasma acute phase proteins, decreases plasma carrier proteins, and increases the number of circulating white blood cells (Deak et al., 1997). Furthermore, although the immediate effects of stressors such as footshock and tailshock are to inhibit macrophage function (Fleshner et al., 1998), the delayed effects are to activate macrophages (Fleshner et al., 1998; Meltzer et al., 1997, 1998). This is not to suggest that the patterns produced by stressors and immune-activating agents are identical, and some differences have been noted (Dunn, 1995). However, the neural and behavioral output patterns produced by different stressors are also not identical, and so the question of degree of similarity between stressor and immune effects is a difficult one. Certainly, the patterns are similar enough to suggest overlapping neural circuitry and mechanisms, at least at the efferent output end of the circuit. However, the afferent part of the circuitry by which stressors and immune activation converge to regulate output control centers such as the hypothalamus are doubtlessly quite different. For example, activation of the PVN following peripheral LPS administration depends on ascending monoaminergic pathways from the brain stem, whereas PVN activation following footshock does not (Nance et al., 1995). PVN activation following footshock depends on circuitry that descends from limbic and forebrain structures (Li, Ericsson, & Sawchenko, 1996, Nance et al., 1995).

Similarities among neural, endocrine, and behavioral outcomes following stress and immune stimuli are perhaps not too surprising. However, why stressors should produce shifts in liver metabolism similar to those observed during infection (increase in positive acute phase reactants such as α-2-glycoprotein and decreases in negative acute phase reactants such as carrier proteins) and delayed macrophage activation is more difficult to understand. It is possible that induction of brain IL-1β is a key overlapping mediator. Icv administration of IL-1β produces not only fever, neurochemical changes similar to those produced by stressors and immune activation, and behaviors characteristic of both stress and infection such as reduced food and water intake, reduced exploration, and the like, but also shifts in liver metabolism such as those occurring during infection and stress (Morimoto, Sakata, Watanabe, & Murakami, 1989; Petit et al., 1994; Rothwell, 1989), as well as altered immune cell function (Sundar et al., 1989; Wan et al., 1993). That is, administration of IL-1β into the brain initiates the activation of autonomic and endocrine outflow systems from brain that impact on the liver, immune cells, and the regulation of peripheral immune function (Brown et al., 1991).

Thus, if stressors were to induce IL-1β in brain, then stressors ought to produce consequences that overlap extensively with those that follow immune activation. The consequences need not be identical, since stressors and infection can activate divergent processes as well. However, there is sufficient similarity between the functional consequences of stressors and immune challenge to warrant an examination of whether stressors do, in fact, induce IL-1β in brain, and importantly whether antagonism of IL-1β in the brain blocks or reduces the physiological and behavioral consequences of stressor exposure. Although not many studies have directly addressed these questions, there are a few reports that support these possibilities. Both IL-1β mRNA (Minami et al., 1991) and protein (Nguyen et al., 1998) levels have been reported to be increased by stressors such as immobilization and tailshock in brain regions such as the hypothalamus. Interpretation of these data is complex and has been discussed by Maier et al. (1999). One difficulty is that corticosteroids inhibit IL-1β gene transcription (Lee et al., 1988), destabilize IL-1β mRNA (Amano, Lee, & Allison, 1993), and inhibit a number of translational and posttranslational processes (Kern, Lamb, Reed, Daniele, & Nowell, 1988) that are involved in IL-1β production. Since stressors elevates corticosteroid levels, the central IL-1β increases observed by Nguyen et al. (1998) were only observable in adrenalectomized subjects, with the exception of the hypothalamus in which IL-1β increases could be detected even in intact animals. However, Nguyen et al. (1998) utilized a 2-h session of intermittent tailshocks, a procedure that produces a very intense and prolonged corticosteroid response (Maier et al., 1986). Using a brief period of social isolation (placement of a rat in a cage by itself) as a stressor, which produces only a modest and brief corticosteroid rise, Pugh et al. (1999) observed large increases in IL-1β in brain in non-adrenalectomized subjects. Although the data are still sparse, there is some support for the argument that stressors induce brain IL-1β. Similarly, data concerning whether antagonism of IL-1 in brain inhibits sequelae of stressor exposure are also not abundant. However, brain injection of IL-1ra has been reported to block or reduce some of the neurochemical (Shintani et al., 1995), endocrine (Shintani et al., 1995), behavioral (Maier & Watkins, 1995), and immunological (Saperstein et al., 1992) responses to stressors. Furthermore, α-MSH, which acts as a functional IL-1β antagonist (Catania & Lipton, 1994), blocks many of the sickness responses produced by exposure to inescapable tailshock such as fever, reduced food and water intake, and shifts in basal corticosteroid levels (Maier et al., 1999; Milligan et al., 1998).

D. Why?

It is always hazardous to ask why a particular process exists, and arguments can be made only in tentative fashion. However, the presence of a cytokine such as IL-1β in brain, and induction in brain by both immune activation and stressors, is sufficiently peculiar to motivate at least an attempt at an answer. Some insight can often be gained by considering more primitive species and what is known concerning the evolution of the processes in question. Even the most primitive species must defend against infection and injury, and contain immune cells and processes (Beck, Cooper, Hobicht, & Harchonis, 1994). Specific immunity is a relatively recent adaptation, but all animals can recognize, process, and eliminate nonself by phagocytosis and can engage in wound healing. Even sponges, the most primitive multicellular organisms, contain phagocytes what recognize pathogens (Johnston & Heldemann, 1982). Amoebocytes are among the most primitive phagocytes, and contain enzymes that are similar to those in mammalian macrophages and are analogous to macrophages in many respects (Bayne, 1990). It is important that amoebocytes in organisms such as mollusks synthesize and release IL-1 (or IL-1-like molecules), TNF, and IL-6, and do so when stimulated by molecules such as LPS (Hughes, Smith, Barnett, Charles, & Stefano, 1991). The cytokines have local functions similar to those in mammals (e.g., attracting other amoebocytes to sites of infection or injury), but also communicate to neural tissue. Indeed, IL-1 receptors have been localized in neural tissue in mollusks (Sawada, Hara, & Maeno, 1991) and IL-1 can alter neural excitability in mollusks (Clatworthy, 1996). Thus, in organisms such as mollusks that do not even have a discrete brain, cytokines communicated with neural tissue for the orchestration of defense against infection and injury. However, primitive organisms such as mollusks do not have a blood-brain barrier, and cytokines have direct access to neural tissue. As nervous systems became more complex they required a more stable ionic environment, leading to the development of a blood-brain barrier (Cserr & Bandgaard, 1988). Unfortunately, now cytokines released by immune cells would no longer have direct access to neural target tissue. Many solutions to this difficulty would be possible—the development of active transport mechanisms, induction of signals at barrier cells that can then enter the brain, the development of transduction mechanisms at regions where the barrier is weak, etc. However, another solution would be to develop mechanisms by which the release of the cytokine outside the blood-brain barrier initiates signals that reach cells inside the brain parenchyma that now manufacture and release the cytokine. Thus, the cytokine signal would still reach the target neural tissue, it is just that it is cytokine that is synthesized in brain, rather than the cytokine released by the immune cell. Of course, neural signals always had direct access to immune cells without a barrier, and IL-1-like molecules have been localized in neural tissue in mollusks (Paeman et al., 1992). Therefore, outflow processes from the brain to the immune system were also needed, thereby making sense of why IL-1 in the brain in mammals leads to outflow from the brain that feeds back to immune cells.

The final question would be why stressors seem to activate this circuitry. One argument focuses on the fact that in species such as the mollusk, IL-1β plays a critical role in initiating energy production during infection and injury. In mammals, the hormones produced by the stress response, namely catecholamines and glucocorticoids, function to liberate energy from bodily stores. These hormones are present in the amoebocyte along with IL-1, and IL-1 initiates the cascade that leads to the release of these hormones to produce energy (see Ottaviani & Franceschi, 1996, for review). Furthermore, there is the same sequence of CRH-to ACTH-to-corticosteroids as is present in mammals, but here within a single cell rather than from hypothalamus-to-pituitary-to-adrenal. In the amoebocyte, the energy production is in the service of fighting infection, namely the sickness response. The stress response in mammals is really a "fight/flight" response (Sapolsky, 1992). Fight/flight requires an organism far more complicated than a primitive invertebrate and evolved much later than did the innate immune response (Maier & Watkins, 1998). It requires an organism complex enough to identify a predator or other threat at a distance, to make organized movements toward or away from a threat, and the sensorimotor integrative capacities to integrate the two. However, fight/flight also requires the production of energy, and so the fight/flight stress response may have coopted (Gould, 1982) the machinery that already existed to produce energy, namely the sickness machinery. All that would be required was to initiate the response from a new source—external threat rather than infection and injury, distal threat rather than proximal threat. This also would have the secondary benefit of priming the innate immune response in case of infection produced during a fight/flight encounter.

V. CONCLUSION

This chapter has focused on multiple routes of action of IL-1 on the nervous system. As complex as the research that has been reviewed might be, the reader should understand that the picture that has been presented is a vast oversimplification of the processes that occur in the whole organism. Cytokines such as IL-1β do not operate in isolation, and their effects may be quite different depending on other events that have or have not occurred. Cytokines are pleotropic (they have multiple functions) and redundant (they have overlapping functions), and so a cytokine such as IL-1 likely never operates by itself to produce a biological outcome. In addition, cytokines induce each other and themselves, as well as other mediators, and so real communication between the immune and central nervous systems must involve complex interactions, allowing for fine-tuned signaling and communication. There will likely be no single mechanism, and message blending and pattern recognition may be the rule. It will be a challenge to determine how the brain decodes and interprets multiple messages arriving over multiple channels, and then in turn regulates outflow back to immune processes and cells. Research to date has focused primarily on early events in the bidirectional signaling process between the brain and the immune system, typically the first few hours after the administration of a cytokine or an immune activating agent. However, there are cytokines that are produced and released by macrophages days after stimulation by agents such as LPS, and communication by these cytokines to the brain has not been studied. Moreover, products of the specific immune response are also known to communicate to the brain at the peak of the specific immune response to an antigen occurring 3–5 days after antigen administration (Besedovsky, 1975). The pathways by which this major arm of the immune system communicates to the brain are even less well understood. Nonetheless, such factors as sensory innervation of sites of antigenic exposure, sympathetic innervation of immune organs, and the neuroendocrine system can all exert profound effects on the specific immune system (Helme, Eglezos, Dandie, Andrews, & Boyd, 1987; Green-Johnson, Zalcman, Vriend, & Greenberg, 1996; Zalcman et al., 1994). It is likely that we have only scratched the surface of the subtleties and complexities of communication pathways between the immune and central nervous systems.

References

Amano, Y., Lee, S. W., & Allison, A. C. (1993). Inhibition by glucocorticoids of the formation of interleukin-1 alpha, interleukin-1 beta, and interleukin-6: Mediation by decreased mRNA stability. *Molecular Pharmacology, 43,* 176–182.

Atkins, E. (1960). Pathogenesis of fever. *Physiological Review, 40,* 580–646.

Avitsur, R., Pollak, Y., & Yirmiya, R. (1997). Different receptor mechanisms mediate the effects of endotoxin and interleukin-1 on female sexual behavior. *Brain Research, 773,* 149–161.

Banks, W. A., & Kastin, A. J. (1987). Minireview: Saturable transport of peptides across the blood-brain barrier. *Life Sciences, 41,* 1319–1338.

Banks, W. A., Kastin, A. J., & Durham, D. A. (1989). Bidirectional transport of interleukin-1 alpha across the blood-brain barrier. *Brain Research Bulletin, 23,* 433–437.

Banks, W. A., Oritz, L., Plotkin, S. R., & Kastin, A. J. (1991). Human IL-1 alpha, murine IL-1 alpha, and murine IL-1 beta are transported from blood to brain in the mouse by a shared saturable mechanism. *Journal of Pharmacology and Experimental Therapeutics, 259,* 988–996.

Baumann, H., & Gauldie, J. (1994). The acute phase response. *Immunology Today, 15,* 74–81.

Bayne, C. J. (1990). Phagocytosis and non-self recognition in invertebrates. *Biological Science, 40,* 723–731.

Beck, G., Cooper, E. L., Hobicht, G. S., & Harchonis, J. J. (1994). Primordeal immunity: Foundations for the vertebrate immune system. *Annals of the New York Academy of Sciences* 712.

Besedovsky, H. O., & Del Rey, A. (1996). Immune-neuroendocrine interactions: Facts and hypotheses. *Endocriology Review, 17,* 64–102.

Besedovsky, H. O., del Rey, A., Sorkin, E., & Dinarello, C. A. (1986). Immunoregulatory feedback between interleukin-1 and glucocorticoid hormones. *Science, 233,* 652–654.

Besedovsky, H. O., Sorkin, E., Keller, M., & Muller, J. (1975). Changes in blood hormone levels during immune response. *Proceedings of the Society for Experimental Biology and Medicine, 150,* 466–470.

Blalock, J. E., Smith, E. S., & Meyer, W. J. (1985). The pituitary-adrenocortical axis and the immune system. *Clinics in Endocrinology and Metabolism, 14,* 1021–1038.

Blatties, C. M. (1974). Influence of body weight and temperature on the pyrogenic effect of endotoxin in guinea pigs. *Toxicology and Applied Pharmacology, 29,* 249–258.

Bluthé, R.-M., Beaudu, C., Kelley, K. W., & Dantzer, R. (1995). Differential effects of IL-1ra on sickness behavior and weight loss induced by IL-1 in rats. *Brain Research, 677,* 171–176.

Bluthe, R.-M., Dantzer, R., & Kelley, K. W. (1992). Effects of interleukin-1 receptor antagonist on the behavioral effects of lipopolysaccharide in rat. *Brain Research, 573,* 318–320.

Bluthé, R.-M., Michaud, B., Kelley, K. W., & Dantzer, R. (1996). Vagotomy blocks behavioural effects of interleukin-1 injected *via* the intraperitoneal route but not via other systemic routes. *NeuroReport, 7,* 2823–2827.

Bluthé, R.-M., Walter, V., Parnet, P., Layé, S., Lestage, J., Verrier, D., Poole, S., Stennig, B. E., Kelley, K. W., & Dantzer, R. (1994). Lipolysaccharide induces sickness behaviour in rats by a vagal mediated mechanism. *C. R. Acad. Sci. Paris, 317,* 499–503.

Brady, L. S., Lynn, A. B., Herkenham, M., & Gottesfeld, Z. (1994). Systemic interleukin-1 induces early and late patterns of c-fos mRNA expression in brain. *Journal of Neuroscience, 14,* 4951–4964.

Breder, C. D., Smith, W. L., Roz, A., & Kasferrer, J. (1992). Distribution and characterization of cyclooxygenase immunoreactivity in the ovine brain. *Journal of Comparative Neurology, 332,* 409–438.

Bret-Dibat, J.-L., Bluthé, R.-M., Kent, S., Kelley, K. W., & Dantzer, R. (1995). Lipopolysaccharide and interleukin-1 depress food-motivated behavior in mice by a vagal-mediated mechanism. *Brain, Behavior, and Immunity, 9,* 242–246.

Brown, R., Li, Z., Vriend, C. Y., Nirula, R., Janz, L., Falk, J., Nance, D. M., Dyck, D. G., & Greenberg, A. H. (1991). Suppression of splenic macrophage interleukin-1 secretion following intracerebroventricular injection of interleukin-1β: Evidence for pituitary-adrenal and sympathetic control. *Cellular Immunology, 132,* 84–93.

Buttini, M., & Boddeke, H. (1995). Peripheral lipopolysaccharide stimulation induces interleukin-1β messenger RNA in rat brain microglial cells. *Neuroscience, 65,* 523–530.

Cao, C., Matsumura, K., Yamagata, K., & Watanabe, Y. (1996). Endothelial cells of the rat brain vasculature express cyclooxygenase 2 mRNA in response to systemic interleukin-1β: A possible site of prostaglandin synthesis responsible for fever. *Brain Research, 73,* 263–272.

Cao, C., Matsumura, K., Yamagata, K., & Watanabe, Y. (1997). Involvement of cyclooxygenase-2 in LPS-induced fever and regulation of its mRNA in the rat brain by LPS. *American Journal of Physiology, 272,* R1712–R1725.

Catania, A., & Lipton, J. M. (1994). The neuropeptide alpha-melanocyte-stimulating hormone: A key component of neuro-immunomodulation. *Neuroimmunomodulation, 1,* 93–99.

Clatworthy, A. L. (1996). A simple systems approach to neural-immune communication. *Comparative Biochemistry and Physiology, 115A*, 1–10.

Cooper, K. E., Cranston, W. I., & Honour, A. M. (1967). Observations on the site and mode of action of pyrogens in the rabbit brain. *Journal of Physiology, 191*, 325–337.

Cserr, H. F., & Bandgaard, M. (1988). The neuronal microenvironment: A comparative view. *Annals of the New York Academy of Sciences, 481*, 1–7.

Cunningham, E. T. Jr. Wada, E., Carter, D. B., Tracey, D. E., Battey, J. F., & De Souza, E. B. (1992). In situ histochemical localization of type 1 interleukin-1 receptor messenger RNA in the central nervous system, pituitary, and adrenal gland of the mouse. *Journal of Neuroscience, 12*, 1101–1114.

Dantzer, R., Bluthé, R.-M., Kent, S., & Goodall, G. (1993). Behavioral effects of cytokines: An insight into mechanisms of sickness behavior. In E. G. DeSouza (Ed.), *Neurobiology of cytokines* (pp. 130–151). San Diego: Academic Press.

Dinarello, C. A. (1991). Interleukin-1 and interleukin-1 antogenism. *Blood, 77*, 1627–1652.

Dinarello, C. A. (1992). ELISA kits based on monoclonal antibodies do not measure total IL-1beta synthesis. *Journal of Immunological Methods, 148*, 255–259.

Dinarello, C. A. (1999). Overview of inflammatory cytokines. In L. R. Watkins & S. F. Maier (Eds.), *Cytokines and pain* (pp. 1–20). Basel: Birkhauser Press.

Dinarello, C. A., Cannon, J. G., Mier, J. W., Bernheim, H. A., Lopreste, G., Lynn, D. L., Love, R. N., Webb, A. C., Auron, P. E., Reuben, R. C., Rich, A., Wolff, S. M., & Putney, S. D. (1986). Multiple biological activities of human recombinant interleukin-1. *Journal of Clinical Investigations, 77*, 1734–1739.

Dunn, A. J. (1995). Interactions between the nervous system and the immune system: Implications for psychopharmacology. In F. E. Bloom & D. J. Kupfer (Eds.), *Psychopharmacology: The fourth generation of progress* (pp. 719–733). New York: Raven Press.

Dunn, A. J., & Swiergiel, A. H. (1998). The role of cytokines in infection-related behavior. *Annals of the New York Academy of Sciences, 840*, 577–585.

Ek, M., Kurosawa, M., Lundeberg, T., & Ericsson, A. (1998). Activation of vagal afferents after intravenous injection of interleukin-1β: Role of endogenous prostaglandins. *Journal of Neuroscience, 18*, 9471–9479.

Elmquist, J. K., Breder, C. D., Sherin, J. E., Scammell, T. E., Hickey, W. F., Dewitt, D., & Saper, C. B. (1997). Intravenous lipopolysaccharide induces cyclooxygenase 2-like immunoreactivity in rat brain perivascular microglia and meningeal macrophages. *Journal of Comparative Neurology, 381*, 119–129.

Ericsson, A., Arias, C., & Sawchenko, P. E. (1997). Evidence for an intramedullary prostaglandin-dependent mechanism in the activation of stress-related neuroendocrine circuitry by intravenous interleukin-1. *Journal of Neuroscience, 17*, 7166–7179.

Ericsson, A., Kovacs, K. J., & Sawchenko, P. E. (1994). A functional anatomical analysis of central pathways subserving the effects of interleukin-1 on stress-related neuroendocrine neurons. *Journal of Neuroscience, 14*, 897–913.

Ericsson, A., Liu, C., Hart, R. P., & Sawchenko, P. E. (1995). Type 1 interluekin-1 receptor in the rat brain: Distribution, regulation, and relationship to sites of IL-1-induced cellular activation. *Journal of Comparative Neurology, 361*, 681–698.

Fleshner, M., Goehler, L. E., Hermann, J., Relton, J. K., Maier, S. F., & Watkins, L. R. (1995). Interleukin-1β induced corticosterone elevation and hypothalamic NE depletion is vagally mediated. *Brain Research Bulletin, 37*, 605–610.

Gaykema, R. P. A., Dijkstra, I., & Tilders, F. J. H. (1995). Subdiaphragmatic vagotomy suppresses endotoxin-induced activation of hypothalamic corticotropin-releasing hormone neurons and ACTH secretion. *Endocrinology, 136*, 4717–4720.

Goehler, L. E., Gaykema, R. P. A., Nguyen, K. T., Lee, J. E., Tilders, F. J. H., Maier, S. F., & Watkins, L. R. (1999). Interleukin-1β in immune cells of the abdominal vagus nerve: An immune to nervous system link? *Journal of Neuroscience, 19*, 2799–2806.

Gould, S. J. (1982). Darwinism and the expansion of evolutionary theory. *Science, 216*, 380–387.

Gourine, A. V., Rudolph, K., Tesfaigzi, J., & Kluger, M. J. (1998). Role of hypothalamic interleukin-1β in fever induced by cecal ligation and puncture in rats. *American Journal of Physiology, 275*, R754–R761.

Green-Johnson, J. M., Zalcman, S., Vriend, C. Y., Nance, D. M., & Greenberg, A. H. (1996). Role of norepinephrine in suppressed IgG production by epilepsy-prone mice. *Life Sciences, 59*, 1121–1132.

Griffiths, R. J., Stam, E. J., Downs, J. T., & Otterness, I. G. (1995). ATP induces the release of IL-1 from LPS-primed cells in vivo. *Journal of Immunology, 154*, 2821–2828.

Gutierrez, E. G., Banks, W. A., & Kastin, A. J. (1993). Murine TNF alpha is transported from blood to brain in the mouse. *Journal of Neuroimmunology, 47*, 169–176.

Habu, S., Watanobe, H., Yasujima, M., & Suda, T. (1998). Different roles of brain interleukin-1 in the adrenocorticotropin response to central versus peripheral administration of lipopolysaccharide in the rat. *Cytokine, 10*, 390–394.

Hansen, M. K., and Kreuger, J. M. (1997). Subdiaphragmatic vagotomy blocks the sleep- and fever-promoting effects of interleukin-1β. *American Journal of Physiology, 273*, R1246–R1253.

Hansen, M. K., Nguyen, K. T., Fleshner, M., Goehler, L. E., & Gaykema, R. P. (1999). Effects of vagotomy on circulating levels of endotoxin cytokines, and corticosterone following intraperitoneal lipopolysaccharide. Manuscript submitted for publication.

Hansen, M. K., Taishi, P., Chen, Z., & Krueger, J. M. (1998). Vagotomy blocks the induction of interleukin-1 beta mRNA in the brain of rats in response to systemic IL-1 beta. *Journal of Neuroscience, 18*, 2247–2253.

Hart, B. L. (1988). Biological basis of the behavior of sick animals. *Neuroscience and Biobehavioral Reviews, 12*, 123–137.

Helme, R. D., Eglezos, A., Dandie, G. W., Andrews, P. V., & Boyd, R. L. (1987). The effect of substance P on the regional lymph node antibody response to antigenic stimulation in capsaicin-pretreated rats. *Journal of Immunology, 139*, 3470–3473.

Herzyk, D. J., Allen, J. N., Marsh, C. B., & Wewers, M. D. (1992). Macrophage and monocyte IL-1 beta regulation differs at multiple sites. mRNA expression, translation, and post-translational processing. *Journal of Immunology, 149*, 3052–3058.

Hughes, T. K., Smith, E. M., Barnett, J. A., Charles, R., & Stefano, G. B. (1991). LPS stimulated invertebrate hemocytes: A role for immunoreactive TNF and IL-1. *Developmental and Comparative Immunology, 15*, 117–122.

Imeri, L., Opp, M. R., & Krueger, J. M. (1993). An IL-1 receptor and an IL-1 receptor antagonist attenuate muramyl dipeptide- and IL-1-induced sleep and fever. *American Journal of Physiology, 265*, R907–R913.

Ishizuka, Y., Ishida, Y., Kunitake, T., Kato, K., Hanamori, T., Mitsuyama, Y., & Kannan, H. (1997). Effects of area postrema lesion and abdominal vagotomy on interleukin-1 beta-induced norepinephrine release in the hypothalamic paraventricular nucleus region in the rat. *Neuroscience Letters, 223*, 57–60.

Ishizuka, Y., Ishida, Y., Qing-Hua, J., Shimokawa, A., Saita, M., Kato, K., Kunitake, T., Hanamori, T., Mitsuyama, Y., & Kannan, H. (1998). Abdominal vagotomy attenuates interleukin-1β-induced nitric oxide release in the paraventricular nucleus region in conscious rats. *Brain Research, 789*, 157–161.

Johnston, I. S., & Heldemann, W. H. (1982). Cellular defense systems in the Porifera. In N. Cohen & M. M. Siegel (Eds.), *The reticuloendotheleal system* (vol. 3, pp. 37–62). New York: Plenum Press.

Kakucska, I., Qi, Y., Clark, B. D., & Lechan, R. M. (1993). Endotoxin-induced corticotropin-releasing hormone gene expression in the hypothalamic paraventricular nucleus is mediated centrally by interleukin-1. *Endocrinology, 133*, 815–821.

Kapás, L., Hansen, M. K., Chang, H.-Y., & Krueger, J. M. (1998). Vagotomy attenuates but does not prevent the somnogenic and febrile effects of lipopolysaccharide in rats. *American Journal of Phsyiology, 274*, R406–R411.

Kapcala, L. P., He, J. R., Gao, Y., Pieper, J. O., & DeTolla, L. J. (1996). Subdiaphragmatic vagotomy inhibits intra-abdominal interleukin-1β stimulation of adrenocorticotropin secretion. *Brain Research, 728*, 247–254.

Katsuura, G., Gottschall, P. E., Dahl, R. R., & Arimura, A. (1988). Adrenocorticotropin release induced by intracerebroventricular injection of recombinant human interleukin-1 in rats: Possible involvement of prostaglandin. *Endocrinology, 122*, 1773–1779.

Kent, S., Bluthé, R.-M., Kelley, K. W., & Dantzer, R. (1992). Sickness behavior as a new target for drug development. *Trends in Pharmacological Science, 13*, 24–28.

Kent, S., Kelley, K. W., & Dantzer, R. (1992). Effects of lipopolysaccharide on food-motivated behavior in the rat are not blocked by an interleukin-1 receptor antagonist. *Neuroscience Letters, 145*, 83–86.

Kent, S., Rodriguez, F., Kelley, K. W., & Dantzer, R. (1994). Anorexia induced by microinjection of interleukin-1β in the ventromedial hypothalamus of the rat. *Physiology and Behavior, 56*, 1031–1036.

Kern, J. A., Lamb, R. J., Reed, J. C., Daniele, R. P., & Nowell, P. C. (1988). Dexamethasone inhibition of interleukin 1 beta production by human monocytes: Posttranscriptional mechanisms. *Journal of Clinical Investigation, 81*, 237–244.

Kluger, M. J. (1979). *Fever: Its biology, evolution and function.* Princeton: Princeton University Press.

Kluger, M. J. (1991). Fever: Role of pyrogens and cryogens. *Physiological Reviews, 71*, 93–127.

Kluger, M. J., Kozak, W., Conn, C. A., Leon, L. R., & Soszynski, D. (1996). The adaptive value of fever. *Infectious Disease Clinics of North America, 10*, 1–21.

Krueger, J. M., & Majde, J. A. (1994). Microbial products and cytokines in sleep and fever regulation. *Critical Reviews in Immunology, 14*, 355–3579.

Lacroix, S., & Rivest, S. (1998). Effect of acute systemic inflammatory response and cytokines on the transcription of the genes encoding cyclooxygenase enzymes (COX-1 and COX-2) in the rat brain. *Journal of Neurochemistry, 70*, 452–466.

Lang, C. H., Cooney, R., & Vary, T. C. (1996). Central interleukin-1 partially mediates endotoxin-induced changes in glucose metabolism. *American Journal of Physiology, 271*, E309–E316.

Lang, C. H., Fan, J., Wojnar, M. M., Vary, T. C., & Cooney, R. (1998). Role of central IL-1 in regulating peripheral IGF-I during endotoxemia and sepsis. *American Journal of Physiology, 274*, R956–R962.

Layé, S., Bluthé, R.-M., Kent, S., Combe, C., Médina, C., Parnet, P., Kelley, K., & Dantzer, R. (1995). Subdiaphragmatic vagotomy blocks induction of IL-1β mRNA in mice brain in response to peripheral LPS. *American Journal of Physiology, 268*, R1327–R1331.

Lechan, R. M., Toni, R., Clark, B. D., Cannon, J. G., Shaw, A. R., Dinarello, C. A., & Reichlin, S. (1990). Immunoreactive interleukin-1β localization in the rat forebrain. *Brain Research, 514*, 135–140.

Lee, H. Y., Whiteside, M. B., & Herkenham, M. (1998). Area postrema removal abolishes stimulatory effects of intravenous IL-1 on HPA activity and c-fos in RNA in the hypothalamic paraventricular nucleus. *Brain Research Bulletin, 46*, 495–503.

Lee, S. W., Tsou, A. P., Chan, H., Thomas, J., Petrie, K., Eugui, E. M., & Allison, A. C. (1988). Glucocorticoids selectively inhibit the transcription of the interleukinl beta gene and decrease the stability of interleukin 1 beta mRNA. *Proceedings of the National Academy of Science, 85*, 1204–1208.

Lenczowski, M. J. P., Van Dam, A.-M., Poole, S., Larrick, J. W., & Tilders, F. J. H. (1997). Role of circulating endotoxin and interleukin-6 in the ACTH and corticosterone response to intraperitoneal LPS. *American Journal of Physiology, 42*, R1870–R1877.

Li, H. Y., Ericsson, A., & Sawchenko, P. E. (1998). Distinct mechanisms underlie activation of hypothalamic neurosecretory neurons and their medullary catecholamingeric afferents in categorically different stress paradigms. *Proceedings of the National Academy of Sciences, 93*, 2359–2364.

Li, Y., Wong, K., Matsumura, L., Bollou, S., Morham, G., & Blatties, C. M. (in press). The febrile response to LPS is blocked in COX-2 but not in COX-1 null mutant mice. *Brain Research.*

Linthorst, A. C., Flachskamm, C., Muller-Preuss, P., Holsboer, F., & Reul, J. M. (1995). Effect of bacterial endotoxin and interleukin-1 beta on hippocampal serotonergic neurotransmission, behavioral activity, and free corticosterone levels: An in vivo microdialysis study. *Journal of Neuroscience, 15*, 2920–2934.

Long, N. C., Otterness, I., Kunkel, S. L., Vander, A. J., & Kluger, M. J. (1990). The roles of interleukin-1β and tumor necrosis factor in lipopolysaccharide fever in rats. *American Journal of Physiology, 259*, R724–R728.

Luheshi, G., Miller, A. J., Brouwer, S., Dascombe, M. J., Rothwell, N. J., & Hopkins, S. J. (1996). Interleukin-1 receptor antagonist inhibits endotoxin fever and systemic interleukin-6 induction in the rat. *American Journal of Physiology, 270*, E91–E95.

Luheshi, G. N., Stefferl, A., Turnbull, A. V., Dascombe, M. J., Brouwer, S., Hopkins, S. J., & Rothwell, N. J. (1997). Febrile response to tissue inflammation involves both peripheral and brain IL-1 and TNF-α in the rat. *American Journal of Physiology, 272*, R862–R868.

MacNeil, B. J., Jansen, A. H., Greenberg, A. H., & Nance, D. M. (1996). Activation and selectivity of splenic sympathetic nerve electrical activity response to bacterial endotoxin. *American Journal of Physiology, 270*, R264–R270.

MacNeil, B. J., Jansen, A. H., Janz, L. J., Greenberg, A. H., & Nance, D. M. (1997). Peripheral endotoxin increases splenic sympathetic nerve activity via central prostaglandin synthesis. *American Journal of Phsyiology, 273*, R609–R614.

Maier, S. F., Nguyen, K. T., Deak, T., Milligan, E. D., & Watkins, L. R. (1998). Stress, learned helplessness, and brain interleukin-1. In R. Dantzer, B. B. Wollmann, & R. Yirmiya (Eds.), *Stress, depression, and cytokines* (pp. 235–250). New York: Plenum Press.

Maier, S. F., & Watkins, L. R. (1998). Cytokines for psychologists: Implications of bidirectional immune-to-brain communication for understanding behavior, mood, and cognition. *Psychological Review, 105*, 83–107.

Mascarucci, P., Perego, C., Terrazzino, S., & De Simoni, M. G. (1998). Glutamate release in the nucleus tractus solitarius induced by peripheral lipopolysaccharide and interleukin-1 beta. *Neuroscience, 86*, 1285–1290.

Matsumura, K., Cao, C., Ozaki, M., Morii, H., Nakadate, K., & Watanabe, Y. (1998). Brain endothelial cells express cyclooxygenase-2 during lipopolysaccharide-induced fever: Light and electron microscopic immunocytochemical studies. *Journal of Neuroscience, 18*, 6279–6289.

Matsumura, K., Watanabe, Y., Imai-Matsumura, K., Connolly, M., Koyama, Y., Onoe, H., & Watanabe, Y. (1992). Mapping of prostaglandin E_2 binding sites in rat brain using quantitative autoradiography. *Brain Research, 581*, 292–298.

Medzhitov, R., & Janeway, C. A., Jr. (1997). Innate immunity: Impact on the adaptive immune response. *Current Opinion in Immunology, 9*, 4–9.

Medzhitov, R., & Janeway, C. A. Jr. (1998). An ancient system of host defense. *Current Opinion in Immunology, 10*, 12–15.

Meltzer, J. C., MacNeil, B. J., Sanders, V., Grimm, P. C., Vriend, J., Jansen, A. H., Greenberg, A. H., & Nance, D. M. (1998). The immunosuppresive effects of stress on splenic cytokine mRNA levels are mediated by adrenal dependent and independent mechanisms. Paper presented at the Society for Neuroscience, Los Angeles, CA.

Meltzer, J. C., MacNeil, B. J., Sanders, V., Vriend, C. A. Y., Jansen, A. H., Greenberg, A. H., & Nance, D. M. (1997). Effects of stress on in vivo splenic TNF-α and IL-1β mRNA levels. Paper presented at the Society for Neuroscience, San Diego, CA.

Miller, A. J., Hopkins, S. J., & Luheshi, G. N. (1997). Sites of action of IL-1 in the development of fever and cytokine responses to tissue inflammation in the rat. *British Journal of Pharmacology, 120*, 1274–1279.

Milligan, E. D., Nguyen, K. T., Deak, T., Hinde, J. L., Fleshner, M., Watkins, L. R., & Maier, S. F. (1998). The long term acute phase-like responses that follow acute stressor exposure are blocked by alpha-melanocyte stimulating hormone. *Brain Research, 810*, 48–58.

Minami, M., Kuraishi, Y., Yagaguchi, T., Nakai, S., Hirai, Y., & Satoh, M. (1991). Immobilization stress induces interleukin-1β mRNA in the rat hypothalamus. *Neuroscience Letters, 123*, 254–256.

Minano, F. J., Sancibrian, M., Vizcaino, M., Paez, X., Davatelis, G., Fahey, T., Sherry, B., Cerami, A., & Myers, R. D. (1990). Macrophage inflammatory protein-1: Unique action on the hypothalamus to evoke fever. *Brain Research Bulletin, 24*, 849–852.

Minor, T. R., & Saade, S. (1997). Poststress glucose mitigates behavioral impairments in rats in the "learned helplessness" model of psychopathology. *Biological Psychiatry, 42*, 324–334.

Morimoto, A., Sakata, Y., Watanabe, T., & Murakami, N. (1989). Characteristics of fever and acute-phase response induced by IL-1 and TNF. *363*, R35–R41.

Myers, R. R., Wagner, R., & Sorkin, L. S. (1999). Hyperalgesic action of cytokines on peripheral nerves. In L. R. Watkins & S. F. Maier (Eds.), *Cytokines and pain* (pp. 133–159). Basel: Birkhauser Press.

Nance, D. M., Greenberg, A. H., & Jackson, A. T. K. (1995). Central catecholamine involvement in the hypothalamic induction of c-fos after endotoxin treatment. Paper presented at the Society for Neuroscience, San Diego, CA.

Niijima, A. (1998). An electrophysiological study on the autonomic innervation of the mesenteric lymph node in the rat. *Neuroscience Letters, 243*, 144–146.

Opp, M. R., Obal, F. Jr., & Krueger, J. M. (1991). Interleukin-1 alters rat sleep: Temporal and dose-related effects. *American Journal of Physiology, 260*, R52–R58.

Opp, M. R., & Toth, L. A. (1997). Circadian modulation of IL-1 induced fever in intact and vagotomized rats. *Annals of the New York Academy of Sciences, 813*, 435–436.

Ottaviani, E., and Franceschi, C. (1996). The neuroimmunology of stress from invertebrates to man. *Progress in Neurobiology, 48*, 421–440.

Paeman, L. R., Porchet-Hennere, E., Masson, M., Leung, M. K., Hughes, T. K., & Stefano, G. B. (1992). Glial localization of interleukin-1 in invertebrate ganglia. *Cellular and Molecular Neurobiology, 12*, 463–472.

Petit, F., Jarous, A., Dickinson, R. D., Molina, P. E., Abumrad, N. N., & Lang, C. H. (1994). Contribution of central and peripheral adrenergic stimulation to IL-1-mediated glucoregulation. *American Journal of Physiology, 267*, E49–E56.

Pitossi, F., Del Rey, A., Kabiersch, A., & Besedovsky, H. (1997). Induction of cytokine transcripts in the CNS and pituitary following peripheral administration of endotoxin to mice. *Journal of Neuroscience Research, 48*, 287–298.

Plata-Salaman, C. R., Oomura, Y., & Kai, Y. (1988). Tumor necrosis factor and interleukin-1β: Suppression of food intake by direct action in the central nervous system. *Brain Research, 448*, 106–114.

Plaza, M. A., Fioramonti, J., & Bueno, L. (1997). Role of central interleukin-1 beta in gastrointestinal motor disturbances induced by lipopolysaccharide in sheep. *Digestive Disease Sciences, 42*, 242–250.

Quan, N., Stern, E. L., Whiteside, M. B., & Herkenham, M. (1999). Induction of pro-inflammatory cytokine mRNAs in the brain after peripheral injection of subseptic doses of lipopolysaccharide in the rat. *Journal of Neuroimmunology, 93*, 72–80.

Quan, N., Whiteside, M., & Herkenham, M. (1998). Time course and localization patterns of interleukin-1β messenger RNA expression in brain and pituitary after peripheral administration of lipopolysaccharide. *Neuroscience, 83*, 281–293.

Quan, N., Zhang, Z., Emery, M., Bosnall, R., & Weiss, J. M. (1996). Detection of interleukin-1 bioactivity in various brain regions of normal healthy rats. *Neuroimmunomodulation, 3*, 47–55.

Rivier, C., Chizzonite, R., & Vale, W. (1989). In the mouse, the activation of the hypothalamic-pituitary-adrenal axis by a lipopolysaccharide (endotoxin) is mediated through interleukin-1. *Endocrinology, 125*, 2800–2805.

Romanovsky, A. A., Kulchitsky, V. A., Simons, C. T., Sugimoto, N., & Szekeley, M. (1997a). Cold defense mechanisms in vagotomized rats. *American Journal of Physiology, 273*, R784–R789.

Romanovsky, A. A., Kulchitsky, V. A., Simons, C. T., Sugimoto, N., & Szekely, M. (1997b). Febrile responsiveness of vagotomized rats is suppressed even in the absence of malnutrition. *American Journal of Physiology, 273*, R777–R783.

Rothwell, N. J. (1989). CRF is involved in the pyrogenic and thermogenic effects of interleukin 1 beta in the rat. *American Journal of Physiology, 256*, E111–E115.

Rothwell, N. J., & Hopkins, S. J. (1995). Cytokines and the nervous system: II. Actions and mechanisms of action. *Trends in Neuroscience, 18*, 130–136.

Saper, C. B., & Breder, C. D. (1994). The neurologic basis of fever. *New England Journal of Medicine, 330*, 1880–1886.

Saperstein, A., Brand, H., Audhya, T., Nobriski, D., Hutchinson, B., Rosenzwieg, J., & Hollander, C. S. (1992). Interleukin-1 beta mediates stress-induced immunosuppression via CRH. *Endocrinology, 130*, 152–158.

Sapolsky, R. M. (1992). *Stress: The aging brain and the mechanisms of neuron death.* Cambridge, MA: MIT Press.

Sawada, M., Hara, N., & Maeno, T. (1991). Ionic mechanism of the outward current induced by extracellular ejection of interleukin-1 onto identified neurons of aplysia. *Brain Research, 545*, 248–256.

Scammell, T. E., Elmquist, J. K., Griffin, J. D., & Saper, C. B. (1996). Ventromedial preoptic prostaglandin E_2 activates fever producing autonomic pathways. *Journal of Neuroscience, 16,* 6246–6254.

Scammell, T. E., Griffin, J. D., Elmquist, J. K., & Saper, C. B. (1998). Microinjection of a cyclooxygenase inhibitor with the anteroventral preoptic region attenuates LPS fever. *American Journal of Physiology, 274,* R783–R789.

Sehic, E., Székely, M., Ungar, A. L., Oladehin, A., & Blatteis, C. M. (1996). Hypothalamic prostaglandin E_2 during lipopolysaccharide-induced fever in guinea pigs. *Brain Research Bulletin, 39,* 391–399.

Shintani, F., Nakaki, T., Kanba, S., Sato, K., Yagi, G., Shiozawa, M., Aiso, S., Kato, R., & Asai, M. (1995). Involvement of interleukin-1 in immobilization stress-induced increase in plasma adrenocorticotropic hormone and in release of hypothalamic monoamines in the rat. *Journal of Neuroscience, 15,* 1961–1970.

Simons, C. T., Kulchitsky, V. A., Sugimoto, N., Homer, L. D., Szekely, M., & Romanovsky, A. A. (1998). Signaling the brain in systemic inflammation: Which vagal branch is involved in fever genesis. *American Journal of Physiology, 275,* R63–R68.

Sperlagh, B., Sershen, H., Lojtha, A., & Vizi, E. S. (1998). Co-release of endogenous ATP and [^{3}H] noradrenaline from rat hypothalamic slices: Origin and modulation of alpha $_2$-adrenoceptors. *Neuroscience, 82,* 511–528.

Sundar, S. K., Becker, K. J., Cierpial, M. A., Carpenter, M. D., Rankin, L. A., Fleener, S. L., Ritchie, J. C., Simson, P. E., & Weiss, J. M. (1989). Intracerebroventricular infusion of interleukin 1 rapidly decreases peripheral cellular immune responses. *Proceedings of the National Academy of Sciences (USA), 86,* 6398–6402.

Tringali, G., Mancuso, C., Mirtella, A., Pozzoli, G., Parente, L., Preziosi, P., & Navarra, P. (1996). Evidence for the neuronal origin of immunoreactive interleukin-1β released by hypothalamic explants. *Neuroscience Letters, 219,* 143–146.

Tringali, G., Mirtella, A., Mancuso, C., Guerriero, G., Preziosi, P., & Navarra, P. (1997). The release of immunoreactive interleukin-1β from rat hypothalamic explants is modulated by neurotransmitters and corticotropin-releasing hormone. *Pharmacological Research, 36,* 269–273.

Turnbull, A. V., Pitossi, F. J., Lebrun, J.-J., Lee, S., Meltzer, J. C., Nance, D. M., del Rey, A., Besedovsky, H. O., & Rivier, C. (1997). Inhibition of tumor necrosis factor-α action within the CNS markedly reduces the plasma adrencorticotropin response to peripheral local inflammation in rats. *Journal of Neuroscience, 17,* 3262–3273.

Turnbull, A. V., & Rivier, C. L. (1999). Regulation of the hypothalamic-pituitary-adrenal axis by cytokines: Actions and mechanisms of action. *Physiological Reviews, 79,* 1–71.

Van Dam, A.-M., Brouns, M., Louisse, S., & Berken-Bosch, F. (1992). Appearance of interleukin-1 in macrophages and in ramified microglia in the brain of endotoxin-treated rats: A pathway for the induction of non-specific symptoms of sickness. *Brain Research, 588,* 291–296.

Van Dam, A.-M., Brouns, M., Man-A-Hing, W., & Berkenbosch, F. (1993). Immunocytochemical detection of prostaglandin E2 in microvasculature and in neurons of rat brain after administration of bacterial endotoxin. *Brain Research, 613,* 331–336.

Wan, W., Vriend, C. Y., Wetmore, L., Gartner, J. G., Greenberg, A. H., & Nance, D. M. (1993). The effects of stress on splenic immune function are mediated by the splenic nerve. *Brain Research Bulletin, 30,* 101–105.

Wan, W., Wetmore, L., Sorensen, C. M., Greenberg, A. H., & Nance, D. M. (1994). Neural and biochemical mediators of endotoxin and stress-induced c-fos expression in the rat brain. *Brain Research Bulletin, 34,* 7–14.

Wang, J., Ando, T., & Dunn, A. J. (1997). Effect of homologous interleukin-1, interleukin-6 and tumor necrosis factor-alpha on the core body temperature of mice. *Neuroimmunomodulation, 4,* 230–236.

Watkins, L. R., Hansen, M. K., Nguyen, K. T., Lee, J. E., & Maier, S. F. (in press). Dynamic regulation of the proinflammatory cytokine, interleukin-1B: Molecular biology for non-molecular biologists. *Life Sciences.*

Watkins, L. R., Maier, S. F., & Goehler, L. E. (1995). Cytokine-to-brain communication: A review and analysis of alternative mechanisms. *Life Sciences, 57,* 1011–1027.

Watkins, L. R., Wiertelak, E. P., Goehler, L. E., Mooney-Heiberger, K., Martinez, J., Furness, L., Smith, K. P., & Maier, S. F. (1994). Neurocircuitry of illness-induced hyperalgesia. *Brain Research, 639,* 283–299.

Wong, M.-L., & Licinio, J. (1994). Localization of interleukin-1 type 1 receptor mRNA in rat brain. *Neuroimmunomodulation, 1,* 110–115.

Yabuuchi, K., Minami, M., Katsumata, S., & Satoh, M. (1994). Localization of type 1 interleukin-1 receptor mRNA in the rat brain. *Molecular Brain Research, 27,* 27–36.

Yao, J., & Johnson, R. W. (1997). Induction of interleukin-1 beta-converting enzyme (ICE) in murine microglia by lipopolysaccharide. *Brain Research: Molecular Brain Research, 51,* 170–178.

Yirmiya, R. (1997). Behavioral and psychological effects of immune activation: Implications for depression due to a general medical condition. *Current Opinion in Psychiatry, 10,* 470–476.

Zalcman, S., Green-Johnson, J. M., Murray, L., Wan, W., Nance, D. M., & Greenberg, A. H. (1994). Interleukin-2 induced enhancement of an antigen-specific IgM response is mediated by the sympathetic nervous system. *Journal of Pharmacology and Experimental Therapeutics, 271,* 977–982.

C H A P T E R

23

Effects of Interleukin-2 and Interferons on the Nervous System

UWE-KARSTEN HANISCH

I. INTRODUCTION

Interleukin-2 (IL-2) and interferon-γ (IFN-γ) are cytokines that participate in the mechanisms of host defense and immune response. Both are produced by T helper cells on antigenic challenges of the immune system. The cytokines of the interferon-α and -β (IFN-α/β) family mainly safeguard the first line of defense against viruses. They differ from IFN-γ by molecular and some functional features and can be produced by many cell types. The primary association of these cytokines with immune cells or defense mechanisms in terms of synthesis and physiological functions does not exclude the notion that they may play additional roles and that cell types outside the hematopoietic system act as sources and targets of their activities. During the last decade, experimental findings and clinical observations supported the concept of certain cytokines being also neuroregulatory factors. Potent effects on neural (neuronal and glial) cells have been described for IL-2 and the interferons (IFNs). Effects also have been noticed at higher levels of complexity. As part of their physiological functions they may modulate the activity of the endocrine axis, induce fever and sleep, or suppress food intake and motor activity. Improved techniques for the molecular detection of cytokine-related mRNAs and proteins allowed for a first correlation of inducible responses with an expression of cytokines and their receptors or binding sites in nervous tissues. In viral infections of the central nervous system (CNS), IFNs will be found inside the brain whereas the endogenous synthesis of certain cytokines within the CNS remains a matter of controversy. Nevertheless, transport across the blood-brain barrier (BBB) may allow circulating cytokines, such as IL-2, to penetrate the brain parenchyma and to gain access to their receptors expressed on neuronal and glial cell populations. Cytokines may therefore serve as humoral mediators in the neuroimmune communication. On the other hand, invasion of nervous tissue by leukocytes under pathophysiological conditions will cause the release of cytokines, such as IFN-γ or IL-2, next to neural cells. Finally, the therapeutic use of some cytokines is accompanied by sometimes markedly increased circulating amounts and tissue levels and can also affect central compartments. Indeed, IFNs and IL-2 belong to the first cytokines that were introduced in clinical practice. Research on the "central" activities of cytokines focused mainly on IL-1, IL-6, or tumor necrosis factor-α (TNF-α). In this chapter, some of the findings are summarized that relate to the effects of IL-2 and IFNs on the nervous system. For both IL-2 and the IFN molecules, this survey cannot acknowledge all contributions to the available literature and the reader may, therefore, be referred to a number of reviews dealing with various aspects of these important factors (Besedovsky & del Rey, 1996; Farrar & Schreiber, 1993; Hanisch & Quirion, 1996; Hopkins & Rothwell, 1995; Merrill, 1991; Merrill & Benveniste, 1996; Otero & Merrill, 1994; Plata Salaman, 1991; Popko, Corbin, Baerwald, Dupree, & Garcia, 1997; Rothwell & Hopkins, 1995; Theze, Alzari, & Bertoglio, 1996; Zhao & Schwartz, 1998). Nevertheless, this chapter may provide enough evidence not only to warrant the scientific interest in neuroregulatory features of IL-2 and IFNs, but also to consider the potential CNS consequences that could arise from their dysregulation and clinical use.

II. IL-2 AND IFNs AS IMMUNOREGULATORY CYTOKINES

A. The IL-2/IL-15 Cytokine System

IL-2 is one of the most intensively investigated cytokines. Described in 1976 (Morgan, Ruscetti, & Gallo, 1976) and cloned in 1983 (Devos et al., 1983; Taniguchi et al., 1983) the knowledge about its functions in the immune system rapidly exceeded the role as the T-cell growth factor (Goldsmith & Greene, 1994; Hatakeyama & Taniguchi, 1991; Morgan et al., 1976; Smith, 1992; Waldmann, 1989). Besides the effects on all T-cell populations IL-2 has biological activities relating to B cells, natural killer (NK) cells, and lymphokine-activated killer (LAK) cells as well as macrophages and monocytes (Goldsmith & Greene, 1994; Hatakeyama & Taniguchi, 1991; Morgan et al., 1976; Smith, 1992; Waldmann, 1989). The term IL-2 was introduced in 1979 to assign the various, independently established biological activities to a single molecule (Taniguchi et al., 1983).

IL-2 is mainly produced by $CD4^+$ T helper cells of the type Th1 (Goldsmith & Greene, 1994; Hatakeyama & Taniguchi, 1991). Other cell types, such as B cells, may also be able to synthesize significant quantities of IL-2 (Goldsmith & Greene, 1994; Kakiuchi, Tamura, Gyotoku, & Nariuchi, 1991). T cells produce IL-2 on antigenic challenge or stimulation with mitogen, but additional signals are needed for maximal synthesis. Parallel induction of the IL-2 receptor subunit α (IL-2Rα) and combination with the constitutive IL-2R chains β and γ results in the formation of trimeric high-affinity receptors. This allows for autocrine and paracrine IL-2 effects that drive the clonal expansion of activated T cells. A subsequent decrease in IL-2 synthesis and the disappearance of the high-affinity IL-2R complexes contribute to the termination of an immune response (Goldsmith & Greene, 1994).

With respect to its molecular features, mature human IL-2 is a polypeptide of 133 amino acids (153 for the precursor) with an apparent molecular weight (MW) of 15 kD (Goldsmith & Greene, 1994; Hatakeyama & Taniguchi, 1991). Sequence comparisons between various mammalian species revealed extensive homology and structural conservation (Goldsmith & Greene, 1994; Mai, Kousoulas, Horohov, & Klei, 1994; McKnight & Classon, 1992). Original concepts of the three-dimensional structure were subsequently corrected (Bazan, 1992; Brandhuber, Boone, Kenney, & McKay, 1987; McKay, 1992; Sprang & Bazan, 1993). The meanwhile established folding topology places IL-2 in the family of the four-core α-helices bundle cytokines that also contains, for example, IL-4 (Davies & Wlodawer, 1995; Goldsmith & Greene, 1994; Theze, 1994).

IL-15 (or "IL-T") was discovered by two groups as a cytokine that binds to IL-2R and exhibits IL-2-like activities (Bamford et al., 1994; Burton et al., 1994; Giri et al., 1994; Grabstein et al., 1994). It was previously noted that a loss of IL-2 in knockout mice did not result in profound immune deficiency and concluded that another factor at least partially covered the functions of IL-2 (Waldmann, Tagaya, & Bamford, 1998). IL-15, like IL-2, is a 15 kD protein and most likely shares with IL-2 a similar folding topology. However, the two cytokines do not show obvious sequence similarity (Waldmann et al., 1998).

Although IL-2 is mainly the product of Th1 cells, IL-15 demonstrates a much broader expression but is, in contrast to IL-2, not synthesized by T cells. Both cytokines have an overlapping—but not identical—spectrum of activities for several cell types. Both stimulate the growth of activated $CD4^+$ and $CD8^+$ as well as $\gamma\delta$ T cells, promote cytolytic activity, including that of cytotoxic T and LAK cells, and support B cell differentiation and immunoglobulin synthesis. In contrast to IL-2, IL-15 is a potent chemoattractant for T cells and has growth factor activity for mast cells (Waldmann et al., 1998). IL-15 may also carry out nonimmune functions as illustrated by its anabolic effects on muscle tissue. IL-2-specific functions that are likely not shared by IL-15 relate to the maintenance of self-tolerance. Mice deficient in IL-2, IL-2Rα, or IL-2Rβ showed increased tendency for inflammatory or autoimmune diseases and spontaneous T-cell activation.

Another difference between the two cytokines relates to the control of their expression. The expression of IL-2 is mainly controlled by transcription and mRNA stabilization whereas IL-15 is regulated post-transcriptionally and via its intracellular trafficking (Bamford, Battiata, Burton, Sharma, & Waldmann, 1996; Bamford, DeFilippis, Azimi, Kurys, & Waldmann, 1998; Nishimura, Washizu, Nakamura, Enomoto, & Yoshikai, 1998; Onu, Pohl, Krause, & Bulfone Paus, 1997; Tagaya et al., 1997; Waldmann et al., 1998). Multiple start codons, alternative splicing and an unusually long N-terminus of the precursor all contribute to this very complex type of regulation.

B. The IFN Family

Virus-infected cells can acquire resistance to other viruses. This observation resulted in the isolation of a protein factor that mediated the phenomenon of viral interference (Isaacs & Lindenmann, 1957). This factor was defined as "interferon." Subsequently, many IFNs were discovered that share to various degree structural similarity and the ability to inhibit viral replication in mammalian cells. On the other hand, IFNs were found to cover a much broader range of biological functions, including antiproliferative and antitumor effects as well as immunomodulatory activities. Today, IFNs are considered as cytokines. The unifying term was introduced to acknowledge common features of lymphokines, interleukins, monokines, and colony-stimulating and growth factors, namely to be synthesized by more than a single nucleated cell type, to act as regulatory peptides with pleiotropic effects on hematopoietic and other cells and to participate in host defense, maintenance and restoration of homeostasis as well as repair (Oppenheim, 1994). Original classifications of the IFN types on the basis of biochemical and serologic properties subsequently have been supported and refined upon cloning and sequencing of the various molecules. The members of this heterogeneous and polymorphic family are accordingly classified as type I and type II IFNs. IFN-α, IFN- ω, IFN-β, and IFN-τ comprise the first group and bind to the same receptor whereas IFN-γ, also referred to as type II IFN, is structurally distinct and interacts with its own binding site (De Maeyer & De Maeyer-Guignard, 1994).

IFN-α, also known as leukocyte interferon, is mainly synthesized by monocytes, macrophages and—to a lesser degree—lymphocytes, but most cells are thought to be potential producers (De Maeyer & De Maeyer-Guignard, 1994; Donnelly, 1994). Besides some constitutive synthesis, IFN-α production depends on induction. Inducers of IFN-α synthesis and secretion are most notably viruses, especially RNA viruses. Certain bacteria and bacterial cell wall components, such as the lipopolysaccharide (LPS) of gram-negative germs, are similarly effective, with macrophages being the major cellular response element. In addition, cytokines, such as IL-1, IL-2, TNF-α or IFN-γ also can stimulate the production of INF-α, at least in some cell types. IFN-α itself comprises a whole family of 16 to 27 kD (glyco)proteins that derive from several intronless genes in both the human and the mouse system (Viscomi, 1997). In these gene clusters, functional IFN-α genes are associated with a number of pseudogenes. The various isoforms show substantial homology (>70% at the protein level) and are thus likely the result of gene duplications and divergence dated to 100 million years ago. Differences in the promoter regions suggest independent regulation of the subtypes and the actual expression pattern may vary with the cell type and/or the respective inducer. IFN-ω [also IFN-α(II)] is another product of the IFN type I gene cluster and has about 60% homology to the IFN-α proteins. It is found in humans and other mammalian species, but seems to be absent in the mouse. Similarly to IFN-α, several isoforms may exist next to each other, as independent genes were found in several species. In addition, IFN-τ (trophoblast IFN) represents a group of related IFN proteins that share almost 80% of their sequence with IFN-ω. However, their function appears developmentally restricted and relates to the implantation of the ovum.

Fibroblasts are the main source of IFN-β, which was therefore also named fibroblast interferon (De Maeyer & De Maeyer-Guignard, 1994; Donnelly, 1994). Monocytes/macrophages and epithelial cells contribute lower quantities and, as for IFN-α, basically all cell types have a potential for IFN-β synthesis. Induction of IFN-β depends on stimulation by viral infection or bacterial challenges. Cytokines can modulate IFN-β production as they do it with IFN-α. IFN-α/β induction, though often in parallel, can also follow independent mechanisms. The decision on preferential synthesis probably depends on the nature of the inducing factor and the cell type. For both IFN-α and -β, the induction of synthesis is controlled on transcriptional and posttranscriptional levels, with a strong but transient synthesis of mRNA followed by an autonomous down-regulation. In contrast to the situation with IFN-α, there is only a single intronless gene in humans and mice coding for IFN-β, the type I IFN showing about 30% homology to both IFN-α as well as IFN-ω sequences. The respective protein is of 20 to 23 kD (human) or 26 to 35 kD (mouse) sizes, depending on glycosylation. Multiple genes were found for the bovine, sheep, and porcine system, suggesting that IFN-β isoforms exist at least in some species. Earlier descriptions as IFN-β1 were used to distinguish between IFN-β and IFN-β2, which is now termed IL-6.

The major functions of the IFN-α/β family relate to the resistance of mammalian cells against viral infection, mainly mediated by interference with the viral protein synthesis within the infected cell. Nevertheless, several pathways exist that together provide antiviral protection by interfering at many stages of viral replication, including the entry and uncoating steps, transcription, initiation of translation, and subsequent processing as well as viral assembly and release (Stark, Kerr, Williams, Silverman, & Schreiber, 1998). The involvement of inducible factors, such as the Mx proteins, that carry antiviral effects is already partially understood. Moreover, these IFNs have strong antiproliferative activities, which involve multiple mechanisms. A major principle is the inhibition of (proto)oncogenes, along with the prolongation of the G1 and a delayed entry of the S-cell cycle phases. IFN-α/β have effects on the major histocompatibility complex (MHC) class I antigen expression, the identification code of the cells, which is also crucial for the cytotoxic removal of infected or malignant cells. These IFNs may also affect MHC class II expression by antigen-presenting cells (APC), but this function is probably more specific for IFN-γ. Some additional overlap in the biological effects of IFNs α/β and γ exists with regard to the enhancement of phagocytic activity of macrophages and an antitumor activity, which is most likely carried by cytotoxic macrophages, T, and NK cells. Enhanced antibody-mediated phagocytosis is induced by the IFN-α/β-triggered enhanced Fc receptor expression. Nevertheless, for macrophage activation, including MHC class II induction, IFN-γ seems to be the more important interferon.

The type II interferon, IFN-γ, also has been described as T cell or immune interferon, due to its production by activated $CD4^+$ and $CD8^+$ T cells as well as NK cells (Boehm, Klamp, Groot, & Howard, 1997; De Maeyer & De Maeyer-Guignard, 1994; Gray, 1994). However, macrophages have recently been found to secrete IFN-γ on combined stimulation with IL-12 and IL-18 (Munder, Mallo, Eichmann, & Modolell, 1998). For the T helper cell system, the population of Th1 cells has been identified as the most relevant source. Th2 cells may produce only small amounts of the interferon. On the other hand, the antiproliferative effect of IFN-γ is stronger for Th2 than for Th1 cells, suggesting that synthesis of this cytokine during an immune system challenge could participate in the decision favoring a Th1 over a Th2 response.

Induction of IFN-γ is mostly triggered by antigenic stimulation and T-cell activation, another feature that distinguishes the IFN-α/β group and IFN-γ. Moreover, IFN-γ is also structurally different from all members of the IFN-α/β family. Despite the lack of obvious evolutionary relations, IFN-α/β and IFN-γ share some biological features and are all together placed—by folding topology—in the α-helical bundle family of cytokines (Davies & Wlodawer, 1995; Nicola, 1994). Occurring as a single copy, the gene contains four exons in the human and mouse systems and codes for a protein with a predicted size of 16 to 17 kD. Higher MW forms are the result of glycosylation, dimerization, and multimeric aggregation. Formation of N-terminal pyroglutamic acid and proteolytic modifications of the C-terminus have been reported as well. The active IFN-γ form is a noncovalent 34 kD homodimer, resulting from an antiparallel interaction of two monomeric subunits. The dimeric form is able to bind two IFN-γ receptors, with the receptor clustering likely being an important event in signal transduction.

In terms of their major functions, type I IFNs are primarily responsible for immediate antiviral protection, before a specific immune response can take over. Similarly, IFN-γ was first discovered in the 1960s as an antiviral agent (Wheelock, 1965). However, its physiologically more prominent functions are associated with immunomodulation and the control of inflammatory processes (Bach, Aguet, & Schreiber, 1997; Boehm et al., 1997). Accordingly, antiviral activity of IFN-γ in vivo may rely more on its assistance in the T-cell stimulation by viral antigens. Moreover, the complex response to IFN-γ—as illustrated by the control of more than 200 genes—has been correlated exclusively with immune regulation (Boehm et al., 1997). IFN-γ is an inducer of MHC class I and class II antigens (even in cells usually not expressing MHC class II), cell adhesion molecules, and several cytokines. By virtue of these features it can support antigen presentation and induction of humoral and cell-mediated immune responses as well as the interaction of lymphocytes with the vascular endothelium. Induction of TNF-α, IL-1, and chemokines, together with synergistic and activity-enhancing actions, will further assist in the triggering and progression of inflammatory events. IFN-γ also has a role in the maturation of B cells, their transformation to antibody-producing plasma cells, and the switch of immunoglobulin classes. In addition to the direct and indirect effects on APC and lymphocyte functions,

IFN-γ activates the cytotoxic potential of macrophages against bacterial infection and intracellular parasites as it stimulates the release of reactive oxygen intermediates and nitric oxide (NO). Stimulation of complement-mediated phagocytosis by IFN-γ is based on enhanced expression of complement C3b receptors as well as the modulation of its binding affinity. IFN-γ effects on macrophages also cover synergistic actions with bacterial stimuli, such as LPS, during the induction of cytokine release (Boehm et al., 1997). Consequently, IFN-γ not only triggers cytokine release in macrophages, but it also modulates the cytokine-inducing efficacy of other factors ("IFN-γ priming"). Similarly, antitumor activities of IFN-γ likely relate to the stimulation of tumoricidal properties of macrophages and NK cells. Other cell types, such as endothelial cells or fibroblasts, respond to this interferon as well. In some cases, the net regulatory effect of IFN-γ activity may be either positive or negative. T suppressor cells, for example, are known to be stimulated under certain conditions although they are inhibited in other situations. However, since cellular responses to a particular cytokine are mostly context-dependent, the effects of IFN-γ (and IFNs in general) are also subject to modulation by other cytokines, such as TNF-α, IL-4, or IFN-α/β (Boehm et al., 1997). Similarly, the physiological impact of IFN-γ-regulated activation of the IL-1β-converting enzyme (ICE) in apoptosis is still less defined whereas ICE is, in turn, needed to process IL-18, the IFN-γ-inducing factor (IGIF) (Dinarello et al., 1998).

III. RECEPTORS AND INTRACELLULAR SIGNALING

A. IL-2/IL-15 Receptors

Biological effects of IL-2 are mediated by specific IL-2 receptors (IL-2R). Three structurally distinct IL-2-binding subunits contribute to the formation of functional di- and trimeric IL-2R but additional molecules are known to associate with the complexes (Goldsmith & Greene, 1994; Hanisch & Quirion, 1996; Minami, Kono, Yamada, & Taniguchi, 1992; Nakamura, Asao, Takeshita, & Sugamura, 1993; Theze et al., 1996; Waldmann et al., 1998; Waldmann, 1991). IL-2Rα (p55, Tac, CD25) binds IL-2 with low affinity ($k_D \sim 10^{-8}$ M) but does not trigger any known intracellular signal. It rather contributes to the formation of high-affinity IL-2R by associating with other IL-2R subunits. Expression of IL-2Rα depends on induction, and the molecule is subject to a rapid turnover (Goldsmith & Greene, 1994; Hanisch & Quirion, 1996; Theze et al., 1996). The alternative name, Tac antigen, is derived from the observation that detection of IL-2Rα depended on T cell activation. A shorter soluble version of IL-2Rα plays a role in controlling the amount of circulating IL-2, a principle common to various cytokines.

IL-2Rβ (p70/75, CD122) and IL-2Rγ (p64, "common γ", γ_c) form together the heterodimeric IL-2R of intermediate affinity ($k_D \sim 10^{-9}$ M) that is expressed constitutively by a number of cell types (Goldsmith & Greene, 1994; Hanisch & Quirion, 1996; Theze et al., 1996; Waldmann et al., 1998) (Figure 1). Both subunits have physical contact to bound IL-2 but their dimerization is required for the cytosolic delivery of the full IL-2 signal. IL-2Rβ or IL-2Rγ alone bind IL-2 only with very low affinity or not at all. The trimeric complex IL-2R$\alpha\beta\gamma$ binds IL-2 with high affinity ($k_D \sim 10^{-11}$ M). Disturbances in the synthesis of IL-2Rγ or its signaling lead to serious impairments in immune functions, clinically manifested as severe combined immunodeficiency disease (SCID) (Leonard, 1996b; Park, Saijo, et al., 1995; Sugamura et al., 1996). IL-2Rγ is also part of other cytokine receptor complexes. Its structural and functional contribution to the receptors of IL-4, IL-7, IL-9, and IL-15 is reflected by similarities in the signaling of these cytokines (Lin et al., 1995). The "common" receptor function of IL-2Rγ has been acknowledged by the term γ_c, although receptor subunit sharing is not an exclusive feature of IL-2, -4, -7, -9, and -15 (Davies & Wlodawer, 1995; Theze, 1994).

IL-15 uses not only γ_c for its signaling but also binds and signals through the IL-2R$\beta\gamma$ dimer (Waldmann et al., 1998). In contrast, it does not bind to IL-2Rα but rather uses its own IL-15Rα subunit (Figure 1). This 60-kD protein is structurally related to IL-2Rα, binds IL-15 as a monomer with high affinity ($k_D \sim 10^{-11}$ M), and contributes to the stable formation of the IL-15·IL-2R$\beta\gamma$ complex (Anderson et al., 1995; de Jong, Farner, Widmer, Giri, & Sondel, 1996; Giri et al., 1995). IL-2Rα and IL-15Rα together represent a new family of cytokine-binding receptors, as they have no obvious relation to other receptor structures. Despite the fact that IL-2 and IL-15 share the IL-2R$\beta\gamma$ in T cells these cytokines do not exhibit an identical spectrum of activities. IL-15Rα having a longer intracellular C-terminal domain, and the individual interactions with the β and γ subunit in the IL-2R complex may result in differences during the signal transduction. On the other hand, there is no evidence directly pointing toward IL-15Rα signaling (Waldmann et al., 1998). IL-15Rα shows a much broader cellular and tissue distribution than IL-2Rα. In combination with the rather widespread presence of

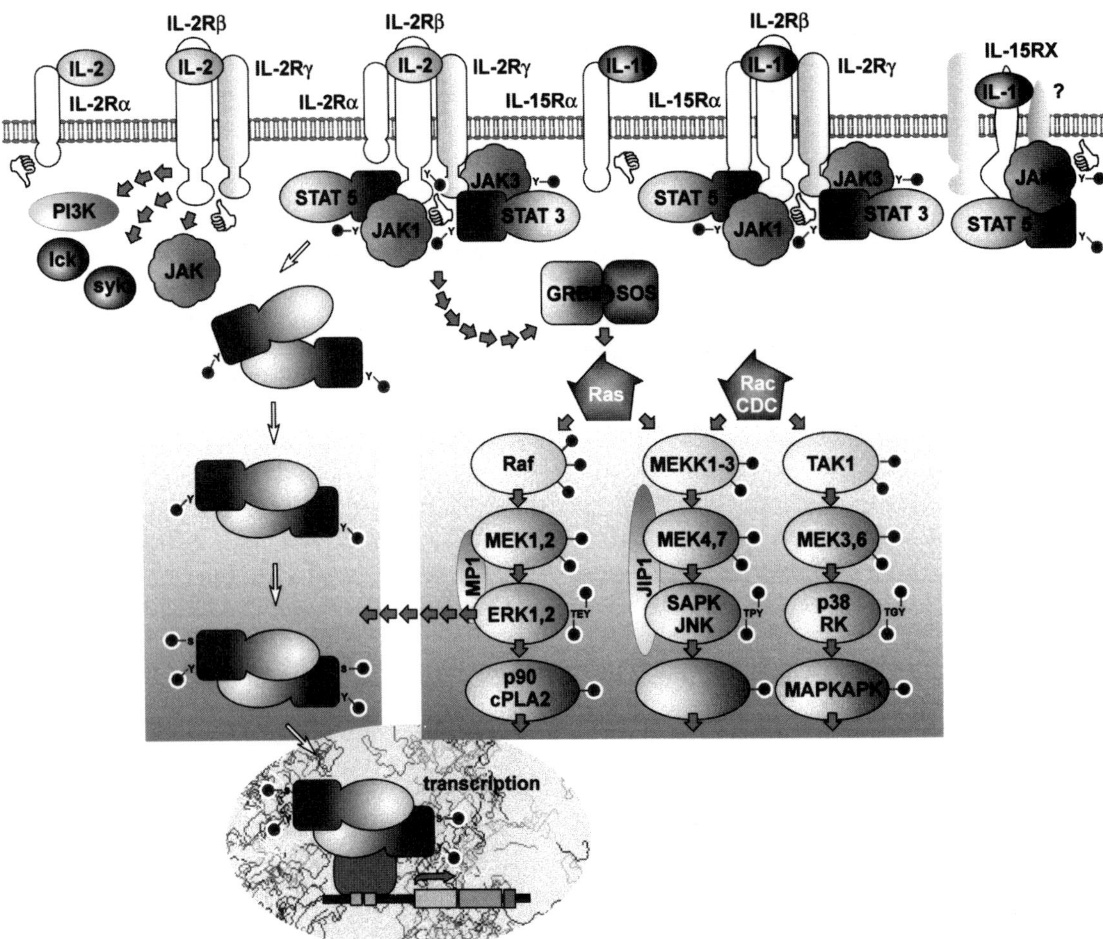

FIGURE 1 Scheme of the molecular components and arrangements of the IL-2 and IL-15 receptors. Their interactions with cytosolic kinases, including lck, syk, and JAK, as well as STAT proteins, is indicated. Binding of IL-2 and IL-15 to the respective α receptor subunits has apparently no consequence for intracellular signaling ("thumb down"). On the other hand, binding of IL-2 or IL-15 to IL-2Rβ and IL-2Rγ in dimeric and trimeric receptor complexes as well as the binding of IL-15 to IL-15RX lead to the activation of, for example, JAK1, JAK3, and JAK2, respectively, followed by the phosphorylation of receptors, kinases, and STAT proteins at Tyr residues (Y) ("thumb up"). Via adapter complexes (GRB2/SOS), IL-2Rβ and IL-2Rγ also may activate phosphorylation cascades of the ERK/MAPK pathways. MAPK, in turn, may catalyze additional phosphorylations of Ser residues (S) in STAT proteins. Thick arrows indicate functional interaction and activation, thin arrows illustrate translocation processes. Additional explanation in the text. (ERK, extracellular signal-activated kinase; JAK, Janus kinase; JNK, c-Jun N-terminal kinase; MAPK, mitogen-activated protein kinase; MAPKAPK, MAPK-activated protein kinase; MEK, MAPK/ERK kinase; MEKK, MEK kinase; p38, p38 MAPK; SAPK, stress-activated protein kinase; STAT, signal transducer and activator of transcription)

IL-2Rβ and IL-2Rγ, trimeric receptors for IL-15 may exist in abundance.

The recent discovery of an alternative IL-15R form, provisionally defined as IL-15RX, may underlie some of the IL-15-specific activities (Tagaya, Burton, Miyamoto, & Waldmann, 1996; Waldmann et al., 1998). This receptor protein with an apparent MW of 60 to 65 kD was determined in mast cells and is able to deliver IL-15 signals in the absence of IL-15Rα/IL-2R$\beta\gamma$ (Tagaya et al., 1996; Waldmann et al., 1998). With this new receptor system, IL-15 may signal independently of IL-2 and may thus execute pleiotropic activities apart from an IL-2-like type (Waldmann et al., 1998) (Figure 1).

B. IFN RECEPTORS

The current model of the functional IFN-α/β receptor depicts the IFNAR1 (α) subunit and the IFNAR2c (β) subunit. Both subunits must cooperate to create the high-affinity binding site for IFN-α/β, and additional factors may interact with the complex

(Langer, Garotta, & Pestka, 1996; Stark et al., 1998). Other forms of IFNAR2 represent a soluble (IFNAR2a) and a truncated (IFNAR2b) version with no or a shortened cytoplasmic domain.

The structure and the signaling of the IFN-γ receptor complex have been subject of intensive investigation since the beginning of the 1980s, with the concepts gaining substantiation in more recent years (Bach et al., 1997; Boehm et al., 1997; De Maeyer & De Maeyer-Guignard, 1994; Langer et al., 1996; Schreiber & Aguet, 1994; Stark et al., 1998). The receptor for IFN-γ consists of two N-glycosylated polypeptides that belong to the class 2 cytokine receptor family. The human and murine α chains have apparent MW of 90 kD and share significant, but moderate homology (52% sequence identity). Similarly, the respective β chains, both in the apparent MW range of 60 to 67 kD, exhibit an overall sequence identity of 58%. IFNγRα binds IFN-γ with high affinity ($k_D \sim 10^{-9}$ to 10^{-10} M). According to a recently refined model of the IFN-γ interaction with its receptor chains the ligand induces the dimerization of α chains by simultaneous binding. The complex is further stabilized by two β chains that are also required for effective intracellular signaling (Bach et al., 1996).

The expression of the two polypeptides is quite different. Whereas the α chain is found on the surface of nearly all cell types, expression of the β chain appears on induction and in some cells only. The actual presence of the β chain seems to be the limiting factor for cellular responsiveness to IFN-γ. For example, the IFN-γ-producing Th1 cells lacking IFNγRβ fail to respond to the cytokine. On the other hand, Th2 cells expressing IFNγRβ, but not synthesizing the ligand, respond to IFN-γ.

IL-2, IL-15, and types I and II IFNs trigger responses in their target cells by protein phosphorylation cascades that finally turn into the ligand-specific activation of subsets of genes. Recently two protein families reshaped the picture of cytokine signaling. The soluble cytosolic (nonreceptor) Janus kinase (JAK) proteins were first structurally identified and subsequently shown to link cytokine receptors to subsequent events by catalyzing the phosphorylation of tyrosine (Tyr) residues on several proteins. Signal transducer and activator of transcription (STAT) proteins were shown to be JAK substrates and to serve as latent cytosolic transcription factors.

The original discovery of the JAK/STAT system was initiated by the investigation of IFN effects on gene regulation (Heim, 1996; Lamb, Tapley, & Rosen, 1998; O'Shea, 1997). Following the identification of characteristic DNA regions in the promoters of IFN-α- and IFN-γ-stimulated genes, STAT1 and STAT2 were isolated as proteins that bound to these sequences on IFN-α or IFN-γ stimulation, respectively. Based on their similarity with the prototypic sequence motifs, more and more DNA sequences were identified, sharing the consensus motif of the interferon-stimulated response element (ISRE) type or that of the gamma-activated sequences (GAS). Tyk2 was found to be a tyrosine kinase that catalyzed STAT phosphorylation. These observations assigned STAT proteins as substrates to the JAK family and established the principle of JAK/STAT pathways. Subsequently, more and more cytokine and growth factor receptors were demonstrated to use primarily or at least partially JAK/STAT pathways. IL-2 and IL-15 are among those that crucially depend on JAK-mediated phosphorylations of Tyr residues and the activation of STAT dimers for transcriptional activation.

C. JAK/STAT Pathways and the Signaling of IL-2, IL-15, IFN-α/β, and IFN-γ

This section briefly illustrates the principle of cytokine signaling as it is mediated through the JAK/STAT system and as it contributes to intracellular consequences initiated by IL-2/IL-15 as well as IFN-α/β and IFN-γ binding to their respective receptors. The discovery of the molecular components and the mechanisms of these pathways had an enormous impact on the understanding of cytokine-induced gene activation. Although the bulk of the experimental studies of JAKs and STATs has been carried out in nonneural cells, the players and rules of this signaling system are also relevant to cytokine functions in the brain, including those carried by IL-2, IL-15, and the IFNs (Berhow, Hiroi, Kobierski, Hyman, & Nestler, 1996; Bonni et al., 1997; Cattaneo et al., 1996; Kahn et al., 1997; Mizuno et al., 1997; Rajan, Stewart, & Fink, 1995; Rajan, Symes, & Fink, 1996; Sanchez et al., 1994; Spleiss, Appel, Boddeke, Berger, & Gebicke Haerter, 1998; Yao, Kato, Khalil, Kiryu, & Kiyama, 1997; Zhou et al., 1998a; Zocchia et al., 1997). Moreover, neuroscience research will address the cell type-specific and integrative aspects of JAK/STAT signaling in neuronal and glial cells.

The family of JAKs comprises the homologous members JAK1, JAK2, JAK3, and Tyk2 in the human and mouse systems which share 42 to 50% of sequence identity (Heim, 1996; Lamb et al., 1998; Leonard, 1996a; Leonard & O'Shea, 1998; O'Shea, 1997). Related structures have been identified in other species, including Hop (Hopscotch) from *Drosophila* as well as JAK-like forms in *Xenopus laevis* and *Caenorhabditis elegans*. JAK1, JAK2 and Tyk2 serve the signaling of various cytokine receptors by associating with different receptor subunits. Recruitment of JAK3 is more restricted. This kinase associates with γ_c, thereby, however, participating in the signaling of several cytokines. JAKs are relatively large kinase molecules with apparent MW of 120 to 130 kD. They contain a C-terminal kinase domain (JH1 domain), next to a pseudokinase (JH2) domain. The structural feature of a dual kinase region inspired the name Janus kinase. Although the role of JH2 is still unknown, it may have some regulatory function (Chen, Gadina, Galon, Chen, & O'Shea, 1998). Similarly, there is currently no functional correlation for the other homology domains, JH3 to JH7, or the various C-terminal splice variants. The N-terminal stretch is, however, thought to participate in the receptor association (O'Shea, 1997).

When cytokines bind to their receptors cytosolic JAKs are recruited to the cytoplasmic receptor portions, whereas constitutively receptor-associated JAKs may become activated by conformational changes of the intracellular receptor tail (Ihle, 1995). Dimerization/oligomerization of the respective receptors may precede or be induced by the occupation of the cytokine binding sites. As a consequence of the receptor-mediated JAK activation, multiple (self- and/or trans-)phosphorylations of Tyr residues on both the kinases and the receptors occur (Ihle, 1995). The respective interactions of JAKs with cytokine receptors show three patterns. There are single-chain receptors that predominantly associate with JAK2, such as the receptor for growth hormone. Another group of receptors consists of the specific ligand-binding subunit complexed with a common signal-transducing protein, a situation found for IL-3, IL-5, or IL-6. JAK1, JAK2, and Tyk2 have been shown to serve as kinases for this type of receptor. Finally, the receptors for IL-2 and IFNs are typical for oligomeric receptor complexes in which two subunits contribute to the triggering of intracellular phosphorylation cascades, each interacting with a JAK.

JAK-mediated Tyr-phosphorylation of cytokine receptors creates specific interaction sites for several cytoplasmic factors, such as Shc, the p85 unit of the PI3K, or STAT proteins (Darnell, 1997; Heim, 1996; Ihle, 1995; Ihle, 1996; Lamb et al., 1998; Leonard & O'Shea, 1998; O'Shea, 1997) (see also Figure 1). STAT1, STAT2, STAT3, STAT4, STAT5A, STAT5B, and STAT6 as well as their variants resulting from alternative splicing are a family of related transcription factors (28 to 54% sequence identity) that are also substrates for JAK activities. STATs and related structures (Wegenka et al., 1994) have been identified not only in humans and mice but also in other taxa (Darnell, 1997). JAK-catalyzed Tyr-phosphorylation of STAT proteins causes their homo- or heterodimerization followed by a translocation to the nucleus and the binding to regulatory segments of cytokine-inducible genes (Figure 1). STAT proteins can also associate with other proteins, such as p48 (member of the IRF-1 family), p300, or CBP (CREB-binding protein) to form DNA-binding complexes, for example, IFN-α-stimulated gene factor 3 (ISGF3), a STAT1·STAT·2p48 heterotrimer (Bhattacharya et al., 1996; Chen et al., 1998; Darnell, 1997; Kanno et al., 1993). STATs also may have adapter functions by interacting with other kinases. Within the STAT proteins, there are domains responsible for dimerization and those conveying DNA binding or interaction with other factors that are involved in transcriptional control. A src-homology 2 (SH2) domain plays a role in the dimerization and is responsible for the recognition of phosphotyrosine (PTyr) on the respective receptors. In these interactions, the sequence context of the PTyr residue as it is recognized by the SH2 domains decides the STAT form that can dock to a particular receptor subunit. Replacing the SH2 domain in a STAT therefore changes its association with receptors. The DNA-binding domain carries the specificity of each STAT protein for the respective DNA sequence and thus bears the key to the various gene promoters. Experimental manipulations of this domain can, for example, switch the specificity of a given STAT protein to that of another one. The Tyr-phosphorylation site of STATs is found close to the C-terminus. In its vicinity, there is also a serine (Ser) residue that can be phosphorylated by other kinases. The double phosphorylated STATs can then develop a higher transcriptional efficacy. Mitogen-activated protein kinases (MAPK), especially the extracellular signal regulated kinases (ERKs), are likely candidates for the Ser-phosphorylation of STATs. Adapter complexes, such as GRB2/SOS, are also thought to link JAKs to Raf/Ras and the kinase cascades of the ERK/MAPK system (Denhardt, 1996; Seger & Krebs, 1995), illustrating the intimate interactions between phosphorylation pathways (Adunyah, Wheeler, & Cooper, 1997; Denhardt, 1996; Waldmann et al., 1998) (Figure 1). Indeed, $p42^{MAPK}$ (ERK2) was shown to be involved in IFN-α/β-stimulated gene expression via STAT (David et al., 1995) p42 even physically interacts with the α subunit of the receptor on one hand and with STAT1 on the other.

The discovery of the JAK/STAT system did more than add another signaling pathway to the already known protein phosphorylation cascades. The specific protein-protein interactions between receptors, JAKs, and STATs and the combinatory variety in the activation of sets of kinases and dimeric STATs that, by themselves, have DNA-recognition domains guarantee some ligand-specific transmission of a signal to the nucleus. Unraveling the mechanisms and elements of the JAK/STAT system also allows for a molecular understanding of cytokine redundancy, synergism and, probably, antagonism (O'Shea, 1997). Cytokine signal integration currently is becoming more transparent as it is based on (i) the principle of receptor subunit sharing, (ii) the use of common kinases and their substrates, and (iii) the reciprocal influences between the JAK/STAT and other phosphorylation cascades. In addition, phosphatases, proteosome activity, and a growing number of regulatory factors and adapter/scaffold proteins have been described that control, route, and terminate kinase signaling (Aman & Leonard, 1997; Barford, 1996; Darnell, Jr., 1997; Elion, 1998; Endo et al., 1997; Fauman & Saper, 1996; Hafen, 1998; Ihle, 1995; Moutoussamy, Kelly, & Finidori, 1998; Naka et al., 1997; Sengupta, Schmitt, & Ivashkiv, 1996; Starr et al., 1997; Ihle, 1995). It has been known that on IL-2 exposure of T cells, phosphorylation of proteins follows, and that kinases contribute to the IL-2 signaling. However, it remained enigmatic which enzymatic activities catalyze all these events that finally lead to the IL-2 activation of transcription, including that of protooncogenes and antiapoptotic factors. Besides protein kinase C (Gomez et al., 1994; Lu & Durkin, 1997), phosphoinositide 3-kinase (PI3K) (Brennan et al., 1997), Raf (Maslinski, Remillard, Tsudo, & Strom, 1993), Ras (Hatakeyama, Kawahara, Mori, Shibuya, & Taniguchi, 1992; Satoh et al., 1992), ERK1 (Adunyah et al., 1997), and several soluble nonreceptor protein tyrosine kinases of the src family, such as $p56^{lck}$ or $p72^{syk}$ (Goldsmith & Greene, 1994; Ihle, 1995; Kirken et al., 1997; Taniguchi, 1995), especially JAKs were shown to mediate the various effects of IL-2 and IL-15 (Johnston et al., 1995; Lai et al.,1996; Taniguchi, 1995; Waldmann et al., 1998; Zhu, Berry, Russell, & Leonard, 1998) (Figure 1). Phosphorylations of the IL-2Rβ and IL-2Rγ chains and the JAKs are crucial steps in the sequence leading to the activation of STAT proteins. IL-2Rβ stimulation was found to activate JAK1. Subsequently, JAK1 triggers by Tyr-phosphorylation the activation of STAT5. The γ chain interacts with JAK3 and leads to activation of STAT3. Although IL-2 and IL-15 signaling also involves other intracellular elements, the JAK1/STAT5 and JAK3/STAT3 pathways together crucially participate in the consequences of IL-2R$\beta\gamma$ activation (Johnston et al., 1995; Lai et al., 1996; Taniguchi, 1995; Waldmann et al., 1998; Zhu et al., 1998). Alternatively, IL-15 signaling through IL-15RX apparently recruits a JAK2/STAT5 route (Waldmann et al., 1998) (Figure 1).

IFN-α/β activate JAK1 via the IFNAR2 (or β) chain and Tyk2 via the IFNAR1 (or α) chain of their receptors. JAK1 deficiency in JAK1$^{-/-}$ mice causes loss of response to IFN-α/β as well as IFN-γ stimulation, whereas JAK2 appears dispensable for IFN-α/β receptor signaling (Chen et al., 1998; Meraz et al., 1996; Rodig et al., 1998). At the level of STATs, IFN-α/β activate STAT1 and STAT2 whereas IFN-γ is linked to the activation of STAT1.

Activation of IFN-α/β-inducible genes via the JAK/STAT system follows a sequence that has been dissected thus far into several molecular events (Ransohoff, 1998; Stark et al., 1998). First, ligand association with the receptor causes IFNAR1·IFNAR2 dimerization. Then Tyk2, which is already associated with INFAR1, becomes Tyr-phosphorylated by JAK1 that is bound to IFNAR2c. In turn, Tyk2 phosphorylates JAK1 and the two activated kinases catalyze the phosphorylation of a Tyr residue on IFNAR1. Subsequently, STAT2, which together with STAT1 preassociates with IFNAR2c, repositions to become the substrate of JAK1-mediated Tyr-phosphorylation. The rearrangement involves the binding of STAT2 via its SH2 domain to the Tyr-phosphorylated site of IFNAR1. Next, STAT1 undergoes phosphorylation at a Tyr residue, a process that also may include a repositioning step. Finally, the STAT1·STAT2 heterodimer disconnects from the receptor and travels to the nucleus. In response to IFN-α/β stimulation, the heterodimer may act on GAS elements or combine with p48 to form ISGF3 that binds to ISRE sites. In addition, homodimeric STAT1, which can also result from type I interferon stimulation, can bind to GAS elements as well, although it will not activate IFN-γ-inducible genes (Stark et al., 1998). Phosphorylation of the dimer at Ser residues may decide whether the STAT1 outcome turns into an IFN-α/β or IFN-γ response pattern.

IFN-γR signaling involves JAK1, which associates with the α chain, JAK2, that interacts with IFNγRβ, and a JAK1-dependent activation of Raf-1/MAPK (Sakatsume et al., 1998). Both kinases are constitutively bound to their respective receptor chain but become active when IFN-γ (dimer) binds to the receptor (Bach et al., 1997). The activation of the kinases is a result of the ligand-induced $\alpha\beta$ association and involves a JAK1-JAK2 transactivation process. The next step in the sequence is the phosphorylation of the two α receptor chains that are contained in the IFNγ_2·IFNγRα_2·IFNγRβ_2 complex that creates docking sites for STAT1 proteins. STAT1 binding to the receptor is thereby mediated by its

SH2 domain. Subsequently, the two IFNγRα-bound STAT1s undergo Tyr-phosphorylation, dissociate from the receptor, and dimerize. Additional Ser-phosphorylation is carried out by a MAPK and is followed by the translocation of the STAT complex to the nucleus, where its selective binding to promoter regions can trigger the transcription of IFN-γ-inducible genes.

IV. EXPRESSION OF IL-2, IL-15, IFNs, AND THEIR RECEPTORS IN THE NERVOUS SYSTEM

Most of the information concerning possible roles of IL-2, IL-15, and IFNs in the nervous system derives from functional studies under experimental conditions or from clinical findings. The demonstration or observation of (cellular) responses to exogenous cytokines can be taken as evidence for the expression of appropriate functional receptor/effector systems. This does not imply that the natural ligands are constitutively present in vivo. However, cytokines may gain access to receptors on neuronal and glial cells by crossing the BBB and blood-cerebrospinal fluid borders that separate central compartments from the circulation or when lymphocytes or macrophages infiltrate the brain.

Cytokine passage of the BBB does not necessarily require a breakdown of its integrity (Banks & Kastin, 1992). Carrier systems and mechanisms have been identified that allow small quantities to enter and penetrate the CNS even under normal conditions, at least at certain sites (Banks & Kastin, 1991; Banks, Kastin, & Durham, 1989; Banks, Kastin, & Gutierrez, 1993; Banks, Ortiz, Plotkin, & Kastin, 1991; Dafny, 1998; Gutierrez, Banks, & Kastin, 1993; Gutierrez, Banks, & Kastin, 1994; Maness, Banks, Zadina, & Kastin, 1995; Mattson et al., 1983; Smith R. A., Landel, Cornelius, & Revel, 1986; Smith, R. A., Norris, Palmer, Bernhardt, & Wills, 1985; Waguespack, Banks, & Kastin, 1994). However, it is still not resolved whether the quantities transferred to the brain in vivo are significant in physiological terms, i.e., sufficient to trigger cellular responses (Hopkins & Rothwell, 1995). On the other hand, impairment of the BBB could facilitate an inundation of the brain by cytokines and even can be the result of high circulating cytokine concentrations, as in the IL-2-induced vascular leak syndrome (Alexander, Saris, & Oldfield, 1989; Funke et al., 1994; Lissoni et al., 1990; Merchant, Ellison, & Young, 1990; Saija et al., 1995; Tjuvajev et al., 1995; Wiranowska et al., 1994). Similarly, massive CNS infiltration of cytokine-producing cells from the periphery under pathophysiological conditions would certainly raise parenchymal levels of cytokines. Nevertheless, endogenous synthesis of cytokines by resident cells, i.e., neurons and glia, may also occur, as few studies identified IL-2, IL-15, and IFN(-like) molecules. Under normal conditions, intrinsic synthesis may occur only at low levels and in restricted anatomical divisions. Production may be induced or augmented by stimulation or disturbances of brain homeostasis. Activated glial cells, especially microglia, could then serve as a cytokine source also in CNS tissue regions that are normally devoid of those molecules.

Cytokines and cytokine receptors in the CNS may be identical to their peripheral counterparts (Petitto & Huang, 1994, 1995; Petitto, Huang, Raizada, Rinker, & McCarthy, 1998; Petitto, Huang, Rinker, & McCarthy, 1997). They may also differ in some structural and functional features (Eitan et al., 1992; Merrill, 1991; Nieto Sampedro & Chandy, 1987; Otero & Merrill, 1995; Otero & Merrill, 1997). The differences may arise from different sequences per se or result from alternative splicing, posttranslational processing, or tissue-specific arrangements and association with other molecules (Eitan & Schwartz, 1993). At present, there is no uniform answer to the question of whether the molecules known from the immune system and CNS-intrinsic IL-2, IL-15, IFNs, and related receptors are structurally identical, similar, or different.

In addition to their specific receptors, cytokines like IL-2 and IFN-α may interact with other receptor systems, due to some structural similarities to the respective ligands. With respect to the IL-2 effects that are apparently mediated by opioid receptors, indirect mechanisms involving the activation by IL-2 of interneurons may be accompanied by direct opioid-like actions of the cytokine itself (Wang et al., 1996, 1997). Similarly, IFN-α has been shown to interfere with the binding of naloxone, dihydromorphine, and enkephalin to rodent brain membrane preparations (Blalock & Smith, 1980; Blalock & Smith, 1981; Menzies, Patel, Hall, O'Grady, & Rier, 1992; Panchenko, Aliab'eva, Malinovskaia, & Balashov, 1987; Smith, E. M., Dion, & Blalock, 1985). Binding of IFN-α to opioid receptors is thereby specific because IFN-β and IFN-γ are devoid of this feature (Dafny, 1998). Some structural relatedness of IL-2 and corticotropin-releasing factor (CRF) (Ottaviani, Franchini, Caselgrandi, Cossarizza, & Franceschi, 1995), as well as IFN-α and adrenocorticotropic hormone (ACTH) and melanocyte-stimulating hormone (MSH) (Blalock & Smith, 1980; Root Bernstein, 1984) may account for some of the endocrine effects of these cytokines, as both are known to modulate adrenocortical secretion (Dafny, 1998; Hanisch & Quirion, 1996; Karanth & McCann, 1991; Kidron, Saphier, Ovadia, Weidenfeld, & Abramsky, 1989).

Currently available data suggest that functional receptors for these cytokines are expressed on neuronal and glial cell populations and that signaling through these receptors can be triggered by recombinant cytokines. Both brain-endogenous cytokines and/or their peripheral counterparts may have access to these receptors in vivo. Whether brain-derived cytokines and their receptors share all structural and pharmacological features with the proteins of extraneural origin or whether they partially represent tissue-specific versions remains to be demonstrated. Some of the findings concerning the demonstration of the molecular elements of the IL-2/IL-15 and the IFN systems are discussed in the following section.

A. Expression of the Cytokines and Their Receptor Molecules

A multitude of functional reports suggests that receptors for IFN molecules are expressed on both glial and neuronal cells (see section V). It can be assumed, for example, that microglial cells, as the CNS equivalent of tissue macrophages, express functional IFN-γ receptors. Moreover, due to the functional nature of IFNs, most of the cell types are thought to be able to produce IFN-α molecules when infection occurs. Nevertheless, the demonstration of IFNs and IFN receptor molecules in the normal brain may further support the concept that the molecular elements of this/these system(s) are involved in CNS functions also under normal conditions.

IFN-γ receptor molecules were found to be expressed in sensory and sympathetic neurons as well as rat brain and spinal cord, especially in the neurons of the hippocampus and the suprachiasmatic nuclei, the latter being a center regulating behavioral, physiological, and hormonal rhythms (Chang, Martin, & Johnson, 1990; Lundkvist, Robertson, Mhlanga, Rottenberg, & Kristensson, 1998; Neumann, Schmidt, Cavalie, Jenne, & Wekerle, 1997; Neumann, Schmidt, Wilharm, Behrens, & Wekerle, 1997; Robertson et al., 1997). Messages for IFN-α/β and IFN-γ receptors were also identified in normal astrocytes and oligodendrocytes, respectively (Tada, Diserens, Desbaillets, & de Tribolet, 1994; Torres, Aranguez, & Rubio, 1995).

IFN-γ expression itself was reported for astrocytes and activated microglia (De Simone, Levi, & Aloisi, 1998; Xiao & Link, 1998) as well as sensory neurons, with a cytoplasmic location of protein via immunocytochemistry and the detection of its message by single-cell reverse transcriptase-polymerase chain reaction (RT-PCR) (Neumann, Schmidt, Wilharm, Behrens, & Wekerle, 1997). Increased CNS levels during infection or other pathophysiological situations can be caused by T cells trafficking into the brain followed by the release of their soluble factors (Popko et al., 1997). Interestingly, an endogenous IFN-γ-like substance—by function and some structural features—seems to be produced by hippocampal, hypothalamic, thalamic, tegmental, sensory, and motor neurons (Bentivoglio, Florenzano, Peng, & Kristensson, 1994; Eneroth, Andersson, Olsson, Orvell, Norrby, & Kristensson, 1992; Eneroth, Kristensson, Ljungdahl, & Olsson, 1991; Kiefer, Haas, & Kreutzberg, 1991; Kiefer & Kreutzberg, 1990; Kristensson et al., 1994; Ljungdahl et al., 1989; Olsson et al., 1989, 1994; Peng, Mohammed, Olsson, Edlund, & Kristensson, 1994). The fact that the molecular properties of this "neuronal" IFN-γ are clearly different from the peripheral form suggests the existence of an independent IFN-γ-like system in the nervous tissue.

First reports on the expression of IL-2 and IL-2-binding structures appeared in the 1980s (for a survey of the related literature see Hanisch & Quirion, 1996). Due to the low tissue levels and technical limitations, information about the presence of an IL-2/IL-2R system initially remained rare. In the 1990s several reports appeared demonstrating the molecular components in cells, tissue homogenates, and brain slices by immunocytochemistry, radioligand binding studies, and biochemical/molecular biology methods for the detection of related mRNA and protein.

These studies have revealed that [^{125}I]-IL-2 binding sites and IL-2R molecules predominantly localize in the frontal cortex, hippocampal formation, septum, striatum, cerebellum, and the locus coeruleus (Araujo & Lapchak, 1994; Araujo, Lapchak, Collier, & Quirion, 1989; Lapchak, 1992; Lapchak, Araujo, Quirion, & Beaudet, 1991; Seto, Hanisch, Villemain, Beaudet, & Quirion, 1993; Seto & Quirion, 1993). Discrete and relatively high-density binding was observed in the pyramidal cell layer of the hippocampal formation, suggesting neuronal localization. Interestingly, relatively strong binding also was seen in major fiber tracts, such as the corpus callosum and the anterior commissure, indicating IL-2 binding to oligodendrocytes (Lapchak et al., 1991).

Studies based on antibodies against the IL-2Rα subunit revealed the presence of the antigen in various regions of the rat brain (Lapchak et al., 1991; Luber-Narod & Rogers, 1988). The neuron-rich cell layers of the hippocampal formation/dentate gyrus and to some extent the cerebellum showed highest density (Lapchak et al., 1991). Other studies confirm these data by providing evidence for an expression of this receptor in microglia, astrocytes, oligodendrocytes, sympathetic neurons, pituitary cells, or brain tissue preparations, using antibodies or mRNA detection (Arzt et al.1992, 1993; Hanisch, Lyons, et al., 1997; Haugen & Letourneau, 1990; McGeer, Itagaki, Tago, & McGeer, 1987; Merrill, 1990; Otero & Merrill, 1994, 1995; Petitto & Huang, 1995; Saneto, Altman, Knobler, Johnson, & De Vellis, 1986; Saneto, Chiapelli, & De Vellis, 1987; Sawada, Suzumura, & Marunouchi, 1995; Shimojo et al., 1993).

The message for the signal-transducing subunit IL-2Rβ was detected in brain preparations as well as in several rodent and/or human brain regions, namely the frontal and parietal cortex, caudate nucleus, hippocampus, amygdala, hypothalamus, thalamus, substantia nigra, cerebellum and the corpus callosum (Hanisch, Lyons, et al., 1997; Hanisch & Quirion, 1996; Otero & Merrill, 1995; Petitto & Huang, 1994; Satoh, Kurohara, Yukitake, & Kuroda, 1998). At cellular level, microglia, astrocytes, oligodendroglioma, and pituitary cells were identified as synthesizing IL-2Rβ molecules (Hanisch, Lyons, et al., 1997; Otero & Merrill, 1995; Petitto, Huang, et al., 1997; Sawada et al., 1995).

The γ chain mRNA similarly has been found in whole brain preparation and various regions, respectively, of the rodent and human brain, including cortical areas, hippocampus, medulla oblongata, and cerebellum, with preliminary evidence pointing to microglial and oligodendroglial (oligodendroglioma)—and probably even some neuronal—cells as sources (Hanisch, Lyons, et al., 1997; Otero & Merrill, 1995; Petitto et al., 1998; Satoh et al., 1998).

The demonstration of IL-2 synthesis by neural cells is a prerequisite when postulating functions of the brain IL-2/IL-2R system that are independent from lymphocytic cytokine production. However, the demonstration of any cytokine synthesis intrinsic to the brain may raise questions about copurification of immune cell-derived material. Nevertheless, identification of IL-2(-like) molecules in neural cell cultures devoid of blood-derived contamination could give additional evidence. The occurrence of CNS-specific (or unusual) molecule forms of IL-2 (transcripts and proteins) especially may support the notion that IL-2-like molecules are produced in the brain (Hanisch & Quirion, 1996).

First evidence for unusual IL-2 proteins emerged from investigations on CNS trauma. The presence of an IL-2-like activity was shown in tissues next to an entorhinal/occipital lesion (Nieto Sampedro & Chandy, 1987). Interestingly, the brain IL-2 activity eluted in two fractions, one being similar to the known MW of splenocyte IL-2, one being apparently a dimer. A lesion-induced dimeric IL-2 also was isolated from regenerating fish optic nerve (Eitan et al., 1992). However, a lesion-induced dimerization of IL-2 apparently occurred at the posttranslational level, being catalyzed by a nervous tissue-specific transglutaminase (Eitan & Schwartz, 1993). Using tissue extracts from normal hippocampus, striatum, and frontal cortex of the rat, IL-2-like material was measured by radioimmunoassay (RIA) in a range of 0.1 – 0.7 ng/mg tissue (Araujo et al., 1989), a rather high and probably overestimated content (Hanisch & Quirion, 1996). Much lower tissue levels of IL-2 were subsequently determined in human hippocampal tissue and corticotrophic adenoma supernatants by means of antihuman IL-2 antibody-based RIAs (Araujo & Lapchak, 1994; Arzt et al., 1992).

Immunocytochemical IL-2 detection in rat brain revealed highest signal densities in the caudate-putamen, frontoparietal extent of the cerebral cortex, preferentially layer IV, lateral septum, pyramidal and granule cell layers of the hippocampus, and dentate gyrus, respectively, and the arcuate nucleus/median eminence of the hypothalamus (Lapchak et al., 1991). The interpenduncular nucleus, locus coeruleus, and the molecular layer of the cerebellum also were clearly labeled. The thalamus was labeled at low level throughout, and more caudal regions of the cerebral cortex also showed only low signal intensity. All other regions were much less stained or showed only background levels of antibody binding. Essentially the same distribution of IL-2-IRM was observed in the mouse CNS (Seto et al., 1993). Cellular localization was reported as perikaryal labeling in the areas observed by immunoautoradiography (Lapchak et al., 1991). Electron microscopy confirmed the association of IL-2 with neuronal cell bodies, especially in the hippocampus and arcuate nucleus. Similarly, in situ hybridization experiments confirmed IL-2 (mRNA) presence in subpopulations of arcuate neurons, over the hippocampal formation, habenula, and cerebral cortex (Villemain, Owens, Renno, & Beaudet, 1991) and, with a patchy distribution, in the striatum (Lapchak, 1992). Others also detected IL-2 mRNA in white and gray matter of rat, mouse, and human brain as well as CRF-stimulated human corticotrophic adenoma and mouse AtT-20 cells (Arzt et al., 1992; Ashman, Bolitho, & Fulurija, 1995; Eizenberg, Faber-Elman, Lotan, & Schwartz, 1995; Lapchak, 1992). Lymphocyte-derived probes identified several IL-2-like transcripts in both human and rodent CNS tissues (Eizenberg, Faber-Elman, Lotan, et al., 1995). On the other hand, an IL-2 mRNA species of unusual size, 5 kb, appeared to be unique to the brain and was not detectable in lymphocyte-derived mRNA (Eizenberg, Faber-Elman, Lotan, et al., 1995).

For IL-15 and its specific α receptor subunit, mRNA data suggest a rather widespread CNS distribution with microglia, astrocytes, and neuronal cells being suggested as cellular sources (Hanisch, Lyons, et al., 1997; Lee, Satoh, Walker, & Kim, 1996; Satoh et al., 1998). As revealed by these studies, the IL-2Rβ and γ_c chain—as part of the IL-15R complex—appeared to be relatively abundant in the CNS (Hanisch, Lyons, et al., 1997).

Nevertheless, an anatomical map of the expression of all respective proteins is far from complete. Initial data on the molecular properties of IL-2/IL-15 and IFN systems in the CNS point to both identity with the sequences as they are known from peripheral (immune) cells as well as to unusual, more tissue-specific versions. Indeed, some distinct features clearly support the notion that the molecular forms or arrangements of the ligands and their receptors within the CNS may differ from their peripheral counterparts (Merrill, 1990, 1991; Otero & Merrill, 1994, 1995, 1997).

B. CNS-Specific Features

For the neuronal version of IFN-γ (N-IFN-γ), the available data suggest structural similarity, as antibodies against classical IFN-γ cross-react (Olsson et al., 1994). On the other hand, Olsson et al. isolated three molecular species from trigeminal ganglia, showing apparent MW of 54, 62, and 66 kD. Others could detect only a 60-kD band in Western blots of ganglia homogenates, the difference probably and partially due to the respective antibodies involved in the isolation and detection (Kiefer et al., 1991). Nevertheless, the MW data and the (only) partial cross-reactivity are strong facts in support of a real brain-specific cytokine form. For other cases, the situation is less clear.

The dimeric IL-2 isolated from injured brain tissue (Eitan & Schwartz, 1993; Eitan et al., 1992; Nieto Sampedro & Chandy, 1987) or the brain-derived 5 kb mRNA of IL-2 (Eizenberg, Faber-Elman, Lotan, et al., 1995) are clearly unusual and point to some tissue-specific version of the cytokine. However, unusual molecular forms can also be isolated from other tissues (Kloth, Flad, & Brandt, 1994). For CNS-specific properties, more information is available regarding IL-2 receptors. First evidence is thereby provided by a rather simple observation. Several cytokines, including IL-2, occasionally show different species restriction with respect to their abilities to bind and stimulate receptors from different tissues (Hanisch & Quirion, 1996; Naito et al., 1989; Tominaga et al., 1991). The observation that a given human recombinant cytokine can evoke responses in, for example, rat CNS, but fail to elicit an effect in peripheral tissue of the animal implies that the respective receptors differ in some pharmacological features. IL-2 binding can also differ from the classical pattern in terms of the respective k_D values (Otero & Merrill, 1994, 1997). Investigating binding and cellular responses to IL-2 by oligodendrocytes, in comparison with T cells, other differences were noted besides the induction of proliferation (Otero & Merrill, 1997). The immunohistochemical staining pattern and the antigenic properties of an IL-2Rα(-like) molecule in oligodendrocytes were clearly distinct. Most notably, immunoblot analysis of the IL-2Rα(-like) molecule with cross-reacting anti-IL-2Rα antibodies revealed three proteins with apparent MWs of 47, 83, and 100 kD, values deviating from the expected 55-kD range.

Another CNS-specific feature of IL-2Rα relates to its expression in brain tissues (Hanisch & Quirion, 1996). Immunhistochemical (Lapchak et al., 1991) and PCR studies (Hanisch, Lyons, et al., 1997) demonstrated a widespread and constitutive presence of IL-2Rα message and immunoreactive material (protein) in the rat and mouse brain. This contrasts with the situation found in the immune system where the synthesis of IL-2Rα strictly depends on induction, as also illustrated by the alternative name, T cell activation antigen (Tac). Studies using antibodies against Tac to inhibit IL-2-evoked effects on cultured oligodendrocytes or hippocampal neurons in slice preparations provide further evidence for a constitutive expression of IL-2Rα or a similar protein on neural cells (Otero & Merrill, 1994, 1997; Seto, Kar, & Quirion, 1997). Finally, the correlation of available anatomical data for the expression of IL-2-binding sites, IL-2Rα-immunoreactive material, IL-2 responsiveness, and IL-2 itself show some mismatches (Hanisch & Quirion, 1996; Lapchak et al., 1991) and suggest that IL-2Rα or a related molecule may have functions in the CNS partially not restricted to the binding of IL-2.

In contrast, several studies confirmed sequence identity for brain-derived and lymphocyte cytokine or cytokine receptor structures. Petitto and colleagues meanwhile isolated cDNA for the IL-2 receptor chains α, β, and γ from mouse and human brain as well as pituitary cells and determined complete identity with the structures obtained from lymphocytes, at least for the isolated segments (Petitto & Huang, 1994, 1995; Petitto et al., 1998; Petitto, Huang, et al., 1997). Similarly, studies on the regional and microglial expression of IL-2Rα, IL-15Rα, IL-2Rβ, and IL-2Rγ in mouse brain—also partially carried out at the single cell level—revealed sequence identity for all PCR amplimers (Hanisch, Lyons, et al., 1997). An alternative splice variant of IL-15 mRNA identified in certain microglial cells (Prinz, Hanisch, Kettenmann, & Kirchhoff, 1998) is similarly found in human lung cancer cell lines (Meazza et al., 1996) and thus does not represent a CNS-specific species. In all the studies that depend on the isolation of RNA material from nervous tissue proper, especially perfusion of the brain is a prerequisite, but is no guarantee for avoiding contamination from blood cells. Coamplification of lymphocyte marker mRNA should therefore serve as a control in future studies, with neural cell cultures and single-cell techniques providing alternative approaches.

V. EFFECTS OF IL-2 AND IFNs ON THE NERVOUS SYSTEM

Several lines of evidence clearly support the notion that IL-2 and IFNs have neuroregulatory activities. Less is known about the effects of IL-15. (It may even prove to be responsible in vivo for some of the IL-2 activities that were discovered by the experimental use of recombinant IL-2.) Work on cell cultures and in vitro tissue preparations demonstrated IL-2 and IFN effects on cell viability and differentiation, transmitter and neurohormone release, and the electrophysiological features of neural cells. Studies performed with laboratory animals confirmed and extended the in vitro data, also revealing neuroendocrine and behavioral consequences of elevated cytokine concentrations in the circulation and within the brain. Some of these findings are listed in the Tables I, II, and III. Nevertheless, besides acting directly on neural cells themselves, peripheral cytokines may also trigger CNS effects indirectly via activation of neuronal afferents (Hopkins & Rothwell, 1995; Rothwell & Hopkins, 1995). These mechanisms, though not yet well understood, may play a role in the induction of fever or the feedback loops regulating the activity of the neuroendocrine axis.

A. Effects on Survival, Growth, Differentiation, and Activation of Neural Cells

IL-2 was found to support the survival of cortical, hippocampal, septal, striatal, cerebellar, and sympathetic neurons as well as neuroblastoma cells (Awatsuji, Furukawa, Nakajima, Furukawa, & Hayashi, 1993; Haugen & Letourneau, 1990; Moroni & Rossi, 1995; Sarder, Saito, & Abe, 1993; Shimojo et al., 1993; Wang, Yao, & Ding, 1994). IL-2 can also modify morphological features of cultured neurons, such as the length and the branching index of the axons. Effects on neurite outgrowth and morphology were suggested to be direct, whereas the survival support appeared to be mediated by glial factors. Reports on the survival-promoting activities of IL-2, especially those for hippocampal cells, contrast with toxic effects observed in high-density cultures of rat hippocampal neurons in which IL-2 attenuated neuronal survival over a dose range found by others to be supportive (Araujo, 1992; Araujo & Cotman, 1991; Awatsuji et al., 1993; Sarder et al., 1993; Wang et al., 1994). Moreover, IL-2 also has been reported to be toxic to neurons in vivo, most likely involving more indirect mechanisms and the contribution of brain macrophages and infiltrating immune cells (Hanisch, Kar, et al., 1993; Hanisch, Neuhaus, et al., 1996, 1997; Hanisch, Rowe, Sharma, Meaney, & Quirion, 1994; Hanisch, Rowe, van Rossum, Meaney, & Quirion, 1996; Nemni et al., 1992).

Both IFN-α/β and IFN-γ can prevent cell death in sympathetic neurons deprived of nerve growth factor (NGF) (Chang et al., 1990), can mimic some NGF effects on neuronal gene induction (Toledo Aral, Brehm, Halegoua, & Mandel, 1995), and facilitate the NGF-induced neuronal differentiation of PC 12 cells (Improta et al., 1988). Like a few other cytokines (e.g., TNF-α), IFN-γ can induce expression of neuronal markers, terminal differentiation, and neuronal commitment in retinoblastoma and neuroblastoma cells (Hooks, Chader, Evans, & Detrick, 1990; Montaldo, Carbone, Corrias, Ferraris, & Ponzoni, 1994; Munoz Fernandez et al., 1994; Ponzoni, Guarnaccia, Corrias, & Cornaglia Ferraris, 1993). The cytokine known to increase NO synthase activity and NO production in glial cells may also influence neuronal NO synthesis (Minc Golomb, Yadid, Tsarfaty, Resau, & Schwartz, 1996; Munoz Fernandez et al., 1994; Sato, Kim, Himi, & Murota, 1995). Most notably, several studies report on the up-regulation or induction of MHC class I antigen in neuronal and neuroblastoma cells (Table I). When electrophysiological recording and sodium channel blockade were combined with the detection of MHC antigen, it was concluded that mainly silent (or silenced) neurons up-regulated expression on IFN-γ treatment and that, therefore, immunsurveillance by cytotoxic T cells would affect functionally impaired cells.

Reports regarding the effects of IL-2 on astrocytic proliferation and properties are heterogeneous (Balasingam, Tejada Berges, Wright, Bouckova, &

TABLE I Effects on the Survival, Growth, Differentiation, and Features of Neural Cells

Effect	Cytokine	Reference
Support of survival of rat hippocampal, cortical, septal, & striatal neurons	IL-2	(Awatsuji, Furukawa, Nakajima, Furukawa, & Hayashi, 1993)
Enhanced neurite outgrowth and support of survival in cultures of rat hippocampal neurons	IL-2	(Wang, Yao, & Ding, 1994)
Support of neurite extension and process morphology in rat hippocampal neurons	IL-2	(Sarder, Saito, & Abe, 1993)
Survival support for rat hippocampal, cortical, septal, and cerebellar neurons in high-density cultures	IL-2	(Sarder et al., 1993)
Reduced survival of cultured rat hippocampal neurons	IL-2	(Araujo, 1992)
Support of survival of rat cortical neurons	IL-2	(Shimojo et al., 1993)
Support of the growth of sympathetic neurites from rat and chicken	IL-2	(Haugen & Letourneau, 1990)
Increases in choline acetyltransferase activity in rat septal cell culture without changes in cell number or morphology	IL-2	(Mennicken, Mazzoni, Kenigsberg, & Quirion, 1994; Mennicken & Quirion, 1995; Mennicken & Quirion, 1997)
Abnormalities in axonal ultrastructure of rat neurons	IL-2	(Ellison & Merchant, 1991)
Suppression of rat anterior pituitary cell growth	IL-2	(Arzt et al., 1993)
Stimulation of GH_3 rat pituitary tumor cell growth	IL-2	(Arzt et al., 1993)
Enhanced proliferation of human pituitary adenoma	IL-2	(Sauer, Rupprecht, Arzt, Stalla, & Rupprecht, 1993)
Axonal degeneration and demyelination in rats	IL-2	(Ellison, Krieg, & Povlishock, 1990)
Stimulation of proliferation and maturation of rat oligodendrocytes	IL-2	(Benveniste & Merrill, 1986)
Enhanced proliferation of human oligodendrocytes	IL-2	(Otero & Merrill, 1997)
Enhanced proliferation of human oligodendroglioma subclones	IL-2	(Otero & Merrill, 1994; Otero & Merrill, 1997)
Suppression of proliferation of rat oligodendrocytes (progenitors)	IL-2	(Saneto, Altman, Knobler, Johnson, & De Vellis, 1986; Saneto, Chiapelli, & De Vellis, 1987)
Toxicity for cultured rat oligodendrocytes	IL-2	(Eitan et al., 1992)
Toxicity for cultured rat oligodendrocytes	IL-2-like factor	(Eitan et al., 1992)
Down-regulation of proteolipid protein mRNA in the mouse brain and up-regulation of mRNA for P0 and myelin-basic protein in the peripheral nervous system	IL-2	(Sessa et al., 1992)
Enhanced mouse astrocytic proliferation	IL-2	(Hunter, Sporn, & Davies, 1993)
Increased experimentally induced astrogliosis in mice	IL-2	(Balasingam, Tejada Berges, Wright, Bouckova, & Yong, 1994)
Promotion of growth of mouse microglia	IL-2	(Sawada, Suzumura, & Marunouchi, 1995)
Promotion of the survival of mouse microglia	IL-15	(Hanisch, Lyons et al., 1997)
Facilitation of nerve growth factor (NGF)-induced neuronal differentiation of PC12 cells	IFN-γ	(Improta et al., 1988)
Prevention of NGF deprivation-induced cell death in cultured rat sympathetic neurons	IFN-α/β IFN-γ	(Chang, Martin, & Johnson, Jr., 1990)
NGF-like effect on sodium channel gene induction in PC12 cells	IFN-γ	(Toledo Aral, Brehm, Halegoua, & Mandel, 1995)
Increased choline acetyltransferase activity in cultured rat septal nuclei, probably via a factor produced by microglia	IFN-γ	(Jonakait, Luskin, Wei, Tian, & Ni, 1996; Jonakait, Wei, Sheng, Hart, & Ni, 1994)
Increases in choline acetyltransferase activity in human spinal cord cell culture (probably indirect)	IFN-γ	(Erkman, Wuarin, Cadelli, & Kato, 1989)
Up-regulation of MHC class I antigen in neuronal cells	IFN-γ	(Linda et al., 1998; Neumann, Cavalie, Jenne, & Wekerle, 1995; Neumann, Schmidt, Cavalie, Jenne, & Wekerle, 1997), (Drew et al., 1993; Joly & Oldstone, 1992; Rensing Ehl et al., 1996)
Induction of neuronal injury in mixed neuron/glia cultures, synergistic effect with lipopolysaccaride or IL-1	IFN-γ	(Hu, Peterson, & Chao, 1997; Jeohn, Kong, Wilson, Hudson, & Hong, 1998)

(*Continues*)

TABLE I (*Continued*)

Effect	Cytokine	Reference
Stimulation of astrocyte proliferation	IFN-γ	(Becher, D'Souza, Troutt, & Antel, 1998; Satoh, Paty, & Kim, 1996)
Induction of differentiation-like morphological changes in cultured embryonic astrocytes	IFN-γ	(Janabi, Mirshahi, Wolfrom, Mirshahi, & Tardieu, 1996)
Increased expression of glial fibrillary acidic protein in astrocytes of human spinal cord cell culture	IFN-γ	(Erkman et al., 1989)
Induction of complex changes in rat astrocytic gene expression	IFN-γ	(Kuchinke, Hart, & Jonakait, 1995)
Enhanced expression of MHC class II antigen and B7 by astrocytes	IFN-γ	(Neumann, Boucraut, Hahnel, Misgeld, & Wekerle, 1996; Nikcevich et al., 1997; Panek, Lee, & Benveniste, 1995; Tan, Gordon, Mueller, Matis, & Miller, 1998; Van Wagoner, O'Keefe, & Benveniste, 1998)
Enhanced production of nitric oxide (NO) and induction of NO synthase in astrocytes	IFN-γ	(Bhat, Zhang, Lee, & Hogan, 1998; Brodie, Blumberg, & Jacobson, 1998; Ding & Merrill, 1997; Hellendall & Ting, 1997; Hu, Sheng, Peterson, & Chao, 1995; Kitamura et al., 1998)
Inhibition of oligodendroglial proliferation and differentiation	IFN-γ	(Agresti, D'Urso, & Levi, 1996)
Induction of apoptosis in cultured oligodendrocytes	IFN-γ	(Vartanian, Li, Zhao, & Stefansson, 1995)
Increased apoptosis in developing oligodendrocytes and increased necrosis in mature oligodendrocytes in culture	IFN-γ	(Baerwald & Popko, 1998)
Induced microglia-mediated toxicity for oligoendrocytes	IFN-γ	(Merrill & Zimmerman, 1991)
Induction of MHC class II antigen in cultured rat oligodendrocytes, synergistic effect with dexamethasone	IFN-γ	(Bergsteindottir, Brennan, Jessen, & Mirsky, 1992)
Induction of MHC antigen in cultured mouse oligodendrocytes	IFN-γ	(Suzumura, Silberberg, & Lisak, 1986)
Induction of MHC class I and II antigens on cultured rat Schwann cells	IFN-γ	(Lisak & Bealmear, 1992; Samuel, Jessen, Grange, & Mirsky, 1987)
Down-regulation of myelin-associated glycoprotein in Schwann cells	IFN-γ	(Schneider Schaulies, Kirchhoff, Archelos, & Schachner, 1991)
Increase in ICAM-1 expression on rat microglia	IFN-γ	(Zielasek, Archelos, Toyka, & Hartung, 1993; Zuckerman, Gustin, & Evans, 1998)
Increased proliferation of rat brain microglia	IFN-γ	(Grau, Herbst, van der Meide, & Steiniger, 1997)
Reduced proliferation of rat brain microglia	IFN-γ	(Kloss, Kreutzberg, & Raivich, 1997)
Induction of MHC class I and II antigens and B7 in microglia	IFN-γ	(Becher & Antel, 1996; Frei et al., 1987; Grau et al., 1997; Loughlin, Woodroofe, & Cuzner, 1992; Loughlin, Woodroofe, & Cuzner, 1993; Menendez Iglesias, Cerase, Ceracchini, Levi, & Aloisi, 1997; Panek & Benveniste, 1995; Sethna & Lampson, 1991; Suzumura, Mezitis, Gonatas, & Silberberg, 1987; Suzumura, Sawada, Yamamoto, & Marunouchi, 1993; Woodroofe, Hayes, & Cuzner, 1989; Xu & Ling, 1994; Xu & Ling, 1995)
Induction of NO synthase/NO release in microglia	IFN-γ	(Corradin, Mauel, Donini, Quattrocchi, & Ricciardi Castagnoli, 1993; Goodwin, Uemura, & Cunnick, 1995; Htain, Leong, & Ling, 1997; Peterson, Hu, Anderson, & Chao, 1994; Zielasek, Tausch, Toyka, & Hartung, 1992)
Enhanced expression of Fc receptor by rat microglia	IFN-γ	(Loughlin, Woodroofe, & Cuzner, 1992; Woodroofe et al., 1989)
Increased scavenger receptor by rat microglia	IFN-γ	(Grewal, Yoshida, Finch, & Morgan, 1997)
Down-regulation of CD14 expression by human microglia	IFN-γ	(Becher, Fedorowicz, & Antel, 1996)

TABLE II Effects on the Release or the Tissue Levels of Transmitters and Hormones

Effects	Cytokine	Reference
Suppression of K^+-evoked acetylcholine (ACh) release from rat hippocampal and cortical tissues at nanomolar doses	IL-2	(Araujo, Lapchak, Collier, & Quirion, 1989)
Potentiated K^+-evoked ACh release from rat hippocampal slices at subpicomolar doses	IL-2	(Hanisch, Seto, & Quirion, 1993; Seto, Kar, & Quirion, 1997)
Inhibited K^+-evoked ACh release from rat hippocampal and frontal cortical tissues at nanomolar doses	IL-2	(Hanisch, Seto, & Quirion, 1993; Seto et al., 1997)
Increased choline acetyltransferase activity in rat septal cell culture	IL-2	(Mennicken & Quirion, 1997)
Enhanced spontaneous and K^+-evoked [^{3}H]dopamine release from rat striatal slices	IL-2	(Lapchak, 1992)
Enhanced N-methyl-D-aspartate (NMDA)- and kainate-induced [^{3}H]dopamine release from rat mesencephalic cultures at picomolar doses	IL-2	(Alonso et al., 1993)
Enhanced K^+-evoked [^{3}H]dopamine release from rat mesencephalic cultures at picomolar doses	IL-2	(Alonso et al., 1993)
Inhibited K^+-evoked [^{3}H]dopamine release from rat mesencephalic cultures at nanomolar doses, but no effect on evoked [^{3}H]GABA release	IL-2	(Alonso et al., 1993)
Increased veratridine-evoked release of dopamine from mouse striatal slices at low doses (0.1 nM)	IL-2	(Petitto, McCarthy, Rinker, Huang, & Getty, 1997)
Decreased veratridine-evoked release of dopamine from mouse striatal slices at higher doses (10 nM)	IL-2	(Petitto et al., 1997)
Decreased dopamine release in the rat nucleus accumbens	IL-2	(Anisman, Kokkinidis, & Merali, 1996)
Inhibited K^+-evoked [^{3}H]noradrenaline, but not 5-HT, GABA, glutamate or dopamine, release in rat hypothalamic slices	IL-2	(Lapchak & Araujo, 1993)
Increased noradrenaline levels in the amygdala of olfactory bulbectomized rats	IL-2	(Song & Leonard, 1995)
Increased 5-HT levels in the rat hypothalamus	IL-2	(Song & Leonard, 1995)
Increased 5-HT levels in the rat hippocampus	IL-2	(Pauli, Linthorst, & Reul, 1998)
Increased K^+-evoked release of Met-enkephalin, β-endorphin, but not Leu-enkephalin from rat hypothalamic slices	IL-2	(Lapchak & Araujo, 1993)
Enhanced expression of proopiomelanocortin (POMC) gene in pituitary cells and pituitary tumor cells of rat and mouse origin	IL-2	(Brown, Smith, & Blalock, 1987)
Elevation of plasma levels of ACTH in rats	IL-2	(Naito et al., 1989)
Induction of ACTH release in rat pituitary cells	IL-2	(Smith, Brown, & Blalock, 1989)
Induction of ACTH release from the rat pituitary	IL-2	(Karanth & McCann, 1991)
Increases in plasma ACTH and corticosterone basal levels in rats; decreases in the plasma levels of corticosterone-binding globulin	IL-2	(Hanisch, Kar, et al., 1993; Hanisch, Neuhaus, et al., 1997; Hanisch, Rowe, Sharma, Meaney, and Quirion, 1994)
Phasic increases in hypothalamic-pituitary-adrenal (HPA) activity	IL-2	(Hanisch, Rowe, van Rossum, Meaney, & Quirion, 1996)
Normalization by increase of corticosteron levels in olfactory bulbectomized rats	IL-2	(Song & Leonard, 1995)
Increased free corticosterone levels in rats	IL-2	(Pauli et al., 1998)
Stimulation of rat ACTH, prolactin (PRL), and thyrotropic hormone (TSH) release; inhibition of rat follicle-stimulating hormone (FSH), luteinizing hormone (LH), and growth hormone (GH) release	IL-2	(McCann et al., 1994)
Induction of corticotropin releasing factor (CRF) release from rat hypothalami	IL-2	(Cambronero, Rivas, Borrell, & Guaza, 1992)
Stimulation of CRF release from medial rat hypothalamic fragments	IL-2	(Karanth, Krzysztof, & McCann, 1993)
Induction of CRF release from the rat hypothalamus and amygdala	IL-2	(Raber, Koob, & Bloom, 1995)

(Continues)

TABLE II (*Continued*)

Effects	Cytokine	Reference
Increases in vasopressin and oxytocin mRNA in the hypothalamus of the nude mouse	IL-2	(Pardy, Murphy, Carter, & Hui, 1993)
Induction of vasopressin release from the rat hypothalamus and the amygdala	IL-2	(Raber & Bloom, 1994; Raber & Bloom, 1996)
Stimulation of arginine vasopressin release from rat hypothalamic preparation	IL-2	(Hillhouse, 1994)
Stimulation of arginine vasopressin release from rat hypothalamic cells	IL-2	(Hillhouse, 1994)
Increased PRL and TSH release from rat hemipituitaries		
Inhibited release of FSH, LH, GH	IL-2	(Karanth, Marubayashi, & McCann, 1992; Karanth & McCann, 1991)
Inhibited release of LH releasing hormone (LHRH) from medial rat hypothalamic fragments	IL-2	(McCann et al., 1994)
Enhanced basal release of somatostatin from rat mediobasal hypothalamus	IL-2	(Karanth, Aguila, & McCann, 1993)
Inhibited K^+-evoked release of somatostatin from mediobasal hypothalamus		
Inhibited K^+-evoked release of GH releasing hormone (GHRH) from mediobasal hypothalamus		
Stimulation of rat microglial nitric oxide (NO) (and biopterin) production in synergism with IFN-γ	IL-2	(Sakai, Kaufman, & Milstien, 1995)
Increase in ACTH and corticosterone levels in rats	IFN-α/β	(Menzies et al., 1996)
Decreased basal levels of corticosterone in rats	IFN-α	(Kidron, Saphier, Ovadia, Weidenfeld, & Abramsky, 1989; Saphier, 1989; Saphier, Ovadia, & Abramsky, 1990)
Inhibition of the hypothalamic-pituitary-adrenocortical activity	IFN-α	(Saphier, 1995; Saphier et al., 1994)
Enhanced release of arginine vasopressin from rat hypothalamus and amygdala	IFN-α	(Raber & Bloom, 1996)
Stimulation of CRF release from the hypothalamus and amygdala	IFN-α	(Raber, Koob, & Bloom, 1997)
Decreased dopamine levels in the mouse brain	IFN-α	(Shuto, Kataoka, Horikawa, Fujihara, & Oishi, 1997)
Stimulation of prolactin secretion by the rat pituitary gland	IFN-α/β IFN-γ	(Yamaguchi et al., 1991)
Stimulation of serotoninergic transmission in the nucleus raphe dorsalis of the rat	IFN-γ	(Clement et al., 1997)
Increased levels of 5-HT in cultured rat pineal gland	IFN-γ	(Withyachumnarnkul, Nonaka, Attia, & Reiter, 1990)
Enhanced melatonin production in the rat pineal gland	IFN-γ	(Withyachumnarnkul, Nonaka , Attia, et al., 1990; Withyachumnarnkul, Nonaka, Santana, & Attia, Reiter, 1990; Withyachumnarnkul, Reiter, Lerchl, Nonaka, & Stokkan, 1991)
Inhibition of IL-1-induced substance P expression in cultured sympathetic ganglia	IFN-γ	(Hart, Shadiack, & Jonakait, 1991)
Increased acetylcholine release from cultured parasympathetic neurons	IFN-γ	(Jacoby, Xiao, Lee, Chan Li, & Fryer, 1998)
Synergistic stimulation of rat microglial NO (and biopterin) production together with IL-2	IFN-γ	(Sakai et al., 1995)
Inhibition of human thyrotropin receptor expression	IFN-γ	(Nishikawa et al., 1993)
Increase in ACTH and corticosterone levels in rats	IFN-γ	(Menzies et al., 1996)
Inhibition of stimulated ACTH, prolactin, and growth hormone release from cultured rat anterior pituitary cells, probably mediated via folliculo-stellate cells	IFN-γ	(Vankelecom, Andries, Billiau, & Denef, 1992; Vankelecom et al., 1990)
Inhibition of prolactin and GHRH-induced growth hormone release from cultured pituitary cells	IFN-γ	(Vankelecom, Matthys, & Denef, 1997b)

TABLE III Effects on Bioelectric Activity and Animal Behavior

Effects	Cytokine	Reference
Decrease in neuronal discharge frequency in the rat ventromedial nucleus of the hypothalamus	IL-2	(Bindoni, Perciavalle, Beretta, Belluardo, & Diamantstein, 1988)
Increase in the neuronal discharge frequency in supraoptic and paraventricula nuclei	IL-2	(Bindoni et al., 1988)
Decreased multiple unit activity in the mouse anterior hypothalamus	IL-2	(Bartholomew & Hoffman, 1993)
Suppression of afferent sensory transmission to neurons of the rat primary somatosensory cortex	IL-2	(Park, Won, Pyun, & Shin, 1995)
Reduced short-term potentiation and inhibition of long-term potentiation (LTP) induction in the rat hippocampus	IFN-	(D'Arcangelo et al., 1991)
Inhibition of LTP induction in the rat hippocampus Suppression of established LTP in the rat hippocampus	IL-2	(Tancredi, Zona, Velotti, Eusebi, & Santoni, 1990)
Depolarization of rat hippocamapal neurons in culture	IL-2	(Wang et al., 1994; Yao, Wang, Ding, Liu, & Ling, 1994)
Hyperpolarization of rat hippocampal neurons in culture	IL-2	(Wang et al., 1994; Yao et al., 1994)
Depression of voltage-dependent guinea pig hippocampal Ca^{2+} currents	IL-2	(Plata Salaman & ffrench Mullen, 1993)
Increased rat body temperature during the light and dark phase of the diurnal circle	IL-2	(Pauli et al., 1998)
Lengthening of acetylcholine (ACh) receptor channel open time in rat and mouse muscle cells	IL-2	(Lorenzon et al., 1991)
Inhibition of Na^+ currents in human muscle cells	IL-2	(Brinkmeier, Kaspar, Wietholter, & Rudel, 1992)
Inhibition of GABA-induced Cl^- currents in Aplysia neurons	IL-2	(Sawada, Hara, & Ichinose, 1992)
Inhibition of GABA-induced Cl^- currents in Lymnaea neurons	IL-2	(S. Rozsa, Rubakhin, Szucs, Hughes, & Stefano, 1997)
Reduction of ACh-induced K^+ currents in Aplysia neurons	IL-2	(Sawada, Hara, & Maeno, 1992)
Inhibition of Na^+ currents in human muscle cells	IL-2	(Kaspar, Brinkmeier, & Rudel, 1994)
Inhition of Na^+ currents neuroblastoma × glioma mouse/rat hybrid cells	IL-2	(Hamm, Rudel, & Brinkmeier, 1996)
Inhibition of calcitonin-induced outward current associated with Na^+ conductance in *Aplysia* neurons	IL-2	(Sawada, Ichinose, & Stefano, 1994)
Impairment of mnesic function associated with neuronal loss in mouse hippocampal but not frontocortical and cerebellar regions	IL-2	(Nemni et al., 1992)
Augmentation os scopolamine-induced amnesia and hyperactivity in mice	IL-2	(Biachi & Panerai, 1993)
Induction of asymmetric body posture and ipsilateral turning behavior in rats	IL-2	(Nistico & De Sarro, 1991a)
Induction of increased locomotor and exploratory activity in rats	IL-2	(Nistico & De Sarro, 1991a)
Induction of epileptiform effects in rats	IL-2	(Nistico, 1993; Nistico & De Sarro, 1991a)
Proconvulsant effects in experimental epilepsy in mice	IL-2	(De Sarro, Rotiroti, Audino, Gratteri, & Nistico, 1994)
Production of increased locomotor activity of mice in an elevated plus-maze	IL-2	(Petito et al., 1997)
Reduced rat locomotor activity (only during the dark phase of the dirunal cycle)	IL-2	(Pauli et al., 1998)
Reduced total behavioral activity of rats	IL-2	(Pauli et al., 1998)
Induction of behavioral sedation, sleep, electrocorticial activity Synchronization and increase in total voltage power in rats	IL-2	(De Sarro, Masuda, Ascioti, Audino, & Nistico, 1990; De Sarro & Nistico, 1990a, 1990b; Nistico & De Sarro, 1991a)
Decreased grooming activity in olfactory bulbectomized rats	IL-2	(Song & Leonard, 1995)
Attenuation of impaired behaviour of olfactory bulbbectomized rats in open field and elevated plus-maze	IL-2	(Song & Leonard, 1995)
Decreased responding for rewarding lateral hypothalamic stimulation in rats	IL-2	(Anisman, Kokkinidis, Borowski, & Merali, 1998; Anisman et al., 1996)

(*Continues*)

TABLE III (*Continued*)

Effects	Cytokine	Reference
Excitation of pyramidal cells in the rat CA3 region of the hippocampus	IFN-α/β IFNγ	(Muller, Fontana, Zbinden, & Gahwiler, 1993)
Excitation of hippocampal neurons and biphasic responses of hypothalamic neurons	IFN-α	(Prieto Gomez, Reyes Vazquez, & Dafny, 1983)
Increased activity of rat and cat cortical and cerebellar neurons	IFN-α	(Calvet & Gresser, 1979)
Altered activity of rat cortical, hippocampal, thalamic, and hypothalamic neurons	IFN-α	(Dafny, Prieto Gomez, & Reyes Vazquez, 1985)
Acceleration of neuronal activity in rat cortex, hippocampus, and amygdala and suppression of hypthalamic neuronal activity	IFN-α	(Dafny, Prieto Gomez, Dong, & Reyes Vazquez, 1996)
Increased discharge of rat cortical and hippocampal neurons	IFN-α	(Reyes Vazquez, Prieto Gomez, Georigades, & Dafny, 1984)
Suppression of the activity of glucose-sensitive neurons in the rat lateral hypothalamus	IFN-α	(Reyes Vazquez, Mendoza Fernandez, Herrera Ruiz, & Dafny, 1997)
Suppression of neuronal activity in the rat lateral hypothalamus	IFN-α	(Reyes Vazquez, prieto Gomez, & Dafny, 1994)
Excitation of the activity of glucose-sensitive neurons in the rat ventromedial hypothalamus	IFN-α	(Kuriyama, Hori, Mori, & Nakashima, 1990; Reyes Vazquez et al., 1997)
Altered activity of glucose-responsive neurons in the ventromedial hypothalamus	IFN-α	(Hori et al., 1991)
Increased activity of cold-sensitive and decreased of warm-sensitive neurons in the preoptic area/hypothalamus of the rat	IFN-α	(Nakashima, Hori, Kuriyama, & Matsuda, 1988)
Altered activity of thermosensitive neurons in the preoptic area and anterior hypothalamus	IFN-α	(Hori et al., 1991)
Decreased multiunit electrical activity in the preoptic area and anterior hypothalamus	IFN-α	(Kidron et al., 1989; Saphier, 1989; Saphier et al., 1988; Saphier et al., 1990)
Suppression of neuronal activity in the rat anterior hypothalamus and increased activity of ventromedial hypothalamic neurons	IFN-α	(Nakashima, Hori, Kuriyama, & Kiyohara, 1987)
Decreased electrical activity of neurons, including putative CRF-secreting cells in the hypothalamic paraventricular nucleus	IFN-α	(Saphier, 1995; Saphier et al., 1994)
Increased cortical electroencephalogram (EEG) synchronization	IFN-α	(Birmanns, Saphier, & Abramsky, 1990; Kidron et al., 1989; Saphier, 1989; Saphier et al., 1990)
Increased electrocortical activity and induction of sedation and sleep in rats	IFN-α	(De Sarro et al., 1990)
Enhanced slow-wave sleep in rabbits/somnogenic effects	IFN-α/β	(Borbely & Tobler, 1989; Kimura, Majde, Toth, Opp, & Krueger, 1994; Krueger et al., 1987; Krueger & Majde, 1994)
Induction of sleep in mice	IFN-α/β IFN-γ	(Deloria & Mannering, 1993)
Modification of ECG and EEG-like activity in rat somatosensory, motor, and limbic structures with increases in the amplitude of the dominating frequency and irregular spiking	IFN-α	(Dafny, 1983)
Decreased motor activity	IFN-α	(Crnic & Segall, 1992a, 1992b; Dunn & Crnic, 1993; Saphier et al., 1988; Segall & Crnic, 1990b)
Decreased food intake or food-related behaviour in mice	IFN-α	(Crnic & Segall, 1992a, 1992b; Plata Salaman, 1989, 1992, 1995; Reyes Vazquez et al., 1994; Segall & Crnic, 1990a)
Induction of "wet dog shaking" followed by decreases locomotor activity	IFN-α	(De Sarro et al., 1990)
Inhibition of induced "wet dog shaking" in rats	IFN-α	(Kugaya, Kagaya, Uchitomi, Yokota, & Yamawaki, 1996)
Induction of K^+ outward currents in rat microglia	IFN-γ	(Elder & Heinemann, 1996; Mc Larnon, Xu, Lee, & Kim, 1997; Nörenberg, Gebicke Haerter, & Illes, 1992; Visentin, Agresti, Patrizio, & Levi, 1995; Visentin & Levi, 1997, 1998)
Decreased food intake or food-related behaviour in mice	IFN-γ	(Crnic & Segall, 1992a; Plata Salaman, 1992)

Yong, 1994; Benveniste, Whitaker, Gibbs, Sparacio, & Butler, 1989; Eitan et al., 1992; Hunter, Sporn, & Davies, 1993; Nieto Sampedro & Chandy, 1987; Selamj, Raine, Farooq, Norton, & Brosnan, 1991; Simmons & Murphy, 1993; Zwain, Grima, & Cheng, 1994). IL-2 was found to promote DNA synthesis and proliferation in cultured mouse astrocytes (Hunter et al., 1993). Similarly, local administration of IL-2 in vivo enhanced experimentally induced astrogliosis in the neonatal mouse (Balasingam et al., 1994). These observations indicate that IL-2, and other cytokines, could modify the proliferative and scar-forming activity of astroglia, for example, during early ontogenesis or after brain lesion, and that this effect is under the control of other cytokines, such as transforming growth factor-β (TGF-β). IL-2 was further reported to increase astrocytic mRNA for clusterin (Zwain et al., 1994), whereas in some studies effects in astrocytes were not seen (Noguchi et al., 1993) or were seen only with partially purified IL-2 (but not recombinant cytokine), suggesting contaminants to be responsible for the response (Simmons & Murphy, 1993). Similarly, astrocytic growth response to injured-brain extracts was reported to be blocked by an anti-IL-2R antibody, suggesting some involvement of the IL-2/IL-2R system but IL-2 itself was found to have no influence on thymidine incorporation in astrocytes (Nieto Sampedro & Chandy, 1987), as was subsequently confirmed by others (Benveniste et al., 1989).

Astrocytes may, along with mocroglia, serve as APC in the brain. Although being less efficient than microglia in T cell activation, they were found to process and present antigen. IFN-γ is a potent astrocyte activator and was shown to induce or increase the expression of MHC classII antigen, B7-1, intercellular adhesion molecule-1 (ICAM-I) and other adhesion molecules (Aloisi et al., 1995; Aloisi, Ria, Penna, & Adorini, 1998; Hellendall & Ting, 1997; Klyushnenkova & Vanguri, 1997; Sun, Coleclough, & Whitaker, 1997; Winkler & Beveniste, 1998) (see Table I). In contrast, IFN-β counteracts the IFN-γ induced effects (Jiang, 1995; Satoh, Paty, & Kim, 1995). Furthermore, IFN-γ can enhance the production of NO and the expression of inducible NO synthase in astrocytes (Table I) while inhibiting the activity of the constitutive NO synthase isoform (Colasanti et al., 1997). These IFN-γ activities seem also to be (selectively) blocked by IFN-α/β (Hua, Liu, Brosnan, & Lee, 1998; Stewart et al., 1997; Stewart, Land, Clark, & Heales, 1998). Stimulation of cultured fetal astrocytes with IFN-γ can result in proliferation (Becher, D'Souza, Troutt, & Antel, 1998; Satoh, Paty, & Kim, 1996), with IFN-α/β having antagonistic effects (Satoh et al., 1996). The opposite effect, i.e., inhibited growth, was noticed for IFN-γ both in vitro and on intracerebral injection in animals following brain injury (DiProspero, Meiners, & Geller, 1997; Pawlinski & Janeczko, 1997). Others obtained evidence that IFN-γ might not be required for posttraumatic astrogliosis (Rostworowski, Balasingam, Chabot, Owens, & Yong, 1997). Nevertheless, IFN-γ can regulate the expression of cytokine receptors, such as IL-1R, thus rendering the cells more susceptible to the influence of activating factors (Rubio, 1994). It should be mentioned that IL-1 is a known astroglial growth factor and stimulator of astrogliosis (Giulian, Woodward, Young, Krebs, & Lachman, 1988; Giulian, Young, Woodward, Brown, & Lachman, 1988). IFN-γ can also induce or modulate the expression, release, and delivery of various factors, including cyto- and chemokines as well as neurotrophic substances (Appel, Kolman, Kazimirsky, Blumberg, & Brodie, 1997; Bhat, Zhang, Lee, & Hogan, 1998; Brodie, 1996; Gasque, Fontaine, & Morgan, 1995; Kuchinke, Hart, & Jonakait, 1995; Lafortune, Nalbantoglu, & Antel, 1996; Lee et al., 1996; Rubio, 1997a; Rubio, 1997b; Schwartz & Nishiyama, 1994; Zhou et al., 1998b).

For microglial cells, correlation of in vitro findings with the situation in vivo are even more difficult to make. Nevertheless, IL-2 was shown to support microglial growth after treatment of the cells with LPS (Sawada et al., 1995). Similarly, IL-15 was recently shown to support microglial survival and growth in culture (Hanisch et al., 1997a) Together with IFN, IL-2 also stimulated microglial NO and tetrahydrobiopterin production (Sakai, Kaufman, & Milstien, 1995). Interestingly, the stimulating effect of IL-2 on microglial NO synthesis is not shared by IL-15. Although IL-2 was found to enhance NO production in cultured microglia, IL-15 showed the opposite influence and rather reduced the nitrite levels in the culture supernatant (Hanisch et al., 1997a). These observations may indicate that microglia activation as a consequence of inflammation or trauma could further be influenced by IL-2, for example, being produced by infiltrating T cells. Considering the sharing of bioactivities and receptor proteins by IL-2 and IL-15, IL-15 mRNA shown to be synthesized by unstimulated microglia (and astrocytes) and at higher levels following cell stimulation with IFN (and IL-1β) suggests that IL-15 may serve as an autocrine and paracrine factor for activated microglia and T cells in the CNS (Hanisch et al., 1997; Lee et al., 1996). IL-15 produced by activated microglia could even serve as a T-cell chemoattractant and thus promote brain infiltration by immune cells (Wilkinson & Liew, 1995).

IFN(γ) has multiple effects on microglia, most notably on the induction or (up)regulation of cell surface molecule expression, the release of cytokines, and the production of NO (Table I). IFN-γ was shown to affect ICAM-1, leukocyte function-associated molecule 1 (LFA-1), CD14, Fc and complement receptors, and MHC class I and II molecules as well as the immune-accessory molecule B7. The type II interferon can also modulate the production of certain—but not all—microglial cytokines and release products, for example, complement factors C1q, C2, C3 or C4, IL-1, IL-6, or TNFα (Bhat et al., 1998; Haga, Aizawa, Ishii, & Ikeda, 1996; Liu, Amaral, Brosnan, & Lee, 1998; McManus, Brosnan, & Berman, 1998; Meda et al., 1995; Xiao, Bai, Zhang, Hojeberg, & Link, 1996), or negatively and positively modulate the cytokine-inducing effects of other stimulating agents (Loughlin & Woodroofe, 1996; Meda et al., 1996). IFN-β or TGF-β, on the other hand, can antagonize some of these effects, one of the mechanisms exploited in the IFN-β treatment of multiple sclerosis (Chabot, Williams, & Yong, 1997; Hall, Wing, Compston, & Scolding, 1997; Liu et al., 1998; Porrini & Reder, 1994; Rothwell & Hopkins, 1995; Suzumura, Sawada, Yamamoto, & Marunouchi, 1993). Together, the effects of IFN-γ on microglial cells resemble those known for other tissue macrophages and most likely contribute to their functions as potentially cytotoxic and antigen-presenting cells (Kreutzberg, 1996; Merrill & Benveniste, 1996; Perry, 1994; Perry, Andersson, & Gordon, 1993; Streit, Graeber, & Kreutzberg, 1988).

The discovery that IL-2 influenced the proliferation of cultured oligodendrocytes represented one of the earliest reports concerning modulatory effects of the cytokine on neural cells. Inhibitory IL-2 effects were observed on the [^{3}H]thymidine incorporation in A2B5$^+$ oligodendrocyte progenitor cells, but growth itself was not affected (Saneto et al., 1986). IL-1 had to be present together with IL-2 to modify cell numbers and the IL-2 effect was mediated by and dependent on IL-2Rα. These results indicated a growth-controlling activity of IL-2 in immature oligodendrocytes that is itself regulated by IL-1. IL-1 is also an astroglial growth factor during development, can induce astrogliosis, and is produced, for example, by activated microglia (Giulian, Woodward, et al., 1988; Giulian, Young, et al., 1988). It also may thus modulate the IL-2-mediated growth of oligodendrocytes during earlier ontogenetic periods and in posttraumatic episodes and diseases characterized by gliosis. Both cytokines, IL-1 and IL-2, might therefore be involved in the process of scar formation by astrocytes or remyelination during tissue repair (Saneto et al., 1986). In contrast to the reports on the progenitor cells, IL-2 exerted a positive effect on the proliferation and maturation of more mature oligodendrocytes (Benveniste & Merrill, 1986; Otero & Merrill, 1994). The same group also reported on the up-regulation of myelin basic protein (MBP) mRNA in IL-2-treated oligodendrocytes (Benveniste, Herman, & Whitaker, 1987). Hence, there seems to be a temporal dependence of cultured oligodendrocytes/precursors with respect to their response to IL-2, with negative growth control at early and positive effects at later stages of development.

An IL-2-like substance isolated from regenerating fish optic nerve and apparently consisting of an IL-2 dimer was shown to be toxic to rat oligodendrocytes (Eitan et al., 1992), the effect apparently being mediated by the tumor suppressor gene product, p53 (Eizenberg, Faber Elman, Gottlieb, et al., 1995). Intracellular effects occurred within 15 min of exposure and the apoptosis-like cell death reached a maximum within a day. It was further demonstrated that a nerve transglutaminase catalyzed the Ca^{2+}-dependent conversion of lymphocyte-derived IL-2 into a 30 kD dimerized form that subsequently also exerted toxic effects (Eitan & Schwartz, 1993). Toxicity was observed at 25 U/mL of dimerized IL-2 whereas much higher doses of unconverted cytokine did not show any toxic properties. On the other hand, a linear version of dimeric IL-2 created by genetic engineering was not toxic to oligodendrocytes although it retained the mitogenic effect on T cells, suggesting that only the enzymatic conversion product possessed the toxicity-inducing activity (Eizenberg, Kaplitt, Eitan, Pfaff, Hirschberg, & Schwartz, 1994). It was concluded that (lesion-induced) conversion of IL-2 into a factor toxic to oligodendroglia might be a mechanism by which outgrowing nerves overcome the growth-inhibiting properties of oligodendrocytes. Interestingly, treatment of injured rat optic nerve with transglutaminase, indeed, resulted in a recovery of visual response (Eitan et al., 1994). The dimeric form of IL-2 characterized in these studies likely relates to the dimeric IL-2 earlier isolated from posttraumatic brain tissue (Nieto Sampedro & Chandy, 1987). On the other hand, dimeric IL-2 does not appear to be an exclusive product of nervous tissue, as nonmonomeric molecules can also be purified from immune cells. Still, the comparative investigations on the dimeric IL-2 molecules indicate that toxicity for oligodendrocytes and the proliferative effect on lymphocytes involve different ligand-receptor interactions.

IFN-γ can also inhibit oligodendroglial and Schwann cell proliferation as well as differentiation and can induce cell death probably by both direct and indirect mechanisms (Agresti, D'Urso, & Levi, 1996; Merrill, Ignarro, Sherman, Melinek, & Lane, 1993; Merrill & Zimmerman, 1991; Schneider Schaulies, Kirchhoff, Archelos, & Schachner, 1991; Vartanian, Li, Zhao, & Stefansson, 1995). Increased levels of IFN-γ during inflammation likely play a deleterious role in demyelination processes (Baerwald & Popko, 1998; Grimaldi & Martino, 1995; McCombe, Nickson, & Pender, 1998). Accordingly, administration of the cytokine augments both myelin injection-induced and T cell-mediated myelin destruction in experimental models (Hartung, Schafer, van der Meide, Fierz, Heininger, & Toyka, 1990). Moreover, transgenic mice expressing IFN-γ under the control of an oligodendrocytic promoter and developing gliosis, MHC class II induction, and lymphocytic infiltration also show demyelination (Corbin et al., 1996; Horwitz, Evans, McGavern, Rodriguez, & Oldstone, 1997). The mechanisms by which IFN-γ contributes to lesions, for example, as seen in multiple sclerosis and experimental allergic encephalomyelitis (EAE) thus include direct effects on myelinating cells and indirect effects via resident glial and infiltrating immune cells (Merrill, 1992; Merrill & Benveniste, 1996; Navikas & Link, 1996; Olsson, 1992; Zhao & Schwartz, 1998). In contrast, IFN-β can have beneficial outcomes on the course of the disease by induction of immunosuppressive cytokines, down-regulation of MHC class II expression, by antagonizing some of the IFN-γ activity as well as by restoration of T cell suppressor function (Arnason, Toscas, Dayal, Qu, & Noronha, 1997; Hall, Compston, & Scolding, 1997; Martin, 1997; Rudick et al., 1998; Ruuls et al., 1996).

B. Effects on Transmitter and Neuropeptide Release

Under experimental conditions, IL-2 was shown in vitro and in vivo to modulate, more or less directly, the release and the tissue levels of various neurotransmitters (Hanisch & Quirion, 1996). Thus far, the cytokine was reported to affect acetylcholine (ACh), dopamine, noradrenaline, and serotonin (5-HT) as well as related metabolites in mainly rodent-based experiments (Alonso et al., 1993; Anisman, Kokkinidis, & Merali, 1996; Araujo et al., 1989; Hanisch, Seto, & Quirion, 1993; Lapchak, 1992; Pauli, Linthorst, & Reul, 1998; Petitto, McCarthy, Rinker, Huang, & Getty, 1997; Seto et al., 1997; Song & Leonard, 1995; Zalcman et al., 1994). IL-2 appears to be a specific and regioselective neuroregulator that can exhibit extremely potent effects on certain release systems, also partially showing biphasic dose-response relations. Major anatomical structures in which IL-2 was found to modify transmitter release are the frontal cortex, hippocampus, striatum, and the hypothalamus (Table II).

Due to its relatively recent discovery, there is currently no information available suggesting transmitter release-modulating activity for IL-15. It can be expected that IL-15 would have similar neuroregulatory properties as found for IL-2, but definitive proof can be obtained only from the experiment. Thus far, administration of recombinant IL-2 to rodent tissue preparations has given functional evidence for the role of IL-2R in the regulation of transmitter release, especially ACh, that can be correlated topographically with the distribution of IL-2 and IL-2R-like molecules as obtained from anatomical studies.

Several studies demonstrated a potent and most likely IL-2R-mediated effect of IL-2 on the release of ACh in the rat hippocampus (Araujo et al., 1989; Hanisch, Seto, & Quirion, 1993; Lapchak et al., 1991; Seto et al., 1997). Using static incubation and superfusion approaches IL-2 was shown to inhibit the K^+- or veratridine-evoked release of ACh at nanomolar concentrations (Hanisch, Seto, & Quirion, 1993; Seto et al., 1997). On the other hand, very low concentrations of the cytokine caused an augmentation of transmitter release. Doses as low as 0.1 pM significantly enhanced ACh release, whereas femtomolar concentrations had no effect (Hanisch, Seto, & Quirion, 1993). The potentiating and inhibitory actions of IL-2 thus resulted in a biphasic dose-response relation, independent of the stimulus involved to evoke ACh release, i.e., 25 mM of K^+ or 30 μM of veratridine. Both the release-potentiating and the inhibitory effects of IL-2 showed a rundown phenomenon (Hanisch, Seto, & Quirion, 1993), suggestive of a desensitization due to the internalization of the ligand-receptor complex as it is known from immune cells (Fung, Ju, & Greene, 1988; Legrue, Sheu, & Chernajovsky, 1991).

Similarly, studies on mesencephalic cell cultures revealed a biphasic IL-2 modulation of K^+-evoked dopamine release, with the extrema of the effects being separated by three to four orders of magnitude (Alonso et al., 1993). Release enhancement was observed with relatively low IL-2 concentrations (1 to 10 pM), whereas treatment with higher doses (1 to 10 nM) resulted in release attenuation. Picomolar IL-2 concentrations also increased the transmitter release as it was triggered by N-methyl-D-aspartate (NMDA), suggestive of an independence of the effect with respect to the release-evoking stimulus. In agreement with these release-modulating effects of IL-2, the cytokine was also shown to suppress noradrenaline release from hypothalamic tissue preparations (Lapchak & Araujo, 1993). Nevertheless, IL-2 had no effect on the basal release of ACh from hippocampal, frontocortical, or striatal tissues, of dopamine from mesencephalic cells or of noradrenaline from hypothalamic slices (Alonso et al., 1993; Hanisch, Seto, & Quirion, 1993; Kumaki et al., 1995). Moreover, other data on dopamine, serotonin, GABA, or glutamate demonstrate that inhibition of evoked release by IL-2 is regionally restricted and specific in terms of the transmitter as well as the cytokine (Hanisch & Quirion, 1996). IL-1α, IL-1β, IL-3, IL-4, IL-5, IL-6, and IFN-α tested in parallel all failed to modify ACh release (Araujo et al., 1989; Hanisch, Seto, & Quirion, 1993).

Modulation of evoked ACh release could also be demonstrated for preparations of rat frontal cortex (Hanisch, Seto, & Quirion, 1993). Nanomolar doses of IL-2 inhibited release from the frontocortical slices but no effect was observed for tissue samples from the parietal cortex or the striatum. From the regional differences it could be deduced that IL-2 modulates the release of ACh from certain cholinergic projections but not from, for example, cholinergic striatal interneurons.

Information about the mechanisms of release modulation by IL-2 derives from studies using tetrodotoxin (TTX), GABA receptor antagonists, and anti-IL-2Rα antibodies (Seto et al., 1997). Stimulation of hippocampal ACh release by IL-2 remained unaffected in the presence of TTX but its inhibitory action was found to be TTX-sensitive. This observation suggests that the release-potentiating effect of IL-2 is due to a more direct effect on cholinergic nerve terminals whereas the inhibition is more indirect and may involve interneurons. GABA, a major inhibitory transmitter in the hippocampus (Thompson, 1994), opioid peptides, and NO are potential candidates for the mediation of IL-2 effects. Opioid receptors have been shown to play a role in the regulation of ACh release not only at the neuromuscular junction but also in the hippocampus (Lapchak, Araujo, & Collier, 1989). In addition, several IL-2 effects are known to be blocked by naloxone (De Sarro, Masuda, Ascioti, Audino, & Nistico, 1990; De Sarro & Nistico, 1990a, 1990b). Most notably, direct actions of IL-2 on δ-opioid receptors are under discussion (Wang et al., 1996) that seem to involve an "analgesic domain" within the cytokine molecule (Wang et al., 1997). With respect to NO, its synthesis and release was demonstrated to participate in the regulation of ACh (Lonart, Wang, & Johnson, 1992) as well as the IL-2 effects in the hypothalamus (Raber & Bloom, 1994; Raber, Koob, & Bloom, 1995), and NO synthase is expressed in the hippocampus (Bredt et al., 1991). Nevertheless, GABA is the most likely mediator of an IL-2 modulation of ACh release (Seto et al., 1997). The $GABA_A$ and $GABA_B$ receptor antagonists, bicucullin and phaclofen, were found to abolish the inhibitory effect of IL-2. In contrast, experiments with naloxone demonstrated that opioid receptors are neither involved in the inhibitory nor in the stimulatory ACh modulation by IL-2. Furthermore, NO synthase-blocking agents also failed to modify the IL-2 effects.

The release-modulating activity at subpicomolar IL-2 concentration points to the involvement of high-affinity receptors. Interactions of IL-2 with the trimeric IL-2R$\alpha\beta\gamma$ complex in immune cells are characterized by a k_D of about 10^{-11} M and [^{125}I]-IL-2 binding studies with rat brain tissue were found to give similar results (Araujo et al., 1989; Hanisch & Quirion, 1996). More direct evidence for the actual involvement of IL-2R in the effects on ACh release were obtained with anti-IL-2Rα antibodies. Both the negative and the positive release modulation by IL-2 could be blocked effectively when the antibody was added to the hippocampal slices (Seto et al., 1997). Anti-IL-2Rα antibodies also inhibited the IL-2-inducible increase of choline acetyltransferase activity in septal cell cultures (Mennicken & Quirion, 1997). These findings imply a constitutive expression of IL-2Rα (or a similar IL-2-binding structure) by neuronal cells of the rat CNS and thus a situation that is different from that known for lymphocytes.

IL-2Rα appears to be expressed in several regions of the normal brain whereas its synthesis in immune cells depends on stimulation (Hanisch & Quirion, 1996; Lapchak et al., 1991; Seto et al., 1993). Binding studies on the basis of rat brain preparations and human post mortem material identified IL-2 binding sites. For the rat hippocampus, B_{max} values of ≤ 1 fmol/mg protein were determined. A value of 0.6 fmol/mg was obtained with human material, however, using a single concentration of IL-2 (Araujo & Lapchak, 1994; Araujo et al., 1989). Autoradiographic analyses of [^{125}I]-IL-2 binding sites in the rat brain also revealed relatively intense labeling of the hippocampal formation, subsequently localized to the pyramidal and granular cell layers of the hippocampus proper and the dentate gyrus, respectively (Araujo et al., 1989; Lapchak et al., 1991). Similarly, "Tac antigen" (IL-2Rα-) like immunoreactive material also was found in these structures, the anatomical distribution of the antigen generally being quite comparable with that of IL-2 (Lapchak et al., 1991; Seto et al., 1993).

Detection by radioimmunochemical techniques revealed the presence of IL-2 in the pyramidal cell layer of the hippocampus and the granule cell layer of the dentate gyrus. Conventional immunocytochemistry and electronmicroscopy supported these findings and localized IL-2-like molecules in neuronal cell bodies. Measurements of the tissue levels by a radioimmune assay showed detectable levels of the cytokine for rat brain material (Araujo et al., 1989). Subsequent analyses using more adequate techniques determined hippocampal IL-2 tissue levels in human post mortem samples in the range of 5 fmol/mg protein, relating to an overall concentration of 0.5 nM (Araujo & Lapchak, 1994).

Cholinergic projections of the rat septum find their targets throughout the hippocampus (Gaykema, Luiten, Nyakas, & Traber, 1990), but the density of terminals is higher in the strata oriens and radiatum of the CA2 and CA3 subdivisions where they meet dendritic processes of the neurons of the pyramidal cell layer (Semba & Fibiger, 1989). These projection are also received in the infra- and supragranular layers of the gyrus dentatus where they can make contact with the granular cells. The close association of IL-2 and IL-2R-like molecules and binding sites with cholinergic terminals provides strong anatomical support for the functional observation that IL-2 can modulate the release of ACh from these fibers.

In the frontoparietal portion of the cerebral cortex, IL-2- and IL-2R-like immunoreactive material concentrates in layer IV, the signal intensity fading in caudal and ventral directions (Lapchak et al., 1991; Seto et al., 1993). Interestingly, [^{125}I]-IL-2 binding was obtained in the cortex but at a much lower level, when compared with the hippocampal formation (Araujo & Cotman, 1992; Araujo et al., 1989). Cholinergic fibers innervating the cortex of the rat originate from cells of the substantia innominata (or neighboring areas) and from ventromedial parts of the globus pallidus (Semba & Fibiger, 1989). Although the cortex contains "intrinsic" cholinergic neurons, especially in layers II/III, the pattern of cholinergic terminals is dominated by the far-projecting fibers (Eckenstein, Baughman, & Quinn, 1988). Accordingly, IL-2 effects on ACh release in the cortex also show some topographic correlation with terminals of cholinergic projections.

Hippocampal ACh release and signaling are known to play a crucial role in learning and memory functions. The modulatory effect of IL-2 on ACh release may thus be of potential interest for the cholinergic deficits observed in Alzheimer's disease (AD) (Muir, 1997; Small, 1998; Whitehouse et al., 1982). Inflammatory processes have been considered to play a role in AD, and antiinflammatory strategies have been discussed for treatment (Griffin et al., 1998; McGeer & McGeer, 1997; McRae, Dahlstrom, & Ling, 1997; Rogers et al., 1996). In association with neurodegenerative plaques and neurofibrillary tangles, several cytokines, complement factors, and other immune-related markers have been detected in brains of AD patients. Besides IL-1 and IL-6, IL-2, IL-2(R) immunoreactive material, and IL-2 binding sites have been found to be elevated, with quantitative analyses of IL-2-like antigen and IL-2 binding sites revealing increases of 130 and 70%, respectively (Araujo & Lapchak, 1994; Huberman et al., 1994; McGeer et al., 1987; Singh, 1994). Increased hippocampal IL-2 and IL-1 levels (Rada et al., 1991) may contribute to decreased hippocampal ACh release. In addition to its demonstrated electrophysiological effects on hippocampal neurons (Plata Salaman & ffrench Mullen, 1993; Tancredi, Zona, Velotti, Eusebi, & Santoni, 1990; Yao, Wang, Ding, Liu, & Ling, 1994), behavioral studies in animals showed that IL-2 treatment can, indeed, interfere with mnesic functions (Bianchi & Panerai, 1993; Hanisch et al., 1997; Nemni et al., 1992). Intracerebroventricular (icv) administration of IL-2 in rats also was found to affect muscarinic receptors. Autoradiographic analyses revealed reduced binding of [^{3}H]pirenzepine and [^{3}H]AFDX 384 to M_1- and M_2-like receptors in the stratum radiatum of the hippocampal CA1 region (Hanisch et al., 1997). Similarly, changes in muscarinic receptors were noticed in the frontoparietal cortex of the IL-2-treated animals. Topical application of IL-2 at cortical sites also have been shown to suppress somatosensory transmission, with the thalamocortical projections reaching layer IV, where IL-2R are expressed (Lapchak et al., 1991; Park, Won, Pyun, & Shin, 1995). Somatosensory gating of afferent signals is thought to contribute to the functional shaping of the body representation within the primary somatosensory (SI) cortex and ACh has been considered to be an essential "permissive agent" in this process (Hanisch, Rothe, Krohn, & Dykes, 1992; Tremblay, Warren, & Dykes, 1990; Webster, Hanisch, Dykes, & Biesold, 1991).

Together, these experimental studies on IL-2-mediated transmitter release modulation suggest that the cytokine plays a role for the cholinergic system in selected regions of the brain. Elevated levels, therefore, may potentially interfere with cognitive performance and memory function. With the introduction of IL-2 as an antitumor agent several side effects have been observed that include cognitive impairment, disorientation, or memory loss. Even following systemic administration in patients, IL-2 levels were determined to reach concentrations in the liquor that were found to be effective for the inhibition of ACh release under experimental conditions (Hanisch, Seto, & Quirion, 1993; Saris et al., 1989).

It is worth emphasizing that the release modulating activities of cytokines—in particular those of IL-2—are extremely potent. For example, ACh release modulation is known from various muscarinic agonists and antagonists (Lapchak, Araujo, Quirion, & Collier, 1989; Raiteri, Leardi, Marchi, Song, & Leonard, 1995), excitatory amino acids (Scatton & Lehmann, 1982), and from neuropeptides such as neurotensin (Lapchak, Araujo, Quirion, & Beaudet, 1990) and somatostatin (Araujo, Lapchak, Collier, & Quirion, 1990). However, significant effects usually require micromolar concentrations of these agents. With a minimal effective dose of less than 10^{-12} M, IL-2 is the most potent molecule known thus far to have an effect on the release activity of cholinergic neurons. Similarly, neuroendocrine effects of IL-2 are elicited at even lower concentrations (Hanisch & Quirion, 1996). Pico- and femtomolar dose ranges were found to modulate pituitary and hypothalamic release of neuropeptides and hormones, such as Arg-vasopressin (AVP), ACTH, or CRF (Hillhouse, 1994; Karanth, Aguila, & McCann, 1993; Karanth, Krzysztof, & McCann, 1993; Karanth, Marubayashi, & McCann, 1992; Karanth & McCann, 1991; McCann et al., 1994).

Cytokines such as IL-1α, IL-1β, IL-2, IL-6, and TNF-α can regulate the release activity of the pituitary and higher hierarchical structures, such as the hypothalamus, and thereby affect the function of peripheral glands and target organs (Besedovsky & del Rey, 1992; Besedovsky & del Rey, 1996; Hanisch & Quirion, 1996; Jones & Kennedy, 1993; Karanth, Aguila, & McCann, 1993; Koenig, 1991; McCann et al., 1994; Tabibzadeh, 1994; Weigent & Blalock, 1995). A single cytokine may trigger complex regulatory networks by affecting different elements of the neuroendocrine axis and by inducing other neuroendocrine factors (including other cytokines). Nevertheless, the main net effect appears to be an activation of hypothalamic-pituitary-adrenocortical (HPA) function and an inhibition of the axis controlling functions of the thyroid gland and the gonades.

Several pituitary hormones and hypothalamic peptides were found to be modulated by IL-2, namely Met-enkephalin, β-endorphin, prolactin (PRL), luteinizing hormone (LH), follicle-stimulating hormone (FSH), thyrotropic hormone (TSH), growth hormone (GH), ACTH, as well as CRF, GH-releasing hormone (GHRH), and somatostatin (Table II). IL-2 can modulate the release of these molecules by acting on putative IL-2R at various levels of the neuroendocrine axis. It may thus influence the secretory activity of a peripheral gland, such as the adrenal gland, either directly (Tominaga et al., 1991) or via the pituitary (Farrar, 1984; Karanth & McCann, 1991; Smith, Brown, & Blalock, 1989), the hypothalamus, or other brain structures known to play a role in controling pituitary and adrenal activities (Cambronero, Rivas, Borrell, & Guaza, 1992; Karanth, Aguila, & McCann, 1993; Raber & Bloom, 1994; Raber et al., 1995). Studies in vivo confirmed the in vitro data by demonstrating that systemic and central injections of IL-2 can acutely and chronically stimulate the HPA axis (Hanisch et al., 1997; Hanisch et al., 1994; Hanisch, Rowe, van Rossum, Meaney, & Quirion, 1996; McCann et al., 1994; Pauli et al., 1998). In addition, IL-2 may act on transmitter release in brain regions that have regulatory influences on hypothalamic secretory neurons (Bodnoff et al., 1995; Hanisch et al., 1994; Hanisch, Seto, & Quirion, 1993; Issa, Rowe, Gauthier, & Meaney, 1990; Lupien et al., 1998; Meaney, Aitken, Sharma, & Viau, 1992). Indeed, IL-2 binding sites and IL-2R proteins have been localized in the pituitary, the hypothalamus, and the hippocampus (Arzt et al., 1993; Hanisch & Quirion, 1996; Lapchak et al., 1991).

Recently, a model has been presented for the mechanism of an IL-2-induced release of CRF (McCann et al., 1994; Raber et al., 1995). Based on the finding that the stimulation of CRF release can be blocked by atropine it was suggested that IL-2 acts on cholinergic neurons (Karanth, Krzysztof, & McCann, 1993). ACh released by an IL-2-receptive cholinergic cell then activates muscarinic cholinergic receptors on an interneuron, activating a constitutive NO synthase (NOS) via $[Ca^{2+}]_i$/calmodulin. This causes the release of NO that can reach CRF-secreting cells. CRF release involves the activating of a sequence comprising cyclooxygenase activation, prostaglandin E_2 synthesis, adenylate cyclase activation and cAMP generation, protein kinase A activation, and finally the exocytosis of CRF-containing granulae (Karanth, Krzysztof, & McCann, 1993; McCann et al., 1994). IL-2-receptive cholinergic neurons could also act on muscarinic receptors expressed on CRF-positive neurons, causing an increase in $[Ca^{2+}]_i$ and thus activating phospholipase A_2. This could cause the generation of arachidonate substrate for the NO-activated cyclooxygenase (Karanth, Krzysztof, & McCann, 1993). It is likely that NO also activates other heme enzymes involved in the metabolism of arachidonate (lipoxygenase, epoxygenase) (McCann et al., 1994). NO was shown to mediate the IL-2-induced release of both CRF and AVP from both the hypothalamus and the amygdala (Raber & Bloom, 1994; Raber et al., 1995). Besides NO, some IL-2-induced CRF release in the hypothalamus and amygdala could also be mediated by carbon monoxide (CO), since the NO/CO inactivator hemoglobin, but not the NOS-specific competitive inhibitor N^G-monomethyl-L-arginine blocked the IL-2 effect (Raber et al., 1995). N^G-monomethyl-L-arginine was observed to block ACh-induced CRF release from both anatomical structures (Raber et al., 1995). Therefore, some IL-2 effect on CRF secretion also might be independent of ACh. In parallel to the model IL-2 $\Rightarrow$ ACh $\Rightarrow$ NO $\Rightarrow$ CRF (Karanth, Krzysztof, & McCann, 1993), there could be a sequence IL-2 $\Rightarrow$ CO $\Rightarrow$ CRF. IL-2 can also modulate CRF secretion by affecting hypothalamic noradrenaline (Lapchak & Araujo, 1993) that can stimulate CRF in a NO-independent manner (Karanth, Krzysztof, & McCann, 1993; Raber et al., 1995). It should be mentioned that an involvement of glial cells in the circuits mediating the IL-2 stimulation of CRF release also has been postulated (Raber et al., 1995) and that a glial contribution to cytokine-mediated CNS effects also may be relevant for physiological as well as pathophysiological conditions.

The concept of neuroimmunendocrine communication suggests the informational exchange among these systems and proposes that direct cellular contacts (innervation of glands and lymphoid organs) as well as humoral factors (neurotransmitters, neuropeptides, hormones, cytokines) coordinate the function of immune cells by endocrine support and the involvement of CNS structures (Besedovsky & del Rey, 1996; Plata Salaman, 1991). Increased levels of circulating IL-2 can result from an activation of the immune system but also—and more massively—during transplant rejection or following peripheral nerve damage (Hanisch & Quirion, 1996). Significant amounts of the cytokine may reach not only the pituitary but also hypothalamic nuclei during an immune response (Banks & Kastin, 1992; Waguespack et al., 1994). In turn, hypothalamic and pituitary hormones and peptides, but especially glucocorticoids, would subsequently act on immune cells and participate in the control of the extent and the duration of the immune response as well as adjust the metabolic and vegetative functions to the needs of the defense system (Hanisch & Quirion, 1996). Glucocorticoids thereby have multiple effects on cellular immune activities (Besedovsky, del Rey, Sorkin, & Dinarello, 1986; Besedovsky & del Rey, 1991; Besedovsky & del Rey, 1996). Normally antiinflammatory and immunosuppressive, these steroids spare already activated T cells and even stimulate activated B cells. Their discriminating influence with suppressive and permissive effects together with a rhythmic and timed induction could thus conceivably participate in the clonal selection of activated T cells, the prevention of immune hyperresponses, the phenomenon of sequential antigen competition, and the decision on favoring either Th1 or Th2 types of immune responses (Constant & Bottomly, 1997; Levi et al. , 1992; Petrovsky & Harrison, 1995; Ramierz, Fowell, Puklavec, Simmonds, & Mason, 1996).

IFNs may affect hormone secretion in a similarly complex manner and by multiple mechanisms (Table II). IFN-α/β was found to modulate the release of ACTH and glucocorticoids in laboratory animals (Menzies et al., 1996) and in humans undergoing immunotherapy (Roosth, Pollard, Brown, & Meyer, 1986). Activation of the HPA axis may involve the stimulation of CRF and AVP in the hypothalamus and amygdala (Raber & Bloom, 1996; Raber, Koob, & Bloom, 1997). On the other hand, acute as well as chronic inhibitory outcomes on HPA activity and decreased levels of corticosterone following peripheral and central administration of IFN-α have been reported as well (Kidron et al., 1989; Saphier, 1989; Saphier, 1995; Saphier, Ovadia, & Abramsky, 1990; Saphier et al., 1994). Suppression of electrical activity of neurons, including putative CRF-secreting cells in the paraventricular nucleus, could correlate with the suppressive effect on HPA release activity (Saphier, 1995; Saphier et al., 1994). Decreased adrenocortical secretion therefore has been suggested to serve in a positive feedback of IFN-α on its immunopotentiating activities (Dafny, 1998). Structural similarity between IFN-α and ACTH could contribute to the endocrine profile of the cytokine (Blalock & Smith, 1980; Root Bernstein, 1984). In addition, lymphocytic factors produced during infection along with IFNs and having affects on hormone secretion themselves may allow for concerted endocrine responses and adjustments (Besedovsky & del Rey, 1996; Plata Salaman, 1991; Smith, Meyer, & Blalock, 1982). However, direct and indirect mechanisms as well as the regulatory feedback loops involved in the IFN-mediated regulation of hormone release are still largely unknown.

IFN-γ has also been observed to affect the release of several hormones in various ways and to modulate the activity of the respective releasing factors, including prolactin, growth hormone, ACTH, and glucocorticoids (Goldstein et al., 1987; Krishnan, Ellinwood, Laszlo, Hood, & Ritchie, 1987; Menzies et al., 1996; Nishikawa et al., 1993; Saphier et al., 1994; Vankelecom et al., 1990; Vankelecom, Matthys, & Denef, 1997a, 1997b; Yamaguchi et al., 1991). The endocrine findings as derived from animal studies, however, may not always allow to predict the endocrine outcomes of clinical IFN-γ treatments (Goldstein et al., 1987).

C. Effects on Electrophysiological Properties

During an immune response electrophysiological changes can be observed in the hypothalamus (Besedovsky & del Rey, 1996). Immunoregulators that are released from activated immune cells can reach certain CNS structures, alter neuronal discharge frequencies, or stimulate the secretion of neuropeptides. The principle of immune-CNS communication via cytokines has been developed especially with respect to IL-1(β), IL-6, and TNF-α, also demonstrating their potent effects on the HPA axis (Besedovsky & del Rey, 1996) Subsequently, systemic and central administrations of IL-2 confirmed that neurons in hypothalamic structures, such as in the supraoptic nucleus and paraventricular nucleus, can also respond to the T cell growth factor by changing their electrical activity (Bartholomew & Hoffman, 1993; Bindoni, Perciavalle, Beretta, Belluardo, & Diamantstein, 1988). The findings together suggest that circulating or brain-endogenous IL-2 can influence hypothalamic functions as they relate to the control of water retention and HPA activity (for a review see Hanisch & Quirion, 1996). Besides influencing hippocampal formation of long-term potentiation (LTP) (Tancredi et al., 1990) and thalamocortical signaling in the somatosensory cortex (Park et al., 1995), several studies have shown that IL-2 can directly affect the properties of ion channels and excitable membranes. Thus far, mostly inhibitory effects have been noticed on voltage- and ligand-evoked Ca^{2+}, K^{+}, Na^{+}, and Cl^{-} currents (Brinkmeier, Kaspar, Wietholter, & Rudel, 1992; Hamm, Rudel, & Brinkmeier, 1996; Kaspar, Brinkmeier, & Rudel, 1994; Lorenzon et al., 1991; Plata Salaman & ffrench Mullen, 1993; Rozsa, Rubakhin, Szucs, Hughes, & Stefano, 1997; Sawada, Hara, & Ichinose, 1992; Sawada, Hara, & Maeno, 1992; Sawada, Ichinose, & Stefano, 1994). Some reports demonstrating effects of IL-2 administration on the electrophysiological properties of neurons and electroencephalogram (EEG) properties are summarized in Table III.

Just as for IL-2, sleep induction and increased cortical EEG synchronization have been observed with IFN-α treatments. IFN-α also has been shown to have a multitude of effects on neuronal activity in several regions of the brain, including cortical and subcortical structures (for a review see Dafny, 1998). Injections or administration of the cytokine cause suppression of hippocampal LTP (D'Arcangelo et al., 1991), changes in EEG, and increased or decreased field potentials and single neuron activities, for example, in the sensory cortex, preoptic area, anterior, ventromedial and lateral hypothalamus, hippocampus, and the cerebellum (Table III). Affecting thermo- and glucose-sensitive neurons in the hypothalamus, IFN can exert fever and participate in the regulation of food intake (Dafny, 1998) (see also below). Fever induction by central mechanisms is thus accompanying the functions of IFN in host defense against infection but also has been noticed in cancer patients as an undesired side effect of immunotherapies (Blatteis, 1990; Dinarello et al., 1984; Dinarello & Bunn, 1997). IFN-α, like IL-1 also considered to be an endogenous pyrogen, apparently affects populations of thermosensitive neurons in an opposite way, increasing the activity of cold-sensitive and decreasing the activity of warm-sensitive neurons (Dafny, 1998; Dinarello, Cannon, & Wolff, 1988; Nakashima, Hori, Kuriyama, & Matsuda, 1988). Pyrogenecity of IFN-α likely involves opioid mechanisms, as naloxone can interfere with the effect of the cytokine on the thermosensitive neurons.

D. Behavioral Effects

Systemic, icv, and intraparenchymal injections of IL-2 lead to behavioral changes in laboratory animals (Anisman, Kokkinidis, Borowski, & Merali, 1998; Anisman et al., 1996; Bianchi, Sacerdote, & Panerai, 1998; Connor, Song, Leonard, Merali, & Anisman, 1998; Hanisch & Quirion, 1996; Petitto et al., 1997; Song & Leonard, 1995) (Table III). Investigating EEG changes and the sleep-inducing properties of IL-2 administration into the locus coeruleus resulted in strong sedative and soporific effects (De Sarro, Rotiroti, Audino, Gratteri, & Nistico, 1994; De Sarro et al., 1990; Nistico, 1993; Nistico & De Sarro, 1991a, 1991b). Asymmetric body posture and ipsilateral turning behavior following IL-2 injections into the nucleus caudatus and substantia nigra/pars compacta (Nistico & De Sarro, 1991a) may reflect interference with the dopaminergic nigrostriatal projection system as the cytokine has modulatory effects on dopamine release in vitro as well as in vivo (Alonso et al., 1993; Anisman et al., 1996; Lapchak, 1992; Nistico & De Sarro, 1991b; Petitto et al., 1997). Effects on locomotor and exploratory activity may differ substantially due to the dose or route (site) of IL-2 administration as well as the experimental paradigms involved (Connor et al., 1998; Nistico & De Sarro, 1991a; Pauli et al., 1998; Petitto et al., 1997). For example, injections of the cytokine into the hippocampus or ventromedial hypothalamus were shown to increase these activities (Nistico & De Sarro, 1991a) whereas other studies showed no (Bianchi & Panerai, 1993; Connor et al., 1998) or opposite effects (Pauli et al., 1998) following icv or systemic IL-2 administration. High-dose treatment of animals using delivery into the third ventricle caused epileptiform effects (Nistico, 1993; Nistico & De Sarro, 1991b), with IL-2 also showing proconvulsant properties in mouse models of epilepsy (De Sarro, Rotiroti, Audino, Gratteri, & Nistico, 1994).

Interference with mnesic functions has been observed in mice systemically treated with IL-2 (Bianchi & Panerai, 1993; Nemni et al., 1992). Chronic injections led to impaired performance in a passive-avoidance task and correlated with neuronal loss in the hippocampus (Nemni et al., 1992). However, these effects were seen only in aged animals, suggesting that IL-2 augmented some latent functional impairment. Similarly, IL-2 only augmented amnesia in mice treated with scopolamine (Bianchi & Panerai, 1993). These effects probably correlate with the reported modulation of ACh release by IL-2, especially in the hippocampal formation (Araujo et al., 1989; Hanisch, Seto, & Quirion, 1993; Seto et al., 1997). Interestingly, chronic icv infusion of IL-2 in rats caused only a transient impairment in a Morris swim maze task; however, the impairment was accompanied by transient changes in muscarinic cholinergic receptors in the hippocampus (Hanisch et al., 1997). In addition, the cytokine was shown to have electrophysiological effects on rat and guinea pig hippocampal neurons (Plata Salaman & ffrench Mullen, 1993; Yao et al., 1994) and, most notably, to inhibit the formation of LTP (Tancredi et al., 1990), as was similarly found for IFN (D'Arcangelo et al., 1991).

Behavioral effects also are noted in rodents following the administration of IFN-α (Dafny, 1998; Plata Salaman, 1991) (Dafny, 1998; Plata Salaman, 1991) (Table III). IFN-α caused a depression in the open field activity of mice as well as in their motor abilities as measured in a test on swim posture and endurance (Dunn & Crnic, 1993). IFN-α-induced and (partly also) IFN-γ-induced suppression in general activity and food-related behavior (food intake) has been subject to various studies in animals and related to the side effects of clinical applications, such as fatigue and anorexia (Crnic & Segall, 1992a, 1992b; Plata Salaman, 1989, 1992, 1995; Reyes Vazquez, Prieto Gomez, & Dafny, 1994; Segall & Crnic, 1990a, 1990b). As to the CNS mechanisms, IFN(α) is thought to affect reciprocally both "feeding" (or "hunger") and "satiety" centers in the lateral and ventromedial hypothalamus by inhibiting glucose-sensitive neurons in the former and exciting respective neuronal populations in the latter structure (for a review see Dafny, 1998). Although anorexigenic effects are not an exclusive feature of IFNs (Plata Salaman, 1996; Plata Salaman & Borkoski, 1994; Plata Salaman, Sonti, & Borkoski, 1995) they may represent an important centrally mediated outcome of elevated IFN levels as they are associated with infection, malignancy, or immunotherapeutic applications.

VI. NEUROPATHOLOGICAL FEATURES AND CLINICAL ASPECTS OF IL-2 AND IFNs

Despite the increasing knowledge about the various nervous system and neuroendocrine effects of IL-2 and IFNs, their actual contribution to the pathogenesis of CNS diseases is still poorly understood. First concepts combine the available clinical findings of changes in peripheral and brain cytokine levels, cytokine receptor expression, and cytokine responsiveness with the experimentally induced effects on neural cells, tissues, and system functions (Kreutzberg, 1996; McGeer & McGeer, 1997; Merrill & Benveniste, 1996; Mrak, Sheng, & Griffin, 1995; Rogers et al., 1996; Rothwell & Relton, 1993; Zhao & Schwartz, 1998). Roles of cytokines, including IL-2 and the IFNs, can be assumed for CNS pathologies involving inflammatory or (auto)immune processes or the hyperactivation of glial cells, such as in AD, multiple sclerosis, stroke, neurodegeneration, and posttraumatic lesions, and, to some extent, psychiatric disorders (Rothwell & Relton, 1993; Zhao & Schwartz, 1998). However, the net effect of a single cytokine is determined by the "signaling context," and interactions within the cytokine network include synergistic as well as antagonistic mechanisms. The observation of an elevated cytokine level in a pathological condition does not automatically contain the information about the causal relationship and whether the change is an aggravating element or part of counteracting mechanisms. Still, a large proportion of the knowledge concerning the powerful actions of IL-2 and IFNs on the nervous system had to be taken from clinical observations. The mechanisms of cytokine effects on nervous system functions and tissue homeostasis mainly involve direct activities on neuronal and glial cells as well as indirect cascades by affecting the vascular conditions, recruitment of myeloic and lymphoid cells, and the challenge of neuroendocrine responses and feedbacks.

IFNs were the first cytokines to be introduced in clinical practice on a broader basis. The antiviral, antiproliferative, oncogene-down-regulating and differentiation-inducing effects found application in the treatment of various forms of cancer. IFN-α has proven to be successful in certain malignancies (Dafny, 1998). IFN-β has been introduced in clinical practice as a promising tool against multiple sclerosis (Hall et al., 1997). IFN-γ may find special application in antiinfective strategies (Jaffe, 1992). However, most if not all behavioral and other CNS effects elicited by experimental IFN application and administration in animals have correlates in patients under cytokine therapies (Adams, Fernandez, & Mavligit, 1988; Dafny, 1998; Meyers & Abbruzzese, 1992; Meyers, Scheibel, & Forman, 1991; Pavol et al., 1995; Segall & Crnic, 1990b; Valentine, Meyers, Kling, Richelson, & Hauser, 1998). Cognitive impairments, confusion, hallucination, abnormal mood states, and psychotic behavior have been reported.

The IL-2/IL-2R system became the focus of intensive clinical research chiefly with respect to the development of IL-2 as an antitumor drug (Janssen, Mulder, The, & de Leij, 1994; Rosenberg, 1990; Rosenberg, Yang, Topalian, Schwartzentruber, Weber, Parkinson, Seipp, Einhorn, & White, 1994; Rubin, 1993; Whittington & Faulds, 1993). IL-2 therapy showed positive results in various types of tumors and proved effective also in neoplasias that did not respond to conventional treatments. However, IL-2 has pleiotropic effects and any disturbance in its synthesis, bioavailability, and responsiveness can lead to multiple systemic consequences (Kroemer, Andreu, Gonzalo, Gutierrez Ramos, & Martinez, 1991). Indeed, adverse side effects are observed during IL-2-based tumor therapies. Capillary leakage syndrome, probably mediated by LAK cell-induced endothelial injury, appears to be the most frequent complication, associated with hypotension and edema (Janssen et al., 1994; Whittington & Faulds, 1993). Nevertheless, the spectrum of undesired effects also covers increased energy expenditure and protein breakdown and cardiovascular, hematological, hepatic, renal, gastrointestinal, pulmonary, dermatological, and (neuro)endocrine, neurological, and neuropsychiatric abnormalities (Caraceni et al., 1993; Cesario et al., 1991; Denicoff et al., 1989; Denicoff et al., 1987; Lotze et al., 1986; Naredi, Hafstrom, Zachrisson, Rudenstam, & Lundholm, 1994; Saris et al., 1989; Tartour, Mathiot, & Fridman, 1992; Vassilopoulou Sellin, Sella, Dexeus, Theriault, & Pololoff, 1992; Vial & Descotes, 1992; Whittington & Faulds, 1993; Winkelhake & Gauny, 1990). Neurological and neuropsychiatric symptoms are common in IL-2-treated patients (up to 50% of the cases) and can also be treatment limiting (Forman, 1994; Michon et al., 1994; Vial & Descotes, 1992). Complications with a central involvement include headache, motor weakness, confusion and disorientation, memory impairment, cognitive failure, somnolence, anxiety, paranoid delusions, hallucinations, and psychotic and combative behavior (for a review see Hanisch & Quirion, 1996). Side effects were usually thought to resolve on termination of IL-2 delivery (Margolin et al., 1989; Oppenheim & Lotze, 1994; Vial & Descotes, 1992; Whittington & Faulds, 1993). However, some long-lasting memory and neuroendocrine disturbances, permanent neurologic damage, or delayed and progressive brain injury have been reported as a consequence of IL-2 in both humans (Denicoff et al., 1989; Karp, Yang, Khorsand, Wood, & Merigan, 1996; Meyers & Yung, 1993; Ravaud et al., 1994; Vecht, Keohane, Menon, Punt, & Stoter, 1990) and laboratory animals (Hanisch, Neuhaus, Quirion, & Kettenmann, 1996; Hanisch et al., 1997; Hanisch et al., 1994; Hanisch, Rowe, van Rossum, Meaney, & Quirion, 1996; Nemni et al., 1992).

Taken together, although the understanding of how IL-2 and IFNs may participate in the onset of certain CNS pathologies is still incomplete, the question of whether they are subsequently part or potential triggers of pathogenic processes can be answered positively.

VII. CONCLUSION

IL-2, the functionally related IL-15, and IFNs have direct effects on cells of the nervous system. The cellular responses likely are triggered by cytokine binding to their specific receptors. These cytokines may participate in the coordination of immune, CNS, and neuroendocrine functions. Elevated levels outside the brain also probably can affect neural cells expressing the respective receptors, as some cytokine amounts may reach the CNS. Alternatively, central responses may be triggered by peripheral stimulation of afferent pathways. Invading immune cells could serve as an intracranial source of cytokine production under pathological conditions, rendering central cytokine receptors likely to function as latent sensors. Cytokine synthesis endogenous to the brain may be challenged by infection, disturbance of the tissue homeostasis, or as a consequence of trauma and diseases. However, IL-2, IL-15, and IFNs may have physiological roles in the nervous system not necessarily related to antiinfectious and immune responses. They may carry out cell-regulatory functions that are independent of a primary association with host defense and that involve receptors also constitutively expressed under normal conditions.

Compared with the immune system, little is known about the constitutive and inducible expression of cytokine receptors and cytokines by the various populations of neural cells. Cytokine receptor-typical signaling elements, such as the JAK/STAT system, are currently gaining neuroscientific attention but their integration in nervous system functions is mostly enigmatic. The implication of nervous tissue-specific cytokine and cytokine receptor molecules needs clarification but may bear the potential for specific pharmacological interference.

Clinical applications of IL-2, IL-15, and IFNs in immunotherapies must take into account the expression of cytokine receptors by neural cells. The use of these response modifiers in the treatment of brain tumors, as has already been the case for IL-2, especially must be based on an evaluation of their potent neuroregulatory and potentially neurotoxic activities. Strategies aiming at a suppression of the immune system, such as in antiautoimmune therapies targeting high-affinity IL-2R (IL-2R α)-expressing immune cells should consider the constitutive expression of these structures by neural cells. Similarly, future therapeutic antisignaling concepts against JAK3 would potentially affect microglia and other IL-2Rγ-expressing cells of the brain. Nevertheless, recent development in the understanding of molecular and physiological aspects concerning IL-2, IL-15, and IFNs in the nervous system makes it possible to foresee and to expect improved clinical applications.

References

Adams, F., Fernandez, F., & Mavligit, G. (1988). Interferon-induced organic mental disorders associated with unsuspected pre-existing neurologic abnormalities. *Journal of Neurooncology, 6,* 355–359.

Adunyah, S. E., Wheeler, B. J., & Cooper, R. S. (1997). Evidence for the involvement of LCK and MAP kinase (ERK-1) in the signal transduction mechanism of interleukin-15. *Biochemical Biophys Research Communications, 232,* 754–758.

Agresti, C., D'Urso, D., & Levi, G. (1996). Reversible inhibitory effects of interferon-gamma and tumour necrosis factor-alpha on oligodendroglial lineage cell proliferation and differentiation in vitro. *European Journal of Neuroscience, 8,* 1106–1116.

Alexander, J. T., Saris, S. C., & Oldfield, E. H. (1989). The effect of interleukin-2 on the blood-brain barrier in the 9L gliosarcoma rat model. *Journal of Neurosurgery, 70,* 92–96.

Aloisi, F., Borsellino, G., Care, A., Testa, U., Gallo, P., Russo, G., Peschle, C., & Levi, G. (1995). Cytokine regulation of astrocyte function: In-vitro studies using cells from the human brain. *International Journal of Developmental Neuroscience, 13,* 265–274.

Aloisi, F., Ria, F., Penna, G., & Adorini, L. (1998). Microglia are more efficient than astrocytes in antigen processing and in Th1 but not Th2 cell activation. *Journal of Immunology, 160,* 4671–4680.

Alonso, R., Chaudieu, I., Diorio, J., Krishnamurthy, A., Quirion, R., & Boksa, P. (1993). Interleukin-2 modulates evoked release of [^{3}H]dopamine in rat cultured mesencephalic cells. *Journal of Neurochemistry, 61,* 1284–1290.

Aman, M. J., & Leonard, W. J. (1997). Cytokine signaling: cytokine-inducible signaling inhibitors. *Current Biology, 7,* R784–8.

Anderson, D. M., Kumaki, S., Ahdieh, M., Bertles, J., Tometsko, M., Loomis, A., Giri, J., Copeland, N. G., Gilbert, D. J., Jenkins, N. A., Valentine, V., Shapiro, D. N., Morris, S. W., Park, L. S., & Cosman, D. (1995). Functional characterization of the human interleukin-15 receptor alpha chain and close linkage of IL15RA and IL2RA genes. *Journal of Biological Chemistry, 270,* 29862–29869.

Anisman, H., Kokkinidis, L., Borowski, T., & Merali, Z. (1998). Differential effects of interleukin (IL)-1beta, IL-2 and IL-6 on responding for rewarding lateral hypothalamic stimulation. *Brain Research, 779,* 177–187.

Anisman, H., Kokkinidis, L., & Merali, Z. (1996). Interleukin-2 decreases accumbal dopamine efflux and responding for rewarding lateral hypothalamic stimulation. *Brain Research, 731,* 1–11.

Appel, E., Kolman, O., Kazimirsky, G., Blumberg, P. M., & Brodie, C. (1997). Regulation of GDNF expression in cultured astrocytes by inflammatory stimuli. *Neuroreport, 8,* 3309–3312.

Araujo, D. M. (1992). Contrasting effects of specific lymphokines on the survival of hippocampal neurons in culture. *Advances in Behavavioral Biology, 40,* 113–122.

Araujo, D. M., & Cotman, C. W. (1991). Effects of lymphokines on glial and neuronal cells in vitro: A role for lymphokines as modulators of neural-glial interactions. *Society for Neuroscience Abstracts, 17,* 1199.

Araujo, D. M., & Cotman, C. W. (1992). Basic FGF in astroglial, microglial, and neuronal cultures: characterization of binding sites and modulation of release by lymphokines and trophic factors. *Journal of Neuroscience, 12,* 1668–1678.

Araujo, D. M., & Lapchak, P. A. (1994). Induction of immune system mediators in the hippocampal formation in Alzheimer's and Parkinson's diseases: Selective effects on specificinterleukins and interleukin receptors. *Neuroscience, 61,* 745–754.

Araujo, D. M., Lapchak, P. A., Collier, B., & Quirion, R. (1989). Localization of interleukin-2 immunoreactivity and interleukin-2 receptors in the rat brain: interaction with the cholinergic system. *Brain Research, 498,* 257–266.

Araujo, D. M., Lapchak, P. A., Collier, B., & Quirion, R. (1990). Evidence that somatostatin enhances endogenous acetylcholine release in the rat hippocampus. *Journal of Neurochemistry, 55,* 1546–1555.

Arnason, B. G., Toscas, A., Dayal, A., Qu, Z., & Noronha, A. (1997). Role of interferons in demyelinating diseases. *Journal of Neural Transmission* (suppl.), *49,* 117–123.

Arzt, E., Buric, R., Stelzer, G., Stalla, J., Sauer, J., Renner, U., & Stalla, G. K. (1993). Interleukin involvement in anterior pituitary cell growth regulation: Effects of IL-2 and IL-6. *Endocrinology, 132,* 459–467.

Arzt, E., Stelzer, G., Renner, U., Lange, M., Muller, O. A., & Stalla, G. K. (1992). Interleukin-2 and interleukin-2 receptor expression in human corticotrophic adenoma and murine pituitary cell cultures. *Journal of Clinical Investigation, 90,* 1944–1951.

Ashman, R. B., Bolitho, E. M., & Fulurija, A. (1995). Cytokine mRNA in brain tissue from mice that show strain-dependent differences in the severity of lesions induced by systemic infection with *Candida albicans* yeast. *Journal of Infectious Diseases, 172,* 823–830.

Awatsuji, H., Furukawa, Y., Nakajima, M., Furukawa, S., & Hayashi, K. (1993). Interleukin-2 as a neurotrophic factor for supporting the survival of neurons cultured from various regions of fetal rat brain. *Journal of Neuroscience Research, 35,* 305–311.

Bach, E. A., Aguet, M., & Schreiber, R. D. (1997). The IFN gamma receptor: A paradigm for cytokine receptor signaling. *Annual Review of Immunology, 15*, 563–591.

Bach, E. A., Tanner, J. W., Marsters, S., Ashkenazi, A., Aguet, M., Shaw, A. S., & Schreiber, R. D. (1996). Ligand-induced assembly and activation of the gamma interferon receptor in intact cells. *Molecular Cell Biology, 16*, 3214–3221.

Baerwald, K. D., & Popko, B. (1998). Developing and mature oligodendrocytes respond differently to the immune cytokine interferon-gamma. *Journal of Neuroscience Research, 52*, 230–239.

Balasingam, V., Tejada Berges, T., Wright, E., Bouckova, R., & Yong, V. W. (1994). Reactive astrogliosis in the neonatal mouse brain and its modulation by cytokines. *Journal of Neuroscience, 14*, 846–856.

Bamford, R. N., Battiata, A. P., Burton, J. D., Sharma, H., & Waldmann, T. A. (1996). Interleukin (IL) 15/IL-T production by the adult T-cell leukemia cell line HuT-102 is associated with a human T-cell lymphotrophic virus type I region /IL-15 fusion message that lacks many upstream AUGs that normally attenuates IL-15 mRNA translation. *Proceedings of the National Academy of Science USA, 93*, 2897–2902.

Bamford, R. N., DeFilippis, A. P., Azimi, N., Kurys, G., & Waldmann, T. A. (1998). The 5′ untranslated region, signal peptide, and the coding sequence of the carboxyl terminus of IL-15 participate in its multifaceted translational control. *Journal of Immunology, 160*, 4418–4426.

Bamford, R. N., Grant, A. J., Burton, J. D., Peters, C., Kurys, G., Goldman, C. K., Brennan, J., Roessler, E., & Waldmann, T. A. (1994). The interleukin (IL) 2 receptor beta chain is shared by IL-2 and a cytokine, provisionally designated IL-T, that stimulates T-cell proliferation and the induction of lymphokine-activated killer cells. *Proceedings of the National Academy of Science USA, 91*, 4940–4944.

Banks, W. A., & Kastin, A. J. (1991). Blood to brain transport of interleukin links the immune and central nervous systems. *Life Sciences, 48*, PL117–PL121

Banks, W. A., & Kastin, A. J. (1992). The interleukins-1 alpha, -1 beta, and -2 do not acutely disrupt the murine blood-brain barrier. *International Journal of Immunopharmacology, 14*, 629–636.

Banks, W. A., Kastin, A. J., & Durham, D. A. (1989). Bidirectional transport of interleukin-1 alpha across the blood- brain barrier. *Brain Research Bulletin, 23*, 433–437.

Banks, W. A., Kastin, A. J., & Gutierrez, E. G. (1993). Interleukin-1 alpha in blood has direct access to cortical brain cells. *Neuroscience Letters, 163*, 41–44.

Banks, W. A., Ortiz, L., Plotkin, S. R., & Kastin, A. J. (1991). Human interleukin (IL) 1 alpha, murine IL-1 alpha and murine IL- 1 beta are transported from blood to brain in the mouse by a shared saturable mechanism. *Journal of Pharmacolology and Experimental Therapeutics, 259*, 988–996.

Barford, D. (1996). Molecular mechanisms of the protein serine/threonine phosphatases. *Trends in Biochemical Sciences, 21*, 407–412.

Bartholomew, S. A., & Hoffman, S. A. (1993). Effects of peripheral cytokine injections on multiple unit activity in the anterior hypothalamic area of the mouse. *Brain Behavior and Immunity, 7*, 301–316.

Bazan, J. F. (1992). Unraveling the structure of IL-2. *Science, 257*, 410–413.

Becher, B., & Antel, J. P. (1996). Comparison of phenotypic and functional properties of immediately ex vivo and cultured human adult microglia. *Glia, 18*, 1–10.

Becher, B., D'Souza, S. D., Troutt, A. B., & Antel, J. P. (1998). Fas expression on human fetal astrocytes without susceptibility to fas-mediated cytotoxicity. *Neuroscience, 84*, 627–634.

Becher, B., Fedorowicz, V., & Antel, J. P. (1996). Regulation of CD14 expression on human adult central nervous system-derived microglia. *Journal of Neuroscience Research, 45*, 375–381.

Bentivoglio, M., Florenzano, F., Peng, Z. C., & Kristensson, K. (1994). Neuronal IFN-gamma in tuberomammillary neurones. *Neuroreport, 5*, 2413–2416.

Benveniste, E. N., Herman, P. K., & Whitaker, J. N. (1987). Myelin basic protein-specific RNA levels in interleukin-2-stimulated oligodendrocytes. *Journal of Neurochemistry, 49*, 1274–1279.

Benveniste, E. N., & Merrill, J. E. (1986). Stimulation of oligodendroglial proliferation and maturation by interleukin-2. *Nature, 321*, 610–613.

Benveniste, E. N., Whitaker, J. N., Gibbs, D. A., Sparacio, S. M., & Butler, J. L. (1989). Human B cell growth factor enhances proliferation and glial fibrillary acidic protein gene expression in rat astrocytes. *International Immunology, 1*, 219–228.

Bergsteindottir, K., Brennan, A., Jessen, K. R., & Mirsky, R. (1992). In the presence of dexamethasone, gamma interferon induces rat oligodendrocytes to express major histocompatibility complex class II molecules. *Proceedings of the National Academy of Science USA, 89*, 9054–9058.

Berhow, M. T., Hiroi, N., Kobierski, L. A., Hyman, S. E., & Nestler, E. J. (1996). Influence of cocaine on the JAK-STAT pathway in the mesolimbic dopamine system. *Journal of Neuroscience, 16*, 8019–8026.

Besedovsky, H., del Rey, A., Sorkin, E., & Dinarello, C. A. (1986). Immunoregulatory feedback between interleukin-1 and glucocorticoid hormones. *Science, 233*, 652–654.

Besedovsky, H. O., & del Rey, A. (1991). Feed-back interactions between immunological cells and the hypothalamus-pituitary-adrenal axis. *Netherlands Journal of Medicine, 39*, 274–280.

Besedovsky, H. O., & del Rey, A. (1992). Immune-neuroendocrine circuits: Integrative role of cytokines. *Frontiers in Neuroendocrinology, 13*, 61–94.

Besedovsky, H. O., & del Rey, A. (1996). Immune-neuroendocrine interactions: facts and hypotheses. *Endocrine Reviews, 17*, 64–102.

Bhat, N. R., Zhang, P., Lee, J. C., & Hogan, E. L. (1998). Extracellular signal-regulated kinase and p38 subgroups of mitogen-activated protein kinases regulate inducible nitric oxide synthase and tumor necrosis factor-alpha gene expression in endotoxin-stimulated primary glial cultures. *Journal of Neuroscience, 18*, 1633–1641.

Bhattacharya, S., Eckner, R., Grossman, S., Oldread, E., Arany, Z., D'Andrea, A., & Livingston, D. M. (1996). Cooperation of Stat2 and p300/CBP in signalling induced by interferon-alpha. *Nature, 383*, 344–347.

Bianchi, M., & Panerai, A. E. (1993). Interleukin-2 enhances scopolamine-induced amnesia and hyperactivity in the mouse. *Neuroreport, 4*, 1046–1048.

Bianchi, M., Sacerdote, P., & Panerai, A. E. (1998). Cytokines and cognitive function in mice. *Biological Signals and Receptors, 7*, 45–54.

Bindoni, M., Perciavalle, V., Beretta, S., Belluardo, N., & Diamantstein, T. (1988). Interleukin 2 modifies the bioelectric activity of some neurosecretory nuclei in the rat hypothalamus. *Brain Research, 462*, 10–14.

Birmanns, B., Saphier, D., & Abramsky, O. (1990). Alpha-interferon modifies cortical EEG activity: Dose-dependence and antagonism by naloxone. *Journal of Neurological Sciences, 100*, 22–26.

Blalock, J. E., & Smith, E. M. (1980). Human leukocyte interferon: Structural and biological relatedness to adrenocorticotropic hormone and endorphins. *Proceedings of the National Academy of Science USA, 77*, 5972–5974.

Blalock, J. E., & Smith, E. M. (1981). Human leukocyte interferon (HuIFN-alpha): Potent endorphin-like opioid activity. *Biochemical and Biophysical Research Communications, 101*, 472–478.

Blatteis, C. M. (1990). Neuromodulative actions of cytokines. *Yale Journal of Biological Medicine, 63*, 133–146.

Bodnoff, S. R., Humphreys, A. G., Lehman, J. C., Diamond, D. M., Rose, G. M., & Meaney, M. J. (1995). Enduring effects of chronic corticosterone treatment on spatial learning, synaptic plasticity, and hippocampal neuropathology in young and mid-aged rats. *Journal of Neuroscience, 15*, 61–69.

Boehm, U., Klamp, T., Groot, M., & Howard, J. C. (1997). Cellular responses to interferon-gamma. *Annual Review of Immunology, 15*, 749–795.

Bonni, A., Sun, Y., Nadal Vicens, M., Bhatt, A., Frank, D. A., Rozovsky, I., Stahl, N., Yancopoulos, G. D., & Greenberg, M. E. (1997). Regulation of gliogenesis in the central nervous system by the JAK-STAT signaling pathway. *Science, 278*, 477–483.

Borbely, A. A., & Tobler, I. (1989). Endogenous sleep-promoting substances and sleep regulation. *Physiological Reviews, 69*, 605–670.

Brandhuber, B. J., Boone, T., Kenney, W. C., & McKay, D. B. (1987). Three-dimensional structure of interleukin-2. *Science, 238*, 1707–1709.

Bredt, D. S., Glatt, C. E., Hwang, P. M., Fotuhi, M., Dawson, T. M., & Snyder, S. H. (1991). Nitric oxide synthase protein and mRNA are discretely localized in neuronal populations of the mammalian CNS together with NADPH diaphorase. *Neuron, 7*, 615–624.

Brennan, P., Babbage, J. W., Burgering, B. M., Groner, B., Reif, K., & Cantrell, D. A. (1997). Phosphatidylinositol 3-kinase couples the interleukin-2 receptor to the cell cycle regulator E2F. *Immunity, 7*, 679–689.

Brinkmeier, H., Kaspar, A., Wietholter, H., & Rudel, R. (1992). Interleukin-2 inhibits sodium currents in human muscle cells. *Pflügers Archiv, 420*, 621–623.

Brodie, C. (1996). Differential effects of Th1 and Th2 derived cytokines on NGF synthesis by mouse astrocytes. *FEBS Letters, 394*, 117–120.

Brodie, C., Blumberg, P. M., & Jacobson, K. A. (1998). Activation of the A2A adenosine receptor inhibits nitric oxide production in glial cells. *FEBS Letters, 429*, 139–142.

Brown, S. L., Smith, L. R., & Blalock, J. E. (1987). Interleukin 1 and interleukin 2 enhance proopiomelanocortin gene expression in pituitary cells. *Journal of Immunology, 139*, 3181–3183.

Burton, J. D., Bamford, R. N., Peters, C., Grant, A. J., Kurys, G., Goldman, C. K., Brennan, J., Roessler, E., & Waldmann, T. A. (1994). A lymphokine, provisionally designated interleukin T and produced by a human adult T-cell leukemia line, stimulates T-cell proliferation and the induction of lymphokine-activated killer cells. *Proceedings of the National Academy of Science USA, 91*, 4935–4939.

Calvet, M. C., & Gresser, I. (1979). Interferon enhances the excitability of cultured neurons. *Nature, 278*, 558–560.

Cambronero, J. C., Rivas, F. J., Borrell, J., & Guaza, C. (1992). Interleukin-2 induces corticotropin-releasing hormone release from superfused rat hypothalami: Influence of glucocorticoids. *Endocrinology, 131*, 677–683.

Caraceni, A., Martini, C., Belli, F., Mascheroni, L., Rivoltini, L., Arienti, F., & Cascinelli, N. (1993). Neuropsychological and neurophysiological assessment of the central effects of interleukin-2 administration. *European Journal of Cancer, 29A*, 1266–1269.

Cattaneo, E., De Fraja, C., Conti, L., Reinach, B., Bolis, L., Govoni, S., & Liboi, E. (1996). Activation of the JAK/STAT pathway leads to proliferation of ST14A central nervous system progenitor cells. *Journal of Biological Chemistry, 271*, 23374–23379.

Cesario, T. C., Vaziri, N. D., Ulich, T. R., Khamiseh, G., Oveisi, F., Rahimzadeh, M., Yousefi, S., & Pandian, M. R. (1991). Functional, biochemical, and histopathologic consequences of high-dose interleukin-2 administration in rats. *Journal of Laboratory and Clinical Medicine, 118*, 81–88.

Chabot, S., Williams, G., & Yong, V. W. (1997). Microglial production of TNF-alpha is induced by activated T lymphocytes. Involvement of VLA-4 and inhibition by interferonbeta-1b. *Journal of Clinical Investigation, 100*, 604–612.

Chang, J. Y., Martin, D. P., & Johnson, E. M. Jr. (1990). Interferon suppresses sympathetic neuronal cell death caused by nerve growth factor deprivation. *Journal of Neurochemistry, 55*, 436–445.

Chen, E. H., Gadina, M., Galon, J., Chen, M., & OShea, J. J. (1998). Not just another meeting: The coming of age of JAKs and STATs. *Immunology Today, 19*, 338–341.

Clement, H. W., Buschmann, J., Rex, S., Grote, C., Opper, C., Gemsa, D., & Wesemann, W. (1997). Effects of interferon-gamma, interleukin-1 beta, and tumor necrosis factor-alpha on the serotonin metabolism in the nucleus raphe dorsalis of the rat. *Journal of Neural Transmission, 104*, 981–991.

Colasanti, M., Cavalieri, E., Persichini, T., Mollace, V., Mariotto, S., Suzuki, H., & Lauro, G. M. (1997). Bacterial lipopolysaccharide plus interferon-gamma elicit a very fast inhibition of a Ca^{2+}-dependent nitric-oxide synthase activity in human astrocytoma cells. *Journal of Biological Chemistry, 272*, 7582–7585.

Connor, T. J., Song, C., Leonard, B. E., Merali, Z., & Anisman, H. (1998). An assessment of the effects of central interleukin-1beta, -2, - 6, and tumor necrosis factor-alpha administration on some behavioural, neurochemical, endocrine and immune parameters in the rat. *Neuroscience, 84*, 923–933.

Constant, S. L., & Bottomly, K. (1997). Induction of Th1 and Th2 $CD4^+$ T cell responses: the alternative approaches. *Annual Review of Immunology, 15*, 297–322.

Corbin, J. G., Kelly, D., Rath, E. M., Baerwald, K. D., Suzuki, K., & Popko, B. (1996). Targeted CNS expression of interferon-gamma in transgenic mice leads to hypomyelination, reactive gliosis, and abnormal cerebellar development. *Molecular and Cellular Neuroscience, 7*, 354–370.

Corradin, S. B., Mauel, J., Donini, S. D., Quattrocchi, E., & Ricciardi Castagnoli, P. (1993). Inducible nitric oxide synthase activity of cloned murine microglial cells. *Glia, 7*, 255–262.

Crnic, L. S., & Segall, M. A. (1992a). Behavioral effects of mouse interferons-alpha and -gamma and human interferon-alpha in mice. *Brain Research, 590*, 277–284.

Crnic, L. S., & Segall, M. A. (1992b). Prostaglandins do not mediate interferon-alpha effects on mouse behavior. *Physiology and Behavior, 51*, 349–352.

D'Arcangelo, G., Grassi, F., Ragozzino, D., Santoni, A., Tancredi, V., & Eusebi, F. (1991). Interferon inhibits synaptic potentiation in rat hippocampus. *Brain Research, 564*, 245–248.

Dafny, N. (1983). Interferon modifies EEG and EEG-like activity recorded from sensory, motor, and limbic system structures in freely behaving rats. *Neurotoxicology, 4*, 235–240.

Dafny, N. (1998). Is interferon-alpha a neuromodulator? *Brain Research Brain Research Reviews, 26*, 1–15.

Dafny, N., Prieto Gomez, B., Dong, W. Q., & Reyes Vazquez, C. (1996). Interferon modulates neuronal activity recorded from the hypothalamus, thalamus, hippocampus, amygdala and the somatosensory cortex. *Brain Research, 734*, 269–274.

Dafny, N., Prieto Gomez, B., & Reyes Vazquez, C. (1985). Does the immune system communicate with the central nervous system? Interferon modifies central nervous activity. *Journal of Neuroimmunology, 9*, 1–12.

Darnell, J. E. Jr. (1997). STATs and gene regulation. *Science, 277*, 1630–1635.

David, M., Petricoin, E., Benjamin, C., Pine, R., Weber, M. J., & Larner, A. C. (1995). Requirement for MAP kinase (ERK2) activity in interferon alpha- and interferon beta-stimulated gene expression through STAT proteins [see comments]. *Science, 269*, 1721–1723.

Davies, D. R., & Wlodawer, A. (1995). Cytokines and their receptor complexes. *FASEB Journal, 9*, 50–56.

de Jong, J. L., Farner, N. L., Widmer, M. B., Giri, J. G., & Sondel, P. M. (1996). Interaction of IL-15 with the shared IL-2 receptor beta and gamma c subunits. The IL-15/beta/gamma c receptor-ligand complex is less stable than the IL-2/beta/gamma c receptor-ligand complex. *Journal of Immunology, 156*, 1339–1348.

De Maeyer, E., & De Maeyer-Guignard, J. (1994). Interferons. In A. Thomsen (Ed.), *The cytokine handbook* (pp. 265–288). London: Academic Press.

De Sarro, G., Rotiroti, D., Audino, M. G., Gratteri, S., & Nistico, G. (1994). Effects of interleukin-2 on various models of experimental epilepsy in DBA/2 mice. *Neuroimmunomodulation, 1*, 361–369.

De Sarro, G. B., Masuda, Y., Ascioti, C., Audino, M. G., & Nistico, G. (1990). Behavioural and ECoG spectrum changes induced by intracerebral infusion of interferons and interleukin 2 in rats are antagonized by naloxone. *Neuropharmacology, 29*, 167–179.

De Sarro, G. B., & Nistico, G. (1990a). Behavioral and electrocortical power spectrum effects after intracerebral microinfusion of interleukin-2 in rats are antagonized by naloxone. *International Journal of Neuroscience, 51*, 209–210.

De Sarro, G. B., & Nistico, G. (1990b). Naloxone antagonizes behavioural and ECoG effects induced by systemic or intracerebral administration of some lymphokines. *Annali dell'Istituto Superiore di Sanita, 26*, 99–106.

De Simone, R., Levi, G., & Aloisi, F. (1998). Interferon gamma gene expression in rat central nervous system glial cells. *Cytokine, 10*, 418–422.

Deloria, L. B., & Mannering, G. J. (1993). Interferon induces sleep and other CNS responses in mice recovering from hexobarbital anesthesia. *Neuropharmacology, 32*, 1433–1436.

Denhardt, D. T. (1996). Signal-transducing protein phosphorylation cascades mediated by Ras/Rho proteins in the mammalian cell: The potential for multiplex signalling. *Biochemical Journal, 318*, 729–747.

Denicoff, K. D., Durkin, T. M., Lotze, M. T., Quinlan, P. E., Davis, C. L., Listwak, S. J., Rosenberg, S. A., & Rubinow, D. R. (1989). The neuroendocrine effects of interleukin-2 treatment. *Journal of Clinical Endocrinology and Metabolism, 69*, 402–410.

Denicoff, K. D., Rubinow, D. R., Papa, M. Z., Simpson, C., Seipp, C. A., Lotze, M. T., Chang, A. E., Rosenstein, D., & Rosenberg, S. A. (1987). The neuropsychiatric effects of treatment with interleukin-2 and lymphokine-activated killer cells. *Annals of Internal Medicine, 107*, 293–300.

Devos, R., Plaetinck, G., Cheroutre, H., Simons, G., Degrave, W., Tavernier, J., Remaut, E., & Fiers, W. (1983). Molecular cloning of human interleukin 2 cDNA and its expression in E. coli. *Nucleic Acids Research, 11*, 4307–4323.

Dinarello, C. A., Bernheim, H. A., Duff, G. W., Le, H. V., Nagabhushan, T. L., Hamilton, N. C., & Coceani, F. (1984). Mechanisms of fever induced by recombinant human interferon. *Journal of Clinical Investigation, 74*, 906–913.

Dinarello, C. A., & Bunn, P. A. Jr. (1997). Fever. *Seminars in Oncology, 24*, 288–298.

Dinarello, C. A., Cannon, J. G., & Wolff, S. M. (1988). New concepts on the pathogenesis of fever. *Reviews of Infectious Diseases, 10*, 168–189.

Dinarello, C. A., Novick, D., Puren, A. J., Fantuzzi, G., Shapiro, L., Muhl, H., Yoon, D. Y., Reznikov, L. L., Kim, S. H., & Rubinstein, M. (1998). Overview of interleukin-18: More than an interferon-gamma inducing factor. *Journal of Leukocyte Biology, 63*, 658–664.

Ding, M., & Merrill, J. E. (1997). The kinetics and regulation of the induction of type II nitric oxide synthase and nitric oxide in human fetal glial cell cultures. *Molecular Psychiatry, 2*, 117–119.

DiProspero, N. A., Meiners, S., & Geller, H. M. (1997). Inflammatory cytokines interact to modulate extracellular matrix and astrocytic support of neurite outgrowth. *Experimental Neurology, 148*, 628–639.

Donnelly, R. J. (1994). The type I ($\alpha/\beta/\omega/\tau$) interferon family. In N. A. Nicola (Ed.), *Guidebook to cytokines and their receptors* (pp. 111–114). Oxford: Oxford University Press.

Drew, P. D., Lonergan, M., Goldstein, M. E., Lampson, L. A., Ozato, K., & McFarlin, D. E. (1993). Regulation of MHC class I and beta 2-microglobulin gene expression in human neuronal cells. Factor binding to conserved cis-acting regulatory sequences correlates with expression of the genes. *Journal of Immunology, 150*, 3300–3310.

Dunn, A. L., & Crnic, L. S. (1993). Repeated injections of interferon-alpha A/D in Balb/c mice: Behavioral effects. *Brain Behavior and Immunity, 7*, 104–111.

Eckenstein, F. P., Baughman, R. W., & Quinn, J. (1988). An anatomical study of cholinergic innervation in rat cerebral cortex. *Neuroscience, 25*, 457–474.

Eder, C., & Heinemann, U. (1996). Proton modulation of outward K^+ currents in interferon-gamma- activated microglia. *Neuroscience Letters, 206*, 101–104.

Eitan, S., & Schwartz, M. (1993). A transglutaminase that converts interleukin-2 into a factor cytotoxic to oligodendrocytes. *Science, 261*, 106–108.

Eitan, S., Solomon, A., Lavie, V., Yoles, E., Hirschberg, D. L., Belkin, M., & Schwartz, M. (1994). Recovery of visual response of injured adult rat optic nerves treated with transglutaminase. *Science, 264*, 1764–1768.

Eitan, S., Zisling, R., Cohen, A., Belkin, M., Hirschberg, D. L., Lotan, M., & Schwartz, M. (1992). Identification of an interleukin 2-like substance as a factor cytotoxic to oligodendrocytes and associated with central nervous system regeneration. *Proceedings of the National Academy of Science USA, 89*, 5442–5446.

Eizenberg, O., Faber-Elman, A., Lotan, M., & Schwartz, M. (1995). Interleukin-2 transcripts in human and rodent brains: Possible expression by astrocytes. *Journal of Neurochemistry, 64*, 1928–1936.

Eizenberg, O., Faber Elman, A., Gottlieb, E., Oren, M., Rotter, V., & Schwartz, M. (1995). Direct involvement of p53 in programmed cell death of oligodendrocytes. *EMBO Journal, 14*, 1136–1144.

Eizenberg, O., Kaplitt, M. G., Eitan, S., Pfaff, D. W., Hirschberg, D. L., & Schwartz, M. (1994). Linear dimeric interleukin-2 obtained by the use of a defective herpes simplex viral vector: Conformation-activity relationship. *Brain Research Molecular Brain Research, 26*, 156–162.

Elion, E. A. (1998). Routing MAP kinase cascades. *Science, 281*, 1625–1626.

Ellison, M. D., Krieg, R. J., & Povlishock, J. T. (1990). Differential central nervous system responses following single and multiple recombinant interleukin-2 infusions. *Journal of Neuroimmunology, 28*, 249–260.

Ellison, M. D., & Merchant, R. E. (1991). Appearance of cytokine-associated central nervous system myelin damage coincides temporally with serum tumor necrosis factor induction after recombinant interleukin-2 infusion in rats. *Journal of Neuroimmunology, 33,* 245–251.

Endo, T. A., Masuhara, M., Yokouchi, M., Suzuki, R., Sakamoto, H., Mitsui, K., Matsumoto, A., Tanimura, S., Ohtsubo, M., Misawa, H., Miyazaki, T., Leonor, N., Taniguchi, T., Fujita, T., Kanakura, Y., Komiya, S., & Yoshimura, A. (1997). A new protein containing an SH2 domain that inhibits JAK kinases. *Nature, 387,* 921–924.

Eneroth, A., Andersson, T., Olsson, T., Orvell, C., Norrby, E., & Kristensson, K. (1992). Interferon-gamma-like immunoreactivity in sensory neurons may influence the replication of Sendai and mumps viruses. *Journal of Neuroscience Research, 31,* 487–493.

Eneroth, A., Kristensson, K., Ljungdahl, A., & Olsson, T. (1991). Interferon-gamma-like immunoreactivity in developing rat spinal ganglia neurons in vivo and in vitro. *Journal of Neurocytology, 20,* 225–231.

Erkman, L., Wuarin, L., Cadelli, D., & Kato, A. C. (1989). Interferon induces astrocyte maturation causing an increase in cholinergic properties of cultured human spinal cord cells. *Developmental Biology, 132,* 375–388.

Farrar, M. A., & Schreiber, R. D. (1993). The molecular cell biology of interferon-gamma and its receptor. *Annual Review of Immunology, 11,* 571–611.

Farrar, W. L. (1984). Endorphine modulations of lymphokine activity. In F. Fraioli, A. Isidori, & M. Mazetti (Eds.), *Opioid peptides in the periphery* (pp. 159–165). Amsterdam: Elsevier.

Fauman, E. B., & Saper, M. A. (1996). Structure and function of the protein tyrosine phosphatases. *Trends in Biochemical Sciences, 21,* 413–417.

Forman, A. D. (1994). Neurologic complications of cytokine therapy. *Oncology (Williston Park), 8,* 105–110.

Frei, K., Siepl, C., Groscurth, P., Bodmer, S., Schwerdel, C., & Fontana, A. (1987). Antigen presentation and tumor cytotoxicity by interferon-gamma-treated microglial cells. *European Journal of Immunology, 17,* 1271–1278.

Fung, M. R., Ju, G., & Greene, W. C. (1988). Co-internalization of the p55 and p70 subunits of the high-affinity human interleukin 2 receptor. Evidence for a stable ternary receptor complex. *Journal of Experimental Medicine, 168,* 1923–1928.

Funke, I., Prummer, O., Schrezenmeier, H., Hardt, D., Weiss, M., Porzsolt, F., Arnold, R., & Heimpel, H. (1994). Capillary leak syndrome associated with elevated IL-2 serum levels after allogeneic bone marrow transplantation. *Annals of Hematology, 68,* 49–52.

Gasque, P., Fontaine, M., & Morgan, B. P. (1995). Complement expression in human brain. Biosynthesis of terminal pathway components and regulators in human glial cells and cell lines. *Journal of Immunology, 154,* 4726–4733.

Gaykema, R. P. A., Luiten, P. -G. M., Nyakas, C., & Traber, J. (1990). Cortical projection patterns of the medial septum-diagonal band comlex. *Journal of Comparative Neurology, 293,* 103–124.

Giri, J. G., Ahdieh, M., Eisenman, J., Grabstein, K. H., Kumaki, S., Namen, A., Park, L. S., Cosman, D., & Anderson, D. (1994). Utilization of the beta and gamma chains of the IL-2 receptor by the novel cytokine IL-15. *EMBO Journal, 13,* 2822–2830.

Giri, J. G., Kumaki, S., Ahdieh, M., Friend, D. J., Loomis, A., Shanebeck, K., DuBose, R., Cosman, D., Park, L. S., & Anderson, D. M. (1995). Identification and cloning of a novel IL-15 binding protein that is structurally related to the alpha chain of the IL-2 receptor. *EMBO Journal, 14,* 3654–3663.

Giulian, D., Woodward, J., Young, D. G., Krebs, J. F., & Lachman, L. B. (1988). Interleukin-1 injected into mammalian brain stimulates astrogliosis and neovascularization. *Journal of Neuroscience, 8,* 2485–2490.

Giulian, D., Young, D. G., Woodward, J., Brown, D. C., & Lachman, L. B. (1988). Interleukin-1 is an astroglial growth factor in the developing brain. *Journal of Neuroscience, 8,* 709–714.

Goldsmith, M. A., & Greene, W. C. (1994). Interleukin-2 and the interleukin-2 receptor. In A. Thomsen (Ed.), *The cytokine handbook* (pp. 57–80). London: Academic Press.

Goldstein, D., Gockerman, J., Krishnan, R., Ritchie, J., Jr., Tso, C. Y., Hood, L. E., Ellinwood, E., & Laszlo, J. (1987). Effects of gamma-interferon on the endocrine system: Results from a phase I study. *Cancer Research, 47,* 6397–6401.

Gomez, J., de la Hera, A., Silva, A., Pitton, C., Garcia, A., & Rebollo, A. (1994). Implication of protein kinase C in IL-2-mediated proliferation and apoptosis in a murine T cell clone. *Experimental Cell Research, 213,* 178–182.

Goodwin, J. L., Uemura, E., & Cunnick, J. E. (1995). Microglial release of nitric oxide by the synergistic action of beta-amyloid and IFN-gamma. *Brain Research, 692,* 207–214.

Grabstein, K. H., Eisenman, J., Shanebeck, K., Rauch, C., Srinivasan, S., Fung, V., Beers, C., Richardson, J., Schoenborn, M. A., Ahdieh, M., Johnson, L., Alderson, M. R., Watson, J. D., Anderson, D. M., & Giri, J. G. (1994). Cloning of a T cell growth factor that interacts with the beta chain of the interleukin-2 receptor. *Science, 264,* 965–968.

Grau, V., Herbst, B., van der Meide, P. H., and Steiniger, B. (1997). Activation of microglial and endothelial cells in the rat brain after treatment with interferon-gamma in vivo. *Glia, 19,* 181–189.

Gray, P. W. (1994). Interferon-gamma (IFNγ). In N. A. Nicola (Ed.), *Guidebook to cytokines and their receptors* (pp. 118–119). Oxford: Oxford University Press.

Grewal, R. P., Yoshida, T., Finch, C. E., & Morgan, T. E. (1997). Scavenger receptor mRNAs in rat brain microglia are induced by kainic acid lesioning and by cytokines. *Neuroreport, 8,* 1077–1081.

Griffin, W. S., Sheng, J. G., Royston, M. C., Gentleman, S. M., McKenzie, J. E., Graham, D. I., Roberts, G. W., & Mrak, R. E. (1998). Glial-neuronal interactions in Alzheimer's disease: The potential role of a 'cytokine cycle' in disease progression. *Brain Pathology, 8,* 65–72.

Grimaldi, L. M., & Martino, G. (1995). Effect of interferon gamma on T lymphocytes from patients with multiple sclerosis. *Multiple Sclerosis, 1*(suppl 1), S38–43.

Gutierrez, E. G., Banks, W. A., & Kastin, A. J. (1993). Murine tumor necrosis factor alpha is transported from blood to brain in the mouse. *Journal of Neuroimmunology, 47,* 169–176.

Gutierrez, E. G., Banks, W. A., & Kastin, A. J. (1994). Blood-borne interleukin-1 receptor antagonist crosses the blood-brain barrier. *Journal of Neuroimmunology, 55,* 153–160.

Hafen, E. (1998). Kinases and phosphatases—a marriage is consummated. *Science, 280,* 1212–1213.

Haga, S., Aizawa, T., Ishii, T., & Ikeda, K. (1996). Complement gene expression in mouse microglia and astrocytes in culture: Comparisons with mouse peritoneal macrophages. *Neuroscience Letters, 216,* 191–194.

Hall, G. L., Compston, A., & Scolding, N. J. (1997). Beta-interferon and multiple sclerosis. *Trends in Neurosciences, 20,* 63–67.

Hall, G. L., Wing, M. G., Compston, D. A., & Scolding, N. J. (1997). beta-Interferon regulates the immunomodulatory activity of neonatal rodent microglia. *Journal of Neuroimmunology, 72,* 11–19.

Hamm, S., Rudel, R., & Brinkmeier, H. (1996). Excitatory sodium currents of NH15-CA2 neuroblastoma x glioma hybrid cells are differently affected by interleukin-2 and interleukin-1beta. *Pflügers Archiv*, *433*, 160–165.

Hanisch, U. K., Kar, S., Rowe, W., Sharma, S., Beffert, U., Meaney, M. J., Poirier, J., & Quirion, R. (1993). Neurotoxic and neuroendocrine consequences of chronic intracerebroventricular administration of the T cell growth factor interleukin-2 in rats. *Society for Neuroscience Abstracts*, *19*, 504.

Hanisch, U. K., Lyons, S. A., Prinz, M., Nolte, C., Weber, J. R., Kettenmann, H., & Kirchhoff, F. (1997a). Mouse brain microglia express interleukin-15 and its multimeric receptor complex functionally coupled to Janus kinase activity. *Journal of Biological Chemistry*, *272*, 28853–28860.

Hanisch, U. K., Neuhaus, J., Quirion, R., & Kettenmann, H. (1996). Neurotoxicity induced by interleukin-2: Involvement of infiltrating immune cells. *Synapse*, *24*, 104–114.

Hanisch, U. K., Neuhaus, J., Rowe, W., van Rossum, D., Moller, T., Kettenmann, H., & Quirion, R. (1997). Neurotoxic consequences of central long-term administration of interleukin-2 in rats. *Neuroscience*, *79*, 799–818.

Hanisch, U. K., & Quirion, R. (1996). Interleukin-2 as a neuroregulatory cytokine. *Brain Research Reviews*, *21*, 246–284.

Hanisch, U. K., Rothe, T., Krohn, K., & Dykes, R. W. (1992). Muscarinic cholinergic receptor binding in rat hindlimb somatosensory cortex following partial deafferentation by sciatic nerve transection. *Neurochemistry International*, *21*, 313–327.

Hanisch, U. K., Rowe, W., Sharma, S., Meaney, M. J., & Quirion, R. (1994). Hypothalamic-pituitary-adrenal activity during chronic central administration of interleukin-2. *Endocrinology*, *135*, 2465–2472.

Hanisch, U. K., Rowe, W., van Rossum, D., Meaney, M. J., & Quirion, R. (1996). Phasic hyperactivity of the HPA axis resulting from chronic central IL-2 administration. *Neuroreport*, *7*, 2883–2888.

Hanisch, U. K., Seto, D., & Quirion, R. (1993). Modulation of hippocampal acetylcholine release: A potent central action of interleukin-2. *Journal of Neuroscience*, *13*, 3368–3374.

Hart, R. P., Shadiack, A. M., & Jonakait, G. M. (1991). Substance P gene expression is regulated by interleukin-1 in cultured sympathetic ganglia. *Journal of Neuroscience Research*, *29*, 282–291.

Hartung, H. P., Schafer, B., van der Meide, P. H., Fierz, W., Heininger, K., & Toyka, K. V. (1990). The role of interferon-gamma in the pathogenesis of experimental autoimmune disease of the peripheral nervous system. *Annals of Neurology*, *27*, 247–257.

Hatakeyama, M., Kawahara, A., Mori, H., Shibuya, H., & Taniguchi, T. (1992). c-fos gene induction by interleukin 2: Identification of the critical cytoplasmic regions within the interleukin 2 receptor beta chain. *Proceedings of the National Academy of Science USA*, *89*, 2022–2026.

Hatakeyama, M., & Taniguchi, T. (1991). Interleukin-2. In M. B. Sporn and A. B. Roberts (Eds.), *Peptide growth factors and their receptors I* (pp. 523–540). New York: Springer Verlag.

Haugen, P. K., & Letourneau, P. C. (1990). Interleukin-2 enhances chick and rat sympathetic, but not sensory, neurite outgrowth. *Journal of Neuroscience Research*, *25*, 443–452.

Heim, M. H. (1996). The Jak-STAT pathway: Specific signal transduction from the cell membrane to the nucleus. *European Journal of Clinical Investigation*, *26*, 1–12.

Hellendall, R. P., & Ting, J. P. (1997). Differential regulation of cytokine-induced major histocompatibility complex class II expression and nitric oxide release in rat microglia and astrocytes by effectors of tyrosine kinase, protein kinase C, and cAMP. *Journal of Neuroimmunology*, *74*, 19–29.

Hillhouse, E. W. (1994). Interleukin-2 stimulates the secretion of arginine vasopressin but not corticotropin-releasing hormone from rat hypothalamic cells in vitro. *Brain Research*, *650*, 323–325.

Hooks, J. J., Chader, G., Evans, C. H., & Detrick, B. (1990). Interferon-gamma enhances the expression of retinal S-antigen, a specific neuronal cell marker. *Journal of Neuroimmunology*, *26*, 245–250.

Hopkins, S. J., & Rothwell, N. J. (1995). Cytokines and the nervous system I: Expression and recognition. *Trends in Neurosciences*, *18*, 83–88.

Hori, T., Nakashima, T., Take, S., Kaizuka, Y., Mori, T., & Katafuchi, T. (1991). Immune cytokines and regulation of body temperature, food intake and cellular immunity. *Brain Research Bulletin*, *27*, 309–313.

Horwitz, M. S., Evans, C. F., McGavern, D. B., Rodriguez, M., & Oldstone, M. B. (1997). Primary demyelination in transgenic mice expressing interferon-gamma. *Nature Medicine*, *3*, 1037–1041.

Htain, W. W., Leong, S. K., & Ling, E. A. (1997). In vivo expression of inducible nitric oxide synthase in supraventricular amoeboid microglial cells in neonatal BALB/c and athymic mice. *Neuroscience Letters*, *223*, 53–56.

Hu, S., Peterson, P. K., & Chao, C. C. (1997). Cytokine-mediated neuronal apoptosis. *Neurochemistry International*, *30*, 427–431.

Hu, S., Sheng, W. S., Peterson, P. K., & Chao, C. C. (1995). Differential regulation by cytokines of human astrocyte nitric oxide production. *Glia*, *15*, 491–494.

Hua, L. L., Liu, J. S., Brosnan, C. F., & Lee, S. C. (1998). Selective inhibition of human glial inducible nitric oxide synthase by interferon-beta: Implications for multiple sclerosis. *Annals of Neurology*, *43*, 384–387.

Huberman, M., Shalit, F., Roth Deri, I., Gutman, B., Brodie, C., Kott, E., & Sredni, B. (1994). Correlation of cytokine secretion by mononuclear cells of Alzheimer patients and their disease stage. *Journal of Neuroimmunology*, *52*, 147–152.

Hunter, K. E., Sporn, M. B., & Davies, A. M. (1993). Transforming growth factor-betas inhibit mitogen-stimulated proliferation of astrocytes. *Glia*, *7*, 203–211.

Ihle, J. N. (1995). Cytokine receptor signalling. *Nature*, *377*, 591–594.

Ihle, J. N. (1996). STATs: Signal transducers and activators of transcription. *Cell*, *84*, 331–334.

Improta, T., Salvatore, A. M., Di Luzio, A., Romeo, G., Coccia, E. M., & Calissano, P. (1988). IFN-gamma facilitates NGF-induced neuronal differentiation in PC12 cells. *Experimental Cell Research*, *179*, 1–9.

Isaacs, A., & Lindenmann, J. (1957). Virus interference. I. The interferon. *Proceedings of the Royal Society London Series B*, *147*, 258–267.

Issa, A. M., Rowe, W., Gauthier, S., & Meaney, M. J. (1990). Hypothalamic-pituitary-adrenal activity in aged, cognitively impaired and cognitively unimpaired rats. *Journal of Neuroscience*, *10*, 3247–3254.

Jacoby, D. B., Xiao, H. Q., Lee, N. H., Chan Li, Y., & Fryer, A. D. (1998). Virus- and interferon-induced loss of inhibitory M2 muscarinic receptor function and gene expression in cultured airway parasympathetic neurons. *Journal of Clinical Investigation*, *102*, 242–248.

Jaffe, H. S. (1992). The interferons: A clinical overview. In H. S. Jaffe, L. R. Bucalo, & S. A. Sherwin (Eds.), *Anti-infective applications of interferon-gamma* (pp. 1–7). New York: Marcel Dekker.

Janabi, N., Mirshahi, A., Wolfrom, C., Mirshahi, M., & Tardieu, M. (1996). Effect of interferon gamma and TNF alpha on the differentiation/activation of human glial cells: Implication for the TNF alpha receptor 1. *Research in Virology*, *147*, 147–153.

Janssen, R. A. J., Mulder, N. H., The, T. H., & de Leij, L. (1994). The immunobiological effects of interleukin-2 in vivo. *Cancer Immunology Immunotherapy, 39*, 207–216.

Jeohn, G. H., Kong, L. Y., Wilson, B., Hudson, P., & Hong, J. S. (1998). Synergistic neurotoxic effects of combined treatments with cytokines in murine primary mixed neuron/glia cultures. *Journal of Neuroimmunology, 85*, 1–10.

Jiang, H., Milo, R., Swoveland, P., Johnson, K. P., Panitch, H., & Dhib Jalbut, S. (1995). Interferon beta-1b reduces interferon gamma-induced antigen-presenting capacity of human glial and B cells. *Journal of Neuroimmunology, 61*, 17–25.

Johnston, J. A., Bacon, C. M., Finbloom, D. S., Rees, R. C., Kaplan, D., Shibuya, K., Ortaldo, J. R., Gupta, S., Chen, Y. Q., Giri, J. D., & O'Shea, J. J. (1995). Tyrosine phosphorylation and activation of STAT5, STAT3, and Janus kinases by interleukins 2 and 15. *Proceedings of the National Academy of Science USA, 92*, 8705–8709.

Joly, E., & Oldstone, M. B. (1992). Neuronal cells are deficient in loading peptides onto MHC class I molecules. *Neuron, 8*, 1185–1190.

Jonakait, G. M., Luskin, M. B., Wei, R., Tian, X. F., & Ni, L. (1996). Conditioned medium from activated microglia promotes cholinergic differentiation in the basal forebrain in vitro. *Developmental Biology, 177*, 85–95.

Jonakait, G. M., Wei, R., Sheng, Z. L., Hart, R. P., & Ni, L. (1994). Interferon-gamma promotes cholinergic differentiation of embryonic septal nuclei and adjacent basal forebrain. *Neuron, 12*, 1149–1159.

Jones, T. H., & Kennedy, R. L. (1993). Cytokines and hypothalamic-pituitary function. *Cytokine, 5*, 531–538.

Kahn, M. A., Huang, C. J., Caruso, A., Barresi, V., Nazarian, R., Condorelli, D. F., & De Vellis, J. (1997). Ciliary neurotrophic factor activates JAK/Stat signal transduction cascade and induces transcriptional expression of glial fibrillary acidic protein in glial cells. *Journal of Neurochemistry, 68*, 1413–1423.

Kakiuchi, T., Tamura, T., Gyotoku, Y., & Nariuchi, H. (1991). IL-2 production by B cells stimulated with a specific antigen. *Cellular Immunology, 138*, 207–215.

Kanno, Y., Kozak, C. A., Schindler, C., Driggers, P. H., Ennist, D. L., Gleason, S. L., Darnell, J. E. Jr., & Ozato, K. (1993). The genomic structure of the murine ICSBP gene reveals the presence of the gamma interferon-responsive element, to which an ISGF3 alpha subunit (or similar) molecule binds. *Molecular Cell Biology, 13*, 3951–3963.

Karanth, S., Aguila, M. C., & McCann, S. M. (1993). The influence of interleukin-2 on the release of somatostatin and growth hormone-releasing hormone by mediobasal hypothalamus. *Neuroendocrinology, 58*, 185–190.

Karanth, S., Krzysztof, L., & McCann, S. M. (1993). Role of nitric oxide in interleukin 2-induced corticotropin-releasing factor release from incubated hypothalami. *Proceedings of the National Academy of Sciences USA, 90*, 3383–3387.

Karanth, S., Marubayashi, U., & McCann, S. M. (1992). Influence of dopamine on the altered release of prolactin, luteinizing hormone, and follicle-stimulating hormone induced by interleukin-2 in vitro. *Neuroendocrinology, 56*, 871–880.

Karanth, S., & McCann, S. M. (1991). Anterior pituitary hormone control by interleukin 2. *Proceedings of the National Academy of Sciences USA, 88*, 2961–2965.

Karp, B. I., Yang, J. C., Khorsand, M., Wood, R., & Merigan, T. C. (1996). Multiple cerebral lesions complicating therapy with interleukin-2. *Neurology, 47*, 417–424.

Kaspar, A., Brinkmeier, H., & Rudel, R. (1994). Local anaesthetic-like effect of interleukin-2 on muscular Na^+ channels: No evidence for involvement of the IL-2 receptor. *Pflügers Archiv, 426*, 61–67.

Kidron, D., Saphier, D., Ovadia, H., Weidenfeld, J., & Abramsky, O. (1989). Central administration of immunomodulatory factors alters neural activity and adrenocortical secretion. *Brain, Behavior, and Immunity, 3*, 15–27.

Kiefer, R., Haas, C. A., & Kreutzberg, G. W. (1991). Gamma interferon-like immunoreactive material in rat neurons: Evidence against a close relationship to gamma interferon. *Neuroscience, 45*, 551–560.

Kiefer, R., & Kreutzberg, G. W. (1990). Gamma interferon-like immunoreactivity in the rat nervous system. *Neuroscience, 37*, 725–734.

Kimura, M., Majde, J. A., Toth, L. A., Opp, M. R., & Krueger, J. M. (1994). Somnogenic effects of rabbit and recombinant human interferons in rabbits. *American Journal of Physiology, 267*, R53–61.

Kirken, R. A., Malabarba, M. G., Xu, J., DaSilva, L., Erwin, R. A., Liu, X., Hennighausen, L., Rui, H., & Farrar, W. L. (1997). Two discrete regions of interleukin-2 (IL2) receptor beta independently mediate IL2 activation of a PD98059/rapamycin/wortmannin-insensitive Stat5a/b serine kinase. *Journal of Biological Chemistry, 272*, 15459–15465.

Kitamura, Y., Furukawa, M., Matsuoka, Y., Tooyama, I., Kimura, H., Nomura, Y., & Taniguchi, T. (1998). In vitro and in vivo induction of heme oxygenase-1 in rat glial cells: Possible involvement of nitric oxide production from inducible nitric oxide synthase. *Glia, 22*, 138–148.

Kloss, C. U., Kreutzberg, G. W., & Raivich, G. (1997). Proliferation of ramified microglia on an astrocyte monolayer: Characterization of stimulatory and inhibitory cytokines. *Journal of Neuroscience Research, 49*, 248–254.

Kloth, S., Flad, H. D., & Brandt, E. (1994). Detection of intracellular interleukin 2: Evidence for novel immunologically related forms of the lymphokine. *Cytokine, 6*, 349–357.

Klyushnenkova, E. N., & Vanguri, P. (1997). Ia expression and antigen presentation by glia: Strain and cell type-specific differences among rat astrocytes and microglia. *Journal of Neuroimmunology, 79*, 190–201.

Koenig, J. I. (1991). Presence of cytokines in the hypothalamic-pituitary axis. *Progress in NeuroEndocrinImmunology, 4*, 143–153.

Kreutzberg, G. W. (1996). Microglia: A sensor for pathological events in the CNS. *Trends in Neurosciences, 19*, 312–318.

Krishnan, R., Ellinwood, E. H. Jr., Laszlo, J., Hood, L., & Ritchie, J. (1987). Effect of gamma interferon on the hypothalamic-pituitary-adrenal system. *Biological Psychiatry, 22*, 1163–1166.

Kristensson, K., Aldskogius, M., Peng, Z. C., Olsson, T., Aldskogius, H., & Bentivoglio, M. (1994). Co-induction of neuronal interferon-gamma and nitric oxide synthase in rat motor neurons after axotomy: A role in nerve repair or death? *Journal of Neurocytology, 23*, 453–459.

Kroemer, G., Andreu, J. L., Gonzalo, J. A., Gutierrez Ramos, J. C., & Martinez, C. (1991). Interleukin-2, autotolerance, and autoimmunity. *Advances in Immunology, 50*, 147–235.

Krueger, J. M., Dinarello, C. A., Shoham, S., Davenne, D., Walter, J., & Kubillus, S. (1987). Interferon alpha-2 enhances slow-wave sleep in rabbits. *International Journal of Immunopharmacology, 9*, 23–30.

Krueger, J. M., & Majde, J. A. (1994). Microbial products and cytokines in sleep and fever regulation. *Critical Reviews of Immunology, 14*, 355–379.

Kuchinke, W., Hart, R. P., & Jonakait, G. M. (1995). Identification of mRNAs regulated by interferon-gamma in cultured rat astrocytes by PCR differential display. *Neuroimmunomodulation, 2,* 347–355.

Kugaya, A., Kagaya, A., Uchitomi, Y., Yokota, N., & Yamawaki, S. (1996). Effect of interferon-alpha on DOI-induced wet-dog shakes in rats. *Journal of Neural Transmission, 103,* 947–955.

Kumaki, S., Ochs, H. D., Timour, M., Schooley, K., Ahdieh, M., Hill, H., Sugamura, K., Anderson, D., Zhu, Q., & Cosman, D. (1995). Characterization of B-cell lines established from two X-linked severe combined immunodeficiency patients: Interleukin-15 binds to the B cells but is not internalized efficiently. *Blood, 86,* 1428–1436.

Kuriyama, K., Hori, T., Mori, T., & Nakashima, T. (1990). Actions of interferon alpha and interleukin-1 beta on the glucose-responsive neurons in the ventromedial hypothalamus. *Brain Research Bulletin, 24,* 803–810.

Lafortune, L., Nalbantoglu, J., & Antel, J. P. (1996). Expression of tumor necrosis factor alpha (TNF alpha) and interleukin 6 (IL-6) mRNA in adult human astrocytes: Comparison with adult microglia and fetal astrocytes. *Journal of Neuropathology and Experimental Neurology, 55,* 515–521.

Lai, S. Y., Xu, W., Gaffen, S. L., Liu, K. D., Longmore, G. D., Greene, W. C., & Goldsmith, M. A. (1996). The molecular role of the common gamma c subunit in signal transduction reveals functional asymmetry within multimeric cytokine receptor complexes. *Proceedings of the National Academy of Science USA, 93,* 231–235.

Lamb, P., Tapley, P., & Rosen, J. (1998). Biochemical approaches to discovering modulators of the JAK-STAT pathway. *Drug Discovery Today, 3,* 122–130.

Langer, J., Garotta, G., & Pestka, S. (1996). Interferon receptors. *Biotherapy, 8,* 163–174.

Lapchak, P. A. (1992). A role for interleukin-2 in the regulation of striatal dopaminergic function. *Neuroreport, 3,* 165–168.

Lapchak, P. A., & Araujo, D. M. (1993). Interleukin-2 regulates monoamine and opioid peptide release from the hypothalamus. *Neuroreport, 4,* 303–306.

Lapchak, P. A., Araujo, D. M., & Collier, B. (1989). Regulation of endogenous acetylcholine release from mammalian brain slices by opiate receptors: Hippocampus, striatum and cerebral cortex of guinea-pig and rat. *Neuroscience, 31,* 313–325.

Lapchak, P. A., Araujo, D. M., Quirion, R., & Beaudet, A. (1990). Neurotensin regulation of endogenous acetylcholine release from rat cerebral cortex: Effect of quinolinic acid lesions of the basal forebrain. *Journal of Neurochemistry, 55,* 1397–1403.

Lapchak, P. A., Araujo, D. M., Quirion, R., & Beaudet, A. (1991). Immunoautoradiographic localization of interleukin 2-like immunoreactivity and interleukin 2 receptors (Tac antigen-like immunoreactivity) in the rat brain. *Neuroscience, 44,* 173–184.

Lapchak, P. A., Araujo, D. M., Quirion, R., & Collier, B. (1989). Binding sites for [^{3}H]AF-DX 116 and effect of AF-DX 116 on endogenous acetylcholine release from rat brain slices. *Brain Research, 496,* 285–294.

Lee, Y. B., Satoh, J.-I., Walker, D. G., & Kim, S. U. (1996). Interleukin-15 gene expression in human astrocytes and microglia in culture. *Neuroreport, 7,* 1062–1066.

Legrue, S. J., Sheu, T. L., & Chernajovsky, Y. (1991). The role of receptor-ligand endocytosis and degradation in interleukin-2 signaling and T-lymphocyte proliferation. *Lymphokine and Cytokine Research, 10,* 431–436.

Leonard, W. J. (1996a). STATs and cytokine specificity. *Nature Medicine, 2,* 968–969.

Leonard, W. J. (1996b). The molecular basis of X-linked severe combined immunodeficiency: Defective cytokine receptor signaling. *Annual Review of Medicine, 47,* 229–239.

Leonard, W. J., & O'Shea, J. J. (1998). Jaks and STATs: Biological implications. *Annual Review of Immunology, 16,* 293–322.

Levi, F., Canon, C., Deprés-Brummer, P., Adam, R., Bourin, P., Pati, A., Florentin, I., Misset, J. L., & Bismuth, H. (1992). The rhythmic organization of the immune network: Implications for the chronopharmacologic delivery of interferons, interleukins and cyclosporin. *Advances in Drug Delivery Reviews, 9,* 85–112.

Lin, J. X., Migone, T. S., Tsang, M., Friedmann, M., Weatherbee, J. A., Zhou, L., Yamauchi, A., Bloom, E. T., Mietz, J., & John, S. (1995). The role of shared receptor motifs and common Stat proteins in the generation of cytokine pleiotropy and redundancy by IL-2, IL-4, IL-7, IL-13, and IL-15. *Immunity, 2,* 331–339.

Linda, H., Hammarberg, H., Cullheim, S., Levinovitz, A., Khademi, M., & Olsson, T. (1998). Expression of MHC class I and beta2-microglobulin in rat spinal motoneurons: Regulatory influences by IFN-gamma and axotomy. *Experimental Neurology, 150,* 282–295.

Lisak, R. P., & Bealmear, B. (1992). Differences in the capacity of gamma-interferons from different species to induce class I and II major histocompatibility complex antigens on neonatal rat Schwann cells in vitro. *Pathobiology, 60,* 322–329.

Lissoni, P., Barni, S., Cattaneo, G., Archili, C., Crispino, S., Tancini, G., D'Angelo, L., Magni, S., & Fiorelli, G. (1990). Activation of the complement system during immunotherapy of cancer with interleukin-2: A possible explanation of the capillary leak syndrome. *International Journal of Biological Markers, 5,* 195–197.

Liu, J. S., Amaral, T. D., Brosnan, C. F., & Lee, S. C. (1998). IFNs are critical regulators of IL-1 receptor antagonist and IL-1 expression in human microglia. *Journal of Immunology, 161,* 1989–1996.

Ljungdahl, A., Olsson, T., van der Meide, P. H., Holmdahl, R., Klareskog, L., & Hojeberg, B. (1989). Interferon-gamma-like immunoreactivity in certain neurons of the central and peripheral nervous system. *Journal of Neuroscience Research, 24,* 451–456.

Lonart, G., Wang, J., & Johnson, K. M. (1992). Nitric oxide induces neurotransmitter release from hippocampal slices. *European Journal of Pharmacology, 220,* 271–272.

Lorenzon, P., Ruzzier, F., Caratsch, C. G., Giovannelli, A., Velotti, F., Santoni, A., & Eusebi, F. (1991). Interleukin-2 lengthens extrajunctional acetylcholine receptor channel open time in mammalian muscle cells. *Pflügers Archiv, 419,* 380–385.

Lotze, M. T., Matory, Y. L., Rayner, A. A., Ettinghausen, S. E., Vetto, J. T., Seipp, C. A., & Roisenberg, S. A. (1986). Clinical effects and toxicity of interleukin-2 in patients with cancer. *Cancer, 58,* 2764–2772.

Loughlin, A. J., & Woodroofe, M. N. (1996). Inhibitory effect of interferon-gamma on LPS-induced interleukin 1 beta production by isolated adult rat brain microglia. *Neurochemistry International, 29,* 77–82.

Loughlin, A. J., Woodroofe, M. N., & Cuzner, M. L. (1992). Regulation of Fc receptor and major histocompatibility complex antigen expression on isolated rat microglia by tumour necrosis factor, interleukin-1 and lipopolysaccharide: Effects on interferon-gamma induced activation. *Immunology, 75,* 170–175.

Loughlin, A. J., Woodroofe, M. N., & Cuzner, M. L. (1993). Modulation of interferon-gamma-induced major histocompatibility complex class II and Fc receptor expression on isolated microglia by transforming growth factor-beta 1, interleukin-4, noradrenaline and glucocorticoids. *Immunology, 79,* 125–130.

Lu, Y., & Durkin, J. P. (1997). Protein kinase C in IL-2 signal transduction. *Immunologic Research, 16,* 355–374.

Luber-Narod, J., & Rogers, J. (1988). Immune system associated antigens expressed by cells of the human central nervous system. *Neuroscience Letters, 94,* 17–22.

Lundkvist, G. B., Robertson, B., Mhlanga, J. D., Rottenberg, M. E., & Kristensson, K. (1998). Expression of an oscillating interferon-gamma receptor in the suprachiasmatic nuclei. *Neuroreport, 9*, 1059–1063.

Lupien, S. J., de Leon, M., de Santi, S., Convit, A., Tarshish, C., Nair, N. P. V., Thakur, M., McEwen, B. S., Hauger, R. L., & Meaney, M. J. (1998). Cortisol levels during human aging predict hippocampal atrophy and memory deficits. *Nature Neuroscience, 1*, 69–73.

Mai, Z., Kousoulas, K. G., Horohov, D. W., & Klei, T. R. (1994). Cross-species PCR cloning of gerbil (*Meriones unguiculatus*) interleukin-2 cDNA and its expression in COS-7 cells. *Veterinary Immunology and Immunopathology, 40*, 63–71.

Maness, L. M., Banks, W. A., Zadina, J. E., & Kastin, A. J. (1995). Selective transport of blood-borne interleukin-1 alpha into the posterior division of the septum of the mouse brain. *Brain Research, 700*, 83–88.

Margolin, K. A., Rayner, A. A., Hawkins, M. J., Atkins, M. B., Dutcher, J. P., Fisher, R. I., Weiss, G. R., Doroshow, J. H., Jaffe, H. S., Roper, M., & et al. (1989). Interleukin-2 and lymphokine-activated killer cell therapy of solid tumors: Analysis of toxicity and management guidelines. *Journal of Clinical Oncology, 7*, 486–498.

Martin, R. (1997). Immunological aspects of experimental allergic encephalomyelitis and multiple sclerosis and their application for new therapeutic strategies. *Journal of Neural Transmission*, 49, (suppl.) 53–67.

Maslinski, W., Remillard, B., Tsudo, M., & Strom, T. B. (1993). Interleukin-2 receptor signal transduction: Translocation of active serine-threonine kinase Raf-1 from IL-2 receptor into cytosol depends on IL-2-induced tyrosine kinase activation. *Transplantation Proceedings, 25*, 109–110.

Mattson, K., Niiranen, A., Iivanainen, M., Farkkila, M., Bergstrom, L., Holsti, L. R., Kauppinen, H. L., & Cantell, K. (1983). Neurotoxicity of interferon. *Cancer Treatment Reports, 67*, 958–961.

McCann, S. M., Karanth, S., Kamat, A., Les Dees, W., Lyson, K., Gimeno, M., & Rettori, V. (1994). Induction by cytokines of the pattern of pituitary hormone secretion in infection. *Neuroimmunomodulation, 1*, 2–13.

McCombe, P. A., Nickson, I., & Pender, M. P. (1998). Cytokine expression by inflammatory cells obtained from the spinal cords of Lewis rats with experimental autoimmune encephalomyelitis induced by inoculation with myelin basic protein and adjuvants. *Journal of Neuroimmunology, 88*, 30–38.

McGeer, E. G., & McGeer, P. L. (1997). The role of the immune system in neurodegenerative disorders. *Movement Disorders, 12*, 855–858.

McGeer, P. L., Itagaki, S., Tago, H., & McGeer, E. G. (1987). Expression of HLA-DR and interleukin-2 receptors on reactive microglia in senile dimentia of the Alzheimer type. *Journal of Neuroimmunology, 16*, 122–129.

McKay, D. B. (1992). Unraveling the structure of IL-2 [Response]. *Science, 257*, 412–413.

McKnight, A. J., & Classon, B. J. (1992). Biochemical and immunological properties of rat recombinant interleukin-2 and interleukin-4. *Immunology, 75*, 286–292.

McLarnon, J. G., Xu, R., Lee, Y. B., & Kim, S. U. (1997). Ion channels of human microglia in culture. *Neuroscience, 78*, 1217–1228.

McManus, C. M., Brosnan, C. F., & Berman, J. W. (1998). Cytokine induction of MIP-1 alpha and MIP-1 beta in human fetal microglia. *Journal of Immunology, 160*, 1449–1455.

McRae, A., Dahlstrom, A., & Ling, E. A. (1997). Microglial in neurodegenerative disorders: Emphasis on Alzheimer's disease. *Gerontology, 43*, 95–108.

Meaney, M. J., Aitken, D. H., Sharma, S., & Viau, V. (1992). Basal ACTH, corticosterone and corticosterone-binding globulin levels over the diurnal cycle, and age-related changes in hippocampal type I and type II corticosteroid receptor binding capacity in young and aged, handled and nonhandled rats. *Neuroendocrinology, 55*, 204–213.

Meazza, R., Verdiani, S., Biassoni, R., Coppolecchia, M., Gaggero, A., Orengo, A. M., Colombo, M. P., Azzarone, B., & Ferrini, S. (1996). Identification of a novel interleukin 15 (IL-15) transcript isoform generated by alternative splicing in human small cell lung cancer cell lines. *Oncogene, 12*, 2187–2192.

Meda, L., Bernasconi, S., Bonaiuto, C., Sozzani, S., Zhou, D., Otvos, L. Jr., Mantovani, A., Rossi, F., & Cassatella, M. A. (1996). Beta-amyloid (25–35) peptide and IFN-gamma synergistically induce the production of the chemotactic cytokine MCP-1/JE in monocytes and microglial cells. *Journal of Immunology, 157*, 1213–1218.

Meda, L., Cassatella, M. A., Szendrei, G. I., Otvos, L. Jr., Baron, P., Villalba, M., Ferrari, D., & Rossi, F. (1995). Activation of microglial cells by beta-amyloid protein and interferon-gamma. *Nature, 374*, 647–650.

Menendez Iglesias, B., Cerase, J., Ceracchini, C., Levi, G., & Aloisi, F. (1997). Analysis of B7-1 and B7-2 costimulatory ligands in cultured mouse microglia: Upregulation by interferon-gamma and lipopolysaccharide and downregulation by interleukin-10, prostaglandin E2 and cyclic AMP-elevating agents. *Journal of Neuroimmunology, 72*, 83–93.

Mennicken, F., Mazzoni, I. E., Kenigsberg, R. L., & Quirion, R. (1994). Interleukin-2 stimulates cholinergic neurons in septal cell cultures. *Society for Neuroscience Abstracts, 20*, 667.

Mennicken, F., & Quirion, R. (1995). Cytokines such as interleukin(IL)-2, IL-4, IL-7, IL-15 and LIF on the expression of the cholinergic phenotype in rat septal neuronal cultures. *Society for Neuroscience Abstracts, 21*, 1051.

Mennicken, F., & Quirion, R. (1997). Interleukin-2 increases choline acetyltransferase activity in septal-cell cultures. *Synapse, 26*, 175–183.

Menzies, R., Phelps, C., Wiranowska, M., Oliver, J., Chen, L., Horvath, E., & Hall, N. (1996). The effect of interferon-alpha on the pituitary-adrenal axis. *Journal of Interferon and Cytokine Research, 16*, 619–629.

Menzies, R. A., Patel, R., Hall, N. R., O'Grady, M. P., & Rier, S. E. (1992). Human recombinant interferon alpha inhibits naloxone binding to rat brain membranes. *Life Sciences, 50*, PL227– 232.

Meraz, M. A., White, J. M., Sheehan, K. C., Bach, E. A., Rodig, S. J., Dighe, A. S., Kaplan, D. H., Riley, J. K., Greenlund, A. C., Campbell, D., Carver Moore, K., DuBois, R. N., Clark, R., Aguet, M., & Schreiber, R. D. (1996). Targeted disruption of the Stat1 gene in mice reveals unexpected physiologic specificity in the JAK-STAT signaling pathway. *Cell, 84*, 431–442.

Merchant, R. E., Ellison, M. D., & Young, H. F. (1990). Immunotherapy for malignant glioma using human recombinant interleukin-2 and activated autologous lymphocytes. A review of pre-clinical and clinical investigations. *Journal of Neurooncology, 8*, 173–188.

Merrill, J. E. (1990). Interleukin-2 effects in the central nervous system. *Annals of the New York Academy of Sciences, 594*, 188–199.

Merrill, J. E. (1991). Bellini, Carpaccio, and receptors in the central nervous system. *Journal of Cell Biochemistry, 46*, 191–198.

Merrill, J. E. (1992). Proinflammatory and antiinflammatory cytokines in multiple sclerosis and central nervous system acquired immunodeficiency syndrome. *Journal of Immunotherapy, 12*, 167–170.

Merrill, J. E., & Benveniste, E. N. (1996). Cytokines in inflammatory brain lesions: Helpful and harmful. *Trends in Neurosciences, 19*, 331–338.

Merrill, J. E., Ignarro, L. J., Sherman, M. P., Melinek, J., & Lane, T. E. (1993). Microglial cell cytotoxicity of oligodendrocytes is mediated through nitric oxide. *Journal of Immunology, 151*, 2132–2141.

Merrill, J. E., & Zimmerman, R. P. (1991). Natural and induced cytotoxicity of oligodendrocytes by microglia is inhibitable by TGF beta. *Glia, 4*, 327–331.

Meyers, C. A., & Abbruzzese, J. L. (1992). Cognitive functioning in cancer patients: Effect of previous treatment. *Neurology, 42*, 434–436.

Meyers, C. A., Scheibel, R. S., & Forman, A. D. (1991). Persistent neurotoxicity of systemically administered interferon-alpha. *Neurology, 41*, 672–676.

Meyers, C. A., & Yung, W. K. (1993). Delayed neurotoxicity of intraventricular interleukin-2: A case report. *Journal of Neurooncology, 15*, 265–267.

Michon, J., Negrier, S., Coze, C., Mathiot, C., Frappaz, D., Oskam, R., Pacquement, H., Quintana, E., Bouffet, E., Bernard, J. L., Floret, D., Cochat, P., Palmer, P., Franks, C. R., Doz, F., Lanier, F., Favrot, M., Zucker, J. M., Fridman, W. H., & Philip, T. (1994). Administration of high-dose recombinant interleukin 2 after autologous bone marrow transplantation in patients with neuroblastoma: Toxicity, efficacy and survival. A Lyon-Marseille-Curie-east of France Group Study. *Progress in Clinical and Biological Research, 385*, 293–300.

Minami, Y., Kono, T., Yamada, K., & Taniguchi, T. (1992). The interleukin-2 receptors: Insights into a complex signalling mechanism. *Biochimica et Biophysica Acta, 1114*, 163–177.

Minc Golomb, D., Yadid, G., Tsarfaty, I., Resau, J. H., & Schwartz, J. P. (1996). In vivo expression of inducible nitric oxide synthase in cerebellar neurons. *Journal of Neurochemistry, 66*, 1504–1509.

Mizuno, M., Kondo, E., Nishimura, M., Ueda, Y., Yoshiya, I., Tohyama, M., & Kiyama, H. (1997). Localization of molecules involved in cytokine receptor signaling in the rat trigeminal ganglion. *Molecular Brain Research, 44*, 163–166.

Montaldo, P. G., Carbone, R., Corrias, M. V., Ferraris, P. C., & Ponzoni, M. (1994). Synergistic differentiation-promoting activity of interferon gamma and tumor necrosis factor-alpha: Role of receptor regulation on human neuroblasts. *Journal of the National Cancer Institute, 86*, 1694–1701.

Morgan, D. A., Ruscetti, F. W., & Gallo, R. C. (1976). Selective in vitro growth of T-lymphocytes from normal human bone marrows. *Science, 193*, 1007–1008.

Moroni, S. C., & Rossi, A. (1995). Enhanced survival and differentiation in vitro of different neuronal populations by some interleukins. *International Journal of Developmental Neuroscience, 13*, 41–49.

Moutoussamy, S., Kelly, P. A., & Finidori, J. (1998). Growth-hormone-receptor and cytokine-receptor-family signaling. *European Journal of Biochemistry, 255*, 1–11.

Mrak, R. E., Sheng, J. G., & Griffin, W. S. (1995). Glial cytokines in Alzheimer's disease: Review and pathogenic implications. *Human Pathology, 26*, 816–823.

Muir, J. L. (1997). Acetylcholine, aging, and Alzheimer's disease. *Pharmacology Biochemistry Behavior, 56*, 687–696.

Muller, M., Fontana, A., Zbinden, G., & Gahwiler, B. H. (1993). Effects of interferons and hydrogen peroxide on CA3 pyramidal cells in rat hippocampal slice cultures. *Brain Research, 619*, 157–162.

Munder, M., Mallo, M., Eichmann, K., & Modolell, M. (1998). Murine macrophages secrete interferon gamma upon combined stimulation with interleukin (IL)-12 and IL-18: A novel pathway of autocrine macrophage activation. *Journal of Experimental Medicine, 187*, 2103–2108.

Munoz Fernandez, M. A., Cano, E., O'Donnell, C. A., Doyle, J., Liew, F. Y., & Fresno, M. (1994). Tumor necrosis factor-alpha (TNF-alpha), interferon-gamma, and interleukin-6 but not TNF-beta induce differentiation of neuroblastoma cells: The role of nitric oxide. *Journal of Neurochemistry, 62*, 1330–1336.

Naito, Y., Fukata, J., Tominaga, T., Masui, Y., Hirai, Y., Murakami, N., Tamai, S., Mori, K., & Imura, H. (1989). Adrenocorticotropic hormone-releasing activities of interleukins in a homologous in vivo system. *Biochemical Biophysical Research Communications, 164*, 1262–1267.

Naka, T., Narazaki, M., Hirata, M., Matsumoto, T., Minamoto, S., Aono, A., Nishimoto, N., Kajita, T., Taga, T., Yoshizaki, K., Akira, S., & Kishimoto, T. (1997). Structure and function of a new STAT-induced STAT inhibitor. *Nature, 387*, 924–929.

Nakamura, M., Asao, H., Takeshita, T., & Sugamura, K. (1993). Interleukin-2 receptor heterotrimer complex and intracellular signaling. *Seminars in Immunology, 5*, 309–317.

Nakashima, T., Hori, T., Kuriyama, K., & Kiyohara, T. (1987). Naloxone blocks the interferon-alpha induced changes in hypothalamic neuronal activity. *Neuroscience Letters, 82*, 332–336.

Nakashima, T., Hori, T., Kuriyama, K., & Matsuda, T. (1988). Effects of interferon-alpha on the activity of preoptic thermosensitive neurons in tissue slices. *Brain Research, 454*, 361–367.

Naredi, P., Hafstrom, L., Zachrisson, H., Rudenstam, C. M., & Lundholm, K. (1994). Whole body energy expenditure protein breakdown and polyamine excretion during high dose treatment with interleukin-2 and interferon-alpha. *European Journal of Surgery, 160*, 67–75.

Navikas, V., & Link, H. (1996). Review: Cytokines and the pathogenesis of multiple sclerosis. *Journal of Neuroscience Research, 45*, 322–333.

Nemni, R., Iannaccone, S., Quattrini, A., Smirne, S., Sessa, M., Lodi, M., Erminio, C., & Canal, N. (1992). Effect of chronic treatment with recombinant interleukin-2 on the central nervous system of adult and old mice. *Brain Research, 591*, 248–252.

Neumann, H., Boucraut, J., Hahnel, C., Misgeld, T., & Wekerle, H. (1996). Neuronal control of MHC class II inducibility in rat astrocytes and microglia. *European Journal of Neuroscience, 8*, 2582–2590.

Neumann, H., Cavalie, A., Jenne, D. E., & Wekerle, H. (1995). Induction of MHC class I genes in neurons [see comments]. *Science, 269*, 549–552.

Neumann, H., Schmidt, H., Cavalie, A., Jenne, D., & Wekerle, H. (1997). Major histocompatibility complex (MHC) class I gene expression in single neurons of the central nervous system: Differential regulation by interferon (IFN)-gamma and tumor necrosis factor (TNF)-alpha. *Journal of Experimental Medicine, 185*, 305–316.

Neumann, H., Schmidt, H., Wilharm, E., Behrens, L., & Wekerle, H. (1997). Interferon gamma gene expression in sensory neurons: Evidence for autocrine gene regulation. *Journal of Experimental Medicine, 186*, 2023–2031.

Nicola, N. A. (1994). An introduction to the cytokines. In N. A. Nicola (Ed.), *Guidebook to cytokines and their receptors* (pp. 1–7). Oxford: Oxford University Press.

Nieto Sampedro, M., & Chandy, K. G. (1987). Interleukin-2-like activity in injured rat brain. *Neurochemical Research, 12*, 723–727.

Nikcevich, K. M., Gordon, K. B., Tan, L., Hurst, S. D., Kroepfl, J. F., Gardinier, M., Barrett, T. A., & Miller, S. D. (1997). IFN-gamma-activated primary murine astrocytes express B7 costimulatory molecules and prime naive antigen-specific T cells. *Journal of Immunology, 158*, 614–621.

Nishikawa, T., Yamashita, S., Namba, H., Usa, T., Tominaga, T., Kimura, H., Izumi, M., & Nagataki, S. (1993). Interferon-gamma inhibition of human thyrotropin receptor gene expression. *Journal of Clinical Endocrinology and Metabolism, 77*, 1084–1089.

Nishimura, H., Washizu, J., Nakamura, N., Enomoto, A., & Yoshikai, Y. (1998). Translational efficiency is up-regulated by alternative exon in murine IL-15 mRNA. *Journal of Immunology, 160*, 936–942.

Nistico, G. (1993). Communications among central nervous system, neuroendocrine and immune systems: Interleukin-2. *Progress in Neurobiology, 40*, 463–475.

Nistico, G., & De Sarro, G. (1991a). Behavioral and electrocortical spectrum power effects after microinfusion of lymphokines in several areas of the rat brain. *Annals of the New York Academy of Sciences, 621*, 119–134.

Nistico, G., & De Sarro, G. (1991b). Is interleukin-2 a neuromodulator in the brain? *Trends in Neurosciences, 14*, 146–150.

Noguchi, M., Nakamura, Y., Russell, S. M., Ziegler, S. F., Tsang, M., Cao, X., & Leonard, W. J. (1993). Interleukin-2 receptor gamma chain: A functional component of the interleukin-7 receptor. *Science, 262*, 1877–1880.

Nörenberg, W., Gebicke Haerter, P. J., & Illes, P. (1992). Inflammatory stimuli induce a new K^+ outward current in cultured rat microglia. *Neuroscience Letters, 147*, 171–174.

O'Shea, J. J. (1997). Jaks, STATs, cytokine signal transduction, and immunoregulation: Are we there yet? *Immunity, 7*, 1–11.

Olsson, T. (1992). Cytokines in neuroinflammatory disease: Role of myelin autoreactive T cell production of interferon-gamma. *Journal of Neuroimmunology, 40*, 211–218.

Olsson, T., Kelic, S., Edlund, C., Bakhiet, M., Hojeberg, B., van der Meide, P. H., Ljungdahl, A., & Kristensson, K. (1994). Neuronal interferon-gamma immunoreactive molecule: Bioactivities and purification. *European Journal of Immunology, 24*, 308–314.

Olsson, T., Kristensson, K., Ljungdahl, A., Maehlen, J., Holmdahl, R., & Klareskog, L. (1989). Gamma-interferon-like immunoreactivity in axotomized rat motor neurons. *Journal of Neuroscience, 9*, 3870–3875.

Onu, A., Pohl, T., Krause, H., & Bulfone Paus, S. (1997). Regulation of IL-15 secretion via the leader peptide of two IL-15 isoforms. *Journal of Immunology, 158*, 255–262.

Oppenheim, J. J. (1994). Foreword. In A. Thomsen (Ed.), *The cytokine handbook* (pp. xvii–xx). London: Academic Press.

Oppenheim, M. H., & Lotze, M. T. (1994). Interleukin-2: Solid-tumor therapy. *Oncology, 51*, 154–169.

Otero, G. C., & Merrill, J. E. (1994). Cytokine receptors on glial cells. *Glia, 11*, 117–128.

Otero, G. C., & Merrill, J. E. (1995). Molecular cloning of IL-2α, IL-2β, and IL-2γ cDNAs from a human oligodendroglioma cell line: Presence of IL-2R mRNAs in the human central nervous system. *Glia, 14*, 295–302.

Otero, G. C., & Merrill, J. E. (1997). Response of human oligodendrocytes to interleukin-2. *Brain, Behavior, and Immunity, 11*, 24–38.

Ottaviani, E., Franchini, A., Caselgrandi, E., Cossarizza, A., & Franceschi, C. (1995). Relationship between corticotropin-releasing factor and interleukin-2: Evolutionary evidence. *FEBS Letters, 351*, 19–21.

Panchenko, L. F., Aliab'eva, T. N., Malinovskaia, V. V., & Balashov, A. M. (1987). Alpha interferon interaction with opiate receptors in the rat brain. *Biulletin Eksperementalnoi Biologii i Medicini, 104*, 87–89.

Panek, R. B., & Benveniste, E. N. (1995). Class II MHC gene expression in microglia. Regulation by the cytokines IFN-gamma, TNF-alpha, and TGF-beta. *Journal of Immunology, 154*, 2846–2854.

Panek, R. B., Lee, Y. J., & Benveniste, E. N. (1995). TGF-beta suppression of IFN-gamma-induced class II MHC gene expression does not involve inhibition of phosphorylation of JAK1, JAK2, or signal transducers and activators of transcription, or modification of IFN-gamma enhanced factor X expression. *Journal of Immunology, 154*, 610–619.

Pardy, K., Murphy, D., Carter, D., & Hui, K. M. (1993). The influence of interleukin-2 on vasopressin and oxytocin gene expression in the rodent hypothalamus. *Journal of Neuroimmunology, 42*, 131–138.

Park, H. J., Won, C. K., Pyun, K. H., & Shin, H. C. (1995). Interleukin 2 suppresses afferent sensory transmission in the primary somatosensory cortex. *Neuroreport, 6*, 1018–1020.

Park, S. Y., Saijo, K., Takahashi, T., Osawa, M., Arase, H., Hirayama, N., Miyake, K., Nakauchi, H., Shirasawa, T., & Saito, T. (1995). Developmental defects of lymphoid cells in Jak3 kinase-deficient mice. *Immunity, 3*, 771–782.

Pauli, S., Linthorst, A. C. E., & Reul, J. M. H. (1998). Tumour necrosis factor-alpha and interleukin-2 differentially affect hippocampal serotonergic neurotransmission, behavioural activity, body temperature and hypothalamic-pituitary-adrenocortical axis activity in the rat. *European Journal of Neuroscience, 10*, 868–878.

Pavol, M. A., Meyers, C. A., Rexer, J. L., Valentine, A. D., Mattis, P. J., & Talpaz, M. (1995). Pattern of neurobehavioral deficits associated with interferon alfa therapy for leukemia. *Neurology, 45*, 947–950.

Pawlinski, R., & Janeczko, K. (1997). Intracerebral injection of interferon-gamma inhibits the astrocyte proliferation following the brain injury in the 6-day-old rat. *Journal of Neuroscience Research, 50*, 1018–1022.

Peng, Z. C., Mohammed, A. H., Olsson, T., Edlund, C., & Kristensson, K. (1994). Interferon-gamma and a factor derived from trypanosomes cause behavioural changes in the rat. *Behavioral Brain Research, 62*, 171–175.

Perry, V. H. (1994). *Macrophages and the nervous system*. Austin, TX: R. G. Landes Company/CRC Press.

Perry, V. H., Andersson, P. B., & Gordon, S. (1993). Macrophages and inflammation in the central nervous system. *Trends in Neurosciences, 16*, 268–273.

Peterson, P. K., Hu, S., Anderson, W. R., & Chao, C. C. (1994). Nitric oxide production and neurotoxicity mediated by activated microglia from human versus mouse brain. *Journal of Infectious Diseases, 170*, 457–460.

Petitto, J. M., & Huang, Z. (1994). Molecular cloning of a partial cDNA of the interleukin-2 receptor-β in normal mouse brain: In situ localization in the hippocampus and expression by neuroblastoma cells. *Brain Research, 650*, 140–145.

Petitto, J. M., & Huang, Z. (1995). Molecular cloning of the coding sequence of an interleukin-2 receptor alpha subunit cDNA in murine brain. *Journal of Neuroimmunology, 59*, 135–141.

Petitto, J. M., Huang, Z., Raizada, M. K., Rinker, C. M., & McCarthy, D. B. (1998). Molecular cloning of the cDNA coding sequence of IL-2 receptor-gamma (gamma c) from human and murine forebrain: Expression in the hippocampus in situ and by brain cells in vitro. *Brain Research Molecular Brain Research, 53*, 152–162.

Petitto, J. M., Huang, Z., Rinker, C. M., & McCarthy, D. B. (1997). Isolation of IL-2 receptor-beta cDNA clones from AtT-20 pituitary cells: Constitutive expression and role in signal transduction. *Neuropsychopharmacology, 17*, 57–66.

Petitto, J. M., McCarthy, D. B., Rinker, C. M., Huang, Z., & Getty, T. (1997). Modulation of behavioral and neurochemical measures of forebrain dopamine function in mice by species-specific interleukin-2. *Journal of Neuroimmunology, 73*, 183–190.

Petrovsky, N., & Harrison, L. C. (1995). Th1 and Th2: Swinging to a hormonal rhythm. *Immunology Today, 16*, 605

Plata Salaman, C. R. (1989). Immunomodulators and feeding regulation: A humoral link between the immune and nervous systems. *Brain, Behavior, and Immunity, 3*, 193–213.

Plata Salaman, C. R. (1991). Immunoregulators in the nervous system. *Neuroscience and Biobehavioral Reviews, 15*, 185–215.

Plata Salaman, C. R. (1992). Interferons and central regulation of feeding. *American Journal of Physiology, 263*, R1222–1227.

Plata Salaman, C. R. (1995). Cytokines and feeding suppression: An integrative view from neurologic to molecular levels. *Nutrition, 11*, 674–677.

Plata Salaman, C. R. (1996). Anorexia induced by activators of the signal transducer gp 130. *Neuroreport, 7*, 841–844.

Plata Salaman, C. R., & Borkoski, J. P. (1994). Chemokines/intercrines and central regulation of feeding. *American Journal of Physiology, 266*, R1711–5.

Plata Salaman, C. R., & ffrench Mullen, J. M. (1993). Interleukin-2 modulates calcium currents in dissociated hippocampal CA1 neurons. *Neuroreport, 4*, 579–581.

Plata Salaman, C. R., Sonti, G., & Borkoski, J. P. (1995). Modulation of feeding by beta 2-microglobulin, a marker of immune activation. *American Journal of Physiology, 268*, R1513–1519.

Ponzoni, M., Guarnaccia, F., Corrias, M. V., & Cornaglia Ferraris, P. (1993). Uncoordinate induction and differential regulation of HLA class-I and class-II expression by gamma-interferon in differentiating human neuroblastoma cells. *International Journal of Cancer, 55*, 817–823.

Popko, B., Corbin, J. G., Baerwald, K. D., Dupree, J., & Garcia, A. M. (1997). The effects of interferon-gamma on the central nervous system. *Molecular Neurobiology, 14*, 19–35.

Porrini, A. M., & Reder, A. T. (1994). IFN-gamma, IFN-beta, and PGE1 affect monokine secretion: Relevance to monocyte activation in multiple sclerosis. *Cellular Immunology, 157*, 428–438.

Prieto Gomez, B., Reyes Vazquez, C., & Dafny, N. (1983). Differential effects of interferon on ventromedial hypothalamus and dorsal hippocampus. *Journal of Neuroscience Research, 10*, 273–278.

Prinz, M., Hanisch, U. K., Kettenmann, H., & Kirchhoff, F. (1998). Alternative splicing of mouse IL-15 is due to the use of an intzernal splice site in exon 5. *Molecular Brain Research, 63*, 155–162.

Raber, J., & Bloom, F. E. (1994). IL-2 induces vasopressin release from the hypothalamus and the amygdala: Role of nitric oxide-mediated signaling. *Journal of Neuroscience, 14*, 6187–6195.

Raber, J., & Bloom, F. E. (1996). Arginine vasopressin release by acetylcholine or norepinephrine: Region-specific and cytokine-specific regulation. *Neuroscience, 71*, 747–759.

Raber, J., Koob, G. F., & Bloom, F. E. (1995). Interleukin-2 (IL-2) induces corticotropin-releasing factor (CRF) release from the amygdala and involves a nitric oxide-mediated signaling; comparison with the hypothalamic response. *Journal of Pharmacology and Experimental Therapeutics, 272*, 815–824.

Raber, J., Koob, G. F., & Bloom, F. E. (1997). Interferon-alpha and transforming growth factor-beta 1 regulate corticotropin-releasing factor release from the amygdala: Comparison with the hypothalamic response. *Neurochemistry International, 30*, 455–463.

Rada, P., Mark, G. P., Vitek, M. P., Mangano, R. M., Blume, A. J., Beer, B., & Hoebel, B. G. (1991). Interleukin-1 beta decreases acetylcholine measured by microdialysis in the hippocampus of freely moving rats. *Brain Research, 550*, 287–290.

Raiteri, M., Leardi, R., Marchi, M., Song, C., & Leonard, B. E. (1995). Heterogeneity of presynaptic muscarinic receptors regulating neurotransmitter release in the rat brain Interleukin-2-induced changes in behavioural, neurotransmitter, and immunological parameters in the olfactory bulbectomized rat. *Journal of Pharmacology and Experimental Therapeutics, 2*, 263–273.

Rajan, P., Stewart, C. L., & Fink, J. S. (1995). LIF-mediated activation of STAT proteins after neuronal injury in vivo. *Neuroreport, 6*, 2240–2244.

Rajan, P., Symes, A. J., & Fink, J. S. (1996). STAT proteins are activated by ciliary neurotrophic factor in cells of central nervous system origin. *Journal of Neuroscience Research, 43*, 403–411.

Ramierz, F., Fowell, D. J., Puklavec, M., Simmonds, S., & Mason, D. (1996). Glucocorticoids promote a TH2 cytokine response by $CD4^+$ T cells in vitro. *Journal of Immunology, 156*, 2406–2412.

Ransohoff, R. M. (1998). Cellular responses to interferons and other cytokines: The JAK-STAT paradigm. *New England Journal of Medicine, 338*, 616–618.

Ravaud, A., Negrier, S., Cany, L., Merrouche, Y., Le Guillou, M., Blay, J. Y., Clavel, M., Gaston, R., Oskam, R., & Philip, T. (1994). Subcutaneous low-dose recombinant interleukin 2 and alpha-interferon in patients with metastatic renal cell carcinoma. *British Journal of Cancer, 69*, 1111–1114.

Rensing Ehl, A., Malipiero, U., Irmler, M., Tschopp, J., Constam, D., & Fontana, A. (1996). Neurons induced to express major histocompatibility complex class I antigen are killed via the perforin and not the Fas (APO-1/CD95) pathway. *European Journal of Immunology, 26*, 2271–2274.

Reyes Vazquez, C., Mendoza Fernandez, V., Herrera Ruiz, M., & Dafny, N. (1997). Interferon modulates glucose-sensitive neurons in the hypothalamus. *Experimental Brain Research, 116*, 519–524.

Reyes Vazquez, C., Prieto Gomez, B., & Dafny, N. (1994). Alpha-interferon suppresses food intake and neuronal activity of the lateral hypothalamus. *Neuropharmacology, 33*, 1545–1552.

Reyes Vazquez, C., Prieto Gomez, B., Georgiades, J. A., & Dafny, N. (1984). Alpha and gamma interferons' effects on cortical and hippocampal neurons: Microiontophoretic application and single cell recording. *International Journal of Neuroscience, 25*, 113–121.

Robertson, B., Xu, X. J., Hao, J. X., Wiesenfeld Hallin, Z., Mhlanga, J., Grant, G., & Kristensson, K. (1997). Interferon-gamma receptors in nociceptive pathways: Role in neuropathic pain-related behaviour. *Neuroreport, 8*, 1311–1316.

Rodig, S. J., Meraz, M. A., White, J. M., Lampe, P. A., Riley, J. K., Arthur, C. D., King, K. L., Sheehan, K. C., Yin, L., Pennica, D., Johnson, E. M. Jr., & Schreiber, R. D. (1998). Disruption of the Jak1 gene demonstrates obligatory and nonredundant roles of the Jaks in cytokine-induced biologic responses. *Cell, 93*, 373–383.

Rogers, J., Webster, S., Lue, L. F., Brachova, L., Civin, W. H., Emmerling, M., Shivers, B., Walker, D., & McGeer, P. (1996). Inflammation and Alzheimer's disease pathogenesis. *Neurobiology of Aging, 17*, 681–686.

Roosth, J., Pollard, R. B., Brown, S. L., & Meyer, W. J. III (1986). Cortisol stimulation by recombinant interferon-alpha 2. *Journal of Neuroimmunology, 12*, 311–316.

Root Bernstein, R. S. (1984). "Molecular sandwiches" as a basis for structural and functional similarities for interferons, MSH, ACTH, LHRH, myelin basic protein, and albumins. *FEBS Letters, 168*, 208–212.

Rosenberg, S. A. (1990). Adoptive immunotherapy for cancer. *Scientific American, 262*, 62–69.

Rosenberg, S. A., Yang, J. C., Topalian, S. L., Schwartzentruber, D. J., Weber, J. S., Parkinson, D. R., Seipp, C. A., Einhorn, J. H., & White, D. E. (1994). Treatment of 283 consecutive patients with metastatic melanoma or renal cell cancer using high-dose bolus interleukin 2. *Journal of the American Medical Association, 271*, 907–913.

Rostworowski, M., Balasingam, V., Chabot, S., Owens, T., & Yong, V. W. (1997). Astrogliosis in the neonatal and adult murine brain post-trauma: Elevation of inflammatory cytokines and the lack of requirement for endogenous interferon-gamma. *Journal of Neuroscience, 17*, 3664–3674.

Rothwell, N. J., & Hopkins, S. J. (1995). Cytokines and the nervous system II: Actions and mechanisms of action. *Trends in Neurosciences, 18*, 130–136.

Rothwell, N. J., & Relton, J. K. (1993). Involvement of cytokines in acute neurodegeneration in the CNS. *Neuroscience and Biobehavioral Reviews, 17*, 217–227.

Rubin, J. T. (1993). Interleukin-2: Its biology and clinical application in patients with cancer. *Cancer Investigation, 11*, 460–472.

Rubio, N. (1994). Demonstration of the presence of an interleukin-1 receptor on the surface of murine astrocytes and its regulation by cytokines and Theiler's virus. *Immunology, 82*, 178–183.

Rubio, N. (1997a). Interferon-gamma induces the expression of immediate early genes c-fos and c-jun in astrocytes. *Immunology, 91*, 560–564.

Rubio, N. (1997b). Mouse astrocytes store and deliver brain-derived neurotrophic factor using the non-catalytic gp95trkB receptor. *European Journal of Neuroscience, 9*, 1847–1853.

Rudick, R. A., Ransohoff, R. M., Lee, J. C., Peppler, R., Yu, M., Mathisen, P. M., & Tuohy, V. K. (1998). In vivo effects of interferon beta-1a on immunosuppressive cytokines in multiple sclerosis. *Neurology, 50*, 1294–1300.

Ruuls, S. R., de Labie, M. C., Weber, K. S., Botman, C. A., Groenestein, R. J., Dijkstra, C. D., Olsson, T., & van der Meide, P. H. (1996). The length of treatment determines whether IFN-beta prevents or aggravates experimental autoimmune encephalomyelitis in Lewis rats. *Journal of Immunology, 157*, 5721–5731.

S. Rozsa, K., Rubakhin, S. S., Szucs, A., Hughes, T. K., & Stefano, G. B. (1997). Opposite effects of interleukin-2 and interleukin-4 on GABA-induced inward currents of dialysed Lymnaea neurons. *General Pharmacology, 29*, 73–77.

Saija, A., Princi, P., Lanza, M., Scalese, M., Aramnejad, E., & De Sarro, A. (1995). Systemic cytokine administration can affect blood-brain barrier permeability in the rat. *Life Sciences, 56*, 775–784.

Sakai, N., Kaufman, S., & Milstien, S. (1995). Parallel induction of nitric oxide and tetrahydrobiopterin synthesis by cytokines in rat glial cells. *Journal of Neurochemistry, 65*, 895–902.

Sakatsume, M., Stancato, L. F., David, M., Silvennoinen, O., Saharinen, P., Pierce, J., Larner, A. C., & Finbloom, D. S. (1998). Interferon gamma activation of Raf-1 is Jak1-dependent and p21ras-independent. *Journal of Biological Chemistry, 273*, 3021–3026.

Samuel, N. M., Jessen, K. R., Grange, J. M., & Mirsky, R. (1987). Gamma interferon, but not *Mycobacterium leprae*, induces major histocompatibility class II antigens on cultured rat Schwann cells. *Journal of Neurocytology, 16*, 281–287.

Sanchez, M. P., Tapley, P., Saini, S. S., He, B., Pulido, D., & Barbacid, M. (1994). Multiple tyrosine protein kinases in rat hippocampal neurons: Isolation of Ptk-3, a receptor expressed in proliferative zones of the developing brain. *Proceedings of the National Academy of Science USA, 91*, 1819–1823.

Saneto, R. P., Altman, A., Knobler, R. L., Johnson, H. M., & De Vellis, J. (1986). Interleukin 2 mediates the inhibition of oligodendrocyte progenitor cell proliferation in vitro. *Proceedings of the National Academy of Science USA, 83*, 9221–9225.

Saneto, R. P., Chiapelli, F., & De Vellis, J. (1987). Interleukin-2 inhibition of oligodendrocyte progenitor proliferation depends on expression of the Tac receptor. *Journal of Neuroscience Research, 18*, 147–154.

Saphier, D. (1989). Neurophysiological and endocrine consequences of immune activity. *Psychoneuroendocrinology, 14*, 63–87.

Saphier, D. (1995). Neuroendocrine effects of interferon-alpha in the rat. *Advances in Experimental Medicine and Biology, 373*, 209–218.

Saphier, D., Kidron, D., Ovadia, H., Trainin, N., Pecht, M., Burstein, Y., & Abramsky, O. (1988). Neurophysiological changes in the brain following central administration of immunomodulatory factors. *Israel Journal of Medical Sciences, 24*, 261–263.

Saphier, D., Ovadia, H., & Abramsky, O. (1990). Neural responses to antigenic challenges and immunomodulatory factors. *Yale Journal of Biological Medicine, 63*, 109–119.

Saphier, D., Roerig, S. C., Ito, C., Vlasak, W. R., Farrar, G. E., Broyles, J. E., & Welch, J. E. (1994). Inhibition of neural and neuroendocrine activity by alpha-interferon: Neuroendocrine, electrophysiological, and biochemical studies in the rat [published erratum appears in Brain, Behavor, and Immunity, 1994, 8, 374]. *Brain, Behavior, and Immunity, 8*, 37–56.

Sarder, M., Saito, H., & Abe, K. (1993). Interleukin-2 promotes survival and neurite extension of cultured neurons from fetal rat brain. *Brain Research, 625*, 347–350.

Saris, S. C., Patronas, N. J., Rosenberg, S. A., Alexander, J. T., Frank, J., Schwartzentruber, D. J., Rubin, J. T., Barba, D., & Oldfield, E. H. (1989). The effect of intravenous interleukin-2 on brain water content. *Journal of Neurosurgery, 71*, 169–174.

Sato, I., Kim, Y., Himi, T., & Murota, S. (1995). Induction of calcium-independent nitric oxide synthase activity in cultured cerebellar granule neurons. *Neuroscience Letters, 184*, 145–148.

Satoh, J., Kurohara, K., Yukitake, M., & Kuroda, Y. (1998). Interleukin-15, a T-cell growth factor, is expressed in human neural cell lines and tissues. *Journal of Neurological Science, 155*, 170–177.

Satoh, J., Paty, D. W., & Kim, S. U. (1995). Differential effects of beta and gamma interferons on expression of major histocompatibility complex antigens and intercellular adhesion molecule-1 in cultured fetal human astrocytes. *Neurology, 45*, 367–373.

Satoh, J., Paty, D. W., & Kim, S. U. (1996). Counteracting effect of IFN-beta on IFN-gamma-induced proliferation of human astrocytes in culture. *Multiple Sclerosis, 1*, 279–287.

Satoh, T., Minami, Y., Kono, T., Yamada, K., Kawahara, A., Taniguchi, T., & Kaziro, Y. (1992). Interleukin 2-induced activation of Ras requires two domains of interleukin 2 receptor beta subunit, the essential region for growth stimulation and Lck-binding domain. *Journal of Biological Chemistry, 267*, 25423–25427.

Sauer, J., Rupprecht, M., Arzt, E., Stalla, G. K., & Rupprecht, R. (1993). Glucocorticoids modulate soluble interleukin-2 receptor levels in vivo depending on the state of immune activation and the duration of glucocorticoid exposure. *Immunopharmacology, 25*, 269–276.

Sawada, M., Hara, N., & Ichinose, M. (1992). Interleukin-2 inhibits the GABA-induced Cl-current in identified *Aplysia* neurons. *Journal of Neuroscience Research, 33*, 461–465.

Sawada, M., Hara, N., & Maeno, T. (1992). Reduction of the acetylcholine-induced K+ current in identified *Aplysia* neurons by human interleukin-1 and interleukin-2. *Cell Molecular Neurobiology, 12*, 439–445.

Sawada, M., Ichinose, M., & Stefano, G. B. (1994). Inhibition of the calcitonin-induced outward current in identified *Aplysia* neurons by interleukin-1 and interleukin-2. *Cellular and Molecular Neurobiology, 14*, 175–184.

Sawada, M., Suzumura, A., & Marunouchi, T. (1995). Induction of interleukin-2 receptor in mouse microglia. *Journal of Neurochemistry, 64*, 1973–1979.

Scatton, B., & Lehmann, J. (1982). N-methyl-C-aspartate-type receptors mediate striatal ^{3}H-acetylcholine release evoked by excitatory amino acids. *Nature, 297*, 422–424.

Schneider Schaulies, J., Kirchhoff, F., Archelos, J., & Schachner, M. (1991). Down-regulation of myelin-associated glycoprotein on Schwann cells by interferon-gamma and tumor necrosis factor-alpha affects neurite outgrowth. *Neuron, 7*, 995–1005.

Schreiber, R. D., & Aguet, M. (1994). The interferon-g receptor. In N. A. Nicola (Ed.), *Guidebook to cytokines and their receptors* (pp. 120–123). Oxford: Oxford University Press.

Schwartz, J. P., & Nishiyama, N. (1994). Neurotrophic factor gene expression in astrocytes during development and following injury. *Brain Research Bulletin, 35*, 403–407.

Segall, M. A., & Crnic, L. S. (1990a). A test of conditioned taste aversion with mouse interferon-alpha. *Brain, Behavior, and Immunity, 4*, 223–231.

Segall, M. A., & Crnic, L. S. (1990b). An animal model for the behavioral effects of interferon. *Behavioral Neurosciences, 104*, 612–618.

Seger, R., & Krebs, E. G. (1995). The MAPK signaling cascade. *FASEB Journal, 9*, 726–735.

Selamj, K., Raine, C. S., Farooq, M., Norton, W. T., & Brosnan, C. F. (1991). Cytokine toxicity against oligodendrocytes. Apoptosis induced by lymphotoxin. *Journal of Immunology, 147*, 1522–1529.

Semba, K., & Fibiger, H. C. (1989). Organization of central cholinergic systems. In A. Nordberg, K. Fuxe, B. Holmstedt, & A. Sundwall (Eds.), *Nicotinic receptors in the CNS: Their role in synaptic transmission* (pp. 37–63). Amsterdam: Elsevier.

Sengupta, T. K., Schmitt, E. M., & Ivashkiv, L. B. (1996). Inhibition of cytokines and JAK-STAT activation by distinct signaling pathways. *Proceedings of the National Academy of Science USA, 93*, 9499–9504.

Sessa, M., Nemni, R., Iannaccone, S., Quattrini, A., Confalonieri, V., & Canal, N. (1992). In vivo modulation of myelin gene expression by human recombinant IL-2. *Brain Research Molecular Brain Research, 12*, 331–334.

Sethna, M. P., & Lampson, L. A. (1991). Immune modulation within the brain: Recruitment of inflammatory cells and increased major histocompatibility antigen expression following intracerebral injection of interferon-gamma. *Journal of Neuroimmunology, 34*, 121–132.

Seto, D., Hanisch, U. K., Villemain, F., Beaudet, A., & Quirion, R. (1993). Anatomical and functional approaches to study of interleukin 2 and its receptors in brain. In E. B. De Souza (Ed.), *Neurobiology of cytokines, part A (methods in neurosciences, vol. 16)* (pp. 173–184). San Diego: Academic Press.

Seto, D., Kar, S., & Quirion, R. (1997). Evidence for direct and indirect mechanisms in the potent modulatory action of interleukin-2 on the release of acetylcholine in rat hippocampal slices. *British Journal of Pharmacology, 120*, 1151–1157.

Seto, D., & Quirion, R. (1993). Receptor-mediated effects of interleukin-2 on hippocampal acetylcholine release. *Society for Neuroscience Abstracts, 19*, 1763.

Shimojo, M., Imai, Y., Nakajima, K., Mizushima, S., Uemura, A., & Kohsaka, S. (1993). Interleukin-2 enhances the viability of primary cultured rat neocortical neurons. *Neuroscience Letters, 151*, 170–173.

Shuto, H., Kataoka, Y., Horikawa, T., Fujihara, N., & Oishi, R. (1997). Repeated interferon-alpha administration inhibits dopaminergic neural activity in the mouse brain. *Brain Research, 747*, 348–351.

Simmons, M. L., & Murphy, S. (1993). Cytokines regulate L-arginine-dependent cyclic GMP production in rat glial cells. *European Journal of Neuroscience, 5*, 825–831.

Singh, V. K. (1994). Studies of neuroimmune markers in Alzheimer's disease. *Molecular Neurobiology, 9*, 73–81.

Small, G. W. (1998). Treatment of Alzheimer's disease: Current approaches and promising developments. *American Journal of Medicine, 104*, 32S–38S.

Smith, E. M., Dion, L. D., & Blalock, J. E. (1985). Opiate receptor mediated effects of IFN-alpha and lymphocyte derived endorphin-like peptides. *Progress in Clinical Biology Research, 192*, 259–264.

Smith, E. M., Meyer, W. J., & Blalock, J. E. (1982). Virus-induced corticosterone in hypophysectomized mice: A possible lymphoid adrenal axis. *Science, 218*, 1311–1312.

Smith, K. A. (1992). Interleukin-2. *Current Opinion in Immunology, 4*, 271–276.

Smith, L. R., Brown, S. L., & Blalock, J. E. (1989). Interleukin-2 induction of ACTH secretion: Presence of an interleukin-2 receptor alpha-chain-like molecule on pituitary cells. *Journal of Neuroimmunology, 21*, 249–254.

Smith, R. A., Landel, C., Cornelius, C. E., & Revel, M. (1986). Mapping the action of interferon on primate brain. *Journal of Interferon Research, 6*, 140

Smith, R. A., Norris, F., Palmer, D., Bernhardt, L., & Wills, R. J. (1985). Distribution of alpha interferon in serum and cerebrospinal fluid after systemic administration. *Clinical Pharmacology and Therapeutics, 37*, 85–88.

Song, C., & Leonard, B. E. (1995). Interleukin-2-induced changes in behavioural, neurotransmitter, and immunological parameters in the olfactory bulbectomized rat. *Neuroimmunomodulation, 2*, 263–273.

Spleiss, O., Appel, K., Boddeke, H. W., Berger, M., & Gebicke Haerter, P. J. (1998). Molecular biology of microglia cytokine and chemokine receptors and microglial activation. *Life Sciences, 62*, 1707–1710.

Sprang, S. R., & Bazan, J. F. (1993). Cytokine structural taxonomy and mechanisms of receptor engagement. *Current Opinion in Structural Biology, 3*, 815–827.

Stark, G. R., Kerr, I. M., Williams, B. R. G., Silverman, R. H., & Schreiber, R. D. (1998). How cells respond to interferons. *Annual Review of Biochemistry, 67*, 227–264.

Starr, R., Willson, T. A., Viney, E. M., Murray, L. J., Rayner, J. R., Jenkins, B. J., Gonda, T. J., Alexander, W. S., Metcalf, D., Nicola, N. A., & Hilton, D. J. (1997). A family of cytokine-inducible inhibitors of signalling. *Nature, 387*, 917–921.

Stewart, V. C., Giovannoni, G., Land, J. M., McDonald, W. I., Clark, J. B., & Heales, S. J. (1997). Pretreatment of astrocytes with interferon-alpha/beta impairs interferon-gamma induction of nitric oxidesynthase. *Journal of Neurochemistry, 68*, 2547–2551.

Stewart, V. C., Land, J. M., Clark, J. B., & Heales, S. J. (1998). Pretreatment of astrocytes with interferon-alpha/beta prevents neuronal mitochondrial respiratory chain damage. *Journal of Neurochemistry, 70*, 432–434.

Streit, W. J., Graeber, M. B., & Kreutzberg, G. W. (1988). Functional plasticity of microglia: A review. *Glia, 1*, 301–307.

Sugamura, K., Asao, H., Kondo, M., Tanaka, N., Ishii, N., Ohbo, K., Nakamura, M., & Takeshita, T. (1996). The interleukin-2 receptor gamma chain: Its role in the multiple cytokine receptor complexes and T cell development in XSCID. *Annual Review of Immunology, 14*, 179–205.

Sun, D., Coleclough, C., & Whitaker, J. N. (1997). Nonactivated astrocytes downregulate T cell receptor expression and reduce antigen-specific proliferation and cytokine production of myelin basic protein (MBP)-reactive T cells. *Journal of Neuroimmunology, 78*, 69–78.

Suzumura, A., Mezitis, S. G., Gonatas, N. K., & Silberberg, D. H. (1987). MHC antigen expression on bulk isolated macrophage-microglia from newborn mouse brain: Induction of Ia antigen expression by gamma-interferon. *Journal of Neuroimmunology, 15*, 263–278.

Suzumura, A., Sawada, M., Yamamoto, H., & Marunouchi, T. (1993). Transforming growth factor-beta suppresses activation and proliferation of microglia in vitro. *Journal of Immunology, 151*, 2150–2158.

Suzumura, A., Silberberg, D. H., & Lisak, R. P. (1986). The expression of MHC antigens on oligodendrocytes: Induction of polymorphic H-2 expression by lymphokines. *Journal of Neuroimmunology, 11*, 179–190.

Tabibzadeh, S. (1994). Cytokines and the hypothalamic-pituitary-ovarian-endometrial axis. *Human Reproduction Update, 9*, 947–967.

Tada, M., Diserens, A. C., Desbaillets, I., & de Tribolet, N. (1994). Analysis of cytokine receptor messenger RNA expression in human glioblastoma cells and normal astrocytes by reverse-transcription polymerase chain reaction. *Journal of Neurosurgery, 80*, 1063–1073.

Tagaya, Y., Burton, J. D., Miyamoto, Y., & Waldmann, T. A. (1996). Identification of a novel receptor/signal transduction pathway for IL-15/T in mast cells. *EMBO Journal, 15*, 4928–4939.

Tagaya, Y., Kurys, G., Thies, T. A., Losi, J. M., Azimi, N., Hanover, J. A., Bamford, R. N., & Waldmann, T. A. (1997). Generation of secretable and nonsecretable interleukin 15 isoforms through alternate usage of signal peptides. *Proceedings of the National Academy of Science USA, 94*, 14444–14449.

Tan, L., Gordon, K. B., Mueller, J. P., Matis, L. A., & Miller, S. D. (1998). Presentation of proteolipid protein epitopes and B7-1-dependent activation of encephalitogenic T cells by IFN-gamma-activated SJL/J astrocytes. *Journal of Immunology, 160*, 4271–4279.

Tancredi, V., Zona, C., Velotti, F., Eusebi, F., & Santoni, A. (1990). Interleukin-2 suppresses established long-term potentiation and inhibits its induction in the rat hippocampus. *Brain Research, 525*, 149–151.

Taniguchi, T. (1995). Cytokine signaling through nonreceptor protein tyrosine kinases. *Science, 268*, 251–255.

Taniguchi, T., Matsui, H., Fujita, T., Takaoka, C., Kashima, N., Yoshimoto, R., & Hamuro, J. (1983). Structure and expression of a cloned cDNA for human interleukin-2. *Nature, 302*, 305–310.

Tartour, E., Mathiot, C., & Fridman, W. H. (1992). Current status of interleukin-2 therapy in cancer. *Biomedical Pharmacotherapy, 46*, 473–484.

Theze, J. (1994). Cytokine receptors: A combinative family of molecules. *European Cytokine Network, 5*, 353–368.

Theze, J., Alzari, P. M., & Bertoglio, J. (1996). Interleukin-2 and its receptors: Recent advances and new immunological functions. *Immunology Today, 17*, 481–486.

Thompson, S. M. (1994). Modulation of inhibitory synaptic transmission in the hippocampus. *Progress in Neurobiology, 42*, 575–609.

Tjuvajev, J., Gansbacher, B., Desai, R., Beattie, B., Kaplitt, M., Matei, C., Gilboa, E., & Blasberg, R. (1995). RG-2 glioma growth attenuation and severe brain edema caused by local production of interleukin-2 and interferon-gamma. *Cancer Research, 55*, 1902–1910.

Toledo Aral, J. J., Brehm, P., Halegoua, S., & Mandel, G. (1995). A single pulse of nerve growth factor triggers long-term neuronal excitability through sodium channel gene induction. *Neuron, 14*, 607–611.

Tominaga, T., Fukata, J., Naito, Y., Usui, T., Murakami, N., Fukushima, M., Nakai, Y., Hirai, Y., & Imura, H. (1991). Prostaglandin-dependent in vitro stimulation of adrenocortical steroidogenesis by interleukins. *Endocrinology, 128*, 526–531.

Torres, C., Aranguez, I., & Rubio, N. (1995). Expression of interferon-gamma receptors on murine oligodendrocytes and its regulation by cytokines and mitogens. *Immunology, 86*, 250–255.

Tremblay, N., Warren, R. A., & Dykes, R. W. (1990). Electrophysiological studies of acetylcholine and the role of the basal forebrain in the somatosensory cortex of the cat. II. Cortical neurons excited by somatic stimuli. *Journal of Neurophysiology, 64*, 1212–1222.

Valentine, A. D., Meyers, C. A., Kling, M. A., Richelson, E., & Hauser, P. (1998). Mood and cognitive side effects of interferon-alpha therapy. *Seminars in Oncology, 25*, 39–47.

Van Wagoner, N. J., O'Keefe, G. M., & Benveniste, E. N. (1998). Kinase inhibitors abrogate IFN-gamma-induced class II transactivator and class II MHC gene expression in astroglioma cell lines. *Journal of Neuroimmunology, 85*, 174–185.

Vankelecom, H., Andries, M., Billiau, A., & Denef, C. (1992). Evidence that folliculo-stellate cells mediate the inhibitory effect of interferon-gamma on hormone secretion in rat anterior pituitary cell cultures. *Endocrinology, 130*, 3537–3546.

Vankelecom, H., Carmeliet, P., Heremans, H., Van Damme, J., Dijkmans, R., Billiau, A., & Denef, C. (1990). Interferon-gamma inhibits stimulated adrenocorticotropin, prolactin, and growth hormone secretion in normal rat anterior pituitary cell cultures. *Endocrinology, 126*, 2919–2926.

Vankelecom, H., Matthys, P., & Denef, C. (1997a). Inducible nitric oxide synthase in the anterior pituitary gland: Induction by interferon-gamma in a subpopulation of folliculostellate cells and in an unidentifiable population of non-hormone-secreting cells. *Journal of Histochemistry and Cytochemistry, 45*, 847–857.

Vankelecom, H., Matthys, P., & Denef, C. (1997b). Involvement of nitric oxide in the interferon-gamma-induced inhibition of growth hormone and prolactin secretion in anterior pituitary cell cultures. *Molecular and Cellular Endocrinology, 129*, 157–167.

Vartanian, T., Li, Y., Zhao, M., & Stefansson, K. (1995). Interferon-gamma-induced oligodendrocyte cell death: Implications for the pathogenesis of multiple sclerosis. *Molecular Medicine, 1*, 732–743.

Vassilopoulou Sellin, R., Sella, A., Dexeus, F. H., Theriault, R. L., & Pololoff, D. A. (1992). Acute thyroid dysfunction (thyroiditis) after therapy with interleukin-2. *Hormone and Metabolism Research, 24*, 434–438.

Vecht, C. J., Keohane, C., Menon, R. S., Punt, C. J., & Stoter, G. (1990). Acute fatal leukoencephalopathy after interleukin-2 therapy. *New England Journal of Medicine, 323*, 1146–1147.

Vial, T., & Descotes, J. (1992). Clinical toxicity of interleukin-2. *Drug Safety, 7*, 417–433.

Villemain, F., Owens, T., Renno, T., & Beaudet, A. (1991). Localization of mRNA for interleukin-2 (IL-2) in mouse brain by in situ hybridization. *Society for Neuroscience Abstracts, 17*, 1199.

Viscomi, G. C. (1997). Structure-activity of type I interferons. *Biotherapy, 10*, 59–86.

Visentin, S., Agresti, C., Patrizio, M., & Levi, G. (1995). Ion channels in rat microglia and their different sensitivity to lipopolysaccharide and interferon-gamma. *Journal of Neuroscience Research, 42*, 439–451.

Visentin, S., & Levi, G. (1997). Protein kinase C involvement in the resting and interferon-gamma-induced K^+ channel profile of microglial cells. *Journal of Neuroscience Research, 47*, 233–241.

Visentin, S., & Levi, G. (1998). Arachidonic acid-induced inhibition of microglial outward-rectifying K^+ current. *Glia, 22*, 1–10.

Waguespack, P. J., Banks, W. A., & Kastin, A. J. (1994). Interleukin-2 does not cross the blood-brain barrier by a saturable transport system. *Brain Research Bulletin, 34*, 103–109.

Waldmann, T., Tagaya, Y., & Bamford, R. (1998). Interleukin-2, interleukin-15, and their receptors. *International Reviews of Immunology, 16*, 205–226.

Waldmann, T. A. (1989). The multi-subunit interleukin-2 receptor. *Annual Review of Biochemistry, 58*, 875–911.

Waldmann, T. A. (1991). The interleukin-2 receptor. *Journal of Biological Chemistry, 266*, 2681–2684.

Wang, F. Z., Yao, H., & Ding, A. S. (1994). Effects of interleukin-1 and interleukin-2 on rat hippocampal neurons in culture. *Society for Neuroscience Abstracts, 20*, 1687.

Wang, Y., Li, L., Liu, J., Wang, Z., Jiang, C., & Liu, X. (1997). The analgesic domain of IL-2. *Biochemical Biophysical Research Communications, 230*, 542–545.

Wang, Y., Pei, G., Cai, Y. C., Zhao, Z. Q., Wang, J. B., Jiang, C. L., Zheng, Z. C., & Liu, X. Y. (1996). Human interleukin-2 could bind to opioid receptor and induce corresponding signal transduction. *Neuroreport, 8*, 11–14.

Webster, H. H., Hanisch, U. K., Dykes, R. W., & Biesold, D. (1991). Basal forebrain lesions with or without reserpine injection inhibit cortical reorganization in rat hindpaw primary somatosensory cortex following sciatic nerve section. *Somatosensory and Motor Research, 8*, 327–346.

Wegenka, U. M., Lutticken, C., Buschmann, J., Yuan, J., Lottspeich, F., Muller Esterl, W., Schindler, C., Roeb, E., Heinrich, P. C., & Horn, F. (1994). The interleukin-6-activated acute-phase response factor is antigenically and functionally related to members of the signal transducer and activator of transcription (STAT) family. *Molecular Cell Biology, 14*, 3186–3196.

Weigent, D. A., & Blalock, J. E. (1995). Associations between the neuroendocrine and immune systems. *Journal of Leukocyte Biology, 58*, 137–150.

Wheelock, E. F. (1965). Interferon-like virus inhibitor induced in human leukocytes by phytohemagglutinin. *Science, 149*, 310–311.

Whitehouse, P. J., Price, D. L., Struble, R. G., Clark, A. W., Coyle, J. T., & Delon, M. R. (1982). Alzheimer's disease and senile dementia: Loss of neurons in the basal forebrain. *Science, 215*, 1237–1239.

Whittington, R., & Faulds, D. (1993). Interleukin-2. A review of its pharmacological properties and therapeutic use in patients with cancer. *Drugs, 46*, 446–514.

Wilkinson, P. C., & Liew, F. Y. (1995). Chemoattraction of human blood T lymphocytes by interleukin-15. *Journal of Experimental Medicine, 181*, 1255–1259.

Winkelhake, J. L., & Gauny, S. S. (1990). Human recombinant interleukin-2 as an experimental therapeutic. *Pharmacological Reviews, 42*, 1–28.

Winkler, M. K., & Beveniste, E. N. (1998). Transforming growth factor-beta inhibition of cytokine-induced vascular cell adhesion molecule-1 expression in human astrocytes. *Glia, 22*, 171–179.

Wiranowska, M., Prockop, L. D., Naidu, A. K., Saporta, S., Kori, S., & Kulkarni, A. P. (1994). Interferon entry through the blood-brain barrier in glioma and its effect on lipoxygenase activity. *Anticancer Research, 14*, 1121–1126.

Withyachumnarnkul, B., Nonaka, K. O., Attia, A. M., & Reiter, R. J. (1990). Changes in indole metabolism in organ cultured rat pineal glands induced by interferon-gamma. *Journal of Pineal Research, 8*, 313–322.

Withyachumnarnkul, B., Nonaka, K. O., Santana, C., Attia, A. M., & Reiter, R. J. (1990). Interferon-gamma modulates melatonin production in rat pineal glands in organ culture. *Journal of Interferon Research, 10*, 403–411.

Withyachumnarnkul, B., Reiter, R. J., Lerchl, A., Nonaka, K. O., & Stokkan, K. A. (1991). Evidence that interferon-gamma alters pineal metabolism both indirectly via sympathetic nerves and directly on the pinealocytes. *International Journal of Biochemistry, 23*, 1397–1401.

Woodroofe, M. N., Hayes, G. M., & Cuzner, M. L. (1989). Fc receptor density, MHC antigen expression and superoxide production are increased in interferon-gamma-treated microglia isolated from adult rat brain. *Immunology, 68*, 421–426.

Xiao, B. G., Bai, X. F., Zhang, G. X., Hojeberg, B., & Link, H. (1996). Shift from anti- to proinflammatory cytokine profiles in microglia through LPS- or IFN-gamma-mediated pathways. *Neuroreport, 7*, 1893–1898.

Xiao, B. G., & Link, H. (1998). IFN-gamma production of adult rat astrocytes triggered by TNF-alpha. *Neuroreport, 9*, 1487–1490.

Xu, J., & Ling, E. A. (1994). Upregulation and induction of major histocompatibility complex class I and II antigens on microglial cells in early postnatal rat brain following intraperitoneal injections of recombinant interferon-gamma. *Neuroscience, 60*, 959–967.

Xu, J., & Ling, E. A. (1995). Induction of major histocompatibility complex class II antigen on amoeboid microglial cells in early postnatal rats following intraperitoneal injections of lipopolysaccharide or interferon-gamma. *Neuroscience Letters, 189*, 97–100.

Yamaguchi, M., Koike, K., Matsuzaki, N., Yoshimoto, Y., Taniguchi, T., Miyake, A., & Tanizawa, O. (1991). The interferon family stimulates the secretions of prolactin and interleukin-6 by the pituitary gland in vitro. *Journal of Endocrinological Investigation, 14*, 457–461.

Yao, G. L., Kato, H., Khalil, M., Kiryu, S., & Kiyama, H. (1997). Selective upregulation of cytokine receptor subchain and their intracellular signalling molecules after peripheral nerve injury. *European Journal of Neuroscience, 9*, 1047–1054.

Yao, H., Wang, F. Z., Ding, A. S., Liu, Z. W., & Ling, S. G. (1994). Effects of interleukin-1 and interleukin-2 on electrophysiological characteristics of rat hippocampal neurons in culture. *Sheng. Li. Hsueh. Pao., 46*, 539–545.

Zalcman, S., Green-Johnson, J. M., Murray, L., Nance, D. M., Dyck, D., Anisman, H., & Greenberg, A. H. (1994). Cytokine-specific central monoamine alterations induced by interleukin-1, -2 and -6. *Brain Research, 643*, 40–49.

Zhao, B., & Schwartz, J. P. (1998). Involvement of cytokines in normal CNS development and neurological diseases: Recent progress and perspectives. *Journal of Neuroscience Research, 52*, 7–16.

Zhou, Z. H., Chaturvedi, P., Han, Y. L., Aras, S., Li, Y. S., Kolattukudy, P. E., Ping, D., Boss, J. M., & Ransohoff, R. M. (1998a). IFN-gamma induction of the human monocyte chemoattractant protein (hMCP)-1 gene in astrocytoma cells: Functional interaction between an IFN-gamma-activated site and a GC-rich element. *Journal of Immunology, 160*, 3908–3916.

Zhou, Z. H., Chaturvedi, P., Han, Y. L., Aras, S., Li, Y. S., Kolattukudy, P. E., Ping, D., Boss, J. M., & Ransohoff, R. M. (1998b). IFN-gamma induction of the human monocyte chemoattractant protein (hMCP)-1 gene in astrocytoma cells: Functional interaction between an IFN-gamma-activated site and a GC-rich element. *Journal of Immunology, 160*, 3908–3916.

Zhu, M. H., Berry, J. A., Russell, S. M., & Leonard, W. J. (1998). Delineation of the regions of interleukin-2 (IL-2) receptor beta chain important for association of Jak1 and Jak3. Jak1-independent functional recruitment of Jak3 to Il-2Rbeta. *Journal of Biological Chemistry, 273*, 10719–10725.

Zielasek, J., Archelos, J. J., Toyka, K. V., & Hartung, H. P. (1993). Expression of intercellular adhesion molecule-1 on rat microglial cells. *Neuroscience Letters, 153*, 136–139.

Zielasek, J., Tausch, M., Toyka, K. V., & Hartung, H. P. (1992). Production of nitrite by neonatal rat microglial cells/brain macrophages. *Cellular Immunology, 141*, 111–120.

Zocchia, C., Spiga, G., Rabin, S. J., Grekova, M., Richert, J., Chernyshev, O., Colton, C., & Mocchetti, I. (1997). Biological activity of interleukin-10 in the central nervous system. *Neurochemistry International, 30*, 433–439.

Zuckerman, S. H., Gustin, J., & Evans, G. F. (1998). Expression of CD54 (intercellular adhesion molecule-1) and the beta 1 integrin CD29 is modulated by a cyclic AMP dependent pathway in activated primary rat microglial cell cultures. *Inflammation, 22*, 95–106.

Zwain, I. H., Grima, J., & Cheng, C. Y. (1994). Regulation of clusterin secretion and mRNA expression in astrocytes by cytokines. *Molecular and Cellular Neuroscience, 5*, 229–237.

CHAPTER

24

The Hypothalamo-Pituitary-Adrenal Axis Response to Immune Signals

CATHERINE RIVIER

I. INTRODUCTION

Homeostasis, which pertains to the requirement that a variety of bodily parameters be maintained within preset limits, is the goal of most of our behavioral, autonomic, immune, and endocrine responses. In other words when faced with a threat, whether real or perceived, the organism will put in place a cascade of well-defined changes aimed at restoring and preserving the consistency of the *milieu intérieur*. The classical stress response involves the activation of the central and peripheral catecholamines systems and the release of hormones belonging to the hypothalamo-pituitary-adrenal (HPA) axis response, in particular adrenocorticotropin hormone (ACTH) and glucocorticosteroids (GC). If the stress includes infection or injury, the immune system will also be activated. Although these three systems (autonomic, endocrine, and immune) can act separately and independently of each other, the mounting of a viable, healthy, and coordinated response requires that they not only communicate with each other, but also regulate each other's activities. The purpose of this chapter is to highlight some of our present understanding of this phenomenon, as well as of the mechanisms underlying interactions among neuroendocrine and immune processes of adaptation. Specifically, we will discuss the influence exerted by immune signals on the HPA axis using paradigms used in our laboratory. This is not intended as a review of the field, which the interested reader can find in many comprehensive recent articles (see for example Besedovsky & DelRey, 1996; Dunn, 1995; Rivest & Rivier, 1995; Shintani, Nakaki, Kanba, Kato, & Asai, 1995; Turnbull, Lee, & Rivier, 1998; Turnbull & Rivier, 1999b; Wilder, 1995), nor is it an attempt to provide an exhaustive review of the literature. Rather, the chapter relies on work published over the last few years to illustrate the points made, knowing full well that in many cases, seminal contributions not quoted here were made at earlier times. Finally, for the most part the discussion is restricted to the rodent (rat and mouse).

The activity of the HPA axis is reflected in the periphery by the release of ACTH from the pituitary, and of GC from the adrenals. At the hypothalamic level, neurons in the paraventricular nucleus (PVN) of the hypothalamus produce corticotropin-releasing factor (CRF) and/or vasopressin (VP), which are secreted from nerve terminals in the median eminence (ME) (Sawchenko et al., 1996; Swanson, 1987; Watts, 1996; Whitnall, 1993). At the pituitary level, CRF and VP bind to their G protein-coupled type 1 receptors (CRF-R_1 and VP-R_{1a}), an event that triggers a cascade of enzymatic reactions that begins with the stimulation of adenylate cyclase and mobilization of intracellular calcium (Howl & Wheatley, 1995; Morel, O'Carroll, Brownstein, & Lolait, 1992; Perrin, Donaldson, Chen, Lewis, & Vale, 1993), and ultimately regulates the gene expression of proopiomelanocortin (POMC), and the release of POMC-derived peptides in the circulation (Behan et al., 1996; Chalmers, Lovenberg, Grigoriadis, Behan, & DeSouza, 1996; DeSouza, 1995; Vale, Vaughan, & Perrin, 1997).

Following exposure to a stressor, the increased levels of GC measured in the general circulation exert a classical feedback influence at the level of the pituitary, where they blunt the ACTH response to CRF (Rivier, C.L., & Plotsky, 1986), and at the level of the PVN, where they interfere with CRF production (Li & Sawchenko, 1998). In general, the ability of VP to release ACTH requires the presence of CRF (Antoni, 1993; Hauger & Aguilera, 1993; Plotsky, P. M., 1985; Plotsky, P. M., Bruhn, & Vale, 1985; Rivier, C., & Vale, 1983, 1984, 1985a, 1985b); it is therefore considered as a relatively weak ACTH secretagogue. However, under chronic immune or nonimmune stress, the enhanced release of PVN CRF is often accompanied by down-regulated pituitary CRF-R_1 (Aubry, Turnbull, Pozzoli, Rivier, & Vale, 1997; Luo, Kiss, Makara, Lolait, & Aguilera, 1994; Makino et al., 1995; Pozzoli, Bilezikjian, Perrin, Blount, & Vale, 1996; Sakai et al., 1996; Turnbull & Rivier, 1997; Zhou, Y., et al., 1996). Under these circumstances, the activity of the corticotrophs can be maintained by VP (Aguilera, Pham, & Rabadan-Diehl, 1994; Scaccianoce et al., 1991), which renders this gland and higher centers less sensitive to GC feedback (see for example Chowdrey, Larsen, Harbuz, Jessop, et al., 1995; deGoeij, Dijkstra, & Tilders, 1992; Ma, Levy, & Lightman, 1997).

II. EXPERIMENTAL MODELS USED TO STUDY THE EFFECT OF IMMUNE SIGNALS ON THE HPA AXIS

A. Single Cytokines

The influence of peripheral immune stimulation originally was studied in animals administered single proinflammatory cytokines such as tumor necrosis factor-α (TNF-α), interleukin-1β (IL-1β), and IL-6 (see Besedovsky et al., 1991; Dunn, 1992b; Harbuz, Stephanou, Sarlis, & Lightman, 1992; Reichlin, 1993; Rivier, C., 1995c; van der Meer et al., 1996). The present consensus is that acutely (systemically) injected proinflammatory cytokines do not act directly on the pituitary, but stimulate ACTH release through

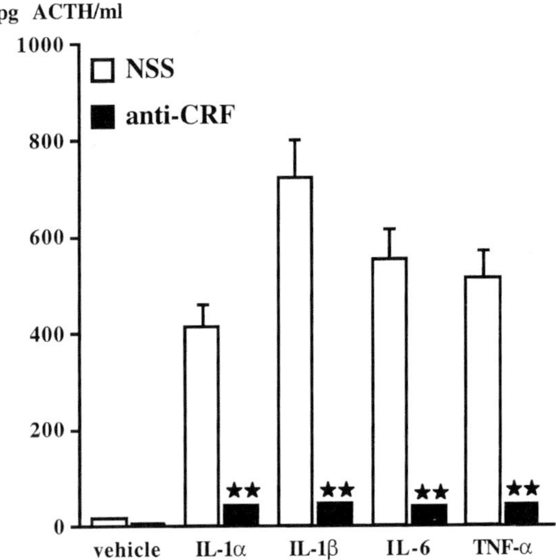

FIGURE 1 Effect of peripheral corticotropin-releasing factor (CRF) immunoneutralization on the adrenocorticotropin hormone (ACTH) response to the iv injection of recombinant human tumor necrosis factor-α (TNF-α) (0.5 μg/kg), interleukin (IL)-1α or β (0.5 μg/kg), and IL-6 (5.0 μg/kg). Blood samples were obtained 30 min after cytokine treatment. Each bar represents the mean ± SEM of 5 intact adult male rats. $^{**}P < 0.01$ vs. NSS (normal sheep serum).

a CRF-dependent mechanism references in (Rivier, C., 1995c; Watanobe, Sasaki, & Takebe, 1991) (Figure 1). That is, removal of endogenous CRF with specific antibodies, or blockade of its pituitary receptors with specific antagonists, significantly blunt the stimulatory effect of these immune signals. VP antibodies also decrease the ACTH response to IL-1β, which supports the concept of a VP-dependent component in this phenomenon. However, the magnitude of this decrease is less than that observed in animals treated with CRF antibodies, indicating that the role of VP is probably secondary (Rivier, C., 1995a). The stimulatory effect exerted on ACTH release by immune proteins present in the peripheral circulation probably initially depends at least in part on CRF and/or VP secretion from nerve terminals. Activation of PVN neurons subsequently takes place as the result of depleted peptide stores. Indeed, the question of whether relatively low doses of TNF-α, IL-1β, and IL-6 are, by themselves and following a single acute systemic injection, capable of activating CRF and/or VP perikarya in the PVN, is still being debated, and may depend on the concentration of cytokine used (Callahan & Piekut, 1997; Ericsson, Kovács, & Sawchenko, 1994; Parsadaniantz, Levin, Lenoir, Roberts, & Kerdelhué, 1994; Rivest, Torres, & Rivier, 1992; Rivier, C., 1995c; Valliéres, Lacroix, & Rivest, 1997). For example, we observed that the intravenous (iv) or intraperitoneal (ip) delivery of 0.5 μg/kg IL-1β

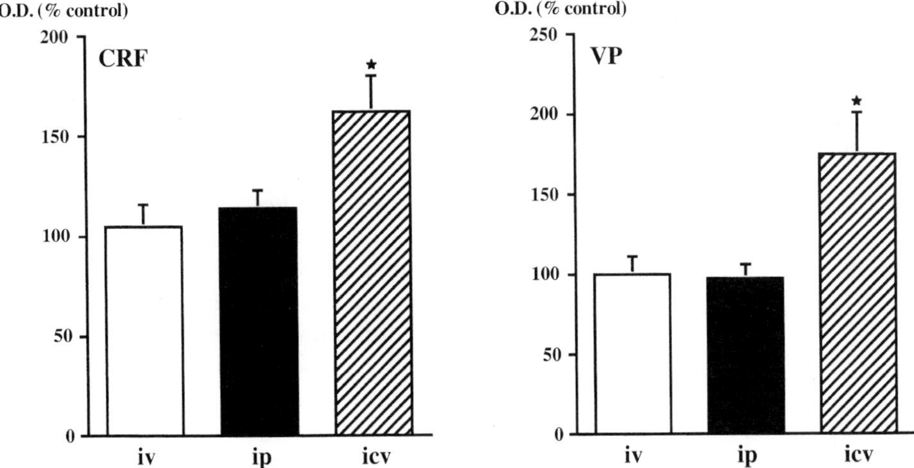

FIGURE 2 Corticotropin-releasing factor (CRF) and vasopressin (VP) mRNA levels measured in the pPVN of intact adult male rats injected with IL-1β ip (0.5 μg/kg), iv (0.5 μg/kg), or icv (0.1 μg/kg). Brains were obtained 2 h after cytokine treatments. For in situ methods, see Lee and Rivier, 1994. Each bar represents the mean ± SEM of four to five duplicates. * $P < 0.01$.

did not significantly increase CRF or VP transcripts in the rat PVN, whereas the intracerebroventricular (icv) administration of 0.2 μg/kg did (Figure 2). Nevertheless, if given at high enough doses, IL-1β in particular can activate PVN neurons and increase CRF synthesis (Brady, Lynn, Herkenham, & Gottesfeld, 1994; Ericsson & Sawchenko, 1993; Ju, Zhang, Jin, & Huang, 1991; Saphier & Ovadia, 1990; Senba & Ueyama, 1997; Suda et al., 1990; Veening et al., 1993). Increased activity of PVN cell bodies, either directly or via their afferent pathways, may also result from the production of cytokine-induced intermediates such as prostaglandins (PGs) and catecholamines (see below), which may be produced by cells in circumventricular organs, in the wall of the ventricles, and/or within brain glial cells and astrocytes (see discussion in (Rivier, C., 1995c). Indeed, the importance of the PVN, which is the site of the CRF and VP neurons whose activity regulates ACTH release (Sawchenko, et al., 1996; Swanson, Sawchenko, Rivier, & Vale, 1983; Watts, 1996), has been shown by the inability of iv TNF-α or IL-1β to stimulate ACTH secretion in PVN-lesioned rats (Kovács & Elenkov, 1995; Rivest & Rivier, 1991).

Although the role played by CRF and VP in mediating the ability of proinflammatory cytokines to activate the HPA axis is crucial, other neurotransmitters and circuitries (Chan, Brown, Ericsson, Kovács, & Sawchenko, 1993; Ericsson et al., 1994) also participate in this response (Li & Sawchenko, 1998). For example PGs are very important, as demonstrated by the ability of indomethacin or ibuprofen to virtually block the immediate ACTH response to these immune challenges (discussed in Ericsson, Arias, & Sawchenko, 1997; Rivier, C., 1995c; Watanobe, Nasushita, Sasaki, & Suda, 1998). However, it has been routinely observed that even in the presence of large and/or repeated doses of the PGs inhibitors indomethacin or ibuprofen, the ACTH response to iv IL-1β began to be restored within 2 h of treatment with these antagonists (Figure 3). It therefore appears that although PGs are very important

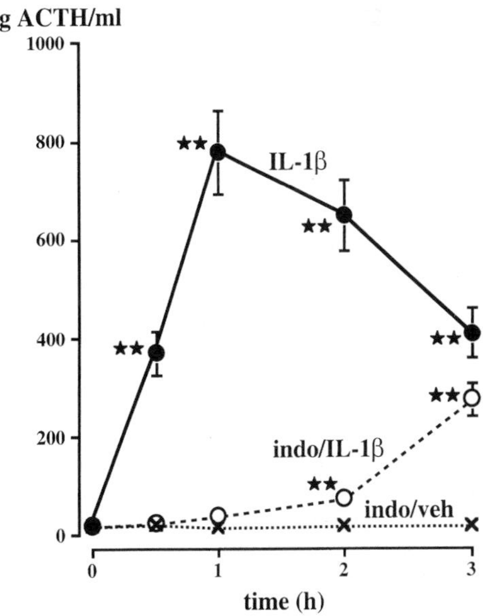

FIGURE 3 Indomethacin (indo, 10 mg/kg, iv 15 min earlier) reduces the adrenocorticotropin hormone (ACTH) response to iv interleukin (IL)-1β (0.5 mg/kg). Veh, vehicle. Each point represent the mean ± SEM of 5 intact adult male rats. ** $P < 0.01$ indo/veh.

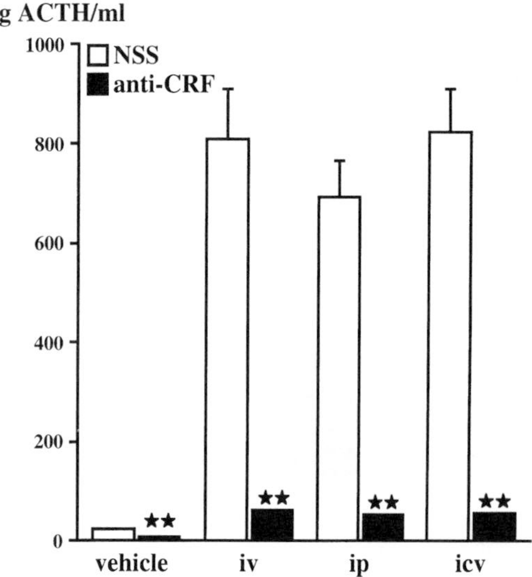

FIGURE 4 Immunoneutralization of endogenous corticotropin-releasing factor (CRF) by the iv injection of specific antibodies significantly (**$P < 0.01$) decreases the adrenocorticotropin hormone (ACTH) response to the iv, ip, or icv injection of interleukin (IL)-1β (doses, see Figure 2). Blood samples were obtained 30 min after cytokine treatment. Each bar represents the mean ± SEM of 5 intact adult male rats.

mediators during the early part of this response, other secretagogues gain importance at later time points. It must also be noted that the route through which cytokines reach the brain influences the effect of PGs (Dunn & Chuluyan, 1992; Ericsson et al., 1997; Rivier, C., 1993). Indeed, there is mounting evidence that the mechanisms responsible for the response of the HPA axis to ip-administered cytokines may be different from those operative in other paradigms. We, as well as many other investigators (references in Rivier, 1995c), have consistently observed that the iv, ip, or icv injection of IL-1β all significantly increase ACTH levels, and that endogenous CRF is essential for these responses (Figure 4). However, vagal afferents appear to be crucial in mediating the brain influence of ip injection of IL-1β, possibly by transmitting a stimulatory signal to the PVN (Fleshner et al., 1997; Hansen, Taishi, Chen, & Krueger, 1998; Kapcala, He, Gao, Pieper, & DeTolla, 1996; Sehic & Blatteis, 1996; Wan, Wetmore, Sorensen, Greenberg, & Nance, 1994; Watkins et al., 1995).

The role of catecholamines is somewhat less clear. There is little doubt that endotoxin and some proinflammatory cytokines activate noradrenergic circuits projecting to the hypothalamus (Terao, Oikawa, & Saito, 1993) and release norepinephrine and related compounds in the brain (see for example Delrue, Deleplanque, Rouge-Pont, Vitiello, & Neveu, 1994; Dunn & Vickers, 1994; Lacosta, Merali, & Anisman, 1998; Lavicky & Dunn, 1995; Rivier, C., Vale, & Brown, 1989; Shintani et al., 1993; Smagin, Swiergiel, & Dunn, 1996; Terao et al., 1993; Zalcman et al., 1994). As these amines stimulate PVN neuronal activity (Al-Damluji, 1993; Cunningham, Bohn, & Sawchenko, 1990; Plotsky, P., Cunningham, & Widmaier, 1989), it would be logical to predict that they participate in the HPA axis response to immune challenges. Experiments carried out with 6-hydroxydopamine lesions or surgical transections of aminergic innervation have usually, but not always, indicated that this procedure indeed interferes with the activation of the HPA axis by cytokines (Chuluyan, Saphier, Rohn, & Dunn, 1992; Li, Ericsson, & Sawchenko, 1996; Matta, Singh, Newton, & Sharp, 1990; Weidenfeld, Abramsky, & Ovadia, 1989). However, surprisingly the administration of adrenergic antagonists is often without effect (Cambronero, Rivas, Borrell, & Guaza, 1992; Rivier, C., et al., 1989; Weidenfeld et al., 1989). The fact that ascending catecholaminergic pathways exert dual and opposite regulatory roles (Weidenfeld et al., 1989), and that the influence of peripheral and central catecholamines is probably different (Zhou, Z. Z., & Jones, 1993), may have relevance for these apparently conflicting data. Also, as in the case of PGs, the influence of these amines may depend at least in part on the route through which cytokines are administered (Barbanel et al., 1993) and the presence of vagal afferents (Fleshner et al., 1995; Ishizuka et al., 1997, 1998), and may be different throughout the time-course of the HPA axis response (Givalois et al., 1995).

Finally, nitric oxide (NO) and carbon monoxide (CO) are unstable gases that have emerged as new brain neurotransmitters (see for example Garthwaite & Boulton, 1995; Maines, 1997; Snyder & Dawson, 1995; Snyder, Jaffrey, & Zakhary, 1998) playing an important role in the endocrine hypothalamus (Amir, 1995; Mancuso, Preziosi, Grossman, & Navarra, 1998). Transcripts for constitutive (c) NO synthase (cNOS), the enzyme responsible for NO formation, are upregulated in the PVN during endotoxemia (Lee, Barbanel, & Rivier, 1995). Although these results could not be duplicated by others, who proposed that LPS-induced corticosteroids might have exerted a negative feedback on NOS synthesis (Satta, Jacobs, Kaltas, & Grossman, 1998), this experiment was repeated recently in adrenalectomized rats and no significant difference was found between levels measured in the presence or absence of corticosterone (Lee and Rivier, unpublished). It should be noted that the gene for cNOS is constitutively expressed in the PVN (see for example Arevalo et al., 1992; Torres, Lee,

& Rivier, 1993), and furthermore that it is not only influenced by immune challenges, but also by non-immune challenges (Calzà, Giardino, & Ceccatelli, 1993; Ceccatelli, 1997; Tsuchiya, Kishimoto, & Nakayama, 1996). This indicates that NO, which is present in PVN CRF and VP neurons (Siaud et al., 1994; Torres et al., 1993) probably plays a wide role with regard to the HPA axis. In further support of this hypothesis, we recently reported that iv LPS stimulated NO production in the PVN along a time-course that coincided with that of the ACTH response (Uribe, Lee, & Rivier, in press).

Using specific NOS antagonists that fully block NOS activity in the hypothalamus (Kim & Rivier, 1998), we showed that NO exerts a dual influence on the stimulatory effect of cytokines. During circumstances accompanied by elevated levels of TNF-α, IL-1β, and/or IL-6 in the peripheral circulation, NO restrains the ACTH response (Kim & Rivier, 1998; Rivier, C., & Shen, 1994; Turnbull & Rivier, 1996a, 1996b). In contrast, it does not significantly alter the effect of icv IL-1β (Turnbull & Rivier, 1996b). On the other hand, NO augments ACTH released by physicoemotional stresses such as mild electrofootshocks, water-avoidance stress, and restraint [(Rivier, C., 1994; Turnbull, Kim, Lee, & Rivier, 1998; and Kim and Rivier, unpublished)]. Although studies on the production of CRF and VP by isolated brain tissues exposed to NO donors or antagonists have yielded contradictory results (Brunetti, Volpe, Ragazzoni, Preziosi, & Vacca, 1996; Costa, Trainer, Besser, & Grossman, 1993; Karanth, Lyson, & McCann, 1993; Kostoglou-Athanassiou et al., 1998; Lutz-Bucher & Koch, 1994; McCann, Kumura, Karanth, Yu, & Rettori, 1997; Pozzoli et al., 1994; Sàndi & Guaza, 1995), experiments conducted in whole animals have provided strong evidence for the concept that NO indeed stimulates PVN neurons that are relevant for ACTH release. In particular, we found that the injection of NO donors into the brain ventricles or the PVN, at doses that did not significantly alter blood pressure, stimulated ACTH release and CRF synthesis in the hypothalamus, and augmented the ACTH response to systemic LPS (Lee, Kim, & Rivier, 1999; Uribe et al., 1999; Uribe and Rivier, unpublished). With regard to CO, we recently reported that systemic administration of the enzyme responsible for CO formation, heme oxygenase (HO), decreased the ACTH response to shocks (Turnbull et al., 1998). These results, which suggest that CO also exerts a stimulatory influence on the intact rat's hypothalamic PVN, have not yet been repeated in animals exposed to immune challenges.

At present, we clearly have a still incomplete and confusing understanding of the role played by NO and CO on the HPA axis. In particular, it is quite intriguing that results obtained from in vitro and in vivo preparations are so consistently conflicting. One possible explanation is that NO and CO exert a variety of opposite effects on the PVN. Isolated systems may allow us to identify some of these components, but the net result of these effects in the whole animal would depend on the nature and intensity of the stimulus to which it is exposed. It also appears that parameters that we have not yet identified may influence the response of NOS transcripts to specific stimuli so that results reported by various laboratories, as well as inconsistencies noticed in the same laboratory, will eventually be explained and understood. There is little doubt that both gases will be found to play an essential role in modulating the functional interactions between the immune system and the HPA axis, though the present state of affair suggests that unraveling it will represent quite a challenge (Jessop, 1999; Mancuso et al., 1998).

B. Endotoxin

In addition to experiments conducted with single proinflammatory cytokines, several investigators have used endotoxin (lipopolysaccharide [LPS]) as a means of mimicking the acute-phase response (Lenczowski, Van Dam, Poole, Larrick, & Tilders, 1997), which is the initial immune response to most antigens. However, LPS administration represents a complicated model that includes the production of hepatic acute-phase proteins, alterations in the plasma concentrations of metals such as iron and zinc, and fever and sickness behaviors (Kent, Bluthe, Kelley, & Dantzer, 1992). The stress that these changes induce might have consequences that are independent of the immune events in the strict sense of the term. Another problem is that although the published literature contains many studies performed with LPS, a significant number of them have relied on enormous doses of this reagent, which not only may damage the blood-brain barrier, but also probably have little physiological relevance. Furthermore, results are rarely reported in terms of LPS units injected, and because commercially available endotoxins are not standarized, comparing studies done in different laboratories can be quite difficult.

This being said, the fact that endotoxemia is characterized by the release of TNF-α, IL-1β, and IL-6 in the plasma (see for example Besedovsky & DelRey, 1992; Givalois et al., 1994; and Figure 5) and in the brain (see for example Klir, McClellan, &

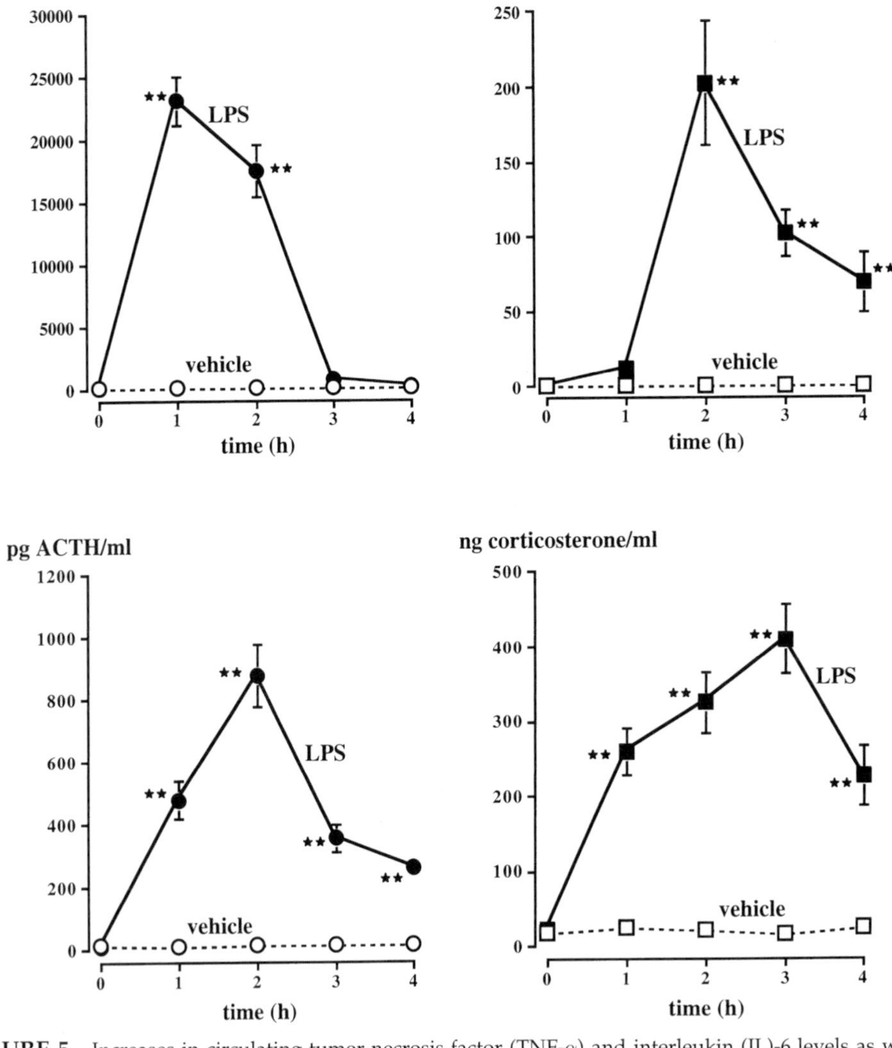

FIGURE 5 Increases in circulating tumor necrosis factor (TNF-α) and interleukin (IL)-6 levels as well as ACTH and corticosterone, after the iv injection of lipopolysaccaride (LPS) (25 μg/kg). Cytokines were measured by bioassay (Turnbull et al., 1996, 1997). Each point represents the mean ± SEM of 5 intact adult male rats. **$P < 0.01$.

Kluger, 1994; Sacoccio, Dornand, & Barbanel, 1998) has been used as a means of determining the endocrine consequence of elevated levels of these proteins. Endotoxemia induces a significant activation of the HPA axis (see for example (Carlson, 1996; Mekaouche et al., 1996; Rivier, C., 1993; Rivier, C., et al., 1989; Tilders et al., 1994)]. As in the case of single cytokines (Rivier, C., & Vale, 1989), LPS stimulates ACTH release whether injected systemically or centrally (Habu, Watanobe, Yasujima, & Suda, 1998). However, the route of LPS injection determines the pattern of PVN response (Wan et al., 1993), with vagal afferents being important for the full response of the HPA axis to ip treatment (Wan et al., 1994). In contrast to single cytokine administration, on the other hand, the systemic injection of LPS is well recognized for its ability to up-regulate the neuronal activity of the PVN and related areas (Dunn, 1992a; Elmquist et al., 1993; Sagar, Price, Kasting, & Sharp, 1995; Vallières & Rivest, 1997), a phenomenon that participates in the subsequent release of ACTH. The hormonal response to endotoxemia depends on the same neurotransmitters shown to be important for single cytokines, namely endogenous CRF, VP, PGs, and NO, though the specific involvement of each of these secretagogues can depend on the dose of LPS used (references in (Rivier, C., 1995c; Schotanus, Makara, Tilders, & Berkenbosch, 1994). The up-regulated production of catecholamines in the periphery (Delrue-Perollet, Li, Vitiello, & Neveu, 1995)

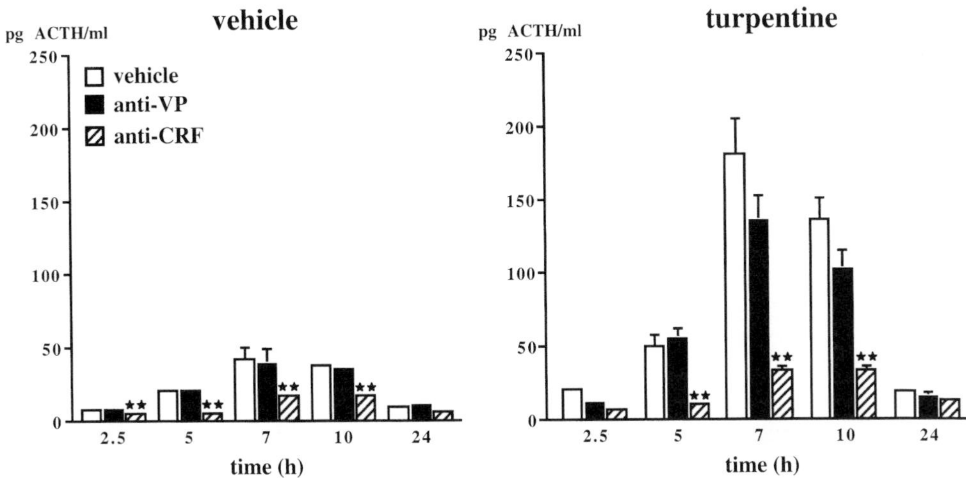

FIGURE 6 Plasma adrenocorticotropin hormone (ACTH) levels in vehicle- or turpentine-injected intact adult male rats. The vehicle or the corticotropin-releasing factor (CRF) or vasopressin (VP) antibodies were injected at the same time as turpentine. Blood samples were obtained through permanent indwelling iv cannulae. Each bar represents the mean ± SEM of 5–6 intact adult male rats. $^{**}P < 0.01$ vs. vehicle.

and the brain (Delrue et al., 1994; Dunn, 1992a; Linthorst, Flachskamm, Holsboer, & Reul, 1996; Tolchard, Hare, Nutt, & Clarke, 1996) is probably also important for the HPA axis response, though serotonin may not be involved (Conde, Renshaw, Lightman, & Harbuz, 1998). What is less clear is the role played by individual cytokines in this response. As discussed in detail elsewhere (Turnbull & Rivier, 1999b), this kind of study is complicated by the presence of potential functional interactions between TNF-α, IL-1β, and IL-6, chaperoning influences of antibodies and the use of icv-injected reagents that may have leaked to the periphery (Bluthé et al., 1994; LeMay, Otterness, Vander, & Kluger, 1990; Perlstein, Whitnall, Abrams, Mougey, & Neta, 1993). Indeed, results obtained with antibodies against one of these proteins, or attempts to correlate temporal changes in plasma cytokines and ACTH levels, have failed to provide solid and convincing evidence that increases in cytokine levels are critically necessary for the full HPA axis response (Dunn, 1992b; Ebisui et al., 1994; Schotanus, Tilders, & Berkenbosch, 1993; Takao et al., 1997).

C. Tissue Injury

Tissue injury can be induced by the injection of small doses of irritants such as turpentine, formaline, Freund's adjuvant, or carrageenan (Aloisi et al., 1995; Sternberg, 1995; Turnbull et al., 1994). It has been shown that the intramuscular administration of turpentine induced a biphasic response of the HPA axis. The first phase corresponds to the stress of the injection and is not accompanied by detectable changes in IL-6 levels, whereas the second phase characterizes the inflammatory process with significant increases in circulating ACTH, corticosterone, and IL-6 concentrations (Cooper et al., 1994; Turnbull & Rivier, 1996a). CRF, VP (Figure 6), and PGs play a stimulatory role in this model, whereas NO restrains the pituitary response (Turnbull & Rivier, 1996a). What triggers the release of these secretagogues? IL-1β may be important, because mice lacking the gene for this cytokine show a blunted corticosterone response to turpentine (Horai et al., 1998). Turnbull and colleagues (1997) showed that brain TNF-α was also important for the ACTH response we measured in this inflammatory model. However, they were unable to detect changes in CNS levels of this cytokine (Turnbull et al., 1997). This fact adds to the list of unresolved issues pertaining to the importance of brain proinflammatory cytokines as mediators of the HPA axis response to various immune challenges.

D. Arthritis

Arthritis is a phenomenon of long-term inflammation, and in rodents it is characteristically induced by the injection of complete Freund's adjuvant or collagen (Cromartie, Craddock, Schwab, Anderle, & Yang, 1977; Durie, Fava, & Noelle, 1994; Wilder & Sternberg, 1990). In this laboratory model, one can demonstrate the presence of increased circulating levels of ACTH and corticosterone and/or a loss of circadian rhythm in the release of these hormones (Sarlis, Chowdrey, Stephanou, & Lightman, 1992; Stephanou, Sarlis, Knight, Lightman, & Chowdrey,

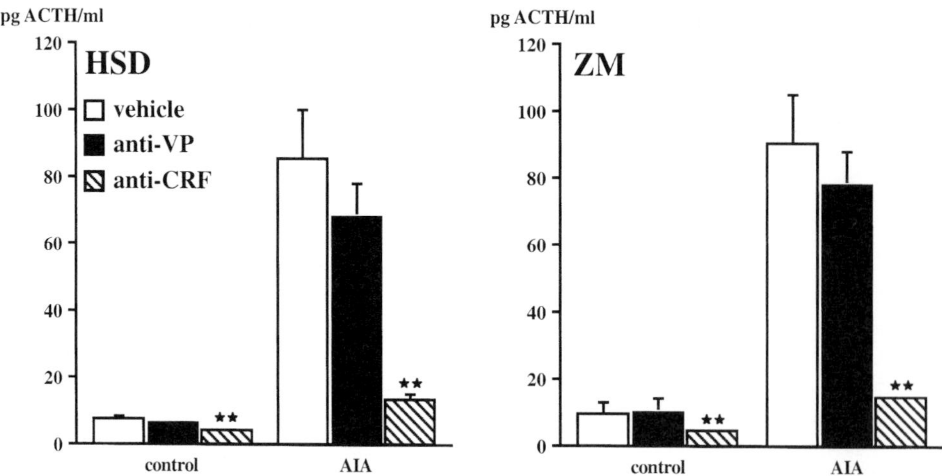

FIGURE 7 Plasma adrenocorticotropin hormone (ACTH) levels in intact adult male Sprague-Dawley rats obtained from Harlan Sprague-Dawley (HSD) or Ziwig Miller (ZM), which were injected with complete Freund's adjuvant 13 days earlier. The vehicle or corticotropin-releasing factor (CRF) antibodies were injected iv 30 min prior to blood sampling. Each bar represents the mean ± SEM of 5 intact adult male rats. ** $P < 0.01$ vs. vehicle. VP, vasopressin.

1992; Tanaka, Ueta, Yamashita, Kannan, & Yamashita, 1996). Even though this type of arthritis is used as a model of pain (Millan, Millan, Czionkowski, Hollt, et al., 1986; Millan, Millan, Czlonkowski, Pilcher, et al., 1986), there is evidence from our laboratory (Rivier, C., 1995b) as well as others' (Sarlis et al., 1992), that increases in plasma ACTH and corticosterone levels precede the appearance of the symptoms and obvious signs of discomfort. Levels of IL-1β and/or IL-6 are significantly elevated in the joints, the circulation, the spleen, and the anterior pituitary (Jessop, Chowdrey, & Lightman, 1993; Sarlis, Stephanou, Knight, Lightman, & Chowdrey, 1993; Stephanou, Sarlis, Knight, Lightman, & Chowdrey, 1992; Sugita et al., 1993). Therefore it is probable that the response of the HPA axis is primarily mediated, at least initially, by increases in peripheral cytokine concentrations. Unfortunately, this is not an easy hypothesis to test, as experimental manipulations that block IL-6 activity or prevent its release significantly reduce the inflammatory process.

The investigation of the role of hypothalamic peptides in the HPA axis response to arthritis has yielded unexpected results. It has been observed that removal of endogenous CRF abolished, whereas blockade of VP reduced, the elevated ACTH levels in the rats tested (Figure 7). Interestingly, some but not all strains of rats display decreased PVN CRF transcripts when rendered arthritic (Chowdrey, Larsen, Harbuz, Jessop, et al., 1995; Chowdrey, Larsen, Harbuz, Lightman, & Jessop, 1995; Harbuz, Rees, et al., 1992; and Figure 8). Some investigators have proposed that in these cases an up-regulated synthesis of PVN VP, and the subsequent release of this peptide in the median eminence, was responsible for the increased ACTH secretory rate (Chowdrey, Larsen, Harbuz, Jessop, et al., 1995; Chowdrey, Larsen, Harbuz, Lightman, et al., 1995; Harbuz and Lightman, 1992; Harbuz, et al., 1992). However, at least in our studies, this was not the case (Figure 8). Furthermore, the development of symptoms and the activation of the HPA axis appeared to be similar in animals in which PVN CRF synthesis was either not altered or significantly blunted (Rivier, unpublished). These results suggest that decreased CRF and increased VP synthesis may not necessarily be general characteristics of inflammatory processes, and that additional work is necessary to understand the functional importance of hypothalamic CRF and VP in inflammatory processes. With regard to the peripheral influence of this peptide, published information was initially controversial. However, the initially reported antiinflammatory effect of CRF (Wei, Kiang, & Tian, 1987; Wei, Serda, & Tian, 1988) may be due at least in part to changes in vascular flow induced by this and related peptides (Torpy, Webster, Zachman, Aguilera, & Chrousos, 1999). Present consensus seems to hold that CRF, which is produced in immune cells (see for example Brouxhon, Prasad, Joseph, Felten, & Bellinger, 1998; Crofford et al., 1992; Mastorakos et al., 1995; Radulovic, Dautzenberg, Sydow, Radulovic, & Spiess, 1999; Van Tol, Petrusz, Lund, Yamauchi, & Sartor, 1996), exerts complex influences on inflammatory processes (Karalis et al.,

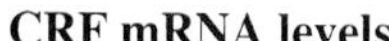

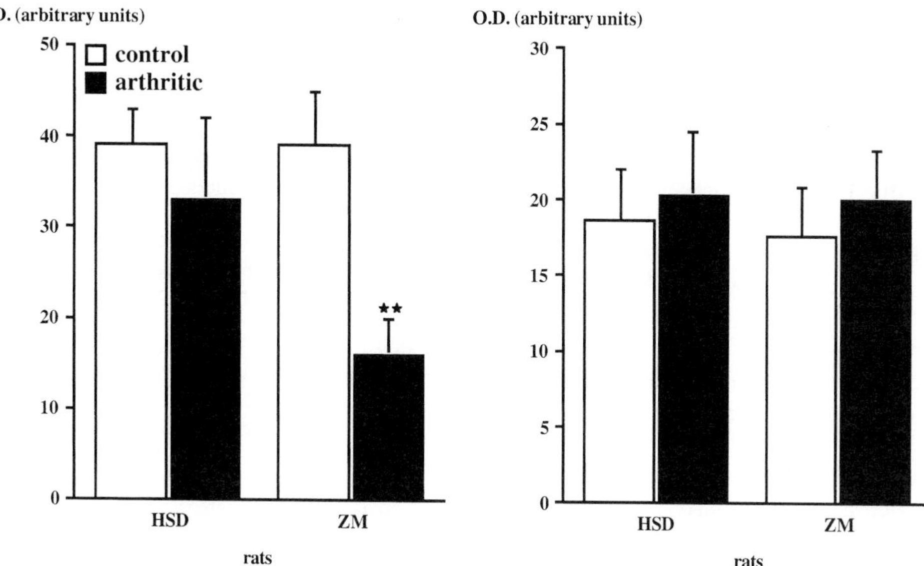

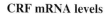

FIGURE 8 Corticotropin-releasing factor (CRF) and vasopressin (VP) mRNA levels measured in the PVN of Harlan Sprague-Dawley (HSD) or Ziwig Miller (ZM) rats (see Figure 7) that had been injected with the vehicle or complete Freund's adjuvant 13 days earlier. For methods, see (Lee et al., 1994; Rivier, 1995). Each bar represents the mean ± SEM of 5 intact adult male rats. $^{**}P < 0.01$.

1991; Theoharides et al., 1997; Vamvakopoulos, 1995). Preliminary data indicated that continuous blockade of CRF receptors with the systemic injection of a potent and long-acting peptidic CRF antagonist injected from the day of MBB injection slightly, but not significantly, reversed the effect of MBB on body weights and arthritic symptoms (scored as described in Lysle, Luecken, & Maslonek, 1992; Santos & Tipping, 1994; Wooley, Dutcher, Widmer, & Gillis, 1993) (Figure 9). If these results are confirmed, they would suggest that the role of peripheral CRF in mediating long-term inflammation remains unclear.

E. Nonimmune Stresses

Finally, it is important to mention that nonimmune stresses also can increase circulating levels of proinflammatory cytokines. Hemorrhage (Abraham,

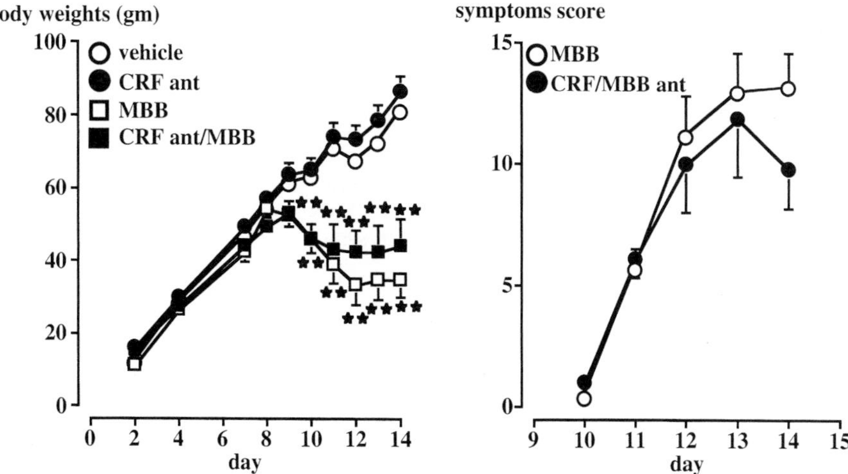

FIGURE 9 Effect of a potent corticotropin-releasing factor (CRF) antagonist (ant), injected twice daily from day 1 of MBB injection, on weight changes and the development of symptoms. The decrease in weight usually precedes the onset of visible symptoms (i.e., blood spots on the leg tissue and swelling of the articulations) by 1–2 days. $^{**}P < 0.01$ vs. vehicle or CRF ant.

Richmond, & Chang, 1988; Komaki et al., 1994) as well as some psychological (Dugue, Leppanen, Teppo, Fyhrquist, & Grasbeck, 1993; LeMay, Vander, & Kluger, 1990; Maes et al., 1998) and physical stresses (Mekaouche et al., 1994; Nukina et al., 1998; Papanicolaou et al. 1996; Pedersen, Ostrowski, Rohde, & Bruunsgaard, 1998; Zhou, D., Kusnecov, Shurin, DePaoli, & Rabin, 1993) all increase these levels through mechanisms that may include catecholamines (DeRijk, Boelen, Tilders, & Berkenbosch, 1994; Takaki, Huang, Somogyvári-Vigh, & Arimura, 1994) and peripheral CRF (Ando, Rivier, Yanaihara, & Arimura, 1998). However, a comparison between plasma ACTH and IL-6 levels in models of immune and nonimmune stresses indicated that the correlation between the two indexes is sometimes poor (Turnbull & Rivier, 1999). Thus, the role played by cytokines in participating in the ACTH response to nonimmune stresses remains to be determined.

III. CONCLUSION

Initially, the concept of a functional interaction between the immune system and the HPA axis was greeted with much skepticism. However, the characterization of the signals that convey to the brain the occurrence of peripheral immune activation, as well as the identification of the molecular mechanisms through which these signals activate the CNS, have provided the basis for our increasing understanding of this bilateral communication pathway. Over the last few years the discovery of the role of neural circuitries such as the vagus, the increasing realization that the route through which cytokines are presented is very important, and the addition of neurotransmitters such as NO and CO to the list of essential intermediates, have vastly expanded our knowledge in the neuroimmunoendocrine field. There is also increased recognition that the abnormal activity of the signaling between the immune system and the HPA axis may underlie numerous pathologies. Finally, the discovery that nonimmune challenges also seem able to induce the production of cytokines has altered our concept of possible interactions between immune and neuroendocrine signals, as well as that of the physiological role played by these proteins. Expanded studies in these areas will undoubtedly be extremely useful and beneficial.

Acknowledgments

Research in the author's laboratory was supported by National Institutes of Health grants DK-26741, MH-51774 and AR (NIAMS)-40770, and by the Clayton Foundation. CR is a senior foundation researcher. The author is indebted to Dr. Soon Lee for the results in Figures 2 and 8, and to Dr. Andrew Turnbull for the results in Figure 5.

References

Abraham, E., Richmond, N. J., & Chang, Y.-H. (1988). Effects of hemorrhage on interleukin-1 production. *Circulatory Shock, 25*, 33–40.

Aguilera, G., Pham, Q., & Rabadan-Diehl, C. (1994). Regulation of pituitary vasopressin receptor during chronic stress: Relationship to corticotroph responsiveness. *Journal of Neuroendocrinology, 6*, 299–304.

Al-Damluji, S. (1993). Adrenergic control of the secretion of anterior pituitary hormones. *Bailliere's Clinical Endocrinology and Metabolism, 7*, 355–392.

Aloisi, A. M., Albonetti, M. E., Muscettola, M., Facchinetti, F., Tanganelli, C., & Carli, G. (1995). Effects of formalin-induced pain on ACTH, beta-endorphin, corticosterone and interleukin-6 plasma levels in rats. *Neuroendocrinology, 62*, 13–18.

Amir, S. (1995). Nitric oxide signalling in the hypothalamus. In *Nitric oxide in the nervous system* (pp. 151–162). San Diego: Academic Press.

Ando, T., Rivier, J., Yanaihara, H., & Arimura, A. (1998). Peripheral corticotropin-releasing factor mediates the elevation of plasma IL-6 by immobilization stress in rats. *American Journal of Physiology—Regulatory Integrative and Comparative Physiology, 44*, R1461–R1467.

Antoni, F. A. (1993). Vasopressinergic control of pituitary adrenocorticotropin secretion comes of age. *Frontiers in Neuroendocrinology, 14*, 76–122.

Arevalo, A., Sanchez, F., Alonso, J. R., Carretero, J., Vazquez, R., & Aijon, J. (1992). NADPH-Diaphorase activity in the hypothalamic magnocellular neurosecretory nuclei of the rat. *Brain Research Bulletin, 28*, 599–603.

Aubry, J.-M., Turnbull, A., Pozzoli, G., Rivier, C., & Vale, W. (1997). Endotoxin decreases corticotropin-releasing factor receptor 1 messenger ribonucleic acid levels in the rat pituitary. *Endocrinology, 138*, 1621–1626.

Barbanel, B., Gaillet, S., Mekaouche, M., Givalois, L., Ixart, G., Siaud, P., Szafarczyk, S., Malaval, F., & Assenmacher, I. (1993). Complex catecholaminergic modulation of the stimulatory effect of interleukin-1β on the corticotropic axis. *Brain Research, 626*, 31–36.

Behan, D. P., Grigoriadis, D. E., Lovenberg, T., Chalmers, D., Heinrichs, S., Liaw, C., & De Souza, E. B. (1996). Neurobiology of corticotropin releasing factor (CRF) receptors and CRF-binding protein: Implications for the treatment of CNS disorders. *Molecular Psychiatry, 1*, 265–277.

Besedovsky, H. O., & DelRey, A. (1992). Immuno-neuroendocrine circuits: Integrative role of cytokines. *Frontiers in Neuroendocrinology, 13*, 61–94.

Besedovsky, H. O., & DelRey, A. (1996). Immune-neuro-endocrine interactions: Facts and hypotheses. *Endocrine Reviews, 17*, 64–102.

Besedovsky, H. O., DelRey, A., Klusman, I., Furukawa, H., Arditi, G. M., & Kabiersch, A. (1991). Cytokines as modulators of the hypothalamus-pituitary-adrenal axis. *Journal of Steroid Biochemistry and Molecular Biology, 40*, 613–618.

Bluthé, R. M., Pawlowski, M., Suarez, S., Parnet, P., Pittman, Q., Kelley, K. W., & Dantzer, R. (1994). Synergy between tumor necrosis factor α and interleukin-1 in the induction of sickenss behavior in mice. *Psychoneuroendocrinology, 19*, 197–207.

Brady, L. S., Lynn, A. B., Herkenham, M., & Gottesfeld, Z. (1994). Systemic interleukin-1 induces early and late patterns of *c-fos* mRNA expression in brain. *Journal of Neuroscience, 14*, 4951–4964.

Brouxhon, S. M., Prasad, A. V., Joseph, S. A., Felten, D. L., & Bellinger, D. L. (1998). Localization of corticotropin-releasing factor in primary and secondary lymphoid organs of the rat. *Brain, Behavior, and Immunity, 12*, 107–122.

Brunetti, L., Volpe, A. R., Ragazzoni, E., Preziosi, P., & Vacca, M. (1996). Interleukin-1β specifically stimulates nitric oxide production in the hypothalamus. *Life Sciences, 58*(25), PL373–PL377.

Callahan, T. A., & Piekut, D. T. (1997). Differential fos expression induced by IL-1β and IL-6 in rat hypothalamus and pituitary gland. *Journal of Neuroimmunology, 73*, 207–211.

Calzà, L., Giardino, L., & Ceccatelli, S. (1993). NOS mRNA in the paraventricular nucleus of young and old rats after immobilization stress. *Neuroendocrinology, 4*, 627–630.

Cambronero, J. C., Rivas, F. J., Borrell, J., & Guaza, C. (1992). Release of corticotropin-releasing factor from superfused rat hypothalami induced by interleukin-1 is not dependent on adrenergic mechanism. *European Journal of Pharmacology, 219*, 75–80.

Carlson, D. (1996). Adrenocorticotropin correlates strongly with endotoxemia after intravenous but not after intraperitoneal inoculations of *E. coli*. *Shock, 6*, 1–9.

Ceccatelli, S. (1997). Expression and plasticity of NO synthase in the neuroendocrine system. *Brain Research Bulletin, 44*, 533–538.

Chalmers, D. T., Lovenberg, T. W., Grigoriadis, D. E., Behan, D. P., & DeSouza, E. B. (1996). Corticotrophin-releasing factor receptors: from molecular biology to drug design. *Trends in Pharmacological Sciences, 17*(4), 166–172.

Chan, R. K. W., Brown, E. R., Ericsson, A., Kovács, K. J., & Sawchenko, P. E. (1993). A comparison of two immediate-early genes, c-fos and NGFI-β, as markers for functional activation in stress-related neuroendocrine circuitry. *Journal of Neuroscience, 13*, 5126–5138.

Chowdrey, H. S., Larsen, P. J., Harbuz, M. S., Jessop, D. S., Aguilera, G., Eckland, D. J. A., & Lightman, S. L. (1995). Evidence for arginine vasopressin as the primary activator of the HPA axis during adjuvant-induced arthritis. *British Journal of Pharmacology, 116*, 2417–2424.

Chowdrey, H. S., Larsen, P. J., Harbuz, M. S., Lightman, S. L., & Jessop, D. S. (1995). Endogenous substance P inhibits the expression of corticotropin-releasing hormone during a chronic inflammatory stress. *Life Sciences, 57*, 2021–2029.

Chuluyan, H. E., Saphier, D., Rohn, W. M., & Dunn, A. J. (1992). Noradrenergic innervation of the hypothalamus participates in adrenocortical responses to interleukin-1. *Neuroendocrinology, 56*, 106–111.

Conde, G. L., Renshaw, D., Lightman, S. L., & Harbuz, M. S. (1998). Serotonin depletion does not alter lipopolysaccharide-induced activation of the rat paraventricular nucleus. *Journal of Endocrinology, 156*, 245–251.

Cooper, A. L., Brouwer, S., Turnbull, A. V., Luheshi, G. N., Hopkins, S. J., Kunkel, S. L., & Rothwell, N. J. (1994). Tumor necrosis factor-α and fever after peripheral inflammation in the rat. *American Journal of Physiology, 36*, R1431–R1436.

Costa, A., Trainer, P., Besser, M., & Grossman, A. (1993). Nitric oxide modulates the release of corticotropin-releasing hormone from the rat hypothalamus in vitro. *Brain Research, 605*, 187–192.

Crofford, L. J., Sano, H., Karalis, K., Webster, E. L., Goldmuntz, E. A., Chrousos, G. P., & Wilder, R. L. (1992). Local secretion of corticotropin-releasing hormone in the joints of Lewis rats with inflammatory arthritis. *Journal of Clinical Investigation, 90*, 2555–2564.

Cromartie, W., Craddock, J., Schwab, J., Anderle, S., & Yang, C.-H. (1977). Arthritis in rats after systemic injection of streptococcal cells or cells walls. *Journal of Experimental Medicine, 146*, 1585–1602.

Cunningham, E., Bohn, M., & Sawchenko, P. (1990). Organization of adrenergic inputs to the paraventricular and supraoptic nuclei of the hypothalamus in the rat. *Journal of Comparative Neurology, 292*, 651–667.

deGoeij, D. C. E., Dijkstra, H., & Tilders, F. J. H. (1992). Chronic psychosocial stress enhances vasopressin, but not corticotropin-releasing factor, in the external zone of the median eminence of male rats: Relationship to subordinate status. *Endocrinology, 131*, 847–853.

Delrue, C., Deleplanque, B., Rouge-Pont, F., Vitiello, S., & Neveu, P. J. (1994). Brain monoaminergic, neuroendocrine, and immune responses to an immune challenge in relation to brain and behavioral lateralization. *Brain, Behavior, and Immunity, 8*, 137–152.

Delrue-Perollet, C., Li, K.-S., Vitiello, S., & Neveu, P. J. (1995). Peripheral catecholamines are involved in the neuroendocrine and immune effects of LPS. *Brain, Behavior, and Immunity, 9*, 149–162.

DeRijk, R. H., Boelen, A., Tilders, F. J. H., & Berkenbosch, F. (1994). Induction of plasma interleukin-6 by circulating adrenaline in the rat. *Psychoneuroendocrinology, 19*, 155–163.

DeSouza, E. B. (1995). Corticotropin-releasing factor receptors: Physiology, pharmacology, biochemistry and role in central nervous system and immune disorders. *Psychoneuroendocrinology, 20*, 789–819.

Dugue, B., Leppanen, E. A., Teppo, A. M., Fyhrquist, F., & Grasbeck, R. (1993). Effects of psychological stress on plasma interleukin-1-beta and interelukin-6-beta, C-reactive protein, tumour necrosis factor-alpha, anti-diuretic hormone and serum cortisol. *Scandinavian Journal of Clinical and Laboratory Investigation, 53*, 555–561.

Dunn, A. (1992a). Endotoxin-induced activation of cerebral catecholamine and serotonin metabolism: Comparison with interleukin-1. *Neuroscience Research Communications, 261*, 964–969.

Dunn, A. (1995). Interactions between the nervous system and the immune system: Implications for psychopharmacology. In F. E. Bloom & D. J. Kupfer (Eds.), *Psychopharmacology* (pp. 719–731). New York: Raven Press.

Dunn, A. J. (1992b). The role of interleukin-1 and tumor necrosis factor α in the neurochemical and neuroendocrine responses to endotoxin. *Brain Research Bulletin, 29*, 807–812.

Dunn, A. J., & Chuluyan, H. E. (1992). The role of cyclo-oxygtenase and lipoxygenase in the interleukin-1-induced activation of the HPA axis: Dependence on the route of injection. *Life Sciences, 51*, 219–225.

Dunn, A., & Vickers, S. (1994). Neurochemical and neuroendocrine responses ot Newcastle disease virus administration in mice. *Brain Research, 645*, 103–112.

Durie, F. H., Fava, R. A., & Noelle, R. J. (1994). Short analytical review: Collagen-induced arthritis as a model of rheumatoid arthritis. *Clinical Immunology and Immunopathology, 73*, 11–18.

Ebisui, O., Fukata, J., Murakami, N., Kobayashi, H., Segawa, H., Muro, S., Hanaoka, I., Naito, Y., Masui, Y., Ohmoto, Y., Imura, H., & Nakao, K. (1994). Effect of IL-1 receptor antagonist and antiserum to TNF-α on LPS-induced plasma ACTH and corticosterone rise in rats. *American Journal of Physiology, 266*, E986–E992.

Elmquist, J. K., Ackermann, M. R., Register, K. B., Rimler, R. B., Ross, L. R., & Jacobson, C. D. (1993). Induction of Fos-like immunoreactivity in the rat brain following *Pasteurella multocida* endotoxin administration. *Endocrinology, 133*, 3054–3057.

Ericsson, A., Arias, C., & Sawchenko, P. (1997). Evidence for an intramedullary prostaglandin-dependent mechanism in the activation of stress-related neuroendocrine circuitry by intravenous interleukin-1. *Journal of Neuroscience, 17*, 166–179.

Ericsson, A., Kovács, K. J., & Sawchenko, P. E. (1994). A functional anatomical analysis of central pathways subserving the effects of interleukin-1 on stress-related neuroendocrine neurons. *Journal of Neuroscience, 14*, 897–913.

Ericsson, A., & Sawchenko, P. E. (1993). c-fos-Based functional mapping of central pathways subserving the effects of interleukin-1 on the hypothalamo-pituitary-adrenal axis. In E. B. DeSouza (Ed.), *Methods in neuroscience* (pp. 155–172). New York: Academic Press.

Fleshner, M., Goehler, L. E., Hermann, J., Relton, J. K., Maier, S. F., & Watkins, L. R. (1995). Interleukin-1β induced corticosterone elevation and hypothalamic NE depletion is vagally mediated. *Brain Research Bulletin, 37*, 605–610.

Fleshner, M., Silbert, L., Deak, T., Goehler, L. E., Martin, D., Watkins, L. R., & Maier, S. F. (1997). TNF-α-induced corticosterone elevation but not serum protein or corticosteroid binding globulin reduction is vagally mediated. *Brain Research Bulletin, 44*, 701–706.

Garthwaite, J., & Boulton, C. L. (1995). Nitric oxide signaling in the central nervous system. *Annual Review of Physiology, 57*, 683–706.

Givalois, L., Dornand, J., Mekaouche, M., Solier, M., Bristow, A., Ixart, G., Siaud, P., Assenmacher, I., & Barbanel, G. (1994). Temporal cascade of plasma level surges in ACTH, corticosterone, and cytokines in endotoxin-challenged rats. *American Journal of Physiology, 267*, R164–R170.

Givalois, L., Gaillet, S., Mekaouche, M., Ixart, G., Bristow, A. F., Siaud, P., Szafarczyk, A., Malaval, F., Assenmacher, I., & Barbanel, G. (1995). Deletion of the ventral noradrenergic bundle obliterates the early ACTH response after systemic LPS, independently from the plasma IL-1β surge. *Endocrine, 3*, 481–486.

Habu, S., Watanobe, H., Yasujima, M., & Suda, T. (1998). Different roles of brain interleukin 1 in the adrenocorticotropin response to central versus peripheral administration of lipopolysaccharide in the rat. *Cytokine, 10*, 390–394.

Hansen, M. K., Taishi, P., Chen, Z., & Krueger, J. M. (1998). Vagotomy blocks the induction of interluekin-1β (IL-1β) mRNA in the brain of rats in response to systemic IL-1β. *Journal of Neuroscience, 18*, 2247–2253.

Harbuz, M. S., & Lightman, S. L. (1992). Stress and the hypothalamo-pituitary-adrenal axis: Acute, chronic and immunological activation. *Journal of Endocrinology, 134*, 327–339.

Harbuz, M. S., Rees, R. G., Eckland, D., Jessop, D. S., Brewerton, D., & Lightman, S. L. (1992). Paradoxical responses of hypothalamic corticotropin-releasing factor (CRF) messenger ribonucleic acid (mRNA) and CRF-41 peptide and adenohypophysial proopiomelanocortin mRNA during chronic inflammatory stress. *Endocrinology, 130*, 1394–1400.

Harbuz, M. S., Stephanou, A., Sarlis, N., & Lightman, S. L. (1992). The effects of recombinant human interleukin (IL)-1α, IL-1β or IL-6 on hypothalamo-pituitary-adrenal axis activation. *Journal of Endocrinology, 133*, 349–355.

Hauger, R. L., & Aguilera, G. (1993). Regulation of pituitary CRH receptors by CRH: Interaction with vasopressin. *Endocrinology, 133*, 1708–1714.

Horai, R., Asano, M., Sudo, K., Kanuka, H., Suzuki, M., Nishihara, M., Takahashi, M., & Iwakura, Y. (1998). Production of mice deficient in genes for interleukin (IL)-1α, IL-1β, IL-α/β, and IL-1 receptor antagonist shows that IL-1β is crucial in turpentine-induced fever development and glucocorticoid secretion. *Journal of Experimental Medicine, 187*, 1463–1475.

Howl, J., & Wheatley, M. (1995). Molecular pharmacology of V_{1a} vasopressin receptors. *General Pharmacology, 26*, 1143–1152.

Ishizuka, Y., Ishida, Y., Jin, Q.-H., Shimokawa, A., Saita, M., Kato, K., Kunitake, T., Hanamori, T., Mitsuyama, Y., & Kannan, H. (1998). Abdominal vagotomy attenuates interleukin-1β-induced nitric oxide release in the paraventricular nucleus region in concious rats. *Brain Research, 789*, 157–161.

Ishizuka, Y., Ishida, Y., Kunitake, T., Kato, K., Hanamori, T., Mitsuyama, Y., & Kannan, H. (1997). Effects of area postrema lesion and abdominal vagotomy on interleukin-1β-induced norepinephrine release in the hypothalamic paraventricular nucleus region in the rat. *Neuroscience Letters, 223*, 57–60.

Jessop, D., Chowdrey, H., & Lightman, S. (1993). Interleukin-1β measured by radioimmunoassay in the rat spleen and thymus is increased during chronic inflammatory stress. *Neuropeptides, 24*, 367–371.

Jessop, D. S. (1999). Central non-glucocorticoid inhibitors of the hypothalamo-pituitary-adrenal axis. *Journal of Endocrinology, 160*, 169–180.

Ju, G., Zhang, X., Jin, B.-Q., & Huang, C.-S. (1991). Activation of corticotropin-releasing factor-containing neurons in the paraventricular nucleus of the hypothalamus by interleukin-1 in the rat. *Neuroscience Letters, 132*, 151–154.

Kapcala, L. P., He, J. R., Gao, Y., Pieper, J. O., & DeTolla, L. J. (1996). Subdiaphragmatic vagotomy inhibits intra-abdominal interleukin-1β stimulation of adrenocorticotropin secretion. *Brain Research, 728*, 247–254.

Karalis, K., Sano, H., Redwine, J., Listwak, S., Wilder, R. L., & Chrousos, G. P. (1991). Autocrine or paracrine inflammatory actions of corticotropin-releasing hormone in vivo. *Science, 254*, 421–423.

Karanth, S., Lyson, K., & McCann, S. M. (1993). Role of nitric oxide in interleukin-2-induced corticotropin-releasing factor release from incubated hypothalami. *Proceedings of the National Academy of Sciences, USA, 90*, 3383–3387.

Kent, S., Bluthe, R., Kelley, K., & Dantzer, R. (1992). Sickness behavior as a new target for drug development. *Trends in Pharmacological Science, 13*, 24–28.

Kim, C. K., & Rivier, C. (1998). Influence of nitric oxide synthase inhibitors on the ACTH and cytokine responses to peripheral immune signals. *Journal of Neuroendocrinology, 10*, 353–362.

Klir, J. J., McClellan, J. L., & Kluger, M. J. (1994). Interleukin-1β causes the increase in anterior hypothalamic interleukin-6 during LPS-induced fever in rats. *American Journal of Physiology, 266*, R1845–R1848.

Komaki, G., Gottschall, P. E., Somogyvári-Vigh, A., Tatsuno, I., Yatohgo, T., & Arimura, A. (1994). Rapid increase in plasma IL-6 after hemorrhage, and posthemorrhage reduction of the IL-6 response to LPS, in conscious rats: Interrelation with plasma corticosterone levels. *Neuroimmunomodulation, 1*, 127–134.

Kostoglou-Athanassiou, I., Costa, A., Navarra, P., Nappi, G., Forsling, M. L., & Grossman, A. B. (1998). Endotoxin stimulates an endogenous pathway regulating corticotropin-releasing hormone and vasopressin release involving the generation of nitric oxide and carbon monoxide. *Journal of Neuroimmunology, 86*, 104–109.

Kovács, K. J., & Elenkov, I. J. (1995). Differential dependence of ACTH secretion induced by various cytokines on the integrity of the paraventricular nucleus. *Journal of Neuroendocrinology, 7*, 15–23.

Lacosta, S., Merali, Z., & Anisman, H. (1998). Influence of interleukin-1β on exploratory behaviors, plasma ACTH, corticosterone, and central biogenic amines in mice. *Psychopharmacology, 137*, 351–361.

Lavicky, J., & Dunn, A. J. (1995). Endotoxin administration stimulates cerebral catecholamine release in freely moving rats as assessed by microdialysis. *Journal of Neuroscience Research, 40*, 407–413.

Lee, S., Barbanel, G., & Rivier, C. (1995). Systemic endotoxin increases steady-state gene expression of hypothalamic nitric oxide synthase: Comparison with corticotropin-releasing factor and vasopressin gene transcripts. *Brain Research, 705*, 136–148.

Lee, S., Kim, C., & Rivier, C. (1999). Nitric oxide stimulates ACTH secretion and the transcription of the genes encoding for NGFI-B, corticotropin-releasing factor, corticotropin-releasing factor receptor type 1 and vasopressin in the hypothalamus of the intact rat. *Journal of Neuroscience, 19*, 7640–7647.

Lee, S., & Rivier, C. (1994). Hypophysiotropic role and hypothalamic gene expression of corticotropin-releasing factor and vasopressin in rats injected with interleukin-1β systemically or into the brain ventricles. *Journal of Neuroendocrinology, 6*, 217–224.

LeMay, L., Otterness, I., Vander, A., & Kluger, M. (1990). In vivo evidence that the rise in plasma IL-6 following injection of a fever-inducing dose of LPS is mediated by IL-1β. *Cytokine, 2*, 199–204.

LeMay, L. G., Vander, A. J., & Kluger, M. J. (1990). The effects of psychological stress on plasma interleukin-6 activity in rats. *Physiology and Behavior, 47*, 957–961.

Lenczowski, M. J. P., Van Dam, A.-M., Poole, S., Larrick, J. W., & Tilders, F. J. H. (1997). Role of circulating endotoxin and interleukin-6 in the ACTH and corticosterone response to intraperitoneal LPS. *American Journal of Physiology—Regulatory Integrative and Comparative Physiology, 42*, R1870–R1877.

Li, H.-Y., Ericsson, A., & Sawchenko, P. E. (1996). Distinct mechanisms underlie activation of hypothalamic neurosecretory neurons and their medullary catecholaminergic afferents in categorically different stress paradigms. *Proceedings of the National Academy of Sciences, USA, 93*, 2359–2364.

Li, H.-Y., & Sawchenko, P. E. (1998). Hypothalamic effector neurons and extended circuitries activated in "neurogenic" stress: A comparison of footshock effects exerted acutely, chronically, and in animals with controlled glucocorticoid levels. *Journal of Comparative Neurology, 393*, 244–266.

Linthorst, A. C. E., Flachskamm, C., Holsboer, F., & Reul, J. M. H. M. (1996). Activation of serotonergic and noradrenergic neurotransmission in the rat hippocampus after peripheral administration of bacterial endotoxin: Involvement of the cyclooxygenase pathway. *Neuroscience, 72*, 989–997.

Luo, X., Kiss, A., Makara, G., Lolait, S. J., & Aguilera, G. (1994). Stress-specific regulation of corticotropin releasing hormone receptor expression in the paraventricular and supraoptic nuclei of the hypothalamus in the rat. *Journal of Neuroendocrinology, 6*, 689–696.

Lutz-Bucher, B., & Koch, B. (1994). Evidence for an inhibitiory effect of nitric oxides on neuropeptide secretion from isolated neural lobe of the rat pituitary gland. *Neuroscience Letters, 165*, 48–50.

Lysle, D. T., Luecken, L. J., & Maslonek, K. A. (1992). Suppression of the development of adjuvant arthritis by a conditioned aversive stimulus. *Brain, Behavior, and Immunity 6*, 64–73.

Ma, X.-M., Levy, A., & Lightman, S. L. (1997). Emergence of an isolated arginine vasopressin (AVP) response to stress after repeated restraint: A study of both AVP and corticotropin-releasing hormone messenger ribonucleic acid (RNA) and heteronuclear RNA. *Endocrinology, 138*, 4351–4357.

Maes, M., Song, C., Lin, A., Jongh, R. D., Gastel, A. V., Kenis, G., Bosmans, E., De Meester, I., Benoy, I., Neels, H., Demedts, P., Janca, A., Scharpé, S., & Smith, R. S. (1998). The effects of psychological stress on humans: Increased production of pro-inflammatory cytokines and a Th1-like response in stress-induced anxiety. *Cytokine, 10*, 313–318.

Maines, M. (1997). The heme oxygenase system: A regulator of second messenger gases. *Annual Review of Pharmacology and Toxicology, 37*, 517–554.

Makino, S., Schulkin, J., Smith, M. A., Pacak, K., Palkovits, M., & Gold, P. W. (1995). Regulation of corticotropin-releasing hormone receptor messenger ribonucleic acid in the rat brain and pituitary by glucocorticoids and stress. *Endocrinology, 136*, 4517–4525.

Mancuso, C., Preziosi, P., Grossman, A. B., & Navarra, P. (1998). The role of carbon monoxide in the regulation of neuroendocrine function. *NeuroImmunoModulation, 4*, 225–229.

Mastorakos, G., Bouzas, E. A., Silver, P. B., Sartani, G., Friedman, T. C., Chan, C.-C., Caspi, R. R., & Chrousos, G. P. (1995). Immune corticotropin-releasing hormone is present in the eyes of and promotes experimental autoimmune uveoretinitis in rodents. *Endocrinology, 136*, 4650–4658.

Matta, S. G., Singh, J., Newton, R., & Sharp, B. M. (1990). The adrenocorticotropin response to interleukin-1β instilled into the rat median eminence depends on the local release of catecholamines. *Endocrinology, 127*, 2175–2182.

McCann, S. M., Kumura, M., Karanth, S., Yu, W. H., & Rettori, V. (1997). Nitric oxide controls the hypothalamo-pituitary response to cytokines. *Neuroimmunomodulation, 4*, 98–106.

Mekaouche, M., Givalois, L., Barbanel, G., Siaud, P., Maurel, D., Malaval, F., Bristow, A. F., Boissin, J., Assenmacher, I., & Ixart, G. (1994). Chronic restraint enhances interleukin-1-beta release in the basal state and after an endotoxin challenge, independently of adrenocorticotropin and corticosterone release. *Neuroimmunomodulation, 1*, 292–299.

Mekaouche, M., Siaud, P., Givalois, L., Barbanel, G., Malaval, F., Maurel, D., Assenmacher, I., & Ixart, G. (1996). Different responses of plasma ACTH and corticosterone and of plasma interleukin-1β to single and recurrent endotoxin challenges. *Journal of Leukocyte Biology, 59*, 341–346.

Millan, M. J., Millan, M. H., Czionkowski, A., Hollt, V., Pilcher, C. W., Herz, A., & Colpaert, F. C. (1986). A model of chronic pain in the rat: response of multiple opioid systems to adjuvant-induced arthritis. *Journal of Neuroscience, 6*, 899–906.

Millan, M. J., Millan, M. H., Czlonkowski, A., Pilcher, C. W. T., Höllt, V., Colpaert, F. C., & Herz, A. (1986). Functional response of multiple opioid systems to chronic arthritic pain in the rat. *Annals of the New York Academy of Science, 467*, 182–193.

Morel, A., O'Carroll, A.-M., Brownstein, M. J., & Lolait, S. J. (1992). Molecular cloning and expression of a rat V1a arginine vasopressin receptor. *Nature, 356*, 523–526.

Nukina, H., Sudo, N., Komaki, G., Yu, X.-N., Mine, K., & Kubo, C. (1998). The restraint stress-induced elevation in plasma interleukin-6 negatively regulates the plasma TNF-α level. *NeuroImmunoModulation, 5*, 323–327.

Papanicolaou, D. A., Petrides, J. S., Tsigos, C., Bina, S., Kalogeras, K. T., Wilder, R., Gold, P. W., Deuster, P. A., & Chrousos, G. P. (1996). Exercise stimulates interleukin-6 secretion: Inhibition by glucocorticoids and correlationwith catecholamines. *American Journal of Physiology—Endocrinology and Metabolism, 34*, E601–E605.

Parsadaniantz, S. M., Levin, N., Lenoir, V., Roberts, J. L., & Kerdelhué, B. (1994). Human interleukin 1β: Corticotropin releasing factor and ACTH release and gene expression in the male rat: in vivo and in vitro studies. *Journal of Neuroscience Research, 37*, 675–682.

Pedersen, B. K., Ostrowski, K., Rohde, T., & Bruunsgaard, H. (1998). The cytokine response to strenuous exercise. *Canadian Journal of Physiology and Pharmacology, 76*, 505–511.

Perlstein, R. S., Whitnall, M. H., Abrams, J. S., Mougey, E. H., & Neta, R. (1993). Synergistic roles of interleukin-6, interleukin-1, and tumor necrosis factor in the adrenocorticotropin response to bacterial lipopolysaccharide in vivo. *Endocrinology, 132*, 946–952.

Perrin, M. H., Donaldson, C. J., Chen, R., Lewis, K. A., & Vale, W. W. (1993). Cloning and functional expression of a rat brain corticotropin releasing factor (CRF) receptor. *Endocrinology, 133*, 3058–3061.

Plotsky, P., Cunningham, E. T. J., & Widmaier, E. P. (1989). Catecholaminergic modulation of corticotropin-releasing factor and adrenocorticotropin secretion. *Endocrine Reviews, 10*, 437–458.

Plotsky, P. M. (1985). Hypophysiotropic regulation of adenohypophysial adrenocorticotropin secretion. *Federation Proceedings, 44*, 207–213.

Plotsky, P. M., Bruhn, T. O., & Vale, W. (1985). Evidence for multifactor regulation of the adrenocorticotropin secretory response to hemodynamic stimuli. *Endocrinology, 116*, 633–639.

Pozzoli, G., Bilezikjian, L. M., Perrin, M. H., Blount, A. L., & Vale, W. W. (1996). Corticotropin-releasing factor (CRF) and glucocorticoids modulate the expression of type 1 CRF receptor messenger ribonucleic acid in rat anterior pituitary cell cultures. *Endocrinology, 137*, 65–71.

Pozzoli, G., Mancuso, C., Mirtella, A., Preziosi, P., Grossman, A. B., & Navarra, P. (1994). Carbon monoxide as a novel neuroendocrine modulator: Inhibition of stimulated corticotropin-releasing hormone release from acute rat hypothalamic explants. *Endocrinology, 135*, 2314–2317.

Radulovic, M., Dautzenberg, F. M., Sydow, S., Radulovic, J., & Spiess, J. (1999). Corticotropin-releasing factor receptor 1 in mouse spleen: Expression after immune stimulation and identification of receptor–bearing cells. *Journal of Immunology, 162*, 3013–3021.

Reichlin, S. (1993). Neuroendocrine-immune interactions. *New England Journal of Medicine, 329*, 1246–1253.

Rivest, S., & Rivier, C. (1991). Influence of the paraventricular nucleus of the hypothalamus in the alteration of neuroendocrine functions induced by physical stress or interleukin. *Endocrinology, 129*, 2049–2057.

Rivest, S., & Rivier, C. (1995). The role of corticotropin-releasing factor and interleukin-1 in the regulation of neurons controlling reproductive functions. *Endocrine Reviews, 16*, 177–199.

Rivest, S., Torres, G., & Rivier, C. (1992). Differential effects of central and peripheral injection of interleukin-1β on brain *c-fos* expression and neuroendocrine functions. *Brain Research, 587*, 13–23.

Rivier, C. (1995a). Blockade of nitric oxide formation augments adrenocorticotropin released by blood-borne interleukin-1β: Role of vasopressin, prostaglandins, and α1-adrenergic receptors. *Endocrinology, 136*, 3597–3603.

Rivier, C. (1995b). Decreased plasma gonadotropin and testosterone levels in arthritic rats: Are corticosteroids involved? *Endocrine, 3*, 383–390.

Rivier, C. (1993). Effect of peripheral and central cytokines on the hypothalamo-pituitary-adrenal axis of the rat. *Annals of the New York Academy of Sciences, 796*, 97–105.

Rivier, C. (1994). Endogenous nitric oxide participates in the activation of the hypothalamo-pituitary-adrenal axis by noxious stimuli. *Endocrine Journal, 2*, 367–373.

Rivier, C. (1995c). Influence of immune signals on the hypothalamo-pituitary axis of the rodent. *Frontiers in Neuroendocrinology, 16*, 151–182.

Rivier, C., Chizzonite, R., & Vale, W. (1989). In the mouse, the activation of the hypothalamo-pituitary-adrenal axis by a lipopolysaccharide (endotoxin) is mediated through interleukin-1. *Endocrinology, 125*, 2800–2805.

Rivier, C., & Shen, G. (1994). In the rat, endogenous nitric oxide modulates the response of the hypothalamo-pituitary-adrenal axis to interleukin-1β, vasopressin and oxytocin. *Journal of Neuroscience, 14*, 1985–1993.

Rivier, C., & Vale, W. (1984). Effect of corticotropin-releasing factor (CRF) on some endocrine functions. *Endocrinology*, 959–962.

Rivier, C., & Vale, W. (1985a). Effects of CRF, neurohypophysial peptides and catecholamines on pituitary function. *Federation Proceedings, 44*, 189–195.

Rivier, C., & Vale, W. (1983). Interaction of corticotropin-releasing factor (CRF) and arginine vasopressin (AVP) on ACTH secretion in vivo. *Endocrinology, 113*, 939–942.

Rivier, C., & Vale, W. (1989). In the rat, interleukin-1α acts at the level of the brain and the gonads to interfere with gonadotropin and sex steroid secretion. *Endocrinology, 124*, 2105–2109.

Rivier, C., & Vale, W. (1985b). Neuroendocrine interaction between CRF and vasopressin on ACTH secretion in the rat. In R. W. Schrier (Ed.), *Vasopressin* (pp. 181–188). New York: Raven Press.

Rivier, C., Vale, W., & Brown, M. (1989). In the rat, interleukin-1α and -β stimulate adenocorticotropin and catecholamine release. *Endocrinology, 125*, 3096–3102.

Rivier, C. L., & Plotsky, P. M. (1986). Mediation by corticotropin-releasing factor (CRF) of adenohypophysial hormone secretion. *Annual Reviews in Physiology, 48*, 475–494.

Sacoccio, C., Dornand, J., & Barbanel, G. (1998). Differential regulation of brain and plasma TNFα produced after endotoxin shock. *Neuroreport, 9*, 309–313.

Sagar, S. M., Price, K. J., Kasting, N. W., & Sharp, F. R. (1995). Anatomic patterns of FOS immunostaining in rat brain following system endotoxin administration. *Brain Research Bulletin, 36*, 381–392.

Sakai, K., Horiba, N., Sakai, Y., Tozawa, F., Demura, H., & Suda, T. (1996). Regulation of corticotropin-releasing factor receptor messenger ribonucleic acid in rat anterior pituitary. *Endocrinology, 137*, 1758–1763.

Sandi, C., & Guaza, C. (1995). Evidence for a role of nitric oxide in the corticotropin-releasing factor release induced by interleukin-1β. *European Journal of Pharmacology, 274*, 17–23.

Santos, L., & Tipping, P. G. (1994). Attenuation of adjuvant arthritis in rats by treatment with oxygen radical scavengers. *Immunology and Cell Biology, 72*, 406–414.

Saphier, D., & Ovadia, H. (1990). Selective facilitation of putative corticotropin-releasing factor-secreting neurons by interleukin-1. *Neuroscience Letters, 114*, 283–288.

Sarlis, N. J., Chowdrey, H. S., Stephanou, A. K., & Lightman, S. L. (1992). Chronic activation of the hypothalamo-pituitary-adrenal axis and loss of circadian rhythm during adjuvant-induced arthritis in the rat. *Endocrinology, 130*, 1775–1779.

Sarlis, N. J., Stephanou, A., Knight, R. A., Lightman, S. L., & Chowdrey, H. S. (1993). Effects of glucocorticoids and chronic inflammatory stress upon anterior pituitary interleukin-6 mRNA expression in the rat. *British Journal of Rheumatology, 32*, 653–657.

Satta, M., Jacobs, R., Kaltas, G., & Grossman, A. (1998). Endotoxin induces interleukin-1β and nitric oxide mRNA in rat hypothalamus and pituitary. *Neuroendocrinology, 67*, 109–116.

Sawchenko, P. E., Brown, E. R., Chan, R. K. W., Ericsson, A., Li, H.-Y., Roland, B. L., & Kovacs, K. J. (1996). The paraventricular nucleus of the hypothalamus and the functional neuroanatomy of visceromotor responses to stress. In G. Holstege, R. Bandler, &

C. B. Saper (Eds.), *Emotional motor system* (pp. 201–222). Amsterdam: Elsevier Science B. V.

Scaccianoce, S. L., Muscolo, A. A., Ciglinana, G., Navarra, D., Nicolai, R., & Angelucci, L. (1991). Evidence for a specific role of vasopressin in sustaining pituitary-adrenocortical stress response in the rat. *Endocrinology, 128*, 3138–3143.

Schotanus, K., Makara, G. B., Tilders, F. J. H., & Berkenbosch, F. (1994). ACTH response to a low dose but not a high dose of bacterial endotoxin in rats is completely mediated by corticotropin-releasing hormone. *Neuroimmunomodulation, 1*, 300–307.

Schotanus, K., Tilders, F., & Berkenbosch, F. (1993). Human recombinant interleukin-1 receptor antagonist prevents adrenocorticotropin, but not interleukin-6 responses to bacterial endotoxin in rats. *Endocrinology, 133*, 2461–2468.

Sehic, E., & Blatteis, C. M. (1996). Blockade of lipopolysaccharide-induced fever by subdiaphragmatic vagotomy in guinea pigs. *Brain Research, 726*, 160–166.

Senba, E., & Ueyama, T. (1997). Stress-induced expression of immediate early genes in the brain and peripheral organs of the rat. *Neuroscience Research, 29*, 183–207.

Shintani, F., Kanba, S., Nakaki, T., Nibuya, M., Kinoshita, N., Suzuki, E., Yagi, G., Kato, R., & Asai, M. (1993). Interleukin-1β augments release of norepinephrine, dopamine, and serotonin in the rat anterior hypothalamus. *Journal of Neuroscience, 13*, 3574–3581.

Shintani, F., Nakaki, T., Kanba, S., Kato, R., & Asai, M. (1995). Role of interleukin-1 in stress responses. *Molecular Neurobiology, 10*, 47–71.

Siaud, P., Mekaouche, M., Ixart, G., Balmefrezol, M., Givalois, L., Barbanel, G., & Assenmacher, I. (1994). A subpopulation of corticotropin-releasing hormone neurosecretory cells in the paraventricular nucleus of the hypothalamus also contain NADPH-diaphorase. *Neuroscience Letters, 170*, 51–54.

Smagin, G. N., Swiergiel, A. H., & Dunn, A. J. (1996). Peripheral administration of Interleukin-1 increases extracellular concentrations of norepinephrine in rat hypothalamus: Comparison with plasma corticosterone. *Psychoneuroendocrinology, 21*, 83–93.

Snyder, S. H., & Dawson, T. M. (1995). Nitric oxide and related substances as neural messengers. In F. E. Bloom & D. J. Kupfer (Eds.), *Psychopharmacology: The fourth generation of progress* (pp. 609–618). New York: Raven Press.

Snyder, S. H., Jaffrey, S. R., & Zakhary, R. (1998). Nitric oxide and carbon monoxide: Parallel roles as neural messengers. *Brain Research Reviews, 26*, 167–175.

Stephanou, A., Sarlis, N. J., Knight, R. A., Lightman, S. L., & Chowdrey, H. S. (1992a). Effects of cyclosporine A on the hypothalamo-pituitary-adrenal axis and anterior pituitary interleukin-6 mRNA expression during chronic inflammatory stress in the rat. *Journal of Neuroimmunology, 41*, 215–222.

Stephanou, A., Sarlis, N. J., Knight, R. A., Lightman, S. L., & Chowdrey, H. S. (1992b). Glucocorticoid-mediated responses of plasma ACTH and anterior pituitary pro-opiomelanocortin, growth hormone and prolactin mRNAs during adjuvant-induced arthritis in the rat. *Journal of Molecular Endocrinology, 9*, 273–281.

Sternberg, E. M. (1995). Neuroendocrine factors in susceptibility to inflammatory disease: Focus on the hypothalamo-pituitary-adrenal axis. *Hormone Research, 43*, 159–161.

Suda, T., Tozawa, F., Ushiyama, T., Sumitomo, T., Yamada, M., & Demura, H. (1990). Interleukin-1 stimulates corticotropin-releasing factor gene expression in rat hypothalamus. *Endocrinology, 126*, 1223–1228.

Sugita, T., Furukawa, O., Ueno, M., Murakami, T., Takata, I., & Tosa, T. (1993). Enhanced expression of interleukin 6 in rat and murine arthritis models. *International Journal of Immunopharmacology, 15*, 469–476.

Swanson, L. W. (1987). The hypothalamus. In A. Bjorklund P. Hokfelt, & L. W. Swanson (Eds.), *Handbook of chemical neuroanatomy* (pp. 1–124). Amsterdam: Elsevier.

Swanson, L. W., Sawchenko, P. E., Rivier, J., & Vale, W. W. (1983). Organization of ovine corticotropin releasing factor (CRF)-immunoreactive cells and fibers in the rat brain: An immunohistochemical study. *Neuroendocrinology, 36*, 165–186.

Takaki, A., Huang, Q.-H., Somogyvári-Vigh, A., & Arimura, A. (1994). Immobilization stress may increase plasma interleukin-6 via central and peripheral catecholamines. *Neuroimmunomodulation, 1*, 335–342.

Takao, T., Nanamiya, W., Takemura, T., Nishiyama, M., Asaba, K., Makino, S., Hashimoto, K., & De Souza, E. B. (1997). Endotoxin induced increases in rat plasma pituitary-adrenocortical hormones are better reflected by alterations in tumor necrosis factor-α than interleukin-1β. *Life Sciences, 61*, PL263–PL268.

Tanaka, H., Ueta, Y., Yamashita, U., Kannan, H., & Yamashita, H. (1996). Biphasic changes in behavioral, endocrine, and sympathetic systems in adjuvant arthritis in Lewis rats. *Brain Research Bulletin, 39*, 33–37.

Terao, A., Oikawa, M., & Saito, M. (1993). Cytokine-induced change in hypothalamic norepinephrine turnover: Involvement of corticotropin-releasing hormone and prostaglandins. *Brain Research, 622*, 257–261.

Theoharides, T. C., Singh, L. K., Boucher, W., Pang, X., Letourneau, R., Webster, E., & Chrousos, G. (1997). Corticotropin-releasing hormone induces skin mast cell degranulation and increased vascular permeability, a possible explanation for its proinflammatory effects. *Endocrinology, 139*, 403–413.

Tilders, F. J. H., DeRijk, R. H., Van Dam, A.-M., Vincent, V. A. M., Schotanus, K., & Persoons, J. H. A. (1994). Activation of the hypothalamus-pituitary-adrenal axis by bacterial endotoxins: routes and intermediate signals. *Psychoneuroendocrinology, 19*, 209–232.

Tolchard, S., Hare, A. S., Nutt, D. J., & Clarke, G. (1996). TNF-α mimics the endocrine but not the thermoregulatory responses of bacterial lipopolysaccharide (LPS): Correlaton with FOS-expression in the brain. *Neuropharmacology, 35*, 243–248.

Torpy, D. J., Webster, E. L., Zachman, E. K., Aguilera, G., & Chrousos, G. P. (1999). Urocortin and inflammation: Confounding effects of hypotension on measures of inflammation. *NeuroImmunoModulation, 6*, 182–186.

Torres, G., Lee, S., & Rivier, C. (1993). Ontogeny of the rat hypothalamic nitric oxide synthase and colocalization with neuropeptides. *Molecular and Cellular Neuroscience, 4*, 155–163.

Tsuchiya, T., Kishimoto, J., & Nakayama, Y. (1996). Marked increases in neuronal nitric oxide synthase (nNOS) mRNA and nadph-diaphorase histostaining in adrenal cortex after immobilization stress in rats. *Psychoneuroendocrinology, 21*, 287–293.

Turnbull, A., Kim, C., Lee, S., & Rivier, C. (1998). Influence of carbon monoxide, and its interaction with nitric oxide, on the ACTH response of the intact rat to a physico-emotional stress. *Journal of Neuroendocrinology, 10*, 793–802.

Turnbull, A., Lee, S., & Rivier, C. (1998). Mechanisms of hypothalamo-pituitary-adrenal axis stimulation by immune signals in the adult rat. In S. McCann, E. Sternberg, J. Lipton, G. Chrousos, P. Gold, and C. Smith (Eds.), *Neuroimmunomodulation: Molecular aspects, integrative systems and clinical advances* (pp. 434–443). New York: New York Academy of Sciences.

Turnbull, A., Pitossi, F., Lebrun, J.-J., Lee, S., Nance, D., Besedovsky, U., & Rivier, C. (1997). Inhibition of tumor necrosis factor-α (TNF-α) action within the CNS reduces the plasma adrenocorticotropin response to peripheral local inflammation in rats. *Journal of Neuroscience, 17*, 3262–3273.

Turnbull, A. V., & Rivier, C. (1997). Corticotropin-releasing factor (CRF) and endocrine responses to stress: CRF receptors, binding protein and related peptides. *Proceedings of the Society for Experimental Biology and Medicine, 215*, 1–10.

Turnbull, A. V., & Rivier, C. (1996a). Corticotropin-releasing factor, vasopressin and prostaglandins mediate, and nitric oxide restrains, the hypothalamo-pituitary-adrenal response to acute local inflammation in the rat. *Endocrinology, 137*, 455–463.

Turnbull, A. V., & Rivier, C. L. (1999). Regulation of the hypothalamo-pituitary-adrenal (HPA) axis by cytokines: Actions and mechanisms of action. *Physiological Reviews, 79*, 1–71.

Turnbull, A. V., & Rivier, C. (1996b). Selective inhibitors of nitric oxide synthase (NOS) implicate a constitutive isoform of NOS in the regulation of interleukin-1-induced ACTH secretion in rats. *Endocrine, 5*, 135–140.

Turnbull, A., & Rivier, C. (1999). Sprague-Dawley rats obtaine from different vendors exhibit different ACTH nd interleukin-6 respones to noxious stimuli. *Neuroendocrinology, 70*, 186–195.

Turnbull, A. V., Dow, R. C., Hopkins, S. J., White, A., Fink, G., & Rothwell, N. J. (1994). Mechanisms of activation of the pituitary-adrenal axis by tissue injury in the rat. *Psychoneuroendocrinology, 19*, 165–178.

Uribe, R. M., Lee, S., & Rivier, C. (1999) Endotoxin stimulates nitric oxide production in the paraventricular nucleus of the hypothalamus through nitric oxide synthase I: Correlation with HPA axis activation. *Endocrinology, 140*, 5971–5981.

Vale, W., Vaughan, J., & Perrin, M. (1997). Corticotropin-releasing factor family of ligands and their receptors. *Endocrinologist, 7*, 3S–9S.

Valliéres, L., Lacroix, S., & Rivest, S. (1997). Influence of interleukin-6 on neural activity and transcription of the gene encoding corticotrophin-releasing factor in the rat brain: An effect depending upon the route of administration. *European Journal of Neuroscience, 9*, 1461–1472.

Vallières, L., & Rivest, S. (1997). Regulation of the genes encoding interleukin-6, its receptor, and gp130 in the rat brain in response to the immune activator lipopolysaccharide and the proinflammatory cytokine interleukin-1β. *Journal of Neurochemistry, 69*, 1668–1683.

Vamvakopoulos, N. V. (1995). Sexual dimorphism of stress response and immune/inflammatory reaction: the corticotropin releasing hormone perspective. *Mediators of Inflammation, 4*, 163–174.

van der Meer, M. J. M., Sweep, C. G. J., Rijnkels, C. E. M., Pesman, G. J., Tilders, F. J. H., Kloppenborg, P. W. C., & Hermus, A. R. M. M. (1996). Acute stimulation of the hypothalamo-pituitary-adrenal axis by IL-1β, TNF-α and IL-6: A dose response study. *Journal of Endocrinological Investigation, 19*, 175–182.

Van Tol, E. A. F., Petrusz, P., Lund, P. K., Yamauchi, M., & Sartor, R. B. (1996). Local production of corticotropin releasing hormone is increased in experimental intestinal inflammation in rats. *Gut, 39*, 385–392.

Veening, J. G., van der Meer, M. J. M., Joosten, H., Hermus, A. R. M. M., Rijnkels, C. E. M., Geeraedts, L. M., & Sweep, C. G. J. (1993). Intravenous administration of interleukin-1β induces fos-like immunoreactivity in corticotropin-releasing hormone neurons in the paraventricular hypothalamic nucleus of the rat. *Journal of Chemical Neuroanatomy, 6*, 391–397.

Wan, W., Janz, L., Vriend, C. Y., Sorensen, C. M., Greenberg, A. H., & Nance, D. M. (1993). Differential induction of *c-Fos* immunoreactivity in hypothalamus and brain stem nuclei following central and peripheral administration of endotoxin. *Brain Research Bulletin, 32*, 581–587.

Wan, W. H., Wetmore, L., Sorensen, C. M., Greenberg, A. H., & Nance, D. M. (1994). Neural and biochemical mediators of endotoxin and stress-induced *c-fos* expression in the rat brain. *Brain Research Bulletin, 34*, 7–14.

Watanobe, H., Nasushita, R., Sasaki, S., & Suda, T. (1998). Evidence that a fast, rate-sensitive negative feedback effect of corticosterone is not a principal mechanism underlying the indomethacin inhibition of interleukin-1β-induced adrenocorticotropin secretion in the rat. *Cytokine, 10*, 377–381.

Watanobe, H., Sasaki, S., & Takebe, K. (1991). Evidence that intravenous administration of interleukin-1 stimulates corticotropin releasing hormone secretion in the median eminence of freely moving rats: Estimation by push-pull perfusion. *Neuroscience Letters, 133*, 7–10.

Watkins, L. R., Goehler, L. E., Relton, J. K., Tortaglia, N., Silbert, L., Martin, D., & Maier, S. F. (1995). Blockade of interleukin-1 induced hyperthermia by subdiaphragmatic vagotomy: Evidence for vagal mediation of immune-brain communication. *Neuroscience Letters, 183*, 27–31.

Watts, A. G. (1996). The impact of physiological stimuli on the expression of corticotropin-releasing hormone (CRH) and other neuropeptide genes. *Frontiers in Neuroendocrinology, 17*, 281–326.

Wei, E. T., Kiang, J. G., & Tian, J. Q. (1987). Anti-inflammatory activity of corticotropin releasing factor: I. Efficacy studies. *Proceedings of the Western Pharmacology Society, 30*, 59–62.

Wei, E. T., Serda, S., & Tian, J. Q. (1988). Protective actions of corticotropin-releasing factor on thermal injury to rat pawskin. *Journal of Pharmacology and Experimental Therapeutics, 247*, 1082–1085.

Weidenfeld, J., Abramsky, O., & Ovadia, H. (1989). Evidence for the involvement of the central adrenergic system in interleukin 1-induced adrenocortical response. *Neuropharmacology, 28*, 1411–1414.

Whitnall, M. H. (1993). Regulation of the hypothalamic corticotropin-releasing hormone neuroscretory system. *Progress in Neurobiology, 40*, 573–629.

Wilder, R. L. (1995). Neuroendocrine-immune system interactions and autoimmunity. *Annual Reviews on Immunology, 13*, 307–308.

Wilder, R. L., & Sternberg, E. M. (1990). Neuroendocrine hormonal factors in rheumatoid arthritis and related conditions. *Current Opinion in Rheumatology, 2*, 436–440.

Wooley, P., Dutcher, J., Widmer, M., & Gillis, S. (1993). Influence of a recombinant human soluble tumor necrosis factor receptor FC fusion protein on type II collagen-induced arthritis in mice. *Journal of Immunology, 151*, 6602–6607.

Zalcman, S., Green-Johnson, J. M., Murray, L., Nance, D. M., Dyck, D., Anisman, H., & Greenberg, A. H. (1994). Cytokine-specific central monoamine alterations induced by interleukin-1, -2 and -6. *Brain Research, 643*, 40–49.

Zhou, D., Kusnecov, A. W., Shurin, M. R., DePaoli, M., & Rabin, B. S. (1993). Exposure to physical and psychological stressors elevates plasma interleukin 6: Relationship to the activation of hypothalamo-pituitary-adrenal axis. *Endocrinology, 133*, 2523–2530.

Zhou, Y., Spangler, R., LaForge, K. S., Maggos, C. E., Ho, A., & Kreek, M. J. (1996). Modulation of CRF-R1 mRNA in rat anterior pituitary by dexamethasone: Correlation with POMC mRNA. *Peptides, 17*, 435–441.

Zhou, Z. Z., & Jones, S. B. (1993). Involvement of central vs. peripheral mechanisms in mediating sympathoadrenal activation in endotoxic rats. *American Journal of Physiology, 265*, R683–R688.

CHAPTER

25

Effects of Cytokines and Infections on Brain Neurochemistry

ADRIAN J. DUNN

A number of observations in the early literature suggested that the metabolism of neurotransmitters in the brain responds to immune stimuli. The major neurotransmitters affected were the catecholamines, dopamine (DA) and norepinephrine (NE), as well as the indoleamine, serotonin (5-hydroxytryptamine, 5-HT). An early study indicated that treatment of rats with endotoxin (lipopolysaccharide, LPS) increased the apparent turnover of NE, but not 5-HT in the brain (Pohorecky, Wurtman, Taam, & Fine, 1972). Later, evidence was presented that the apparent turnover of NE in the hypothalamus decreased following administration of an antigen, sheep red blood cells (SRBC), to rats (Besedovsky et al., 1983). A subsequent study found that SRBC administration decreased the NE content of the hypothalamic paraventricular nucleus (PVN) and the 5-HT content of the hypothalamic paraventricular and supraoptic nuclei, but no changes were observed in the other hypothalamic or extrahypothalamic regions studied (Carlson, Felten, Livnat, & Felten, 1987). The changes occurred only at the peak of the immune response to SRBC. There was no known mechanism for these responses, but because cytokines were known to be synthesized and secreted by immune cells following activation, they became prime candidates as immune cell-to-brain messengers.

Studies with purified cytokines have suggested that peripheral administration can indeed affect brain neurochemistry, opening up a new field of investigation. The majority of studies has focused on changes in neurotransmission, and this has proved to be particularly sensitive to the action of cytokines. Thus, this chapter mainly addresses the effects on brain neurotransmitters.

I. MEASUREMENT OF NEUROTRANSMITTER FUNCTION

Studies of neurotransmission focus on the messenger rather than the message, thus it is important to understand what those measures mean. This section will describe the kinds of measurements that are made of neurotransmission. For most neurotransmitters, the neuronal stores are significant, so that the measurement of the total content of neurotransmitters reveals little of their function, although increases in neurotransmitter release that outpace replenishment by synthesis or accumulation will result in measurable depletions. For this reason, techniques were developed to assess the neurotransmitter function by measuring the *turnover* rate of neurotransmitters, a loosely defined term indicating rates of synthesis or depletion. The first attempts to measure turnover exploited the use of specific inhibitors of neurotransmitter synthesis or degradation. Thus, for catecholamines, inhibitors of the critical synthetic enzyme tyrosine hydroxylase, such as α-methyl-para-tyrosine (metyrosine), were used to block synthesis, and the subsequent decline in concentrations of the amines was used to estimate the rate of turnover. For serotonin, the inhibitor of choice was para-chlorophenylalanine, a relatively specific inhibitor of tryptophan hydroxylase. The synthesis blockade technique was favored because assays for the measurement of neurotransmitter content were available. The problems with this strategy are that only the initial rate of decline is useful (because the rate of release may depend on available stores), and that the inhibitors used are unlikely to be absolutely specific and will have side effects or even be toxic. Inhibition of degradation is less useful, because the accumulation of the neurotransmitter tends to inhibit its own synthesis by negative feedback, and the inhibitors themselves are rather ineffective (probably because the major mechanism of inactivation of many neurotransmitters involves reuptake by neurotransmitter transporters, rather than degradation).

Turnover also can be estimated using radiolabeled tracer techniques. Most often a labeled precursor of the neurotransmitter such as [^{3}H]tyrosine, [^{3}H]tryptophan, or [^{3}H]choline is used. To estimate synthesis rates accurately, it is important to know the specific radioactivity of the precursor in the appropriate cellular compartment, because the administered radiolabeled precursor will be diluted by endogenous precursors. This is not an easy task. Methods have been developed to overcome many of the problems (Neff, Spano, Groppetti, Wang, & Costa, 1971), but they are insensitive and cumbersome. An alternative procedure involves administration of a labeled neurotransmitter (usually intracerebroventricularly [icv], because most neurotransmitters do not cross the blood-brain barrier) and following its subsequent accumulation (by reuptake) and its clearance.

Later studies exploited the measurement of catabolites as an index of the amount of neurotransmitter lost after release. For DA the major catabolites are 3,4-dihydroxyphenylacetic acid (DOPAC) and homovanillic acid (HVA); for NE, 3,4-dihydroxyphenylethyleneglycol (DHPG) and 3-methoxy,4-hydroxyphenylethyleneglycol (MHPG); and for 5-HT, 5-hydroxyindoleacetic acid (5-HIAA). Because the parent amines and their catabolites can be determined in small amounts by high-performance liquid chromatography with electrochemical detection, this approach became very popular (Dunn, 1993a). However, the concentration of catabolites depends on the balance between synthesis of the catabolite and its clearance, and thus may not be related in a simple way to release, although changes in release generally are associated with changes in catabolites in the same direction. The technique is sensitive because many of the catabolites are acidic, slowing their clearance from nervous tissue (because of the bidirectional blood-brain barrier), so that the measured concentrations of catabolites reflect an integral of past neurotransmitter release. A particularly often used measure is the ratio of a catabolite to the parent amine (proposed as a "utilization index," Lavielle et al., 1979). In practice this ratio provides very stable data, in part because it tends to minimize variability caused by variations in tissue dissection.

More recently developed techniques attempt to estimate the extracellular concentrations of the neurotransmitters. Extracellular concentrations of neurotransmitters are thought to reflect overflow, or what is lost from synapses. This is not likely to be the concentration in the synaptic cleft, but presumably bears some relationship to it. Note, however, that many neurotransmitters, especially the catecholamines and serotonin, do not appear to be released at synapses, and may diffuse significant distances through the extracellular space to activate their target receptors (Descarries, Seguela, & Watkins, 1991). This phenomenon is known as volume transmission. The most frequently used technique for measuring extracellular concentrations of neurotransmitters is in vivo microdialysis, which involves insertion of a dialysis probe into the brain to allow sampling of the small molecules that pass through the dialysis membrane (Benveniste, 1989; Parsons & Justice, 1994; see Figure 1). The presence of the dialysis membrane diminishes tissue damage caused by the fluid flow in the "push-pull" techniques used earlier (but see Myers, Adell, & Lankford, 1998). Microdialysis requires very sensitive assays for the neurotransmitters themselves and much patience to work with unanesthetized (so-called freely moving) animals. The principal problems with microdialysis are the tissue damage caused by inserting the relative large probes (typically 0.17–0.5 mm diameter, see Figure 1) and the lack of anatomical selectivity, because the length of the dialysis membrane is typically 1–4 mm. The extent of the tissue damage can be quite substantial, providing a significant local source of cytokines (see Section

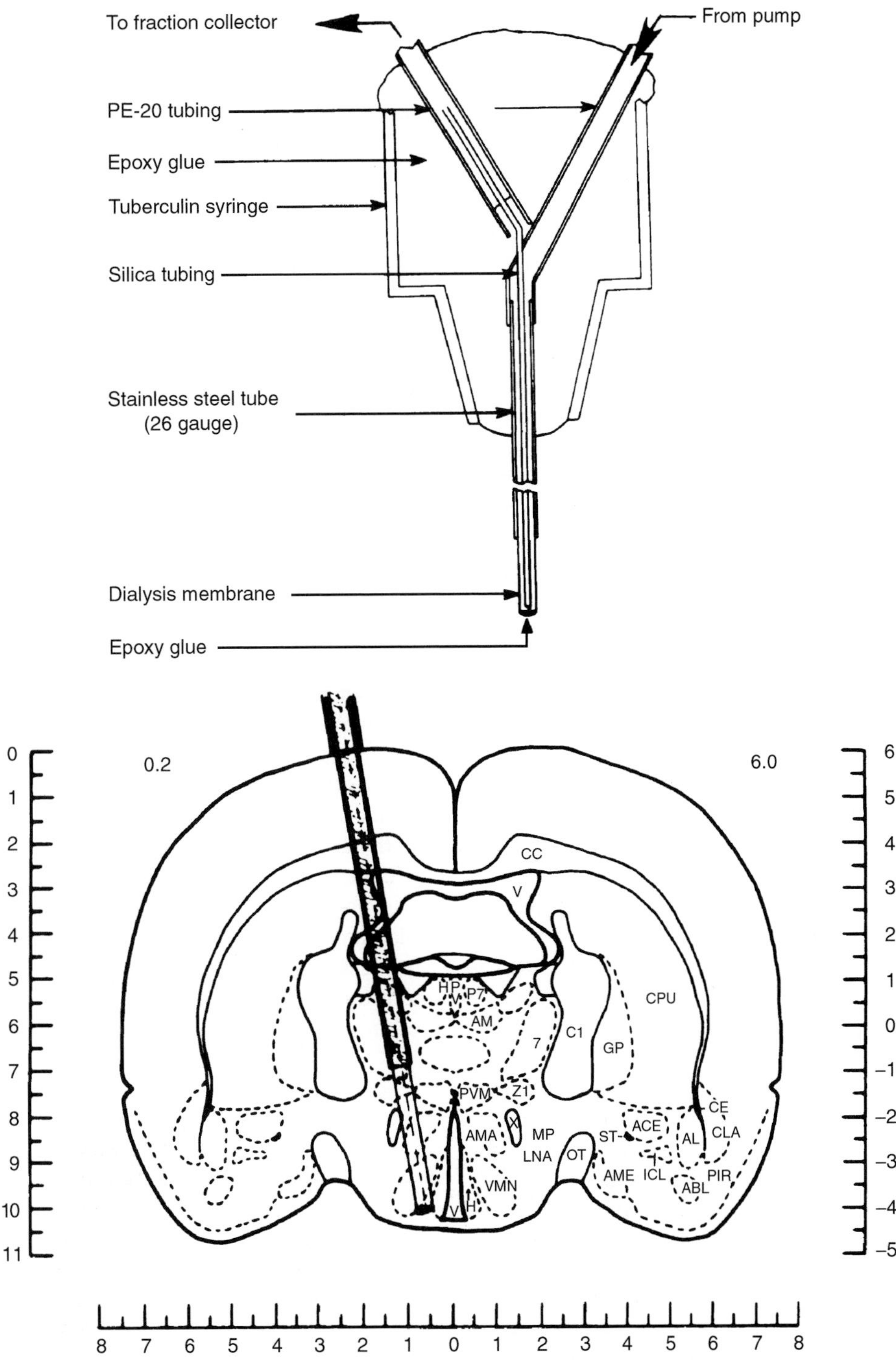

FIGURE 1 Diagrams of a typical microdialysis probe (top), and the same probe placed in the rat medial hypothalamus (bottom). Reproduced from Lavicky & Dunn (1993).

IV,G). Microdialysis is most useful for relatively small molecules such as amino acids, catecholamines, serotonin, acetylcholine, etc., for which recoveries in the range 10 to 30% or so can be achieved. Microdialysis can be used for larger molecules, such as peptides, but recoveries can be quite low (typically 1–2% or less), requiring very sensitive assays. Most microdialysis studies are performed in rats or larger animals, because the mouse brain is rather small, and there are problems securing the probe guides to the thin mouse skull. Microdialysis assesses extracellular concentrations of metabolites over a large volume, and it should not be conceived that neurotransmitter concentrations in area of the target receptors are being approximated.

A related methodology uses in vivo voltammetry in which carbon fiber electrodes are inserted into brain tissue. With appropriate external electronic controls, it is possible to estimate extracellular concentrations of oxidizable molecules, such as the catecholamines and serotonin (Boulton, Baker, & Adams, 1995). A major advantage of in vivo voltammetry is that the electrodes are much smaller (the tips can be as small as 8 μm) so that less tissue damage is caused than with microdialysis probes, and more discrete structures can be probed because the active area of the electrode is the cut surface of the tip of the carbon fiber. A second major advantage is that measurements can be made in close to real time, up to around 10 times per second. A major disadvantage of the technique is the lack of chemical specificity, and the limited number of neurotransmitters that can be measured in this way.

II. NEUROCHEMICAL RESPONSES TO VIRAL INFECTION

Elevations of plasma corticosterone associated with sickness are consistent with earlier reports in the literature, and with our own previous observations of animals that became sick for a variety of reasons (often unknown). In an early study, administration of Newcastle disease virus (NDV) to mice was shown to elevate plasma concentrations of corticosterone, indicating an activation of hypothalamo-pituitary-adrenocortical (HPA) axis (Smith, Meyer, & Blalock, 1982). NDV administration also caused neurochemical changes. MHPG and MHPG:NE ratios, an index of activation of NE neurons, DOPAC and DOPAC:DA ratios, an index of activation of DA neurons, and 5-HIAA and 5-HIAA : 5-HT ratios, an index of activation of 5-HT neurons, were all increased in a number of brain regions (Dunn, Powell, Moreshead, Gaskin, & Hall, 1987; Dunn & Vickers, 1994). Tryptophan was also elevated throughout the brain. The HPA and neurochemical changes were short-lived. However, NDV does not cause a true infection in mice; although the viral RNA is copied, there is no production of infective virus.

Bacterial infections have long been known to activate the HPA axis (Beisel, 1981; Kass & Finland, 1958). Thus, infection of mice with influenza virus was studied. Infusion of the virus into the lungs (the natural site of influenza virus infection) induced a chronic elevation of plasma corticosterone (Dunn, Powell, Meitin, & Small, 1989), which contrasts with the temporary elevation seen with most commonly studied stressors. The corticosterone changes were accompanied by neurochemical ones. MHPG and MHPG:NE ratios were elevated in all brain regions studied, but the magnitude of the response was greater in the hypothalamus than in the other brain regions (Dunn et al., 1989). DOPAC and DOPAC:DA ratios, and HVA and HVA : DA ratios were not significantly altered. Tryptophan concentrations were elevated in all regions studied, and 5-HIAA and 5-HIAA : 5-HT ratios, too. These changes appeared around 24–36 h after infection with influenza virus and continued as long as the animals appeared sick.

Similar HPA and neurochemical changes have been associated with infection with other viruses (Ben Hur, Rosenthal, Itzik, & Weidenfeld, 1996; Guo, Qian, Peters, & Liu, 1993; Miller et al., 1997; Weidenfeld, Wohlman, & Gallily, 1995). It is likely that infections are rather generally associated with activation of the HPA axis, as well as activation of brain noradrenergic systems, and brain tryptophan and serotonin.

There is clearly great similarity between the neurochemical and physiological responses to infections and other stressors commonly used, such as footshock or restraint (see Table I). Stress is associated with the peripheral coactivation of the sympathoadrenal system (sympathetic nervous system plus the adrenal medulla) and the HPA axis, increasing the plasma concentrations of corticotropin-releasing factor (CRF), adrenocorticotropin (ACTH), and corticosteroids (corticosterone in rodents; cortisol in most other animals, including man). In the central nervous

TABLE I Physiological Responses to Physical Stressors and Viral Infection (Immune Stress)*

	Footshock or restraint	Viral infection
HPA axis (plasma ACTH and corticosterone)[a]	++	++
Sympathetic nervous system	++	+
Adrenal medulla	++	+
Brain norepinephrine	++	++
Brain dopamine	+	0
Brain 5-hydroxytryptamine	+	+
Brain tryptophan	++	++

*Note: + indicates an increase in activity, ++ a large increase in activity, and 0 no change.

[a]HPA = hypothalamo-pituitary-adrenal axis; ACTH = adrenocorticotropic hormone.

system, the major response occurs in noradrenergic neurons, but responses also occur in dopaminergic and serotonergic (5-HT) systems (Dunn & Kramarcy, 1984; Stone, 1975). The noradrenergic response is widespread and appears to affect similarly both the locus coeruleus (A6) system innervating dorsal structures, such as the cortex, hippocampus, and cerebellum, and the nucleus tractus solitarius (NTS) A1/A2 system innervating ventral structures, such as the hypothalamus, via the ventral noradrenergic ascending bundle (VNAB). The dopaminergic response is also widespread such that all the major neuronal systems show responses (nigrostriatal, mesolimbic, mesocortical), but the magnitude of the response is much greater in the mesocortical system (i.e., in the prefrontal and cingulate cortices) compared with the other systems. The 5-HT response is not markedly regionally specific, although some have reported regional differences (e.g., Kirby, Allen, & Lucki, 1995). There is also a robust elevation of concentrations of tryptophan (the natural precursor of 5-HT) in all regions of the brain. This increase is quite uniform in magnitude, and does not appear to be related in any obvious way to the extent of the serotonergic innervation of a region (Curzon, Joseph, & Knott, 1972; Dunn, 1988a). The responses associated with what have been called immune stressors are not identical to those associated with physical and psychological stressors. A major difference is that the HPA activation associated with infection is continuous and not transient as it is to stressors such as electric shock. A major neurochemical difference is that infections and illness are associated with larger noradrenergic responses in the hypothalamus (the A1/A2, VNAB system) relative to other brain regions, whereas the responses to footshock and restraint are relatively uniform on a regional basis. The second important difference is the lack of dopaminergic responses associated with infections, especially in the prefrontal cortex. However, small dopaminergic responses are observed throughout the brain after LPS administration (see next section).

III. NEUROCHEMICAL RESPONSES TO ENDOTOXIN (LPS)

It has long been known that administration of LPS activates the HPA axis (Bliss, Migeon, Eik-Nes, Sandberg, & Samuels, 1954). As already indicated, an early study suggested that noradrenergic utilization was activated by high doses of LPS (Pohorecky et al., 1972). Administration of LPS (2.5 mg/rat ip or 50 μg icv) significantly decreased the brain content of NE, but did not affect that of 5-HT. LPS also accelerated the disappearance of [^{3}H]NE administered icv. Low doses of LPS (1 μg/mouse ip) induced rapid elevations of plasma ACTH and corticosterone reaching peaks at around 2 h (Dunn, 1992a). Increased concentrations of MHPG and MHPG:NE ratios also appear throughout the brain with a similar time course (Delrue, Deleplanque, Rouge-Pont, Vitiello, & Neveu, 1994; Dunn, 1992a; Lacosta, Merali, & Anisman, 1999; Masana, Heyes, & Mefford, 1990; Mefford & Heyes, 1990). Like the response to influenza virus infection, the response was greatest in the hypothalamus, suggesting a relatively greater activation of the ventral than the dorsal ascending noradrenergic bundle. LPS also induces small increases of DOPAC in most brain regions, including prefrontal cortex, hypothalamus, and brain stem (Delrue et al., 1994; Dunn, 1992a; Lacosta et al., 1999; Masana et al., 1990; Mefford, & Heyes, 1990; Molina-Holgado, & Guaza, 1996). The peak responses for both catecholamines (DA and NE) occurred around 2 h (Dunn, 1992a). Tryptophan and 5-HIAA were also increased in a regionally nonspecific manner (Delrue et al., 1994; Dunn, 1992a; Heyes, Quearry, & Markey, 1989; Mefford & Heyes, 1990; Molina-Holgado & Guaza, 1996). However, these latter changes reached a peak much later at around 8 h (Dunn, 1992a). Very similar changes were observed following icv LPS and the effective doses were quite similar (Dunn, 1992a).

In vivo microdialysis studies have indicated increased extracellular concentrations of DA, DOPAC, NE, DHPG, MHPG, and 5-HIAA (5-HT was not measurable) in the medial prefrontal cortex and hypothalamus following ip LPS administration in rats (Lavicky & Dunn, 1995), and of 5-HT in the hippocampus (Linthorst, Flachskamm, Holsboer, & Reul, 1996; Linthorst, Flachskamm, Müller-Preuss, Holsboer, & Reul, 1995), and of NE, MHPG, 5-HT, and 5-HIAA in the preoptic area (Linthorst, Flachskamm, Holsboer, & Reul, 1995). In the nucleus accumbens, LPS injection (100 μg ip) increased DA and 5-HIAA (Borowski, Kokkinidis, Merali, & Anisman, 1998). Thus, administration of LPS induces a pattern of neuroendocrine and neurochemical responses rather similar to those described above for influenza virus infection, but with the addition of some changes in cerebral DA.

IV. NEUROCHEMICAL RESPONSES TO CYTOKINES

Cytokines are produced by immune cells following activation. They are proteins or glycoproteins whose primary function is to coordinate immune responses. Following infections a cascade of different cytokines appears in various tissues and in the circulation. The specific cytokines and the temporal characteristics depend on the nature of the infection. The following review focuses on the effects of peripherally administered cytokines, because there are serious problems interpreting the results of studies in which cytokines are administered into the brain.

A. Interleukin-1 (IL-1)

1. The Catecholamines, DA, and NE

IL-1 was studied first because it had been cloned and characterized, and appears shortly after most infections and tissue damage (Dinarello, 1988). More important, it had been shown to be a potent stimulator of the HPA axis (Besedovsky, del Rey, Sorkin, & Dinarello, 1986). IL-1 administration to mice markedly increased plasma concentrations of ACTH and corticosterone and brain concentrations of MHPG and MHPG : NE ratios (Dunn, 1988b, 1992a) (Figures 2 and 3). The anatomic pattern of activation showed the greatest response in the hypothalamus, significantly greater than in the cortex and other brain regions studied. Within the hypothalamus, the greatest response was found medially. This anatomic specificity suggested that it reflected a preferential activation of the ventral noradrenergic system, which originates largely from NTS, although it receives some contribution from the locus coeruleus. This response closely paralleled in dose and time the HPA activation, indicated by elevation of plasma corticosterone (see Figures 2 and 3). These results were subsequently replicated in rats (Kabiersch, del Rey, Honegger, & Besedovsky, 1988) and in mice (Zalcman et al., 1994). The ability of IL-1β to increase hypothalamic NE turnover and its selectivity for the hypothalamus was confirmed when the cytokine accelerated the loss of NE following metyrosine-inhibited synthesis in rats (Terao, Oikawa, & Saito, 1993). Also in rats, IL-1 decreased the hypothalamic content of NE (Fleshner et al., 1995), suggesting that release was accelerated beyond the synthetic capacity. Depletions of NE associated with stress are observed more often in rats than in mice (Stone, 1975), and rarely have significant depletions in mice been observed. Most studies have not detected effects on DA metabolism (increases in DOPAC or HVA) (Dunn, 1988b; Kabiersch et al., 1988). However, Zalcman et al. (1994) reported increases in DOPAC in mouse prefrontal cortex and other brain regions. In a large number of experiments with ip IL-1 administration to mice, our laboratory has occasionally observed statistically significant increases of DOPAC or DOPAC:DA ratios, but such responses were rare and were not observed consistently. When they did occur they did not follow the anatomical pattern typical of responses to stressors; increases in the prefrontal cortex were much greater than in other brain regions, in agreement with Zalcman et al. (1994). Interestingly, administration of low doses of IL-1β to rats in the first few days of life results in permanent decreases in DA in the hypothalamus and superior cervical ganglion (Kabiersch, Furukawa, del Rey, & Besedovsky, 1998).

The neurochemical and HPA-activating effects of IL-1 occur with various forms of IL-1. Most authors report similar responses to IL-1α and IL-1β (Dunn, 1988b, 1992a), although some have found IL-1α to be less potent than IL-1β in activating the HPA axis (Matta, Linner, & Sharp, 1993; Uehara, Gottschall, Dahl, & Arimura, 1987). Similar responses also have been observed using IL-1 from different species (mouse, rat, or human). These observations are consistent with the similar binding affinities of the various forms of IL-1 for the IL-1 type I receptor (Liu, Takao, Hashimoto, & De Souza, 1996). Similar activity of IL-1 partially purified from the same strain of mouse (Dunn, 1988b, 1992a) also has been observed. The HPA and neurochemical responses are observed in response to ip or subcutaneous injections, and to icv administration at considerably lower doses (Dunn, 1992a). Intravenous administration induces a more rapid and short-lived HPA response and elicits smaller neurochemical effects (Dunn & Chuluyan, 1992; van der Meer et al., 1996). The HPA and neurochemical effects are not due to contamination with endotoxin because heat-denatured IL-1 lacks all these activities (Dunn, 1988b).

Subsequent studies have indicated that the effect of IL-1 on NE most likely reflects increased synaptic release, because in vivo microdialysis studies have indicated increased extracellular concentrations of NE in the medial hypothalamus in the region of the paraventricular nucleus (Ishizuka et al., 1997; Merali, Lacosta, & Anisman, 1997; Smagin, Swiergiel, & Dunn, 1996). A study with push-pull cannulation of the hypothalamus also suggested increased NE release (MohanKumar & Quadri, 1993). DA was not altered in dialysates from prefrontal cortex, nucleus accumbens, or hippocampus by ip IL-1β (Merali et al., 1997). IL-1β has also been reported to increase tyrosine hydroxylase activity in the median eminence of rats (Abreu, Llorente, Hernández, & González, 1994).

The cyclooxygenase inhibitor, indomethacin, prevented the increases in MHPG (Dunn & Chuluyan,

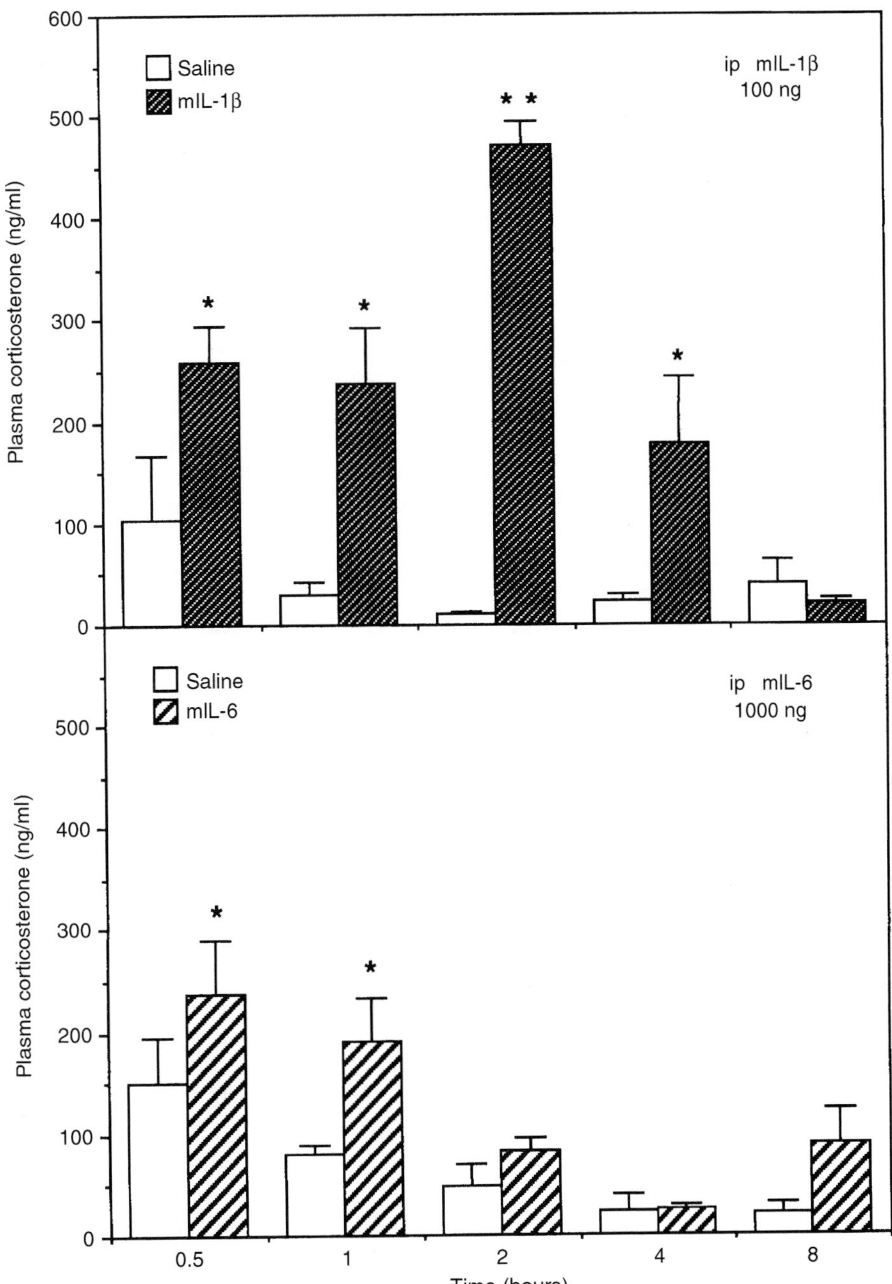

FIGURE 2 Time course of the plasma corticosterone responses of mice to mouse interleukin (IL)-1β and IL-6. Mouse IL-1β (100 ng/mouse; upper figure) or mouse IL-6 (1 µg/mouse; lower figure) was injected ip, and samples were collected at various subsequent times. Plasma corticosterone was determined by radioimmunoassay. The data from the lower figure are taken from Wang & Dunn (1998). *Significantly different from the saline group ($^*p < 0.05$, $^{**}p < 0.01$).

1992) and NE turnover (Terao, Kitamura, Asano, Kobayashi & Saito, 1995; Terao et al., 1993). The opiate receptor antagonist naloxone had no effect, but an antibody to CRF attenuated the response (Terao et al., 1993). However, a normal neurochemical response has been observed to ip mIL-1β in mice lacking the gene for CRF (Dunn, unpublished observations). Lesions of the area postrema attenuated the IL-1β-induced increase in NE in hypothalamic dialysates (Ishizuka et al., 1997). The vagus nerve may play a major role in the effects of ip IL-1 on the neurochemical responses, because subdiaphragmatic, but not hepatic, vagotomy prevented the decrease in hypothalamic NE caused by ip IL-1β (Fleshner et al.,

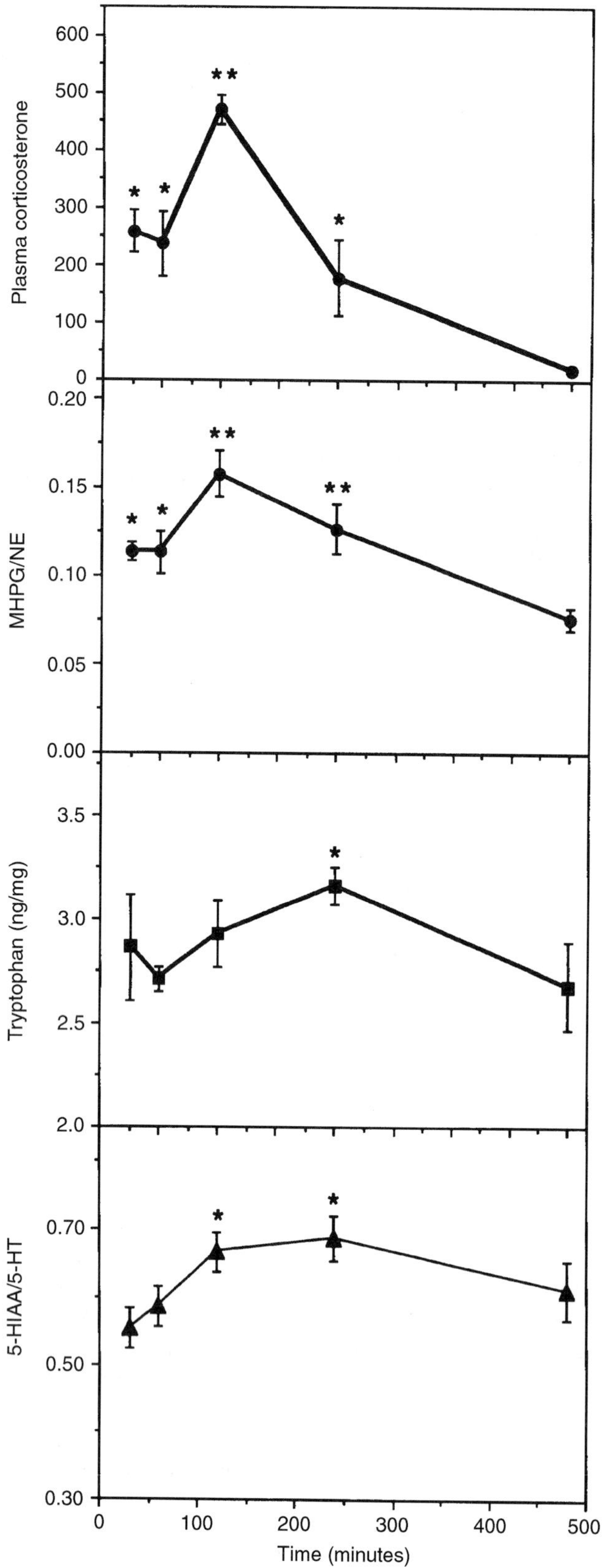

FIGURE 3 Time course of the neurochemical responses to IL-1β. Mice were injected with 100 ng mIL-1β in the same experiment as the upper panel of Figure 2. Top panel: plasma corticosterone. Second panel: (circles) hypothalamic MHPG:NE ratio. Third panel: (squares) hypothalamic tryptophan. Bottom panel: (triangles) hypothalamic 5-HIAA:5-HT ratios. *Significantly different from saline-treated mice at the same time after injection (*$p < 0.05$, **$p < 0.01$).

1995), and abdominal vagotomy attenuated the IL-1β-induced increase in hypothalamic dialysate NE (Ishizuka et al., 1997).

IL-1 administration also activates the adrenal medulla and the sympathetic nervous system, although this response is weaker than that induced by commonly used laboratory stressors (Berkenbosch, De Goeij, del Rey, & Besedovsky, 1989; Kannan et al., 1996; Niijima, Hori, Aou, & Oomura, 1991). Intravenous IL-1β increases the activity of vagal nerves innervating the thymus (Niijima, Hori, Katafuchi, & Ichijo, 1995). NE turnover in the spleen and pancreas was increased by ip IL-1β, but not IL-6 (Akiyoshi, Shimizu, & Saito, 1990; Terao, Oikawa, & Saito, 1994). NE release also was increased in a splenic dialysis study (Shimizu, Hori, & Nakane, 1994). However, in vitro studies have shown that IL-1β decreased NE release from the rat myenteric nerves (Hurst and Collins, 1993), from the perfused spleen (Bognar et al., 1994), and from the heart (Foucart & Abadie, 1996).

2. *Tryptophan and 5-HT*

IL-1 administration also induces an increase in tryptophan concentrations in most brain regions (Figure 3) (Dunn, 1988b; Mefford & Heyes, 1990). It also increases 5-HIAA, best observed by an increase in 5-HIAA:5-HT ratios (Figure 3) (Dunn, 1988b; Mefford & Heyes, 1990; Zalcman et al., 1994). Increases in 5-HIAA in push-pull samples from the hypothalamus were detected after intrahypothalamic injection of IL-1β (Mohankumar, Thyagarajan, & Quadri, 1993). Microdialysate concentrations of 5-HT from the hippocampus were not altered, but 5-HIAA was increased in nucleus accumbens and hippocampus (Merali et al., 1997). However, icv IL-1β increased 5-HT in dialysates from the hippocampus (Linthorst et al., 1995). A voltammetric study noted increases in 5-HIAA in the dorsal raphe nucleus after peripheral or icv IL-1β (Clement et al., 1997).

Increases in the brain content of tryptophan have been observed in response to a variety of stimuli, including a number of psychotropic drugs, increases in body temperature, and many stressors (Chaouloff,

1993; Curzon et al., 1972; Dunn, 1988a; Dunn & Welch, 1991; Tagliamonte, Tagliamonte, Perez-Cruet, Stern, & Gessa, 1971). Increases in brain tryptophan have been found to be a very sensitive index of an animal's health. Illness associated with infection, wounds or surgery, or food or water deprivation are almost always associated with increases of brain tryptophan. These increases are often accompanied by increases in 5-HIAA, which may be driven by the increased tryptophan. Peripheral administration of relatively high doses of tryptophan results in increases in brain tryptophan and 5-HIAA (Lookingland, Shannon, Chapin, & Moore, 1986; Dunn, unpublished observations), although it is not clear that the increased 5-HIAA reflects increased synaptic release (De Simoni, Sokola, Fodritto, Dal Toso, & Algeri, 1987; Joseph & Kennett, 1983). The increases in tryptophan and 5-HIAA in response to footshock, restraint, IL-1, and LPS may depend on peripheral sympathetic activity, because they can be blocked by pretreatment with the ganglionic blocker, chlorisondamine, and largely prevented by the β-adrenergic receptor antagonist propranolol, but not by the α-adrenergic receptor antagonist phentolamine, or the muscarinic receptor antagonist scopolamine (Dunn & Welch, 1991). Thus, the increases in brain tryptophan may reflect sympathetic activation.

The noradrenergic and indoleamine responses to IL-1 appear to be distinct. The NE response to ip IL-1 reaches a peak at around 2 h along with the increases in plasma ACTH and corticosterone, whereas the peak responses in tryptophan and 5-HIAA appear at around 4 h (Figure 3; Dunn, 1992a). The peak responses to LPS are even later (around 8 h; Dunn, 1992a). Pretreatment with nitric oxide synthase (NOS) inhibitors prevents the tryptophan and 5-HIAA response to IL-1 and LPS, with no effects detected on the HPA or NE responses (Dunn, 1993b). Other evidence for the dissociation was derived from studies with endotoxin-resistant (C3H/HeJ) mice, which exhibit very small HPA responses to LPS and no changes in MHPG, whereas the increases in tryptophan and 5-HIAA were similar to those in a control (C3H/HeN) strain (Dunn and Chuluyan, 1994). The HPA and neurochemical responses to IL-1 were similar in both endotoxin-resistant and normal strains. Thus, the NE and indoleamine responses can be independently manipulated and are activated by distinct mechanisms.

3. *Other Neurotransmitters*

Ip administration of hIL-1β decreased the secretion of acetylcholine from the hippocampus, as measured by microdialysis in freely moving rats (Rada et al., 1991). This effect occurred only at doses of 20 or 50 μg/kg; 7.5 μg/kg was ineffective. Consistent with indirect cholinergic effects, iv IL-1β increased the activity of vagal nerves (Niijima et al., 1995). Histamine turnover (assessed by accumulation following inhibition of degradation by pargyline) was reported to be increased in the rat hypothalamus by IL-1β 25 ng icv (Kang et al., 1994), and increased release of histamine from the rat hypothalamus was observed following intrahypothalamic injection of IL-1β in a microdialysis study (Niimi, Mochizuki, Yamamoto, & Yamatodani, 1994). Ip injection of hIL-1β (20 μg/kg, but not 10 μg/kg) decreased hippocampal concentrations of glutamate, glutamine, and gamma-aminobutyric acid (GABA) 1 h later (Bianchi, Ferrario, Zonta, & Panerai, 1995). Most authors have found 3–5 μg/kg IL-1 to induce maximal HPA activation in the rat, so the physiological significance of these effects at substantially higher doses is not clear. Ip IL-1β (4 μg/rat) also induced a short-lived increase in dialysate concentrations of glutamate from the nucleus troetus solitarius (Mascarucci, Perego, Terrazzino, & De Simoni, 1998).

4. *Other Neurochemical Responses*

The most commonly studied nonneurotransmitter-related neurochemical response is Fos. Peripheral administration of IL-1 increases the expression of Fos protein in a number of brain regions (Chang, Ren, & Zadina, 1993; Ericsson, Kovács, & Sawchenko, 1994; Veening et al., 1993). The most prominent structure affected is the PVN, the site of the cell bodies of neurons that synthesize CRF and initiate the activation of the HPA axis. Typically, increases in Fos also are observed in the central amygdaloid nucleus, the medial preoptic area, the bed nucleus of the stria terminalis, and the NTS. The mRNA for Fos (c-fos) is also induced in most of the same structures (Brady, Lynn, Herkenham, & Gottesfeld, 1994; Day & Akil, 1996; Rivest & Rivier, 1994). This Fos response appears to depend on activation of the PVN by noradrenergic neurons because it is markedly attenuated in mice depleted of NE with 6-hydroxydopamine (6-OHDA) (Swiergiel, Dunn, & Stone, 1996).

Interestingly, the rate of protein synthesis in the brain is altered by subcutaneous injection of hIL-1β in the rat (Williams, Ballmer, Hannah, Grant, & Garlick, 1994). Increases were observed in the subfornical organ, choroid plexus, medial habenula, dentate gyrus, and the anterior and posterior lobes of the pituitary, and decreases in the cingulate cortex and the pineal gland.

B. Interleukin-2 (IL-2)

IL-2 (200 ng ip) was reported to increased MHPG concentrations and MHPG : NE ratios in the hypothalamus of BALB/c mice 2 h after injection (Zalcman et al., 1994). DOPAC : DA ratios also were increased in the prefrontal cortex, but plasma corticosterone was unaffected. Interestingly, a microdialysis study showed decreased release of DA from the nucleus accumbens following systemic administration of IL-2 (Anisman, Kokkinidis, & Merali, 1996). Icv IL-2 (500, but not 50 ng) markedly increased 5-HT and 5-HIAA in hippocampal dialysates (Pauli, Linthorst, & Reul, 1998). Peripheral IL-2 administration reversed the decreases in brain NE and 5-HT in olfactory bulbectomized rats as well as the behavioral and immunological deficits (Song & Leonard, 1995). Ip injection of human IL-2 (5 μg/kg) induced small increases in glutamine in the cortex and hippocampus of mice 1 h later (Bianchi et al., 1995).

C. IL-6

IL-6 administration has been widely reported to activate the HPA axis as indicated by elevations of plasma ACTH and corticosterone. Zalcman et al. (1994) reported that hIL-6 (200 ng, ip) injected into mice elevated 5-HIAA in the hippocampus, and 5-HIAA and DOPAC in the prefrontal cortex. Injection of mIL-6 into mice iv or ip elicited modest increases in plasma ACTH and corticosterone; maximal concentrations were much lower than observed with IL-1 (Figure 2) (Wang & Dunn, 1998). The corticosterone elevations were maximal at 30–60 min and were no longer evident by 2 h. In an earlier study no effects of IL-6 on cerebral biogenic amines were observed (Dunn, 1992b), consistent with the report of Terao et al. (1993), who found no effects on NE turnover (using metyrosine). However, in a more recent study mIL-6 (iv or ip) consistently elevated tryptophan in all brain regions at around 2 h and 5-HIAA in the brain stem at the same time, but had no effect on MHPG or DOPAC in any brain region (Wang & Dunn, 1998). Icv mIL-6 had similar endocrine and neurochemical effects. Because IL-1 and LPS administration both stimulate the synthesis and secretion of IL-6, it is possible that IL-6 mediates the indoleamine responses to IL-1 and LPS. The effects of IL-6 on serotonin have been confirmed in a preliminary microdialysis study, which showed increases in dialysate 5-HT and 5-HIAA from the hypothalamus of rats injected ip with rat IL-6 (2 μg per rat) (Barkhudaryan & Dunn, 1999). A similar response to rat IL-6 was observed in striatal dialysates (Ma & Dunn, unpublished observations).

Fos responses have also been reported to peripheral administration of IL-6, but the results have been varied. The PVN was affected in some studies (Niimi, Wada, Sato, Takahara, & Kawanishi, 1997), but not others (Callahan and Piekut, 1997; Tinsley and Dunn, unpublished observations). Other structures that have been involved include the central amygdala, bed nucleus of stria terminalis, the superoptic nuclei, NTS, and the superchiasmatic nucleus.

D. Tumor Necrosis Factor α

Human tumor necrosis factor α (hTNF-α) administration activates the HPA axis in man (Michie et al., 1988) and rodents (Besedovsky et al., 1991; Perlstein, Whitnall, Abrams, Mougey, & Neta, 1993; Sharp & Matta, 1993). In most cases, TNF-α was reported to be significantly less potent than IL-1 in rats (Besedovsky et al., 1991; del Rey & Besedovsky, 1992; van der Meer et al., 1996) and mice (Dunn, 1992b), but in one study in rats, hTNF-α was almost equipotent with hIL-1β (Sharp et al., 1989). hTNF-α did not elevate plasma corticosterone in mice, except when it was injected iv (Dunn, 1992b). However, mouse TNF-α iv and ip elicited modest increases in plasma corticosterone; 1 μg was necessary to produce an elevation of plasma corticosterone (Ando & Dunn, 1999). mTNF-α increased brain MHPG and tryptophan, but only at the higher doses (1 μg or more), thus this result is not inconsistent with an earlier study (Dunn, 1992b), nor that of Terao et al. (1993), who observed no effects on NE turnover. Injection of mTNF-α (50 or 100 ng) icv did not alter hippocampal dialysate concentrations of 5-HT or 5-HIAA, but did elevate body temperature and plasma corticosterone (Pauli et al., 1998). A recent report indicated that hTNF-α (4 μg ip) increased hypothalamic MHPG in mice, and that chronic treatment sensitized this response (Hayley, Brebner, Lacosta, Merali, & Anisman, 1999).

In contrast, TNF-α inhibited NE release from the median eminence (Elenkov, Kovacs, Duda, Stark, & Vizi, 1992). Similarly TNF-α inhibited NE release from hippocampal slices (Ignatowski & Spengler, 1994). Interestingly, chronic treatment with the antidepressant desmethylimipramine reversed this effect, such that TNF-α stimulated NE release (Ignatowski & Spengler, 1994).

In the periphery, TNF-α inhibited NE release from the rat myenteric plexus (Hurst & Collins, 1994) and the mouse heart (Foucart & Abadie, 1996).

E. Interferons

No significant changes in plasma corticosterone or cerebral biogenic amines were observed following ip injection of human interferon-α (hIFN-α: 1000 or 10000 U; Dunn, 1992b). Mouse IFN-α (mIFN-α) administration at doses and times when the mice were behaviorally active (Crnic & Segall, 1992) did not result in significant changes in plasma corticosterone or catecholamine or 5-HT metabolism in any of five brain regions 2 h following ip administration of 400, 800, or 1600 U of mIFN-α (Leenhouwers, Crnic, & Dunn, unpublished observations). However, chronic treatment of mice with IFN-γ increased brain concentrations of quinolinic acid and the activity of the enzyme indoleamine-2,3-dioxygenase (IDO), a key enzyme in indoleamine degradation (Saito, Markey, & Heyes, 1991). Peripheral administration of IFN-γ to rats did not alter 5-HIAA in the dorsal raphe, but local administration increased 5-HT activity assessed by voltammetry (Clement et al., 1997). In cultured immune cells, IFN-γ stimulates the activity of GTP cyclohydrolase, a critical enzyme for the synthesis of tetrahydrobiopterin (Werner, Werner-Felmayer, & Wachter, 1993). Tetrahydrobiopterin is an essential cofactor for NOS and also for the biosynthesis of catecholamines and 5-HT.

F. Other Cytokines

Granulocyte/macrophage colony-stimulating factor (GM-CSF) administration to rats (5 and 10 µg ip) significantly reduced hypothalamic glutamate, glutamine, aspartate, and GABA, as well as NE and 5-HT, but not DA (Bianchi, Clavenna, Bondiolotti, Ferrario, & Panerai, 1997).

G. Effects of Intracerebral Administration of Cytokines

Many studies have examined responses to intracerebral administration of IL-1 (and other cytokines and LPS). Such studies often have been performed to demonstrate direct actions on brain tissue, but they are very difficult to interpret because of the tissue damage inherent in the introduction of the injector, as well as the microdialysis probes, the push-pull cannulae, or the electrodes, if used. Not only will the lesion create a site for macrophage and lymphocyte invasion and microglial and astroglial proliferation, but also there will be substantial local production of cytokines and many other factors. There is thus the potential for interaction of the introduced (injected) substances with any of these factors. Intracerebral administration of IL-1 (icv or into tissue) has been shown in numerous studies to increase HPA activity, as well as the extracellular concentrations and metabolism of NE (e.g., Shintani et al., 1993; Terrazzino, Perego, & De Simoni, 1995) and increased extracellular concentrations of hypothalamic 5-HIAA (Gemma, De Luigi, & De Simoni, 1994).

This problem has important implications for those who wish to propose an intracerebral function for IL-1. For example, Shintani et al. (1993) reported that anterior hypothalamic infusion of IL-1β increased dialysate concentrations of DA, NE, and 5-HT from the anterior hypothalamus. In a subsequent report, they showed that infusion of the IL-1-receptor antagonist (IL-1ra) into this same region attenuated the plasma ACTH and dialysate DA, NE, and 5-HT responses to immobilization (Shintani et al., 1995). They concluded that hypothalamic IL-1 plays a role in the HPA and neurochemical responses to the stressor. The problem is that the insertion of microdialysis probes creates a massive lesion and thus a site for the local production of cytokines, such as IL-1 and IL-6, as demonstrated by Woodroofe et al. (1991). Thus, the net effect on plasma ACTH and dialysate amines reflects the sum of the effect of the stressor and the local cytokine activity. Therefore an attenuation of the response to immobilization may indicate only the removal of contribution of local IL-1, rather than an attenuation of the response to the stressor. In simple terms, the intracerebral antagonists may merely be antagonizing the artifacts of the cannulae and probe insertions. Dunn (2000) observed no attenuation by icv IL-1ra of the neurochemical responses to footshock or restraint in mice.

H. Mechanism(s) of the Effects of the Cytokines

The above sections have described a variety of effects of cytokines on the brain and its neurochemistry. An important question is how these effects are produced. Cytokines are too large to readily pass the blood-brain barrier. They could act on one or other of the brain regions that lack a blood-brain barrier, the so-called circumventricular organs, such as the median eminence, organum vasculosum laminae terminalis (OVLT), or the area postrema. Some authors believe that IL-1, especially when administered intravenously, may act directly on CRF-containing terminals in the median eminence to initiate HPA axis activation (Rivier, 1995). Local application of IL-1 in the median eminence has been shown to elevate plasma ACTH and corticosterone in rats, and these responses are prevented by local administration of α- and β-adrenergic receptor antagonists (Matta, Singh, Newton, & Sharp, 1990) or indomethacin (McCoy, Matta, & Sharp, 1994).

Another possibility is that cytokines may cross the blood-brain barrier using specific uptake systems.

Banks and co-workers have shown that there appear to be specific uptake systems for many cytokines from the blood to the brain (Banks, Ortiz, Plotkin, & Kastin, 1991). Uptake has been demonstrated for IL-1α, IL-1β, IL-1ra, IL-2, IL-6, and TNF-α, as well as the soluble receptors for IL-1 and TNF-α. However, the capacity of these uptake systems is quite low, and it is not clear whether the concentrations of the cytokines achieved would be adequate to induce significant effects (Banks, Kastin, & Broadwell, 1995).

A third mechanism involves the vagus nerve, and possibly other afferent nerves. Initially, it was demonstrated that lesioning the vagus nerve below the diaphragm prevented the cerebral Fos response to ip LPS (Wan, Wetmore, Sorensen, Greenberg, & Nance, 1994). Subsequently, several groups have demonstrated that vagal lesions may prevent the CNS effects of ip IL-1 or LPS on behavior (Bret-Dibat, Bluthé, Kent, Kelley, & Dantzer, 1995; Watkins et al., 1994), as well as attenuating the HPA response and preventing the decrease in hypothalamic NE (Fleshner et al., 1995; for review, see Watkins, Maier, & Goehler, 1995). The current view is that IL-1 binds to receptors on paraganglion cells associated with the vagus (Goehler et al., 1999). The vagal afferents terminate in the NTS in the brain stem, which also contains the cell bodies of the A1/A2 noradrenergic projection system.

The fourth possibility is that cytokines bind to receptors on cerebral endothelial cells. These in turn may activate cyclooxygenases to produce prostaglandins, leukotrienes, thromboxanes, and other lipid mediators that can easily cross into the brain. This mechanism is particularly appealing, because despite the extreme sensitivity of the brain to IL-1, the brain contains very few receptors for IL-1. In fact, binding sites for IL-1 have not been clearly demonstrated in the rat, and in the mouse they appear only in the hippocampus (Haour, Ban, Marquette, Milon, & Fillion, 1992; Takao, Tracey, Mitchell, & De Souza, 1990). mRNA for IL-1 receptors has also been difficult to demonstrate in the parenchyma of normal brain. However, IL-1-receptors are common in the capillary endothelium and choroid plexus.

It is likely is that these distinct mechanisms operate in parallel, so that when cytokines are administered, more than one mechanism operates, especially for the HPA-activating effects.

V. PARTICIPATION OF CYTOKINES IN THE RESPONSES TO LPS AND VIRAL INFECTION

Because the responses to IL-1 resemble so closely those to influenza virus infection and LPS, an obvious question is the extent to which this cytokine accounts for the HPA and neurochemical responses. Surprisingly, studies with antibodies to IL-1 and IL-1ra suggest that IL-1 is not critical for the responses to LPS (Dunn, 2000). It is important that whereas LPS is a potent stimulator of IL-1 production, little appears in less than 1 h, and the peak response in the plasma is around 2 h. Therefore, if IL-1 were the mediator, the endocrine and neurochemical responses to LPS should be delayed more than is actually observed (Dunn, 1992a; Dunn, 2000). Studies with antibodies to IL-1 and with IL-1ra failed to show blockade of either the increases in plasma ACTH and corticosterone, or those in MHPG or tryptophan (Dunn, 1992b). More recent studies using higher doses of IL-1ra produced similar results, although there was a trend toward an attenuation of the HPA activation at 3–4 h (Dunn, 2000), as would be expected from the time considerations indicated above. These results are consistent with the observation of a normal response to LPS in mice that lack the gene for IL-1β (Fantuzzi et al., 1996). Because LPS is a potent stimulator of IL-1β synthesis and secretion, it is unlikely that IL-1 does not contribute to the HPA and neurochemical responses to LPS. However, IL-1β is clearly not the only factor.

Studies with antibodies to IL-6 have suggested a role for IL-6 in the HPA responses to both the administration of LPS (Perlstein et al., 1993; Wang & Dunn, 1999) and IL-1 (Wang & Dunn, 1999). Treatment with the IL-6 antibody attenuates the response only in the later phases of the HPA response, consistent with the delay necessary for the production and secretion of IL-6. Pretreatment with a neutralizing monoclonal antibody to mouse IL-6 also attenuated the increases in tryptophan and 5-HIAA following LPS administration to mice, but not that to IL-1, suggesting that IL-6 contributes only to the indoleamine responses to LPS, and is not involved in those to IL-1 (Wang & Dunn, 1999). Treatment with a neutralizing antibody to TNF-α also failed to prevent the HPA and neurochemical responses to LPS, even when supplemented with IL-1ra (Dunn, 1992b).

VI. THE FUNCTIONAL SIGNIFICANCE OF THE NEUROCHEMICAL RESPONSES TO CYTOKINES

An important question is whether any of the neurochemical responses observed following cytokine administration can be linked to a functional response. The most useful functional responses in this respect are the HPA responses and various behavioral responses.

A. Neurotransmitter Involvement in HPA Responses

Both NE and 5-HT have been implicated in HPA activation (Plotsky, Cunningham, & Widmaier, 1989), and thus are obvious candidates for mediating the responses to IL-1 (see chapter by C. Rivier). As described above, the NE response and that of plasma ACTH and corticosterone are closely linked in time, and have been highly correlated over a large number of experiments involving a large number of different manipulations. A microdialysis study in freely moving rats also indicated a very close temporal relationship between extracellular concentrations of NE in the hypothalamus and plasma concentrations of corticosterone following both iv and ip IL-1β (Smagin et al., 1996). When the noradrenergic neurotoxin 6-OHDA was injected into the VNAB or the PVN of rats, resulting in depletions of PVN NE of 75% or more, the plasma corticosterone response to ip IL-1 was largely prevented (Chuluyan, Saphier, Rohn, & Dunn, 1992). A similar result was obtained using icv IL-1 in 6-OHDA-treated rats (Weidenfeld, Abramsky, & Ovadia, 1989). A similar 6-OHDA lesion prevented the increase in plasma corticosterone following infection with herpes simplex virus, whereas a serotonergic lesion with 5,7-dihydroxytryptamine (5,7-DHT) did not (Ben Hur et al., 1996). Surprisingly, however, when whole brain NE was depleted by around 98% using 6-OHDA in mice, no impairment of the plasma corticosterone response to IL-1β was observed (Swiergiel et al., 1996, and other unpublished observations). Also, α- and β-adrenergic receptor antagonists have little effect on the response to IL-1 in rats (Rivier, 1995), and the α_1-adrenergic receptor antagonist prazosin attenuates the response in mice only at high doses (Dunn, Wang, & Ando, 1999). Thus, it is likely that brain NE is involved in the HPA response to IL-1, but it does not appear to be essential.

B. Neurotransmitter Involvement in the Behavioral Responses

Many authors have demonstrated IL-1-induced reductions of food intake (see chapter by R. Dantzer). This cytokine-induced hypophagia is sensitive to cyclooxygenase inhibitors (Swiergiel, Smagin, & Dunn, 1997). Because the peak of this hypophagia just like the peak increase in MHPG occurs around 2 h, the ability of adrenergic receptor antagonists to reverse the hypophagia has been tested. However, neither α_1-, α_2-, nor nonspecific α- or β-adrenergic receptor antagonists, alone or in combination, induced significant reductions in IL-1-induced hypophagia in mice (Swiergiel, Burunda, Peterson, & Dunn, 1999). Likewise, pretreatment with 6-OHDA or (N-2-chloroethyl)-N-ethyl-2-bromobenzylamine (DSP-4) to deplete cerebral NE failed to alter the hypophagic response to IL-1 (Swiergiel et al., 1999). Surprisingly, no effects were observed of cerebral 5-HT depletion (with 5,7-DHT) or pretreatment with a variety of 5-HT-receptor antagonists (Swiergiel & Dunn, 2000). The role of histamine in the IL-1- and LPS-induced hypophagia also has been examined. Pretreatment with histamine H_1, H_2, and H_3 antagonists and the histamine synthesis inhibitor α-fluoromethylhistidine all failed to alter the feeding responses to IL-1β (Swiergiel et al., 1999).

However, studies of other cytokine-induced behaviors has produced some evidence implicating noradrenergic mechanisms. For example, Ovadia, Abramsky, and Weidenfeld (1989) found that pretreatment with 6-OHDA, the β-adrenoreceptor blocker propranolol, or the α_2-adrenoreceptor blocker yohimbine, prevented IL-1-induced fever. Also, 6-OHDA pretreatment or prazosin prevented the antinociceptive effect of icv hIL-1α determined in the hot-plate test (Bianchi & Panerai, 1995). In this latter study, icv administration of the CRF antagonist alpha-helical $CRF_{9\text{-}41}$ also was effective.

The effects of IL-6 on cerebral 5-HT are interesting in that mice lacking the gene for IL-6 (IL-6 knockout mice) show a high degree of aggressive behavior, whereas mice overexpressing IL-6 show more social interactions (Alleva, 1998). IL-6 administration has no dramatic effects on behavior in mice and does not reduce food intake (Swiergiel & Dunn, 1999). However, Zalcman, Murray, Dyck, Greenberg, & Nance (1998) reported modest increases in locomotor activity, exploratory activity, and grooming when hIL-6 was administered to mice. Chronic IL-6 treatment exacerbated the locomotor activating effects of amphetamine (Zolcman, Savina, & Wise, 1999).

VII. SUMMARY

Table II summarizes the reported HPA and catecholamine and indoleamine responses to cytokines, as well as to endotoxin and influenza virus infection.

Cytokine administration to animals can elicit a number of effects on the brain, including neuroendocrine and behavioral effects, and also alters the metabolism of neurotransmitters. The best-documented effect is the activation by IL-1 of the HPA axis, which is accompanied by a stimulation of cerebral NE metabolism, probably reflecting increased NE secretion. IL-1 also stimulates indoleamine metabolism,

TABLE II Comparison of Hypothalamo-Pituitary-Adrenal and Brain Neurochemical Responses to Viral Infection, Lipopolysacharide (LPS), and Some Cytokines*

Stimulus	Corticosterone	NE	DA	Tryptophan	5-HT
Influenza virus	+	+	0	+	+
LPS	+	+	+	+	+
IL-1α/IL-1β	+	+	0	+	+
IL-2	0	+	+	nd	0
IL-6	+	0	0	+	+
TNF-α	+	(+)	0	(+)	0
IFN-α	0	0	0	0	0

* Note: +, increased; 0, no change; (+) indicates increases only at the highest doses of TNF-α (1 μg or more); nd, not determined. Abbreviations: NE, norepinephrine; DA, dopamine; 5-HT, serotonin; IL, interleukin; TNF-α, tumor necrosis factor-alpha; IFN, interferon.

most prominently increasing concentration of tryptophan, and increasing the catabolism of serotonin. IL-6 induces a short-lived activation of the HPA axis and has effects on tryptophan and 5-HT similar to those of IL-1. TNF-α has effects on the HPA axis similar to those of IL-6, but affects NE and tryptophan only at high doses. INF-α had no effects on the parameters studied. The effects of IL-1 are remarkably similar to those observed following administration of endotoxin and infections, such as influenza virus. They also resemble quite closely the responses that are observed to stressors commonly studied in laboratory animals, such as electric shock or restraint (Table I). The major differences are that the NE response to shock or restraint is very uniform throughout the brain, whereas that to IL-1, LPS, or infection is significantly greater in the hypothalamus. Also, responses of dopaminergic systems are normally observed to shock or restraint, with especially prominent responses in the limbic cortex, whereas dopaminergic responses are rarely observed in response to IL-1 and immune stimuli, and when they do occur, the response in the limbic cortex is similar to that in other brain regions. A small dopaminergic response occurs throughout the brain to peripheral administration of LPS. The neurochemical responses to cytokines may underlie some of the endocrine and behavioral responses. The noradrenergic response to IL-1 is apparently related to the HPA activation, but may not be essential for it. Neither the noradrenergic nor the serotonergic systems appear to be involved in the hypophagic responses. The significance of the indoleaminergic responses is not known.

Acknowledgments

The author's research described in this review was supported by the Office of Naval Research (N0001-4-85K-0300), the U.S. National Institute of Mental Health (MH46261), and the U.S. National Institute of Neurological Diseases and Stroke (NS25370). I am grateful for the excellent technical assistance of Bunney Powell, Sandra Vickers, Michael Adamkiewicz, and Lynn Pittman-Cooley, and the clerical assistance of Rhonda Hiers, Sharon Farrar, and Karen Scott.

References

Abreu, P., Llorente, E., Hernández, M. M., & González, M. C. (1994). Interleukin-1β stimulates tyrosine hydroxylase activity in the median eminence. *NeuroReport, 5*, 1356–1358.

Akiyoshi, M., Shimizu, Y., & Saito, M. (1990). Interleukin-1 increases norepinephrine turnover in the spleen and lung in rats. *Biochemical, Biophysical Research Communications, 173*, 1266–1270.

Alleva, E., Cirulli, F., Bianchi, M., Bondiolotti, F. P., Chiarotti, F., De Acetis, L., & Panerai, A. E. (1998). Behavioural characterization of interleukin-6 overexpressing or deficient mice during agonistic encounters. *European Journal of Neuroscience, 10*, 3664–3672.

Ando, T., & Dunn, A. J. (1999). Mouse tumor necrosis factor-α increases brain tryptophan concentrations and norepinephrine metabolism while activating the HPA axis in mice. *Neuroimmunomodulation, 6*, 319–329.

Anisman, H., Kokkinidis, L., & Merali, Z. (1996). Interleukin-2 decreases accumbal dopamine efflux and responding for rewarding lateral hypothalamic stimulation. *Brain Research, 731*, 1–11.

Banks, W. A., Kastin, A. J., & Broadwell, R. D. (1995). Passage of cytokines across the blood-brain barrier. *Neuroimmunomodulation, 2*, 241–248.

Banks, W. A., Ortiz, L., Plotkin, S. R., & Kastin, A. J. (1991). Human interleukin (IL)1α, murine IL-1α and murine IL-1β are transported from blood to brain in the mouse by a shared saturable mechanism. *Journal of Pharmacology and Experimental Therapeutics, 259*, 988–996.

Barkhudaryan, N., & Dunn, A. (1999). Molecular mechanisms of actions of interleukin-6 on the brain, with special reference to serotonin and the hypothalamo-pituitary-adrenocortical axis. *Neurochemical Research, 24*, 1169–1180.

Beisel, W. R. (1981). Alterations in hormone production and utilization during infection. In M. C. Powanda & P. G. Canonico (Eds.), *Infections: The physiologic and metabolic responses of the host*, (pp. 147–172). Amsterdam: Elsevier/North-Holland Biomedical Press.

Ben Hur, T., Rosenthal, J., Itzik, A., & Weidenfeld, J. (1996). Adrenocortical activation by herpes virus: Involvement of IL-1β and central noradrenergic system. *NeuroReport, 7*, 927–931.

Benveniste, H. (1989). Brain microdialysis. *Journal of Neurochemistry, 52*, 1667–1679.

Berkenbosch, F., De Goeij, D. E. C., del Rey, A., & Besedovsky, H. O. (1989). Neuroendocrine, sympathetic and metabolic responses induced by interleukin-1. *Neuroendocrinology, 50*, 570–576.

Besedovsky, H. O., del Rey, A., Klusman, I., Furukawa, H., Monge Arditi, G., & Kabiersch, A. (1991). Cytokines as modulators of the hypothalamus-pituitary-adrenal axis. *Journal of Steroid Biochemistry and Molecular Biology, 40*, 613–618.

Besedovsky, H. O., del Rey, A., Sorkin, E., & Dinarello, C. A. (1986). Immunoregulatory feedback between interleukin-1 and glucocorticoid hormones. *Science, 233*, 652–654.

Besedovsky, H. O., del Rey, A. E., Sorkin, E., Da Prada, M., Burri, R., & Honegger, C. (1983). The immune response evokes changes in brain noradrenergic neurons. *Science, 221*, 564–566.

Bianchi, M., Clavenna, A., Bondiolotti, G. P., Ferrario, P., & Panerai, A. E. (1997). GM-CSF affects hypothalamic neurotransmitter levels in mice: Involvement of interleukin-1. *NeuroReport, 10*, 3587–3590.

Bianchi, M., Ferrario, P., Zonta, N., & Panerai, A. E. (1995). Effects of interleukin-1β and interleukin-2 on amino acids levels in mouse cortex and hippocampus. *NeuroReport, 6*, 1689–1692.

Bianchi, M., & Panerai, A. E. (1995). CRH and the noradrenergic system mediate the antinociceptive effects of central interleukin-1α in the rat. *Brain Research Bulletin, 36*, 113–117.

Bliss, E. L., Migeon, C. J., Eik-Nes, K., Sandberg, A. A., & Samuels, L. T. (1954). The effects of insulin, histamine, bacterial pyrogen, and the antabuse-alcohol reaction upon the levels of 17-hydroxycorticosteroids in the peripheral blood of man. *Metabolism, 3*, 493–501.

Bognar, I. T., Albrecht, S.-A., Farasaty, M., Schmitt, E., Seidel, G., & Fuder, H. (1994). Effects of human recombinant interleukins on stimulation-evoked noradrenaline overflow from the rat perfused spleen. *Naunyn-Schmiedeberg's Archives of Pharmacology, 349*, 497–502.

Borowski, T., Kokkinidis, L., Merali, Z., & Anisman, H. (1998). Lipopolysaccharide, central in vivo amine variations, and anhedonia. *NeuroReport, 9*, 3797–3802.

Boulton, A. A., Baker, G. B., & Adams, R. N. (1995). *Voltammetric methods in brain systems.* Totowa, NJ: Humana Press.

Brady, L. S., Lynn, A. B., Herkenham, M., & Gottesfeld, Z. (1994). Systemic interleukin-1 induces early and late patterns of *c-fos* mRNA expression in brain. *Journal of Neuroscience, 14*, 4951–4964.

Bret-Dibat, J.-L., Bluthé, R.-M., Kent, S., Kelley, K. W., & Dantzer, R. (1995). Lipopolysaccharide and interleukin-1 depress food-motivated behavior in mice by a vagal-mediated mechanism. *Brain, Behavior, and Immunity, 9*, 242–246.

Callahan, T. A., & Piekut, D. T. (1997). Differential Fos expression induced by IL-1β and IL-6 in rat hypothalamus and pituitary gland. *Journal of Neuroimmunology, 73*, 207–211.

Carlson, S. L., Felten, D. L., Livnat, S., & Felten, S. Y. (1987). Alterations of monoamines in specific central autonomic nuclei following immunization in mice. *Brain, Behavior, and Immunity, 1*, 52–63.

Chang, S. L., Ren, T., & Zadina, J. E. (1993). Interleukin-1 activation of Fos proto-oncogene protein in the rat hypothalamus. *Brain Research, 617*, 123–130.

Chaouloff, F. (1993). Physiopharmacological interactions between stress hormones and central serotonergic systems. *Brain Research Reviews, 18*, 1–32.

Chuluyan, H., Saphier, D., Rohn, W. M., & Dunn, A. J. (1992). Noradrenergic innervation of the hypothalamus participates in the adrenocortical responses to interleukin-1. *Neuroendocrinology, 56*, 106–111.

Clement, H. W., Buschmann, J., Rex, S., Grote, C., Opper, C., Gemsa, D., & Wesemann, W. (1997). Effects of interferon-γ, interleukin-1β, and tumor necrosis factor-α on the serotonin metabolism in the nucleus raphe dorsalis of the rat. *Journal of Neural Transmission, 104*, 981–991.

Crnic, L. S., & Segall, M. A. (1992). Behavioral effects of mouse interferon-α and interferon-γ and human interferon-α in mice. *Brain Research, 590*, 277–284.

Curzon, G., Joseph, M. H., & Knott, P. J. (1972). Effects of immobilization and food deprivation on rat brain tryptophan metabolism. *Journal of Neurochemistry, 19*, 1967–1974.

Day, H. E. W., & Akil, H. (1996). Differential pattern of *c-fos* mRNA in rat brain following central and systemic administration of interleukin-1-beta: Implications for mechanism of action. *Neuroendocrinology, 63*, 207–218.

De Simoni, M. G., Sokola, A., Fodritto, F., Dal Toso, G., & Algeri, S. (1987). Functional meaning of tryptophan-induced increase of 5-HT metabolism as clarified by in vivo voltammetry. *Brain Research, 411*, 89–94.

del Rey, A., & Besedovsky, H. O. (1992). Metabolic and neuroendocrine effects of pro-inflammatory cytokines. *European Journal of Clinical Investigation, 22* (suppl. 1), 10–15.

Delrue, C., Deleplanque, B., Rouge-Pont, F., Vitiello, S., & Neveu, P. J. (1994). Brain monoaminergic, neuroendocrine, and immune responses to an immune challenge in relation to brain and behavioral lateralization. *Brain, Behavior, and Immunity, 8*, 137–152.

Descarries, L., Seguela, P., & Watkins, K. C. (1991). Nonjunctional relationships of monamine axon terminals in the cerebral cortex. In K. Fuxe and L. F. Agnati (Eds.), *Volume transmission in the brain. Novel mechanism for neural transmission* (vol. 1,). New York: Raven Press.

Dinarello, C. A. (1988). Biology of interleukin 1. *FASEB Journal, 2*, 108–115.

Dunn, A. J. (1988a). Changes in plasma and brain tryptophan and brain serotonin and 5-hydroxyindoleacetic acid after footshock stress. *Life Sciences, 42*, 1847–1853.

Dunn, A. J. (1988b). Systemic interleukin-1 administration stimulates hypothalamic norepinephrine metabolism parallelling the increased plasma corticosterone. *Life Sciences, 43*, 429–435.

Dunn, A. J. (1992a). Endotoxin-induced activation of cerebral catecholamine and serotonin metabolism: Comparison with interleukin-1. *Journal of Pharmacology and Experimental Therapeutics, 261*, 964–969.

Dunn, A. J. (1992b). The role of interleukin-1 and tumor necrosis factor α in the neurochemical and neuroendocrine responses to endotoxin. *Brain Research Bulletin, 29*, 807–812.

Dunn, A. J. (1993a). Neurochemical methods for evaluating cerebral biogenic amine responses to cytokines and their involvement in the central actions of interleukin-1. In E. B. De Souza (Ed.), *Neurobiology of Cytokines* (vol. 17, part B, pp. 209–222). San Diego: Academic Press.

Dunn, A. J. (1993b). Nitric oxide synthase inhibitors prevent the cerebral tryptophan and serotonergic responses to endotoxin and interleukin-1. *Neuroscience Research Communications, 13*, 149–156.

Dunn, A. J. (2000). Effects of the interleukin-1 (IL-1) receptor antagonist on the IL-1- and endotoxin-induced activation of the HPA axis and cerebral biogenic amines in mice. *Neuroimmunomodulation 7*, 36–45.

Dunn, A. J., & Chuluyan, H. (1992). The role of cyclo-oxygenase and lipoxygenase in the interleukin-1-induced activation of the HPA axis: Dependence on the route of injection. *Life Sciences, 51*, 219–225.

Dunn, A. J., & Chuluyan, H. E. (1994). Endotoxin elicits normal tryptophan and indolamine responses but impaired catecholamine and pituitary-adrenal responses in endotoxin-resistant mice. *Life Sciences, 54*, 847–853.

Dunn, A. J., & Kramarcy, N. R. (1984). Neurochemical responses in stress: relationships between the hypothalamic-pituitary-adrenal and catecholamine systems. In L. L. Iversen, S. D. Iversen, & S. H. Snyder (Eds.), *Handbook of psychopharmacology*, (vol. 18, pp. 455–515). New York: Plenum Press.

Dunn, A. J., Powell, M. L., Meitin, C., & Small, P. A. (1989). Virus infection as a stressor: Influenza virus elevates plasma concentrations of corticosterone, and brain concentrations of MHPG and tryptophan. *Physiology and Behavior, 45*, 591–594.

Dunn, A. J., Powell, M. L., Moreshead, W. V., Gaskin, J. M., & Hall, N. R. (1987). Effects of Newcastle disease virus administration to mice on the metabolism of cerebral biogenic amines, plasma corticosterone, and lymphocyte proliferation. *Brain, Behavior, and Immunity, 1*, 216–230.

Dunn, A. J., & Vickers, S. L. (1994). Neurochemical and neuroendocrine responses to Newcastle disease virus administration in mice. *Brain Research, 645*, 103–112.

Dunn, A. J., Wang, J.-P., & Ando, T. (1999). Effects of cytokines on central neurotransmission: Comparison with the effects of stress. In R. Dantzer, E. E. Wollman, & R. Yirmiya (Eds.), *Cytokines, stress and depression*, (pp. 117–127). New York: Kluwer Academic/Plenum Publishers.

Dunn, A. J., & Welch, J. (1991). Stress- and endotoxin-induced increases in brain tryptophan and serotonin metabolism depend on sympathetic nervous system activation. *Journal of Neurochemistry, 57*, 1615–1622.

Elenkov, I. J., Kovacs, K., Duda, E., Stark, E., & Vizi, E. S. (1992). Presynaptic inhibitory effect of TNF-α on the release of noradrenaline in isolated median eminence. *Journal of Neuroimmunology, 413*, 117–120.

Ericsson, A., Kovács, K. J., & Sawchenko, P. E. (1994). A functional anatomical analysis of central pathways subserving the effects of interleukin-1 on stress-related neuroendocrine neurons. *Journal of Neuroscience, 14*, 897–913.

Fantuzzi, G., Zheng, H., Faggioni, R., Benigni, F., Ghezzi, P., Sipe, J. D., Shaw, A. R., & Dinarello, C. A. (1996). Effect of endotoxin in IL-1β-deficient mice. *Journal of Immunology, 157*, 291–296.

Fleshner, M., Goehler, L. E., Hermann, J., Relton, J. K., Maier, S. F., & Watkins, L. R. (1995). Interleukin-1β induced corticosterone elevation and hypothalamic NE depletion is vagally mediated. *Brain Research Bulletin, 37*, 605–610.

Foucart, S., & Abadie, C. (1996). Interleukin-1β and tumor necrosis factor-α inhibit the release of [3H]-noradrenaline from mice isolated atria. *Naunyn Schmiedebergs Archives of Pharmacology, 354*, 1–6.

Gemma, C., De Luigi, A., & De Simoni, M. G. (1994). Permissive role of glucocorticoids on interleukin-1 activation of the hypothalamic serotonergic system. *Brain Research, 651*, 169–173.

Goehler, L. E., Gaykema, R. P. A., Nguyen, K. T., Lee, J. E., Tilders, F. J. H., Maier, S. F., & Watkins, L. R. (1999). Interleukin-1β in immune cells of the abdominal vagus nerve: A link between the immune and nervous systems? *Journal of Neuroscience, 19*, 2799–2806.

Guo, Z. M., Qian, C. G., Peters, C. J., & Liu, C. T. (1993). Changes in platelet-activating factor, catecholamine, and serotonin concentrations in brain, cerebrospinal fluid, and plasma of Pichinde virus-infected guinea pigs. *Laboratory Animal Science, 43*, 569–574.

Haour, F., Ban, E., Marquette, C., Milon, G., & Fillion, G. (1992). Brain Interleukin-1 receptors: Mapping, characterization and modulation. In N. J. Rothwell and R. D. Dantzer (Eds.), *Interleukin-1 in the brain*, (pp. 13–25). Oxford: Pergamon Press.

Hayley, S., Brebner, K., Lacosta, S., Merali, Z., & Anisman, H. (1999). Sensitization to the effects of tumor necrosis factor-α: Neuroendocrine, central monoamine, and behavioral variations. *Journal of Neuroscience, 19*, 5654–5665.

Heyes, M. P., Quearry, B. J., & Markey, S. P. (1989). Systemic endotoxin increases L-tryptophan, 5-hydroxyindoleacetic acid, 3-hydroxykynurenine and quinolinic acid content of mouse cerebral cortex. *Brain Research, 491*, 173–179.

Hurst, S., & Collins, S. M. (1993). Interleukin-1β modulation of norepinephrine release from rat myenteric nerves. *American Journal of Physiology, 264*, G30–35.

Hurst, S. M., & Collins, S. M. (1994). Mechanism underlying tumor necrosis factor-α suppression of norepinephrine release from rat myenteric plexus. *American Journal of Physiology, 266*, G1123–1129.

Ignatowski, T. A., & Spengler, R. N. (1994). Tumor necrosis factor-α: Presynaptic sensitivity is modified after antidepressant drug adminstration. *Brain Research, 665*, 293–299.

Ishizuka, Y., Ishida, Y., Kunitake, T., Kato, K., Hanamori, T., Mitsuyama, Y., & Kannan, H. (1997). Effects of area postrema lesion and vagotomy on interleukin-1β-induced norepinephrine release in the hypothalamic paraventricular nucleus region in the rat. *Neuroscience Letters, 223*, 57–60.

Joseph, M. H., & Kennett, G. A. (1983). Stress-induced release of 5-HT in the hippocampus and its dependence on increased tryptophan availability: An in vivo electrochemical study. *Brain Research, 270*, 251–257.

Kabiersch, A., del Rey, A., Honegger, C. G., & Besedovsky, H. O. (1988). Interleukin-1 induces changes in norepinephrine metabolism in the rat brain. *Brain, Behavior, and Immunity, 2*, 267–274.

Kabiersch, A., Furukawa, H., del Rey, A., & Besedovsky, H. O. (1998). Administration of interleukin-1 at birth affects dopaminergic neurons in adult mice. *Annals of the New York Academy of Sciences, 840*, 123–127.

Kang, M., Yoshimatsu, H., Ogawa, R., Kurokawa, M., Oohara, A., Tamari, Y., & Sakata, T. (1994). Thermoregulation and hypothalamic histamine turnover modulated by interleukin-1 beta in rats. *Brain Research Bulletin, 35*, 299–301.

Kannan, H., Tanaka, Y., Kunitake, T., Ueta, Y., Hayashida, T., & Yamashita, H. (1996). Activation of sympathetic outflow by recombinant human interleukin-1β in conscious rats. *American Journal of Physiology, 270*, R479–R485.

Kass, E. H., & Finland, M. (1958). Corticosteroids and infections. *Advances in Internal Medicine, 9*, 45–80.

Kirby, L. G., Allen, A. R., & Lucki, I. (1995). Regional differences in the effects of forced swimming on extracellular levels of 5-hydroxytryptamine and 5-hydroxyindoleacetic acid. *Brain Research, 682*, 189–196.

Lacosta, S., Merali, Z., & Anisman, H. (1999). Behavioral and neurochemical consequences of lipopolysaccharide in mice: anxiogenic-like effects. *Brain Research, 818*, 291–303.

Lavicky, J., & Dunn, A. J. (1993). Corticotropin-releasing factor stimulates catecholamine release in hypothalamus and prefrontal cortex in freely moving rats as assessed by microdialysis. *Journal of Neurochemistry, 60*, 602–612.

Lavicky, J., & Dunn, A. J. (1995). Endotoxin administration stimulates cerebral catecholamine release in freely moving rats as assessed by microdialysis. *Journal of Neuroscience Research, 40*, 407–413.

Lavielle, S., Tassin, J.-P., Thierry, A.-M., Blanc, G., Herve, D., Barthelemy, C., & Glowinski, J. (1979). Blockade by benzodiazepines of the selective high increase in dopamine turnover induced by stress in mesocortical dopaminergic neurons of the rat. *Brain Research, 168*, 585–594.

Linthorst, A. C. E., Flachskamm, C., Holsboer, F., & Reul, J. M. H. M. (1995). Intraperitoneal administration of bacterial endotoxin enhances noradrenergic neurotransmission in the rat preoptic area: relationship with body temperature and hypothalamic-pituitary-adrenocortical axis activity. *European Journal of Neuroscience, 7*, 2418–2430.

Linthorst, A. C. E., Flachskamm, C., Holsboer, F., & Reul, J. M. H. M. (1996). Activation of serotonergic and noradrenergic neurotransmission in the rat hippocampus after peripheral administration of bacterial endotoxin: Involvement of the cyclooxygenase pathway. *Neuroscience, 72*, 989–997.

Linthorst, A. C. E., Flachskamm, C., Müller-Preuss, P., Holsboer, F., & Reul, J. M. H. M. (1995). Effect of bacterial endotoxin and interleukin-1β on hippocampal serotonergic neurotransmission, behavioral activity, and free corticosterone levels: An in vivo microdialysis study. *Journal of Neuroscience, 15*, 2920–2934.

Liu, C., Takao, T., Hashimoto, K., & De Souza, E. B. (1996). Interleukin-1 receptors in the nervous system. In N. J. Rothwell (Ed.), *Cytokines in the nervous System* (pp. 21–40). Austin, TX: R. G. Landes.

Lookingland, K. J., Shannon, N. J., Chapin, D. S., & Moore, K. E. (1986). Exogenous tryptophan increases synthesis, storage, and intraneuronal metabolism of 5-hydroxytryptamine in the rat hypothalamus. *Journal of Neurochemistry, 47*, 205–212.

Mascarucci, P., Perego, C., Terrazzino, S., & De Simoni, M. (1998). Glutamate release in the nucleus tractus solitarius induced by peripheral lipolysaccharide and interleukin-1β. *Neuroscience, 86*, 1285–1290.

Masana, M. I., Heyes, M. P., & Mefford, I. N. (1990). Indomethacin prevents increased catecholamine turnover in rat brain following systemic endotoxin challenge. *Progress in Neuro-Psychopharmacology and Biological Psychiatry, 14*, 609–621.

Matta, S. G., Linner, K. M., & Sharp, B. M. (1993). Interleukin-1-α and interleukin-1-β stimulate adrenocorticotropin secretion in the rat through a similar hypothalamic receptor(s): Effects of interleukin-1 receptor antagonist protein. *Neuroendocrinology, 57*, 14–22.

Matta, S. G., Singh, J., Newton, R., & Sharp, B. M. (1990). The adrenocorticotropin response to interleukin-1β instilled into the rat median eminence depends on the local release of catecholamines. *Endocrinology, 127*, 2175–2182.

McCoy, J. G., Matta, S. G., & Sharp, B. (1994). Prostaglandins mediate the ACTH response to interleukin-1-beta instilled into the hypothalamic median eminence. *Neuroendocrinology, 60*, 426–435.

Mefford, I. N., & Heyes, M. P. (1990). Increased biogenic amine release in mouse hypothalamus following immunological challenge: Antagonism by indomethacin. *Journal of Neuroimmunology, 27*, 55–61.

Merali, Z., Lacosta, S., & Anisman, H. (1997). Effects of interleukin-1β and mild stress on alterations of norepinephrine, dopamine and serotonin neurotransmission: A regional microdialysis study. *Brain Research, 761*, 225–235.

Michie, H. R., Spriggs, D. R., Manogue, K. R., Sherman, M. L., Revhaug, A., O'Dwyer, S. T., Arthur, K., Dinarello, C. A., Cerami, A., Wolff, S. M., Kufe, D. W., & Wilmore, D. W. (1988). Tumor necrosis factor and endotoxin induce similar metabolic responses in human beings. *Surgery, 104*, 280–286.

Miller, A. H., Spencer, R. L., Pearce, B. D., Pisell, T. L., Tanapat, P., Leung, J. J., Dhabhar, F. S., McEwen, B. S., & Biron, C. A. (1997). Effects of viral infection on corticosterone secretion and glucocorticoid receptor binding in immune tissues. *Psychoneuroendocrinology, 22*, 455–474.

Mohankumar, P. S., Thyagarajan, S., & Quadri, S. K. (1993). Interleukin-1β increases 5-hydroxyindoleacetic acid release in the hypothalamus in vivo. *Brain Research Bulletin, 31*, 745–748.

Mohankumar, P. S., & Quadri, S. K. (1993). Systemic administration of interleukin-1 stimulates norepinephrine release in the paraventricular nucleus. *Life Sciences, 52*, 1961–1967.

Molina-Holgado, F., & Guaza, C. (1996). Endotoxin administration induced differential neurochemical activation of the rat brain stem nuclei. *Brain Research Bulletin, 40*, 151–156.

Myers, R. D., Adell, A., & Lankford, M. F. (1998). Simultaneous comparison of cerebral dialysis and push-pull perfusion in the brain of rats: A critical review. *Neuroscience and Biobehavioral Reviews, 22*, 371–387.

Neff, N. H., Spano, P. F., Groppetti, A., Wang, C. T., & Costa, E. (1971). A simple procedure for calculating the synthesis rate of norepinephrine, dopamine and serotonin in rat brain. *Journal of Pharmacology and Experimental Therapeutics, 176*, 701–710.

Niijima, A., Hori, T., Aou, S., & Oomura, Y. (1991). The effects of interleukin-1β on the activity of adrenal, splenic and renal sympathetic nerves in the rat. *Journal of the Autonomic Nervous System, 36*, 183–192.

Niijima, A., Hori, T., Katafuchi, T., & Ichijo, T. (1995). The effect of interleukin-1β on the efferent activity of the vagus nerve to the thymus. *Journal of the Autonomic Nervous System, 54*, 137–144.

Niimi, M., Mochizuki, T., Yamamoto, Y., & Yamatodani, A. (1994). Interleukin-1 beta induces histamine release in the rat hypothalamus in vivo. *Neuroscience Letters, 181*, 87–90.

Niimi, M., Wada, Y., Sato, M., Takahara, J., & Kawanishi, K. (1997). Effect of continuous intravenous injection of interleukin-6 and pretreatment with cyclooxygenase inhibitor on brain c-fos expression in the rat. *Neuroendocrinology, 66*, 47–53.

Ovadia, H., Abramsky, O., & Weidenfeld, J. (1989). Evidence for the involvement of the central adrenergic system in the febrile response induced by interleukin-1 in rats. *Journal of Neuroimmunology, 25*, 109–116.

Parsons, L. H., & Justice, J. B. (1994). Quantitative approaches to in vivo brain microdialysis. *Critical Reviews of Neurobiology, 8*, 189–220.

Pauli, S., Linthorst, A. C., & Reul, J. M. (1998). Tumour necrosis factor-α and interleukin-2 differentially affect hippocampal serotonergic neurotransmission, behavioural activity, body temperature and hypothalamic-pituitary-adrenocortical axis activity in the rat. *European Journal of Neuroscience, 10*, 868–878.

Perlstein, R. S., Whitnall, M. H., Abrams, J. S., Mougey, E. H., & Neta, R. (1993). Synergistic roles of interleukin-6, interleukin-1, and tumor necrosis factor in the adrenocorticotropin response to bacterial lipopolysaccharide in vivo. *Endocrinology, 132*, 946–952.

Plotsky, P. M., Cunningham, E. T., & Widmaier, E. P. (1989). Catecholaminergic modulation of corticotropin-releasing factor and adrenocorticotropin secretion. *Endocrine Reviews, 10*, 437–458.

Pohorecky, L. A., Wurtman, R. J., Taam, D., & Fine, J. (1972). Effects of endotoxin on monoamine metabolism in the rat. *Proceedings of the Society for Experimental Biology and Medicine, 140*, 739–746.

Rada, P., Mark, G. P., Vitek, M. P., Mangano, R. M., Blume, A. J., Beer, B., & Hoebel, B. G. (1991). Interleukin-1β decreases acetylcholine measured by microdialysis in the hippocampus of freely moving rats. *Brain Research, 550*, 287–290.

Rivest, S., & Rivier, C. (1994). Stress and interleukin-1β-induced activation of *c-fos*, NGFI-B and CRF gene expression in the hypothalamic PVN: Comparison between Sprague-Dawley, Fisher-344 and Lewis rats. *Journal of Endocrinology, 6*, 101–117.

Rivier, C. (1995). Influence of immune signals on the hypothalamic-pituitary axis of the rodent. *Frontiers of Neuroendocrinology, 16*, 151–182.

Saito, K., Markey, S. P., & Heyes, M. P. (1991). Chronic effects of y-interferon on quinolinic acid and indoleamine-2,3-dioxygenase in brain of C57BL6 mice. *Brain Research, 546*, 151–154.

Sharp, B. M., & Matta, S. G. (1993). Prostaglandins mediate the adrenocorticotropin response to tumor necrosis factor in rats. *Endocrinology, 132*, 269–274.

Sharp, B. M., Matta, S. G., Peterson, P. K., Newton, R., Chao, C., & McAllen, K. (1989). Tumor necrosis factor-α is a potent ACTH secretagogue: Comparison to interleukin-1β. *Endocrinology, 124*, 3131–3133.

Shimizu, N., Hori, T., & Nakane, H. (1994). An interleukin-1β-induced noradrenaline release in the spleen is mediated by brain corticotropin-releasing factor: An in vivo microdialysis study in conscious rats. *Brain, Behavior, and Immunity, 8,* 14–23.

Shintani, F., Kanba, S., Nakaki, T., Nibuya, M., Kinoshita, N., Suzuki, E., Yagi, G., Kato, R., & Asai, M. (1993). Interleukin-1β augments release of norepinephrine, dopamine, and serotonin in the rat anterior hypothalamus. *Journal of Neuroscience, 13,* 3574–3581.

Shintani, F., Nakaki, T., Kanba, S., Sato, K., Yagi, G., Shiozawa, M., Aiso, S., Kato, R., & Asai, M. (1995). Involvement of interleukin-1 in immobilization stress-induced increase in plasma adrenocorticotropic hormone and in release of hypothalamic monoamines in the rat. *Journal of Neuroscience, 15,* 1961–1970.

Smagin, G. N., Swiergiel, A. H., & Dunn, A. J. (1996). Peripheral administration of interleukin-1 increases extracellular concentrations of norepinephrine in rat hypothalamus: Comparison with plasma corticosterone. *Psychoneuroendocrinology, 21,* 83–93.

Smith, E. M., Meyer, W. J., & Blalock, J. E. (1982). Virus-induced corticosterone in hypophysectomized mice: A possible lymphoid adrenal axis. *Science, 218,* 1311–1312.

Song, C., & Leonard, B. E. (1995). Interleukin-2-induced changes in behavioural, neurotransmitter, and immunological parameters in the olfactory bulbectomized rat. *Neuroimmunomodulation, 2,* 263–273.

Stone, E. A. (1975). Stress and catecholamines. In A. J. Friedhoff (Ed.), *Catecholamines and behavior. Neuropsychopharmacology* (vol. 2, pp. 31–72). New York: Plenum Press.

Swiergiel, A. H., Burunda, T., Peterson, B., & Dunn, A. J. (1999). Endotoxin- and interleukin-1-induced hypophagia are not affected by noradrenergic, dopaminergic, histaminergic and muscarinic antagonists. *Pharmacology Biochemistry and Behavior, 63,* 629–637.

Swiergiel, A. H., & Dunn, A. J. (1999). The roles of IL-1, IL-6 and TNF-α in the feeding responses to endotoxin and influenza virus infection in mice. *Brain, Behavior, and Immunity, 13,* 252–265.

Swiergiel, A. H., & Dunn, A. J. (2000). Lack of evidence for a role of serotonin in interleukin-1-induced hypophagia. *Pharmacology, Biochemistry and Behavior, 65,* 531–537.

Swiergiel, A. H., Dunn, A. J., & Stone, E. A. (1996). The role of cerebral noradrenergic systems in the Fos response to interleukin-1. *Brain Research Bulletin, 41,* 61–64.

Swiergiel, A. H., Smagin, G. N., & Dunn, A. J. (1997). Influenza virus infection of mice induces anorexia: Comparison with endotoxin and interleukin-1 and the effects of indomethacin. *Pharmacology, Biochemistry and Behavior, 57,* 389–396.

Tagliamonte, A., Tagliamonte, P., Perez-Cruet, J., Stern, S., & Gessa, G. L. (1971). Effect of psychotropic drugs on tryptophan concentration in rat brain. *Journal of Pharmacology and Experimental Therapeutics, 177,* 475–480.

Takao, T., Tracey, D. E., Mitchell, W. M., & De Souza, E. B. (1990). Interleukin-1 receptors in mouse brain: Characterization and neuronal localization. *Endocrinology, 127,* 3070–3078.

Terao, A., Kitamura, H., Asano, A., Kobayashi, M., & Saito, M. (1995). Roles of prostaglandins D_2 and E_2 in interleukin-1-induced activation of norepinephrine turnover in the brain and peripheral organs of rats. *Journal of Neurochemistry, 65,* 2742–2747.

Terao, A., Oikawa, M., & Saito, M. (1993). Cytokine-induced change in hypothalamic norepinephrine turnover: Involvement of corticotropin-releasing hormone and prostaglandins. *Brain Research, 622,* 257–261.

Terao, A., Oikawa, M., & Saito, M. (1994). Tissue-specific increase in norepinephrine turnover by central interleukin-1, but not by interleukin-6, in rats. *American Journal of Physiology, 266,* R400–404.

Terrazzino, S., Perego, C., & De Simoni, M. G. (1995). Noradrenaline release in hypothalamus and ACTH secretion induced by central interleukin-1β. *NeuroReport, 6,* 2465–2468.

Uehara, A., Gottschall, P. E., Dahl, R. R., & Arimura, A. (1987). Stimulation of ACTH release by human interleukin-1β, but not by interleukin-1α, in conscious, freely moving rats. *Biochemical and Biophysical Research Communications, 146,* 1286–1290.

Veening, J. G., van der Meer, M. J. M., Joosten, H., Hermus, A. R. M. M., Rijnkels, C. E. M., Geeraedts, L. M., & Sweep, C. G. J. F. (1993). Intravenous administration of interleukin-1β induces fos-like immunoreactivity in corticotropin-releasing hormone neurons in the paraventricular hypothalamic nucleus of the rat. *Journal of Chemistry and Neuroanatomy, 6,* 391–397.

Wan, W., Wetmore, L., Sorensen, C. M., Greenberg, A. H., & Nance, D. M. (1994). Neural and biochemical mediators of endotoxin and stress-induced *c-fos* expression in the rat brain. *Brain Research Bulletin, 34,* 7–14.

Wang, J. P., & Dunn, A. J. (1998). Mouse interleukin-6 stimulates the HPA axis and increases brain tryptophan and serotonin metabolism. *Neurochemistry International, 33,* 143–154.

Wang, J. P., & Dunn, A. J. (1999). The role of interleukin-6 in the activation of the hypothalamo-pituitary-adrenocortical axis induced by endotoxin and interleukin-1β. *Brain Research, 815,* 337–348.

Watkins, L. R., Maier, S. F., & Goehler, L. E. (1995). Cytokine-to-brain communication: A review and analysis of alternative mechanisms. *Life Sciences, 57,* 1011–1026.

Watkins, L. R., Wiertelak, E. P., Goehler, L. E., Mooney-Heiberger, K., Martinez, J., Furness, J., Smith, K. P., & Maier, S. F. (1994). Neurocircuitry of illness-induced hyperalgesia. *Brain Research, 639,* 283–299.

Weidenfeld, J., Abramsky, O., & Ovadia, H. (1989). Evidence for the involvement of the central adrenergic system in interleukin 1-induced adrenocortical response. *Neuropharmacology, 28,* 1411–1414.

Weidenfeld, J., Wohlman, A., & Gallily, R. (1995). Mycoplasma fermentans activates the hypothalamo-pituitary adrenal axis in the rat. *NeuroReport, 6,* 910–912.

Werner, E. R., Werner-Felmayer, G., & Wachter, H. (1993). Tetrahydrobiopterin and cytokines. *Proceedings of the Society of Experimental and Biological Medicine, 203,* 1–12.

Williams, L. M., Ballmer, P. E., Hannah, L. T., Grant, I., & Garlick, P. J. (1994). Changes in regional protein synthesis in rat brain and pituitary after systemic interleukin-1β administration. *American Journal of Physiology, 267,* E915–920.

Woodroofe, M. N., Sarna, G. S., Wadhwa, M., Hayes, G. M., Loughlin, A. J., Tinker, A., & Cuzner, M. L. (1991). Detection of interleukin-1 and interleukin-6 in adult rat brain, following mechanical injury, by in vivo microdialysis: Evidence of a role for microglia in cytokine production. *Journal of Neuroimmunology, 33,* 227–236.

Zalcman, S., Green-Johnson, J. M., Murray, L., Nance, D. M., Dyck, D., Anisman, H., & Greenberg, A. H. (1994). Cytokine-specific central monoamine alterations induced by interleukin-1, -2 and -6. *Brain Research, 643,* 40–49.

Zalcman, S., Murray, L., Dyck, D. G., Greenberg, A. H., & Nance, D. M. (1998). Interleukin-2 and -6 induce behavioral-activating effects in mice. *Brain Research, 811,* 111–121.

Zalcman, S., Savina, I., & Wise, R. A. (1999). Interleukin-6 increases sensitivity to the locomotor-stimulating effects of amphetamine in rats. *Brain Research, 841,* 276–283.

C H A P T E R

26

Sleep in Health and Disease

JAMES M. KRUEGER, JIDONG FANG, JEANNINE A. MAJDE

I. INTRODUCTION

Sleep is a complex neurological process essential for the survival of warm-blooded animals. Humans spend about 27 years in the course of life sleeping, but the function of sleep is unknown. One approach to understanding normal sleep is to characterize pathological sleep. Investigating sleep changes during infections and other inflammatory states has revealed that critical interactions occur between the immune system and the brain. Much evidence suggests that the same immune system mediators that regulate pathological sleep in response to systemic inflammation also regulate physiological sleep. This chapter outlines the neuroimmune interactions that have been demonstrated in inflammatory disease states and our current knowledge of how these interactions influence sleep in healthy individuals.

A. How Sleep is Measured in Humans and Animals

Sleep is associated with many changes in the brain and body, including reduced responses to stimuli, reduced motor activities, and changes in metabolic rates, body temperature, heart rate, breathing activities, hormone release, brain waves, neuronal activities, and mental activities. Since all of these changes associated with sleep, including unconsciousness, are generated or regulated by the brain, it is reasonable to think that sleep is a brain state different from wakefulness. Given the complexity of the brain, it is not surprising that there is no direct measure of sleep. Nevertheless, sleep as a brain state can be distinguished reliably from wakefulness in mammals using several measurements in combination, such as the electroencephalography (EEG), the electromyography (EMG), the electroocculography (EOG), and brain temperature. There are two different types of sleep in mammals and birds: rapid eye movement sleep (REMS) and non-REMS (NREMS). NREMS sleep is characterized by high amplitude EEG slow waves (.5–4 Hz) (also called synchronized EEG or delta waves), reduced muscle activities, and reduced brain and body temperature compared with wakefulness. In contrast, REMS is characterized by low amplitude fast EEG activities (also called EEG desynchronization) similar to wakefulness, loss of muscle tone (muscle atonia), rapid eye movement, and rapid increases in brain temperature after entry into REMS. In humans, NREMS can be further divided into different stages: stage I is associated with sleep onset, stage II is characterized by the presence of sleep spindles in EEG recordings, and stages III and IV are dominated by EEG slow wave activities (SWA) and collectively called slow wave sleep (SWS) or delta sleep. In animal studies, NREMS and SWS often are used interchangeably. It is clear that sleep as a brain state can be determined only by the combination of several key parameters but not by any single parameter mentioned above. For instance, EEG desynchronization occurs both during wakefulness and REMS, whereas REMS without muscle atonia can be produced in animals with localized brain stem lesions.

Sleep identified by the above parameters can be quantified in many ways. First, the total amount and percentage of each sleep stage can be determined. Each species requires different amounts of sleep. Sleep occupies about one third of time in humans but about 50% of time in rats and mice. NREMS occupies most of the time during sleep in all species. The percentage of REMS in total sleep time is about 20–25% in humans, 15% in rodents, and less than 5% in birds. Secondly, the depth of sleep can be routinely and objectively measured using modern computer technologies. Since the EEG SWA increases as a result of sleep deprivation and is associated with increases in arousal threshold, it is often used as an indicator the depth or intensity of NREMS. The increases in EEG SWA after sleep deprivation also are reflected in the increases in total time spent in stages III and IV, in which SWA dominates EEG recordings. Sleep also can be quantified in other ways, such as latencies to NREMS and REMS, REMS–REMS cycle length, the number and duration of each sleep stage, and so on. These measures are useful in characterizing the effects of different substances on sleep. However, the amounts and intensity of sleep are most relevant to the present discussion and are also the most reliable and objective measures of sleep.

In cold-blooded animals, such as reptiles, changes in behavioral state are not correlated with characteristic changes in EEG activities. In the case of insects, the EEG cannot be recorded using current technology. Since EEG signals are largely generated by orderly packed neurons and their dendrites in the neocortex, which is only present in the mammals and birds, the use of EEG loses its structural rationale in cold-blooded animals. However, this does not exclude the possibility that the cold-blooded animals have sleep. Many cold-blooded animals display behavioral states that are distinct from wakefulness and simple rest and are similar to sleep found in mammals and birds. Behavioral sleep has been observed in *Aplysia* (Strumwasser, 1971), honey bees (Kaiser, 1985), cockroaches (Tobler, 1983), amphibians, and reptiles (Hartse, 1994). Common phenomena associated with sleep in different species include reduced physical activity, reduced responsiveness to external stimuli, characteristic posture, and rebound of the state after deprivation.

B. Regulation of Sleep

The rebound of sleep and EEG SWA after sleep loss leads to the concept of sleep homeostasis. This concept emphasizes the influence of the duration of prior wakefulness on subsequent sleep. However, the need for sleep is further regulated by many other factors such as ambient temperature, thermal regulation, food intake, immune responses, stress responses, and learning and memory. These processes are all integral parts of normal life and have been posited to play important roles in the homeostatic regulation of sleep in different theories. For instance, it has been suggested that the function of NREMS is to save energy (Berger & Phillips ;1995) or to cool the brain (Nakao, McGinty, Szymusiak, & Yamamoto 1995). These suggestions are supported by the enhancement of NREMS after warming the body or the brain, by the decreases in metabolic rates and temperature in the brain and the body during sleep, and by the presence of warm-sensitive neurons in the brain that increase their firing rate during sleep. However, there is ample evidence indicating that the coupling between sleep and thermal regulation is not absolute. Increases in brain and body temperature are not always followed by increases in sleep, and many substances promote sleep without effects on body temperature. Immune responses also play important roles in sleep regulation, and the same molecules that mediate immune responses are also involved in the regulation of physiological sleep. The immune system is constantly stimulated by various types of microbial products derived from the gut under physiological conditions. Cytokines like interleukin-1 (IL-1) and tumor necrosis factor (TNF) are produced in the normal brain and body partially as a result of such stimulation. The above examples illustrate the point that daily sleep is regulated by multiple physiological processes in a dynamic fashion with one or more processes playing a role in sleep regulation depending on the needs of the organism.

The dynamic nature of sleep regulation is also reflected at the levels of neuronal networks, single neurons, and molecules. It is clear that none of the neuronal circuits involved in sleep regulation is unique for sleep regulation. For instance, the preoptic area plays an important role in sleep regulation and also in thermal regulation and sexual behaviors. In addition, single neurons in the brain respond to multiple stimuli and take part in multiple physiological processes. All of the neurotransmitters and humoral factors that are involved in sleep regulation also have other biological effects. For example, IL-1 and TNF are involved in the regulation of physiological sleep, food intake, thermal regulation, and host defense. Further, no individual neural circuit seems to be necessary for sleep to occur; no matter what area of brain is lesioned, if the animal survives, it sleeps. The above observations raise a fundamental question: how can normal sleep arise as the result of interactions of multiple nonspecific physiological processes, networks, neuronal groups, and molecules? Although the regulation of sleep is far from being completely understood, growing evidence suggests that neuronal activities during wakefulness lead, through multiple neurotransmitter systems, to the production and accumulation of multiple humoral factors such as hormones, cytokines, and other growth factors that promote induction or maintenance of sleep. Thus, although the contribution of individual networks, neurons, and molecules to sleep can be very large, no single network, neuron, or sleep regulatory molecule is necessary for sleep to occur.

The distribution of daily sleep is strongly modulated by the circadian rhythm. Diurnal animals such as humans sleep during the night, whereas nocturnal animals such as rats and mice sleep most of time during the day. In mammals the circadian clock is localized in the suprachiasmatic nucleus (SCN), which is entrained primarily by the daily light–dark cycles. Lesions of the SCN in rats result in an even distribution of sleep across the light–dark cycles but have no effect on the total amounts of sleep (Ibuka, Inouye, & Kawamura, 1977). In humans, the multiple sleep latency test indicates that subjects fall into sleep more easily during the morning than during the night even when the subject has slept overnight. These observations suggest that the circadian regulation of sleep can be separated from homeostatic regulation of sleep.

Clearly, sleep is a complex process involving numerous regulatory inputs. Those that form the focus of this chapter are immune system inputs. The sections that follow briefly review the effects on sleep of inflammatory and infectious diseases involving the immune system. Then we examine the molecular basis for the relationship of sleep and immunity, and what it tells us about immune regulation of sleep.

II. CHANGES IN SLEEP DURING CHRONIC INFLAMMATORY DISEASES

Sleep disorders have been observed in a number of chronic inflammatory diseases. Those best studied are rheumatoid arthritis, fibromyalgia, and chronic fatigue syndrome.

A. Rheumatic Disorders

Fatigue is experienced in most chronic inflammatory diseases, and the association of fatigue with changes in the quantity and/or quality of sleep has been examined. Sleep in rheumatoid arthritis is characterized by sleep fragmentation with frequent movement of the extremities and frequent arousal (Mahowald, Mahowald, Bundlie, & Ytterberg, 1989). Alpha-delta sleep patterns (in which alpha EEG NREM sleep intrudes on delta sleep) are frequent. A similar sleep pattern is seen in juvenile rheumatoid arthritis (Zamir, Press, Tal, & Tarasiuk, 1998). Primary Sjogren's syndrome also is characterized by sleep fragmentation that is more severe than in rheumatoid arthritis. The disrupted sleep patterns associated with these rheumatic diseases, rather than reduced total amounts of sleep, correlate with complaints of fatigue (Mahowald et al., 1989). Treating rheumatoid arthritis patients with the hypnotic drug triazolam fails to improve sleep fragmentation but does improve morning stiffness and reduce daytime sleepiness (Walsh, Muehlbach, Lauter, Hilliker, and Schweitzer, 1996).

Rheumatic diseases are marked by either generalized or localized pain, and the role of pain in altering sleep has been examined. No correlation exists between the severity of arthritis symptoms and the sleep disorders detected (Hirsch et al., 1994), although patients with the most abnormal sleep patterns experience the most morning stiffness, pain and joint tenderness (Drewes et al., 1998). Successful treatment of rheumatic pain with a nonsteroidal antiinflammatory does not improve sleep patterns (Lavie, Nadir, Lorer, & Scharf, 1991). Although there is no evidence that pain contributes to sleep changes, there are indications that the sleep disorders associated with rheumatic diseases contribute to the pain experienced by these patients. Specifically, the condition termed fibrositis may be caused by disrupted sleep (Moldofsky, Leu, & Smythe, 1993; Moldofsky, 1989).

B. Chronic Fatigue Disorders

Syndromes associated with chronic fatigue, subjective cognitive impairment, and diffuse myalgia rather than focal inflammation (joint swelling) of the type seen in rheumatic diseases include fibromyalgia and chronic fatigue syndrome. Fibromyalgia is distinguished from chronic fatigue syndrome clinically by its associated marked fibrositis. Depression also is commonly associated with these disorders. Recently the depression in chronic fatigue syndrome was shown to be associated with a characteristic REMS latency that has been associated with other depressive disorders (Morehouse, Flanigan, MacDonald, Braha, & Shapiro, 1998). Most patients with these syndromes complain of nonrestorative sleep. One study has indicated that the association of these two syndromes with sleep disorders is not greater than in patients with psychiatric disorders not associated with pain (Buchwald, Pascualy, Bombardier, & Kith, 1994). Both syndromes are frequently preceded by a febrile illness, but fibromyalgia is also commonly associated with both psychological distress and primary sleep disorders such as sleep apnea and periodic limb movement (Moldofsky, 1993). The association of fibromyalgia and sleep apnea is much stronger in males (44%) than in females (2.2%) and may contribute to the pain syndrome in males with this disorder (May, West, Baker, & Everett, 1993).

Sleep fragmentation similar to that seen in rheumatic diseases is the most common sleep disorder documented in fibromyalgia patients. Some, but not all of the frequent arousals seen are due to the high frequency of sleep apnea in these patients (Jennum, Drewes, Andreasen, & Nielsen, 1993). As in rheumatic disorders, alpha-delta sleep occurs in fibromyalgia and increases over the course of the night (Branco, Atalaia, & Paiva, 1994). The sleep disorder in chronic fatigue syndrome is essentially the same as that in fibromyalgia (Moldofsky, 1993), although the association with primary sleep disorders such as sleep apnea is not seen. Circadian rhythm disruption of melatonin secretion and core temperature is seen in chronic fatigue syndrome, which may or may not be a consequence of the sleep disorder (Williams et al., 1996). It has been proposed that fibromyalgia and chronic fatigue are both clinical manifestations of the reciprocal relationship between the immune and sleep–wake systems, and interference with either the immune system (by an infection generating large amounts of cytokines) or the sleep–wake system (by sleep deprivation) affects the other system and will be accompanied by symptoms of chronic fatigue (Moldofsky, 1993). Interestingly, a study of the chronic fatigue and arthralgia syndrome that commonly follows infection with Lyme disease, known to be caused by a tick-borne spirochete, reveals sleep features similar to other chronic inflammatory diseases (Bujak, Weinstein, & Dornbush, 1996).

C. Summary

Sleep changes in distinct chronic inflammatory disorders appear to be quite similar. Sleep fragmentation is characteristic, as is alpha-delta sleep. These sleep changes appear intrinsic to the inflammatory state and are not a result of pain, but instead may contribute to pain. So far sleep changes in chronic inflammatory diseases have been described only in clinical settings and have provided little insight into the mediators or functions of sleep. More mechanistic investigations have been undertaken in animal models of acute infectious illness. These will be discussed in sections III and V.

III. CHANGES IN SLEEP DURING ACUTE INFECTIONS

The need to lie down and sleep is often overwhelming at the onset of an acute infection such as influenza, and the total amount of sleep may increase two- to threefold over normal. This excess sleep is now recognized to be a component of the acute phase response (APR), or the complex array of stereotypic behavioral, hematological, endocrine, and biochemical changes that accompany acute systemic infections. In addition to excess sleep, the behavioral changes include fever, anorexia, and social withdrawal. This complex of behaviors has been termed sickness behavior (Hart, 1988), and like other elements of the APR is generally considered adaptive. Sleep has been intensively investigated in acute infections in an effort to better understand its physiological as well as its pathological role.

Sleep during acute infections is not only increased in quantity but also is changed in quality. Compared with healthy animals or humans, acutely infected individuals demonstrate increased NREMS and diminished REMS (Krueger & Majde, 1994). Increased amplitudes of EEG slow waves also are seen, which are considered an index of the intensity of sleep (Krueger & Majde, 1994). Sleep changes have been investigated in acute bacterial, viral, and fungal infections (reviewed Toth, 1999). The microbial factors that trigger the proinflammatory cytokines mediating these sleep changes have been characterized for some of these agents. From these studies has evolved a theory of how microbial factors and immune mediators regulate sleep in health and disease. Because these observations have provided such valuable insights into sleep regulation, they will be discussed in detail in section V. Sleep alterations in acute bacterial, fungal, and viral infections recently have been reviewed (Toth, 1999) and will only be summarized here.

A. Bacterial Infections

The most extensive studies of sleep in response to bacterial infections have been conducted in rabbits. Several species of viable bacteria inoculated intravenously cause increases in NREMS, increased EEG SWA, and reduced or absent REMS (Toth & Krueger, 1989). Altered sleep occurs simultaneously with fever, lymphopenia, and neutrophilia but does not persist as long as the fever response (Toth & Krueger, 1988). Sleep changes are apparent by 4 h postchallenge with viable *Staphylococcus aureus* and much more rapidly following challenge with killed *S. aureus*. The response to live bacteria persists longer, is biphasic, and is characterized by decreased EEG SWA and NREMS bout length after 20 h. The response to viable *Streptococcus pyogenes* is less persistent, and killed *S. pyogenes* is inert. The response to both viable and killed *Escherichia coli* persists for only a few hours, is manifested primarily in EEG amplitude changes, and is the same whether the bacteria are alive or dead. When a rabbit pathogen (*Pasteurella multocida*) is employed using more natural routes of infection, a biphasic response is seen with initial increases and later decreases in NREMS; REMS is profoundly suppressed throughout the 48-h observation period (Toth & Krueger, 1990).

B. Fungal Infections

Challenge of rats with baker's yeast or rabbits with *Candida albicans* induces sleep alterations similar to those seen in animals challenged with gram-positive bacteria (Toth, 1999). *Candida*-challenged rabbits demonstrate an initial increase followed by a decrease in the amount of time spent in NREMS with parallel changes in sleep intensity (Toth, 1999). Light conditions modulate the sleep response of rabbits to *Candida*; constant light induced more prolonged increases in NREMS (Toth & Krueger, 1995).

C. Viral Infections

Studies of sleep in acute viral infections have focused on respiratory viruses, primarily influenza virus. Smith and colleagues at the British Common Cold Unit examined subjective assessments of sleep quality and length by volunteers challenged with influenza B, influenza A, or rhinovirus. Volunteers with both subclinical and clinical disease slept less during the prodrome and more during the symptomatic period following influenza challenge (Smith, 1992). Those who subsequently developed clinical influenza slept less during the prodrome than those who resisted clinical disease (Smith, 1992). Symptomatic rhinovirus colds also tended to increase sleep duration and reduce sleep quality, but the effect was not significant (Smith, 1992).

Animal studies of influenza demonstrate a clear impact of more severe viral challenges on sleep. In rabbits given a large intravenous challenge with influenza A, which produces an abortive infection and a brief febrile illness in this species, NREMS and EEG SWA are increased and REMS decreased during the febrile period (Kimura-Takeuchi, Majde, Toth, & Krueger, 1992). An abortive infection of mice with Newcastle disease virus also demonstrates a similar brief increase in NREMS and reduction in REMS (Toth, 1999). A similar but more prolonged sleep alteration is seen in an active influenza infection in mice when virus is administered in such a manner as to cause a pneumonitis, whether or not a lethal infection ensues (Fang, Sanborn, Renegar, Majde, & Krueger, 1995; Toth, 1999). When the same amount of virus is delivered only to the upper respiratory tract, no changes in sleep or other symptoms are seen (Fang et al., 1996).

Other acute viral infections studied for their sleep effects include feline herpes virus in kittens (which causes a respiratory infection) and rabies encephalitis in mice. Feline herpes virus causes an age-dependent increase in auditory arousability from sleep and a reduction in EEG delta-wave amplitudes (Toth, 1999). Rabies encephalitis in mice results in a generalized EEG slowing, flattening of cortical activity, and replacement of normal sleep with abnormal sleep (Toth, 1999). These changes are similar to those seen in animals becoming moribund following infections or experiencing chronic sleep deprivation, and may reflect a generalized neurological change more than sleep alterations per se (Toth, 1999).

IV. CHANGES IN SLEEP DURING CHRONIC INFECTIONS

The chronic infections that have been most extensively investigated with respect to sleep changes are immunodeficiency viruses of humans and cats; trypanosome infections of rabbits, rats, and humans; and prion infections of mice, rats, cats, and humans.

Sleep changes in human immunodeficiency virus type 1 (HIV-1) infections have been studied during asymptomatic and symptomatic phases. Asymptomatic HIV-1-infected men express increased SWS during the second half of the night, sleep fragmentation, and abnormal REMS architecture (reviewed Toth, 1999). These altered sleep patterns precede neurological involvement or onset of secondary infections (Darko, Mitler, & Henriksen, 1995). Progression to overt AIDS is marked by reduced SWS, marked sleep fragmentation, and profound disruption of sleep architecture (Wiegand et al., 1991).

Feline immunodeficiency virus, a retrovirus similar to HIV that is a natural pathogen of cats, causes an unusual NREMS pattern, an increased frequency of arousal and, a decrease in the amount of REMS (Toth, 1999).

Chronic infections with the parasite *Trypanosoma brucei*, the causative agent of human "sleeping sickness," result in increased sleep coincident with the onset of fever and other symptoms (Toth, 1999). Increased somnolence persists in association with episodic recrudescence of parasitemia, and loss of the normal circadian organization of sleep gradually develops during chronic trypanosomiasis in rabbits, rats, and humans (Toth, 1999).

Prions, the agents associated with chronic dementia, also cause alterations in sleep. Rats inoculated with the prion scrapie demonstrate unusual spiking patterns in the EEG during wakefulness 4 months after inoculation (Toth, 1999). Later NREMS and active wakefulness are reduced and drowsiness is increased (Toth, 1999). Cats challenged with Creutzfeldt-Jakob brain homogenate demonstrate increased NREMS, reduced wakefulness, and abnormal REMS 20 months after inoculation (Toth, 1999). The condition known as fatal familial insomnia is associated with prion-related thalamic neurodegeneration (Toth, 1999). Deletion of the prion protein gene results in altered sleep and circadian rhythms in mice (Toth, 1999).

V. TRIGGERS OF THE APR IN ACUTE INFECTIONS (MICROBIAL PRODUCTS AND MACROPHAGE PROCESSING)

Probably the most significant advance in conceptualizing the interaction of sleep and the immune system resulted from observations of sleep changes in animals and humans inoculated with purified microbial products (reviewed Krueger & Majde, 1994). These studies have resulted in the well-supported theory that during infections immune recognition of chemically unique microbial products by phagocytes results in the induction of cytokines, which in turn modulate sleep (Krueger & Majde, 1990). The role of cytokines in both pathological and physiological sleep will be discussed in section VI. Here we briefly review the chemical basis for cytokine induction by various microorganisms.

A. Bacteria

The first insights into the relationship of microbial products to sleep were gained from structural studies on a sleep factor isolated from human urine (Krueger, Pappenheimer, & Karnovsky, 1982b). This factor proved to share the unique chemical properties of the peptidoglycans found in the cell walls of bacteria (Krueger et al., 1982a). Peptidoglycans comprise 90% of the cell wall of gram-positive bacteria and 5–20% of the cell wall of gram-negative bacteria (Krueger & Majde, 1990). Subsequent sleep studies with various natural and synthetic peptidoglycans revealed that the minimally active unit is a glycopeptide consisting of the sugar N-acetylmuramic acid (found only in bacteria) and the dipeptide L-alanine-D-alanine, termed muramic acid dipeptide or MDP (Krueger, Pappenheimer, & Karnovsky, 1982a). MDP and certain derivatives have immunological adjuvant properties. Peptidoglycans also contain the bacterially unique amino acids D-glutamic acid (eukaryotes employ primarily L-amino acids) and diaminopimelic acid as well as L-lysine. Many peptidoglycan derivatives are pyrogenic as well as somnogenic.

The other bacterial cell wall product that has been extensively analyzed with respect to somnogenicity is the lipopolysaccharide (LPS) found in gram-negative bacterial endotoxin. LPS, like peptidoglycans, is comprised, in part, of chemical components that are unique to bacteria. The polysaccharide at one end of the molecule determines the antigenic specificity of the bacterium, whereas the complex phosphorylated lipid at the other end, lipid A, is responsible for the toxicity of endotoxin. LPSs and their lipid A moieties also function as immunological adjuvants and are pyrogenic and somnogenic. As with peptidoglycans, subtle structural differences in the lipid A affect both its toxicity and its somnogenicity. More details on the structure-function relationships of bacterial products with respect to sleep are discussed in Krueger and Majde (1994).

Recently it has been recognized that structural differences in bacterial DNA are recognized by the immune system with the production of cytokines (Sweet, Stacey, Kakuda, Markovich, & Hume, 1998). It is not yet known if bacterial DNA plays a role in bacterial illness or in the sleep responses to bacteria.

Animals are constantly exposed to bacterial products produced by endogenous flora. It has been demonstrated that, as expected on chemical grounds, macrophages that ingest bacteria are incapable of degrading those structures for which eukaryotes lack enzymes. For instance, peptidoglycans are incompletely degraded and fragments comprised of bacterially unique components (particularly muramic acid) are released extracellularly by macrophages (Vermeulen & Gray, 1984). Animals with reduced endogenous flora have lower body temperatures and sleep less (Krueger & Majde, 1994). Therefore, it has been proposed that the immune response (primarily phagocyte-produced cytokines) to bacterial products plays a role in both physiological body temperature maintenance and in physiological sleep as well as pathological changes (Krueger & Majde, 1994). At present, support for this hypothesis is indirect.

B. Fungi

Like bacteria, fungi also have cell walls. However, the structural components are distinct from those of bacteria and more closely resemble the scaffolding of plants and insects. Certain fungal polysaccharide components, particularly glucan and mannan, function as immune modulators (Krueger & Majde, 1994). As with bacterial cell walls, the cell walls of fungi are resistant to mammalian enzymes and stimulate inflammation. As discussed in section III.B, fungi can cause altered sleep. However, the specific components involved in their somnogenicity have not been elucidated (Krueger & Majde, 1994).

C. Viruses

Viruses are structurally distinct from other microbes, although the immune responses they trigger are very similar. Viruses lack chemically unique structural elements capable of stimulating cytokine production. However, viruses produce double-stranded RNA (dsRNA) that is capable of inducing cytokines in much the same manner as microbial cell walls (Krueger & Majde, 1994), and evidence is accumulating that viral dsRNA plays a role in viral cytokine induction. Viral dsRNA is produced either as a byproduct of replication (in the case of RNA viruses), as genomic RNA (reoviruses), or as secondary structure in viral mRNAs (all viruses) (Krueger & Majde, 1994). In addition to cytokine induction, viral dsRNA activates certain enzymes in the cell that, in turn, down-regulate viral protein synthesis or degrade viral mRNA (Krueger & Majde, 1994); these enzymes contribute to host defense by limiting viral replication. A common pathway for viruses and other microbes is activation of proinflammatory transcription factors such as nuclear factor kappa B (NFκB) in phagocytes. The relationship of proinflammatory transcription factors, the cytokines they regulate, and the sleep response is discussed in section VII.

D. Model of Microbial Activation of the Acute Phase Response

The current model for microbial activation of excess sleep, fever, and other acute phase responses invokes the release of a microbial substance that resists biodegradation by phagocytes and triggers proinflammatory cytokine production (particularly IL-1 and TNF) by those phagocytes through activation of immunoregulatory transcription factors. Cytokines so produced may enter the blood or lymph and act on the brain by crossing the blood-brain barrier through specific transporters (Banks, Ortiz, Plotkin, & Kastin, 1991) or at sites lacking the blood-brain barrier (Blatteis & Sehic, 1997). Alternatively, they may act locally on vagal afferents (see section VII). Cytokines produced by other sources of inflammation are similar and take similar paths. The remainder of this chapter addresses what is known about the cytokine-stimulated events in the brain that ultimately result in altered sleep.

VI. HUMORAL REGULATION OF SLEEP THE INVOLVEMENT OF IMMUNE SYSTEM PRODUCTS

Sleep is regulated by neural and humoral mechanisms; these mechanisms interact and are inseparable. Neural mechanisms of sleep regulation have been extensively reviewed elsewhere (Steriade & McCarley, 1990); this chapter focuses on humoral mechanisms. The involvement of specific neurotransmitters in sleep regulation often is included within the concept of humoral regulation of sleep; almost all well-characterized neurotransmitters have been implicated in one or more aspects of sleep-wake regulation. For the purposes of this chapter, we will focus on neuromodulator involvement in sleep regulation. That there are relatively stable (half-life lasting minutes or more) long-acting sleep regulatory substances (SRSs) was first demonstrated at the turn of the century when it was shown that cerebrospinal fluid (CSF) taken from sleep-deprived dogs and given to normal dogs induced excess sleep in the recipients (reviewed Krueger & Majde, 1994). This observation has been replicated many times in the intervening years and there are now several well-documented SRSs, all of which also have actions within the immune system. In this chapter we focus on the involvement of IL-1β, TNF-α, growth hormone releasing hormone (GHRH), and adenosine in physiological NREMS regulation, and prolactin (PRL) and vasoactive intestinal peptide (VIP) in REMS regulation. We also briefly discuss the notion that IL-1, TNF, and other somnogenic growth factors such as nerve growth factor, induce sleep via NFκB-dependent mechanisms; several events downstream from NFκB activation, e.g., cyclooxygenase-2 (COX-2) and inducible-nitric oxide synthase (NOS) induction also seem to be involved in sleep regulation.

A. IL-1β and TNF-α

Systemic or central injection of either IL-1β or TNF-α is followed by prolonged pronounced increases in the amount of time spent in NREMS. For example, mice receiving 3 µg of TNF intraperitoneally (ip) spend about 1.5 extra hours in NREMS during the first 9 h postinjection (Fang, Wang, & Krueger, 1997). The somnogenic actions of IL-1β have been demonstrated in rats, rabbits, mice, monkeys, and cats, whereas TNF-α is somnogenic in mice, rats, rabbits, and sheep; negative results have not been reported for any species. The excess NREMS induced by IL-1β or TNF-α is associated with supranormal EEG slow waves (Krueger, Walter, Dinarello, Wolff, & Chedid, 1984). Similar supranormal EEG slow waves occur after sleep deprivation (Pappenheimer, Koski, Fencl, Karnovsky, & Krueger, 1975) or during the initial sleep responses to infectious challenge (Toth & Krueger, 1988) and are posited to reflect a higher intensity of NREMS (Borbély & Tobler, 1989). Low somnogenic doses of IL-1β and TNF-α have little effect on REMS, whereas doses that induce large increases in NREMS often reduce duration of REMS. In rats (Lancel, Mathias, Faulhaber, & Schiffelholz, 1996; Opp, Obál, & Krueger, 1991) and cats (Susic & Totic, 1989) higher doses of IL-1β inhibit, rather than promote, sleep.

Inhibition of either IL-1 or TNF is associated with a reduction of spontaneous NREMS; these data strongly implicate these substances in physiological sleep regulation. Thus, anti-TNF or IL-1 antibodies, soluble IL-1 or TNF receptors, and the IL-1 receptor antagonist all inhibit spontaneous NREMS (reviewed Krueger & Majde, 1994). These inhibitors also inhibit the expected NREMS rebound that normally would occur after sleep deprivation, thereby suggesting that IL-1 and TNF also are involved in sleep deprivation-induced excess NREMS. Other inhibitors of IL-1 or TNF also inhibit spontaneous sleep; the list includes IL-4 (Kushikata, Fang, Wang, & Krueger, 1998), IL-10 (Opp, Smith, & Hughes, 1995), prostaglandin-E_2, α-melanocyte stimulating hormone, glucocorticoids, and corticotropin releasing hormone (reviewed Krueger & Obál, 1997) (Figure 1).

Within brain there are diurnal variations of IL-1β mRNA (Taishi, Bredow, Guha-Thakurta, Obál & Krueger, 1997) and TNF mRNA levels (Bredow, Taishi, Guha-Thakurta, Obál, & Krueger, 1997) as well as IL-1β (Nguyen et al., 1998) and TNF-α (Floyd & Krueger, 1997) protein levels. These diurnal variations occur in several areas of brain including the hypothalamus (an area involved in sleep regulation), the hippocampus, and the cerebral cortex. Further, after sleep deprivation hypothalamic IL-1β mRNA levels (Mackiewicz, Sollars, Ogilvie, & Pack, 1996; Taishi et al., 1998) and TNF mRNA levels (Taishi & Krueger, unpublished) increase. Related molecules such as the IL-1 receptor accessory protein are not affected by sleep deprivation (Taishi et al., 1998). Central IL-1β also seems to be involved in the excess NREMS associated with excess food intake; rats on a cafeteria diet express increased IL-1β mRNA in brain during peak food-induced sleep responses (Hansen, Taishi, Chen, & Krueger, 1998). Collectively, the data showing change in IL-1β and TNF-α expression are consistent with the hypothesis that they are involved in physiological sleep regulation.

The receptors responsible for the somnogenic actions of IL-1β and TNF-α have been identified. Mutant mice lacking the TNF 55 kD receptor do not elicit sleep responses if given TNF-α, although they are responsive to IL-1β (Fang et al., 1997). In contrast, mutant mice lacking the IL-1 type I receptor are unresponsive if given IL-1β, but do have robust NREMS responses if given TNF-α (Fang, Wang, & Krueger, 1998).

Although the data discussed in preceding paragraphs strongly implicate IL-1β and TNF-α in physiological sleep regulation, there is substantially less data demonstrating their involvement in the sleep responses occurring after infectious challenge. The only data we are aware of in this regard is the finding that muramyl dipeptide (a bacterial cell wall product) induced NREMS responses are attenuated if animals are pretreated with inhibitors of IL-1 (Takahashi, Kapás, Fang, et al., 1996) or TNF (Takahashi, Kapás, & Krueger, 1996). Regardless, since increases in proinflammatory cytokines such as IL-1 and TNF are hallmarks of the response to microbial challenge and these substances are involved in physiological sleep

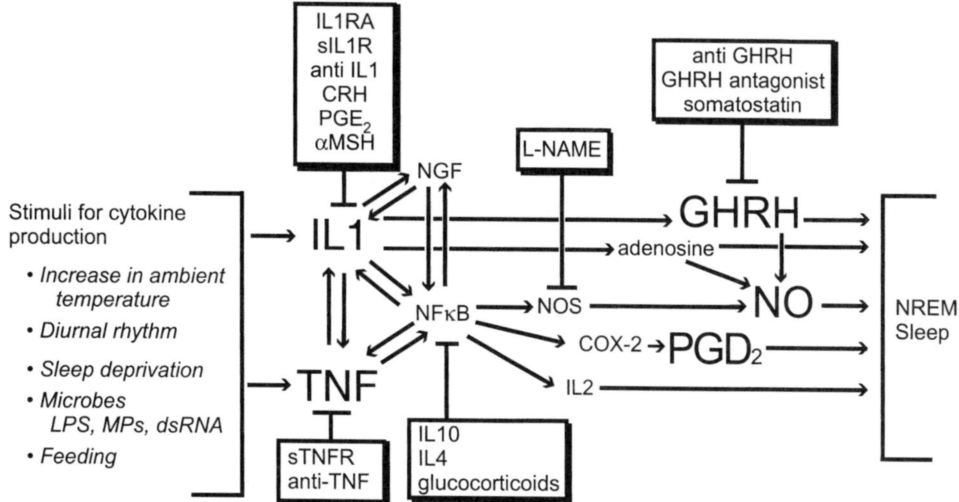

FIGURE 1 Substances involved in sleep regulation form biochemical regulatory cascades. Substances in boxes inhibit sleep and inhibit the production or actions of the sleep-promoting substances illustrated. Inhibition of one step does not completely block sleep, because parallel somnogenic pathways also exist. These redundant pathways provide stability to the sleep regulatory mechanism. Our knowledge of the biochemical events involved in sleep regulation is greater than that illustrated, e. g., see Figure 2. Abbreviations are: IL1RA: IL-1 receptor antagonist; sILIR: soluble IL-1 receptor; anti-IL-1: anti-IL-1 antibodies; CRH: corticotropin releasing hormone; PGD_2: prostaglandin D_2; αMSH: alpha melanocyte stimulating hormone; NGF: nerve growth factor; NFκB: nuclear factor kappa B; sTNFR: soluble TNF receptor; anti-TNF: anti-TNF antibodies; IL-10: interleukin10; IL-4: interleukin-4; L-NAME: an arginine analog; NOS: inducible nitric oxide synthase; COX-2 cyclooxygenase 2; IL-2: interleukin-2; NO: nitric oxide; GHRH: growth hormone releasing hormone. → indicates stimulation; ⊣ indicates inhibition.

regulation, it seems highly likely that IL-1 and TNF play roles in the NREMS responses occurring during infection.

Multiple cytokines and growth factors are likely involved in the host's NREMS responses to microbial challenge. For example, rabbits challenged with influenza virus have increased plasma antiviral activity (likely representing interferon [IFN] activity) during peak sleep responses (Kimura-Takeuchi et al., 1992). Several additional cytokines and growth factors have the capacity to enhance NREMS; the list includes IL-2, IFN-α, neurotrophin-1, neurotrophin-2, epidermal growth factor, fibroblast growth factor, IL-1α, and TNF-β (reviewed in Krueger & Obál, 1997). However, currently there is insufficient data to implicate any of these substances in physiological sleep regulation.

B. The Somatotrophic Axis

An association between the somatotrophic axis and sleep was first demonstrated when it was shown that a major peak in growth hormone (GH) release in humans occurred during the first period of deep, slow-wave sleep (Sassin et al., 1969; Takahashi, Kipnis, & Daughaday, 1968). In humans, abnormal GH secretory patterns are associated with sleep disorders (Aström & Linhölm, 1990; DeBoer, Roelfsema, Frölich, Kamphussen, & Van Sefers, 1989; Ehlers & Kupfer, 1987; Goldstein et al., 1987; Wolff & Money, 1973). Further, during sleep deprivation GH release is suppressed and when subjects are allowed to sleep excess GH secretion occurs (Jacoby, Smith, Sassin, Greenstein, & Weitzman, 1975; Kawakami, Kimura, & Tsai, 1983; Moldofsky, Davidson, & Lue, 1988; Sassin et al., 1979). Nevertheless, dissociation between GH release and sleep can occur (Carlson, Gillin, Gordon, & Snyder, 1972), and it is now posited that GHRH provides the link between GH release and sleep (Obál et al., 1988).

Central or systemic administration of GHRH induces increases in the amount of time spent in NREMS in several species including rats, rabbits, and humans (reviewed in Krueger & Obál, 1997). The GHRH-induced sleep is associated with supranormal EEG slow waves and thus thought to be of greater intensity (Borbély & Tobler, 1989). GHRH also can induce increases in REMS (Obál et al., 1988). However, in hypophysectomized animals, GHRH only induces NREMS (Obál, Floyd, Kapás, Bodosi, & Krueger, 1996). The sleep induced by GHRH appears normal in the sense that it is readily reversible if animals are disturbed and no abnormal behaviors are evident.

Inhibition of GHRH using either anti-GHRH antibodies or a GHRH peptide antagonist inhibits spontaneous NREMS and sleep rebound after sleep deprivation (Obál, Payne, Kapás, Opp, & Krueger, 1991; Obál, Payne, et al., 1992; Zhang, Obál Jr, Zheng, Fang, Taishi, & Krueger, 1999). NREMS, but not REMS, is depressed in a transgenic strain of mice that overexpress GH in brain; thus, these mice have less GHRH and more somatostatin (SRIH) in brain (Zhang, Obál, Fang, Collins, & Krueger, 1996). Further, dwarf rats, which underexpress GHRH receptors, also have reduced NREMS and REMS (Krueger, Obál, & Fang, 1999). Inhibition of GHRH using antibodies also attenuates IL-1β-induced increases in NREMS (Obál, Fang, Payne, & Krueger, 1995), thereby suggesting that IL-1β elicits its effects on sleep in part via GHRH.

Within the hypothalamus, there are two pools of GHRH-containing neurons; those in the arcuate nucleus and those around the ventral medial nucleus. The former project to the median eminence and are thought to be involved in GH release. The GHRHergic neurons around the ventromedial nucleus, including those in the paraventricular nucleus, project to both the median eminence and to the basal forebrain. There are GHRH receptors in both the pituitary and basal forebrain. The preoptic area–basal forebrain is well known for its role in NREMS regulation, e.g., lesions of this area are associated with insomnia (von Economo, 1930) and rapid electrical stimulation of this area induces NREMS. Microinjection of GHRH into the basal forebrain induces excess NREMS, whereas injection of the GHRH peptide antagonist into the same area reduces NREMS and attenuates sleep rebound after sleep deprivation (Zhang et al., 1999). Within the hypothalamus, but not other areas of brain, there is a diurnal rhythm of GHRH mRNA; highest levels occur during the onset of daylight hours, which is the peak sleep period in rats (Bredow, Taishi, Obál, Guha-Thakurta, & Krueger, 1996), and after sleep deprivation there is an increase in GHRH mRNA levels in the hypothalamus (Zhang et al., 1998). These changes in GHRH mRNA are restricted to the extra-arcuate GHRHergic neurons (Toppila et al., 1997). GHRH stores in the hypothalamus also have a diurnal rhythm, with highest values at the beginning of the dark period, and are decreased during sleep deprivation (Gardi, Obál, Fang, Zhang, & Krueger, 1998). Such data are consistent with the notion that GHRH release is associated with higher sleep propensity.

Other members of the somatotrophic axis also can influence sleep and GHRH secretion. SRIH inhibits both GHRH and GH release (Figure 2). It also inhibits

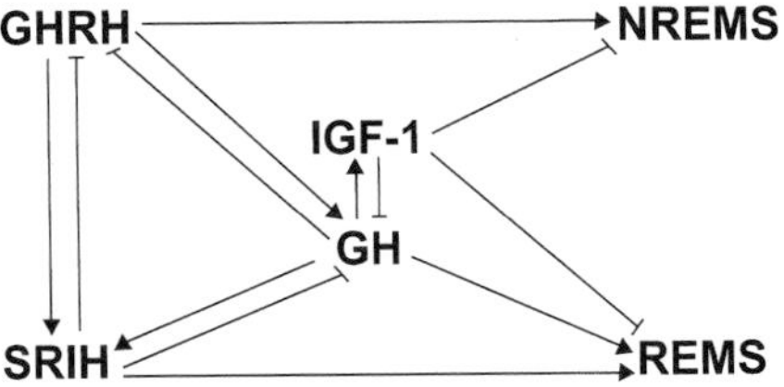

FIGURE 2 The somatotrophic axis is involved in sleep regulation. There is substantial evidence that growth hormone releasing hormone (GHRH) is involved in NREMS (nonrapid eye movement sleep) regulation (see text). Other members of the somatotrophic axis also affect sleep; their sleep actions appear to parallel their regulatory actions on the somatotrophic axis and occur within the anterior hypothalamus/basal forebrain. Abbreviations are: SRIH: somatostatin; GH: growth hormone; IGF-1: insulin-like growth factor-1. → indicates stimulation; ⊣ indicates inhibition.

NREMS, presumably via its effects on GHRH. In contrast, even though SRIH inhibits GH release, it stimulates REMS (Beranek et al., 1997). GH itself stimulates REMS (reviewed Krueger & Obál, 1997), and the promotion of REMS by GHRH is thought to be mediated via GH because in hypophysectomized rats, only NREMS is promoted (Obál et al., 1996). Further, after microinjection of GHRH into the basal forebrain, NREMS but not REMS is promoted (Zhang et al., 1999). GH also, may have via its metabolic action, an NREMS-promoting activity, because sleep is reduced in rats treated with anti-GH antibodies (Obál, Bodosi, Szilágyi, Kacsóh, & Krueger, 1997). In contrast, GH stimulates insulin-like growth factor-1 (IGF-1); IGF-1 has a rapid, but brief, inhibitory action on both REMS and NREMS (Obál, Kapás, Bodosi, & Krueger, 1998).

The role of the somatotrophic axis in sleep responses elicited by infectious agents remains uninvestigated. However, GH release is increased during infection and is induced by cytokines such as IL-1 and TNF. Further, GH has many direct actions on immunocytes, and the effects of IL-1 on sleep involve, in part, GHRH. Collectively, such information suggests a role for the somatotrophic axis hormones in sleep regulation, in health, and in disease.

C. PRL

The first anecdotal account implicating PRL in the regulation of REMS came from Jouvet"s laboratory: the French group reported that REMS was enhanced in response to systemic administration of PRL in pontine cats from which the pituitary had been removed (Jouvet et al., 1986). Thereafter, several lines of evidence implicated PRL in the regulation of REMS (reviewed Roky, et al., 1995). The major observations were as follows: (1) exogenous PRL stimulates REMS in three species: cats, rabbits, and rats; (2) the increases in REMS develop slowly, over 2 to 3 h, and are maintained for several hours; (3) PRL-induced changes in sleep are selective for REMS, i.e., NREMS is not altered after a single injection of PRL; (4) PRL enhances REMS only during the light period in the rat; (5) in contrast, REMS is suppressed during the light period and is enhanced at night in mutant, PRL-deficient rats (Valatx, Roky, & Paut-Pagano, 1990); and (6) rats rendered chronically hyperprolactinemic by means of grafting pituitaries under the kidney capsule exhibited increases in REMS during the light period of the day over a 6-week observation period (Obál Jr., Kacsóh, Bredow, Guha-Thakurta, & Krueger, 1997). Interestingly, slight enhancements in NREMS also were observed in these animals. Both REMS and NREMS are enhanced in hyperprolactinemic pseudopregnant rats (Zhang, Kimura & Inoue, 1995). Slight increases in NREMS might be attributed to a GH-like effect of the chronically increased PRL.

Intracerebral administration of PRL or antibodies to PRL stimulates or inhibits REMS, respectively (Roky, Valatx, & Jouvet, 1993; Roky, Valatx, Paut-Pagano, & Jouvet, 1994). The modulation of REMS, therefore, is a central action of PRL. PRL may come from two sources: it is produced by neurons in the hypothalamus, and PRL is released into the blood from the anterior pituitary. Circulating PRL is transported into the brain via specific receptor-mediated transport mechanisms residing in the choroid plexus (Walsh, Slaby, & Posner, 1987). The REMS-promoting activity of blood-borne PRL is supported by the observations that REMS is enhanced in response to systemically injected PRL (Jouvet et al., 1986; Obál, Opp, Cady, Johannsen, & Krueger, 1989), excess PRL released from pituitary grafts (Obál et al., 1989), or stimulation of endogenous PRL secretion from the pituitary (Obál et al., 1994). Nevertheless, only slight decreases in REMS are observed when basal, nonstimulated blood PRL is suppressed by means of immunoneutralization (Obál, Kacsoh, et al., 1992). In conclusion, increases in blood PRL stimulate REMS, but at normal concentrations in the blood, circulating PRL has only a small significant effect on the regulation of REMS. The impact of the increased blood PRL concentrations on REMS is attributed in part, to a stimulation of the expression of PRL receptors in the choroid plexus whereby PRL enhances its own transport into the brain. It seems likely that intracerebral PRL modulates REMS under normal conditions whereas pituitary PRL provides additional stimulating influence when PRL secretion is high, e.g, in stress. Further, intracerebroventricular (Icv) injections of VIP and pituitary adenylate cyclase activating peptide, which promote REMS (Fang, Payne, & Krueger, 1995; Obál, Sary, Alföldi, Rubicsek, & Obál, 1986), elicit expression of PRL mRNA in the hypothalamus (Bredow, Kacsoh, Obál, Fang, & Krueger, 1994). Although only circumstantial evidence may implicate PRL in the mediation of the effects of VIP on REMS, this finding at least indicates a correlation between changes in intracerebral PRL and REMS.

D. NFκB and NO

The biochemical regulation of NREMS is undoubtedly complex, involving numerous biochemical cascades. Nevertheless, an important component of that process seems to involve IL-1, TNF, GHRH, and several downstream events, including NFκB, NOS, and COX-2 (Figure 1). IL-1 and TNF, as well as other somnogenic substances (e.g., nerve growth factor [NGF]) activate the transcription factor NFκB. NFκB is activated (i.e., translocated to the nucleus) during sleep deprivation and during daylight hours (Chen, Gardi, Fang and Krueger, 1999); NFκB activation is thus higher when sleep propensity is high. NFκB is a DNA binding protein; it usually acts as an enhancer element. IL-1, TNF, and NGF genes have NFκB binding sites and each stimulates activation of NFκB protein, thereby forming a complex positive feedback loop. Several substances are capable of dampening that positive feedback loop, including IL-4, IL-10, α-melanocyte stimulating hormone, etc., all of which inhibit sleep (Figure 1). Several downstream events also seem to form part of the biochemical cascade involved in NREMS regulation. Thus, NFκB promotes COX-2 production; COX-2 is involved in prostaglandin D_2 production; and PGD_2 is involved in sleep regulation (Terao, Matsumura, & Saito, 1998). NFκB also promotes production of NOS, and NO is also implicated in NREMS regulation (reviewed Krueger and Obál, 1997). IL-2 production is also enhanced by NFκB; IL-2 promotes NREMS (Nistico, DeSarro, & Rotiroti, 1992). NFκB is involved in the production of several other transcription factors that also could be involved in sleep regulation, e.g., c-Fos (Shiromani, Basheer, Greco, Ramanathan, & McCarley, 1998). Finally, oxidative stress-induced expression of adenosine A1 receptors, which are thought to be involved in sleep regulation (see Section VI,E) is mediated, in part, via a NFκB mechanism (Nie et al., 1998).

E. Adenosine

It is hypothesized that increases in adenosine levels as a result of increased energy consumption during wakefulness may convey a feedback signal to induce sleep, which is associated with low consumption of energy. It was further proposed that the function of sleep is to restore brain energy supplies (Benington & Heller, 1995). Whether this theory is correct or not, there is substantial evidence supporting the involvement of adenosine in sleep regulation. The arousal effects of caffeine, which blocks adenosine receptors, are widely experienced in daily life and are experimentally confirmed. In humans, caffeine (100 mg) administered at bedtime prolongs sleep latency, reduces sleep efficiency, stage 4 of NREMS, and EEG SWA (Landolt, Dijk, Gaus, & Borbély, 1995). Caffeine (200 mg) given in the morning has similar effects on subsequent sleep during the night (Landolt, Werth, Borbély, & Dijk, 1995). In rats, ip injection of caffeine induces a dose-dependent increase in waking followed by a prolonged increase in EEG SWA during NREMS and attenuates the sleep rebound after sleep deprivation (Schwierin, Borbély, & Tobler, 1996).

Adenosine receptors are divided into A1, A2a, A2b, and A3 according to pharmacological and structural characteristics. Somnogenic effects of adenosine A1 or A2a receptor agonists are observed in many experiments. For instance, N6-cyclopentyladenosine (CPA), an A1 adenosine receptor agonist, increases EEG SWA in NREMS when administered either systemically or intracerebroventricularly in the rat. The power spectrum of EEG changes induced by CPA is similar to the alterations produced by total sleep deprivation in the rat (Benington, Kodali, & Heller, 1995). Bilateral microinjection of CPA into the preoptic area also increases total sleep time in rats, primarily by increasing deep NREMS, whereas adenosine also increases REMS. In contrast, the adenosine A2 receptor agonist CV-1808 has no effects on sleep. It is thus suggested that the effects of adenosine on sleep are mediated by A1 receptors (Ticho & Radulovacki, 1991). However, administration of selective A2a receptor agonists, CGS21680 and APEC, and the nonselective A1/A2 receptor agonist NECA in the subarachnoid space underlying the rostral basal forebrain of rats significantly increases in the total amounts of NREMS and REMS. In contrast, CPA was ineffective in inducing sleep and inhibited REMS at higher doses by this route of administration (Satoh, Matsumura, & Hayaishi, 1998). The somnogenic action of CGS21680 after infusion into the subarachnoid space underlying the ventral surface region of the rostral basal forebrain can be abolished by pretreatment with an ip injection of KF17837, a selective A2-adenosine antagonist. Above the subarachnoid space is a sensitive zone for prostaglandin D_2 (PGD_2), another well-known sleep-promoting substance. KF17837 (ip injections) also attenuated the increases of NREMS induced by the infusion of PGD_2 into the subarachnoid space of the sleep-promoting zone (Satoh, Matsumura, Suzuki, & Hayaishi, 1996). These results indicate that adenosine may enhance sleep in the basal forebrain through A2a receptors and further indicate that the sleep-promoting effects of PGD_2 are also mediated by A2a adenosine receptors.

The effects of adenosine on sleep are thought to be mediated in part by basal forebrain and brain stem cholinergic neurons, which are involved in waking mechanisms. In cats, microdialysis infusion of adenosine into the cholinergic zones of the substantia innominata of the basal forebrain enhances REMS and EEG SWA, and enhances both NREMS and REMS after infusion into the cholinergic laterodorsal tegmental nucleus (Portas, Thakkar, Rainnie, Greene, & McCarley, 1997). Microinjection of the adenosine receptor agonist, cyclohexyladenosine, into the pontine reticular formation enhances REMS. This effect can be attenuated by the adenosinergic receptor antagonist 8-cyclopentyltheophylline (Marks & Birabil, 1998).

In the basal forebrain cholinergic region, the extracellular concentration of adenosine progressively increases during spontaneous wakefulness and decreases during sleep in freely moving cats (Porkka-Heiskanen et al., 1997). In the hippocampus and neostriatum of freely moving rats, the extracellular adenosine levels are higher during the dark period, the active period of rats, than during the light period. The adenosine levels increase toward the end of dark period, reach the peak at light onset, and decline during the following light hours in the hippocampus, but not in the neostriatum (Huston et al., 1996). In the rat cerebral cortex, the pattern of purine compounds such as adenosine, inosine, and hypoxanthine is bimodal, with high levels during the light period reaching their peak at 12.00 h, 08.00 h, and 16.00 h, respectively, and small increments during the night between 02.00 h and 04.00 h. The adenosine-associated enzymatic activities, in general, have a unimodal profile with low activity during the day and high activities at night. The adenine nucleotide profile has a significant dimunition between 12.00 h and 24.00 h (Chagoya de Sanchez et al., 1993).

VII. ROLE OF THE VAGUS IN TRANSMITTING PERIPHERAL INFLAMMATORY SIGNALS

Systemic administration of a variety of microbial products such as LPS, muramyl peptides, and poly

I:C or cytokines such as IL-1β or TNF-α induces many of the acute phase responses including excess NREMS (reviewed Krueger & Majde, 1994). The excess NREMS, fever, and other behavioral responses induced by systemic LPS, muramyl peptides, or IL-1β are attenuated by central inhibition of IL-1β (Kent, Bluthé, Kelly, & Dantzer, 1992; Klir, McClellan, & Kluger, 1994; Takahashi, Kapás, Fang, et al., 1996). It is likely that these systemic signals can reach the brain by several routes including passage via transport mechanisms (Banks et al., 1991) or at places that lack the blood-brain barrier (Blatteis & Sehic, 1997). In addition, vagal afferents seem to play a critical role in transmitting peripheral inflammatory signals to the brain. Thus, IL-1 increases vagal afferent activity (Niijima, 1996). The liver paraganglia contain IL-1 receptors (Goehler et al., 1997). Subdiaphragmatic vagotomy inhibits NREMS (Hansen & Krueger, 1997; Kapás, Hansen, Chang, & Krueger, 1998), fever (Goldbach, Roth, & Zeisberger, 1997; Opp & Toth, 1997; Romanovsky, Simons, Székely, & Kulchitsky, 1997; Sehic & Blatteis 1996; Watkins et al., 1995), hyperalgesia (Watkins et al., 1994), decreased social interaction (Bluthé, Michaud, Kelley, and Dantzer, 1996), and decreased food intake (Bret-Dibat, Bluthé, Kent, Kelley, & Dantzer, 1995) in response to systemic IL-1β or LPS. Vagotomy also inhibits increases in c-Fos expression in brain (Wan, Wetmore, Sorensen, Greenberg, & Nance, 1994), decreased adrenocorticotropic hormone, and corticosteroid secretion and hypothalamic norepinephrine depletion induced by peripheral immune stimuli (Fleshner et al., 1995; Gaykema, Kijkstra, & Tilders, 1995). Furthermore, CNS production of IL-1β mRNA is enhanced in response to inflammatory signal stimulation of vagal afferents. Systemic LPS and IL-1 induce increased IL-1β mRNA production in the brain, and this effect is blocked by vagotomy (Hansen, Taishi, Chen, & Krueger, 1998b; Layé et al., 1995). Promotion of NREMS by other conditions, such as excessive food intake, also depends on vagal inputs (Hansen, Kapás, Fang, & Krueger, 1997) and is paralleled by enhanced brain IL-1β mRNA prodution (Hansen, Taishi, Chen & Krueger, 1998a).

VIII. SLEEP DEPRIVATION AND IMMUNE CONSEQUENCES

Rats deprived of sleep for 2–3 weeks die (Rechtschaffen, Gilliland, Bergmann, & Winter, 1983). The probable cause of death is septicemia; the bacteria cultured from the blood were primarily facultative anaerobes indigenous to the host (Everson, 1993). Whether death or septicemia occurs in other species after sleep deprivation has not been determined. Regardless, the results with rats suggest that loss of sleep leads to host defense breakdown. Consistent with this notion are the more recent findings that after just a few days of sleep deprivation viable bacteria can be cultured from organs of filtration such as mesenteric lymph nodes (Everson & Toth, 1997; Landis, Pollack, & Helton, 1997) and the number of bacteria in the intestine increases (Bergman, Gilliland, et al., 1996; Everson, 1993). The mechanisms responsible for these effects remain unknown although, as will be described, several immune system measures are altered by sleep deprivation. Further, these sleep-linked changes in bacteria could be related to a normal endosymbiotic relationship between bacteria and hosts. Rats treated with antibiotics (neomycin and metronidazole) have reduced NREMS but normal REMS (Brown, Price, King, & Husband, 1990), thereby suggesting that bacterial products could affect everyday sleep (reviewed in Krueger & Majde, 1994).

In contrast to long-term sleep deprivation, short-term sleep deprivation does not result in death and, under some circumstances, may even enhance host-defense mechanisms. For example, in one study, rats deprived of sleep had smaller tumors than corresponding control animals (Bergmann, Rechtschaffen, Gilliland, & Quintans, 1996). Other studies suggest that short-term sleep deprivation has little consequence on infection. In human studies of sleep deprivation, there has been a failure to demonstrate an increased incidence of infection. However, most of these studies involve healthy young volunteers in unchallenging environmental conditions. In fact, if studies were designed to increase the probability of infection, they likely would not be approved. Consistent with these human studies is a report that sleep deprivation of rabbits failed to exacerbate *E. coli*-induced clinical illness (Toth, Opp, & Mao, 1995). Nevertheless, there is a wealth of data indicating that short-term sleep deprivation is associated with changes in immune system parameters.

Several laboratories have measured natural killer cell (NK) activity in conjunction with sleep and sleep loss. In several of these studies, circulating NK activity decreased after sleep deprivation (Irwin et al., 1994; Moldofsky, Lue, Davidson, & Gorczynski, 1989). In other studies, circulating NK activity increased after sleep deprivation (Born, Lange, Hansen, Molle, & Fehm, 1997; Dinges et al., 1994). Although in depressed insomniac patients there is a reduction of NK activity (Irwin, Smith, & Gillin, 1992), in normal individuals NK activity may decrease during sleep (Moldofsky, Lue, Davidson, Saskin, & Gorczynski, 1989). In summary, it seems likely that sleep or sleep loss may affect NK activity but the magnitude and direction of such effects is sensitive to specific experimental conditions and subject population.

Sleep deprivation affects several other facets of the immune system, including, antigen uptake (Casey, Eisenberg, Peterson, & Pieper, 1974), lymphocyte DNA synthesis (Palmblad, Petrini, Wasserman, & Akerstedt, 1979), phagocytosis (Palmbald et al., 1976), mitogen responses (Moldofsky, Lue, Davidson, & Gorczynski, 1989), circulating immune complexes (Isenberg, Crisp, Morrow, Newham, & Snaith, 1981), circulating IgG levels (Renegar, Floyd, & Krueger, 1998), secondary antibody responses (Brown, Price, King, & Husband, 1989), and a variety of lymphocyte subsets (Dinges et al., 1994). Sleep deprivation also is associated with changes in cytokines. Sleep loss is associated with an enhanced ability of lymphocytes to produce IFN (Palmblad et al., 1976), increased white blood cell and monocyte TNF production (Uthgenannt, Schoolmann, Pietrowsky, Fehm, & Born, 1995; Yamasu, Shimada, Sakaizumi, Soma, & Mizuno, 1992), increased production of IL-1β and IFN-α by cultures of whole blood (Hohagen et al., 1993) and increased plasma IL-1 activity in humans and rats (Moldofsky, Lue, Davidson, & Gorczynski, 1989; Opp & Krueger, 1994). In normal people, and in people with sleep disorders, plasma levels of cytokines are related to the sleep–wake cycle or sleep disturbance. For example, IL-1 plasma levels peak at the onset of NREMS (Moldofsky, Lue, Eisen, Keystone, & Gorczynski, 1986) and TNF levels vary with EEG SWA (Darko et al., 1995). Patients with obstructive sleep apnea syndrome have altered plasma TNF (Entzian, Linnemanna, Schlaak, & Zobal, 1996; Vgontzus et al., 1997). Patients with psychoses, who have reduced sleep, have enhanced IL-1β plasma levels (Appelberg, Katila, & Rimon, 1997).

Collectively, the data cited above strongly suggest that sleep and sleep loss affect immune function. Nevertheless, few studies have directly measured the effects of sleep on the outcome of host defense. Thus, often results leave one uninformed as to whether the effects of sleep or sleep loss are adverse or beneficial for the host. Despite such limitations, it does appear that sleep influences immune function. Further, currently, it appears that short-term sleep loss may enhance host defenses whereas long term-sleep loss is devastating.

IX. RECUPERATIVE PROPERTIES OF SLEEP

There is no direct evidence that sleep per se aids in recuperation from infectious diseases or inflammation due primarily to the difficulty of isolating sleep as an independent variable. Thus, during manipulations of sleep, such as sleep deprivation, many physiological parameters vary. For example, sleep deprivation is associated with changes in hormonal and cytokine production, body temperature, food intake, metabolic rate, etc. Regardless, there are some data consistent with the notion that sleep is beneficial during infectious disease. After microbial challenge, rabbits that had robust NREMS responses within the first 12 h had a higher probability of survival than animals that failed to exhibit NREMS responses (Toth, Tolley, & Krueger, 1993). Although this evidence is correlative in nature, it suggest that perhaps our grandmothers' folk wisdom of the curative and preventative properties of sleep may, in fact, be correct. Regardless, it is likely that physicians will continue to prescribe bed rest and sleep, because this is often just what the patient wants to do.

Acknowledgments

This work was supported in part by the National Institutes of Health, grant numbers HD 36520, NS25378, NS 27250, NS31453.

References

Appelberg, B., Katila, H., & Rimon, R. (1997). Plasma interleukin-1 beta and sleep architecture in schizophrenia and other non-affective psychoses. *Psychosomatic Medicine, 59* 529–532.

Aström, C., & Linhölm, J. (1990). Growth hormone-deficient young adults have decreased sleep. *Neuroendocrinology, 51*, 82–84.

Banks, W. A., Ortiz, L., Plotkin, S. R., & Kastin, J. A. (1991). Human interleukin (IL)-1α, murine IL-1α and murine IL-1β are transported from blood to brain in the mouse by a shared saturable mechanism. *Journal of Pharmacology and Experimental Therapeutics, 259*, 988–996.

Benington, J. H., & Heller, H. C. (1995). Restoration of brain energy metabolism as the function of sleep. *Progress in Neurobiology, 45*, 347–360.

Benington, J. H., Kodali, S. K., & Heller, H. C. (1995). Stimulation of A1 adenosine receptors mimics the electroencephalographic effects of sleep deprivation. *Brain Research, 692*, 79–85.

Beranek, L., Obál Jr., F., Taishi, P., Bodosi, B., Laczi, F., & Krueger, J. M. (1997). Changes in rat sleep after single and repeated injections of long-acting somatostatin analog, octreotide. *American Journal of Physiology, 42*, R1484–R1491.

Berger, R. J., & Phillips, N. H. (1995). Energy conservation and sleep. *Behavioral Brain Research, 69*, 65–73.

Bergmann, B. J., Rechtschaffen, A., Gilliland, M. A., & Quintans, J. (1996). Effect of extended sleep deprivation on tumor growth in rats. *American Journal of Physiology, 271*, R1460–R1464.

Bergmann, B. M., Gilliland, M. A., Feng, P.-F., Russell, D. R., Shaw, P., Wright, M., Rechtschaffen, A., & Alverdy, J. C. (1996). Sleep deprivation and sleep extension: Are physiological effects of sleep deprivation in the rat mediated by bacterial invasion? *Sleep, 19*, 554–562.

Blatteis, C. M., & Sehic, E. (1997). Fever: How may circulating pyrogens signal the brain? *News of Physiological Science, 12*, 1–9.

Bluthé, R.-M., Michaud B., Kelley, K. W., & Dantzer, R. (1996). Vagotomy blocks behavioural effects of interluekin-1 injected via the intraperitoneal route but not via other systemic routes. *NeuroReport, 7*, 2823–2827.

Borbély, A., & and Tobler, I. (1989). Endogenous sleep-promoting substances and sleep regulation. *Physiological Reviews, 69*, 605–670.

Born, J., Lange, T., Hansen, K., Molle, M., & Fehm, H. L. (1997). Effects of sleep and circadian rhythm on human circulating immune cells. *Journal of Immunology, 158*, 4454–4464.

Branco, J., Atalaia, A., & Paiva, T. (1994). Sleep cycles and alpha-delta sleep in fibromyalgia syndrome. *Journal of Rheumatology, 21*, 1113–1117.

Bredow, S., Kacsoh, B., Obál, F., Jr., Fang, J., & Krueger J. M. (1994). Increase of prolactin mRNA in the rat hypothalamus after intracerebroventricular injection of VIP or PACAP. *Brain Research, 660*, 301–308.

Bredow, S., Taishi, P., Guha-Thakurta, N., Obál, F., Jr., & Krueger, J. M. (1997). Diurnal variations of tumor necrosis factor α mRNA and α-tubulin mRNA in rat brain. *Journal of NeuroImmuno Modulation 4*, 84–90.

Bredow, S., Taishi, P., Obál, F. Jr., Guha-Thakurta, N. & Krueger, J. M. (1996). Hypothalamic growth hormone-releasing hormone mRNA varies across the day in rat. *NeuroReport, 7*, 2501–2503.

Bret-Dibat, J. L., Bluthé, R-M, Kent, S., Kelley, K. W., & Dantzer, R. (1995). Lipopolysaccharide and interleukin-1 depress food-motivated behavior in mice by a vagal-mediated mechanism. *Brain, Behavior, and Immunity, 9*, 242–246.

Brown, R., Price, J. R., King, M. G., & Husband, A. J. (1990). Are antibiotic effects on sleep behavior in the rat due to modulation of gut bacteria? *Physiology and Behavior, 48*, 561–565.

Brown, R., Price, R. J., King, M. G., & Husband, A. J. (1989). Interleukin-1β and muramyl dipeptide can prevent decreased antibody response associated with sleep deprivation. *Brain, Behavior, and Immunity, 3*, 320–330.

Buchwald, D., Pascualy, R., Bombardier, C., & Kith, P. (1994). Sleep disorders in patients with chronic fatigue. *Clinical Infectious Disease, 18*(Suppl. 1), S68–S72.

Bujak, D. I., Weinstein, A., & Dornbush, R. L. (1996). Clinical and neurocognitive features of the post Lyme syndrome. *Journal of Rheumatology, 23*, 1392–1397.

Carlson, H. E., Gillin, J. C., Gorden P., & Snyder F. (1972). Absence of sleep-related growth hormone peaks in aged normal subjects and in acromegaly. *Journal of Clinical Endocrinology and Metabolism, 34*, 1102–1105.

Casey, F. B., Eisenberg, J., Peterson, D., & Pieper, O. (1974). Altered antigen uptake and distribution due to exposure to extreme environmental temperatures or sleep deprivation. *Reticuloendothelial Society Journal, 15*, 87–90.

Chagoya de Sanchez, V., Hernandez Muronz, R., Suarez, J., Vidrio S., Yanez, L., & Diaz Munoz, M. (1993). Day-night variations of adenosine and its metabolizing enzymes in the brain cortex of the rat—possible physiological significance for the energetic homeostasis and the sleep-wake cycle. *Brain Research, 612*, 115–121.

Chen, Z., Gardi, J., Fang, J., & Krueger, J. M. (1999). Nuclear factor-κB-like activity increases in murine cerebral cortex after sleep deprivation. *American Journal of Physiology, 276*, R1812–R1818.

Darko, D. F., Miller, J. C., Gallen, C., White, W., Koziol, J., Brown, S. J., Hayduk, R., Atkinson, J., Assmus, J., Munnell, D. T., Naitoh, P., McCutchen, J. A., & Mitler, M. M. (1995). Sleep electroencephalogram delta frequency amplitude, night plasma levels of tumor necrosis factor α and human immunodeficiency virus infection. *Proceedings of the National Academy of Science, USA, 92*, 12080–12086.

Darko, D. F., Mitler, M. M., & Henriksen, S. J. (1995). Lentiviral infection, immune response peptides and sleep. *Advances in Neuroimmunology, 5*, 57–77.

DeBoer, H., Roelfsema, F., Frölich, M., Kamphuisen, A. C., & Van Seters, A. P. (1989). Plasma growth hormone profiles and sleep: A study of 13 treated acromegalics. *Clinical Endocrinology, 30*, 256–262.

Dinges, D. F., Douglas, S. D., Zaugg, L., Campbell, D. E., McMann, J. M., Whitehouse, W. G., Orene, E. C., Kapoor, S. C., Icaza, E., & Orene, M. T. (1994). Leukocytosis and natural killer cell function parallel neurobehavioral fatigue induced by 64 hours of sleep deprivation. *Journal of Clinical Investigation, 93*, 1930–1939

Drewes, A. M., Svendsen, L., Taagholt, S. J., Bjerregard, K., Nielsen, K. D., & Hansen, B. (1998). Sleep in rheumatoid arthritis: A comparison with healthy subjects and studies of sleep/wake interactions. *British Journal of Rheumatology, 37*, 71–81.

Ehlers, C. L., & Kupfer, D. J. (1987). Hypothalamic peptide modulation of EEG sleep in depression: A further application of the S-process hypothesis. *Biological Psychiatry, 22*, 513–517.

Entzian, P., Linnemann, K., Schlaak, M., & Zabel, P. (1996). Obstructive sleep apnea syndrome and circadian rhythms of hormones and cytokines. *American Journal of Respiratory Critical Care Medicine, 153*, 1080–1086.

Everson, C. A. (1993). Sustained sleep deprivation impairs host defense. *American Journal of Physiology, 265*, R1148–R1154.

Everson, C. A., & Toth, L. A. (1997). Abnormal control of viable bacteria in body tissues during sleep deprivation in rats. *APSS Abstracts*, 254.

Fang, J., Payne, L., & Krueger, J. M. (1995). Pituitary adenylate activating polypeptide enhances rapid eye movement sleep in rats. *Brain Research, 686*, 23–28.

Fang, J., Sanborn, C. K., Renegar, K. B., Majde, J. A., & Krueger, J. M. (1995). Influenza viral infections enhance sleep in mice. *Proceedings of the Society for Experimental Biology and Medicine, 210*, 242–252.

Fang, J., Tooley, D., Gatewood, C., Renegar, K. B., Majde, J. A., & Krueger, J. M. (1996). Differential effects of total and upper airway influenza viral infection on sleep in mice. *Sleep, 19*, 337–342.

Fang, J., Wang, Y., & Krueger, J. M. (1997). Mice lacking the TNF 55-kD receptor fail to sleep more after TNFα treatment. *Journal of Neuroscience, 17*, 5949–5955.

Fang, J., Wang, Y., & Krueger, J. M. (1998). The effects of interleukin-1β on sleep are mediated by the type I receptor. *American Journal of Physiology, 274*, R655–R660.

Fleshner, M., Goehler, L. E., Hermann, J., Relton, J. K., Maier, S. F., & Watkins, L. R. (1995). Interleukin-1β induced corticosterone elevation and hypothalamic NE depletion is vagally mediated. *Brain Research Bulletin, 37*, 605–610.

Floyd, R. A., & Krueger, J. M. (1997). Diurnal variations of TNFα in the rat brain. *Neuro Report, 8*, 915–918.

Gardi, J., Obál F. Jr., Fang, J., Zhang, J., & Krueger, J. M. (1998). Diurnal variations and sleep-deprivation-induced changes in GHRH contents of the rat hypothalamus. *Journal of Sleep Research, 7*, 97.

Gaykema, R. P. A., Kijkstra, I., & Tilders, F. J. H. (1995). Subdiaphragmatic vagotomy suppresses endotoxin-induced activation of hypothalamic corticotropin-releasing hormone neurons and ACTH secretion. *Endocrinology, 136*, 4717–4720.

Goehler, L. E., Relton, J. K., Dripps, D., Kiechle, R., Tartaglia, N., Maier, S. F., & Watkins, L. R. (1997). Vagal paraganglia bind biotinylated interleukin-1 receptor antagonist: A possible mechanism for immune-to-brain communication. *Brain Research Bulletin, 43*, 357–364.

Goldbach, J.-M., Roth, J., & Zeisberger, E. (1997). Fever suppression by subdiaphragmatic vagotomy in guinea pigs depends on the route of pyrogen administration. *American Journal of Physiology, 272*, 675–681.

Goldstein, S. J., Wu, R. H. K., Thorpy, M. J., Shprintzen, R. J., Marion, R. E., & Saenger P. (1987). Reversibility of deficient sleep entrained growth hormone secretion in a boy with achondroplasia and obstructive sleep apnea. *Acta Endocrinology, 116*, 95–101.

Hansen, M. K., Kapás, L., Fang, J., & Krueger, J. M. (1998). Cafeteria diet-induced sleep is blocked by subdiaphragmatic vagotomy in rats. *American Journal of Physiology, 274*, R168–R174.

Hansen, M. K., & Krueger, J. M. (1997). Subdiaphragmatic vagotomy blocks the sleep-and fever-promoting effects of interleukin-1β. *American Journal of Physiology, 273*, 1246–1253.

Hansen, M. K., Taishi, P., Chen Z., & Krueger, J. M. (1998a). Cafeteria-feeding induces interleukin-1β mRNA expression in rat liver and brain. *American Journal of Physiology, 43*, R1734–R1739.

Hansen, M. K., Taishi, P., Chen, Z., and Krueger J. M. (1998b). Vagotomy blocks the induction of interleukin-1β (IL-1β) mRNA in the brain of rats in response to systemic IL-1β. *Journal of Neuroscience, 18*, 2247–2253.

Hart, B. L. (1988). Biological basis of the behavior of sick animals. *Neuroscience and Biobehavioral Reviews, 12*, 123–137.

Hartse, K. M. (1994). Sleep in insects and nonmammalian vertebrates. In M. H. Kryger, T. Roth, & W. C. Dement (Eds.), *Principles and practice of sleep medicine* (pp. 95–104). Philadelphia: WB Saunders.

Hirsch, M., Carlander, B., Verge, M., Tafti, M., Anaya, J. M., Billiard, M., & Sany, J. (1994). Objective and subjective sleep disturbances in patients with rheumatoid arthritis. A reappraisal. *Arthritis and Rheumatism, 37*, 41–49.

Hohogen, F., Timmer, J., Weyerbrock, A., Firtsch-Montero, R., Ganter, U., Krieger, S., Berger, M., & Bauer, J. (1993). Cytokine production during sleep and wakefulness and its relationship to cortisol in healthy humans. *Neuropsychobiology, 28*, 9–16.

Huston, J. P., Haas, H. L., Boix, F., Pfister, M., Decking, U., Schrader, J., & Schwarting, R. K. (1996). Extracellular adenosine levels in neostriatum and hippocampus during rest and activity periods of rats. *Neuroscience, 73*, 99–107.

Ibuka, N., Inouye, S. -I., & Kawamura, H. (1977). Analysis of sleep-wakefulness rhythms in male rats after suprachiasmatic nucleus lesions and ocular enucleation. *Brain Research, 122*, 33–47.

Irwin, M., Mascovich, A., Gillin, J. C., Willoughby, R., Pike, J., & Smith, T. L. (1994). Partial sleep deprivation reduces natural killer cell activity in humans. *Psychosomatic Medicine, 56*, 493–498.

Irwin, M., McClintick, J., Costlow, C., Fortner, M., White, J., & Gillin, J. C. (1996). Partial night sleep deprivation reduces natural killer and cellular immune responses in humans. *FASEB Journal, 10*, 643–653.

Irwin, M., Smith T. L., & Gillin J. C. (1992). Electroencephalographic sleep and natural killer activity in depressed patients and control subject. *Psychosomatic Medicine, 54*, 10–21.

Isenberg, D. A., Crisp, A. J., Morrow, W. J., Newham, D., & Snaith, M. L. (1981). Variation in circulating immune complex levels with diet, exercise, and sleep: A comparison between normal controls and patients with systemic lupus erythematosus. *Annals of Rheumatic Diseases, 40*, 466–469.

Jacoby, J. H., Smith E., Sassin, J. F., Greenstein, M., & Weitzman E. D. (1975). Altered growth hormone secretory pattern following prolonged sleep deprivation in the rhesus monkey. *Neuroendocrinology, 18*, 9–15.

Jennum, P., Drewes, A. M., Andreasen, A., & Nielsen, K. D. (1993). Sleep and other symptoms in primary fibromyalgia and in healthy controls. *Journal of Rheumatology, 20*, 1756–1759.

Jouvet, M., Buda, C., Cespuglio, R., Chastrette, N., Denoyer, M., Sallanon, M., & Sastre J. P. (1986). Hypnogenic effects of some hypothalamo-pituitary peptides. *Clinical Neuropharmacology, 9*, 465–467.

Kaiser, W. (1985). Comparative neurobiology of sleep—the honey bee model. In W. P. Koella, E. Ruther, & H. Schulz (Eds.), *Sleep '84* (pp. 225–227) Stuttgart: Gustav Fischer Verlag.

Kapás, L., Hansen, M. K., Chang, H.-Y., & Krueger, J. M. (1998). Vagotomy attenuates but does not prevent the somnogenic and febrile effects of lipopolysaccharide in rats. *American Journal of Physiology, 274*, R406–R411.

Kawakami, M., Kimura F., & Tsai, C.-W. (1983). Correlation of growth hormone secretion to sleep in the immature rat. *Journal of Physiology (London), 339*, 325–337.

Kent, S., Bluthé, R-M, Kelley, K. W., & Dantzer, R. (1992). Sickness behavior as a new target for drug development. *Trends in Pharmacological Sciences, 13*, 24–28.

Kimura-Takeuchi, M., Majde, J. A., Toth, L. A., & Krueger, J. M. (1992). Influenza virus-induced changes in rabbit sleep and acute phase responses. *American Journal of Physiology, 263*, R1115–R1121.

Klir, J. J., McClellan, J. L., & Kluger M. J. (1994). Interleukin-1β causes the increase in anterior hypothalamic interleukin-6 during LPS-induced fever in rats. *American Journal of Physiology, 266*, 1845–1848.

Krueger, J. M., & Majde, J. A. (1990). Sleep as a host defense: Its regulation by microbial products and cytokines. *Clinical Immunology and Immunopathology, 57*, 188–199.

Krueger, J. M., & Majde, J. A. (1994). Microbial products and cytokines in sleep and fever regulation. *Critical Reviews of Immunology, 14*, 355–379.

Krueger, J. M., & Obál, F. Jr. (1997). Sleep regulatory substances. In W. J. Schwartz (Ed.), *Sleep science: Integrating basic research and clinical practice* (pp. 175–194). Basel: Karger.

Krueger, J. M., Obál, F. Jr., & Fang, J. (1999). Humoral regulation of physiological sleep: Cytokines and GHRH. *Journal of Sleep Research, 8*(suppl. 1), 53–59.

Krueger, J. M., Pappenheimer, J. R., & Karnovsky, M. L. (1982a). Sleep-promoting effects of muramyl peptides. *Proceedings of the National Academy of Science, USA, 79*, 6102–6106.

Krueger, J. M., Pappenheimer, J. R., & Karnovsky, M. L. (1982b). The composition of sleep-promoting factor isolated from human urine. *Journal of Biological Chemistry, 257*, 1664–1669.

Krueger, J. M., Walter, J., Dinarello, C. A., Wolff, S. M., & Chedid, L. (1984). Sleep-promoting effects of endogenous pyrogen (interleukin-1). *American Journal of Physiology, 246*, R994–999.

Kushikata, T., Fang, J., Wang, Y., & Krueger, J. M. (1998). Interleukin-4 inhibits spontaneous sleep in rabbits. *American Journal of Physiology, 275*, R1185–R1191.

Lancel, M., Mathias, S., Faulhaber, J., & Schiffelholz, T. (1996). Effect of interleukin-1 beta on EEG power density during sleep depends on circadian phase. *American Journal of Physiology, 270*, R830–R835.

Landis, C., Pollack, S., & Helton, W. S. (1997). Microbial translocation and NK cell cytotoxicity in female rats sleep deprived on small platforms. *Sleep Research, 26*, 619.

Landolt, H. P., Dijk, D. J., Gaus, S. E., & Borbély, A. A. (1995). Caffeine reduces low-frequency delta activity in the human sleep EEG. *Neuropsychopharmacology, 12,* 229–238.

Landolt, H. P., Werth, E., Borbély, A. A., & Dijk, D. J. (1995). Caffeine intake (200 mg) in the morning affects human sleep and EEG power spectra at night. *Brain Research, 675,* 67–74.

Lavie, P., Nadir, M., Lorer, M., & Scharf, Y. (1991). Nonsteroidal antiinflammatory drug therapy in rheumatoid arthritis patients. Lack of association between clinical improvement and effects on sleep. *Arthritis and Rheumatism, 34,* 655–659.

Layé, S., Bluthé, R-M., Kent, S., Combe, C., Médina, C., Parnet, P., Kelley, K., & Dantzer, R. (1995). Subdiaphragmatic vagotomy blocks the induction of interleukin-1β mRNA in the brain of mice in response to peripherally administered lipopolysaccharide. *American Journal of Physiology, 268,* 1327–1331.

Mackiewicz, M., Sollars, P. J., Ogilvie, M. D., & Pack, A. I. (1996). Modulation of IL-1β gene expression in the rat CNS during sleep deprivation. *NeuroReport, 7,* 529–533.

Mahowald, M. W., Mahowald, M. L., Bundlie, S. R., & Ytterberg, S. R. (1989). Sleep fragmentation in rheumatoid arthritis. *Arthritis and Rheumatism, 32,* 974–983.

Marks, G. A., & Birabil, C. G. (1998). Enhancement of rapid eye movement sleep in the rat by cholinergic and adenosinergic agonists infused into the pontine reticular formation. *Neuroscience, 86,* 29–37.

May, K. P., West, S. G., Baker, M. R., & Everett, D. W. (1993). Sleep apnea in male patients with fibromyalgia syndrome. *American Journal of Medicine, 94,* 505–508.

Moldofsky, H. (1993). Fribromyalgia, sleep disorder and chronic fatigue syndrome. *CIBA Foundation Symposium, 173,* 262–271.

Moldofsky, H. (1989). Sleep influences on regional and diffuse pain syndromes associated with osteoarthritis. *Seminars in Arthritis and Rheumatism, 18,* 18–21.

Moldofsky, H., Davidson, J. R., & Lue F. A. (1988). Sleep-related patterns of plasma growth hormone and cortisol following 40 hours of wakefulness. *Sleep Research, 17,* 69.

Moldofsky, H., Lue, F. A., Davidson, J. R., & Gorczynski, R. (1989). Effects of sleep deprivation on human immune functions. *FASEB Journal, 3,* 1972–1977.

Moldofsky, H., Lue, F. A., Davidson, J., Saskin, P., & Gorczynski, R. (1989). Comparison of sleep-wake circadian immune function in women vs men. *Sleep Research, 18,* 431.

Moldofsky, H., Leu, F. A., & Smythe, H. A. (1993). Alpha EEG sleep and morning symptoms in rheumatoid arthritis. *Journal of Rheumatology, 10,* 373–379.

Moldofsky, H., Lue, F. A., Eisen, J., Keystone, E., & Gorczynski, R. M. (1986). The relationship of interleukin-1 and immune functions to sleep in humans. *Psychosomatic Medicine, 48,* 309–318.

Morehouse, R. L., Flanigan, M., MacDonald, D. D., Braha, D., & Shapiro, C. (1998). Depression and short REM latency in subjects with chronic fatigue syndrome. *Psychosomatic Medicine, 60,* 347–351.

Nakao, M., McGinty, D., Szymusiak, R., & Yamamoto, M. (1995). Dynamical features of thermoregulatory model of sleep control. *Japanese Journal of Physiology, 45,* 311–326.

Nguyen, K. T., Deak, T., Owens, S. M., Kohno, T., Fleshner, M., Watkins, L. R., & Maier, S. F. (1998). Exposure to acute stress induces brain interleukin-1β protein in the rat. *Journal of Neuroscience, 18,* 2239–2246.

Nie, Z., Mei, Y., Ford, M., Rybak, L., Marcuzzi, A., Ren, H., Stiles, G. L., & Ramkumar, V. (1998). Oxidative stress increases A1 adenosine receptor expression by activating nuclear factor kappa B. *Molecular Pharmacology, 53,* 663–669.

Niijima, A. (1996). The afferent discharges from sensors for interleukin-1β in the hepatoportal system in the anesthetized rat. *Journal of the Autonomic Nervous System, 61,* 287–291.

Nistico, G., DeSarro, G., & Rotiroti, D. (1992). Behavioral and electrocortical spectrum power changes of interleukins and tumor necrosis factor after microinjection into different areas of the brain. In S. Smirne, M. Francesch, L. Ferini-Strambi, & M. Zucconi (Eds.), *Sleep hormones, and immunological system* (pp. 11–18). Masson: Milan.

Obál, F. Jr., Alföldi, P., Cady, A. B., Johannsen, L., Sáry, G., & Krueger, J. M. (1988). Growth hormone releasing factor enhances sleep in rats and rabbits. *American Journal of Physiology, 255,* R310–R316.

Obál, F. Jr., Bodosi, B., Szilágyi, A., Kacsóh, B., & Krueger, J. M. (1997). Antiserum to growth hormone decreases sleep in the rat. *Neuroendocrinology, 66,* 9–16.

Obál, F. Jr., Floyd R., Kapás, L., Bodosi, B., & Krueger J. M. (1996). Effects of systemic GHRH on sleep in intact and hypophysectomized rats. *American Journal of Physiology, 270,* E230–E237.

Obál, F. Jr., Fang, J., Payne, L. C., & Krueger, J. M. (1995). Growth hormone-releasing hormone (GHRH) mediates the sleep promoting activity of interleukin-1 (IL1) in rats. *Neuroendocrinology, 61,* 559–565.

Obál, F. Jr., Kacsóh, B., Alföldi, P., Payne, L., Markovic, O., Grosvenor, C., & Krueger, J. M. (1992). Antiserum to prolactin decreases rapid eye movement sleep (REM sleep) in the male rat. *Physiology and Behavior, 52,* 1063–1968.

Obál, F. Jr., Kacsóh, B., Bredow, S., Guha-Thakurta, N., & Krueger, J. M. (1997). Sleep in rats rendered chronically hyperprolactinemic with anterior pituitary grafts. *Brain Research, 755,* 130–136.

Obál, F. Jr., Kapás, L. Bodosi, B., & Krueger, J. M. (1998). Changes in sleep in response to intracerebral injection of insulin-like growth factor-1 (IGF-1) in the rat. *Sleep Research Online, 2,* 87–91.

Obál, F. Jr., Opp, M., Cady, A. A., Johannsen, L., & Krueger, J. M. (1989). Prolactin, vasoactive intestinal peptide, and peptide histidine methionine elicit selective increases in REM sleep in rabbits. *Brain Research, 490,* 292–300.

Obál, F. Jr., Payne, L., Kacsóh, B., Opp, M., Kapás, L., Grosvenor, C. E., & Krueger, J. M. (1994). Involvement of prolactin in the REM sleep-promoting activity of systemic vasoactive intestinal peptide (VIP). *Brain Research, 645,* 143–149.

Obál, F. Jr., Payne, L., Kapás, L., Opp, M., & Krueger J. M. (1991). Inhibition of growth hormone-releasing hormone suppresses both sleep and growth hormone secretion in the rat. *Brain Research, 557,* 149–153.

Obál, F. Jr., Payne, L., Opp, M., Alföldi, P., Kapás, L., & Krueger, J. M. (1992). Growth hormone-releasing hormone antibodies suppress sleep and prevent enhancement of sleep after sleep deprivation. *American Journal of Physiology, 263,* R1078–R1085.

Obál, F. Jr., Sary, G., Alföldi, P., Rubicsek, G., & Obál, F. (1986). Vasoactive intestinal polypeptide promotes sleep without effects on brain temperature in rats at night. *Neuroscience Letters, 64,* 236–240.

Opp, M. R., & Krueger, J. M. (1994). Anti-interleukin-1β reduces sleep and sleep rebound after sleep deprivation in rats. *American Journal of Physiology, 266,* R688–R695.

Opp, M. R., Obál F. Jr., & Krueger, J. M. (1991). Interleukin-1 alters rat sleep: Temporal and dose-related effects. *American Journal of Physiology, 260,* R52–R58.

Opp, M. R., Smith, E. M., & Hughes, T. K. (1995). Interleukin-10 acts in the central nervous system of rats to reduce sleep. *Journal of Neuroimmunology, 60,* 165–168.

Opp, M. R., & Toth, L. A. (1997). Circadian modulation of interleukin-1-induced fever in intact and vagotomized rats. *Annals of the New York Academy of Sciences, 813*, 435–436.

Palmblad, J., Cantell, K., Strander, H., Fröberg, J., Karlsson, C. G., Levi, L., Granström, M., & Unger, P. (1976). Stressor exposure and immunological response in man: Interferon producing capacity and phagocytosis. *Psychosomatic Research, 20*, 193–199.

Palmblad, J., Petrini, B., Wasserman, J., & Akerstedt, T. (1979). Lymphocyte and granulocyte reactions during sleep deprivation. *Psychosomatic Medicine, 41*, 273–278.

Pappenheimer, J. R., Koski, G., Fencl, V., Karnovsky, M. L., & Krueger, J. M. (1975). Extraction of sleep-promoting factor S from cerebrospinal fluid and from brains of sleep-deprived animals. *Journal of Neurophysiology, 38*, 1299–1311.

Porkka-Heiskanen, T., Strecker, R. E., Thakkar, M., Bjorkum, A. A., Greene, R. W., & McCarley, R. W. (1997). Adenosine: A mediator of the sleep-inducing effects of prolonged wakefulness. *Science, 276*, 1265–1268.

Portas, C. M., Thakkar, M., Rainnie, D. G., Greene, R. W., & McCarley, R. W. (1997). Role of adenosine in behavioral state modulation: A microdialysis study in the freely moving cat. *Neuroscience, 79*, 225–235.

Rechtschaffen, A., Gilliland, M. A., Bergmann, B. M., & Winter J. B. (1983). Physiological correlation of prolonged sleep deprivation in rats. *Science, 221*, 182–184.

Renegar, K. B., Floyd, R., & Krueger, J. M. (1998). Effect of sleep deprivation on serum influenza-specific IgG. *Sleep, 21*, 19–24.

Roky, R., Obál F. Jr., Valatx, J. L., Bredow, S., Fang, J., Pagano, L. P., & Krueger, J. M. (1995). Prolactin and rapid eye movement sleep regulation. *Sleep, 18*, 536–542.

Roky, R., Valatx, J. L., & Jouvet, M. (1993). Effect of prolactin on the sleep-wake cycle in the rat. *Neuroscience Letters, 156*, 117–120.

Roky, R., Valatx, J. L., Paut-Pagano, L., & Jouvet, M. (1994). Hypothalamic injection of prolactin or its antibody alters the rat sleep-wake cycle. *Physiology and Behavior, 55*, 1015–1019.

Romanovsky, A. A., Simons, C. T., Székely, M., & Kulchitsky, V. A. (1997). The vagus nerve in the thermoregulatory response to systemic inflammation. *American Journal of Physiology, 273*, 407–414.

Sassin, J. F., Parker, D. C., Mace, J. W., Gotlin, R. W., Johnson, L. C., & Rossman, L. G. (1969). Human growth hormone release: Relation to slow-wave sleep and sleep-waking cycles. *Science, 165*, 513–515.

Satoh, S., Matsumura, H., & Hayaishi, O. (1998) Involvement of adenosine A2a receptor in sleep promotion. *European Journal of Pharmacology, 351*, 155–162.

Satoh, S., Matsumura, H., Suzuki, F., & Hayaishi, O. (1996). Promotion of sleep mediated by the A2a-adenosine receptor and possible involvement of this receptor in the sleep induced by prostaglandin D2 in rats. *Proceedings of the National Academy of Science, USA, 93*, 5980–5984.

Schwierin, B., Borbély, A. A., & Tobler, I. (1996). Effects of N6-cyclopentyladenosine and caffeine on sleep regulation in the rat. *European Journal of Pharmacology, 300*, 163–171.

Sehic, E., & Blatteis, C. M. (1996). Blockade of lipopolysaccharide-induced fever by subdiaphragmatic vagotomy in guinea pigs. *Brain Research, 726*, 160–166.

Shiromani, P. J., Basheer, R., Greco, M. A., Ramanathan, L., & McCarley, R. W. (1998). Emerging evidence on the role of transcription factors in sleep. *Journal of Sleep Research, 7*, 248.

Smith, A. (1992). Sleep, colds, and performance. In R. J. Broughton & R. D. Ogilvie (Eds.), *Sleep, arousal and performance* (pp 233–242) Boston: Birkhauser.

Steriade, M., & McCarley, R. W. (1990). *Brainstem control of wakefulness and sleep*. New York: Plenum Press.

Stumwasser, F. (1971). The cellular basis of behavior in *Aplysia*. *Journal of Psychiatric Research, 8*, 237–257.

Susic, V., & Totic, S. (1989). "Recovery" function of sleep: Effects of purified human interleukin-1 on the sleep and febrile response of cats. *Metabolic Brain Disease, 4*, 73–80.

Sweet, M. J., Stacey, K. J., Kakuda, D. K., Markovich, D. & Hume, D. A. (1998). IFN-γ primes macrophage responses to bacterial DNA. *Journal of Interferon and Cytokine Research, 18*, 263–271.

Taishi, P., Bredow, S., Guha-Thakurta, N., Obál, F. Jr., & Krueger, J. M. (1997). Diurnal variations of interleukin-1β mRNA and β-actin mRNA in rat brain. *Journal of Neuroimmunology, 75*, 69–74.

Taishi, P., Chen, Z., Obál, F. Jr., Zhang, J., Hansen, M., Fang, J., & Krueger, J. M. (1998). Sleep associated changes in interleukin-1β mRNA in the brain. *Journal of Interferon Cytokine Research, 18*, 793–798.

Takahashi, S., Kapás, L., Fang, J., Wang, Y., Seyer, J. M., & Krueger, J. M. (1996). An interleukin-1 receptor fragment inhibits spontaneous sleep and muramyl dipeptide-induced sleep in rabbits. *American Journal of Physiology, 271*, R101–R108.

Takahashi, S., Kapás, L., & Krueger, J. M. (1996). A tumor necrosis factor (TNF) receptor fragment attenuates TNF-α and muramyl dipeptide-induced sleep and fever in rabbits. *Journal of Sleep Research, 5*, 106–114.

Takahashi, Y., Kipnis, D. M., & Daughaday, W. H. (1968). Growth hormone secretions during sleep. *Journal of Clinical Investigation, 47*, 2079–2090.

Terao, A., Matsumura, H., & Saito, M. (1998). Interleukin-1 induces slow wave sleep at the prostaglandin D_2-sensitive sleep-promoting zone in the rat brain. *Journal of Neuroscience, 18*, 6599–6607.

Ticho S. R., & Radulovacki, M. (1991). Role of adenosine in sleep and temperature regulation in the preoptic area of rats. *Pharmacology, Biochemistry and Behavior, 40*, 33–40.

Tobler, I. (1983). Effect of forced locomotion on the rest-activity cycle of the cockroach. *Behavioral Brain Research, 8*, 351–360.

Toppila, J., Alanko, L., Asikainen, M., Tobler, I., Stenberg, D., & Porkka-Heiskanen, T. (1997). Sleep deprivation increases somatostatin and growth hormone releasing hormone messenger RNA in the rat hypothalamus. *Journal of Sleep Research, 6*, 171–178.

Toth, L. A. (1999). Microbial modulation of sleep. In R. Lydic & H. Baghdoyan (Eds.), *Handbook of behavioral state control: Cellular and molecular mechanisms* (pp. 641–657). Boca Raton, FL: CRC Press.

Toth, L. A., & Krueger, J. M. (1988). Alterations of sleep in rabbits by *Staphylococcus aureus* infection. *Infection and Immunity, 56*, 1785–1791.

Toth, L. A., & Krueger, J. M. (1989). Effects of microbial challenge on sleep in rabbits. *FASEB Journal, 3*, 2062–2066.

Toth, L. A., & Krueger, J. M. (1995). Lighting conditions alter *Candida albicans*-induced sleep responses in rabbits. *American Journal of Physiology, 269*, R1441–R1447.

Toth, L. A., & Krueger, J. M. (1990). Somnogenic, pyrogenic, and hematologic effects of experimental pasteurellosis in rabbits. *American Journal of Physiology, 258*, R536–R542.

Toth, L. A., Opp, M. R., & Mao, L. (1995). Somnogenic effects of sleep deprivation and *Escherichia coli* inoculation in rabbits. *Journal of Sleep Research, 4*, 30–40.

Toth, C. A., Tolley, E. A., & Krueger, J. M. (1993). Sleep as a prognostic indicator during infectious disease in rabbits. *Proceedings of the Society for Experimental Biological Medicine, 203*, 179–192.

Uthgenannt, D., Schoolmann, D., Pietrowsky, R., Fehm, H. L., & Born, J. (1995). Effects of sleep on the production of cytokines in humans. *Psychosomatic Medicine, 57*, 97–104.

Valatx, J. L., Roky, R., & Paut-Pagano, L. (1990). Prolactin and sleep regulation. In J. Horne (Ed.), *Sleep '90*, (pp. 346–348). Bochum, Germany: Pontenagel Press.

Vermeulen, M. W., & Gray, G. R. (1984). Processing of *Bacillus subtilis* peptidoglycan by a mouse macrophage cell line. *Infection and Immunity, 46*, 476–483.

Vgontzas, A. N., Papanicolaou, D. A., Bixler, E. O., Kales, A., Tyson, K., & Chrousos, G. P. (1997). Elevation of plasma cytokines in disorders of excessive daytime sleepiness: Role of sleep disturbance and obesity. *Journal of Clinical Endocrinology Metabolism, 82*, 1313–1316.

von Economo, C. (1930). Sleep as a problem of localization. *Journal of Nervous and Mental Disorders, 71*, 249–259.

Walsh, J. K., Muehlbach, M. J., Lauter, S. A, Hilliker, N. A., & Schweitzer, P. K. (1996). Effects of triazolam on sleep, daytime sleepiness, and morning stiffness in patients with rheumatoid arthritis. *Journal of Rheumatology, 23*, 245–252.

Walsh, R. J., Slaby, F. J., & Posner, B. I. (1987). A receptor-mediated mechanism for the transport of prolactin from blood to cerebrospinal fluid. *Endocrinology, 120*, 1846–1850.

Wan, W., Wetmore, L., Sorensen, C. M., Greenberg, A. H., & Nance, D. M. (1994). Neural and biochemical mediators of endotoxin and stress-induced c-fos expression in the rat brain. *Brain Research Bulletin, 34*, 7–14.

Watkins, L. R., Goehler, L. E., Relton, J. K., Tartaglia, N., Gilbert, L., Martin, D., & Maier. S. F. (1995). Blockade of interleukin-1-induced hyperthermia by subdiaphragmatic vagotomy: Evidence for vagal mediation of immune-brain communication. *Neuroscience Letters, 183*, 27–31.

Watkins, L. R., Wiertelak, E. P., Goehler, L. E., Smith, K. P., Martin, D., & Maier S. F. (1994). Characterization of cytokine-induced hyperalgesia. *Brain Research, 654*, 15–26.

Wiegand, M., Möller, A. A., Schreiber, W., Krieg, J. C., & Holsboer, F. (1991). Alterations of nocturnal sleep in patients with HIV infection. *Acta Neurologica Scandinavica, 83*, 141–142.

Williams, G., Pirmohamed, J., Minors, D., Waterhouse, J., Buchan, I., Arendt, J., & Edwards, R. H. (1996). Dissociation of body-temperature and melatonin secretion circadian rhythms in patients with chronic fatigue syndrome. *Clinical Physiology, 16*, 327–337.

Wolff, G., & Money J. (1973). Relationship between sleep and growth in patients with reversible somatotropin deficiency (psychosocial dwarfism). *Psychological Medicine, 3*, 18–27.

Yamasu, K., Shimada, Y., Sakaizumi, M., Soma, G., & Mizuno, D. (1992). Activation of the systemic production of tumor necrosis factor after exposure to acute stress. *European Cytokine Network, 3*, 391–398.

Zamir, G., Press, J., Tal, A., & Tarasiuk, A. (1998). Sleep fragmentation in children with juvenile rheumatoid arthritis. *Journal of Rheumatology, 25*, 1191–1197.

Zhang, J., Chen, Z., Taishi, P., Obál, F. Jr., Fang, J., & Krueger, J. M. (1998). Sleep deprivation increases rat hypothalamic growth hormone-releasing hormone mRNA. *American Journal of Physiology, 44*, R1755–R1761.

Zhang, J., Obál, F. Jr., Fang, J., Collins, B. J., & Krueger, J. M. (1996). Sleep is suppressed in transgenic mice with a deficiency in the somatotropic system. *Neuroscience Letters, 220*, 97–100.

Zhang, J., Obál F. Jr., Zheng, T., Fang, J., Taishi, P., & Krueger, J. M. (1999). Effects of intrapreoptic microinjection of GHRH and its antagonist on sleep in rats. *Journal of Neuroscience, 19*, 2187–2194.

Zhang, S. Q., Kimura, M., & Inoue, S. (1995). Sleep patterns in cyclic and pseudopregnant rats. *Neuroscience Letters, 193*, 125–128.

C H A P T E R

27

Fever and Immunity

MATTHEW J. KLUGER, WIESLAW KOZAK, KIMBERLY P. MAYFIELD

Fever is a common response to infection and a classic example of brain–immune interaction (Figure 1). Infection results in the release of proinflammatory cytokines such as IL-1β and in turn an elevation of hypothalamic prostaglandin $E_2(PGE_2)$. The thermoregulatory set point is elevated, which results in the central nervous system (CNS) orchestrating physiological and behavioral responses, leading to a rise in body temperature. Many hormones under the control of the CNS (e.g., corticosteroids, arginine vasopressin), as well as some cytokines (e.g., IL-10), act as endogenous antipyretics or cryogens and prevent fever from reaching extremely high levels (e.g., Coehlo, Souza, & Pela, 1992; Kasting, 1989; Leon, Kozak, & Kluger, 1999; Morrow, McClellan, Conn, & Kluger, 1993).

During the past several decades, considerable data have emerged supporting the hypothesis that fever evolved as a host defense response, which helps to resolve infection. Thus, the *immune system* is involved in initiating and regulating the magnitude of fever. The CNS is involved in coordinating the many effector responses necessary to regulate the rise in body temperature. As will be argued in this chapter, the *immune system* is accelerated as a result of this elevation in body temperature.

I. WHAT IS THE EVIDENCE THAT FEVER IMPROVES HOST DEFENSES DURING INFECTION?

We present five types of arguments supporting the hypothesis that fever is a host defense response. Next, we describe several specific aspects of immunity, which are enhanced as a result of an elevation in body temperature, all of which may be responsible for fever's protective function.

Experiments that relate to investigations of the function of fever can be divided into five general categories—(A) evolutionary, (B) correlational, and (C) antipyretic, (D) hyperthermia and hypothermia studies, and (E) those that are homeostatically controlled. In evolutionary studies, the phylogeny of fever is investigated. The argument is made that it is unlikely that the energetically expensive increase in body temperature associated with most infections would have evolved and been retained without this rise in temperature benefiting the host in some way. In correlational studies, the magnitude of the febrile response of some organism to an infectious agent is compared to the mortality or morbidity rate. As in all correlative studies, it is impossible to determine whether the correlated variables have a causal relationship (e.g., people with the likelihood of developing lung cancer also have a tendency to smoke).

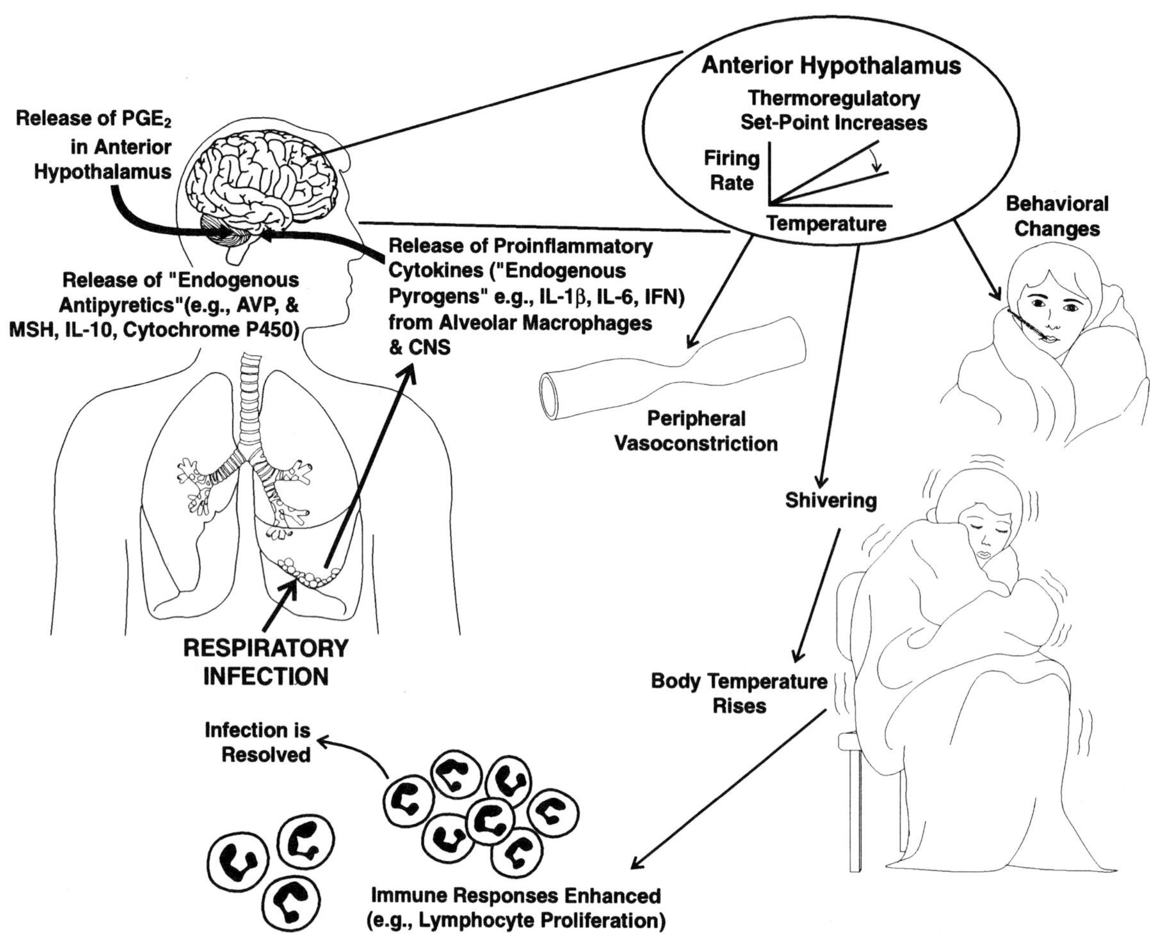

FIGURE 1 Model of fever showing interaction between the brain and immune system.

The third type of study involves the use of antipyretic agents to reduce the fever of an organism (lower its thermoregulatory "set point"); then, as in the correlational studies, the magnitude of the fever is compared with some aspect of the host's physiological state such as the mortality or morbidity rate. The problem with these studies is that in the process of producing antipyresis, drugs are used that have many side-effects, some undoubtedly helpful and others harmful. As such, the results of these studies are difficult to interpret. The fourth type of study involves altering the body temperature of infected organisms by physical means (e.g., using high or low environmental temperatures). These infected organisms will be either "hypothermic" (body temperature below the thermoregulatory set point) or "hyperthermic" (body temperature above the thermoregulatory set point) and will attempt to raise or lower their body temperatures to achieve an equilibrium between their core temperature and their set point temperature. Because hypothermia and hyperthermia lead to an increase in various autonomic reflexes (e.g., peripheral vasoconstriction or vasodilation) not found in animals that are normothermic (body temperature equivalent to the thermoregulatory set point), the results of these investigations are also difficult to interpret. The last type of evidence used to support the hypothesis that fever is beneficial relates to the highly regulated nature of this response. That is, fever is not due to a breakdown in the body's ability to thermoregulate. Rather fever is a highly coordinated response modulated by many hormones and cytokines, a response that almost never results in body temperature reaching dangerously high levels. With this brief introduction into the hazards of interpreting data obtained from investigations into the role of fever in disease, the results of these five types of experiments are described below.

A. Evolutionary Studies

Have physiological/behavioral responses that are not adaptive been retained throughout long evolutionary periods? Although there may be some (we

TABLE I Febrile Responses of Ectothermic Vertebrates and Invertebrates

Reptiles	Activator of fever	Reference
Dipsosaurus dorsalis	Bacteria, endogenous pyrogen	Vaughn, Bernheim, & Kluger, 1974; Bernheim & Kluger, 1977
Iguana iguana	Bacteria	Kluger, 1977
Crotaphytus collaris	Bacteria	Firth, Ralph, & Boardman, 1980
Terrepene carolina	Bacteria	Monagas & Gatten, 1983
Chrysemys picta	Bacteria	Monagas & Gatten, 1983
Sauromalus obesus	Bacteria	Muchlinski, Stoutenburgh, & Hogan, 1989
Alligator mississippiensis	Bacteria	Lang, 1987
Callopistes maculatus	Bacteria	Hallman, Ortega, & Towner, 1990
Amphibians		
Hyla cinerea	Bacteria	Kluger, 1977
Rana pipiens	Bacteria	Casterlin & Reynolds, 1977
Rana catesbeiana	Bacteria	Casterlin & Reynolds, 1977
Rana esculenta	Bacteria, PGE_1, endog. pyrogen	Myhre, Cabanac, & Myhre, 1977
Necturus maculosus	PGE_1	Hutchison & Erskine, 1981
Bufo marinus	LPS	Sherman, Baldwin, Fernandez, & Duerello, 1991
Fishes		
Micropterus salmoides	Bacteria	Reynolds, Casterlin, & Covert, 1976
Lepomis macrochirus	Endotoxin, bacteria	Reynolds, Casterlin, & Covert, 1978
Carassius auratus	Endotoxin, bacteria	Reynolds, Casterlin, & Covert, 1976; Reynolds & Covert, 1978
Invertebrates		
Cambarus bartoni (crayfish)	Bacteria	Casterlin & Reynolds, 1980
Gromphadorhina portentosa (cockroach)	Endotoxin, bacteria	Bronstein & Conner, 1984
Gryllus bimaculatus (cricket)	*Rickettsiella grylli*	Louis, Jourdan, & Cabanac, 1986
Acheta domesticus (cricket)	*Rickettsiella grylli*	Adamo, 1998
Melanoplus sanguinipes (grasshoppers)	*Nosema acridophagus*	Boorstein & Ewald, 1987
Homarus americanus (lobster)	PGE_1	Casterlin & Reynolds, 1979
Penaeus duorarum (shrimp)	PGE_1	Casterlin & Reynolds, 1979
Limulus polyphemus (horseshoe crab)	PGE_1	Casterlin & Reynolds, 1979
Buthus occitanus (scorpion)	PGE_1	Cabanac & Guelte, 1980
Androctonus australis (scorpion)	PGE_1	Cabanac & Guelte, 1980
Onymacris plana (tenebrionid beetle)	Endotoxin	McClain, Magnuson, & Warner, 1988

Note: LPS, lipopolysaccharide; PGE, prostaglandin E.

can't identify any), the probability of finding one decreases as the actual "cost" of the physiological/behavioral response increases.

With few exceptions, both endothermic and ectothermic vertebrates (as well as invertebrates) develop fevers in response to injections of endotoxin or other substances that cause fever in mammals (Table I). The body temperature of cold-blooded animals rises as a result of their "feeling" cold and therefore selecting a warmer microclimate.

How might the seemingly long evolutionary history of fever relate to its role in disease? There is a large metabolic cost to generate and maintain a fever. In endotherms such as birds and mammals, the maintenance of a body temperature of 2 or 3°C above afebrile levels often results in a 20% or more increase in their energy consumption. This is the result of the Q_{10} effect of increased temperature on various biochemical reactions. In ectothermic vertebrates, the amount of excess energy expended during a fever is largely unknown. However, as in endothermic vertebrates, the maintenance of an elevated body temperature will likely also result in an approximately 20% increase in energy consumption. If fever did not have an adaptive function, then this energetically expensive phenomenon would not have persisted for millions of years in so many groups of organisms.

In addition to the metabolic argument, there is another cost to developing fever, particularly in ectothermic organisms. Fever requires them to move to a warmer microclimate, often resulting in their being in the sunlight for extended periods of time. Although there are no studies, to my knowledge, on the effects of basking on increased susceptibility to predation, it is plausible that this would lead to increased mortality. If so, there would be a selective pressure against the development of fever. Because fever is so common throughout the animal kingdom, this is another argument in favor of fever having a *net* beneficial role.

In addition to the above "economic" and increased likelihood of predation arguments for a beneficial role for fever in the vertebrates, several studies have appeared that specifically involve the role of fever in disease in reptiles, fishes, and insects, as well as mammals. The results of these investigations are described below.

B. Correlational Studies

Clinical studies involving human beings generally have shown that the magnitude of the fever is associated with the severity of the infection (Bennett & Nicastri, 1960). As a result, patients with the highest fevers tend to have the highest mortality rate. The difficulty with the studies involving human beings is that the studies are completely uncontrolled. Often the results are confounded because some patients receive certain drugs and others do not. Furthermore, the patients clearly have not been infected with identical doses of pathogens. From a purely scientific viewpoint, to properly perform survival studies on human beings, the subjects must be infected with identical doses of pathogens, administered no drugs, then their resultant fevers compared with their mortality or morbidity rates. These unethical experiments have fortunately not been conducted. What is available in the medical literature tends to be clinical impressions and, as such, it is difficult to assess objectively whether fever has a beneficial role.

In studies that have correlated body temperature with survival rate, several investigators have found that fever is associated with better prognoses during bacterial infections (Bryant, Hood, Hood, & Koenig, 1971; Hallman, Ortega, Towner, & Muchlinski 1990; Mackowiak, Browne, Southern, & Smith, 1980; Weinstein, Iannin, Stratton, & Eickhoff 1978). One study found no correlation between fever and survival rate, but simply that hypothermia in adults or newborns was associated with a higher mortality rate (DuPont & Spink, 1969). In studies involving children who had "febrile" convulsions, high fevers ($>40°C$) were associated with lower incidence of subsequent "febrile" convulsions (El-Radhi & Banajeh, 1989; El-Radhi, Withana, & Banajeh, 1986).

New Zealand white rabbits respond to infection with *Pasteurella multocida* by developing large fevers. Most rabbits developed a fever of less than 2.25°C, and within this temperature range, there is an increase in survival rate as body temperature is elevated (Kluger & Vaughn, 1982). A small number of animals developed fevers above 2.25°C and showed a decrease in survival rate.

Another correlational study was reported by Toms, Davies, Woodward, Sweet, and Smith (1977). In this study, ferrets (*Mustela sp.*) were infected with different strains of influenza viruses, and the resultant fever was correlated with the presence of live viruses in their nasal passages. Groups of three to six ferrets were inoculated intranasally with a constant dose of virus. At 4-h intervals, the nasal passages were washed, and the fluid was collected and assayed for the presence of live virus. Statistically significant ($p < 0.01$) negative correlations were found between the ferrets' rectal temperatures and the presence of live viruses in the nasal washes, suggesting that fever might lead to the inactivation of viruses. In vitro observations from this same laboratory, in which organ cultures of ferret nasal turbinates were grown in the presence of influenza virus, are consistent with the in vivo data described above (Sweet, Cavanagh, Collie, & Smith, 1978). That is, an elevation in temperature of the cultures decreased the replication of the viruses. Interestingly, the more virulent strain of virus was less sensitive to the effects of temperature.

In summary, the results of correlational studies with human and animal subjects are consistent with the theory that fever has a beneficial function.

C. Antipyretic Studies

There have been several studies in which a population of mammals has been infected with identical amounts of pathogens and the effects of antipyresis on mortality or morbidity quantified. Some of these studies have combined antipyretic drug therapy with the use of other drugs (e.g., glucocorticoids or antibiotics) and, thus, the results are difficult to interpret (e.g., Klastersky, 1971). Others have used antipyretic drugs such as aspirin, acetaminophen, or ibuprofen (e.g., Graham, Burrell, Douglas, Debelle, & Davies, 1990), but no temperature measurements were noted and, thus, it is impossible to relate morbidity to temperature.

Van Miert et al. (1978) studied the effects of flurbiprofen, a nonsteroidal anti-inflammatory/antipyretic, on *Trypanosoma vivax* infection in goats. They found that this drug blocked the febrile responses during the acute phase of the infection, with the antipyretic drug alone having no effect on afebrile body temperature. Sixteen of 17 goats given the *T. vivax* without the flurbiprofen had a mild infection. All five infected goats treated with an antipyretic dosage of flurbiprofen died. Vaughn, Veale, and Cooper (1980) studied the effect of administration of an antipyretic drug directly into an area of the brain of rabbits implicated in the control of fever, the preoptic-anterior hypothalamus, on mortality rate during infection of rabbits with *Pasteurella multocida*. The fevers in the rabbits infused with the antipyretic drug were reduced by about 50%. This group of infected rabbits had a significant increase in mortality compared to the group of infected rabbits infused with control solution. Husseini, Sweet, Collie, and Smith (1982) studied the effects of suppression of fever on influenza in ferrets using sodium salicylate and found that treatment with the antipyretic drug results in attenuation of fever and an increased concentration of virus in washes as well as an increase in the duration of illness.

Small, Tauber, Hackbarth, and Sande (1986) investigated the effects of body temperature on bacterial growth rates in experimental pneumococcal infection. Rabbits were injected with *Streptococcus pneumoniae* intracisternally and developed fevers averaging 1.5°C. To lower body temperature, the rabbits were anesthetized with pentobarbital or urethane. Body temperature was controlled by varying ambient temperature. The growth rate of bacteria was significantly higher in anesthetized rabbits maintained at afebrile body temperatures. The correlation between changes in bacterial titer in the cerebrospinal fluid and body temperatures (from 38.5 to 41°C) was −0.70 ($p < 0.001$), suggesting that elevated temperatures suppressed the growth rate of the bacteria. Kurosawa, Kobune, Okuyama, and Sugiura (1987) studied the effects of antipyretics in rinderpest infection in rabbits. Rabbits were infected with the lapinized Nakamura III strain of RPV (L strain) and then treated with mefanamic acid or acetylsalicylic acid or were untreated. The antipyretic drugs led to varying reductions in body temperature. Treatment with either drug led to increased mortality rate and slower recovery among the survivors.

Ectothermic vertebrates have also been used to study the role of fever in disease. Bernheim and Kluger (1976) studied the effects of sodium salicylate-induced antipyresis on survival of the lizard *Dipsosaurus dorsalis*. Lizards were injected with the live bacteria (*Aeromonas hydrophila*) along with a dose of sodium salicylate. Seven of the 12 animals treated with the antipyretic drug failed to select a febrile temperature in a thermal gradient. All febrile lizards survived, while the afebrile lizards died. To determine whether the dose of sodium salicylate used in these experiments was toxic, eight lizards were injected with live bacteria and sodium salicylate and placed inside a constant temperature chamber. Their body temperatures were maintained at the febrile level by adjusting the chamber temperature to about 41°C during the day (about the average temperature selected by febrile lizards in the simulated natural environment) and at low temperatures at night (again, as in the simulated natural environment). Only one of these eight lizards died, indicating that the dose of sodium salicylate used in these experiments was not toxic. These data indicated to us that the administration of sodium salicylate to these infected lizards was harmful only when it resulted in a reduction in body temperature to the afebrile level. When sodium salicylate failed to produce antipyresis (as in the five lizards in the simulated desert environment or in the eight lizards maintained in the constant temperature chamber), the drug did not affect their rate of survival.

Thus, the increase in morbidity and mortality in studies using antipyretic drugs to attenuate fever supports the hypothesis that fever is a host-defense response.

D. Hyperthermia and Hypothermia Studies

The effects of hyperthermia and hypothermia on the course of infection through the year 1960 is discussed in greater detail in the excellent review by Bennett and Nicastri (1960). While it is difficult to draw definitive conclusions concerning the role of fever in disease-based on hyper- or hypothermia studies, the weight of the evidence supports an adaptive function for fever during infections with certain bacterial or viral pathogens (Table II).

Klastersky (1971) performed survival studies on rabbits that were made hypothermic by shaving their fur. Klastersky injected these rabbits with pneumococcal bacteria and then treated them with penicillin. Those rabbits developed considerably lower fevers than did the control rabbits that were not shaved. The

TABLE II Effects of Lowered Body Temperature on Morbidity and Mortality to Disease

Species	Pathogen	Effect of lowered temperature	Authors
Rabbit	Pneumococci	Protective	Klastersky, 1971
Rabbit	Pneumococci	Harmful	Muschenheim et al., 1943
Mouse	Malaria	Protective	Cooper, Dascombe, Rothwell, & Vale, 1989
Mouse	Influenza	Protective	Klein, Conn, & Kluger, 1992
Pigeon	Pneumococci	Harmful	Strouse, 1909
Rabbit	*P. multocida*	Protective	Vaughn et al., 1987
Rat	*S. enteritidis*	Protective	Banet, 1981a,b
Mouse pups	Coxsackie virus	Harmful	Teisner & Haahr, 1974
Dog pups	Herpesvirus	Harmful	Carmichael et al., 1969
Mouse	Rabies	Harmful	Bell & Moore, 1974
Humans	Acute rhinitis	Harmful	Yerushalmi & Lwoff, 1980
Humans	Acute rhinitiis	Protective	Macknin et al., 1990
Lizards	*A. hydrophila*	Harmful	Kluger et al., 1975
Goldfish	*A. hydrophila*	Harmful	Covert & Reynolds, 1977
Sockeye salmon	Sockeye virus	Harmful	Watson, Guenther, & Rucker, 1954
Sockeye salmon	IHN virus	Harmful	Amend, 1970
Rainbow trout	IHN virus	Harmful	Amend, 1976
Crickets	*Rickettsiella grylli*	Harmful	Louis et al., 1986
Grasshoppers	*N. acridophagus*	Harmful	Boorstein & Ewald, 1987
Bumblebees	Conopid fly parasite	Protective	Muller & Schmid-Hempel, 1993
Guinea pigs	*E. coli*	Harmful	Sheffield, Sessler, & Hunt, 1994

Note: IHN, Infections hematopoietic necrosis.

mortality rate of the control rabbits was 46% and that of the shaved rabbits only 31%. However, as noted earlier, all the rabbits received penicillin, thus making interpretation difficult.

Many other studies that involved the induction of hypothermia or hyperthermia in pneumococcal-infected animals have led to essentially opposite results of those reported by Klastersky. For example, in 1909, Strouse demonstrated that the natural resistance of pigeons to pneumococci was related to their normal body temperature of about 41.5°C. When their body temperatures were reduced by ice or by the administration of drugs, they became susceptible to the infection and died. Similar findings were reported by Muschenheim, Duerschrer, Hardy, and Stoll (1943) for pneumococcal infections in rabbits. These animals were infected with pneumococci, and hypothermia was induced by one of several methods so that the rectal temperatures of these rabbits were maintained between 30° and 34°C. Control rabbits were infected and their body temperature maintained at normal to low febrile levels, between 39° and 41°. All of the hypothermic rabbits died, whereas only five of the 31 control rabbits died. These investigators concluded that hypothermia was clearly harmful to the infected host and that the development of fever led to an enhancement of the host defense mechanism.

Vaughn, Veale, and Cooper (1987) found that even though treatment of rabbits with antipyretic drugs increased the mortality rate to *P. multocida*, physical cooling of rabbits *decreased* mortality rate. In this study, rabbits were cooled for 48 h after injection with bacteria by passing cold fluid through a small cuff surgically placed around the abdominal vena cavae. The cooled rabbit maintained average body temperature at about the normal afebrile temperature for rabbits (38.98°C) and the noncooled rabbits had body temperatures averaging 40.92°C. The cooled rabbits would presumably have a body temperature below their thermoregulatory set point, and as a result would be activating a variety of heat conservation and production effector responses. The authors of this study suggested that thermoregulatory effector mechanisms involved in cold defense may enhance survival. These data are similar to those by Banet (1981b) for rats infected with *Salmonella enteritidis*. In this study, the spinal cord of rats was cooled, resulting in an increased metabolic rate (oxygen uptake) and a survival rate that was borderline significantly higher than in infected animals that did not have their spinal cords cooled (p=.06). Interestingly, there were no differences in core temperatures between the control and experimental rats. Banet (1983) then showed a correlation between survival rate and the increase in metabolic rate during the rising phase of fever in rats infected with *S. enteritidis*. In rats infected with an LD_{50} of bacteria, there was a negative correlation between the highest fever obtained and the survival rate at fevers above 38.7°C. What this might mean, however, is that the sickest animals mounted the greatest febrile responses, and despite any beneficial effect of fever, these animals had a higher mortality rate. Banet (1983) hypothesized that some of the effects of endogenous pyrogens on the altering metabolism, presumably the neuroendocrine changes, are beneficial, and that the elevation in temperature, itself, may often be harmful.

The febrile responses of newborns is an area that has received considerable attention. It has been known for a long time that many newborn mammals have a labile body temperature during their first few days of life (Pembrey, 1895). Furthermore, in response to infection, newborn human infants (Haahr & Mogensen, 1977), or other infant mammals such as rabbits (Satinoff, McEwen, & Williams, 1976), tend to have a limited febrile response. Satinoff and colleagues have shown, however, that newborn rabbits, while not raising their body temperature by physiological means following an injection of endotoxin, will raise their body temperature by behavioral means. When injected with *Pseudomonas* endotoxins and allowed to select a range of environmental temperatures, these rabbits selected a warmer environment, resulting in an elevation in their body temperatures. Haahr & Mogensen (1977) suggested that a rise in body temperature during certain viral infections was beneficial to newborns. To support their claim, they cited several studies that demonstrated that elevations in body temperature during various viral infections have reduced the mortality rate in newborn mice, dogs, and human beings. For example, Teisner and Haahr (1974) found that when 2- to-3-day-old mice were infected with Coxsackie virus and held at an environmental temperature of 34°C, they had a mean body temperature of 35.8°C, some 2 to 3°C higher than control mice held at room temperature of 22 to 24°C. Those mice held at 34°C had a considerably lower mortality rate than did the control mice. Carmichael, Barnes, and Percy (1969) reported similar findings for 2- to-5-day-old dog pups that were inoculated with canine herpesvirus. When the pups were held at an environmental temperature of 28 to 30°C, they had a rectal temperature of about 35 to 37°C; those held at an environmental temperature of 36.7 to 37.7°C had a rectal temperature of 38.3 to 39.4°C, approximately normal rectal temperatures for adult dogs. Following inoculation with herpesvirus, those dogs with the lower rectal temperatures died within 8 days, whereas those with the higher rectal temperatures survived 9 days or longer. The authors of this study concluded that the elevation of the body temperature to the adult level was beneficial to the infected pups. Based on these data, Haahr & Mogensen (1977) suggested that a reason that generalized herpes-simplex infections are greatly overrepresented in premature babies may be their restricted temperature regulation and poor febrile response. Thus, although newborns might not be able to develop fevers due to inadequate metabolic machinery or the ability to behaviorally thermoregulate, an elevated body temperature during infections appears to be protective.

Bell and Moore (1974) have found that housing of mice in a warm ambient temperature (35°C) led to decreased mortality due to inoculation with rabies virus. The average body temperatures of mice in the warm environmental temperature was 2°C higher than those in the control environment (20°C).

Yerushalmi and Lwoff (1980) found that treatment of human subjects with local hyperthermia (i.e., inhalation of warm humidified air) decreased the magnitude of acute rhinitis ("infective Coryza"). However, in a followup study, Macknin, Mathew, and Medenforp (1990) found a slight improvement in rhinitis in patients provided with *cool* vapor compared to the warmed air.

Mice infected with influenza develop a regulated hypothermia, rather than a fever (Klein, Conn, & Kluger, 1992). This regulated reduction in body temperature appears to be protective. A large literature base shows that hypoxia induces a reduction in body temperature that enhances host survival (Wood & Malvin, 1992). Pilot data by Kozak et al. support the hypothesis that the reduction in body temperature in the influenza-infected mice is, at least in part, attributable to hypoxia. Thus, this may be a case where an infection-induced fall in body temperature, rather than the development of fever, is beneficial.

Many hypothermia/hyperthermia studies have also been designed to investigate the role of fever using ectothermic species. For example, to investigate whether the rise in body temperature in the bacterially infected desert iguana (*Dipsosaurus dorsalis*) had survival value, lizards were injected with live *A. hydrophila* and placed in incubators at 34, 36, 38, 40, and 42°C (Kluger, Ringler, & Anver, 1975). Control lizards were inoculated with saline and placed into the incubators. The relation between the lizards' temperatures and percentage survival following bacterial infection was highly significant ($p < .005$). Within 24 h, approximately 50% of the infected lizards maintained at the afebrile temperature of 38° were dead. However, lizards maintained at the febrile temperatures of 40° and 42°C had only 14 and 0% mortality, respectively. Conversely, infected lizards maintained at 36 and 34°C, temperatures that are hypothermic for this species of lizard, experienced mortalities of 66 and 75%, respectively. After $3\frac{1}{2}$ days, all the lizards at 34°C were dead. After 7 days the percentage mortalities were as follows: 34°C, 100%; 38 and 36°C, 75%; 40°C, 33%; 42°C, 25%. In contrast, lizards injected with saline and maintained at 34, 38, and 42°C for 7 days experienced 0, 0, and 34% mortality, respectively. At the highest temperature tested, the pattern of deaths was similar for the controls and the infected lizards. Whereas most deaths occurred within $3\frac{1}{2}$ days in infected lizards maintained at 34 to 40°C, virtually all deaths at 42°C occurred after $3\frac{1}{2}$ days. Apparently, maintenance at 42°C for a period exceeding $3\frac{1}{2}$ days is harmful in itself. This suggests that the deaths at 42°C were due to some undetermined adverse effect of long-term elevation in body temperature in lizards, rather than to the bacterial infection.

Several studies have involved the effects of temperature on the mortality rate of fishes. One of these, by Covert and Reynolds (1977), involved infecting goldfish with live *A. hydrophila* and monitoring their survival rate over a period of 3 days at temperatures of 25.5, 28.0, or 30.5°C. These represented, respectively, hypothermic, normothermic, and febrile temperatures. Goldfish that are maintained at a febrile temperature of 30.5°C had a survival rate of 84%; those held at 28.0°C had a survival rate of 64%; those at 25.5°C had a survival rate of 24%. Another 10 fish were injected with the same dose of live *A. hydrophila* and allowed to thermoregulate in a shuttlebox. These fish selected an ambient temperature that allowed them to develop a fever averaging almost 5°C and had a mean body temperature of 32.7°C. None of these fish died. Covert and Reynolds concluded that a fever in response to infection with *A. hydrophila* increases the survival rate of goldfish.

Several studies have involved the effects of elevations in water (= body) temperature on the mortality rate of various species of freshwater fishes infected with viruses. For example, Watson, Guenther, and Rucker (1954) reported that sockeye salmon (*Oncorhynchus nerka*) infected with sockeye salmon virus experienced fewer deaths when held at a water temperature of 20°C than when held at 15.5°C or lower. In 1970, Amend reported similar findings for sockeye salmon infected with hematopoietic necrosis virus (IHN). The mortality rate of salmon held between 12 and 16°C was about 66%, whereas for those held between 18 and 20°C, it was only about 30%. Even with a delay of up to 24 h before the infected fishes were placed in the warmer environment, the mortality rate decreased substantially. Similar results were reported for IHN-infected rainbow trout (*Salmo gairdneri*) (Amend, 1976).

The above studies are somewhat difficult to interpret because it is unknown whether these fishes develop fevers in response to viral infections. Thus, it is unclear whether raising their body temperatures simulates hyperthermia (body temperature > set point) or fever (an elevated body temperature in which set point = body temperature). If the fish were simply hyperthermic, then the beneficial effect of raising their body temperatures would simply be a form of fever therapy. Therefore, these results would not be applicable to a discussion of the role of fever in disease. Because several species of freshwater fishes develop fevers in response to bacterial infection, it is likely that, given the opportunity, the species of fishes used in the viral studies would also behaviorally select warmer environmental temperatures. If this turns out to be the case, then these results will support the thesis that fever has an adaptive function in fishes.

Louis and colleagues (1986) infected crickets (*Gryllus bimaculatus*) with the intracellular parasite *Rickettsiella grylli*. The crickets were reared at different ambient temperatures and those crickets reared at warmer temperatures (higher than 29°C) survived this infection. It should be noted that when these crickets were infected and allowed to select a preferred body temperature in a temperature gradient, they selected a temperature averaging 33.0°C. The average body temperature of non-infected crickets was 26.6°C.

Boorstein and Ewald (1987) inoculated grasshoppers (*Melanoplus sanguinipes*) with the protozoan *Nosema acridophagus* and found that this resulted in an increase in preferred body temperature of about 6°C (to ca. 40°C). Maintenance of grasshoppers at febrile and afebrile temperatures demonstrated that fever enhances both survival rate and growth. Infected grasshoppers maintained at febrile temperatures demonstrated increased fecundity, as quantified by numbers of eggs laid, compared to infected grasshoppers maintained at afebrile temperatures.

E. The Highly Regulated Nature of Fever

As shown in Figure 1, fever is a highly coordinated response. Fevers are triggered by the release of "endogenous pyrogens" from a large number of different types of macrophage-like cells. These endogenous pyrogens include the cytokines interleukin-1 (IL-1), IL-6, and others. The cytokines act at the level of the anterior hypothalamus to raise the thermoregulatory set point, thus initiating a large number of physiological and behavioral responses, which result in the elevation of body temperature (e.g., see Kluger, 1991). In addition to the release of endogenous pyrogens, endogenous antipyretics or cryogens act to modulate the febrile rise in body temperature, thus generally preventing body temperature from rising to dangerous levels. Over the past 10 years, investigators have shown that arginine vasopressin, α-melanocyte stimulating hormone, glucocorticoids, and, in some cases, tumor necrosis factor may act as endogenous antipyretics. This highly regulated nature of fever, which involves numerous cytokines and hormones, supports the argument that fever has evolved as a host defense response.

II. WHAT ARE THE MECHANISMS BEHIND A PROTECTIVE EFFECT OF FEVER?

A. Enhancing Specific Components of Host Defense

Wang et al. (1998) studied the effect of temperatures in the normal fever range of 38 to 41°C on the adhesion potential of lymphocytes. They found that elevated temperatures significantly enhance L-selectin-mediated adhesion of human lymphocytes to lymph nodes (*in vitro*) in a time- and temperature-dependent manner. Adhesion of leukocytes to and transmigration across the vascular endothelium constitute the first steps in the pathogenesis of inflammation—processes indispensable for resolving an infection. Fever appears to facilitate these processes. There are numerous other examples of the effects of an increase in temperature on specific and nonspecific components of host defense caused by subtle changes in temperature (Table III). Hasday (1997) wrote an excellent review of the specific effects of temperature on host defenses. Some components of immunity are enhanced at febrile temperature, and others are inhibited. In general, it is our impression that an elevation in temperature tends to increase immune responses.

Sherman and Stephens (1998) showed that the combination of injection with lipopolysaccharide (LPS) and maintenance at a febrile temperature of 32°C leads to an increase in metabolic rate in the toad, *Bufo marinus*, compared to that seen in toads injected with saline and maintained at 32°C. The metabolic rate of LPS- and saline-injected toads was the same when they were maintained at the nonfebrile temperature of 25°C. These investigtors suggested that this elevation in metabolic rate is the result of the "cost of the stimulation of the immune system," which is only seen at febrile temperatures. Table III summarizes a large amount of data, and the interested reader should refer to the references cited below this table.

TABLE III Some Effects of Febrile Temperatures on Host Defense Responses

- Generally, enhanced neutrophil migration
- Increased neutrophil bactericidal activity
- Reduced Natural Killer activity
- Increased L-selectin-dependent adhesion of lymphocytes to vascular endothelium
- Generally increased production of interferon; decreased production of TNF
- Cytokine production may be increased or decreased depending on the study
- Increased biological activities of TNF, IL-1, and IFN
- Increased T-cell proliferation
- Decreased growth of microorganisms in iron-poor environment

Note: For more detailed information, see Hasday, 1997; Kluger, 1991; Mackowiak, 1997; Roberts, 1991; Wang and colleagues, 1998. TNF, tumor necrosis factor; IL, interleukin; IFN, interferon.

B. Protection against Pathogen-Induced Disturbances in Homeostasis

Kozak (1993) proposed an additional rationale for the protective effect of fever. He hypothesized that in addition to the effect of temperature on various host defense responses (Table III), fever could be considered a homeostatic process in maintaining a constancy of the cell membrane of the infected organism. The membrane "condition" is a physical state of the cell surface based on the functional interrelationship of two essential factors: (1) composition of the membrane's lipids and (2) actual temperature of the membrane. The specific physiological interplay of these two factors accounts for a dynamic equilibrium of the membrane with its environment and as, a consequence, the functioning of the cell. During infection, the structural elements of the membrane undergo changes, mostly due to induction of certain phospholipid degradation by phospholipases and the liberation of arachidonic acid. The resultant release of potent mediators of inflammation and infection, such as eicosanoids and platelet-activating factors from the membrane, leads to depletion of double bonds (i.e., decreases the unsaturation index) of the membrane. This, in turn, results in phase shifting in the thermodynamic properties of the membrane (i.e., phase-transition temperature, viscosity/fluidity) toward higher temperatures. Increasing body temperature during infection is hypothesized to result in a compensation for these disturbances in membrane structure and may restore membrane conditions essential for signal transduction, expression of receptors, and the controlled running of metabolic processes, thus maintaining homeostasis.

An elevation in body temperature, therefore, may have two types of effects. One attenuates the viability of some pathogenic microorganisms by enhancing specific components of specific and nonspecific immunity. The other is speculated to help to restore disturbances in membrane properties.

III. POTENTIAL HARMFUL EFFECTS OF DRUGS ON HOST DEFENSE: EXAMPLE—MORPHINE AND FEVER

Based on the data presented in this chapter, a case can be made for the protective role of fever. As a result, any drug that directly or indirectly suppresses fever may result in increased morbidity and mortality. Morphine is one example of how a reduced fever may suppress immunity. Morphine worsens disease outcome and impairs immune function in humans. These effects of morphine have been studied in healthy volunteers (Yeager et al., 1995), as well as in patients who are frequently prescribed morphine such as those suffering with chronic pain (Palm et al., 1998) and cancer (Provinciali et al., 1991). Similar effects of morphine have been found in laboratory studies of disease. Morphine decreases survival time of laboratory animals with different types of infections such as *K. pneumoniae*, *C. albicans* (Tubaro, Borelli, Croce, Cavallo, & Santiangeli, 1983), and *T. gondii* (Chao, Sharp, Pomeroy, Filice, & Peterson 1990).

Morphine suppresses the immune system directly and indirectly. Morphine *directly* acts upon many types of immune cells to impair their function. For example, morphine applied to macrophages in vitro decreases their phagocytic activity (Rojavin et al., 1993). Morphine also acts indirectly (i.e., not directly binding to and affecting immune cells). For example, morphine activates the hypothalamo-pituitary-adrenal axis, resulting in elevated circulating levels of immunosuppressive glucocorticoids (Bryant, Bernton, Kenner, & Holaday, 1991). Only a few examples of the immunosuppressive properties of morphine are listed here as this area has been reviewed extensively elsewhere (Eisenstein and Hilburger, 1998; Mellon and Bayer, 1998; Madden, Whaley, and Ketelsen, 1998).

Suppressing the development of fever is another mechanism by which morphine may decrease immune function. Morphine injected 3 h prior to injection of LPS greatly diminishes the development of fever (Mayfield, Kozak, Rudolph, and Kluger, 1998). The dose of morphine used for this experiment (30 mg/kg, ip) is sufficient to induce analgesia in rats (Porreca, Cowan, & Tallarida, 1981) and has been used as an "immunosuppressive" dose of morphine (e.g., Fecho, Dykstra, & Lysle, 1993). Initially, within 1 h following morphine injection, body temperature rises. This hyperthermic response lasts approximately 2 h. Subsequent to this initial increase in body temperature, the morphine-treated rats do not develop a fever to LPS injection. Studies to understand the mechanism(s) by which morphine suppresses fever are underway; we hypothesize that one of morphine's immunosuppressive actions may be the result of its suppression of fever.

IV. STRESS, FEVER, AND IMMUNITY

Psychological stress may be another example of an association between reduced fever and dampened immunity. Psychological stress increases susceptibility to or worsens prognosis of disease. For example, psychological stress is associated with higher rates of recurrent respiratory infections (Drummond & Hewson-Bower, 1997), mononucleosis (Kasl et al., 1979), streptococcus infections (Meyer & Haggerty, 1962), and tuberculosis (Holmes, 1962). Psychological stress increases susceptibility to infection upon controlled exposure to viruses. In one study, human subjects were maintained under controlled living conditions and exposed to different types of viruses associated with the common cold. The participants were also evaluated by standard psychological tests. Those subjects who experienced more psychological stress had increased susceptibility to developing illness upon exposure to the same amount and type of virus (Cohen, Tyrrell, & Smith, 1991). Stress reactivates latent herpes simplex virus infection (Friedmann Katcher, & Brightman, 1977; Glaser et al., 1987, Glaser, 1991; Goldmeier & Johnson, 1982; Katcher, Brightman, Luborsky, & Ship, 1973; Glaser, Kiecolt-Glaser, Speicher, & Holliday, 1985). Psychological stress is also a risk factor for developing cancer (Chen et al., 1995; Ginsberg, Price, Ingram, & Nottage, 1996), and it hastens the progression of HIV

(Evans et al., 1995, 1997; Goodkin, Fuchs, Feaster, Leeka, & Rishel, 1992). Many epidemiological studies suggest that severe stress precedes the onset and can precipitate relapses of multiple sclerosis (Grant et al., 1989; Warren, Greenhill, & Warren 1982; Warren, Warren, & Cockerill, 1991).

Importantly, measures that alleviate stress, such as exercise or counseling, attenuate the adverse physical effects of stress (Fawzy et al., 1990; LaPerriere et al., 1990). It is necessary to note that not all studies have found a detrimental effect of stress on disease outcome (Cassileth, 1996; Johansen & Olsen, 1997; Perry, Fishman, Jacobsberg, & Frances 1992; Sahs et al., 1994). The discrepancies in this area could be due to many factors including differences in the assessment or definition of stress, the timing of the stress in relationship to time of disease progression, or differences in the subjects' ability to cope with stress.

The effects of psychological stress on disease susceptibility and progression may be related to specific changes in immune function. Numerous immune parameters are affected by psychological stress (reviewed by Kusnecov & Rabin, 1994; Palmblad, 1987). Stress has been found to decrease some aspects of immune function and increase others. We hypothesize that one factor contributing to whether stress increases or decreases immune function is the timing of the stress in relation to the time of measuring immune function. For example, in a study by Schedlowski et al. (1993), stress induced by a parachute jump causes an initial increase in NK cell activity followed by a subsequent depression of NK cell activity.

The effects of stress on immune function seem to parallel the effects of stress on body temperature. Psychological stress induced by many different methods increases body temperature in rats and humans. Rats exposed to handling (Briese & DeQuidada, 1970), to a novel environment (Kluger, O'Reilly, Shope, & Vander, 1987; Kluger et al., 1989; Long, Kluger, & Vander, 1989; Singer, Harker, Vander, & Kluger 1986), or to restraint (Long, Morimoto, Nakamori, & Murakami 1991a Long, Morimoto, Nakamori, Yamashiro, & Murakami, 1991b) have increased body temperature. Medical students preparing for academic exams have elevated body temperatures (Marazziti, Di Muro, & Catrogiovanni, 1992), as do athletes psychologically (not physically) preparing for a competition (Renbourn, 1960). In contrast to this acute effect of stress increasing body temperature, stress also prevents complete development of the febrile response to infectious stimuli. Hamsters subjected to psychological stress by housing them in small cages develop smaller fevers to injection of LPS (Kuhnen, 1998). Rats that are restrained develop smaller fevers to injected LPS, the inflammatory cytokine interleukin-1β, and prostaglandin (Long et al., 1991a,b). Continuous infusion of corticotropin-releasing hormone into the lateral ventricles of rats simulates chronic stress and also blocks the development of the febrile response to LPS (Linthorst et al., 1997). The effect of stress on the febrile response is apparently long-lasting. Pregnant rhesus monkeys injected with adrenocorticotropin-releasing hormone (again another way to endocrinologically simulate stress) give birth to animals that have diminished febrile responses to the inflammatory cytokine (IL-1β). This diminished response lasts for as long as 2 years after birth (Reyes & Coe, 1997). Based on these associations, we hypothesize that one mechanism by which stress decreases immune function is by depressing the febrile response to inflammatory stimuli.

It is interesting to note that both stress and morphine cause an initial increase in body temperature and an apparent immune activation (e.g., both stress and morphine stimulate increased levels of IL-6 in the plasma). This initial increase in body temperature and immune function is followed by a period of time that seems to be refractory to infectious/inflammatory stimuli in that submaximal responses to these stimuli are elicited. While stress and morphine undoubtedly cause many physiological changes, it is possible that some of the changes in immune function are mediated by the failure to develop full febrile responses.

V. SUMMARY AND CONCLUSION

The results of the studies of the survival value of fever in ectothermic vertebrates indicate that following an infection, a rise in body temperature results in decreased mortality and morbidity. These data further support the hypothesis that fever in endotherms is also beneficial because it is unlikely that fever would be adaptive in insects, fishes and reptiles and would have become maladaptive in birds and mammals.

Based on the data reviewed here, it can be concluded that fever has evolved as a host defense mechanism. However, it is also clear that not all fevers are beneficial. Why should this be the case? Mackowiak (1994) suggested that because some data point toward a beneficial role for fever and others support the hypothesis that fever is maladaptive (e.g., in association with hypoglycemia and shock), this apparent paradox can be resolved "if one accepts preservation of the species rather than survival of the individual as the essence of evolution." Mackowiak then states: "the febrile response and its mediators may have evolved both as a mechanism for accelerating the recovery of infected individuals with localized or mild to moderately severe systemic infections and for hastening the demise of hopelessly infected individuals, who pose a threat of epidemic disease to the species." This hypothesis has an inherent problem—evolution works on the level of the individual, not the species. With the rare exception of "kin" selection, organisms are not altruistic, sacrificing themselves for the good of the community.

So, why should there be circumstances in which cytokines and other inflammatory mediators are overproduced (which lead to massive fevers as well as other potentially harmful effects such as vascular leakage)? These instances represent a breakdown in host defenses, and so, why do they occur? One possible explanation is that, unlike specific immune responses, nonspecific host defense responses are highly stereotypical. Infection with any number of different organisms will produce similar acute-phase responses characterized by loss of food appetite, lethargy, increased sleep, fever, hypoferremia, hypozincemia, synthesis of a wide array of acute phase proteins, etc. If we assume that for some large percentage of the time (e.g., 95%) the acute phase responses induced by infection, injury, or trauma are beneficial, one can readily see why the stereotyped acute phase responses would have evolved and been retained. So long as the cost-benefit ratio is weighted toward the benefit side, fever (and other host defense responses) would be selected, even if this occasionally leads to increased morbidity and mortality.

Another explanation for the occasional maladaptive role for fever (or other acute phase responses) is that host–pathogen interactions continues to evolve. As the host evolves new mechanisms for combating infection (e.g., antibody production, elevation in body temperature, etc.), the pathogen also evolves new mechanisms for successfully parasitizing the host. A symbiotic relationship undoubtedly develops between the host and its parasite with, in most cases, a balance being achieved. This balance keeps the host immunologically "primed" or prepared in the event that it is exposed to some new pathogen. Although we believe that the balance is skewed toward fever being adaptive, a "smart" pathogen may develop mechanisms to use the host's elevated temperature to facilitate its own growth or survival.

If fever is, overall, beneficial, then why doesn't the organism maintain a fever continually, even when not infected? First, there is the metabolic cost of fever. As described earlier, simply elevating and maintaining a body temperature at an elevated level cost considerable energy. Another hypothesis to explain this failure to continually maintain a febrile body temperature was raised by Sohnle and Gambert (1982). They proposed that the maintenance of a body temperature below the optimum temperature for immunological defenses may be a mechanism for reducing the "contribution of the immune system to ageing." The maintenance of a body temperature that reduces overall host defenses would reduce the amount of cytotoxic agents (e.g., free radicals) released by neutrophils and macrophages and thus reduce tissue damage unrelated to fighting infection. Sohnle and Gambert (1982) argued that support for their intriguing hypothesis comes from data indicating that fish living in cooler water live longer than those at higher temperatures, and that dietary restriction in rats and mice was associated with lower body temperatures and greater longevity. There is also anecdotal evidence that hibernating species (e.g., microchiropteran bats) live longer than other small nonhibernating species of mammals.

Another possible explanation for short-acting fevers is that *a change in body temperature*, itself, may be beneficial to the host. Most living organisms have had to adapt their structural and biochemical characteristics to a given temperature in order to function at the lowest possible thermodynamic cost. Invading microorganisms acclimated to a given ambient temperature may encounter unfavorable conditions if the temperature of the host changes rapidly either upward or downward. The invading microbe may suffer "thermal shock," which might contribute to reduced growth.

Overall, we believe that the evidence is overwhelming in favor of fever being an adaptive host response to infection that has persisted throughout the animal kingdom for hundreds of millions of years. As such, it is probable that the use of antipyretic/antiinflammatory/analgesic drugs, when they lead to the suppression of fever, results in increased morbidity and mortality during most infections. The reason that this increased morbidity and mortality may not be readily apparent to most healthcare workers is that we are armed with dozens of host defense responses, with fever being only one of them. Furthermore, most infections are not life-threatening, and subtle changes in morbidity are not easily detected, particularly, in "experiments" that are not carefully controlled.

Acknowledgment

Research supported by NIH AI 27556, MH 48609.

References

Adamo, S. A. (1998). The specificity of behavioral fever in the cricket *Acheta domesticus*. *Journal of Parasitology, 84*, 529–533.

Amend, D. F. (1976). Prevention and control of viral diseases of salmonids. *Journal of Fisheries Research Board Canada, 33*, 1059–1066.

Amend, D. F. (1970). Control of infectious hematopoietic necrosis virus disease by elevating the water temperature. *Journal of Fisheries Research Board Canada, 27*, 265–270.

Banet, M. (1981a). Fever and survival in the rat. Metabolic versus temperature response. *Experientia, 37*, 1302–1304.

Banet, M. (1981b). Fever and survival in the rat. The effect of enhancing the cold defense response. *Experientia, 37*, 985–986.

Banet, M. (1983). The biological function of fever: An alternative view. *Functional Biology and Medicine, 2*, 211–218.

Bell, J. F., & Moore, G. J. (1974). Effects of high ambient temperature on various stages of rabies virus infection in mice. *Infection and Immunity, 10*, 510–515.

Bennett, I. L., & Nicastri, A. (1960). Fever as a mechanism of resistance. *Bacteriological Reviews, 24*,16–34.

Bernheim, H. A., & Kluger, M. J. (1976). Fever: Effect of drug-induced antipyresis on survival. *Science, 193*, 237–239.

Bernheim, H. A., & Kluger, M. J. (1977). Endogenous pyrogen-like substance produced by reptiles. *Journal of Physiology (London), 267*, 659–666.

Boorstein, S. M., & Ewald, P. W. (1987). Costs and benefits of behavioral fever in *Melanoplus sanuinipes* infected by *Nosema acridophagus*. *Physiological Zoology, 60*, 586–595.

Briese, E., & DeQuijada, M. G. (1970). Colonic temperature of rats during handling. *Acta physiologica Latinoam, 20*, 97–102.

Bronstein, S. M., & Conner, W. E. (1984). Endotoxin-induced behavioural fever in the Madagascar cockroach, *Gromphadorhina portentosa*. *Journal of Insect Physiology, 30*, 327–330.

Bryant, H. U., Bernton, E. W., Kenner, J. R., & Holaday, J. W. (1991). Role of adrenal cortical activation in the immunosuppressive effects of chronic morphine treatment. *Endocrinology, 128*(6), 3253–3258.

Bryant, R. E., Hood, A. F., Hood, C. E., & Koenig, M. G. (1971). Factors affecting mortality of gram-negative rod bacteremia. *Archives of Internal Medicine, 127*, 120–128.

Cabanac, M., & Guelte, L. L. (1980). Temperature regulation and prostaglandin E_1 fever in scorpions. *Journal of Physiology (London), 303*, 365–370.

Carmichael, L. E., Barnes, F. D., & Percy, D. H. (1969). Temperature as a factor in resistance of young puppies. *Journal of Infectious Diseases, 120*, 669–678.

Cassileth, B. R. (1996). Stress and the development of breast cancer: A persistent and popular link despite contrary evidence. *Cancer, 77*(6), 1015–1016.

Casterlin, M. E., & Reynolds, W. W. (1977). Behavioral fever in anuran amphibian larvae. *Life Sciences, 20*, 593–596.

Casterlin, M. E., & Reynolds, W. W. (1979). Fever induced in marine arthropods by prostaglandin E_1. *Life Sciences, 25*, 1601–1604.

Casterlin, M. E., & Reynolds, W. W. (1980). Fever and antipyresis in the crayfish *Cambarus bartoni*. *Journal of Physiology (London), 303*, 417–421.

Chao, C. C., Sharp, B. M., Pomeroy, C., Filice, G. A., & Peterson, P. K. (1990). Lethality of morphine in mice infected with Toxoplasma gondii. *Journal of Pharmacology and Experimental Therapeutics, 252*(2), 605–609.

Chen, C. C., David, A. S., Nunnerley, H., Michell, M., Dawson, J. L., Berry, H., Dobbs, J., & Fahy, T. (1995). Adverse life events and breast cancer: Case–control study. *British Medical Journal, 311*, 1527–1530.

Coehlo, M. M., Souza, G. E. P., & Pela, I. R. (1992) Endotoxin-induced fever is modulated by endogenous glucocorticoids in rats. *American Journal of Physiology, 263*, R423–R427.

Cohen, S., Tyrrell, D. A. J., & Smith, A. P. (1991). Psychological stress and susceptibility to the common cold. *New England Journal of Medicine, 325*(9), 606–612.

Cooper, A. L., Dascombe, M. J., Rothwell, N. J., & Vale, M. J. (1989). Effects of malaria on O_2 consumption and brown adipose tissue activity in mice. *Journal of Applied Physiology, 67*, 1020–1023.

Covert, J. B., & Reynolds, W. W. (1977) Survival value of fever in fish. *Nature, 267*, 43–45.

Drummond, P. D., Hewson-Bower, B. (1997). Increased psychosocial stress and decreased mucosal immunity in children with recurrent upper respiratory tract infections. *Journal of Psychosomatic Research, 43*(3), 271–278.

DuPont, H. G., & Spink, W. W. (1969). Infections due to gram-negative organisms: An analysis of 860 patients with bacteremia at the University of Minnesota Medical Center, 1958–1966. *Medicine, 48*, 307–332.

Eisenstein, T. K., & Hilburger, M. E. (1998). Opioid modulation of immune responses: effects on phagocyte and lymphoid cell populations. *Journal of Neuroimmunol, 83*, 36–44.

El-Radhi, A. S., & Banajeh, S. (1989). Effect of fever on recurrence of febrile convulsions. *Archives of Diseases of Childhood, 64*, 869–870.

El-Radhi, A. S., Withana, K., & Banajeh, S. (1986). Recurrence rate of febrile convulsion related to the degree of pyrexia during the first attack. *Clinical Pediatrics, 25*, 311–313.

Evans, D. L., Leserman, J., Perkins, D. O., Stern, R. A., Murphy, C., Tamul, K., Liao, D., van der Horst, C. M., Hall, C. D., Folds, J. D., Golden, R. N., & Petitto, J. M. (1995). Stress-associated reductions of cytotoxic T lymphocytes and natural killer cells in asymptomatic HIV infection. *American Journal of Psychiatry, 152*, 543–550.

Evans, D. L., Leserman, J., Perkins, D. O., Stern, R. A., Murphy, C., Zheng, B., Gettes, D., Longmate, J. A., Silva, S. G., van der Horst, C. M., Hall, C. D., Folds, J. D., Golden, R. N., & Petitto, J. M. (1997). Severe life stress as a predictor of early disease progression in HIV infection. *American Journal of Psychiatry, 154*, 630–634.

Fawzy, F. I., Kemeny, M. E., Fawzy, N. W., Elashoff, R., Morton, G., Cousins, N., & Fahey, J. L. (1990). A structured psychiatric intervention for cancer patients. *Archives of General Psychiatry, 47*, 729–735.

Fecho, K., Dykstra, L. A., & Lysle, D. T. (1993). Evidence for beta adrenergic receptor involvement in the immunomodulatory effects of morphine. *Journal of Pharmacology and Experimental Therapeutics, 265*, 1079–1087.

Firth, B. T., Ralph, C. L., & Boardman, T. J. (1980). Independent effects of the pineal and a bacterial pyrogen in behavioural thermoregulation in lizards. *Nature, 285*, 399–400.

Friedmann, E., Katcher, A. H., & Brightman, V. J. (1977). Incidence of recurrent herpes labialis and upper respiratory infection: A prospective study of the influence of biologic, social, and psychologic predictors. *Oral Medicine, 43*, 873–878.

Ginsberg, A., Price, S., Ingram, D., & Nottage, E. (1996). Life events and the risk of breast cancer: A case–control study. *European Journal of Cancer, 32A* (12), 2049–2052.

Glaser, R., Kiecolt-Glaser, J. K., Speicher, C. E., & Holliday, J. E. (1985). Stress, loneliness, and changes in herpesvirus latency. *Journal of Behavioral Medicine, 8*, 249–260.

Glaser, R., Pearson, G. R., Jones, J. F., Hillhouse, J., Kennedy, S., Mao, H., & Kiecolt-Glaser, J. (1991). Stress-related activation of Epstein-Barr virus. *Brain Behavior and Immunity, 5*, 219–232.

Glaser, R., Rice, J., Sheridan, J., Fertel, R., Stout, J., Speicher, C., Pinsky, D., Kotur, M., Post, A., Beck, M., & Kiecolt-Glaser, J. (1987). Stress-related immune suppression: Health Implications. *Brain Behavior and Immunity, 1,* 7–20.

Goldmeier, D., & Johnson, A. (1982). Does psychiatric illness affect the recurrence rate of genital herpes? *British Journal of Venereal Diseases, 54,* 40–43.

Goodkin, K., Fuchs, I., Feaster, D., Leeka, J., & Rishel, D. D. (1992). Life stressors and coping style are associated with immune measures in HIV-1 infection—A preliminary report. *International Journal of Psychiatry in Medicine, 22*(2), 155–172.

Graham, N. M. H., Burrell, C. J., Douglas, R. M., Debelle, P., & Davies, L. (1990). Adverse effects of aspirin, acetaminophen, and ibuprofen on immune function, viral shedding, and clinical status in rhinovirus-infected volunteers. *Journal of Infectious Diseases, 162,* 1277–1282.

Grant, I., Brown, G. W., Harris, T., McDonald, W. I., Patterson, T., Trimble, M. R. (1989). Severely threatening events and marked life difficulties preceding onset or exacerbation of multiple sclerosis. *Journal of Neurology, Neurosurgery and Psychiatry, 52,* 8–13.

Haahr, S., & Mogensen, S. (1977). Function of fever. *The Lancet, ii,* (No. 8038), 613.

Hallman, G. M., Ortega, C. E., Towner, M. C., & Muchlinski, A. E. (1990). Effect of bacterial pyrogen on three lizard species. *Comparative Biochemistry and Physiology, 96A,* 383–386.

Hasday, J. D. (1997). The influence of temperature on host defenses. In P. A. Mackowiak (Ed.), *Fever: Basic mechanisms and management* (pp. 177–196). Philadelphia, PA: Lippincott-Raven.

Holmes, T. H. (1962). Psychosocial and psychophysiological studies of tuberculosis. In (R. Roessler, Ed.), *Physiological corrections of psychological disorders* (pp. 239–255).

Husseini, R. H., Sweet, C., Collie, M. H., & Smith, H. (1982). Elevation of nasal viral levels by suppression of fever in ferrets infected with influenza viruses of differing virulence. *Journal of Infectious Diseases, 145,* 520–524.

Hutchison, V. H., & Erskine, D. J. (1981) Thermal selection and prostaglandin E_1 fever in the salamander *Necturus maculosus. Herpetologica, 37,* 195–198.

Johansen, C., & Olsen, J. H. (1997). Psychological stress, cancer incidence and mortality from non-malignant diseases. *British Journal of Cancer, 75*(1), 144–148.

Kasl, S. V., Evans, A. S., & Niederman, J. C. (1979). Psychosocial risk factors in the development of infectious mononucleosis. *Psychosomatic Medicine, 41*(6), 445–466.

Kasting, N. W. (1989). Criteria for establishing a physiological role for brain peptides. A case in point: The role of vasopressin in thermoregulation during fever and antipyresis. *Brain Research Reviews, 14,* 143–153.

Katcher, A. H., Brightman, V. J., Luborsky, L., & Ship, I. (1973). Prediction of the incidence of recurrent herpes labialis and systemic illness from psychosocial measures. *Journal of Dental Research, 52,* 49–58.

Klastersky, J. (1971). Etude experimentale et clinique des effets favorables et defavorables de la fievre et de l'administration de corticoides au cours d'infections bacteriennes. *Acta Clinica Belgica, 26* (Suppl. 6).

Klein, M. S., Conn, C. A., Kluger, M. J. (1992). Behavioral thermoregulation in mice inoculated with influenza virus. *Physiology and Behavior, 52,* 1133–1139.

Kluger, M. J. (1977) Fever in the frog Hyla cinerea. *Journal of Thermal Biology, 2,* 79–81.

Kluger, M. J. (1978). The evolution and adaptive value of fever. *American Scientist, 66,* 38–43.

Kluger, M. J. (1991). Fever: Role of pyrogens and cryogens. *Physiological Reviews, 71,* 93–127.

Kluger, M. J., O'Reilly, B. O., Shope, T. R., & Vander, A. J. (1987). Further evidence that stress hyperthermia is a fever. *Physiology and Behavior, 39,* 763–766.

Kluger, M. J., O'Reilly, B., & Vander, A. J. (1989). Polymyxin attenuates stress induced hyperthermia. In Lomax and Schonbaum (Eds.), *Thermoregulation: Research and clinical applications, 7th International Symposium of Thermoregulation, Odense, Denmark, 1988* (pp. 171–175). Basel: Karger.

Kluger, M. J., Ringler, D. H., & Anver, M. R. (1975). Fever and survival. *Science, 188,* 166–168.

Kluger, M. J., & Vaughn, L. K. (1982). Fever and survival in rabbits infected with *Pasteurella multocida. Journal of Physiology (London), 282,* 243–251.

Kozak, W. (1993). Fever: A possible strategy for membrane homeostasis during infection. *Perspectives in Biology and Medicine, 37,* 14–34.

Kuhnen, G. (1998). Reduction of fever by housing in small cages. *Laboratory Animals, 32,* 42–45.

Kurosawa, S., Kobune, F., Okuyama, K., & Sugiura, A. (1987). Effects of antipyretics in rinderpest virus infection in rabbits. *Journal of Infectious Diseases, 155,* 991–997.

Kusnecov, A. W., & Rabin, B. S. (1994). Stressor-induced alterations of immune function: Mechanisms and issues. *International Archives of Allergy and Immunology, 105,* 107–121.

Lang, J. W. (1987). Crocodilian thermal selection. In G. J. W. Webb, S. C. Manolis, & P. J. Whitehead (Eds.), *Wildlife Management: Crocodiles and Alligators.* (pp. 301–317) Surrey Beatty and Sons.

LaPerriere, A. R., Antoni, M. H., Schneiderman, N., Ironson, G., Klimas, N., Caralis, P., & Fletcher, M. A. (1990). Exercise intervention attenuates emotional distress and natural killer cell decrements following notification of positive serologic status for HIV-1. *Biofeedback and Self-Regulation, 15*(3), 229–242.

Leon, L. R., Kozak, W., & Kluger, M. J. (1999). An antipyretic role for IL–10 in LPS fever in mice. *American Journal of Physiology, 276,* R81–89.

Linthorst, A. C. E., Flachskamm, C., Hopkins, S. J., Hoadley, M. E., Labeur, M. S., Holsboer, F., & Reul, J. M. H. M. (1997). Long-term intracerebroventricular infusion of corticotropin-releasing hormone alters neuroendocrine, neurochemical, autonomic, behavioral, and cytokine responses to a systemic inflammatory challenge. *Journal of Neuroscience, 17*(11), 4448–4460.

Long, N. C., Kluger, M. J., & Vander, A. J. (1989). Antiserum against mouse IL-1 alpha does not block stress hyperthermia or LPS fever in the rat. In Lomax and Schonbaum (Eds.), *Thermoregulation: Research and clinical Applications, 7th International Symposium of Thermoregulation, Odense, Denmark, 1988* (pp. 78–84). Basel: Karge.

Long, N. C., Morimoto, A., Nakamori, T., & Murakami, N. (1991a). The effect of physical restraint on IL-1β- and LPS-induced fever. *Physiology and Behavior, 50,* 625–628.

Long, N. C., Morimoto, A., Nakamori, T., Yamashiro, O., & Murakami, N. (1991b). Intraperitoneal injections of prostaglandin E_2 attenuate hyperthermia induced by restraint or interleukin-1 in rats. *Journal of Physiology (London), 444,* 363–373.

Louis, C., Jourdan, M., & Cabanac, M. (1986). Behavioral fever and therapy in a rickettsia-infected Orthoptera. *American Journal of Physiology, 250,* R991–R995.

Macknin, M. L., Mathew, S., & Medenforp, S. V. (1990). Effect of inhaling heat vapor on symptoms of the common cold. *Journal of American Medical Association, 264,* 989–991.

Mackowiak, P. A. (1994) Fever: Blessing or curse? A unifying hypothesis. *Annals of International Medicine, 120,* 1037–1040.

Mackowiak, P. A. (1997). *Fever: Basic mechanisms and management (2nd ed.).* Philadelphia: Lippincott-Raven.

Mackowiak, P. A., Browne, R. H., Southern, P. M., Jr., & Smith, J. W. (1980). Polymicrobial sepsis: An analysis of 184 cases using log linear models. *American Journal of Medical Science, 280,* 73–80.

Madden, J. J., Whaley, W. L., & Ketelsen, D. (1998). Opiate binding sites in the cellular immune system: Expression and regulation. *Journal of Neuroimmunology, 83,* 57–62.

Marazziti, D., Di Muro, A., & Castrogiovanni, P. (1992). Psychological stress and body temperature changes in humans. *Physiology and Behavior, 52,* 393–395.

Mayfield, K. P., Kozak, A., Rudolph, K., & Kluger, M. J. (1998). Morphine suppresses development of fever to lipopolysaccharide in rats. *New York Academy of Sciences, 856,* 281–285.

McClain, E., Magnuson, P., & Warner, S. J. (1988). Behavioural fever in a Namibia desert tenebrionid beetle, *Onymacris plana. Journal of Insect Physiology, 34,* 279–284.

Mellon, R. D., & Bayer, B. M. (1998). Evidence for central opioid receptors in the immunomodulatory effects of morphine: Review of potential mechanism(s) of action. *Journal of Neuroimmunology, 83,* 19–28.

Meyer, R. J., & Haggerty, R. J. (1962). Streptococcal infections in families: Factors altering individual susceptibility. *Pediatrics, April,* 539–549.

Monagas, W. R., & Gatten, R. E., Jr. (1983). Behavioural fever in the turtles *Terrapene carolina* and *Chrysemys picta. Journal of Thermal Biology, 8,* 285–288.

Morrow, L. E., McClellan, J. L., Conn, C. A., & Kluger, M. J. (1993). Glucocorticoids alter fever and IL-6 responses to psychological stress and to lipopolysaccharide. *American Journal of Physiology, 264,* R1010–R1016.

Muchlinski, A. E., Stoutenburgh, R. J., & Hogan, J. M. (1989). Fever response in laboratory-maintained and free-ranging chuckwallas (*Sauromalus obesus*). *American Journal of Physiology, 257,* R150–R155.

Muller, C. B., & Schmid-Hempel, P. (1993). Exploitation of cold temperature as defence against parasitoids in bumblebees. *Nature, 363,* 65–67.

Muschenheim, C., Duerschrer, D. R., Hardy, J. D., & Stoll, A. M. (1943). Hypothermia in experimental infections. III. The effect of hypothermia on resistance to experimental pneumococcus infection. *Journal of Infectious Diseases, 72,* 187–196.

Myhre, K. M., Cabanac, M., & Myhre, G. (1977). Fever and behavioural temperature regulation in the frog *Rana esculenta. Acta Physiologica Scandinavia, 101,* 219–229.

Palm, S., Lehzen, S., Mignat, C., Steinmann, J., Leimenstoll, G., & Maier, C. (1998). Does prolonged oral treatment with sustained-release morphine tablets influence immune function? *Anesthesia and Analgesia, 86*(1), 166–172.

Palmblad, J. E. W. (1987). Stress-related modulation of immunity. *Cancer Detection and Prevention, Suppl. 1, 57–64.*

Pembrey, M. S. (1985). The effect of variations in external temperature upon the output of carbonic acid and the temperature of young animals. *Journal of Physiology (London), 18,* 364–379.

Perry, S., Fishman, B., Jacobsberg, L., & Frances, A. (1992). Relationships over 1 year between lymphocyte subsets and psychosocial variables among adults with infection by human immunodeficiency virus. *Archives of General Psychiatry, 49,* 396–401.

Porreca, F., Cowan, A., & Tallarida, R. J. (1981). Time course of antagonism of morphine antinociception by intracerebroventricularly administered naloxone in the rat. *European Journal of Pharmacology, 76,* 55–59.

Provinciali, M., DiStefano, G., Raffaeli, W., Pari, G., Desiderio, F., & Fabris, N. (1991). Evaluation of NK and LAK cell activities in neoplastic patients during treatment with morphine. *International Journal of Neuroscience, 59*(1–3), 127–133.

Renbourn, E. T. (1960). Body temperature and pulse rate in boys and young men prior to sporting contests. A study in emotional hyperthermia: with a review of the literature. *Journal of Psychosomatic Research, 4,* 149–175.

Reyes, T. M., & Coe, C. L. (1997). Prenatal manipulations reduce the prinflammatory response to a cytokine challenge in juvenile monkeys. *Brain Research, 769,* 29–35.

Reynolds, W. W., Casterlin, M. E., & Covert, J. B. (1976). Behavioural fever in teleost fishes. *Nature, 259,* 41–42.

Reynolds, W. W., Casterlin, M. E., & Covert, J. B. (1978). Febrile responses of bluegill (*Lepomis macrochirus*) to bacterial pyrogens. *Journal of Thermal Biology, 3,* 129–130.

Reynolds, W. W., & Covert, J. B. (1978). Febrile responses of goldfish *Carassius auratus* to *Aeromonas hydrophila* and to *Escherichia coli* endotoxin. *Journal of Fish Diseases, 1,* 271–273.

Roberts, N. J., Jr. (1991). Impact of temperature elevation on immunologic defenses. *Review of Infectious Diseases, 13,* 462–472.

Rojavin, M., Szabo, I., Bussiere, J. L., Rogers, T. J., Adler, M. W., & Eisenstein, T. K. (1993) Morphine treatment in vitro or in vivo decreases phagocytic functions of murine macrophages. *Life Sciences, 53,* 997–1006.

Sahs, J. A., Goetz, R., Reddy, M., Rabkin, J. G., Williams, J. B. W., Kertzner, R., & Gorman, J. M. (1994). Psychological distress and natural killer cells in gay men with and without HIV infection. *American Journal of Psychiatry, 151,* 1479–1484.

Satinoff, E., McEwen, G. N., Jr., & Williams, B. A. (1976). Behavioral fever in newborn rabbits. *Science, 193,* 1139–1140.

Schedlowski, M., Jacobs, R., Stratmann, G., Richter, S., Hadicke, A., Tewes, U., Wagner, T. O. F., & Schmidt, R. E. (1993). Changes of natural killer cells during acute psychological stress. *Journal of Clinical Immunology, 13*(2), 119–126.

Sheffield, C. W., Sessler, D. I., & Hunt, T. K. (1994). Mild hypothermia during isoflurane anesthesia decreases resistance to *E. coli* dermal infection in guinea pigs. *Acta Anaesthesiologica Scandinavia, 38,* 201–205.

Sherman, E., Baldwin, L., Fernandez, G., & Deurell, E. (1991) Fever and thermal tolerance in the toad *Bufo marinus. Journal of Thermal Biology, 16,* 297–301.

Sherman, E., & Stephens, A. (1998). Fever and metabolic rate in the toad *Bufo marinus. Journal of Thermal Biology, 23,* 49–52.

Singer, R., Harker, C. T., Vander, A. J., & Kluger, M. J. (1986). Hyperthermia induced by open-field stress is blocked by salicylate. *Physiology and Behavior, 36,* 1179–1182.

Small, P. M., Tauber, M. G., Hackbarth, C. J., & Sande, M. A. (1986). Influence of body temperature on bacterial growth rates in experimental pneumococcal meningitis in rabbits. *Infection and Immunity, 52,* 484–487.

Sohnle, P. G., & Gambert, S. R. (1982). Thermoneutrality: An evolutionary advantage against ageing? *The Lancet,* 1099–1101.

Strouse, S. (1909). Experimental studies on pneumococcus infections. *Journal of Experimental Medicine, 11,* 743–761.

Sweet, C., Cavanagh, D., Collie, M. H., & Smith, H. (1978). Sensitivity to pyrexial temperatures: A factor contributing to the virulence differences between two clones of influenza virus. *British Journal of Experimental Pathology, 59,* 373–380.

Teisner, B., & Haahr, S. (1974). Poikilothermia and susceptibility of suckling mice to Coxsackie B_1 virus. *Nature, 247,* 568.

Toms, G. L., Davies, J. A., Woodward, C. G., Sweet, C., & Smith, H. (1977). The relation of pyrexia and nasal inflammatory response to virus levels in nasal washings of ferrets infected with influenza viruses of differing virulence. *British Journal of Experimental Pathology, 58*, 444–458.

Tubaro, E., Borelli, G., Croce, C., Cavallo, G., & Santiangeli, C. (1983). Effect of morphine on resistance to infection. *Journal of Infectious Diseases, 148*(4), 656–666.

Van Miert, A. S. J. P. A. M., Van Duin, C. Th., Busser, F. J. M., Perie, N., Van Den Ingh, T. S. G. A. M., & Neys-Backers, M. H. H. (1978). The effect of flurbiprofen, a potent non-steroidal anti-inflammatory agent, upon *Trypansosoma vivax* infection in goats. *Journal of Veterinary Pharmacology and Therapeutics, 1*, 69–76.

Vaughn, L. K., Bernheim, H. A., & Kluger, M. J. (1974). Fever in the lizard *Dipsosaurus dorsalis. Nature, 252*, 473–474.

Vaughn, L. K., Veale, W. L., & Cooper, K. E. (1980). Antipyresis: Its effect on mortality rate of bacterially infected rabbits. *Brain Research Bulletin, 5*, 69–73.

Vaughn, L. K., Veale, W. L., & Cooper, K. E. (1987). The effect of venous blood stream cooling on survival of bacterially infected rabbits. *Pflugers Arch, 409*, 635–637.

Wang, W-C., Goldman, L. M., Schleider, D. M., Appenheimer, M. M., Subjeck, J. R., Repasky, E. A., & Evans, S. S. (1998). Fever-range hyperthermia enhances L-selectin-dependent adhesion of lymphocytes to vascular endothelium. *Journal of Immunology, 160*, 961–969.

Warren, S., Greenhill, S., & Warren, K. G. (1982). Emotional stress and the development of multiple sclerosis: Case-control evidence of a relationship. *Journal of Chronic Diseases, 35*, 821–831.

Warren, S., Warren, K. G., & Cockerill, R. (1991). Emotional stress and coping in multiple sclerosis (MS) exacerbations. *Journal of Psychosomatic Research, 35*(1), 37–47.

Watson, S. W., Guenther, R. W., & Rucker, R. R. (1954). A virus disease of sockeye salmon: Interim Report. *US Fisheries and Wildlife Services Science Report Fish, 138*, 36.

Weinstein, M. P., Iannin, P. B., Stratton, C. W., & Eickhoff, T. C. (1978). Spontaneous bacterial peritonitis. A review of 28 cases with emphasis on improved survival and factors influencing prognosis. *American Journal of Medicine, 64*, 592–598.

Wood, S. C., & Malvin, G. M. (1992). Behavioral hypothermia: an adaptive stress response. In S. C. Wood, A. R. Hargens, R. W. Millard & R. Weber (Eds). *Strategies of physiological adaptation: Respiration, circulation and metabolism* (pp. 295–314). New York: Dekker, Inc.

Yeager, M. P., Colacchio, T. A., Yu, C. T., Hildebrandt, L., Howell, A. L., Weiss, J., & Guyre, P. M. (1995). Morphine inhibits spontaneous and cytokine-enhanced natural killer cell cytotoxicity in volunteers. *Anesthesia, 83*(3), 500–508.

Yerushalmi, A., & Lwoff, A. (1980). Traitement du coryza infectieux et des rhinites persistantes allergiques pra la thermotherapie. *Comptes Rendus Seances de l' Academie des Sciences D, 291*(12), 957–959.

C H A P T E R

28

Cytokine Effects on Behavior

ROBERT DANTZER, ROSE-MARIE BLUTHÉ, NATHALIE CASTANON, NATHALIE CHAUVET, LUCILE CAPURON, GLYN GOODALL, KEITH W. KELLEY, JAN-PETER KONSMAN, SOPHIE LAYÉ, PATRICIA PARNET, FLORENCE POUSSET

I. INTRODUCTION

Sickness is a common if not trivial experience, especially during the course of an infectious process. At the behavioral level, a sick individual typically displays depressed activity and little or no interest in the environment. Body care activities are usually absent and ingestive behavior is profoundly depressed despite the increased metabolism that is necessary for the fever response. At the subjective level, a sick person experiences malaise, fatigue, and apathy and sometimes mental confusion. Since the initial demonstration in the late 1980s that the symptoms of sickness are induced in healthy subjects by peripheral and central injection of the proinflammatory cytokines that are released by activated monocytes and macrophages during the host response to infection (Dantzer & Kelley, 1989), the mechanisms of cytokine-induced sickness behavior have been the subject of intense research, carried out at several levels of investigation. The purpose of the present chapter is to review the results that have been obtained in this field during the past decade. At the behavioral level, there is now clear evidence showing that cytokine-induced sickness behavior is not the result of weakness and physical debilitation affecting the sick individual, but the expression of a central motivational state that reorganizes the organism's priorities in order to cope with infectious microorganisms. At the organ level, this motivational aspect of sickness behavior is important since it implies that the endogenous signals of sickness act on the brain to activate neural structures that are at the origin of the subjective, behavioral, and physiological components of sickness. Cytokine receptors are present in the brain, and they are activated not by peripheral cytokines entering the brain, but by cytokines that are produced locally in the brain in response to peripheral cytokines. At the cellular level, there is still some uncertainty concerning the identification of the exact cell types that are the source of cytokines in the brain, and those that are the targets of brain-released cytokines. At the molecular level, the cytokines that are behaviorally active and the receptor mechanisms that mediate their effects are not yet fully understood. Because sickness behavior dissipates gradually during recovery, it has been proposed that the production and effects of cytokines are opposed by endogenous regulatory factors. These factors have been termed cryogens, by analogy with pyrogens, and they include a wide variety of bioactive molecules, from glucocorticoids to anti-inflammatory cytokines. However, their exact mechanisms of action have not yet been fully elucidated.

II. THE CYTOKINE NETWORK

The main proinflammatory cytokines that are responsible for the initial host response to infection are interleukin-1 (IL-1), interleukin-6 (IL-6), and tumor necrosis factor-α (TNF-α) (Nicola, 1994). At the periphery, these cytokines are synthesized and released by activated monocytes and macrophages and play a pivotal role in inflammation. A convenient way of inducing the expression of these cytokines in healthy subjects is to inject lipopolysaccharide (LPS), the active fragment of endotoxin from Gram-negative bacteria. LPS activates macrophages and monocytes by binding to the CD14 receptor.

Although the biological actions of proinflammatory cytokines widely overlap, each cytokine has its own characteristic properties. IL-1 can be considered as a prototypical proinflammatory cytokine (Dinarello, 1996). It exists in two molecular forms, IL-1α and IL-1β, which are encoded by two different genes. Another member of the IL-1 family is the IL-1 receptor antagonist (IL-1ra). This last cytokine behaves as a pure endogenous antagonist of IL-1 receptors and blocks most biological effects of IL-1α and IL-1β in vitro and in vivo. IL-6 is mainly responsible for the synthesis of acute phase proteins by hepatocytes. TNF-α plays a major role in the pathogenesis of the septic shock syndrome.

IL-1 binds to two types of receptors belonging to the immunoglobulin superfamily and representing two separate gene products. The type I IL-1 receptor transduces the signal to the cell nucleus via the activation of the nuclear transcription factor NFκB. This results in the activation of several genes, including the genes for the inducible form of the nitric oxide synthase (iNOS) and the inducible form of cyclooxygenase (COX-2). In contrast, the type II IL-1 receptor does not transduce the signal and certainly functions as a "decoy" receptor that binds the excess of IL-1 to downregulate its actions. The ability of the type I IL-1 receptor to transduce a signal is dependent on the formation of an heterodimeric complex with an IL-1 receptor accessory protein (IL-1R AcP). IL-1ra behaves as an antagonist of IL-1 receptors by preventing the formation of this complex after binding to the type I IL-1 receptor.

III. BEHAVIORAL EFFECTS OF CYTOKINES

A. Human Studies

The recourse to interferon-α (IFN-α) and IL-2 as immunomodulator agents for the medical treatment of malignancies and chronic viral infection is plagued by many adverse effects, including neurotoxicity. Cytokine therapy is associated with the development of cognitive and psychiatric disorders that range from subtle impairment of attention and everyday memory undetectable on routine medical evaluation to frank delirium and psychosis (Meyers, 1999). Depressive symptoms induced by cytokine immunotherapy include dysphoria, anhedonia, and helplessness in addition to constitutional symptoms of fatigue, apathy, and mental slowing. Guilt, delusions, and suicidal ideation are rarely encountered. Although it is not easy to separate the effects of cytokines on the mood of cancer patients from other factors that might precipitate depression in these patients, the fact that depressive symptoms spontaneously regress when the treatment is interrupted provides good evidence for a causal role of cytokines. Since cytokine therapy is still experimental, there are not many examples of controlled clinical trials with cytokines in cancer patients. However, a recent study on patients with advanced colorectal cancer revealed that compared to chemotherapy alone, immunotherapy resulted in reduced energy, impaired confidence, higher depressed mood and more confusion (Walker et al., 1997).

The time course of the development of depressive symptoms in response of cancer patients to cytokine therapy, and the associated risk factors, have been assessed in recent studies. IL-2, administered alone or in combination with INF-α, was found to induce the rapid development of depressive symptoms (Capuron, Ravaud, & Dantzer, 2000). The depressive effects of IFN-α developed only after several weeks of treatment, and they were a positive function of the patient's initial mood in the sense that patients with a relatively elevated score on a psychological scale of depressed mood were more likely to develop high depression scores in response to the treatment than patients with low initial scores (Capuron & Ravaud, 1999). It is worth noting that in a case-report study, the antidepressant drug nortriptyline was found to improve INF-α-induced depressed mood that developed 1 month after the initiation of cytokine treatment in a patient diagnosed with chronic active hepatitis C (Goldman, 1994).

The effects of cytokines other than IL-2 and IFN-α on behavior, affect, and cognition have been less well studied. Acute administration of a low dose of IL-6 in the evening to healthy young men induced tiredness and feelings of being inactive and less capable of concentrating (Späth-Schwalbe et al., 1998). Endotoxin administered during the daytime induced subjective sleepiness (Hermann et al., 1998). In seven drug-free severely depressed patients, administration of a low dose of LPS significantly improved mood on the next day following the treatment but this effect was transient and dissipated during the next days (Bauer et al., 1995).

B. Animal Studies

Peripheral and central administration of IL-1α, IL-1β, and TNF-α to healthy laboratory animals induce fever (Kluger, 1991), activation of the hypothalamo-pituitary-adrenal axis (Besedovsky, del Rey, Sorkin, & Dinarello, 1986), and behavioral symptoms of sickness (Kent, Bluthé, Kelley, & Dantzer, 1992b). Depressed activity and apathy are commonly observed, together with decreases in food intake and the adoption of a curled posture. The two behavioral endpoints that have been mostly used to investigate the mechanisms of cytokine-induced sickness behavior are social exploration and food intake. In the first case, the effects of cytokines are assessed by measuring changes in the duration of exploration of a conspecific juvenile that is temporarily introduced into the home cage of the animal under test. This social stimulus normally induces a full sequence of close following and olfactory investigation that is profoundly depressed in a time- and dose-dependent manner in mice and rats injected with LPS and recombinant proinflammatory cytokines (Kent et al., 1992b).

Changes in ingestive behavior that develop in sick animals can be measured by the disruption of food intake in animals provided with free food or the decrease in operant responding in animals trained to press a lever or to poke their nose in a hole for a food reward (Kent, Bret-Dibat, Kelley, & Dantzer, 1996; Plata-Salaman, 1995, 1997). In both cases, LPS and recombinant proinflammatory cytokines have profound depressive effects on ingestive behavior whether injected peripherally or centrally. Anorexigenic cytokines include IL-1, IL-6, IL-8, TNF-α, and IFN-α. Based on computerized analysis of meal pattern, IL-1β at relatively low doses reduced meal size and meal duration and decreased feeding rate. Higher doses of IL-1β also decreased meal frequency and prolonged intermeal intervals (Plata-Salaman, 1999). In contrast, IFN-α induced anorexia by reducing meal size and meal duration but had no effect on meal frequency. In terms of macronutrient intake, rats treated by LPS or IL-1β have been found to decrease their caloric intake, but to ingest relatively more carbohydrate and less protein, while keeping their fat intake constant (Aubert, Goodall, & Dantzer, 1995). This pattern of macronutrient differs from what is observed in rats exposed to cold, which increase their caloric intake mainly by consuming more fat. This difference between cytokine-treated rats and cold-exposed rats is congruent with the metabolic consequences of the cytokine treatment. Cytokines impair lipid metabolism by decreasing lipoprotein lipase activity and lipolysis (Grunfeld & Feingold, 1996). They also increase glycogenolysis and glucose oxidation and utilization and enhance protein breakdown and synthesis of acute-phase proteins (Spurlock, 1997).

It is important to note that decreased behavioral activities are not always observed in cytokine-treated animals. For instance, IL-2 and IL-6 can have behavioral activating effects in mice, in the form of an increase in digging, rearing, exploration of a new object, and, for IL-6, locomotion and grooming (Zalcman, Murray, Dyck, Greenberg, & Nance, 1998).

During the recent years, there has been a surge of interest for the investigation of a possible role of cytokines in the pathophysiology of depression (Maes, Smith, & Scharpe, 1995; Dantzer, Wollman, & Yirimiya, 1999). In the forced swimming test, a preclinical test of depression used to screen antidepressants drugs, human interferons increased the immobility time in a dose-dependent manner (Makino, Kitano, Hirohashi, & Takasuna, 1998). This activity was not shared by natural interferon-β nor by recombinant interferon-γ 1a and was inhibited by treatment with the anti-depressants imipramine and mianserin. To avoid possible biases related to the behaviorally depressing effects of cytokines, a few experimental studies have concentrated on the possible relationship between the behavioral effects of cytokines and anhedonia. Anhedonia refers to the inability to experience pleasure and is operationally defined by a decreased preference for sweet solutions, an attenuated responding for rewarding intracranial self-stimulation, and an impairment of sexual behavior (Yirmiya, 1997). LPS administration decreased free consumption of saccharin but not water in nondeprived rats, and attenuated the preference for saccharin in fluid-deprived rats (Yirmiya, 1996). This effect was attenuated by chronic but not acute treatment with imipramine. Similar depressing effects of LPS treatment were observed on intake of sweetened milk (Swiergel, Smagin, & Dunn,1996; Swiergel, Smagin, Johnson, & Dunn, 1997). LPS and IL-2 decreased responding for rewarding lateral hypothalamic stimulation, but IL-1β and IL-6 had no effect (Anisman, Kokkinidis, Borowski, & Merali, 1998). Intracerebroventicular administration of IL-2 decreased self-stimulation from the dorsal and ventral aspects of the ventral tegmental area, but had no effect on self-stimulation from the ventral A10 area, indicating that the anhedonic effects of IL-2 are certainly not homogenous across different reward systems (Hebb, Zacharko, & Anisman, 1998). Although the previously described effects of cytokines on self-stimulation were obtained at pharmacological doses, they could be relevant to more physiological conditions of immune activation, as antigenic challenge of rats with sheep red blood cells attenuated intracranial self-stimulation from the nucleus accumbens at times that approximated the peak of immune response (Zacharko et al., 1997). Sexual behavior was also disrupted by systemic administration of LPS and IL-1β, and this effect was more marked in female than in male rats (Avitsur, Pollak, & Yirmiya, 1997b; Avitsur, Cohen, & Yirmiya, 1998). All components of sexual behavior were affected, including sexual motivation, proceptive behavior (soliciting), receptivity, and attractivity.

The possibility that proinflammatory cytokines have anxiogenic effects has been investigated using various tests of anxiety (Anisman & Merali, 1999). In the elevated plus-maze, mice treated with LPS displayed a reduced frequency of open-arm visits, whereas visits to the closed arms were unaffected. Similarly, in the light–dark box, LPS increased the tendency to avoid the illuminated region. These behavioral alterations were not due to motor deficiency since LPS-treated mice escaped very quickly the open arms and the illuminated compartment when they were directly exposed to them. Acute administration of IL-2 had no obvious anxiogenic effect, whereas chronic IL-2 attenuated exploration. IL-1β had anxiogenic effects at low doses when injected either systemically or centrally, whereas these effects were replaced by a general depression of activity at higher doses. The same effects as those obtained with low doses of IL-1β were observed with TNF-α. Increased levels of anxiety-like behavior in the elevated plus-maze were also observed in mice infected orally with the Gram-negative pathogen *Campylobacter jejuni* at a dose that induced a subclinical infection but no immune activation, at least based on circulating IL-6 levels (Lyte, Varcoe, & Bailey, 1998).

Since cytokine treatment in human subjects can cause mental confusion, the possibility that cytokines alter cognition has been investigated in various learning and memory paradigms. LPS and IL-1β administration were found to impair performance in various learning tasks, including autoshaping (Aubert, Vega, Dantzer, & Goodall, 1995) and spatial learning in the radial arm maze and the Morris water maze (Gibertini, 1996; Gibertini, Newton, Friedman, & Klein, 1995; Oitzl, van Oers, Schobitz, & de Kloet, 1993). Gibertini (1998) investigated the critical factors for the IL-1-induced impairment in spatial learning in a series of experiments carried out with female mice. He showed that the impairing effect of IL-1β on learning of the Morris water maze disappeared when mice were subjected to a spaced as opposed to a massed learning protocol, when mice were tested in a cold-water maze as opposed to a warm-water maze and when higher doses of IL-1β were administered.

The effect of IL-1 on learning has been tentatively related to the ability of this cytokine to inhibit long-term potentiation in the hippocampus. Since neurodegeneration and aging are associated with increased levels of brain IL-1β, Murray and Lynch (1998) tried to relate increased levels of IL-1β in the hippocampus to impaired long-term potentiation. Using aged rats, stressed rats, and rats pretreated with IL-1β, they observed an inverse relationship between concentrations of IL-1β in the dentate gyrus and long-term potentiation in the pathway running from perforant path to granule cell synapses.

In a fear conditioning task, LPS administered after conditioning impaired contextual but not auditory-cue fear conditioning (Pugh et al., 1998). Preexposure to the context eliminated the effects of LPS on contextual fear conditioning, and in addition, LPS given after context preexposure negated the beneficial effect of preexposure on contextual fear. These results suggest that LPS disrupts posttrial memory consolidation processes. Repeated central administration of IL-2 to rats disrupted performance in a Morris water maze (Hanisch & Quirion, 1996). Repeated systemic administration of IL-2 to mice disrupted performance in this spatial learning test only when the position of the safe platform varied over days, so that mice had to learn a new strategy every day (Anisman & Merali, 1999). Interestingly, IL-2-treated mice did not differ from saline-treated mice on the first trial of each daily session, indicating that IL-2 did not alter the ability to swim and employ a search strategy to find the platform. The difference between the two groups was that saline-treated mice showed marked between-trial improvement, whereas IL-2-treated mice did not.

Mice overexpressing or not expressing a cytokine or the receptor of a cytokine have been used to assess the way cytokines affect brain function. Mice overexpressing proinflammatory cytokines in astrocytes or in neurons often develop severe neuropathological alterations (Campbell, 1998), which make the study of behavioral activities not very pertinent, except when focusing on early signs of disease progression. Mice in which the gene for a given proinflammatory cytokine or its receptors has been deleted by homologous recombination do not show any obvious behavioral alterations, which is in agreement with the redundancy characterizing the biological activity of these molecules. However, subtle behavioral alterations can sometimes be observed. For example, IL-6 knockout mice were found to display a higher degree of aggressive behavior and a lower frequency of affiliative interactions (Alleva et al., 1998). Although the results of behavioral observations in knockout mice are not easy to interpret due to the fact that the expressed phenotype varies according to the genetic background, the fact that in this study mice overexpressing IL-6 specifically in the central nervous system displayed more intense affiliative interactions than their wild-type counterparts can be interpreted to suggest that IL-6 might be involved in the regulation of agonistic behavior. In a different experiment controlling for the effect of the genetic background, IL-6($-/-$) mice were observed to be less emotional than wild-type mice in the holeboard and the elevated plus-maze, suggesting that IL-6 is involved in the control of emotionality (Armario, Hernandez, Bluethmann, & Hidalgo, 1998). Mice overexpressing TNF-α in the neurons of the central nervous system displayed alterations of exploration in the holeboard and black/white box and increased grooming when exposed to highly unfamiliar environmental stimuli (Fiore et al., 1998).

Because of the redundancy in the biological actions of most proinflammatory cytokines, the injection of a given cytokine in association with another cytokine usually results in potentiation and even sensitization. As a typical example, the combined administration of a behaviorally inactive dose of IL-1β and an inactive dose of TNF-α significantly depressed social exploration (Bluthé et al., 1994). For the same reason, animals with a sustained chronic inflammatory state respond in an exaggerated manner to the behaviorally depressing effects of proinflammatory cytokines. This is the case, for example, for cerebellar mutant mice. These animals develop a cerebellar atrophy that is associated with a chronic inflammatory state both at the periphery and in the brain. Cerebellar mutant mice were found to be more sensitive to the behaviorally depressing effects of intraperitoneal (ip) and intracerebroventricular (icv) administration of LPS and IL-1β (Bluthé, Michaud, Delhaye-Bouchaud, Mariani, & Dantzer, 1997). A similar increased sensitivity to the behavioral effects of IL-1β was observed in prediabetic nonobese diabetic mice (Bluthé et al., 1999).

IV. SICKNESS BEHAVIOR AS THE EXPRESSION OF A CENTRAL MOTIVATIONAL STATE

Most of the symptoms of cytokine-induced sickness behavior resemble the expression of physical debilitation and general weakness. During an infection episode, sick individuals usually remain prostrated and engage in little physical activity. However, this interpretation is not tenable (Figure 1). Hart (1988) has convincingly argued that sickness behavior supports the metabolic and physiological changes occurring in the infected organism and increases their efficiency. The reduced behavioral activities that occur in ill individuals would therefore be the expression of a highly organized strategy that is critical to the survival of the organism. A typical example of such a reorganization of behavioral activities is provided by the effect of IL-1 on agonistic behavior in mice. When confronted by an adult conspecific, mice typically engage in offensive behavioral patterns, and this phase of attack is followed by defensive behavior if they are likely to lose the fight. In contrast, IL-1-treated mice displayed no offensive behavioral elements, but still responded to the opponent's attacks with defensive elements such as upright defensive posture, upright submissive posture, crouching, and fleeing (Cirulli, De Acetis, & Alleva, 1998). This reorganization of behavioral activities under the influence of proinflammatory cytokines is characteristic of what psychologists call motivational changes. A motivation can be defined as a central state that reorganizes perception and action (Bolles, 1970). In the case of fear, for instance, the individual confronted with a threat focuses his attention on all potential sources of danger and, at

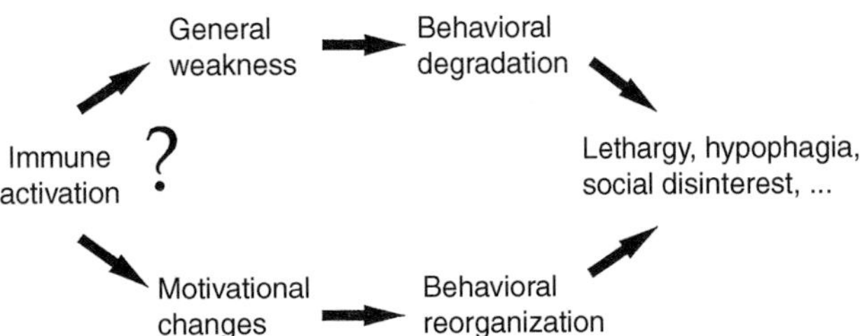

FIGURE 1 The behavioral symptoms of sickness that develop during an infectious episode can be the result of physical debilitation and weakness (upper pathway) or the expression of a reorganization of the organism's priorities in face of the pathogen challenge (lower pathway). The evidence collected during the recent years supports this last interpretation.

the same time, gets ready to engage in the most appropriate defensive behavioral pattern that is available in his behavioral repertoire. In other words, a motivational state does not trigger an inflexible behavioral pattern in response to an internal or external stimulus. Instead, it enables the uncoupling of perception from action and, therefore, selection of the appropriate strategy in relation to the eliciting situation (Bolles, 1970).

The first evidence that sickness behavior is the expression of a motivational state rather than the consequence of weakness was provided by Miller in a review paper (Miller, 1964). While he was initially searching for endogenous signals of the thirst motivational system, Miller observed that endotoxin administration made rats stop bar pressing for water. However, this motivational effect was not specific to thirst since the same endotoxin treatment also reduced bar pressing for food and for intracranial self-stimulation in the lateral hypothalamus. This decrease in response rate was not generalized since rats placed in a rotating drum that they could stop for brief periods by pressing a lever, increased their bar pressing rate in response to endotoxin instead of decreasing it. The mere fact that endotoxin treatment decreased or increased behavioral output depending on its consequences was for Miller a strong indication in favour of a motivational effect of this treatment.

An important characteristic of a motivational state is that it competes with other motivational states for behavioral output. As a typical example, it is difficult if not impossible to search for food and at the same time court a sexual partner, as the behavioral patterns of foraging and courtship are not compatible with each other. The normal expression of behavior therefore requires a hierarchical structure of motivational states which is continuously updated according to variations in the external and internal milieux. When an infection occurs, the sick individual is at a life-or-death juncture and he needs to adjust his physiology and behavior so as to overcome the disease. However, this is a relatively long-term process which must make room for more urgent needs when necessary. If a sick person lying in his bed hears a fire alarm ringing in his house and sees flames and smoke coming out of the basement, he must be able to momentarily overcome his sickness behavior to escape danger. Translated into motivational terms, this means that fear competes with sickness, and fear-motivated behavior takes precedence over sickness behavior.

To show that sickness does not interfere with the subject's ability to adjust his behavioral strategies with regard to his needs and capacities, Aubert and colleagues (Aubert, Kelley, & Dantzer, 1997) assessed the effects of LPS on food hoarding and food consumption in rats receiving or not a food supplement in addition to the amount of food they obtained in the situation. Briefly, rats were trained to get food for 30 min in an apparatus consisting of a cage connected to an alley with free food at its end. In this apparatus, rats normally bring back to their home cage the food that is available at the end of the alley, and the amount of food they hoard is lower when they receive a food supplement than when they have no supplement. In response to LPS, food intake was decreased to the same extent whether rats received a food supplement or not. However, food hoarding was less affected in rats that did not receive a food supplement compared to rats provided with the food supplement. These results are important because they indicate that the internal state of sickness induced by LPS is more effective in suppressing the immediate response to food than the anticipatory response to future needs.

Another example of the motivational aspects of sickness behavior is provided by a study of the effects of cytokines on maternal behavior. Rat and mouse neonates are poikilotherm, and they need the thermoregulatory protection of a nest. Maternal behavior is therefore critical for the survival of the progeny. In accordance with the motivational priority of maternal behavior, lactating mice that were made sick by an appropriate dose of LPS were still able to retrieve their pups which had been removed from the nest, but did not engage in nest building when tested at 24°C. However, when the dams and their litters were placed at 6°C to increase the survival value of nest building, this last behavior was no longer impaired (Figure 2) (Aubert, Goodall, Dantzer, & Gheusi, 1997).

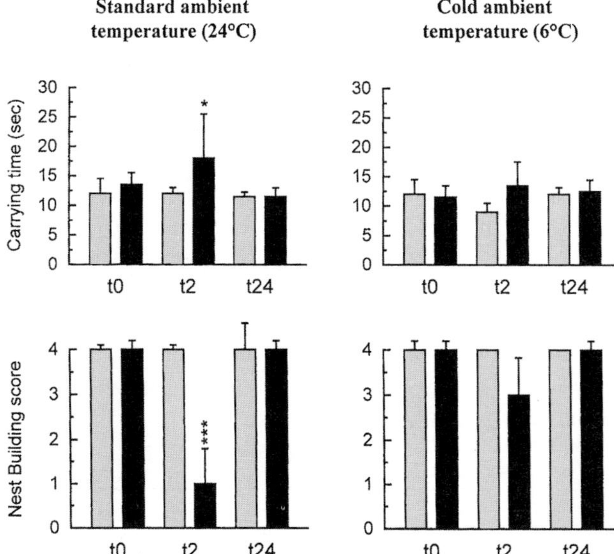

FIGURE 2 Interactions between LPS-induced sickness behavior and maternal behavior in lactating mice. Lactating mice were injected with LPS (400 µg/kg, ip) (black columns) or apyrogenic saline (grey columns) at time 0 (t0). Two and 24 h later, their nest was removed and they were given surgical cotton to build another nest. Then their pups were removed and aligned along the wall on the opposite side from the nest. Dependent variables were the time needed to retrieve all the pups and the quality of the nest built by the dam (from 1, no nest, to 4, fully enclosed nest). * $p < .05$, *** $p < .001$ compared with saline (from Aubert et al., 1997a).

V. MODES OF ACTION OF CYTOKINES ON THE BRAIN

The fact that sickness is a central motivational state implies that the endogenous signals of sickness act on the brain. However, cytokines are relatively large protein molecules, about 15 kDa for IL-1, and their hydrophilic nature does not allow them to easily cross the blood-brain barrier. It has therefore been proposed that cytokines, like many other centrally acting peptides, enter the brain at the sites at which the blood-brain barrier is deficient. These privileged sites for communication with the internal milieu are known as the circumventricular organs, because of their anatomical location around the brain ventricles. Based on results of lesion and knife-cut experiments, the organum vasculosum of the lamina terminalis (OVLT) has long been considered as the site of action of peripherally released cytokines (Blatteis, 1990). Blood-borne cytokines were initially assumed to diffuse into the brain side of the blood-brain barrier through fenestrated capillaries, and act on parenchymal astrocytes to induce the synthesis and release of prostaglandins of the E2 series. Prostaglandins then would freely diffuse to nearby target brain areas, such as the median preoptic area of the hypothalamus in the case of fever. However, there are at least two problems with this proposed mechanism. First, most cytokines have a very limited range of diffusion and are more tuned to act locally in an autocrine and paracrine manner than to act at distance in an hormonal manner. Second, fully functional cytokine receptors are expressed in the brain (see below), and they mediate the effects of peripherally released or exogenously injected cytokines. For example, blockade of brain IL-1 receptors has been found to abrogate the effects of peripheral immune stimuli on behavior (Kent et al., 1992a), corticotropin-releasing hormone gene expression in the hypothalamus (Kakucska, Qi, Clark, & Lechan, 1993), and body temperature (Klir, McClellan, & Kluger, 1994). The simplest interpretation for these findings is that cytokines are actively transported into the brain, as proposed for other peptides. For example, insulin enters the brain by a receptor-mediated, saturable transport process across brain capillary endothelial cells (Baura et al., 1993; Wu, Yang, & Pardridge, 1997). Pharmacokinetic data with radiolabeled cytokines have revealed the existence of specific saturable transport systems for a number of proinflammatory cytokines (Banks, Ortiz, Plotkin, & Kastin, 1991). In the case of insulin, the transporter is nothing other than the insulin receptor. However, the molecular identity of cytokine transporters is still unknown. In addition, the existence of a transport system is not sufficient to explain how peripheral cytokines act on the brain. There is still the problem that in order to be transported, cytokines need to be present in the general blood circulation, or synthesized and released close to their transporter systems. Furthermore, the help of a transport process is apparently not necessary for peripheral cytokines to enter the brain, since independent experiments have provided evidence for the existence of a brain compartment of cytokines that is inducible by peripheral cytokines (Figure 3) (Gatti & Bartfai, 1993; Layé, Parnet, Goujon, & Dantzer, 1994).

Systemic administration of LPS induces the coordinated expression of IL-1β, TNF-α, IL-6, and IL-1ra in various brain structures at the mRNA and protein levels (Gatti & Bartfai, 1993; Layé, Parnet, Goujon, & Dantzer, 1994). The same effect is obtained when IL-1β is injected in place of LPS (Hansen, Taishi, Chen, & Krueger, 1998), which is consistent with the concept that IL-1β induces its own synthesis and the synthesis of other cytokines in cascade. The same cascade of cytokines can be activated when LPS or proinflammatory cytokines are injected directly into the lateral ventricle of the brain (Plata-Salaman, 1999).

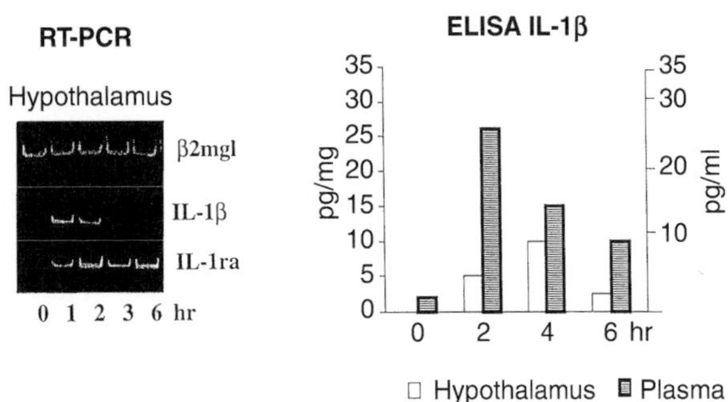

FIGURE 3 Systemic administration of LPS induces the expression of IL-1β and IL-1ra in the brain of mice. Mice were injected intraperitoneally with LPS (10 µg/mouse) and killed just before or at different times after injection. Total RNA was extracted from the hypothalamus and submitted to comparative RT-PCR to determine transcripts for IL-1β and IL-1ra, using β2-microglobulin (β2mgl) as an internal standard. Levels of IL-1β were measured in the hypothalamus (pg/mg protein) and plasma (pg/ml) using a validated ELISA (mean of five different experiments).

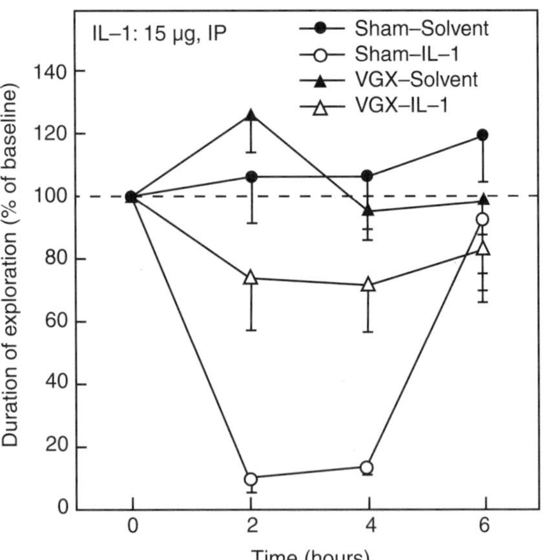

FIGURE 4 Vagotomy attenuates the depressing effects of systemic IL-1β on social exploration of a juvenile conspecific introduced into the home cage of the test animal. The experiment was carried out on rats that had been submitted to vagotomy (VGX) or sham surgery (sham) 4 weeks before the test. Solvent or recombinant rat IL-1β (15 µg/rat) was injected ip immediately after the first behavioral session that took place at time 0 (baseline), and the same animals were tested again with different juveniles 2, 4, and 6 h later ($n = 5$ for each experimental group). Duration of exploration was expressed as percentage of baseline (81 to 100 s for 4 min of test) (from Bluhté et al., 1996b).

In order to produce cytokines in a coordinated manner in response to peripheral cytokines, brain cells need a communication pathway for transmission of immune information from the periphery to the brain (Dantzer, 1994). As proposed by Kent and colleagues (Kent et al., 1992), neural afferents are good candidates for this role, since they already transmit the two sensory components of inflammation, *calor* and *dolor* (heat and pain). When LPS or cytokines are injected into the abdominal cavity, an inflammatory response develops locally. The main afferent pathway from the abdominal cavity to the brain is the vagus nerve. The role of vagus nerves in the transmission of the immune information from the periphery to the brain has first been demonstrated based on *c-fos* mapping experiments. The immediate–early gene *c-fos* is differentially expressed in many regions of the central nervous system following various physiological challenges and can be used as a marker of neuronal activation. Intraperitoneal administration of LPS to rats induced the expression of Fos, the protein product of the *c-fos* gene, in the primary and secondary projections areas of the vagus nerve. This labeling was completely abrogated by subdiaphragmatic section of the vagus nerves (Wan, Wetmore, Sorensen, Greenberg, & Nance, 1994). Vagotomy also blocked the depressing effects of LPS and IL-1β on behavior in rats and mice (Figure 4) (Bluthé et al., 1994; Bret-Dibat, Bluthé, Kent, Kelley, & Dantzer, 1995). This protecting effect of vagotomy was not due to an impaired peripheral immune response since vagotomy had no effect on the increases in the levels of IL-1β that were induced in peritoneal macrophages and plasma in response to an intraperitoneal injection of LPS (Bluthé et al., 1994; Layé et al., 1995). The involvement of the vagus nerves in the behavioral effects of cytokines is specific to cytokines that are released in the abdominal cavity and sensed by afferent vagal terminals since vagotomy did not block sickness behavior induced by subcutaneous and intravenous injections of IL-1β (Bluthé, Michaud, Kelley & Dantzer, 1996a) and had no effect on sickness behavior induced by central injection of IL-1β (Figure 5) (Bluthé, Michaud, Kelley, & Dantzer, 1996b).

According to the hypothesis of a neural transmission pathway of immune signals from the periphery to the brain, the sectioning of vagal afferents should abrogate the induction of brain cytokines in response to intraperitoneal administration of LPS and IL-1β. In accordance with this prediction, vagotomy abrogated LPS- and IL-1β-induced increases in IL-1β mRNA in the hypothalamus and hippocampus but not in the pituitary (Layé et al., 1995; Hansen et al., 1998).

The involvement of vagal afferents in the transmission of information from the peripheral cytokine

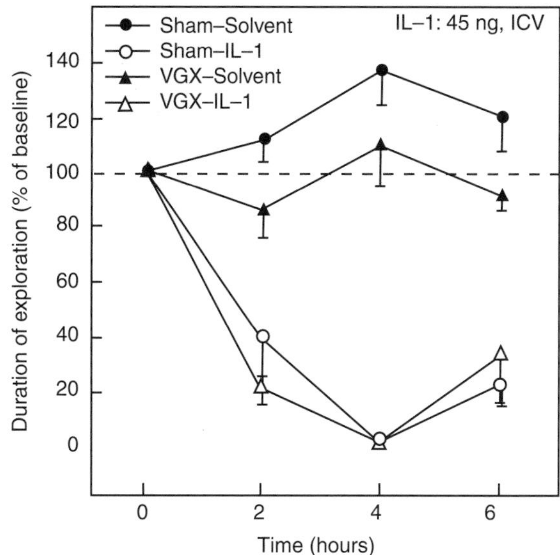

FIGURE 5 Vagotomy does not block the depressing effect of icv IL-1β on social exploration. Solvent or recombinant rat IL-1β (45 ng/rat) was injected icv immediately after the first behavioral session that took place at time 0 (baseline). Same conventions as in Fig. 4 ($n = 5$ for each experimental group). Baseline values varied from 96 to 127 s for 4 min of test) (from Bluthé et al., 1996b).

compartment to the brain is not restricted to the behavioral effects of cytokines, since vagotomy also attenuated LPS-induced hyperalgesia and LPS-induced fever and increase in plasma ACTH levels (Watkins, Maier, & Goehler, 1995).

A potential problem with all these experiments is that the vagotomy procedure eliminates vagal afferent as well as efferent fibers. Furthermore, the vagotomy surgical procedure often includes stripping the oesophagus from all its nerves, which is likely to remove nonvagal, myenteric nerve fibers that are at the origin of the splanchnic visceral nerves. Although surgical transection of the celiac superior mesetenric complex failed to attenuate the hyperalgic effects of LPS in contrast to section of the vagus nerves (Watkins et al., 1995), the effects of this surgical manipulation on the inhibitory effects of LPS and IL-1β on behavior have received little attention. In the only experiment that specifically addressed the question of the role of vagal afferents in the behavioral effects of cytokines, selective vagal rootlet deafferentation of the left vagus nerve associated with subdiapragmatic section of the right vagus nerve did not alter the feeding-suppressive effects of LPS and IL-1β in rats (Schwartz, Plata-Salaman, & Langhans, 1997). Negative results were also obtained when vagal deafferentation was combined with celiac superior mesenteric ganglionectomy (Porter, Hrupka, Langhans, & Schwartz, 1998). However, in the absence of a positive control for the effects of conventional vagotomy on the action of LPS and IL-1β, these last results are difficult to interpret.

In conclusion, the results of neuroanatomy and vagotomy experiments support the hypothesis that vagal afferents transmit the immune message from the abdominal cavity to the brain. The likely involvement of other neural afferent fibers in the transmission of the immune message originating from other bodily sites, such as the derm, remains to be demonstrated. In the same way, it is still necessary to determine the relative contribution of nonneural routes, including brain penetration via the circumventricular organs.

VI. CELLULAR ORGANIZATION OF THE CYTOKINE NETWORK IN THE BRAIN

The concept that peripheral immune activation induces the expression of cytokines at the mRNA and protein levels in the brain was initially based on the observation that intraperitoneal administration of the cytokine inducer, LPS, induces IL-1β synthesis in the brain (Hopkins & Rothwell, 1995). The brain cells at the origin of this synthesis are meningeal and perivascular macrophages and ramified microglial cells (Buttini & Boddeke, 1995; Van Dam, Brouns, Louisse & Berkenbosch, 1992). However, IL-1 is not the sole cytokine to be induced in the brain by peripheral immune stimuli. TNF-α is also expressed at the mRNA and protein levels (Gatti & Bartfai, 1993; Breder, Hazuka, Ghayur, Klug, Huginin, Yasuda, Teno & Saper, 1994), and its cellular sources are represented by perivascular cells and neurons. There is still some controversy as to whether IL-6 is synthesized in the brain or imported from the periphery in response to peripheral LPS (Gatti & Bartfai, 1993; Layé et al., 1994; Schöbitz, de Kloet, & Holsboer, 1994), although the appearance of IL-6 mRNA with a peak of production occurring later than that of IL-1β is in accordance with the first possibility (Layé et al., 1994).

IL-1β presents the peculiarity of being produced in the form of a biologically inactive precursor, known as proIL-1β, that needs to be cleaved at an aspartate residue by a specific enzyme, known as interleukin-1β converting enzyme or ICE, to provide biologically active IL-1β. Despite ICE being colocalized with IL-1β in microglial cells, proIL-1β is the predominant form that is secreted by stimulated microglial cells (Chauvet, Lestage, & Dantzer, unpublished data), suggesting that the precursor might actually regulate the availability of IL-1 receptors for mature IL-1β.

At the periphery, LPS induces first the expression of TNF-α, which is responsible for the synthesis of IL-1. IL-1 itself triggers the synthesis and release of IL-6. RT-PCR studies of brain transcripts for these different cytokines at various intervals following intraperitoneal administration of LPS revealed that the same sequence of events occurs in the brain. TNF-α and IL-1β appeared first and were followed by IL-1ra and IL-6 (Layé et al., 1994). The importance of IL-1β in this cascade was apparent from the observation that icv IL-1ra to LPS-treated mice blocked the induction of expression of IL-1β, IL-6, and TNF-α in the hypothalamus and attenuated it in the hippocampus (Layé et al., 2000). Based on in situ hybridization studies, IL-1ra appears to be mainly expressed in the meninges, choroid plexus, and perivascular cells (Wong, Bongiorno, Rettori, McCann, & Licinio, 1997). At the cellular level, IL-1ra is produced by microglial cells, although it is also present in astrocytes and neurones, perhaps secondary to an internalization process, the nature of which still needs to be elucidated.

The exact cellular targets of proinflammatory cytokines in the brain are still elusive. IL-1 receptors have been identified in brain tissues, using radioligand-binding studies, immunocytochemistry, or expression of receptor mRNA. Equilibrium binding of [^{125}I]-IL-1α by brain membrane homogenates and brain slices was the first technique that was used to demonstrate the presence of binding sites for IL-1 in the mouse brain (Haour, Ban, Milon, Baran, & Fillion, 1990; Parnet et al., 1994; Takao, Tracey, Mitchell, & De Souza, 1991). These binding sites are located almost exclusively in the anterior pituitary, choroid plexus and dentate gyrus of the hippocampus. However, these findings are inconsistent with proposed sites of action of IL-1 receptor agonists in such areas as the hypothalamus and brain stem. In situ hybridization identified the type I IL-1 receptor mRNA in several regions of the rat brain, including the anterior olfactory nucleus, medial thalamic nucleus, posterior thalamic nucleus, basolateral amygdaloid nucleus, ventromedial hypothalamus nucleus, arcuate nucleus, median eminence, mesencephalic trigeminal nucleus, motor trigeminal nucleus, facial nucleus, and Purkinje cells of the cerebellum (Ericsson, Liu, Hart, & Sawchenko, 1995).

Despite their importance for the understanding of the way that IL-1 affects brain functions, the mechanisms of IL-1-mediated cell-to-cell communication in the nervous system have not yet been elucidated. IL-1RI is present on neurons, astrocytes, epithelial cells of the choroid plexus and ventricles, and endothelial cells. Using a rat anti-mouse type I IL-1 receptor monoclonal antibody, neurons and oligodendrocytes have been found to express type I IL-1 receptor protein (Parnet et al., 1994). In addition, transcripts for the type I, but not the type II, IL-1 receptors are expressed in murine neuronal cell lines, whereas transcripts for both types of receptors are present in mouse brain (Figure 6). Northern blot analysis indicates that IL-1R AcP is constitutively expressed at high levels in mouse brain (Greenfeder et al., 1995), but its cellular localization and coexpression with IL-1RI are still unknown. Little information is available on the factors that regulate IL-1 receptors in the nervous system. IL-1 receptor expression on the cell surface is negatively regulated by IL-1 in monocytes and fibroblasts. Indirect evidence in favor of a similar mechanism in the brain comes from experiments showing a decrease in the number of IL-1 binding sites in the hippocampus of mice administered an intraperitoneal injection of LPS (Haour et al., 1990). The same phenomenon occurs in astrocytes and could be due to internalization of the ligand–receptor complex.

Currently, relatively little information is available as to whether IL-1 receptors in the nervous system are the same as those identified in other tissues. Bristulf and colleagues (Bristulf et al., 1994) PCR-cloned a type II IL-1 receptor cDNA from an excitable rat insulinoma cell line. This receptor has structural features that are not found in the previously identified type II IL-1 receptor, suggesting that different subtypes of type II IL-1 receptors could be expressed in the CNS.

VII. MECHANISMS OF ACTION OF CYTOKINES ON THEIR BRAIN TARGETS

The exact way by which cytokines act on their brain targets is still elusive. There are several aspects to this question. The first one concerns the brain circuitry that is involved in the response to proinflammatory cytokines. The second one concerns the respective role of brain cytokines and intermediate molecules, such as prostanoids and nitric oxide (NO), in the activation of this circuitry.

A. Functional Neuroanatomy

The neuronal circuits that underlie the response to immune stimuli have mainly been studied with regard to the activation of the hypothalamo-pituitary-adrenal axis, the fever response, and the altera-

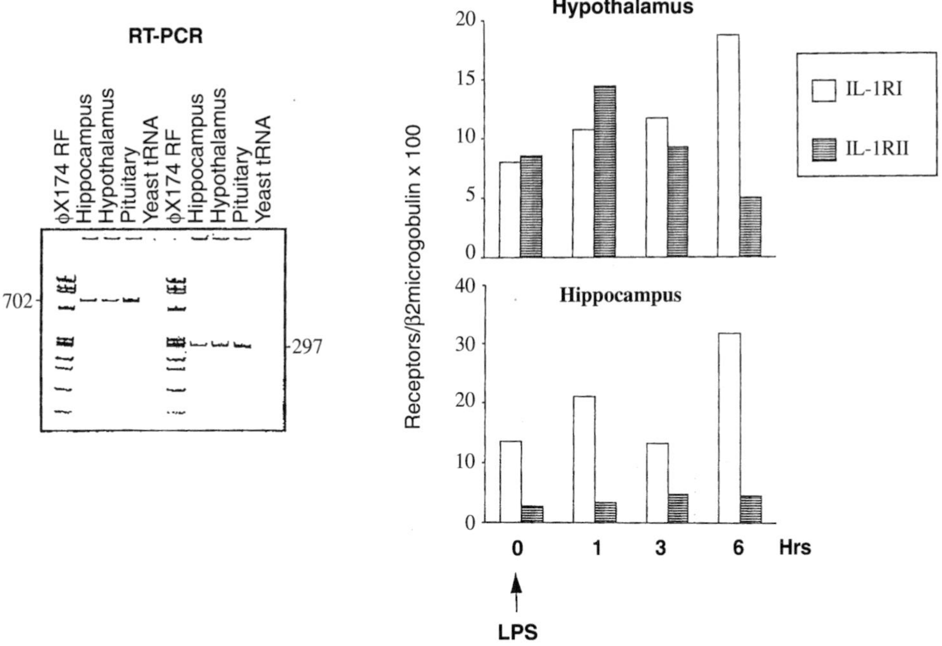

FIGURE 6 RT-PCR demonstration of the expression of type I and type II IL-1 receptors in the pituitary, hippocampus, and hypothalamus of mice and its regulation by systemic administration of LPS. Mice were killed either before or at different times after ip injection of LPS (10 μg/mouse) and total RNA was extracted from various tissues and brain structures for RT-PCR analysis. Yeast total RNA served as a negative control. (Left) A typical acrylamide gel showing transcripts for the type I IL-1 receptor (702 bp) and the type II IL-1 receptor (297 bp). (Right) Variations of IL-1 receptor mRNA in the hypothalamus and hippocampus (expressed as percentage of β2-microglobulin mRNA, mean of three experiments) in response to ip LPS.

tions in food intake that develop in animals injected with LPS and IL-1β. Ericsson and colleagues (Ericsson, Kovacs, & Sawchenko, 1994) have examined the pathways that mediate activation of the hypothalamo-pituitary-adrenal axis in response to an intravenous injection of IL-1β. Using Fos immunohistochemistry, they found that Fos was induced in C1 noradrenergic neurons in the ventrolateral medulla. These neurons project to the corticotropin-releasing hormone (CRH)-containing neurons of the paraventricular nucleus of the hypothalamus (PVN). Interruption of the input from the C1 cells to the PVN by knife cuts prevented the CRH response to IL-1β. In the case of fever, Saper and colleagues (Elmquist, Scammel, & Saper, 1997) observed that intravenously injected LPS activated Fos in the ventromedial preoptic area of the hypothalamus (VMPO). Using retrograde tracing, they found that the VMPO has both direct and indirect (via the anterior perifornical area and parastrial nucleus) projections to the autonomic parvicellular divisions of the PVN. They proposed that activation of VMPO efferents following LPS disinhibits PVN neurons that are involved in thermogenesis by inhibition of warm sensitive neurons that are located in the anterior perifornical area, therefore raising the thermostatic set point for thermoregulation (Elmquist et al., 1997). In the case of food intake, Plata-Salaman and colleagues (Plata-Salaman, Oomura, & Kai, 1988) showed that IL-1β suppressed the neuronal activity of the glucose-sensitive neurons in the lateral hypothalamic area, while activating glucose-sensitive neurons in the hypothalamic ventromedial nucleus (VMH). However, the evidence for a direct involvement of these hypothalamic neural structures in the anorexia induced by immune stimuli is still lacking.

Rather than using functional neuroanatomy techniques to identify the neural structures that mediate the behavioral effects of cytokines, some investigators have microinjected minute amounts of cytokines in specific brain areas. Bilateral infusion of IL-1β into the VMH of rats depressed food-motivated behavior in rats (Kent, Rodriguez, Kelley, & Dantzer, 1994). These effects required a lower dose than that injected into the lateral ventricle of the brain. However, the same effect was observed when the cannula did not hit the VMH. In a different experiment, IL-1β was found to decrease locomotor activity, and food and saccharin consumption when injected into the PVN, whereas administration into adjacent thalamic locations had no effect (Avitsur, Pollak, & Yirmiya, 1997a). These limited findings indicate that the techniques of micropharmacology are certainly useful for dissecting out the sites of action of cytokines in the brain. However, more systematic investigations are clearly needed.

B. Molecular Intermediates

Whether cytokines directly act on the above-described neural pathways or activate them via intermediates such as prostaglandins and NO is still a matter of controversy. There is no doubt that cytokines are powerful inducers of the expression of cyclooxygenase-2 (COX-2) (Breder & Saper, 1996; Cao, Matsumura, Yamagata, & Watanabe, 1996) in the brain. COX-2 is the rate-limiting enzyme in the conversion of arachidonic acid to prostanoids. This enzyme is induced in brain vascular- and perivascular-associated cells in response to systemic administration of LPS and IL-1β, but not IL-6 (Lacroix & Rivest, 1998). Cytokines also induce NO synthase in the brain (Wong et al., 1996). The inducible form of NO synthase (iNOS), also called type II NOS, is synthesized by macrophages in response to inflammatory stimuli. Using in situ hybridization, Wong and colleagues (1996) reported that there is no detectable expression of iNOS in the brain under basal conditions, but that this enzyme is rapidly induced in vascular, glial, and neuronal structures of the rat brain in response to ip LPS. The induction of this enzyme in the hypothalamus was confirmed by Satta and colleagues (Satta, Jacobs, Kaltsas, & Grossman, 1998) using RT-PCR.

Since many of the functional neuroanatomical studies on the brain effects of immune stimuli were carried out using the intravenous route and endothelial cells of the brain microvasculature respond to intraluminar cytokines by producing prostaglandins, Elmquist and colleagues (1997) proposed that these intermediates mediate the CRH and fever responses to immune stimuli. These actions of prostaglandins would take place in different regions of the brain, the C1 noradrenergic neurons for the CRH reponse, and the VMPO neurons for fever. Stimulation of COX-2 in the brain microvasculature of the MPOA results in an increased local production of prostaglandins. These intermediates would bind to specific receptors expressed on nearby neurons to promote the fever in response to peripheral immune stimuli (Elmquist et al., 1997; Lacroix & Rivest, 1998). In the case of a local inflammation, prostaglandins released at the site of inflammation would activate local sensory fibers, resulting in the transmission of the peripheral immune message to the brain. The way activation of vagal sensory fibers and brain production of IL-1β combine with each other to allow the development of the host response to infection has been examined by Konsman and colleagues (Konsman, Kelley, & Dantzer, 1999), using immunohistochemistry for Fos and IL-1β and in situ hybridization for the expression of iNOS mRNA, taken as a marker of IL-1β bioactivity. In this study, rats were killed at different times after ip administration of a behaviorally active dose of LPS. IL-1β-positive cells were found 2 h after LPS in circumventricular organs and the choroid plexus. The cells that expressed IL-1β were isolectin-positive cells and their shape allowed to identify them as perivascular phagocytic cells. Fos expression was restricted at that time to brain parenchymal structures such as the nucleus tractus solitarius, medial preoptic area, paraventicular nucleus, supraoptic nucleus, and central amygdala. Eight hours after LPS, Fos became apparent in circumventricular organs. This was associated with a shift of expression of IL-1β from circumventricular organs to adjacent brain structures such as the nucleus tractus solitarius and medial preoptic area. Since this was accompanied by an expression of iNOS at the interface between circumventricular organs and adjacent brain nuclei, these results were interpreted as suggesting that IL-1β functions as a volume transmision signal, which originates from perivascular cells at the blood side of the circumventricular organs, is passively conveyed through the interstitium of circumventricular organs by pulsations of nearby arterioles, and acts on microglial cells that are located on the neural side of the circumventricular organs. From there, the IL-1β message would propagate itself throughout the brain parenchyma by recruiting adjacent microglial cells (Konsman et al., 1999) (Figure 7). It is important to note that a similar picture was obtained by Quan and colleagues (Quan, Whiteside, Kim, & Herkenham, 1997), based on the induction of IκBα expression in the brain in response to LPS. IκB is an inhibitory intracellular protein that binds to the nuclear transcription factor NFκB, preventing its translocation to the nucleus. Upon cellular activation by immune signals, IκB is phosphorylated and dissociates itself from NFκB. NFκB is then able to enter the nucleus and stimulate transcription of a wide array of genes, including those responsible for COX-2 and iNOS. Since activation of NFκB is followed by induction of IκB, the detection of IκB induction in the brain reveals the extent and cellular location of brain-derived immune molecules in response to peripheral immune stimuli. In response to ip LPS, IκB mRNA was first

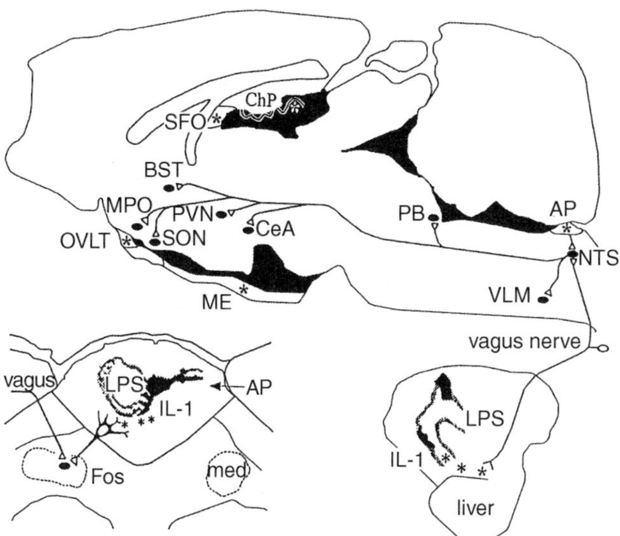

FIGURE 7 Schematic drawing of the way IL-1β is synthesized in the brain in response to ip LPS and its mechanisms of action. (Top) a sagittal section of the rat brain. (Bottom left) A coronal section of the brain at the level of the area postrema (AP). (Bottom right) The liver. Intraperitoneally administered LPS induces the release of IL-1β by Kupffer cells in the liver, resulting in the activation of vagal afferents. This neural message is transmitted to the NTS, and from there to the parabrachial nuclei (PB), the ventrolateral medulla (VLM), and the forebrain nuclei that are implicated in the metabolic, neuroendocrine, and behavioral components of the systemic host response to infection (medial preoptic area, MPO; paraventricular nucleus, PVN; supraoptic nucleus of the hypothalamus, SON; central nucleus of the amygdala, CeA; Bed nucleus of the Stria Terminalis, BST). Neural activation of these structures is apparent from Fos expression. IL-1β, represented by asteriks, is first synthesized and released in the circumventricular organs (organum vasculosum of the lamina terminalis, OVLT; area postrema, AP; subfornical organ, SFO; median eminence, ME) and the choroid plexus (ChP). In the AP, IL-1β is synthesized and released by perivascular phagocytic cells and then diffuses throughout the interstitium to act on IL-1 type I receptors that are present on AP neurons and project to the nucleus tractus solitarius (NTS). This results in a second wave of FOS expression in the NTS and its projection structures. The NTS plays therefore a pivotal role in the integration of peripheral and central IL-1β. A second wave of IL-1β expression occurs on the neural side of the blood-brain barrier and corresponds to the sequential activation of ramified microglial cells. Not represented in this figure is the fact that the actions of IL-1β on many of its target structures are mediated by intermediates such as prostaglandins and NO (from Konsman et al., 1999).

expressed in cells lining the blood side of the blood-brain barrier and progressed to glial cells inside the brain (Quan et al., 1997).

C. Role of Neurotransmitters and Neuropeptides

Administration of LPS or cytokines to laboratory animals induces profound alterations in neurotransmitter metabolism in various areas of the brain. LPS, IL-1, and IL-6 stimulate brain noradrenaline (NA) metabolism and increase tryptophan concentrations and serotonin (5-HT) metabolism (Dunn, Wang, & Ando, 1999). Dopamine is rarely affected by cytokines, except IL-2 which modulates veratrine-evoked release of endogenous dopamine from striatal slices in a biphasic pattern, increasing release at low concentrations and decreasing it at high concentrations (Petitto, McCarthy, Rinker, Huang, & Getty, 1997). TNF-α affects noradrenaline and tryptophan but only at high doses, whereas INF-α has no effect. While the neurochemical response to physical stressors is normally distributed in a relative uniform manner throughout the brain, the neurochemical response to cytokines is more localized and observed mainly in the hypothalamus (Dunn et al., 1999).

In view of the various biological effects of cytokines, it is not easy to relate these changes to specific behavioral effects of cytokines. An attempt to do so has been made by Linthorst and colleagues in an elegant series of studies carried out with in vivo microdialysis techniques in animals of which the core temperature, corticosterone, and behavior were monitored continuously (Linthorst, Flachskmann, Holsboer, & Reul, 1995; Linthorst, Flachskmann, Müller-Preuss, Holsboer, & Reul, 1995). These studies focused on 5-HT and NA neurotransmission in the hippocampus and the hypothalamic preoptic area of rats injected intraperitoneally with LPS. LPS induced a dose-dependent increase in hippocampal extracellular levels of 5-HT and its metabolite 5-hydroxyindoleacetic acid (5-HIAA). In contrast to what was observed in the hippocampus, ip LPS had no effect on preoptic extracellular levels of 5-HT. Intraperitoneal LPS also increased hippocampal extracellular levels of NA and its major metabolite MHPG (Linthorst, Flachskmann, Holsboer, & Reul, 1996), but this effect was small compared to the huge increase of NA and MHPG that was observed in the preoptic area (Figure 8) (Linthorst et al., 1995). Intracerebroventricular administration of IL-1β mimicked the effects of LPS on 5-HT neurotransmission in the hippocampus, whereas ICV TNF-α had no effect on behavior and neurotransmitters. Intracerebroventricular IL-2 affected hippocampal 5-HT neurotransmission only at doses that depressed locomotor activity (Pauli, Linthorst, & Reul, 1998). Based on these findings and the neuroanatomical connectivity of these brain structures, Linthorst and colleagues proposed that the increase in preoptic NA is involved in fever and/or activation of the hypothalamoc-pituitary-adrenal axis, whereas the rise in hippocampal 5-HT is associated with the development of sickness behavior (Linthorst

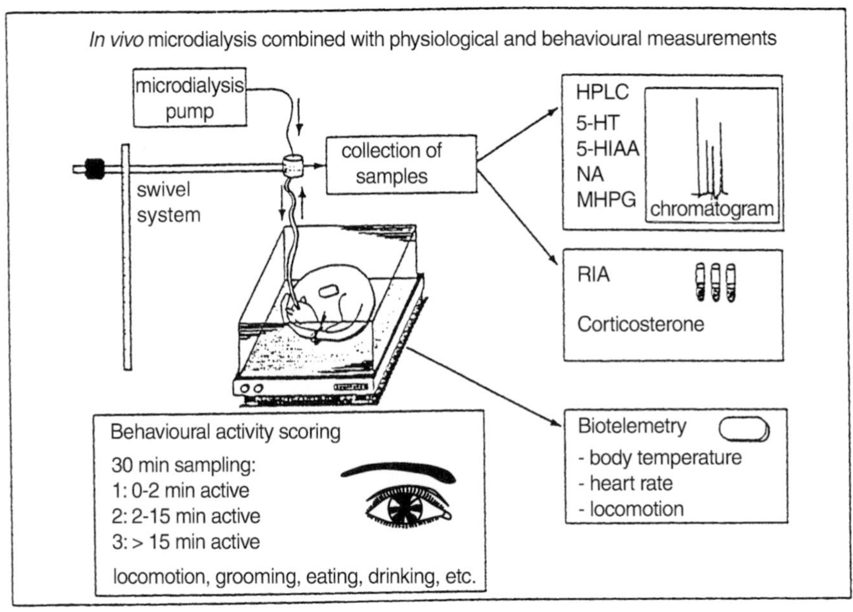

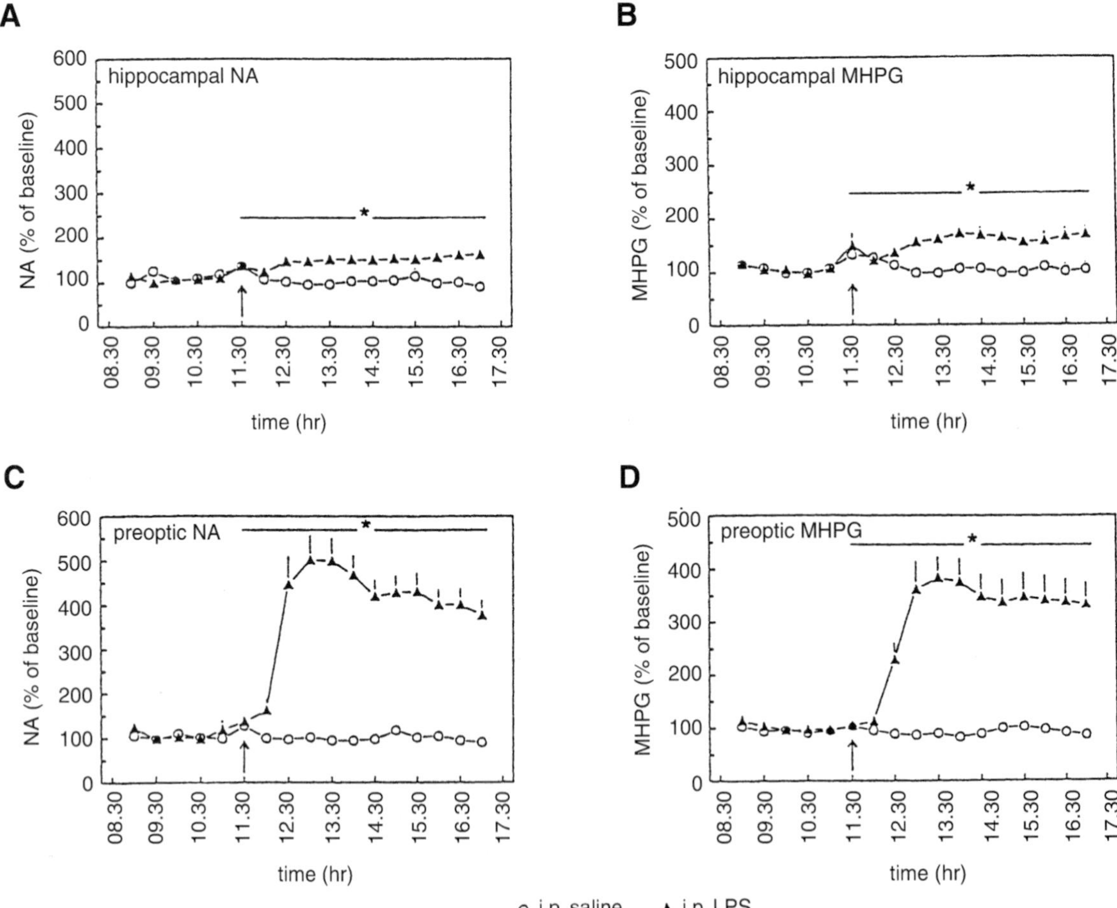

FIGURE 8 Effects of ip administration of saline or LPS (100 μg/kg) on extracellular levels of noradrenaline (NA) and its main metabolite, MHPG, in the hoppocampus (A, B) and the preoptic area (C, D) of the rat. The time point of injection is indicated by the arrow. The asteriks indicate the time periods during which data from saline- and LPS-treated animals differ significantly. (Top) The experimental setup (from Linthorst & Reuls, 1999).

& Reul, 1999). This hypothesis still needs to be tested using local infusion of specific agonists and antagonists of 5-HT and NA.

Studies on the role of neuropeptides in the behavioral effects of cytokines have mainly concentrated on CRH, cholecystokinin (CCK, a feeding inhibitory factor) , neuropeptide Y (NPY, a feeding stimulatory factor), and leptin (a feeding inhibitory factor). Since IL-1 is a potent activator of the hypothalamo-pituitary-adrenal axis, the possibility that CRH mediates some of the effects of this cytokine on anxiety-like behaviors has been assessed, using immunoneutralization of CRH by icv administration of CRH receptor antagonists and neutralizing antibodies directed against CRH. The results of these experiments have not been very conclusive, and the same applies to the depressing effects of IL-1 on food intake. In one experiment, immunoneutralization of endogenous CRF in the brain attenuated the anorexic effect of ip IL-1β (Uehara, Sekiya, Takasugi, Namiki, & Arimura, 1989), whereas, in another experiment, this treatment did not alter the disrupting effect of icv and ip IL-1β on food-motivated behavior (Bluthé, Crestani, Kelley, & Dantzer, 1992). Discrepant results were also obtained with CCK receptor antagonists since administration of a CCK-A receptor antagonist blocked the effects of IL-1α on food intake and gastric emptying in rats in one experiment (Daun & McCarthy, 1993), whereas, in another experiment, antagonism of peripheral or CCK-A or CCK-B receptors had no effect at all on the behavioral effects of IL-1 (Bluthé, Michaud, Kelley & Dantzer, 1997). The recent observation that both leptin and IL-1 are able to inhibit the potent orexigenic effects of NPY and, conversely, that NPY can reverse IL-1-induced anorexia (Sonti, Ilyin, & Plata-Salaman, 1996) led some authors to speculate that a disregulation of leptin–NPY–cytokine interactions might play a pivotal role in the pathophysiology of feeding disorders (Plata-Salaman, 1996). IL-1β and other proinflammatory cytokines act on adipocytes and induce the synthesis of leptin (Faggioni et al., 1998; Sarraf et al., 1997). The in vivo effects of LPS on leptin are likely to be mediated by TNF-α since LPS had no effect on leptin secretion by adipocytes whereas TNF-α increased it (Finck, Kelley, Dantzer, & Johnson, 1998). Leptin per se, however, does not appear to be responsible for cytokine-induced anorexia since leptin deficient (ob/ob) and leptin receptor-deficient (db/db) mice were found to be still sensitive to the anorexic effects of LPS (Faggioni, Fuller, Moser, Feingold, & Grunfeld, 1997). Because the leptin receptor is closely related to glycoprotein 130 (gp130), a common signal transducer among receptors for cytokines of the IL-6 family (IL-6, ciliary neurotrophic factor (CNTF), leukemia inhibitory factor (LIF)), the possibility that CNTF-induced anorexia is mediated by leptin was investigated in rats treated with ip leptin and CNTF (Xu et al., 1998). Both molecules induced anorexia and suppressed NPY-induced feeding. However, CNTF decreased leptin mRNA in adipocytes and had a depressing effect on hypothalamic NPY gene expression only at high dosages, suggesting that the effects of CNTF are not mediated by interactions with these endogenous signals.

VIII. SPECIFICITY OF THE INVOLVEMENT OF PERIPHERAL AND CENTRAL CYTOKINES IN DIFFERENT COMPONENTS OF SICKNESS BEHAVIOR

Although most of the work on the behavioral effects of proinflammatory cytokines has concentrated on IL-1, the different components of the behavioral syndrome that develop in sick individuals do not necessarily have an identical molecular basis. Moreover, the role of a given cytokine in sickness is likely to depend on the compartment, peripheral or central, in which it exerts its effects. The evidence that supports this interpretation is based on time course studies of the effect of IL-1β on social exploration and food-motivated behavior, on experiments examining the behavioral effects of LPS in animals pretreated with various cytokine and cytokine receptor antagonists, and on investigation of the effects of immune stimulation in mice in which the gene coding for a specific cytokine or its receptor has been deleted by the technique of homologous recombination.

Time course studies of the behavioral effects of IL-1β show that the changes in social exploration gradually develop within 2 h following peripheral administration of this cytokine, whereas the changes in food-motivated behavior reach a maximum by 1 h following treatment (Kent et al., 1996). The behavioral alterations that are induced by central administration of IL-1β usually develop more slowly than those induced by peripheral administration of this cytokine, which certainly reflects the time that is necessary for the progression of the cytokine message from the lateral ventricle of the brain to its neural targets.

The identification and cloning of IL-1ra provide a powerful pharmacological tool for attempting to resolve the role of IL-1 in sickness behavior. This cytokine blocks the in vivo biological effects of IL-1 when coadministered at a 100- to 1000-fold excess dose with IL-1. To determine the importance of IL-1 in the behavioral effects of LPS, rats were injected with ip IL-1ra before being administered ip LPS. This treatment abrogated the depressing effect of LPS on social behavior (Bluthé, Dantzer, & Kelley, 1992) but not on food-motivated behavior (Kent, Kelley, & Dantzer, 1992c) nor on female sexual behavior (Avitsur et al., 1997). IL-1ra was not more effective in antagonizing the decrease in milk intake induced by LPS administration in mice (Swiergel et al., 1997). These results can be interpreted to suggest that IL-1 is a key cytokine in the network of proinflammatory cytokines that is induced by LPS when it comes to social activities, but not to food intake.

To determine the importance of brain IL-1 in the depressing effects of peripherally administered IL-1 on social behavior and food-motivated behavior, rats were pretreated with an icv injection of IL-1ra before being injected with IP IL-1β. The depression of social exploration of a conspecific juvenile that normally occurs within 2–6 h following IL-1β injection was totally blocked in IL-1ra-pretreated rats. However, in rats trained to press a bar for a food reward in a Skinner box, the same treatment only partially attenuated the decrease in bar pressing that normally occurs within 1–8 h following IL-1β injection (Kent et al., 1992a). This did not appear to be a dose-dependent effect since increasing the dose of IL-1ra by nearly ninefold did not augment this partial blockade. These results indicate that among the different cytokines that are induced in the brain in response to peripheral IL-1, IL-1 is certainly the predominant molecular signal for the depression in social behavior but not for the decrease in food-motivated behavior. This effect of IL-1 appears to be mediated by the type I IL-1 receptor since icv administration of a neutralizing antibody directed against this receptor blocked the decrease in social behavior that was induced in mice by IP IL-1β (Cremona, Goujon, Kelley, Dantzer, & Parnet, 1998). In accordance with this result, mice in which the gene for the type I IL-1 receptor or the accessory protein of the IL-1 receptor had been deleted by homologous recombination no longer responded to icv IL-1β (Bluthé, Parnet, & Dantzer, unpublished observations).

The importance of a given cytokine depends not only on the compartment, peripheral or central, and on the behavior under consideration, but also on the immune stimulus. As described above, brain IL-1 mediates the effects of ip IL-1 on social behavior. However, when LPS was injected in place of IL-1 to suppress social behavior, icv IL-1ra was no longer able to abrogate the depressing effect of LPS (Bluthé et al., 1992), whereas it still attenuated the LPS-induced reduction in food intake (Layé et al., 2000).

The involvement of brain IL-1β in the depressing effects of LPS on food intake was confirmed in an experiment using mice in which the gene coding for ICE has been deleted (ICE($-/-$)). These mice do not produce bioactive IL-1β. Both wild-type and ICE($-/-$) mice responded to ip and icv IL-1β injection by a decrease in food intake, indicating that the effector mechanisms of this cytokine were not affected by the mutation. However, ICE($-/-$) mice were less sensitive than wild-type mice to the depressing effects of icv LPS on food intake and food-motivated behavior, whereas they did not differ in their response to ip LPS (Burgess et al., 1998).

In general, the presence of a network of cytokines acting in a cascade fashion does not make easy the task of assessing the relative importance of individual molecules in the induction of the behavioral symptoms that are characteristic of sick individuals. Since cytokines act in the context of other cytokines, which have agonist and antagonist activities, the conclusions that can be drawn from a particular combination of cytokines induced by a specific immune stimulus do not necessarily apply to a different combination of the same and possibly other cytokines induced by a different immune stimulus. Even apparently straightforward pharmacological experiments in which the concentration of a given cytokine is artificially modified can lead to erroneous conclusions. For example, icv and ip administration of recombinant rat IL-6 to rats failed to cause any alteration in social behavior, whereas the same treatments reliably induced fever and activation of the pituitary-adrenal axis (Lenczowski et al., 1999). These results could be interpreted to suggest that IL-6 plays no role in sickness behavior. However, icv IL-6 was found to potentiate the effects of a subthreshold dose of icv IL-1β on social behavior in rats. In accordance with their attenuated sensitivity to sickness associated with influenza pneumonitis (Kozak et al., 1997), mice which are deficient in IL-6 were found to be less sensitive to the depressing effects of both IL-1 and LPS on social behavior when these molecules were administered either ip or icv. Moreover, their sensitivity to these treatments was entirely due to IL-1 since pretreatment with icv IL-1ra abrogated the depressing effects of ip LPS on social behavior in IL-6 knockout mice (Bluthé, Michaud, Poli, & Dantzer, in preparation). These results indicate that IL-6 is behaviorally active only in the context of other proinflammatory cytokines.

The problem of identifying a major molecular signal for sickness behavior mirrors the difficulties experienced by pathologists in the selection of an appropriate molecular target for developing potential therapies for the treatment of septic shock and other pathological conditions in which cytokines play a critical role. This does not imply that proinflammatory cytokines are not important for the condition under examination; it just indicates that the redundant nature of the cytokine network imposes the choice of alternative strategies, based on the investigation of the mechanisms that are responsible for the commonality of action of proinflammatory cytokines, e.g., postreceptor mechanisms, and processes that regulate cytokine expression and actions.

IX. MOLECULAR FACTORS OPPOSING THE EXPRESSION AND ACTION OF PROINFLAMMATORY CYTOKINES IN THE BRAIN

Proinflammatory cytokines are often viewed as a two-edged sword. At low concentrations, they have potent biological effects that play a key role in the development of the host response to infection. However, at high concentrations, they can lead to cell death by necrosis or apoptosis. It is therefore important that the activity of proinflammatory cytokines is tightly regulated. Two main categories of molecules oppose the expression and action of proinflammatory cytokines, molecules that are part of the cytokine network and are called anti-inflammatory cytokines and molecules that are exogenous to the cytokine network and are called cryogens (Kluger, 1991). Cryogens include vasopressin and glucocorticoids.

A. Anti-inflammatory Cytokines

Anti-inflammatory cytokines belong to a very heterogenous family of secreted signaling molecules that all have in common the property of inhibiting to some extent the expression and/or action of proinflammatory cytokines. These cytokines include IL-4, IL-10, IL-13, and transforming growth factors-β (TGF-β). Although the biological activity of these molecules was initially defined on peripheral immune and nonimmune cells, there is evidence that they are also able to regulate the effects of proinflammatory cytokines in the nervous system. Most of the studies on anti-inflammatory cytokines in the nervous system have been carried out in the context of neuropathology (Owens, Renno, Taupin, & Krakowski, 1994). During the course of an immune response in the brain, anti-inflammatory cytokines are mainly produced by T helper 2 lymphocytes and they downregulate proinflammatory cytokines produced by T helper 1 lymphocytes (INF-γ and TNF-α). However, anti-inflammatory cytokines can also be produced by macrophages, monocytes, and glial cells, and therefore play a physiological role in the regulation of sickness behavior. TGF-β is constitutively expressed in the brain and is certainly an important factor for the maintenance of the immune privilege of this organ. Whether it is the same for other anti-inflammatory cytokines is still uncertain. Although IL-10 for example is expressed at the mRNA level in the human pituitary and hypothalamus (Rady et al., 1995), its expression and that of IL-13 do not appear to be very sensitive to the inducing effects of systemic LPS in comparison to that seen with IL-1β (Wong et al., 1997). This does not mean that IL-10 has no effect on the brain action of cytokines. In accordance with its ability to protect from the lethal effects of endotoxemia, systemic administration of IL-10 was found to abrogate the fever induced in mice by low doses of LPS (Leon, Kozak, Rudolph, & Kluger, 1999). In addition, IL-10 knockout mice developed an exacerbated and prolonged fever and a more marked suppression of food intake in response to a low dose of LPS, when compared to their wild-type counterparts. Intracerebroventral IL-10 abrogated the depressing effects of ip LPS on locomotor activity but not on water intake in rats (Nava et al., 1997). Intracerebroventricular IL-10 also abrogated the depressing effects of ip and icv LPS on social exploration in rats (Bluthé et al., 1999). The reduction of endotoxin-induced hyperalgesia by ip IL-10 in mice was associated with a downregulation of LPS-induced increases in levels of TNF-α and IL-1β in the skin of injected hind paws (Kanaan, Poole, Saadé, Jabbur, & Safieh-Garabedian, 1998), suggesting that IL-10 acts by inhibiting production of proinflammatory cytokines.

Since many anti-inflammatory cytokines play an important role in growth and development, it is possible that more traditional growth factors actually behave as anti-inflammatory cytokines; This was found to be the case for insulin-like growth factor I, which is abundantly expressed in the brain and, when administered icv, attenuates the behavioral depression induced by icv LPS (Dantzer, Gheusi, Johnson, & Kelley, 1999). These still very scarce data point to a regulatory role of anti-inflammatory cytokines on the behavioral effects of proinflammatory cytokines, but the generality of this action and its mechanisms remain to be elucidated.

B. Vasopressin

Vasopressin (VP) plays a key role in the regulation of water metabolism. It is produced by hypothalamic magnocellular neurons and accumulates in the terminals of these neurons in the posterior pituitary. It is released in the general circulation and acts as an antidiuretic hormone in response to water deprivation. The release of VP is enhanced during the febrile response, and this enhanced release can be of such a degree that miction does not occur before defervescence. VP also acts as a neurotransmitter in the brain. It is particularly present in neurons whose cell bodies are located in the bed nucleus of the stria terminalis (BNST) and whose terminals project to the lateral septum. This vasopressinergic pathway is highly sensitive to circulating androgens in rodents. Castration leads to a dramatic reduction in the content of VP mRNA in the BNST neuronal cell bodies and to a reduction in immunoreactive VP in the terminal areas of the septum. This androgen-dependent pathway is also activated during fever.

Central administration of VP attenuated the depressing effects of centrally injected IL-1β on social exploration. Conversely, central injection of an antagonist of vasopressin receptors, which has no biological activity on its own but prevents endogenously released vasopressin to reach its receptors, sensitized rats to the behavioral effects of IL-1 (Dantzer, Bluthé, & Kelley, 1991). These last results are important since they suggest that endogenous VP plays a physiological modulatory role in the behavioral effects of IL-1. To determine whether this phenomenon is mediated by an androgen-dependent or independent pathway, castrated male rats were compared to intact male rats for their sensitivity to the modulatory role of the VP receptor antagonist. Castration by itself potentiated the depressing effects of IL-1β on social exploration. Central administration of VP was more effective in attenuating the behavioral effects of IL-1 in castrated than in intact male rats and, conversely, icv administration of the VP receptor antagonist was no longer active in potentiating the behavioral effects of IL-1 in castrated male rats lacking vasopressinergic innervation of the lateral septum (Dantzer et al., 1991). The mechanisms by which the brain vasopressinergic system is activated by cytokines and the way vasopressin interacts with the effect of cytokines on their target cells remain to be elucidated.

C. Glucocorticoids

The potent activating effects of proinflammatory cytokines on pituitary-adrenal activity have already been mentioned. Glucocorticoids represent another class of key molecules in the regulation of sickness behavior. In immune cells, proinflammatory cytokine gene expression is mainly regulated by glucocorticoids. Glucocorticoids downregulate the synthesis and secretion of IL-1, IL-6, and TNF-α by activated monocytes and macrophages (Lee et al., 1988). LPS-induced increases in plasma levels of TNF-α and IL-6 are much higher in adrenalectomized (ADX) than in sham-operated animals (Zuckerman, Shellhaas, & Butler, 1989). The enhanced release of these cytokines is inhibited by administration of glucocorticoids. At the molecular level, glucocorticoids inhibit transcriptional and posttranscriptional expression of the IL-1β gene and decrease stability of IL-1β mRNA. Regulation of the synthesis and release of proinflammatory cytokines by glucocorticoids has marked functional consequences since adrenalectomy sensitizes experimental animals to the septic shock syndrome whereas administration of glucocorticoids has the opposite effect (Bertini, Bianchi, & Ghezzi, 1988; Rachamandra, Sehon, & Berczi, 1992).

To assess the possible influence of endogenous glucocorticoids on cytokine expression in the brain, ADX mice and sham-operated mice were injected with saline or LPS, and the levels of transcripts for IL-1α, IL-1β, IL-1ra, IL-6, and TNF-α were subsequently determined in the spleen, pituitary, hypothalamus, hippocampus, and striatum, using comparative reverse transcription polymerase chain reaction (RT-PCR) (Goujon, Parnet, Layé, Combe, & Dantzer, 1996). Levels of IL-1β were also measured by a specific ELISA in the plasma and tissues of experimental animals. In accordance with the results of previous investigations, LPS induced the expression of proinflammatory cytokines at the mRNA level in most tissues under investigation. This effect was potentiated by adrenalectomy in the plasma and other tissues, including several brain structures (Figure 9). However, the magnitude of this enhancement differed according to the tissue under investigation. LPS increased plasma and tissue levels of IL-1β, as determined by ELISA, and this effect was potentiated by adrenalectomy, in the plasma and tissues other than the spleen. Since IL-1β and other proinflammatory cytokines are mainly synthesized in the brain by microglial cells and meningeal and perivascular macrophages, and since glucocorticoids have been shown to inhibit in vitro the synthesis and secretion of IL-1, IL-6, and TNF-α by activated monocytes and macrophages, it is tempting to propose that the enhancing effects of adrenalectomy on cytokine gene expression in peripheral and central tissues is the result of the lack of glucocorticoids.

This interpretation is strengthened by the observation that the effects of stress are contrary to those of adrenalectomy on the LPS-induced expression of

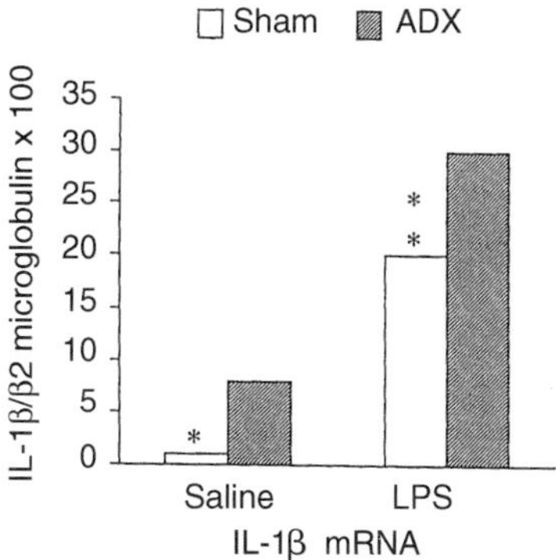

FIGURE 9 Adrenalectomy increases expression of IL-1β mRNA in mice. Adrenalectomized (ADX) and sham-operated mice were injected subcutaneously with saline or LPS (10 μg/mouse) and killed 2 h later. Total RNA was extracted from the hypothalamus and IL-1β mRNA, expressed as percentage of β2-microglobulin mRNA, was measured by comparative RT-PCR. The figure represents the mean results of three different experiments. Note that LPS increased hypothalamic IL-1β mRNA and adrenalectomy increased the expression of this cytokine in saline- and LPS-treated mice (From Goujon et al., 1996).

cytokines in the brain (Goujon, Parnet, Layé, Combe, Kelley, & Dantzer, 1995c). In this experiment, mice injected with LPS or saline, were submitted to a 15-min restraint stress which resulted in a significant increase in plasma corticosterone levels. They were subsequently sacrificed to assess the effects of this stressor on the induction of proinflammatory cytokines in the spleen, pituitary, hypothalamus, hippocampus, and striatum. LPS-induced cytokine gene expression, as determined by comparative RT-PCR, was lower in restrained than in nonrestrained mice. LPS increased plasma and tissue IL-1β levels, as determined by ELISA. This effect of LPS was also less marked in restrained than in nonrestrained mice. In contrast with these findings, stress has been reported to induce an increase in IL-1β mRNA levels in the hypothalamus of rats (Minami et al., 1991) and an enhancement of plasma levels of IL-6 (Le May, Vander & Kluger, 1990; Zhou, Kusnecov, Shurin, DePaoli, & Rabin, 1993). The reason for these contradictory results is not known (Watkins, Nguyen, Lee, & Maier, 1999).

As already mentioned, IL-1β is synthesized as an inactive precursor which needs to be cleaved to be secreted in an active form. The enzyme which is responsible for this cleavage is a protease called ICE. To determine whether those factors which regulate the expression of IL-1 in immune and nonimmune tissues are also able to regulate the expression of ICE, mice were injected with LPS and the levels of ICE mRNA in the spleen, pituitary, and brain of experimental animals were measured by comparative RT-PCR. ICE mRNAs were more abundant in the spleen and hippocampus than in the pituitary and hypothalamus, but they were not significantly altered by LPS treatment. In another experiment, mice were submitted to adrenalectomy or a 15-min restraint stress and injected with saline or LPS. ADX mice had significantly higher ICE mRNA levels whereas stressed mice had significantly lower ICE mRNA levels than their respective controls. These results can be interpreted to suggest that endogenous glucocorticoids regulate the expression of ICE in peripheral and brain tissues, in a manner which is commensurate to their effects on IL-1β gene expression (Layé et al., 1996).

In addition to their action on the synthesis of proinflammatory cytokines in the periphery and the brain, glucocorticoids are also able to modulate the expression of IL-1 receptors. Although glucocorticoids induce the expression of IL-1 receptors in various immune and nonimmune tissues, mixed results have been reported in the brain (Ban et al., 1993; Betancur, Lledo, Borrell, & Guaza, 1994). The problem with the radioligand binding techniques which have been used for these studies is that they do not allow an accurate description of what is going on at the molecular level, since the same effect, e.g., decreased binding, can be seen as a result of very different processes, e.g., downregulation of receptors, or activation of receptors with internalization of receptor–ligand complexes. Studies at the mRNA level revealed that ADX was accompanied by a decrease in the levels of IL-1RI and IL-1RII transcripts in the mouse pituitary and brain, whereas stress had the opposite effects (Goujon, Layé, Parnet, & Dantzer, unpublished observations). When ADX mice were implanted with a corticosterone pellet to induce plasma levels of corticosterone intermediate between baseline and stress levels, IL-1RI and IL-1RII mRNAs were increased above baseline levels. In all cases, the effects of corticosterone supplementation and stress were more marked for IL-1RII than for IL-1RI mRNA, which would fit with the downregulatory effects of glucocorticoids on IL-1 biological activity.

The downregulatory effects of glucocorticoids on the proinflammatory cytokine network at the periphery and in the brain should lead to an increased sensitivity of ADX animals to the brain actions of these cytokines. This appears to be the case since adrenalectomy increased the febrile response to LPS whereas administration of glucocorticoids had the opposite effect (Coehlo, Souza, & Pela, 1982; Morrow, McClellan, Conn, & Kluger, 1993). In the same manner, adrenalectomy enhanced the depression of social exploration induced by peripheral injection of IL-1β or LPS (Goujon, Parnet, Aubert, Goodall, &

Dantzer, 1995a). This effect was mimicked by administration of the glucocorticoid type II receptor antagonist, RU 38486. Chronic replacement with a 15-mg corticosterone pellet which yielded plasma corticosterone levels intermediate between baseline and stress levels, abrogated the enhanced susceptibility of ADX mice to the lower dose of IL-1β but had only partial protective effects on the response to a higher dose of IL-1β and to LPS.

Taken together, these findings can be interpreted to suggest that the phasic response of the pituitary-adrenal axis to cytokines has an important regulatory role on the neural effects of cytokines. However, they do not reveal at what level (peripheral or central) glucocorticoids are acting. Central sites of action appear to be involved in the regulatory effects of glucocorticoids on the neural effects of cytokines, since central injection of RU 38486 potentiates fevers induced by a peripheral injection of LPS to rats (McClellan, Klir, Morrow, & Kluger, 1994). In the same manner, adrenalectomy sensitized mice to the depressing effects of intracerebroventricular administration of IL-1β on social exploration, and this effect was attenuated by corticosterone compensation (Goujon, Parnet, Crémona & Dantzer, 1995). Central administration of RU 38486 mimicked the effect of adrenalectomy.

X. CONCLUSION

Although the scope of this chapter has been restricted mainly to the involvement of members of the interleukin-1 family in sickness behavior, sufficient evidence is now available to indicate that the proinflammatory cytokines, which are released at the periphery by activated monocytes and macrophages, activate peripheral afferent nerves to induce the synthesis and release of proinflammatory cytokines in the brain. These centrally released cytokines act probably by volume transmission on those neural structures that are involved in the control of thermoregulation, metabolism and behavior, resulting in the development of the brain components of the host response to infection. Glucocorticoids that are released by the adrenal cortex in response to the hypothalamic effects of proinflammatory cytokines regulate the expression and actions of cytokines not only in the periphery but also in the brain.

Acknowledgments

Supported by INRA, INSERM, DRET, Commission of the European Communities (BIOMED 1 PL93-1450, BIOMED 2 CT97-2492, and TMR CT97-0149), and the National Institutes of Health (MH-51569 and DK-49311 to K.W.K.).

References

Alleva, E., Cirulli, F., Bianchi, M., Bondiolotti, G. P., Chiarotti, F., De Acetis, L., & Panerai, A.E. (1998). Behavioral characterization of interleukin-6 overexpressing or deficient mice during agonistic encounters. *European Journal of Neuroscience, 10*, 3664–3672.

Anisman, H., Kokkinidis, L., Borowski, T., & Merali, Z. (1998). Differential effects of interleukin (IL)-1beta, IL-2 and IL-6 on responding for rewarding lateral hypothalamic stimulation. *Brain Research, 779*, 177–187.

Anisman, H., & Merali, Z. (1999). Anxiogenic and anhedonic effects of cytokine exposure. In R. Dantzer, E. E. Wollman, & R. Yirmiya (Eds.), *Cytokines, stress, and depression*. New York: Kluwer-Academic/Plenum.

Armario, A., Hernandez, J., Bluethmann, H., & Hidalgo, J. (1998). IL-6 deficiency leads to increased emotionality in mice: Evidence in transgenic mice carrying a null mutation for IL-6. *Journal of Neuroimmunology, 92*, 160–169.

Aubert, A., Goodall, G., & Dantzer, R. (1995). Compared effects of cold ambient temperature and cytokines on macronutrient intake in rats. *Physiology and Behavior, 57*, 869–873.

Aubert, A., Goodall, G., Dantzer, R., & Gheusi, G. (1997). Differential effects of lipopolysaccharide on pup retrieving and nest building in lactating mice. *Brain Behavior, and Immunity, 11*, 107–118.

Aubert, A., Kelley, K. W., & Dantzer, R. (1997). Differential effect of lipopolysaccharide on food hoarding behavior and food consumption in rats. *Brain, Behavior, and Immunity, 11*, 229–238.

Aubert, A., Vega, C., Dantzer, R., & Goodall, G. (1995). Pyrogens specifically disrupt the acquisition of a task involving cognitive processes in the rat. *Brain, Behavior, and Immunity, 9*, 129–148.

Avitsur, R., Cohen, E., & Yirmiya, R. (1997). Effects of interleukin-1 on sexual attractivity in a model of sickness behavior. *Physiology and Behavior, 63*, 25–30.

Avitsur, R., Pollak, Y., & Yirmiya, R. (1997a). Administration of interleukin-1 into the hypothalamic paraventricular nucleus induces febrile and behavioral effects. *Neuroimmunomodulation, 4*, 258–265.

Avitsur, R., Pollack, Y., & Yirmiya, R. (1997b). Different receptor mechanisms mediate the effects of endotoxin and interleukin-1 on female sexual behavior. *Brain Research, 773*, 149–161.

Ban, E., Marquette, C., Sarrieau, A., Fitzpatrick, F., Fillion, G., Millon, G., Rostène, W., & Haour, F. (1993). Regulation of interleukin-1 receptor expression in mouse brain and pituitary by lipopolysaccharide and glucocorticoids. *Neuroendocrinology, 58*, 581–587.

Banks, W. A., Ortiz, L., Plotkin, S. R., & Kastin, A. J. (1991). Human interleukin (IL) 1 alpha, murine IL-1 alpha and murine IL-1 beta are transported from blood to brain in the mouse by a shared saturable mechanism. *Journal of Pharmacology and Experimental Therapeutics, 259*, 988–996.

Bauer, J., Hohagen, F., Gimmel, E., Bruns, F., Lis, S., Krieger, S., Ambach, W., Guthmann, A., Grunze, H., & Fritsch-Montero, R. (1995). Induction of cytokine synthesis and fever suppresses REM sleep and improves mood in patients with major depression. *Biological Psychiatry, 38*, 611–621.

Baura, G. D., Foster, D. M., Porte, D., Jr., Kahn, S. E., Bergman, R. N., Cobelli, C., & Schwartz, M. W. (1993). Saturable transport of insulin from plasma into the central nervous system of dogs in vivo. A mechanism for regulated insulin delivery to the brain. *Journal of Clinical Investigation, 92*, 1824–1830.

Bertini, R., Bianchi, M., & Ghezzi, P. (1988). Adrenalectomy sensitizes mice to lethal effects of interleukin-1 and tumor necrosis factor. *Journal of Experimental Medicine, 167*, 1708–1712.

Besedovsky, H. O., del Rey, A., Sorkin, E., & Dinarello, C. A. (1986). Immunoregulatory feedback between interleukin-1 and glucocorticoid hormones. *Science, 233*, 652–654.

Betancur, C., Lledo, A., Borrell, J., & Guaza, C. (1994). Corticosteroid regulation of IL-1 receptors in the mouse hippocampus: Effects of glucocorticoid treatment, stress and adrenalectomy. *Neuroendocrinology, 59*, 120–128.

Blatteis, C. M. (1990). Neuromodulative actions of cytokines. *Yale Journal of Biological Medicine, 63*, 133–142.

Bluthé, R. M., Castanon, N., Pousset, F., Bristow, A., Ball, C., Lestage, J., Michaud, B., Kelley, K. W., & Dantzer, R. (1999). Central injection of IL-10 antagonizes the behavioral effects of lipopolysaccharide in rats, *Psychoneuroendocrinology, 24*, 301–311.

Bluthé, R. M., Crestani, F., Kelley, K. W., & Dantzer, R. (1992). Mechanisms of the behavioral effects of interleukin-1. Role of prostaglandins and CRF. *Annals of the New York Academy of Sciences, 650*, 268–275.

Bluthé, R. M., Dantzer, R., & Kelley, K. W. (1992). Effects of interleukin-1 receptor antagonist on the behavioral effects of lipopolysaccharide in rat. *Brain Research, 573*, 318–320.

Bluthé, R. M., Jafarian-Tehrani, M., Michaud, B., Haour, F., Dantzer, R., & Homo-Delarche, F. (1999). Increased sensitivity of prediabetic nonobese diabetic mouse to the behavioral effects of IL-1. *Brain, Behavior, and Immunity, 13*, 303–314.

Bluthé, R. M., Michaud, B., Dantzer, R., & Kelley, K. W. (1997). Central mediation of the effects of interleukin-1 on social exploration and body weight in mice. *Psychoneuroendocrinology, 22*, 1–11.

Bluthé, R. M., Michaud, B., Delhaye-Bouchaud N., Mariani, J., & Dantzer, R. (1997). Hypersensitivity of lurcher mutant mice to the depressing effects of lipopolysaccharide and interleukin-1 on behavior. *NeuroReport, 8*, 1119–1122.

Bluthé, R. M., Michaud, B., Kelley, K. W., & Dantzer, R. (1996a). Vagotomy blocks behavioral effects of interleukin-1 injected via the intraperitoneal route but not via other systemic routes. *NeuroReport, 7*, 2823–2827.

Bluthé, R. M., Michaud, B., Kelley, K. W., & Dantzer, R. (1996b). Vagotomy attenuates behavioral effects of interleukin-1 injected peripherally but not centrally. *NeuroReport, 7*, 1485–1488.

Bluthé, R. M., Michaud, B., Kelley, K. W., & Dantzer, R. (1997). Cholecystokinin receptors do not mediate behavioral effects of lipopolysaccharide in mice. *Physiology and Behavior, 62*, 385–389.

Bluthé, R. M., Michaud, B., Poli, V., & Dantzer, R. (2000). Role of IL-6 in cytokine-induced sickness behavior: A study with IL-6 deficient mice. *Physiology and Behavior*, in press.

Bluthé, R. M., Pawlowski, M., Suarez, S., Parnet, P., Pittman, Q., Kelley, K. W., & Dantzer, R. (1994a). Synergy between tumor necrosis factor α and interleukin-1 in the induction of sickness behavior in mice. *Psychoneuroendocrinology, 19*, 197–207.

Bluthé, R. M., Walter, V., Parnet, P., Layé, S., Lestage, J.,Verrier, D., Poole, S., Stenning, B. E., Kelley, K. W., & Dantzer, R. (1994). Lipopolysaccharide induces sickness behavior in rats by a vagal mediated mechanism. *Comptes Rendus de l'Académie des Science (Paris), 317*, 499–503.

Bolles, R. C. (1970). Species-specific defense reactions and avoidance learning. *Psychological Review, 77*, 32–48.

Breder, C. D., Hazuka, C., Ghayur, T., Klug, C., Huginin, M., Yasuda, K., Teno, M., & Saper, C. B. (1994). Regional induction of tumor necrosis factor α expression in the mouse brain after systemic lipopolysaccharide administration. *Proceedings of the National Academy of Sciences USA, 91*, 11393–11397.

Breder, C. D., & Saper, C. B. (1996). Expression of inducible cyclooxygenase mRNA in the mouse brain after systemic administration of bacterial lipopolysaccharide. *Brain Research, 713*, 64–69.

Bret-Dibat, J. L., Bluthé, R. M., Kent, S., Kelley, K. W., & Dantzer, R. (1995). Lipopolysaccharide and interleukin-1 depress food-motivated behavior in mice by a vagal-mediated mechanism. *Brain, Behavior and Immunity, 9*, 242–246.

Bristulf, J., Gatti, S., Malinowsky, D., Bjork, L., Sundgren A. K., & Bartfai, T. (1994). Interleukin-1 stimulates the expression of type I and type II interleukin-1 receptors in the rat insulinoma cell line Rinm5F: Sequencing a rat type II interleukin-1 receptor cDNA. *European Cytokine Network, 5*, 319–330.

Burgess, W., Gheusi, G., Yao, J., Johnson, R. W., Dantzer, R., & Kelley, K. W. (1998). Interleukin-1β converting enzyme (ICE)-deficient mice are resistant to central but not systemic lipopolysaccharide-induced aphagia. *American Journal of Physiology, 274*, R1829–R1833.

Buttini, M., & Boddeke, H. (1995). Peripheral lipopolysaccharide stimulation induces interleukin-1β messenger RNA in rat brain microglial cells. *Neuroscience, 65*, 523–530.

Campbell, I. L. (1998). Transgenic mice and cytokine actions in the brain: Bridging the gap between structural and functional neuropathology. *Brain Research Reviews*, 26, 327–336.

Cao, C. Y., Matsumura, K., Yamagata, K., & Watanabe, Y. (1996). Endothelial cells of the rat-brain vasculature express cyclooxygenase-2 messenger-RNA in response to systemic interleukin-1: A possible site of prostaglandin synthesis responsible for fever. *Brain Research, 733*, 263–272.

Capuron, L., & Ravaud, A. (1999). Prediction of the depressive effects of interferon-alpha therapy by the patient initial affective state. *New England Journal of Medicine, 340*, 1370.

Capuron, L., Ravaud, A., & Dantzer, R. (2000). Early depressive symptoms in cancer patients receiving interleukin-2 and/or interferon-alfa-2b therapy. *Journal of Clinical Oncology, 18*, 2143–2151.

Cirulli, F., De Acetis, L., & Alleva, E. (1998). Behavioral effects of peripheral interleukin-1 administration in adult CD1 mice: Specific inhibition of the offensive components of intermale agonistic behavior. *Brain Research, 791*, 308–312.

Coehlo, M. M., Souza, G. E. P., & Pela, I. R. (1982). Endotoxin-induced fever is modulated by endogenous glucocorticoids in rats. *American Journal of Physiology, 263*, R423–R427.

Cremona S., Goujon, E., Kelley, K. W., Dantzer, R. & Parnet, P. (1998). Brain type I but not type II interleukin-1 (IL-1) receptors mediate the effects of IL-1β on behavior in mice. *American Journal of Physiology, 274*, R735–R740.

Dantzer, R. (1994). How do cytokines say hello to the brain? Neural versus humoral mediation. *European Cytokine Network, 5*, 271–273.

Dantzer R., Bluthé, R. M., & Kelley, K. W. (1991). Androgen-dependent vasopressinergic neurotransmission attenuates interleukin-1-induced sickness behavior. *Brain Research, 557*, 115–120.

Dantzer, R., Gheusi, G., Johnson, R. W., & Kelley, K. W. (1999). Central administration of insulin-like growth factor-1 inhibits lipopolysaccharide-induced sickness behavior in mice. *NeuroReport*, in press.

Dantzer, R., & Kelley, K. W. (1989). Stress and immunity: An integrated view of relationships between the brain and the immune system. *Life Sciences, 44*, 1995–2008.

Dantzer, R., Wollman, E. E., & Yirmiya, R. (Eds.) (1999). Cytokines, stress, and depression. New York: Kluwer-Academic/Plenum.

Daun, J. M., & McCarthy, D. O. (1993). The role of cholecystokinin in interleukin-1-induced anorexia. *Physiology, & Behavior, 54*, 237–241.

Dinarello, C. A. (1996). Biologic basis for interleukin-1 in disease. *Blood, 87*, 2095–2147.

Dunn, A. J., Wang, J., & Ando, T. (1999). Effects of cytokines on cerebral neurotransmission: Comparison with the effects of stress. In R. Dantzer, E. E. Wollman, & R. Yirmiya (Eds.), *Cytokines, stress, and depression*. New York: Kluwer-Academic/ Plenum.

Elmquist, J. K., Scammell, T. E., & Saper, C. B. (1997). Mechanisms of CNS response to systemic immune challenge: The febrile response. *Trends in Neuroscience, 20*, 565–570.

Ericsson, A., Kovacs, K. J., & Sawchenko, P. E. (1994). A functional anatomical analysis of central pathways subserving the effects of interleukin-1 on stress-related neuroendocrine neurons. *Journal of Neuroscience, 14*, 897–913.

Ericsson, A., Liu, C., Hart, R. P., & Sawchenko, P. E. (1995). Type 1 interleukin-1 receptor in the rat brain: Distribution, regulation, and relationship to sites of IL-1 induced cellular activation. *Journal of Comparative Neurology, 361*, 681–698.

Faggioni, R., Fantuzzi, G., Fuller, J., Dinarello, C. A., Feingold, K. R., & Grunfeld, C. (1998). IL-1 beta mediates leptin induction during inflammation. *American Journal of Physiology, 274*, R204–R208.

Faggioni, R., Fuller, J., Moser, A., Feingold, K. R., & Grunfeld, C. (1997). LPS-induced anorexia in leptin-deficient (ob/ob) and leptin receptor-deficient (db/db) mice. *American Journal of Physiology, 273*, R181–R186.

Finck, B. N., Kelley, K. W., Dantzer, R., & Johnson, R. W. (1998). In vivo and in vitro evidence for the involvement of tumor necrois factor-α in the induction of leptin by lipopolysaccharide. *Endocrinology, 139*, 2278–2283.

Fiore, M., Alleva, E., Probert, L., Kollias, G., Angelucci, F., & Aloe, L. (1998). Exploratory and displacement behavior in transgenic mice expressing high levels of brain TNF-alpha. *Physiology and Behavior, 63*, 571–576.

Gatti, S., & Bartfai, T. (1993). Induction of tumor necrosis factor α mRNA in the brain after peripheral endotoxin treatment: Comparison with interleukin-1 family and interleukin-6. *Brain Research, 624*, 291–295.

Gibertini, M. (1996). IL-1 beta impairs relational but not procedural rodent learning in a water-maze task. *Advances in Experimental Biology and Biology, 402*, 207–217.

Gibertini, M. (1998). Cytokines and cognitive behavior. *Neuroimmunomodulation, 5*, 160–165.

Glbertini, M., Newton, C., Friedman, H., & Klein, T. W. (1995). Spatial learning impairment in mice infected with Legionella pneumophila or administered exogenous interleukin-1 beta. *Brain, Behavior and Immunity, 9*, 113–128.

Goldman, L. S. (1994). Successful treatment of interferon alfa-induced mood disorder with nortriptyline. *Psychosomatics, 35*, 412–413.

Goujon, E., Parnet, P, Aubert, A., Goodall, G., & Dantzer, R. (1995a). Corticosterone regulates behavioral effects of lipopolysaccharide and interleukin-1β in mice. *American Journal of Physiology, 269*, R154–R159.

Goujon, E., Parnet, P., Crémona, S., & Dantzer, R. (1995b). Endogenous glucocorticoids downregulate central effects of interleukin-1β on body temperature and behavior in mice. *Brain Research, 702*, 173–180.

Goujon, E., Parnet, P., Layé, S., Combe, C., Kelley, K. W., & Dantzer, R. (1995c). Stress downregulates lipopolysaccharide-induced expression of proinflammatory cytokines in the spleen, pituitary and brain of mice. *Brain, Behavior, and Immunity, 9*, 292–303.

Goujon, E., Parnet, P., Layé, S., Combe, C., & Dantzer, R. (1996). Adrenalectomy enhances proinflammatory cytokine gene expression in the spleen, pituitary and brain of mice in response to lipopolysaccharide. *Molecular Brain Research, 36*, 53–62.

Greenfeder, S. A., Nunes, P., Kwee, L., Labow, M., Chizzonite, R. A., & Ju, G. (1995). Molecular cloning and characterization of a second subunit of the interleukin-1 receptor complex. *Journal of Biological Chemistry, 270*, 13757–13765.

Grunfeld, C., & Feingold, K. R. (1996). Regulation of lipid metabolism by cytokines during host defense. *Nutrition, 12*, S24–S26.

Hanisch, U. W., & Quirion, R. (1996). Interleukin-2 as a neuroregulatory cytokine. *Brain Research Reviews, 21*, 246–284.

Hansen, M. K., Taishi, P., Chen, Z., & Krueger, J. M. (1998). Vagotomy blocks the induction of interleukin-1β (IL-1β) mRNA in the brain of rats in response to systemic IL-1β. *Journal of Neuroscience, 18*, 2247–2253.

Haour, F. G., Ban, E. M., Milon, G. M., Baran, D., & Fillion G. M. (1990). Brain interleukin-1 receptors. Characterization and modulation after lipopolysaccharide injection. *Progress in Neuro-EndocrinoImmunology, 3*, 196–204.

Hart, B. L. (1988). Biological basis of the behavior of sick animals. *Neuroscience and Biobehavioral Reviews, 12*, 123–137.

Hebb, A. L., Zacharko, R. M., & Anisman, A. H. (1998). Self-stimulation from the mesencephalon following intraventricular interleukin-2 administration. *Brain Research Bulletin, 45*, 549–556.

Hermann, D. M., Mullington, J., Hinze-Selch, D., Schreiber, W., Galanos, C., & Pollmächer, T. (1998). Endotoxin-induced changes in sleep and sleepiness during the day. *Psychoneuroendocrinology, 23*, 427–437.

Hopkins, S. J., & Rothwell, N. J. (1995). Cytokines and the nervous system. I. Expression and recognition. *Trends in Neurosciences, 18*, 83–87.

Kanaan, S. A., Poole, S., Saadé, N. E., Jabbur, S., & Safieh-Garabedian, B. (1998). Interleukin-10 reduces the endotoxin-induced hyperalgesia in mice. *Journal of Neuroimmunology, 86*, 142–150.

Kakucska, I., Qi, Y., Clark, B. D., & Lechan, R. M. (1993). Endotoxin-induced corticotropin-releasing hormone gene expression in the hypothalamic paraventricular nucleus is mediated centrally by interleukin-1. *Endocrinology, 133*, 815–821.

Kent S., Bluthé, R. M., Dantzer, R., Hardwick, A. J., Kelley, K. W., Rothwell, N. J., & Vannice, J. L. (1992a). Different receptor mechanisms mediate the pyrogenic and behavioral effects of interleukin-1. *Proceedings of the National Academy of Sciences USA, 89*, 9117–9120.

Kent, S., Bluthé, R. M., Kelley, K. W., & Dantzer, R. (1992b). Sickness behavior as a new target for drug development. *Trends in Pharmacological Sciences, 13*, 24–28.

Kent, S., Bret-Dibat, J. L., Kelley, K. W., & Dantzer, R. (1996). Mechanisms of sickness-induced decreases in food-motivated behavior. *Neuroscience and Biobehavioral Reviews, 20*, 171–175.

Kent, S., Kelley, K. W., & Dantzer, R. (1992c). Effects of lipopolysaccharide on food-motivated behavior are not blocked by an interleukin-1 receptor antagonist. *Neuroscience Letters, 145*, 83–86.

Kent, S., Rodriguez, F, Kelley, K. W., & Dantzer, R. (1994). Anorexia induced by microinjection of interleukin-1β in the ventromedial hypothalamus of the rat. *Physiology and Behavior, 56*, 1031–1036.

Klir, J. J., McClellan, J. L., & Kluger, M. J. (1994). Interleukin-1β causes the increase in anterior hypothalamic interleukin-6 during LPS-induced fever in rats. *American Journal of Physiology, 266*, R1845–R1848.

Kluger, M. J. (1991). Fever: Role of pyrogens and cryogens. *Physiological Reviews, 71,* 93–127.

Konsman, J. P., Kelley, K. W., & Dantzer, R. (1999). Temporal and spatial relationships between lipopolysaccharide-induced expression of Fos, interleukin-1β and inducible NO synthase in rat brain. *Neuroscience, 89,* 535–548.

Kozak, W., Poli, V., Soszynski, D., Conn, C. A., Leon, L. R., & Kluger, M. J. (1997). Sickness behavior in mice deficient in interleukin-6 during turpentine abscess and influenza pneumonitis. *American Journal of Physiology, 272,* R621–R630.

Lacroix, S., & Rivest, S. (1998). Effect of acute systemic inflammatory response and cytokines on the transcription of the genes encoding cycloxygenase enzymes (COX-1 and COX-2) in the rat brain. *Journal of Neurochemistry, 70,* 452–466.

Layé S., Bluthé, R. M., Kent, S., Combe, C., Médina, C., Parnet, P., Kelley, K. W., & Dantzer, R. (1995). Subdiaphragmatic vagotomy blocks induction of IL-1β mRNA in mice brain in response to peripheral LPS. *American Journal of Physiology, 268,* R1327–R1331.

Layé, S., Gheusi, G., Cremona, S., Combe, C., Kelley, K. W., Dantzer, R., & Parnet, P. (2000). Endogenous interleukin-1 mediates lipopolysaccharide-induced anorexia and brain cytokine expression. *American Journal of Physiology,* in press.

Layé, S., Goujon, E., Combe, C., VanHoy, R., Kelley K. W., Parnet, P., & Dantzer, R. (1996). Effects of lipopolysaccharide and glucocorticoids on expression of interleukin-1β converting enzyme in the pituitary and brain of mice. *Journal of Neuroimmunology, 68,* 61–66.

Layé, S., Parnet, P., Goujon, E., & Dantzer, R. (1994). Peripheral administration of lipopolysaccharide induces the expression of cytokine transcripts in the brain and pituitary of mice. *Molecular Brain Research, 27,* 157–162.

Lee, S. W., Tsou, A. P., Chan, H., Thomas, J., Petrie, K., Eugui, E. M., & Allison, C. A. (1988). Glucocorticoids selectively inhibit the transcription of the interleukin-1β gene and decrease the stability of interleukin-1β mRNA. *Proceedings of the National Academy of Sciences USA, 85,* 1204–1208.

Lenczowski, M. J. P., Bluthé, R. M., Roth, J., Rees, G. S., Rushforth, D. A., Van Dam, A. M., Tilders, F. J. H., Dantzer, R., Rothwell, N. J., & Luheshi, G. (1999). Central administration of recombinant rat interleukin-6 induces hypothalamic-pituitary-adrenal activation and fever, but not sickness behavior. *American Journal of Physiology, 276,* R652–R658.

Leon, L. R., Kozak, W., Rudolph, K., & Kluger, M. J. (1999). An antipyretic role for interleukin-10 in LPS fever in mice. *American Journal of Physiology, 276,* R81–R89.

Le May, L. G., Vander, A. J., & Kluger, M. J. (1990). The effect of psychological stress on plasma interleukin-6 activity in rats. *Physiology and Behavior, 47,* 957–961.

Linthorst, A. C. E., Flachskmann, C., Holsboer, F., & Reul, J. M. H. M. (1995). Intraperitoneal administration of bacterial endotoxin enhances noradrenergic neurotransmission in the rat preoptic area: Relationship with body temperature and hypothalamic-pituitary-adrenocortical axis activity. *European Journal of Neuroscience, 7,* 2418–2430.

Linthorst, A. C. E., Flachskmann, C., Holsboer, F., & Reul, J. M. H. M. (1996). Activation of serotoninergic and noradrenergic neurotransmission in the rat hippocampus after peripheral administration of bacterial endotoxin: Involvement of the cyclooxygenase pathway. *Neuroscience, 72,* 989–997.

Linthorst, A. C. E., Flachskmann, C., Müller-Preuss, P., Holsboer, F., & Reul, J. M. H. M. (1995). Effect of baacterial endotoxin and interleukin-1 beta on hippocampal serotoninergic neurotransmission, behavioral activity, and free corticosterone levels: An in vivo microdialysis study. *Journal of Neuroscience, 15,* 2920–2934.

Linthorst, A. C. E., & Reul, J. M. H. M. (1999). Inflammation and brain function under basal conditions and during long-term elevation of brain corticotrophin-releasing hormone levels. In R. Dantzer, E.E. Wollman, & R. Yirmiya (Eds.), *Cytokines, stress, and depression.* New York: Kluwer-Academic/Plenum.

Lyte, M., Varcoe, J. J., & Bailey, M. T. (1998). Anxiogenic effect of subclinical bacterial infection in mice in the absence of overt immunee activation. *Physiology and Behavior, 65,* 63–68.

McClellan, J. L., Klir, J. J., Morrow, L. E., & Kluger, M. J. (1994). Central effects of glucocorticoid receptor antagonist RU-38486 on lipopolysacharide and stress-induced fever. *American Journal of Physiology, 267,* R705–R711.

Maes, M., Smith, R., & Scharpe, S. (1995). The monocyte-T-lymphocyte hypothesis of major depression. *Psychoneuroendocrinology, 20,* 111–116.

Makino, M., Kitano, Y., Hirohashi, M., & Takasuna, K. (1998). Enhancement of immobility in mouse forced swimming test by treatment with human interferon. *European Journal of Pharmacology, 356,* 1–7.

Meyers, C. A. (1999). Mood and cognitive disorders in cancer patients receiving cytokine therapy. In R. Dantzer, E. E. Wollman, & R. Yirmiya (Eds.), *Cytokines, stress, and depression.* New York: Kluwer-Academic/Plenum.

Miller, N. E. (1964). Some psychophysiological studies of motivation and of the behavioral effects of illness. *Bulletin of the British Psychology Society, 17,* 1–20.

Minami, M., Kuraishi, Y., Yamaguchi, T., Nakai, S., Hirai, Y., & Satoh, M. (1991). Immobilization stress induces interleukin-1 beta mRNA in the hypothalamus. *Neuroscience Letters, 123,* 254–256.

Morrow, L. E., McClellan, J. L., Conn, C. A., & Kluger M. J. (1993). Glucocorticoids alter fever and IL-6 responses to psychological stress and to lipopolysaccharide. *American Journal of Physiology, 264,* R1010–R1016.

Murray, C. A., & Lynch, M. A. (1998). Evidence that increased hippocampal expression of the cytokine interleukin-1 beta is a common trigger for age- and stress-induced impairments in long-term potentiation. *Journal of Neuroscience, 18,* 2974–2981.

Nava, F., Calapai, G., Facciola, G., Cuzzocrea, S., Marciano, M. C., De Sarro, A., & Caputi, A. P. (1997). Effects of interleukin-10 on water intake, locomotor activity, and rectal temperature in rat treated with endotoxin. *International Journal of Immunopharmacology, 19,* 31–38.

Nicola, N. A. (Ed.) (1994). *Guidebook to cytokines and their receptors.* Oxford: Oxford University Press.

Oitzl, M. S., van Oers, H., Schöbitz, B., & de Kloet, E. R. (1993). Interleukin-1β but not interleukin-β, impairs spatial navigation learning. *Brain Research, 613,* 160–163.

Owens, T., Renno, T., Taupin, V., & Krakowski, M. (1994). Inflammatory cytokines in the brain: Does the CNS shape immune responses? *Trends in Immunology, 15,* 566–571.

Parnet P., Amindari, S., Wu, C., Brunke-Reese, D., Goujon, E., Weyhenmeyer, J. A., Dantzer, R., & Kelley, K. W. (1994). Expression of type I and type II interleukin-1 receptors in mouse brain. *Molecular Brain Research, 27,* 63–70.

Pauli, S., Linthorst, A. C., & Reul, J. M. (1998). Tumour necrosis factor alpha and interleukin-2 differentially affect hippocampal serotoninergic neurotransmission, behavioral activity, body temperature and hypothalamic-pituitary-adrenocorticoal axis activity in the rat. *European Journal of Neuroscience, 10,* 868–878.

Petitto, J. M., McCarthy, D. B., Rinker, C. M., Huang, Z., & Getty, T. (1997). Modulation of behavioral and neurochemical measures of forebrain dopamine fucntion in mice by species-specific interleukin-2. *Journal of Neuroimmunology, 73*, 183–190.

Plata-Salaman, C. R. (1995). Cytokines and feeding suppression: An integrative view from neurological to molecular levels. *Nutrition, 11*, 674–677.

Plata-Salaman, C. R. (1996). Leptin (OB protein), neuropeptide Y, and interleukin-1 interactions as interface mechanisms for the regulation of feeding in health and disease. *Nutrition, 12*, 718–723.

Plata-Salaman, C. R. (1997). Anorexia during acute and chronic disease. Relevance of neurotransmitter-peptide-cytokine interactions. *Nutrition, 13*, 159–160.

Plata-Salaman, C. R. (1999). Brain mechanisms in cytokine-induced anorexia. *Psychoneuroendocrinology, 24*, 25–41.

Plata-Salaman, C. R., Oomura, Y., & Kai, Y. (1988). Tumor necrosis factor and interleukin-1β suppression of food intake by direct action in the central nervous system. *Brain Research, 448*, 106–114.

Porter, M. H., Hrupka, B. J., Langhans, W., & Schwartz, G. J. (1998). Vagal and splanchnic afferents are not necessary for the anorexia produced by peripheral IL-1beta, LPS, and MDP. *American Journal of Physiology, 275*, R384–R389.

Pugh, C. R., Kumagawa, K., Fleshner, M., Watkins, L. R., Maier, S. F., & Rudy, J. W. (1998). Selective effects of peripheral lipopolysaccharide administration on contextual and auditory-cue fear conditioning. *Brain, Behavior, and Immunity, 12*, 212–229.

Quan, N., Whiteside, M., Kim, L., & Herkenham, M. (1997). Induction of inhibitory factor kappaBalpha mRNA in the central nervous system after peripheral lipopolysaccharide administration: an in situ hybridization histochemistry study in the rat. *Proceedings of the National Academy of Sciences USA, 94*, 10985–10990.

Rachamandra, R. N., Sehon A. H., & Berczi, I. (1992). Neurohormonal host defence in endotoxin shock. *Brain, Behavior, and Immunity, 6*, 157–169.

Rady, P. L., Smith, E. M., Cadet, P., Opp, M. R., Tyring, S. K., & Hughes, T. K. Jr. (1995). Presence of interleukin-10 transcripts in human pituitary and hypothalamus. *Cellular and Molecular Neurobiology, 15*, 289–296.

Sarraf, P., Frederich, R. C., Turner, E. M., Ma, G., Jaskowiak, N. T., Rivet, D. J. III, Flier, J. S., Lowell, B. B., Fraker, D. L., & Alexander, H. R. (1997). Multiple cytokines and acute inflammation raise mouse leptin levels: Potential role in inflammatory anorexia. *Journal of Experimental Medicine, 185*, 171–175.

Satta, M. A., Jacobs, R. A., Kaltsas, G. A., & Grossman, A. B. (1998). Endotoxin induces interleukin-1β and nitric oxide synthase mRNA in rat hypothalamus and pituitary. *Neuroendocrinology, 67*, 109–116.

Schöbitz, B., de Kloet, E. R., & Holsboer, F. (1994). Gene expression and function of interleukin 1, interleukin 6 and tumor necrosis factor in the brain. *Progress in Neurobiology, 44*, 397–432.

Schwartz, G. J., Plata-Salaman, C. R., & Langhans, W. (1997). Subdiaphragmatic vagal deafferentation fails to block feeding-suppressive effects of LPS and IL-1β in rats. *American Journal of Physiology, 273*, R1193–R1198.

Sonti, G., Ilyin, S.E., & Plata-Salaman, C. R. (1996). Neuropeptide Y blocks and reverses interleukin-1 beta-induced anorexia in rats. *Peptides, 17*, 517–520.

Späth-Schwalbe, E., Hansen, K., Schmidt, F., Schrezenmeier, H., Marshall, L., Burger, K., Fehm, H.L., & Born, J. (1998). Acute effects of recombinant human interleukin-6 on endocrine and central nervous sleep functions in healthy men. *Journal of Clinical Endocrinology and Metabolism, 83*, 1573–1579.

Spurlock, M. E. (1997). Regulation of metabolism and growth during immune challenge: An overview of cytokine function. *Journal of Animal Science, 75*, 1773–1783.

Swiergiel, A. H., Smagin, G. N., & Dunn, AJ. (1996). Influenza virus infection of mice induces anorexia: Compariosn with endotoxin and interleukin-1 and the effects of indomethacin. *Pharmacology, Biochemistry and Behavior, 57*, 389–396.

Swiergiel, A. H., Smagin, G. N., Johnson, L. J., & Dunn, A. J. (1997). The role of cytokines in the behavioral responses to endotoxin and influenza virus infection in mice: Effects of acute and chronic administration of the interleukin-1-receptor antagonist (IL-1ra). *Brain Research, 776*, 96–104.

Takao, T., Tracey, D. E., Mitchell, W. M., & De Souza, E. B. (1991). Interleukin-1 receptors in mouse brain: Characterization and neuronal localization. *Endocrinology, 127*, 3070–3078.

Uehara, A., Sekiya, C., Takasugi, Y., Namiki, M., & Arimura, A. (1989). Anorexia induced by interleukin-1: Involvement of corticotropin-releasing factor. *American Journal of Physiology, 257*, R613–R617.

Van Dam A. M., Brouns, M., Louisse, S., & Berkenbosch, F. (1992). Appearance of interleukin-1 in macrophages and in ramified microglia in the brain of endotoxin-treated rats: A pathway for the induction of non-specific symptoms of sickness. *Brain Research, 588*, 291–296.

Walker, L. G., Walker, M. B., Heys, S. D., Lolley, J., Wesnes, R., & Eremin, O. (1997). The psychological and psychiatric effects of rIL-2 therapy: A controlled clinical trial. *Psychooncology, 6*, 290–301.

Wan, W., Wetmore, W., Sorensen, C. M., Greenberg, A. H., & Nance, D. M. (1994). Neural and biochemical mediators of endotoxin and stress-induced c-fos expression in the rat brain. *Brain Research Bulletin, 34*, 7–14.

Watkins, L. R., Maier, S. F., & Goehler, L. E. (1995). Cytokine-to-brain communication: A review, & analysis of alternative mechanisms. *Life Sciences, 57*, 1011–1026.

Watkins, L. R., Nguyen, K. T., Lee, J. E., & Maier, S. F. (1999). Dynamic regulation of proinflammatory cytokines. In R. Dantzer, E.E. Wollman, & R. Yirmiya (Eds.), *Stress, cytokines, and depression*. New York: Kluwer-Academic/Plenum.

Wong, M. L., Bongiorno, P. B., Rettori, V., McCann, S. M., & Licinio, J. (1997). Interleukin (IL) 1β, IL-1 receptor antagonist, IL-10, and IL-13 gene expression in the central nervous system and anterior pituitary during systemic inflammation: Pathophysiological implications. *Proceedings of the National Academy of Sciences USA, 94*, 227–232.

Wong, M. L., Rettori, V., Al-Shekhlee, A., Bongiorno, P. B., Canteros, G., McCann, S. M., Gold, P. W., & Licinio, J. (1996). Inducible nitric oxide synthase gene expression in the brain during systemic inflammation. *Nature Medicine, 2*, 581–584.

Wu, D., Yang, J., & Pardridge, W. M. (1997). Drug targeting of a peptide radiopharmaceutical through the primate blood-brain barrier in vivo with a monoclonal antibody to the human insulin receptor. *Journal of Clinical Investigation, 100*, 1804–1812.

Xu, B., Dube, M. G., Kalra, P. S., Farmerie, W. G., Kaibara, A., Moldawer, L. L., Martin, D., & Kalra, S. P. (1998). Anorectic effects of the cytokine, ciliary neutropic factor, are mediated by hypothalamic neuropeptide Y: Comparison with leptin. *Endocrinology, 139*, 466–473.

Yirmiya, R. (1996). Endotoxin produces a depressive-like syndrome in rats. *Brain Research, 711*, 163–174.

Yirmiya, R. (1997). Behavioral and psychological effects of immune activation: Implications for depression due to a general medical condition. *Current Opinions in Psychiatry, 10*, 470–476.

Zacharko, R. M., Zalcman, S., Macneil, G., Andrews, M., Mendella, P. D., & Anisman, H. (1997). Differential effects of immunologic challenge on self-stimulation from the nucleus accumbens and the substantia nigra. *Pharmacology, Biochemistry and Behavior, 58,* 881–886.

Zalcman, S., Murray, I., Dyck, D. G., Greenberg, A. H., & Nance, D. M. (1998). Interleukin-2 and -6 induce behavioral activating effects in mice. *Brain Research, 811,* 111–121.

Zhou, D., Kusnecov, A. W., Shurin, M. R., DePaoli, M., & Rabin, B. S. (1993). Exposure to physical and psychological stressors elevates plasma interleukin-6: Relationship to the activation of hypothalamic-pituitary-adrenal axis. *Endocrinology, 133,* 2523–2530.

Zuckerman, S. H., Shellhaas, J., & Butler, L. D. (1989). Differential regulation of lipopolysacharide-induced interleukin-1 and tumor necrosis factor synthesis: Effects of endogenous glucocorticoids and the role of pituitary-adrenal axis. *European Journal of Immunology, 19,* 301–305.

ISBN 0-12-044315-5